Piyush Gupta's

Learning Through MCQs in PEDIATRICS for MD and DM Students

Piyush Gupta's

Learning Through MCQs in PEDIATRICS for MD and DM Students

VOLUME 2

Systemic Pediatrics and Pediatric Subspecialities

Piyush Gupta
MD FAMS FRCPCH
Former Principal, Professor and Head
Department of Pediatrics
University College of Medical Sciences
New Delhi, India
President, Indian Academy of Pediatrics (2021)

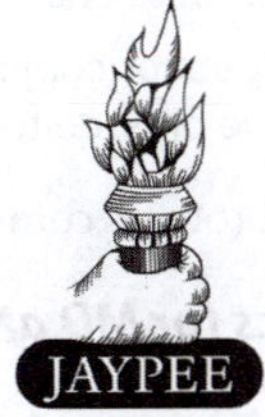

JAYPEE BROTHERS MEDICAL PUBLISHERS
The Health Sciences Publisher
New Delhi | London

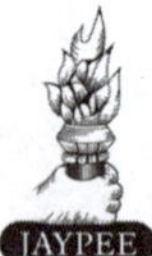

Jaypee Brothers Medical Publishers (P) Ltd.

Headquarters
EMCA House, 23/23-B
Ansari Road, Daryaganj
New Delhi 110 002, India
Landline: +91-11-23272143, +91-11-23272703
+91-11-23282021, +91-11-23245672
e-mail: jaypee@jaypeebrothers.com

Corporate Office
4838/24, Ansari Road, Daryaganj
New Delhi 110 002, India
Phone: +91-11-43574357
Fax: +91-11-43574314
e-mail: jaypee@jaypeebrothers.com

Overseas Office
JP Medical Ltd.
83, Victoria Street, London
SW1H 0HW (UK)
Phone: +44-20 3170 8910
e-mail: info@jpmedpub.com

EU GPSR Authorised Representative
Logos Europe, 9 rue Nicolas Poussin
17000, La Rochelle, France
Phone: +33 (0) 6 67 93 73 78
e-mail: contact@logoseurope.eu

Website: www.jaypeebrothers.com
Website: www.jaypeedigital.com

Piyush Gupta's Learning Through MCQs in Pediatrics for MD and DM Students (2 Volumes)

First Edition: **2025**

Reprint : **2026**

ISBN: 978-93-5696-762-5

Printed in India at Sterling Graphics Pvt. Ltd.

Dedicated to

Children of the Country and all those
Who take care of them
(Parents, Caregivers, Pediatricians, and all caders of Health Workers)

Section Editors (Volume 2)

Endocrinology
Aashima Dabas MD
Professor
Department of Pediatrics
Maulana Azad Medical College
and Lok Nayak Hospital
New Delhi, India

Gastroenterology and Hepatology
Moinak Sen Sarma MD DM
Additional Professor
Department of Pediatric Gastroenterology
Sanjay Gandhi Postgraduate Institute
of Medical Sciences
Lucknow, Uttar Pradesh, India

Nephrology
Priyanka Khandelwal MD DM
Clinical Fellow in Complement-mediated
Diseases, Division of Nephrology
Department of Pediatrics
The Hospital for Sick Children
University of Toronto
Toronto, Ontario, Canada

Cardiology
Sakshi Sachdeva MD DNB FNB DM
Assistant Professor
Division of Pediatric Cardiology
Department of Pediatrics
Atal Bihari Vajpayee Institute of Medical
Sciences and Dr Ram Manohar Lohia Hospital
New Delhi, India

Hematology
Sidharth Totadri MD DM
Associate Professor
Department of Pediatric
Hematology-Oncology
St John's Medical College and Hospital
Bengaluru, Karnataka, India

Contributing Authors (Volume 2)

Aaradhana MD
Professor
Department of Pediatrics
University College of Medical Sciences
and Guru Teg Bahadur Hospital
New Delhi, India

Aashima Dabas MD
Professor
Department of Pediatrics
Maulana Azad Medical College
and Lok Nayak Hospital
New Delhi, India

Aathira Ravindranath MD DM
Consultant Pediatric Gastroenterology
and Hepatology
Apollo BGS Hospitals
Mysuru, Karnataka, India

Abhijeet Saha MD MNAMS FRCPCH
Director–Professor
Department of Pediatrics
Division of Pediatric Nephrology
Lady Hardinge Medical College and
Kalawati Saran Children's Hospital
New Delhi, India

Aditi Sinha MD
Additional Professor
Department of Pediatrics
All India Institute of Medical Sciences
New Delhi, India

Amrit Gopan MD DM
Clinical Fellow
Division of Gastroenterology, Hepatology
and Advanced Clinical Nutrition
The Hospital for Sick Children
University of Toronto
Toronto, Ontario, Canada

Ankit Agrawal MD DM
Assistant Professor
Department of Pediatric Gastroenterology
Postgraduate Institute of Child Health
Noida, Uttar Pradesh, India

Anuradha Rai MD FNB MRCPCH
Consultant
Department of Pediatrics
Chacha Nehru Bal Chikitsalaya
New Delhi, India

Anusha Hegde MD FNB
Assistant Professor
Department of Pediatric Hematology
Oncology
Zulekha Yenepoya Institute of Oncology
Mangaluru, Karnataka, India

Arghya Samanta MD DNB DM
Assistant Professor
Department of Pediatric Gastroenterology
Sanjay Gandhi Postgraduate Institute
of Medical Sciences
Lucknow, Uttar Pradesh, India

Arti Pawaria MD DM
Clinical Lead, Senior Consultant
Assistant Professor
Department of Pediatric Hepatology,
Gastroenterology and Liver
Transplant Physician
Amrita Institute of Medical Sciences
Faridabad, Haryana, India

Arun Danewa MD FNB
Senior Consultant
Department of Pediatric Hematology
Oncology and Bone Marrow Transplantation
Fortis Memorial Research Institute
Gurugram, Haryana, India

Bishnupriya Sahoo MD FPGHN
Associate Professor
Department of Pediatrics
Faculty of Medicine and Health Sciences
SGT University
Gurugram, Haryana, India

Bobbity Deepthi MD
Associate Professor
Department of Pediatrics
Jawaharlal Institute of Medical Education
and Research
Puducherry, India

Deepika Harit MD
Professor
Department of Pediatrics
University College of Medical Sciences
and Guru Teg Bahadur Hospital
New Delhi, India

Divij Sachdeva MD FIAP
Associate Consultant
Department of Pediatric Hematology
Oncology and BMT Unit
Sir Ganga Ram Hospital
New Delhi, India

Ganesh Jevalikar
MD DNB (Ped) PDCC (Ped Endocrinology)
Principal Consultant
Department of Endocrinology
and Diabetes
Max Healthcare
New Delhi, India

Gayathri Sreedhar MD
Pediatric Radiologist
Associate Professor of Radiology
North-East Ohio Medical School
(NEOMED)
Rootstown, Ohio, USA

Girish C Bhatt
MD FISN FASN FRCP
Professor
Division of Pediatric Nephrology
Department of Pediatrics
All India Institute of Medical Sciences
Bhopal, Madhya Pradesh, India

Hema Gupta Mittal MD
Professor and In-charge
Division of Pediatric Pulmonology
Department of Pediatrics
Atal Bihari Vajpayee Institute of
Medical Sciences and Dr Ram Manohar
Lohia Hospital
New Delhi, India

Jagadeesh Menon VR MD DM
Consultant
Pediatric Gastroenterology
and Hepatology
Dr Rela Institute and Medical Centre
Chennai, Tamil Nadu, India

Jagdish P Goyal MD MAMS
Professor
Department of Pediatrics
All India Institute of Medical Sciences
Jodhpur, Rajasthan, India

Janaki Rajagopalan MD DNB
Consultant Psychiatrist
Gleneagles Hospital
Promed Hospital
Chennai, Tamil Nadu, India

Jatinder S Goraya MD FRCPC
Professor
Department of Pediatric Neurology
Dayanand Medical College and Hospital
Ludhiana, Punjab, India

Jayendra Seetharaman MD DM
Assistant Professor
Division of Pediatric Gastroenterology
and Hepatology
Department of Pediatrics
Christian Medical College
Vellore, Tamil Nadu, India

Jijo Joseph John MD FPRD DAA
Professor and Head
Department of Pediatrics
Believers Church Medical College Hospital
Thiruvalla, Kerala, India

Kamal Kumar Singhal DCH MD DM
Professor (Pediatric Pulmonology)
Department of Pediatrics
Lady Hardinge Medical College and
Kalawati Saran Children's Hospital
New Delhi, India

Kanika Kapoor MD FIPNA
Associate Professor
Department of Pediatrics
Vardhman Mahavir Medical College
and Safdarjung Hospital
New Delhi, India

Kavita Srivastava MD FRCPCH
Professor in Pediatrics and
Pediatric Neurologist
Bharati Vidyapeeth's Medical College
Pune, Maharashtra, India

Kirtisudha Mishra MD DNB FIPNA FISPN
Associate Professor
Department of Pediatrics
Chacha Nehru Bal Chikitsalaya
New Delhi, India

Lamak Kadiyani MD DM
Assistant Professor
Department of Cardiology
All India Institute of Medical Sciences
New Delhi, India

Lokesh Guglani MD FAAP
Associate Professor
Division of Pulmonology
Department of Pediatrics
Children's Healthcare of Atlanta
Emory University School of Medicine
Atlanta, Georgia, USA

Lokesh Saini MD DM
Associate Professor
Department of Pediatric Neurology
All India Institute of Medical Sciences
Jodhpur, Rajasthan, India

M Vijayakumar MD DNB FRCP
Professor and Head
Department of Pediatrics
Government Medical College
Kozhikode, Kerala, India

Madhumita Nandi MD FIAP
Professor and Head
Department of Pediatrics
North Bengal Medical College
and Hospital
Darjeeling, West Bengal, India

Maharshi Trivedi MD DM
Senior Associate Specialist
Department of Pediatric Hematology
Oncology and Bone Marrow
Transplantation
Bristol Royal Hospital for Children
Bristol, UK

Mahesh Kamate MD DM
Professor and Head
Department of Pediatric Neurology
KLE Academy of Higher Education
and Research (KAHER)
Jawaharlal Nehru Medical College
Belagavi, Karnataka, India

Manas Kalra MD DNB FNB
Senior Consultant
Department of Pediatric Hematology
Oncology and BMT Unit
Sir Ganga Ram Hospital
New Delhi, India

Manish Kumar MD
Professor
Department of Pediatrics
Chacha Nehru Bal Chikitsalaya
New Delhi, India

Mily Ray MD FNB
Consultant
Department of Pediatric Cardiology
Max Health Care
New Delhi, India

Moinak Sen Sarma MD DM
Additional Professor
Department of Pediatric Gastroenterology
Sanjay Gandhi Postgraduate Institute
of Medical Sciences
Lucknow, Uttar Pradesh, India

Mrigank Choubey MD DM
Associate Professor
Department of Pediatrics
Command Hospital (Eastern Command)
Kolkata, West Bengal, India

Mukta Mantan MD DNB
Director–Professor
Department of Pediatrics
Maulana Azad Medical College
New Delhi, India

Narendra Bagri MD
Additional Professor
Division of Pediatric Rheumatology
and Clinical Immunology
Department of Pediatrics
All India Institute of Medical Sciences
New Delhi, India

Naresh Shanmugam DNB FRCPCH
Senior Consultant and Clinical Lead
Department of Pediatric Gastroenterology and Hepatology
Dr Rela Institute and Medical Centre
Chennai, Tamil Nadu, India

Nidhi Rawal MD FNB
Chief (Pediatric Cardiology)
Department of Pediatric Cardiology
Artemis Hospital
Gurugram, Haryana, India

Nidhi Srivastava MD FNB
Senior Resident
Department of Pediatrics
University College of Medical Sciences and Guru Teg Bahadur Hospital
New Delhi, India

Nishant Wadhwa DCH DNB
Senior Consultant and Chief
Division of Pediatric Gastroenterology and Hepatology
Sir Ganga Ram Hospital
New Delhi, India

NK Subramanya MD MBA
Professor (Pediatrics) and Medical Superintendent
PES Institute of Medical Sciences and Research
Chittoor, Andhra Pradesh, India

OP Mishra MD FIAP FAMS
Dean (Research) and Head
Department of Pediatrics
Heritage Institute of Medical Sciences
Varanasi, Uttar Pradesh, India

Parijat Ram Tripathi MD PDCC DM
Consultant
Department of Pediatric Gastroenterology and Hepatology
Ankura Hospital for Women and Children
Hyderabad, Telangana, India

Pavneet Kaur MD
Senior Resident
Department of Pediatrics
All India Institute of Medical Sciences
New Delhi, India

Payal DVD
Specialist
Department of Dermatology
Vardhman Mahavir Medical College and Safdarjung Hospital
New Delhi, India

Payal Gupta MBBS DNB
Consultant
Department of Ophthalmology
Fortis Hospital
Greater Noida, Uttar Pradesh, India

Prawin Kumar MD
Additional Professor
Department of Pediatrics
All India Institute of Medical Sciences
Jodhpur, Rajasthan, India

Priyanka Khandelwal MD DM
Clinical Fellow in Complement-mediated Diseases
Division of Nephrology
Department of Pediatrics
The Hospital for Sick Children
University of Toronto
Toronto, Ontario, Canada

Priyankar Pal MD MNAMS FRCPCH
Professor and Head
Department of Pediatrics
Institute of Child Health
Kolkata, West Bengal, India

Purva Kanvinde MD FNB
Consultant
Department of Pediatric Hematology-Oncology
BJ Wadia Hospital for Children
Mumbai, Maharashtra, India

Rajesh Kumar Meena MD
Associate Professor
Department of Pediatrics
Vardhman Mahavir Medical College and Safdarjung Hospital
New Delhi, India

Rajiv Sinha MD FRCPCH
Professor and Head
Department of Pediatric Nephrology
Institute of Child Health
Kolkata, West Bengal, India

Ravali Pratima Goud MD
Fellow
Department of Pediatric Rheumatology
Institute of Child Health
Kolkata, West Bengal, India

Reny Joseph MD MRCPCH
Consultant Pediatrician
Rajagiri Hospital
Kochi, Kerala, India

Rishi Bolia MD DM FRACP
Consultant Pediatric Gastroenterologist
Queensland Children's Hospital
Brisbane, Queensland, Australia

Ritika Khurana MD FNB
Junior Consultant
Pediatric Hematology-Oncology
BJ Wadia Hospital for Children
Mumbai, Maharashtra, India

Rohit Khandelwal MD
Professor
Department of Pediatrics
Vydehi Institute of Medical Sciences and Research Centre
Bengaluru, Karnataka, India

Sakshi Sachdeva MD DNB FNB DM
Assistant Professor
Division of Pediatric Cardiology
Department of Pediatrics
Atal Bihari Vajpayee Institute of Medical Sciences and Dr Ram Manohar Lohia Hospital
New Delhi, India

Sangeeta Mudaliar DNB MRCPCH
Head
Department of Pediatric Hematology-Oncology
BJ Wadia Hospital for Children
Mumbai, Maharashtra, India

Sangeetha Yoganathan MD DNB DM
Professor
Pediatric Neurology Unit
Department of Neurological Sciences
Christian Medical College
Vellore, Tamil Nadu, India

Sanghamitra Ray MD
Assistant Professor
Department of Pediatrics
Vardhman Mahavir Medical College
and Safdarjung Hospital
New Delhi, India

Sataroopa Mishra MD DM
Assistant Professor
Department of Cardiology
Jawaharlal Institute of Postgraduate
Medical Education and Research
Puducherry, India

Shilpa Sharma MCh DrNB PhD FAMS
Professor
Department of Pediatric Surgery
All India Institute of Medical Sciences
New Delhi, India

Shrish Bhatnagar MD
Professor and Head
Department of Pediatrics
Era's Lucknow Medical College
and Hospital
Lucknow, Uttar Pradesh, India

Shruti Kakkar MD
Professor
Department of Pediatrics
Consultant
Clinical Hematology, Hemato-oncology,
and Stem Cell Transplant Unit
Christian Medical College and Hospital
Ludhiana, Punjab, India

Sidharth Totadri MD DM
Associate Professor
Department of Pediatric
Hematology-Oncology
St John's Medical College and Hospital
Bengaluru, Karnataka, India

Srinivas Srinidhi Vadlapudi MD DM
Assistant Professor
Department of Pediatric Gastroenterology
Sanjay Gandhi Postgraduate Institute
of Medical Sciences
Lucknow, Uttar Pradesh, India

Sriram Krishnamurthy MD FIPNA FIAP
Professor
Department of Pediatrics
Jawaharlal Institute of Postgraduate
Medical Education and Research
Puducherry, India

Suvasini Sharma MD DM FRCPCH
Professor
Department of Pediatrics
Lady Hardinge Medical College and
Kalawati Saran Children's Hospital
New Delhi, India

Swati Kanakia MD DCH PhD
Consultant Pediatric Hematologist
Oncologist
Lilavati Hospital and Research Centre
SRCC Children's Hospital
Blood and Cancer Clinic for Children
Kanakia Health Care
Mumbai, Maharashtra, India

Tushar Godbole DCH DNB
Consultant Pediatric Endocrinology
Director
Harmony Health Specialty Clinic
Associate Professor of Pediatrics
Dr Vasantrao Pawar Medical College
Nashik, Maharashtra, India

Uma Devi Karuru MD DM
Assistant Professor
Department of Cardiology
ESIC Medical College and Super
Specialty Hospital
Hyderabad, Telangana, India

Vikrant Sood MD DM
Associate Professor
Department of Pediatric Hepatology
and Liver Transplantation
Institute of Liver and Biliary Sciences
New Delhi, India

Vipul Gautam MD DM
Consultant Pediatric Gastroenterologist
and Hepatologist
Centre for Liver and Biliary Sciences
Max Superspecialty Hospital
New Delhi, India

Vishal Sondhi MD DM
Professor (Pediatric Neurology)
Department of Pediatrics
Armed Forces Medical College
Pune, Maharashtra, India

Preface

Welcome to the world of multiple-choice questions (MCQs), where every right answer holds the key to your dreams. As you embark on your journey toward a successful competitive examination, this book aims to be your trusted companion—a compass guiding you through the vast ocean of knowledge. MCQs are not mere puzzles to solve; they are gateways to understanding. They challenge your critical thinking, test your recall abilities, and assess your application of concepts. Each correct answer brings you closer to your goal, while each incorrect choice teaches you valuable lessons.

Learning Through MCQs in Pediatrics for MD and DM Students is not just another question bank. It is a strategic toolkit designed to elevate your performance. Here is what sets it apart:

Comprehensive Coverage: We have meticulously curated MCQs across all topics of pediatrics ranging from General Pediatrics, Neonatology, and Systemic Pediatrics.

Conceptual Clarity: Our questions are not random; they are carefully crafted to reinforce fundamental concepts. Expect clarity, not confusion.

Strategic Insights: We will unravel the art of tackling MCQs strategically. Learn how to eliminate distractors, and approach questions systematically.

Practice, Practice, Practice: Repetition breeds mastery. With hundreds of MCQs, you will hone your skills and build confidence.

Our aim in writing this book is not just to get you to the right answer, but to find a logical way to it. The journey is as important as the destination. A major objective of any assessment is "ongoing learning" besides instigating critical thinking requiring interpretation, integration, synthesis and analysis of medical knowledge and facts. Each MCQ (Stem and 4 discriminators) is followed by the following elements to facilitate learning:

- *Explanation:* Describes how the student should analyze the question and synthesize the reply in a logical manner. A stepwise approach to arrive at the correct answer is provided along with reasons why the other distractors are not correct.
- *Correct answer* (key)
- *Knowledge-boosters:* Provide additional knowledge relevant to the questions being asked and the options given. This can be helpful to the students for solving other questions related to similar topics.
- *Source(s) of the text on which the question is based:* To verify the answer if needed and facilitate further learning from the source provided.

The book is divided into two volumes with *Volume 1* pertaining to General Pediatrics, Neonatology, Adolescent Health, and Social Pediatrics; while *Volume 2* contains questions related to Systemic Pediatrics and Pediatric Subspecialities. Overall, there are 2400+ MCQs contributed by more than 150 Faculty members in Pediatrics from all parts of the country, who are experts in their respective fields. I am grateful to them for their whole-hearted support and valuable contributions. We have taken care that the questions should check the analytical ability rather than rote memory. They should assess factual recall, problem solving, and reasoning. Most questions are based on case scenarios with a difficulty index ranging from moderate to difficult. We have tried to avoid "None of the above" or "All of the above" type distractors since they usually carry poor discriminating value.

As you turn the pages, remember that each question is an opportunity—an opportunity to learn, to grow, and to inch closer to your dream. Embrace the challenge, celebrate the correct answers, and learn from the incorrect ones. So, dear student, best wishes on your quest—you hold a steady aid in your hands. May these MCQs be your compass, guiding you toward that coveted knowledge. The book will be useful for most entrance examinations in the medical field, including MBBS, postgraduation (MD/DNB), and super-specialty (DM/MCh/FNB) courses pertaining to the field of pediatrics.

Wishing you success and resilience. Feedback, criticism, and queries are welcome at *prof.piyush.gupta@gmail.com.*

Piyush Gupta

Acknowledgments

For Review of Literature and Author Database

Professor Nidhi Bedi

Secretarial for Editor-in-Chief

Anju Kumari

Publishers' Editorial Team

We also express our thanks to M/s Jaypee Brothers Medical Publishers (P) Ltd, New Delhi, India, for publishing this book so well. We also thank Shri Jitendar P Vij (Group Chairman), Mr Ankit Vij (Managing Director), Mr MS Mani (Group President), Ms Chetna Malhotra (Senior Director—Professional Publishing, Marketing, and Business Development), Ms Pooja Bhandari [Director—Production (Books and Journals)], Ms Asmi Bharati (Development Editor), Ashwani Kumar Singh (Senior Manager), Mr Yogeshwar Pal (Editor/Assistant Manager), Ms Neha Verma (Cover Visualizer), Mr Gurnam Singh (Quality Controller), Mr Mohd Iqbal (Typesetter), and Mr Manoj Pahuja (Graphic Designer) for their help, guidance, and timely active intervention in composing, designing, and editing of the book.

Contents

VOLUME 1

General Pediatrics, Neonatology, Adolescent Health, and Social Pediatrics

SECTION 5 FLUID AND ELECTROLYTE

SECTION 6 DRUGS

SECTION 7 EMERGENCIES

SECTION 8 INTENSIVE CARE

SECTION 9 NEWBORN AND NEONATOLOGY

SECTION 10 GROWTH, DEVELOPMENT, AND BEHAVIOR

SECTION 11 NUTRITION

SECTION 12 IMMUNIZATION

SECTION 13 INFECTIONS

VOLUME 2

Systemic Pediatrics and Pediatric Subspecialities

SECTION 16 GASTROENTEROLOGY

Section Editor: **Moinak Sen Sarma**

SECTION 17 HEPATOLOGY

Section Editor: **Moinak Sen Sarma**

SECTION 18 HEMATOLOGY

Section Editor: **Sidharth Totadri**

SECTION 19 RESPIRATORY DISEASES

SECTION 20 CARDIOLOGY

Section Editor: **Sakshi Sachdeva**

SECTION 21 NEPHROLOGY

Section Editor: **Priyanka Khandelwal**

SECTION 22 NEUROLOGY

SECTION 23 ENDOCRINOLOGY

Section Editor: **Aashima Dabas**

SECTION 24 RHEUMATOLOGY

SECTION 25 SPECIALITIES

SECTION 16

Gastroenterology

Section Editor: Moinak Sen Sarma

CHAPTER 16.1

Anatomy and Physiology of Gastrointestinal Tract and Anorectal Disorders

Anuradha Rai

1. Which of the following leads to development of Hirschsprung disease (HD)?

A. Failure of rupture of cloacal membrane
B. Failure of rotation of midgut
C. Failure of migration of neural crest cells
D. Fixation of gut

EXPLANATION

During the early stage of fetal development, the cells of the neural crest migrate into the wall of the gut and form the enteric nervous system (ENS). Migration of neural crest tissue is complete by the 24th week of gestation. Hirschsprung disease, achalasia cardia, and congenital megacolon occur due to the failure of migration of neural crest cells to form the nerve plexuses in respective parts of the gut. Failure of rupture of the cloacal membrane leads to imperforate anus. Failure of return of midgut to the abdominal cavity leads to omphalocele or exomphalos. Fixation of the gut maintains its appropriate position in the abdominopelvic cavity and prevents intestinal obstruction due to volvulus.

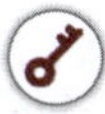

Key: C

BOOST YOUR KNOWLEDGE

Hirschsprung disease is the result of an absence of ganglion cells in the bowel wall, extending proximally and continuously from the anus for a variable distance. Absence of myenteric and submucosal plexus leads to inadequate relaxation of bowel wall and bowel wall hypertonicity which leads to intestinal obstruction. The aganglionic segment is limited to rectosigmoid in 80%, 10–15% cases may have long segment disease, and in 5% cases, aganglionic segment includes terminal ileum in addition to entire length of colon. Rectal suction biopsy is gold standard to diagnose HD.

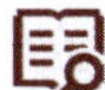

REFERENCE/SOURCE

- Kliegman RM, St Geme III JW, Blum NJ, Shah SS, Tasker RC, Wilson KM. Nelson Textbook of Pediatrics, 21st edition. Elsevier; 2019. p. 10349.

2. A neonate born at 40-week gestation has frothing at mouth and nose as well as coughing, cyanosis, and respiratory distress on feeding. Plain X-ray in the evaluation of respiratory distress revealed a coiled feeding tube in the esophagus and gasless abdomen. What is most likely diagnosis?

A. Esophageal atresia (EA)
B. EA with distal tracheoesophageal fistula (TEF)
C. Diaphragmatic hernia
D. Laryngotracheoesophageal cleft

EXPLANATION

The inability to pass a nasogastric or orogastric tube in the newborn and an airless scaphoid abdomen suggests esophageal atresia. A coiled feeding tube in the esophageal pouch and an air-distended stomach, indicates the presence of a coexisting TEF. Respiratory distress is cardinal sign in babies with congenital diaphragmatic hernia, it can present at birth, may have scaphoid abdomen, bowel sound may be heard in chest with decreased breath sound bilaterally. Chest radiograph will show herniated bowel loops in thoracic cavity which is not the case here.

Laryngotracheoesophageal cleft leads to a common channel defect between esophagus and laryngotracheal lumen, thus makes laryngeal closure incompetent during swallowing or reflux. Infant presents with stridor, choking, cyanosis, aspiration of feedings, and recurrent chest infections. The diagnosis requires direct endoscopic visualization of the larynx and esophagus. When contrast radiography is used, material is often seen in the esophagus and trachea both.

Key: A

BOOST YOUR KNOWLEDGE

Esophageal atresia is the most common congenital anomaly of the esophagus, with a prevalence of 1.7 per 10,000 live births. 50% of infants are nonsyndromic without other anomalies, and the rest have associated anomalies, most often associated with the vertebral, anorectal (cardiac), tracheal, esophageal, renal, radial (limb) (VACTERL) syndrome.

Initial management involves keeping airway patent, preoperative proximal pouch decompression to prevent aspiration of secretions and use of antibiotic to prevent consequent pneumonia. This is followed by standard surgical ligation of TEF and primary end to end anastomosis of the esophagus. If the gap between atretic end of esophagus is >3–4 cm, primary repair cannot be done. Following image shows five most encountered esophageal atresia and TEF and their frequency.

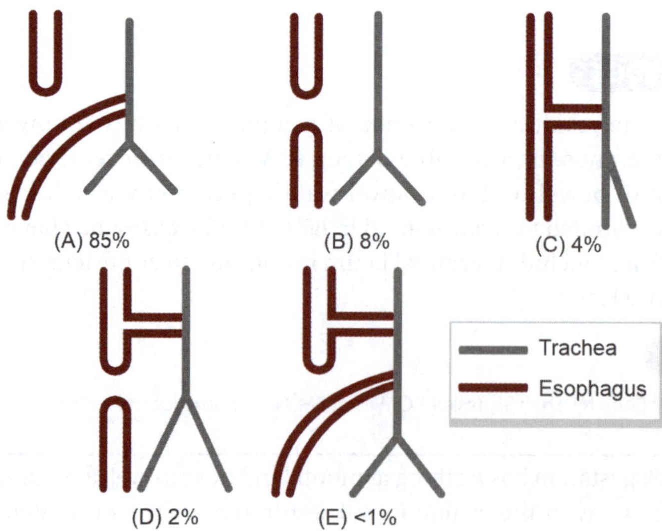

REFERENCE/SOURCE

- Kliegman RM, St Geme III JW, Blum NJ, Shah SS, Tasker RC, Wilson KM. Nelson Textbook of Pediatrics, 21st edition. Elsevier; 2019. Chapter 345. p. 10258.

3. After acute insult to intestinal mucosa, how many days it takes for renewal of mucosa?

A. 4–5 B. 7–10

C. 12–14 D. 20–22

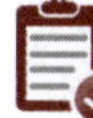

EXPLANATION

Small bowel mucosa is completely renewed in 4–5 days but in young infants or malnourished children this process may get delayed.

Key: A

BOOST YOUR KNOWLEDGE

The cells of the villi originate in adjacent crypts and become functional as they migrate from the crypt up the villus. Crypt cells also secrete fluid and electrolytes. Villi are present by 8-week gestation in duodenum and by 11 weeks in ileum.

REFERENCE/SOURCE

- Kliegman RM, St Geme III JW, Blum NJ, Shah SS, Tasker RC, Wilson KM. Nelson Textbook of Pediatrics, 21st edition. Elsevier; 2019. p. 10350.

4. A 6-week-old infant is brought to emergency because he is having recurrent nonbilious vomiting for last 1 week, which has increased in frequency and have become projectile for last 3 days. Mother describes vomitus to be non-bloody and nonbilious, and child continues to breastfeed hungrily after vomiting. Child appears to be dehydrated. He is at 50th percentile for length and 10th percentile for weight. What will be the biochemical abnormality in this case?

A. Hypochloremic metabolic alkalosis B. Hypochloremic metabolic acidosis

C. Hyperchloremic metabolic acidosis D. Hyperchloremic metabolic alkalosis

EXPLANATION

Nonbilious and projectile vomiting is symptom of pyloric stenosis. Vomiting usually starts after 3 weeks but may present as late as 5 months. Initially 20% infants may have intermittent vomiting from birth which later progresses to classical picture. Infant feels hungry after vomiting and want to feed again. As vomiting continues, a progressive loss of fluid, hydrogen ion, potassium, and chloride lead to hypochloremic hypokalemic metabolic alkalosis.

Key: A

BOOST YOUR KNOWLEDGE

Diagnosis of hypertrophic pyloric stenosis can be established by palpating pyloric mass, which is firm, movable approximately 2 cm in length, olive shaped, hard, and located above and to the right of the umbilicus in mid epigastrium beneath the liver edge and is easiest palpable after an episode of vomiting. Ultrasonography (USG) confirms the diagnosis in the majority and carries sensitivity of 95%. Criteria for diagnosis include pyloric thickness 3–4 mm, an overall pyloric length 15–19 mm, and pyloric diameter of 10–14 mm.

Hyperbilirubinemia is the most common clinical association of pyloric stenosis, also known as icteropyloric syndrome which resolves with surgical correction. Unconjugated hyperbilirubinemia is more common than conjugated.

REFERENCE/SOURCE

- Kliegman RM, St Geme III JW, Blum NJ, Shah SS, Tasker RC, Wilson KM. Nelson Textbook of Pediatrics, 21st edition. Elsevier; 2019. p. 10355.

5. A 2-month-old male infant presents in dehydrated state in pediatric emergency and mother gives history of progressively increasing vomiting for last 2 weeks and significant weight loss. History reveals projectile nature of vomiting, nonbilious which occur after feeding and infant demands breastfeed immediately after vomiting. Contrast studies performed showed string and shoulder sign. What is the most probable diagnosis?

A. Hypertrophic pyloric stenosis
B. Antral web
C. Duodenal stenosis
D. Esophageal stenosis

EXPLANATION

Nonbilious, projectile vomiting, occurring after feed, which usually start after 3 weeks of age are pointers to a diagnosis of hypertrophic pyloric stenosis. Contrast studies demonstrate an elongated pyloric channel which is string sign and bulge of pyloric muscle into the antrum which is shoulder sign. Parallel streaks of barium seen in the narrowed channel produce double track sign. Antral web appears as thin septum near the pyloric channel and presents with failure to thrive and vomiting. Presentation depends on degree of obstruction. Hallmark of duodenal atresia is bilious vomiting without abdominal distension which is usually noted on first day of life. Esophageal atresia will present at birth, neonate typically has frothing and bubbling at the mouth and nose after birth as well as episodes of coughing, cyanosis, and respiratory distress. Feeding will exacerbate these symptoms, cause regurgitation, and can precipitate aspiration.

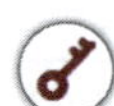

Key: A

BOOST YOUR KNOWLEDGE

Hypertrophic pyloric stenosis occurs in 1–3/1,000 infants. Males are affected 4–6 times as often as females. Incidence is high in infants with B and O blood group and in offspring of mother who had pyloric stenosis. It is characterized by abnormal thickening of the pylorus muscles in the stomach which causes gastric outlet obstruction. Infants are well at birth, then, at 3–6 weeks of age, they develop "projectile" vomiting, potentially leading to dehydration, and weight loss. Subsequently, they can develop profound hypochloremic hypokalemic metabolic alkalosis. Infantile hypertrophic pyloric stenosis is associated with macrolide use in young infants, especially in those <14 days old, with highest risk in those receiving erythromycin versus azithromycin. Preoperative treatment includes correction of fluid, acid base, and electrolyte losses. Correction of alkalosis is important to prevent postoperative apnea. Surgical treatment is definitive and pyloromyotomy (Ramstedt) is procedure of choice.

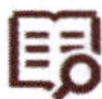

REFERENCE/SOURCE

- Kliegman RM, St Geme III JW, Blum NJ, Shah SS, Tasker RC, Wilson KM. Nelson Textbook of Pediatrics, 21st edition. Elsevier; 2019. pp. 10359, 10367.

6. A newborn is referred to emergency department of hospital with a diagnosis of intestinal atresia. Which of the following statements is true regarding the condition?

A. Type III has mucosal web
B. Type III accounts for 20% of intestinal atresia
C. Type III B has multiple atresia
D. Type III B produce "apple peel" appearance

EXPLANATION

Type I has mucosal web. Type II contributes 30–35% of intestinal atresia. Type IV has multiple atresia not type III B. Type III B jejunoileal atresia is associated with an extensive mesenteric defect and loss of normal blood supply to distal bowel. The distal ileum coils around the ileocolic artery from which it derives its entire blood supply producing an apple peel appearance.

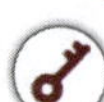

Key: D

BOOST YOUR KNOWLEDGE

Five types of jejunal and ileal atresia are there. In type I (20%), a mucosal web occludes the lumen, but continuity is maintained between the proximal and distal bowel. Type II involves a small-diameter solid cord that connects the proximal and distal bowel. Type III is divided into two subtypes: Type III A occurs when both ends of the bowel end in blind loops, accompanied by a small mesenteric defect. Type IV involves multiple atresia. Type II (30–35%) and III A (30–35%) are most common. III B is least common.

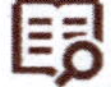

REFERENCE/SOURCE

- Kliegman RM, St Geme III JW, Blum NJ, Shah SS, Tasker RC, Wilson KM. Nelson Textbook of Pediatrics, 21st edition. Elsevier; 2019. p. 10381.

7. A newborn with a birth weight of 1.8 kg, born at 34-week gestation was breastfed within 4 hours after delivery. In 30 minutes, significant amount of vomiting with bile was observed. Physical examination did not show distended abdomen. Abdominal X-ray showed double-bubble sign in epigastrium with otherwise gasless abdomen. What is the most probable diagnosis?

A. Esophageal atresia
B. Pyloric stenosis
C. Biliary atresia
D. Duodenal atresia

EXPLANATION

Approximately 50% infants with duodenal atresia are premature. The hallmark of duodenal obstruction is bilious vomiting without abdominal distention, which is usually noted on the first day of life. History of polyhydramnios is present in half of pregnancies due to inadequate absorption of amniotic fluid in the distal intestine. Plain abdominal radiograph shows double-bubble sign due to distended and gas filled stomach and proximal duodenum.

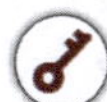

Key: D

BOOST YOUR KNOWLEDGE

Duodenal atresia accounts for 25–40% of all intestinal atresia and occurs in 1/10,000 live births. It results from failed recanalization of intestinal lumen. Prenatal diagnosis can be made by fetal ultrasound which shows sonographic double bubble. Initial treatment includes nasogastric or orogastric decompression and intravenous fluid replacement. Typical surgical repair is duodenoduodenostomy.

REFERENCE/SOURCE

- Kliegman RM, St Geme III JW, Blum NJ, Shah SS, Tasker RC, Wilson KM. Nelson Textbook of Pediatrics, 21st edition. Elsevier; 2019. p. 10376.

8. A 2-year-old female child is brought with issue of passing brick-colored stools. On examination, she appears pale. Otherwise, she is playful and does not cry during abdominal examination. What should be the next most sensitive investigation to be performed in this case?

A. Erect X-ray abdomen
B. Barium study
C. Red blood cell scan
D. Radionuclide scan

EXPLANATION

We are dealing with a case of painless rectal bleeding; color of stool indicates toward higher location of onset of bleeding and it is significant enough to lead to anemia. Most likely this is a case of Meckel's diverticulum. Symptoms of Meckel's diverticulum usually arise in first 2 years of life. It accounts for 50% of all lower gastrointestinal (GI) bleeds in children younger than 2 years of age. Majority presents with intermittent painless rectal bleeding. The stool is typically described as brick-colored or currant jelly colored.

The most sensitive study is radionuclide scan, which is performed after intravenous infusion of technetium-99m pertechnetate. Uptake of this agent by mucus secreting cells of gastric mucosa cells can be enhanced by ranitidine, cimetidine, glucagon, and pentagastrin. Sensitivity reaches 85% and specificity 95% after enhancement.

Plain radiograph is of no value, routine barium study rarely fills the diverticulum. For red blood cell (RBC), scan patient must be actively bleeding.

Key: D

BOOST YOUR KNOWLEDGE

Meckel's diverticulum is most common congenital anomaly of GI tract and is caused by the incomplete obliteration of the omphalomesenteric duct during the 7th week of gestation. Meckel diverticulum has been conveniently referred to by the "rule of 2s", found in approximately 2% of the general population, are usually located 2 feet proximal to the ileocecal valve and are approximately 2 inches in length, can contain two types of ectopic tissue (pancreatic or gastric), generally present before the age of 2 years, and are found twice as commonly in females. Surgical excision of diverticulum is treatment of choice.

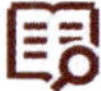

REFERENCE/SOURCE

- Kliegman RM, St Geme III JW, Blum NJ, Shah SS, Tasker RC, Wilson KM. Nelson Textbook of Pediatrics, 21st edition. Elsevier; 2019. Chapter 357. p. 10399.

9. Which of the following statements is *true* regarding development of gut?

A. Cells of the enteric nervous system are generated from the gut
B. Midgut gives rise to biliary system
C. Foregut gives rise to liver
D. Hindgut gives rise to cecum

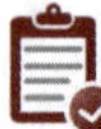

EXPLANATION

Cells of the enteric nervous system are not generated from the gut, instead, they arise from the migration of somatic neural crest cells from the vagal region of the hindbrain into the developing esophagus and subsequently migrate caudally to populate the gut to the anal canal. This process is completed by 12 weeks of gestation. Foregut give rise to pharynx, lower respiratory system, esophagus, stomach, and proximal duodenum down to the level of bile duct, liver, pancreas, and biliary system. Liver develops as a diverticulum (hepatic bud), extending from the lower part of foregut. Midgut give rise to small intestine beyond the opening of bile duct, cecum, appendix, and ascending and proximal transverse colon. Hindgut gives rise to distal third of the transverse colon, descending colon, sigmoid, rectum, and rostral portion of anal canal.

Key: C

BOOST YOUR KNOWLEDGE

Gut develops during 4th week of gestation by division of primitive yolk sac into primitive gut and yolk sac proper. Bile enters duodenum after 13th week of gestation. Blood supply to foregut derived structures is through celiac artery. Blood supply of midgut derived structures is from superior mesenteric artery. Organs derived from hind gut are supplied by inferior mesenteric artery.

Hepatic bud bifurcates into pars cystica and pars hepatica. Pars cystica forms gallbladder and pars hepatica expands to form parenchyma of liver. The proximal part of hepatic duct forms biliary ducts. Stroma of the liver such as sinusoids, Kupffer cells, and capsule develop from septum transversum that also forms part of diaphragm, fibrous pericardium, and ventral mesentery.

REFERENCE/SOURCE

- Wilkinson DJ, Kenny SE. Congenital anomalies including hernias (Chapter 13). In: Kleinman RE, Goulet O-J, Mieli-Vergani G, Sanderson IR, Sherman PM, Shneider BL. Walker's Pediatric Gastrointestinal Disease, 6th edition, Volume 1. USA: People's Medical Publishing House; 2018. p. 319.

10. Which of the following statements are correct regarding small intestine?

A. Meissner's plexus is present between circular and longitudinal muscle layer
B. Auerbach's plexus is present in submucosa
C. Small bowel mucosa is renewed in 4–5 days
D. Paneth cells are present at tip of villi

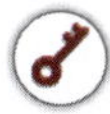

EXPLANATION

Submucosa contains large blood vessels, lymphatic plexus, and submucosal enteric nervous plexus which is called Meissner's plexus. Large cluster of enteric nervous cells called myenteric, or Auerbach's plexus are found between circular and longitudinal muscle layer. The small bowel mucosa is completely renewed in 4–5 days, providing a mechanism for rapid repair after injury, but in young infants or malnourished children, the process may be delayed. Paneth cells are present at the bottom of small intestinal crypt and secrete anti-microbial peptides (defensins) contributing to host defense in the small intestine against microbes.

Key: C

BOOST YOUR KNOWLEDGE

The epithelial cells of intestine are highly specialized and metabolically active, undergo extremely rapid turnover and new cells are continuously generated throughout life from stem cells that are in the middle of each crypt. These cells become functional as they migrate from the crypt up the villus. Four main cell types are produced: (1) enterocytes, (2) enteroendocrine cells, (3) Paneth cells, and (4) goblet cells. Apart from these, microfold cells (M. cells), cup cells, and tuft cells are also present in intestine. Mature colon epithelium has mainly enterocytes and goblet cells.

REFERENCE/SOURCE

- De Santa Barbara P. Anatomy and embryology (Chapter 12). In: Kleinman RE, Goulet OJ, Mieli-Vergani G, Sanderson IR, Sherman PM, Shneider BL. Walker's Pediatric Gastrointestinal Disease, 6th edition, Volume 1. USA: People's Medical Publishing House; 2018. p. 306.

11. A 1-month-old infant presents with large volume watery diarrhea since birth which persists on fasting. Stool examination reveals watery stool with normal stool osmolality, ion gap <100 mOsm/kg, no RBCs, WBCs in stool. Which is the most likely diagnosis?

A. Glucose-galactose malabsorption
B. Lactase deficiency
C. Congenital chloride diarrhea
D. Congenital sucrase isomaltase deficiency

EXPLANATION

The age of onset points toward congenital diarrhea. Persistent on fasting, ion gap <100 indicates secretory diarrhea. The absence of RBC/WBC rules out infectious or inflammatory causes. Glucose-galactose malabsorption and congenital sucrase-isomaltase deficiency shall respond to fasting. Lactase deficiency will also respond to fasting and the ion gap will be more than 100. Congenital chloride diarrhea is secretory diarrhea, persists on fasting, and ion gap will be <100.

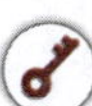

Key: C

BOOST YOUR KNOWLEDGE

Secretory diarrhea occurs when intestinal epithelial cell solute transport system is in an active state of secretion. It is often caused by a secretagogue, such as cholera toxin, some intraluminal fatty acids, and when bile salts stimulate colonic mucosa. Congenital microvillous inclusion disease also causes secretory diarrhea. Secretory diarrhea is usually of large volume and persists with fasting. The stool osmolality is predominantly indicated by the electrolytes and the ion gap is 100 mOsm/kg or less. The ion gap is calculated by subtracting the concentration of electrolytes from total osmolality: Ion gap = Stool osmolality – [(stool Na + stool K) × 2]. Osmotic diarrhea occurs after ingestion of poorly absorbed solute. The solute may be one that is normally not well absorbed (magnesium, phosphate, lactulose, or sorbitol) or one that is not well absorbed because of a disorder of the small bowel. Malabsorbed carbohydrate is fermented in the colon, and short-chain fatty acids (SCFAs) are produced. Although SCFAs can be absorbed in the colon and used as an energy source, the net effect is an increase in the osmotic solute load. Osmotic diarrhea is usually of lesser volume and stops with fasting and the anion gap is >100 mOsm.

REFERENCE/SOURCE

- Kliegman RM, St Geme III JW, Blum NJ, Shah SS, Tasker RC, Wilson KM. Nelson Textbook of Pediatrics, 21st edition. Elsevier; 2019. Chapter 332. p. 10141.

12. A 10-year-old child suffered accident and undergoes resection of terminal ileum. Which nutrient's absorption will suffer most after this?

A. Iron
B. Folate
C. Zinc
D. Vitamin B_{12}

EXPLANATION

Bile salts and vitamin B_{12} are selectively absorbed in distal ileum. Iron, folate, and zinc are absorbed predominantly in proximal small intestine.

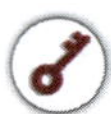

Key: D

BOOST YOUR KNOWLEDGE

Following ileal resection, intestinal transit speeds up. Ileum is the only site of active intestinal bile acid absorption. Following ileal resection, bile acid enters colon where they are deconjugated by colonic bacteria. Deconjugated bile acids directly stimulate colon to secrete fluid and electrolytes and cause secretory watery diarrhea. Resection of ileocecal valve results in small bowel bacterial overgrowth (SBBO) as it prevents movement of colonic microorganisms into distal small bowel. SBBO further causes deconjugation of bile salts leading to reduced absorption of fat and fat-soluble vitamins. Bacteria use intraluminal vitamin B_{12}, limiting vitamin B_{12} for absorption.

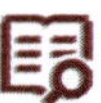

REFERENCES/SOURCES

- Kleinman RE, Goulet OJ, Mieli Vergani G, Sanderson IR, Sherman PM, Shneider BL. (2018). Walker's Pediatric Gastrointestinal Disease: physiology, diagnosis, management, 6th edition. USA: People's Medical Publishing House; 2018. p. 880-1.
- Kliegman RM, St Geme III JW, Blum NJ, Shah SS, Tasker RC, Wilson KM. Nelson Textbook of Pediatrics, 21st edition. Elsevier; 2019. p. 13359.

13. A 3-year-old child is brought to the hospital with explosive watery diarrhea for 2 weeks. He has perianal excoriation, his stool pH is acidic and the reducing substance is >2+ positive. Which of the following statements is true?

A. Rise in breath hydrogen of 10 ppm above baseline shows carbohydrate malabsorption
B. Reducing substance >2+ suggests carbohydrate malabsorption
C. Breath hydrogen test is for protein malabsorption
D. Antibiotic prescription is recommended before breath hydrogen test

EXPLANATION

The increased hydrogen concentration in the breath samples suggests carbohydrate malabsorption. A rise in breath hydrogen of 20 ppm above the baseline preferably with associated symptoms is considered a positive test for carbohydrate malabsorption. Children should not be on antibiotics at the time of the test, because colonic flora is essential for fermenting the sugar. An acidic stool with >2+ reducing substance suggests carbohydrate malabsorption.

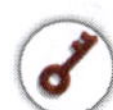

Key: B

BOOST YOUR KNOWLEDGE

A breath hydrogen test is used to identify the specific carbohydrate that is malabsorbed. After an overnight fast, the suspected sugar (lactose, sucrose, fructose, or glucose) is administered as an oral solution, carbohydrate load of up to 2 g/kg, maximum total of 25 g, depending on the specific carbohydrate type. In case of malabsorption, the sugar is not digested or absorbed in the small bowel; it passes on to the colon and is metabolized by the normal gut microflora. One of the products of this process is hydrogen gas, which is absorbed through the colon mucosa and excreted in the breath.

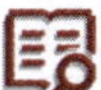

REFERENCE/SOURCE

- Kliegman RM, St Geme III JW, Blum NJ, Shah SS, Tasker RC, Wilson KM. Nelson Textbook of Pediatrics, 21st edition. Elsevier; 2019. Chapter 364. p. 10607.

14. A newborn is diagnosed with congenital glucose-galactose malabsorption. Which of the following statements are true regarding the condition?

A. Mutation in gene coding SGTL-1 causes this condition
B. Mutation in gene coding GLUT 5 causes this condition
C. Transporter is equally distributed in small intestine
D. Entry of glucose-galactose and Na occurs against electrochemical gradient

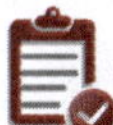

EXPLANATION

Glucose and galactose are actively transported from the small intestine lumen by the sodium glucose transporter (SGLT-1) located in the brush border of the small intestine. The transporter is more prevalent in the duodenum and jejunum. Mutation of gene coding for SGTL-1 is cause of congenital glucose galactose malabsorption. Entry of fructose in enterocytes occurs through glucose transporter 5 (GLUT 5) by facilitated diffusion. The sodium is transported from high to low concentration (with concentration gradient) and at the same time allows the carrier to transport glucose against its concentration gradient.

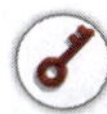

Key: A

BOOST YOUR KNOWLEDGE

Glucose transport is driven by a sodium gradient across the apical cell membrane generated by the Na^+, K^+-ATPase pump located in the basolateral membrane of the enterocyte. The Na^+, K^+-ATPase pump creates a low intracellular sodium concentration by transporting 3 Na^+ ions out of the cell and 2 K^+ ions into the cell. The SGLT-1 transporter utilizes the sodium gradient. Two Na^+ ions bind to the outer face of the SGLT-1 transporter which results in a conformational change permitting subsequent glucose binding. The two Na^+ ions and the glucose molecule are then transferred to the cytoplasmic side of the membrane following another conformational change that involves rotation of the receptor. The glucose is released first followed by the sodium ions. The Na^+ ion is subsequently expelled by Na^+, K^+-ATPase pump to maintain the gradient. The SGLT-1 transporter undergoes another conformational change resulting in the binding sites again being exposed at the apical surface. Exit from the cell of both glucose and fructose occurs via facilitated transport system GLUT 2. Sodium ions and accompanying anions and water follow the glucose, maintaining iso-osmolarity. Fructose transport is not Na-dependent.

REFERENCE/SOURCE

- Cezard JP. Absorption and digestion (Chapter 15). In: Kleinman RE, Goulet OJ, Mieli-Vergani G, Sanderson IR, Sherman PM, Shneider BL. Walker's Pediatric Gastrointestinal Disease, 6th edition, Volume 1. USA: People's Medical Publishing House; 2018. p. 363.

15. A 5-year-old child is brought to the hospital with persistent explosive diarrhea, perianal excoriation, distended gaseous abdomen for the last 1 month following episode of viral acute gastroenteritis. Which of the following is responsible for diarrhea in this child?

A. Exocrine pancreatic insufficiency
B. Congenital glucose-galactose malabsorption
C. Ulcerative colitis
D. Carbohydrate malabsorption

EXPLANATION

Explosive diarrhea, perianal excoriation, and gaseous abdomen indicate fermentative diarrhea due to carbohydrate malabsorption. Partial villous atrophy occurs in post-gastroenteritis syndrome. Disaccharidase activity decreases because of mucosal damage resulting in sugar intolerance and fermentation leading to increased osmotic load in the small intestine and frequently elevated SCFA production in the colon.

Exocrine pancreatic insufficiency will have predominantly steatorrhea. Congenital glucose-galactose malabsorption shall present from the newborn period as life-threatening diarrhea. Ulcerative colitis is an inflammatory condition, that presents with symptoms of colitis such as urgency, tenesmus, and commonly have bloody diarrhea.

Key: D

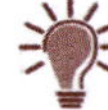

BOOST YOUR KNOWLEDGE

Carbohydrates not digested in the small intestine pass into the large intestine where they are digested by colonic bacteria. This results in the release of SCFA (propionate, butyrate, and acetate) along with methane. The SCFA provides vital nutrition to colonocytes, but excess volumes induce diarrhea and abdominal cramping. Exclusion of the malabsorbed carbohydrate from the diet stops diarrhea in few hours and it is again triggered in a short period of time if reintroduced in the diet.

REFERENCE/SOURCE

- Cezard JP. Absorption and digestion (Chapter 15). In: Kleinman RE, Goulet OJ, Mieli-Vergani G, Sanderson IR, Sherman PM, Shneider BL. Walker's Pediatric Gastrointestinal Disease, 6th edition, Volume 1. USA: People's Medical Publishing House; 2018. p. 364.

16. Which of the following enzymes is *not* upregulated by carbohydrate-rich diet?

A. Sucrase-isomaltase
B. Maltase-glucoamylase
C. Trehalase
D. Lactase

EXPLANATION

Sucrase-isomaltase (SI) and maltase-glucoamylase levels increase in response to high carbohydrate intake. Lactase production is not affected by diet.

Key: D

BOOST YOUR KNOWLEDGE

Sucrose-isomaltase is encoded for by a gene located on chromosome 3. Downregulation of this enzyme occurs in the presence of glucose. The lactase gene is located on chromosome 2. Rate limiting step for lactose digestion is the hydrolysis of lactose.

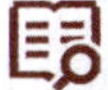

REFERENCE/SOURCE

- Kleinman RE, Goulet OJ, Mieli Vergani G, Sanderson IR, Sherman PM, Shneider BL. (2018). Walker's Pediatric Gastrointestinal Disease: physiology, diagnosis, management, 6th edition. USA: People's Medical Publishing House; 2018. p. 421.

17. An infant, product of consanguineous marriage, is brought to emergency department with osmotic diarrhea and significant failure to thrive since weaning was started. Examination showed perianal redness and acidic pH of stool. His diarrhea subsides on removal of sugars from the diet within few hours. Which of the following is true regarding this condition?

A. Autosomal dominant
B. Commonly presents at birth
C. Treatment involves elimination of sucrose from diet
D. Hydrogen breath test is the gold standard for diagnosis

EXPLANATION

This is most likely congenital sucrase-isomaltase deficiency. This is autosomal recessive disease, which occurs due to homozygous or heterozygous mutation in the sucrase-isomaltase gene resulting in maldigestion of sucrose. Presentation is usually after weaning when sucrose-containing foods are introduced in diet. It leads to osmotic diarrhea, abdominal pain, and failure to thrive. Treatment requires elimination of sucrose from diet and initially restriction of starch too. Gold standard for diagnosis is demonstration of complete or near complete absence of enzyme activity in biopsy tissue of small bowel.

Key: C

BOOST YOUR KNOWLEDGE

Sucrase-isomaltase deficiency is a rare autosomal recessive disorder with a complete absence of sucrase and reduced maltase digestive activity. To identify reducing substances, acid hydrolysis of stool is required as sucrose is a nonreducing sugar. Diagnosis can be achieved with a hydrogen breath test, a direct enzyme assay of small bowel biopsy, or genetic testing. The mainstay of treatment is lifelong dietary restriction of sucrose-containing foods, although symptoms may diminish with age. Enzyme replacement with a purified yeast enzyme, sucrosidase (sucraid) is effective adjunct to dietary restriction.

REFERENCE/SOURCE

- Kliegman RM, St Geme III JW, Blum NJ, Shah SS, Tasker RC, Wilson KM. Nelson Textbook of Pediatrics, 21st edition. Elsevier; 2019. Chapter 364.9. p. 10715.

18. A newborn presented with severe life-threatening diarrhea at birth, with stool osmolality of >100 and 2+ reducing sugar present in watery stool. Diarrhea stops on fasting within few hours and start on even introduction of oral rehydration solution (ORS). What is not true regarding this condition?

A. Genetic mutation affecting SGLT-1 is involved
B. Fructose containing formula should be introduced
C. Diarrhea is osmotic in nature
D. Genetic mutation affecting GLUT5 is involved

EXPLANATION

The presence of diarrhea at birth indicates toward congenital nature of disease. Response to fasting and stool osmolality >100 indicates osmotic diarrhea. Diarrhea even on ORS indicates toward glucose malabsorption. Most likely we are dealing with congenital glucose-galactose malabsorption in this baby. A very rare mutation of SGLT-1 results in glucose-galactose malabsorption. It presents with severe life-threatening diarrhea at birth. The diarrhea is osmotic in nature due to glucose and galactose malabsorption. Treatment is fructose-containing formula and avoidance of glucose and galactose, diarrhea immediately ceases. GLUT5 is carrier protein for facilitated absorption of fructose.

Key: D

BOOST YOUR KNOWLEDGE

Glucose-galactose malabsorption is autosomal recessive condition. Diarrhea follows the ingestion of glucose, breast milk, or conventional lactose-containing formulas. Dehydration and acidosis can be severe, resulting in death. Stools are acidic and contain sugar. Small bowel function and structure is normal in all other aspect. Transport defect is also present in kidney, so intermittent or permanent glycosuria can be seen. Presence of reducing sugar in watery stool and glycosuria despite low blood sugar level is highly suggestive. Diagnosis can be made by hydrogen breath test. Small bowel biopsy will document normal villi and normal disaccharidase activity. Prenatal screening is possible by identification of mutation of SGLT-1.

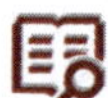

REFERENCE/SOURCE

- Kliegman RM, St Geme III JW, Blum NJ, Shah SS, Tasker RC, Wilson KM. Nelson Textbook of Pediatrics, 21st edition. Elsevier; 2019. Chapter 364.9. p. 10717.

19. A 3-year-old child presents with chronic diarrhea, malnutrition, unexplained anorexia, and worsening of symptoms consisting of vomiting after intake of protein-rich diet. Which of the following could be the most possible diagnosis?

A. Hartnup disease
B. Cystinuria
C. Prolinuria
D. Lysinuric protein intolerance

EXPLANATION

Specific absorption defects involving neutral amino acids as Hartnup disease, basic amino acids as cystinuria, or imino acids as prolinuria does not cause digestive symptoms. Because of associated specific aminoaciduria, it reflects defective tubular reabsorption of the homologous amino acids by the kidney. The only known disease that affects amino acid absorption in which diarrhea is a real problem and is osmotic in nature, often associated with severe malnutrition is lysinuric protein intolerance.

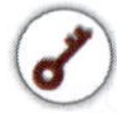

Key: D

BOOST YOUR KNOWLEDGE

Lysinuric protein intolerance is an autosomal recessive disease that results from mutation in *SLC7A7* gene, which encodes for the cationic amino acid transporter y+LAT-1, present on basolateral membrane of enterocytes and renal tubules. In lysinuric protein intolerance, congenital defect affects the exit of arginine, lysine, and ornithine out of the cell through the basolateral membrane. Neutral AA enter the enterocytes through the B, Na-dependent system, whose defect is responsible for Hartnup disease. Bicarboxylic acids enter through a specific Na-dependent, electroneutral X ag system whose defect leads to carboxylic aminoaciduria. Proline uses Na, Cl dependent IMINO carrier, basic AA use B^+, 0 Na-independent and Na-dependent channel whose defect results in type 1 cystinuria. No specific congenital defect of peptide digestion or absorption by the intestinal mucosa is known.

REFERENCE/SOURCE

- Cezard JP. Absorption and digestion (Chapter 15). In: Kleinman RE, Goulet OJ, Mieli-Vergani G, Sanderson IR, Sherman PM, Shneider BL. Walker's Pediatric Gastrointestinal Disease, 6th edition, Volume 1. USA: People's Medical Publishing House; 2018. p. 366.

20. Which of the following statements is true in reference to bile acids and bile salts?

A. Chenodeoxycholic acid is synthesized in the liver
B. Deoxycholic acid is synthesized in liver
C. Bile acids are reabsorbed in the jejunum
D. 95% of bile acids are excreted in stool

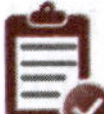

EXPLANATION

Cholic and chenodeoxycholic acids are primary bile acids and are synthesized in liver from cholesterol. They are glycol and tauroconjugated, excreted, and later get transformed by colonic bacteria into deoxycholic acids and lithocholic acids which are secondary acids. Pool of bile acids amounts to 1–2.5 g and they are efficiently reabsorbed in the distal ileum by a Na-dependent, carrier-mediated process leading to the reabsorption of 95% of bile salts secreted in bile.

Key: A

BOOST YOUR KNOWLEDGE

Fats must be wrapped in outwardly hydrophilic, inwardly lipophilic particles—bile salt micelles in the gut lumen, and chylomicrons in the absorbing cell and circulation to reach their site of metabolic use.

REFERENCE/SOURCE

- Cezard JP. Absorption and digestion (Chapter 15). In: Kleinman RE, Goulet OJ, Mieli-Vergani G, Sanderson IR, Sherman PM, Shneider BL. Walker's Pediatric Gastrointestinal Disease, 6th edition, Volume 1. USA: People's Medical Publishing House; 2018. p. 366.

21. A 3-year-old female child is referred with diagnosis of intestinal lymphangiectasia. Which of the following statements is correct?

A. Absence of microsomal TG transfer protein subunit is the defect responsible for this condition
B. Hypoalbuminemia will be present
C. Low protein and high fat diet is recommended
D. Poor micellar solubilization causes steatorrhea in this condition

EXPLANATION

Microsomal TG transfer protein (MTP) transfers resynthesized triglycerides (TG) in the rough endoplasmic reticulum where, together with phospholipids and cholesterol, TG is joined by newly synthesized apolipoproteins AI, AIV, and B48. The absence of one of the MTP subunits, but not of B48, is responsible for abetalipoproteinemia, not intestinal lymphangiectasia. In intestinal lymphangiectasis hypoalbuminemia is present along with steatorrhea, so high protein and low-fat medium chain triglyceride (MCT)-based diet is recommended.

Poor micellar solubilization causes steatorrhea in conditions such as bile acid synthesis defect, abnormal biliary excretion in biliary atresia or progressive loss of bile salt pool due to interrupted bile acid enterohepatic circulation because of bacterial overgrowth, ileal resection, Crohn's disease, or congenital bile acid malabsorption. Poor micellar solubilization does not lead to steatorrhea in intestinal lymphangiectasia.

Key: B

BOOST YOUR KNOWLEDGE

In intestinal lymphangiectasia, reflux of absorbed fat into the intestinal lumen occurs because of blocked lymph flow. Steatorrhea is moderate, and it is associated with enteric loss of other constituents of intestinal lymph including albumin, immunoglobulins, and T lymphocytes. On intestinal biopsy, villi will appear distorted by ecstatic lymphatics.

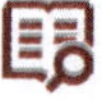

REFERENCE/SOURCE

- Cezard JP. Absorption and digestion (Chapter 15). In: Kleinman RE, Goulet OJ, Mieli-Vergani G, Sanderson IR, Sherman PM, Shneider BL. Walker's Pediatric Gastrointestinal Disease, 6th edition, Volume 1. USA: People's Medical Publishing House; 2018. p. 368.

22. A male baby is brought in emergency at 24 hours of life with absence of anal opening. Examination of perineum showed well-formed buttocks and black bulge at the site of anus. Which of the following statements is true regarding the condition?

A. Invertogram is the radiological investigation of choice
B. Immediate perineal manipulation is advisable followed by dilation program
C. A prone cross table X-ray film is not supportive
D. Extraintestinal anomalies are seen in >10%

EXPLANATION

Imperforate anus can be divided into low lesions, where the rectum has descended through the sphincter complex, and high lesions, where it has not. In males, low lesions usually manifest with meconium staining somewhere on the perineum along median raphe. This baby has low lesion. A high imperforate anus in a male has no apparent cutaneous opening or fistula, perineum appears flat, but it usually has a fistula to the urinary tract, either the urethra or the bladder and may be air or meconium passed via the urethra. Children with a low lesion can usually be treated initially with perineal manipulation to perforate the skin and proceed with dilation or do a simple perineal anoplasty. One should avoid passing a nasogastric tube for the first 24 hours to allow the abdomen and bowel to distend, pushing meconium down into the distal rectum. A prone cross table X-ray at 24 hours of life with a radiopaque marker on perineum helps in identifying low lesion. Extraintestinal anomalies are seen in <10% of these patients.

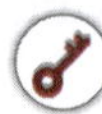

Key: B

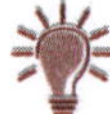

BOOST YOUR KNOWLEDGE

The normal position of the anus on the perineum is approximately halfway (0.5 ratio) between the coccyx and the scrotum or introitus. Although symptoms, primarily constipation, have been attributed to anterior ectopic anus (ratio: <0.34 in females, <0.46 in males), many patients have no symptoms.

The invertogram or upside-down X-ray is of little value, but a prone cross table lateral plain X-ray at 24 hours of life (to allow time for bowel distention from swallowed air) with a radiopaque marker on the perineum can demonstrate a low lesion by showing the rectal gas bubble <1 cm from the perineal skin.

REFERENCE/SOURCE

- Kliegman RM, St Geme III JW, Blum NJ, Shah SS, Tasker RC, Wilson KM. Nelson Textbook of Pediatrics, 21st edition. Elsevier; 2019. Chapter 371. pp. 10954, 10959, 10960.

23. Which of the anomalies does not make part of "Currarino triad"?

A. Ectopic anus
B. Tracheoesophageal fistula
C. Sacral bone hypoplasia
D. Anterior meningocele

EXPLANATION

Currarino triad includes anorectal malformations (ectopic anus, anal stenosis, and imperforate anus), sacral bone anomalies (hypoplasia, poor segmentation), and presacral anomaly (anterior meningoceles, teratoma, and cyst). Tracheoesophageal fistula is not part of this triad.

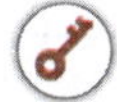

Key: B

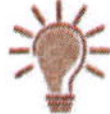

BOOST YOUR KNOWLEDGE

It is an autosomal dominant disorder due in most patients to a mutation in the *MNX1* gene. Patients have funnel-appearing anus, sacral bony defects on X-ray and presacral mass seen on examination or imaging.

REFERENCE/SOURCE

- Kliegman RM, St Geme III JW, Blum NJ, Shah SS, Tasker RC, Wilson KM. Nelson Textbook of Pediatrics, 21st edition. Elsevier; 2019. Chapter 358. pp. 10440, 10959.

24. A 10-year-old girl presents with refractory constipation for 2 years. She undergoes rectal suction biopsy which shows presence of ganglion cells and normal acetylcholinesterase (AChE) activity. Her anal manometry shows absence of rectoanal inhibitory reflex (RAIR). What is the most probable diagnosis?

A. Hirschsprung disease
B. Internal anal sphincter achalasia
C. Intestinal neuronal dysplasia type B
D. Chronic intestinal pseudo-obstruction

EXPLANATION

In Hirschsprung disease, there will be absence of ganglion cells and increased AChE activity. In intestinal neuronal dysplasia type B, there will be submucosal hyperganglionosis with giant ganglia and ectopic ganglion cells with increased AChE activity. Presence of ganglion cells with absence of RAIR is classic of internal anal sphincter achalasia. In chronic intestinal pseudo-obstruction, RAIR will be present.

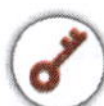

Key: B

BOOST YOUR KNOWLEDGE

Internal anal sphincter achalasia or anal achalasia is also called ultra short segment Hirschsprung disease, where aganglionic segment is limited to the internal sphincter. Clinical symptoms are similar to functional constipation. Current treatment, although controversial, includes anal botulism injection to relax the anal sphincter and anorectal myectomy if indicated. Anorectal manometry evaluates the internal anal sphincter while a balloon is distended in the rectum. In healthy individuals, rectal distention initiates relaxation of the internal anal sphincter in response to rectal distention known as the RAIR.

REFERENCE/SOURCE

- Kliegman RM, St Geme III JW, Blum NJ, Shah SS, Tasker RC, Wilson KM. Nelson Textbook of Pediatrics, 21st edition. Elsevier; 2019. p. 10441.

25. Which segment of the gastrointestinal tract has valves of Houston and columns of Morgagni?

A. Duodenum and jejunum
B. Appendix and ascending colon
C. Transverse colon and sigmoid
D. Rectum and anal canal

EXPLANATION

Lumen of rectum has two to three lateral curves which is known as valves of Houston. Columns of Morgagni are longitudinal folds of mucosa at the dentate line. Dentate line is located 1–2 cm proximal to the external orifice of anus and it marks transition from columnar epithelium of rectum to squamous epithelium of the anal canal. Duodenum and jejunum have villi (tiny finger-like projections) and crypts of Lieberkühn.

Key: D

BOOST YOUR KNOWLEDGE

The colon is a 75–100 cm sacculated tube formed by three strips of longitudinal muscle called Taenia coli that traverse its length and fold the mucosa into haustra. Anterior portion of rectum is covered by peritoneal reflection, posterior rectum is free of peritoneum. The most distal third of rectum is devoid of peritoneum circumferentially.

REFERENCE/SOURCE

- Fisher J, Modi BP, Johson S, Jaksic A. Benign perianal legions (Chapter 18). In: Kleinman RE, Goulet OJ, Mieli-Vergani G, Sanderson IR, Sherman PM, Shneider BL. Walker's Pediatric Gastrointestinal Disease, 6th edition, Volume 1. USA: People's Medical Publishing House; 2018. p. 559.

26. An 18-month-old child is brought with complaint of small amount of red blood streak over stool for the first time. Mother also gives history of him crying during defecation and of passing type 1 stool as per Bristol stool chart. Perianal examination shows a fresh tear at posterior midline and no skin tag. What could be most possible diagnosis in this child?

A. Acute anal fissure
B. Chronic anal fissure
C. Perirectal ulcer
D. Anal fistula

EXPLANATION

Anal fissure is the most frequent cause of anorectal bleeding in the first 2 years of life. It commonly presents with pain, which may last for minutes to hours after defecation and small amount of blood with stooling. Most cases of anal fissure are associated with constipation and are often noted after passage of a large, hard stool. A chronic fissure is defined by symptom that persist longer than 6 weeks after treatment and presence of fibrosis at the base of the fissure. This is rare in children. Acute anal fissure appears as a fresh laceration, while a chronic anal fissure has raised edges exposing the internal anal sphincter muscle fibers. Perirectal abscess is a localized, purulent fluid collection in the tissues surrounding the rectum. *Fistula in ano* may be result of spontaneous or operative drainage of perirectal abscess, which then forms a chronic inflammatory tract from the dentate line to the skin. In contrast to the transient pain of an anal fissure, the pain of a perirectal abscess is constant, and examination reveals tender perirectal swelling and possibly a fever. In *fistula in ano*, a single cutaneous orifice is evident, it communicates directly with the rectum at the level of crypts of Morgagni, persistent drainage is often seen.

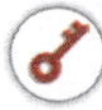

Key: A

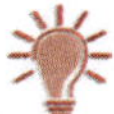

BOOST YOUR KNOWLEDGE

Anal fissure is a tear in the epithelium and superficial tissues of anal canal. It is usually linear, extending from just below the dentate line to the anal verge. First, it forms as simple crack in the anoderm, with subsequent infection and poor healing it develops into chronic fissure identified by a sentinel tag of skin, fibrotic edges, and exposure of the internal sphincter. 90% of anal fissures are in the posterior midline followed by anterior midline. Diagnosis can be made after inspection of anal canal. Treatment includes stool softener, diet change, anal hygiene, and warm baths. In chronic fissure, which does not respond to medical management, lateral internal sphincterotomy is the procedure of choice.

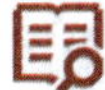

REFERENCE/SOURCE

- Fisher J, Modi BP, Johson S, Jaksic A. Benign perianal legions (Chapter 18). In: Kleinman RE, Goulet OJ, Mieli-Vergani G, Sanderson IR, Sherman PM, Shneider BL. Walker's Pediatric Gastrointestinal Disease, 6th edition, Volume 1. USA: People's Medical Publishing House; 2018. p. 559.

27. A 12-year-old boy is referred to pediatric gastroenterology clinic for evaluation of internal hemorrhoids. During the examination, on performing Valsalva, internal hemorrhoid prolapses and the prolapse requires manual reduction to go back. Based on this finding, what will be grade of internal hemorrhoid?

A. I
B. II
C. III
D. IV

EXPLANATION

Internal hemorrhoids are graded on ascending scale of severity form I to IV. With grade I hemorrhoids, anal cushions are present on rectal examination on the left lateral, right posterolateral, and right anterolateral which corresponds to the locations of the venous plexuses. Grade II hemorrhoids prolapse below the dentate line but reduce spontaneously. Grade III hemorrhoids are also prolapsed but must be manually reduced. Grade IV hemorrhoids are irreducibly prolapsed and may result in chronic soilage and spotting of blood.

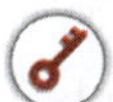

Key: C

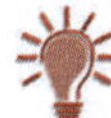

BOOST YOUR KNOWLEDGE

Internal hemorrhoids are dilated blood vessel, specifically a varicosity of the tributaries of the superior rectal vein. They are located above the dentate line and deep to the columnar epithelium lining of the rectum, are viscerally innervated and thus are not painful.

REFERENCE/SOURCE

- Fisher J, Modi BP, Johson S, Jaksic A. Benign perianal legions (Chapter 18). In: Kleinman RE, Goulet OJ, Mieli-Vergani G, Sanderson IR, Sherman PM, Shneider BL. Walker's Pediatric Gastrointestinal Disease, 6th edition, Volume 1. USA: People's Medical Publishing House; 2018. p. 563.

28. A 10-year-old girl complains of pain on defecation for 1 week. She also complains of pain on cleaning after bowel movement as well as on sitting. Perianal examination reveals a tender grape-like protrusion at the anal verge. Based on these findings, which of the following is most likely diagnosis?

A. Rectal prolapse
B. Simple external hemorrhoid
C. Grade IV internal hemorrhoids
D. Thrombosed external hemorrhoid

EXPLANATION

Simple external hemorrhoids (EH) rarely cause symptoms, some may have pruritus. When it becomes very large, then becomes difficult to clean after bowel movements. External hemorrhoids involve skin of the anoderm and therefore are innervated with cutaneous nerve. Sudden acute pain occurs when external hemorrhoid thromboses, and a tender grape-like protrusion is noted on examination. Hence, newly thrombosed EH are associated with acute pain. Internal hemorrhoids (IH) are viscerally innervated, so are not painful. IH may present with painless protruding rectal mass or rectal bleeding. Rectal prolapse is a protrusion of the entire circumference of the rectal mucosa, thus concentric rings of mucosa are seen on examination. While with grade III or IV hemorrhoids, the protrusion occurs only in a defined sector of the anus (usually lateral).

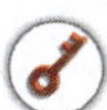

Key: D

BOOST YOUR KNOWLEDGE

Hemorrhoids are varicose veins from either the internal or external rectal plexus of veins and are generally classified in external and internal hemorrhoids. Internal hemorrhoids are above dentate line, external are below. Internal hemorrhoids should be differentiated from anorectal varices seen in cases of chronic liver disease and portal hypertension. These are thought to result from chronic constipation and excessive straining on defecation. Without intervention, external hemorrhoids will drain spontaneously after few days and pain will stop.

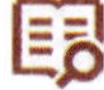

REFERENCE/SOURCE

- Fisher J, Modi BP, Johson S, Jaksic A. Benign perianal legions (Chapter 18). In: Kleinman RE, Goulet OJ, Mieli-Vergani G, Sanderson IR, Sherman PM, Shneider BL. Walker's Pediatric Gastrointestinal Disease, 6th edition, Volume 1. USA: People's Medical Publishing House; 2018. p. 563.

29. A newborn girl is brought in emergency with discharge of meconium from the vagina. Which of the following statement is correct regarding the condition?

A. This is a "low" lesion
B. This is a "high" lesion
C. This is amenable to straightforward perineal reconstructive procedure
D. Postsurgical fecal incontinence is an unlikely complication

EXPLANATION

Newborn has rectovaginal fistula. Anorectal malformations, where rectum has not passed completely through the anal sphincter are considered intermediate or high lesions. So, this is an example of high lesion. Cutaneous fistula is an example of low lesion, where rectum has passed through the anal sphincter. Only infants presenting with low lesion such as cutaneous fistula, are amenable to relatively straightforward perineal reconstructive procedures without a diverting colostomy. In all other cases and so in this case, temporary diverting colostomy followed by a staged reconstructive procedure after the infant has been fully assessed is advisable. The definitive repair or posterior sagittal anorectoplasty (PSARP) is performed at about 1 year of age. Children with high malformations have poorer outcome with higher rates of fecal incontinence post repair.

Key: B

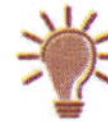

BOOST YOUR KNOWLEDGE

Anorectal malformations occur in one in 2,500 live births. Krickenbeck classification is used to aid both research and prognostic stratification. Anorectal anomalies are most often detected during routine postnatal examination. Anatomically, the lesion is usually associated with a fistulous communication between the rectum and either the genitourinary tract or perineum. About 60% of infants have associated malformation of other organ system, most common is VACTERL (vertebral, anorectal, cardiac, tracheoesophageal, renal, and limb) sequence of anomalies. The infant should have urinary tract antibiotic prophylaxis until vesicoureteric reflux has been excluded. In low lesions, parents are taught to dilate the infant's anus to avoid stenosis. Constipation is a postsurgical complication in low lesions and fecal incontinence in high.

REFERENCE/SOURCE

- Wilkinson DJ, Kenny SE. Congenital anomalies including hernias (Chapter 13). In: Kleinman RE, Goulet OJ, Mieli-Vergani G, Sanderson IR, Sherman PM, Shneider BL. Walker's Pediatric Gastrointestinal Disease, 6th edition, Volume 1. USA: People's Medical Publishing House; 2018. p. 335.

CHAPTER 16.2

Common Surgical Conditions

Rajesh Kumar Meena

1. A 35-days old infant presents with recurrent episodes of forcible, projectile, nonbilious vomiting for 10 days. On examination, the baby is dehydrated and has tachycardia with slow, shallow breathing. Baby appears alert, anxious and hungry, and appearance of the abdomen after feeding is shown in the given picture. What is the most possible diagnosis?

A. Gastric volvulus
B. Gastroesophageal reflux
C. Septicemia
D. Hypertrophic pyloric stenosis

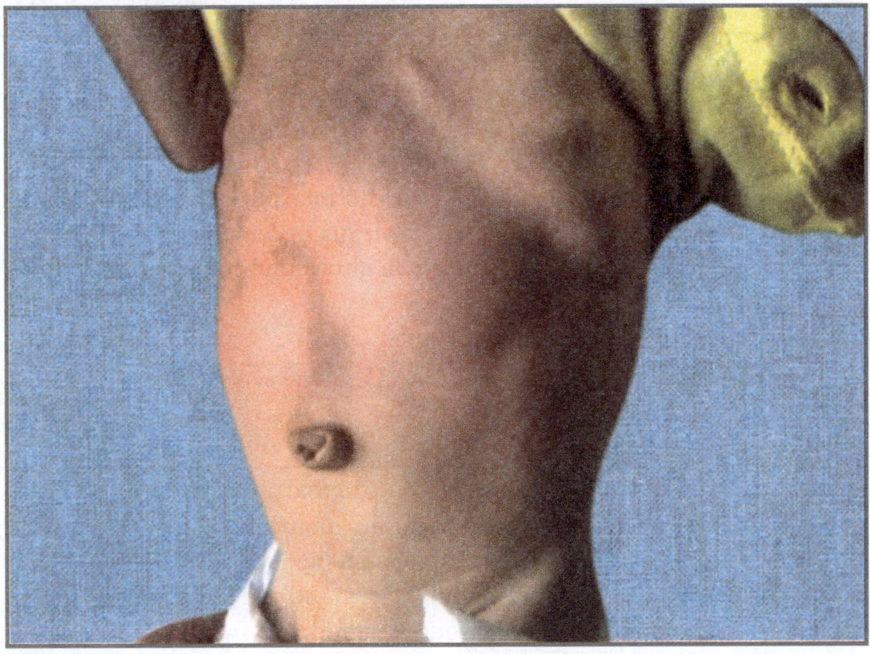

EXPLANATION

The key points in the clinical presentation are: (1) age 35 days; (2) recurrent, forcible, projectile, nonbilious vomiting; (3) dehydration; (4) tachycardia with slow, shallow breathing; (5) alert, anxious, and hungry baby. Findings in abdomen are: (1) distended stomach and (2) visible peristalsis from left to right. Let us analyze these characteristics for each of the four options:

	Gastric volvulus	*Gastroesophageal reflux*	*Septicemia*	*Hypertrophic pyloric stenosis*
Age 35 days at presentation	Rare condition	+	+	+
Recurrent, forcible, projectile, and nonbilious vomiting	Persistent regurgitation, unproductive vomiting, and occasionally projectile	Recurrent regurgitations/small volume vomiting	±	++
Dehydration	±	–	±	++
Tachycardia with slow, shallow breathing	±	Presents with tachycardia and tachypnea especially after the episode of reflux	Presents with tachycardia and tachypnea	Have tachycardia due to dehydration, and slow, shallow breathing due to metabolic alkalosis secondary to persistent vomiting
Alert, anxious, and hungry baby	–	Anxious and irritable	Sick, lethargic with poor feeding	++
Distended stomach	+ (abnormal position of stomach)		±	++
Visible peristalsis (L >R)	–	–	Usually peristalsis is reduced/absent	++

 **Key: D**

BOOST YOUR KNOWLEDGE

Nitric oxide is an essential transmitter responsible for the relaxation of pyloric sphincter muscle. There is a deficiency of nitric oxide synthase in the myenteric plexus in patients with HPS. The presence of pyloric muscle thickness >4 mm and channel length of ≥16 mm on ultrasound confirms the diagnosis of HPS.

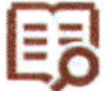

REFERENCE/SOURCE

- Gupta P, Menon PSN, Ramji S, Lodha R. PG Textbook of Pediatrics, 3rd edition. New Delhi: Jaypee Brothers Medical Publishers; 2022.

2. Which of the following statements is *correct* regarding hypertrophic pyloric stenosis?

A. The diagnosis has traditionally been established by observation/inspection of the pyloric mass
B. The mass is firm, movable, olive-shaped, and best palpated from the right side
C. The mass is located below and to the left of the umbilicus in the mid abdomen
D. The pyloric mass is easiest palpated after an episode of vomiting

EXPLANATION

The age-old method to diagnose hypertrophic pyloric stenosis is by palpating the pyloric mass. The mass is firm, movable, olive-shaped, and best palpated from the left side as it is located above and to the right of the umbilicus in the mid epigastrium. The pyloric mass is best palpated after an episode of vomiting. After feed, there may be a visible gastric peristaltic wave that progresses across the abdomen which is often noticed and reported by mother while feeding.

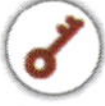 **Key: D**

BOOST YOUR KNOWLEDGE

Differential diagnosis of hypertrophic pyloric stenosis:

Condition	Important points to be considered
Gastroesophageal reflux disease (GERD)	Differentiated from pyloric stenosis by radiographic studies
Adrenal insufficiency	Has projectile vomiting. Absence of a metabolic acidosis, elevated serum potassium, and urinary sodium concentrations of adrenal insufficiency aid in differentiation
Inborn errors of metabolism	Recurrent emesis with alkalosis (urea cycle) or acidosis (organic acidemia), lethargy, coma, or seizures
Pyloric membrane or pyloric duplication	Visible peristalsis and in duplication, a palpable mass
Duodenal stenosis	Proximal to the ampulla of Vater results in clinical features of pyloric stenosis. Differentiated by the presence of a pyloric mass on physical examination or ultrasonography

REFERENCE/SOURCE

- Kliegman RM. Nelson Textbook of Pediatrics, 1st South Asia edition. Amsterdam, Netherlands: Elsevier; 2015.

3. An 8-month-old male child was brought with complaints of irregular passage of hard stools since 1 month of age which resolves intermittently after enema. He is now having progressive abdominal distension for 2 weeks, foul-smelling loose stools, fever, and lethargy for 5 days. A similar episode occurred at 3 months of age requiring hospitalization and enema for 1 week. On examination, child is thin built and pale, having both weight-for-age and weight-for-length between <–2 standard deviation (SD) and >–3 SD. Abdomen is distended (left more than right side), nontender, and no organomegaly. What is the most likely diagnosis?

A. Idiopathic constipation
B. Acute colitis
C. Hypothyroidism with constipation
D. Hirschsprung's disease

EXPLANATION

The key points in the clinical presentation are: (1) age at onset 1 month; (2) irregular passage of hard stools which resolves intermittently after enema; (3) progressive abdominal distension for 2 weeks; (4) foul-smelling loose stools, fever, and lethargy for 5 days; and (5) similar episode at 1 months age requiring hospitalization. Findings on examination: (1) pallor, (2) weight for age and weight for height between <–2 SD and >–3 SD, and (3) abdominal distension (left more than right side) without organomegaly. Let us analyze these characteristics for each of the four options:

	Idiopathic constipation	*Acute colitis*	*Hypothyroidism with constipation*	*Hirschsprung's disease*
Onset at 1 month's age	–	–	Onset at birth	++ (can present at any age)
Irregular hard stools requiring enema	+	–	+	+
Progressive abdominal distension	+	–	+	++ (due to dilated colon)
Foul-smelling loose stools	Encopresis can present as loose stools but not foul smelling	+	–	++ (diarrhea is symptom of enterocolitis)
Fever with lethargy	–	+	–	++ (enterocolitis)
Pallor	+	–	+	+

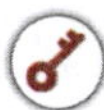

Key: D

BOOST YOUR KNOWLEDGE

The presence of empty rectum on per rectal examination and explosive passage of flatus and feces on withdrawal of the examining finger suggest high probability of Hirschsprung's disease. Full thickness rectal biopsy is the gold standard—absence of ganglion cells in both the myenteric and submucosal plexus, hypertrophic nerve fibers, and presence of increased acetylcholinesterase staining in mucosa and submucosa is confirmatory of Hirschsprung's disease.

REFERENCE/SOURCE

- Gupta P, Menon PSN, Ramji S, Lodha R. PG Textbook of Pediatrics, 3rd edition. New Delhi: Jaypee Brothers Medical Publishers; 2022.

4. A 12-month-old well-nourished infant presents with two episodes of loose stool containing blood, and intermittent episodes of excessive irritability and crying associated with loose stools. Child is having preceding history of coryza, which was started 1 day back only. There is no history of fever, vomiting, or decreased urine output. Mother has started complementary feeding since last 2 weeks in form of few glucose biscuits and undiluted cow milk. On examination, the child is anxious, alert without any features of dehydration. On examination, a small mass is felt in the right inguinal region in a soft, nontender abdomen. Rest of the systemic examination is unremarkable. Picture of the stool is given. What is the most likely diagnosis?

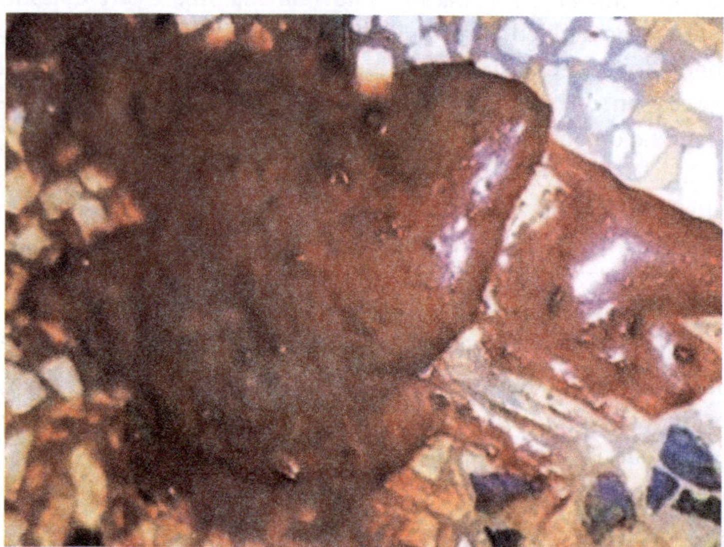

A. Cow milk protein allergy
B. Acute dysentery
C. Intussusception
D. Malrotation

EXPLANATION

The key points in the clinical presentation are: (1) well-nourished infant; (2) age at presentation 12 months; (3) loose stools containing blood and intermittent episodes of excessive irritability and crying; (4) preceding history of coryza; (5) cow milk intake for 2 months; (6) stool mainly consist of blood without any fecal matter. Findings on examination are: (1) alert, anxious without dehydration and (2) small mass is felt in right inguinal region. Let us analyze these characteristics for each of the four options:

	Cow milk protein allergy	*Acute dysentery*	*Intussusception*	*Malrotation*
Well-nourished baby	+	±	+	+
Age 12 months	+	+	+	+ (~50% within 1st month)
Loose stools containing blood	±	++ (contains fecal matter also)	++ (without any fecal matter) red currant jelly stools	– (bilious emesis and acute obstruction are main presentation)
Intermittent episodes of excessive irritability and crying	–	+	++	+
Preceding coryza	±	±	±	–
History of cow milk intake	++	±	±	±
Alert and anxious	+	±	+	±
Mass in right inguinal region	–	–	++	–

Key: C

BOOST YOUR KNOWLEDGE

Passage of red currant jelly stool with negligible amount of fecal matter is hallmark of intussusception. Per abdomen examination reveals presence of banana-shaped mass with concavity toward the umbilicus. Presence of *pseudokidney sign* or *bowel-in-bowel sign* on ultrasound is diagnostic of intussusception.

REFERENCE/SOURCE

- Gupta P, Menon PSN, Ramji S, Lodha R. PG Textbook of Pediatrics, 3rd edition. New Delhi: Jaypee Brothers Medical Publishers; 2022.

5. In the pathophysiology of intestinal obstruction in a case with dynamic obstruction, what is the correct sequence of the events preceding the intestinal perforation?

1. Progressive dilatation
2. Bacterial overgrowth
3. Hyperperistalsis
4. Reverse peristalsis

A. 3, 1, 4, 2
B. 1, 2, 3, 4
C. 1, 3, 4, 2
D. 3, 4, 1, 2

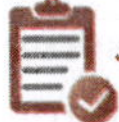

EXPLANATION

Initially in a case with dynamic obstruction there is dilatation of proximal bowel with hyperperistalsis to overcome the obstruction. Persistence of obstruction and progressive dilatation initiate reverse peristalsis in the proximal segment. Later intestinal commensals overgrow in the stagnant intestinal content leading to mucosal inflammation, increased gas production, gut wall ischemia, and subsequently to perforation.

Key: A

BOOST YOUR KNOWLEDGE

Mechanical obstruction of gastrointestinal (GI) tract due to intraluminal occlusion, extraluminal compression, gut wall anomaly, or combination of these is known as dynamic obstruction. It is caused by multiple conditions such as atresia, stenosis, intestinal malrotation with volvulus, peritoneal band and adhesion, and meconium ileus. While obstruction caused by conditions such as hypokalemia, sepsis, and enterocolitis leading to ineffective propulsive peristalsis is known as adynamic obstruction.

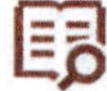

REFERENCE/SOURCE

- Gupta P, Menon PSN, Ramji S, Lodha R. PG Textbook of Pediatrics, 3rd edition. New Delhi: Jaypee Brothers Medical Publishers; 2022.

6. A 5-month-old girl is brought to the pediatric emergency with complaints of loose stools for 15 days which are 8–10 episodes per day watery without any blood or mucus in stools. Child had history of fever and coryza which lasted for 2 days at the onset of illness. Now the child has presented with decreased oral intake for 2 days. Mother feeds undiluted cow's milk with bottle. On examination, vitals are stable, there are no features of dehydration, and child's weight-for-age z-score (WAZ), length-or height-for-age z-score (LAZ), and weight-for-height z-score (WFHZ) are at –2z-score. On systemic examination, abdomen is slightly distended soft, nontender with no palpable organomegaly. Which of the following is not a part of the routine management of this illness?

A. Oral rehydration solution
B. Vitamins and minerals
C. Nutritional therapy
D. Antibiotics

EXPLANATION

This is a case of acute onset diarrhea of infectious etiology (as there is history of fever and coryza at the onset of illness) lasting for >14 days thus meeting the criteria of persistent diarrhea (PD). Age below 6 months and feeding history of undiluted cow's milk with bottle are the underlying risk factor for PD in this child. The routine management of a child with PD involves assessment and management of dehydration, dietary management (in form of reduced lactose diet/lactose free diet/monosaccharide-based diet), and supplementation of vitamins and minerals as most of these children are malnourished. Antibiotics are not routinely recommended in children with PD.

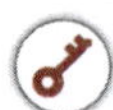

Key: D

BOOST YOUR KNOWLEDGE

Following are the indications for using antibiotics in a case with PD—presence of gross blood in stools, presence of *Shigella*, *Giardia*, and *Cryptosporidium* on stool examination, and features of systemic infection and severe malnutrition.

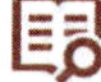

REFERENCE/SOURCE

- Gupta P, Menon PSN, Ramji S, Lodha R. PG Textbook of Pediatrics, 3rd edition. New Delhi: Jaypee Brothers Medical Publishers; 2022.

7. A 9-month-old boy is brought with the complaints of excessive crying/irritability which increase after feeding since 1 month age and sometimes these episodes were associated with vomiting. His symptoms showed some improvement after oral antiemetics but no relieved completely. His mother has noticed that he is not gaining weight since last 4 months. There is no history of coughing, choking during feeds, or swallowing difficulty. On examination, vitals are stable, and no abnormality was detected on systemic examination. Interpretation of anthropometric measurements suggests child is having severe underweight and moderate stunting. In the past, he had been admitted once at the age of 4 months for pneumonia. A provisional diagnosis of pathologic GERD was made. Among the following investigations, which one is least preferred for confirming the diagnosis in this child?

A. Upper GI endoscopy
B. Intraluminal impedance monitoring
C. Bronchoscopy with lavage
D. Contrast radiographic study

EXPLANATION

Excessive irritability/crying, recurrent regurgitation with or without vomiting, and poor growth are the most common symptoms and signs of GERD. Presence of these along with normal systemic examination points toward the high possibility of GERD. Following investigations help in diagnosis of GERD: (1) Upper GI (UGI) endoscopy helps in determining the presence and severity of esophagitis, strictures, and Barrett's esophagus; (2) intraluminal impedance monitoring helps in determining the esophageal function by bolus flow, volume clearance time, and acid exposure by the help of its multiple channels; (3) bronchoscopy with lavage helps in diagnosing GERD by demonstrating the lipid laden macrophages in bronchoalveolar lavage (BAL) sample; and (4) contrast radiographic study has poor sensitivity and specificity, it can be of help only in cases with suspected achalasia cardia, esophageal stricture/stenosis, hiatal hernia or gastric outlet obstruction. Based on these points, contrast radiographic study is the least preferred method for diagnosis of GERD.

Key: D

BOOST YOUR KNOWLEDGE

Gastroesophageal reflux disease is the most common esophageal disorder in children of all ages. It peaks at 4 months of age and resolves in nearly all infants by 24 months of age. Infant gastroesophageal reflux questionnaire (I-GERQ) and its revised version (I-GERQ-R) are two observer-reported outcome measures-based questionnaires which can be used to facilitate and standardized the history in suspected cases.

REFERENCES/SOURCES

- Kliegman RM. Nelson Textbook of Pediatrics, 1st South Asia edition. Amsterdam, Netherlands: Elsevier; 2015.
- Rudolph CD, Hassall E. Gastroesophageal reflux. In: Kleinman RE, Goulet OJ, Mieli-Vergani G, Sanderson IR, Sherman PM, Shneider BL (Eds). Walker's Pediatric Gastrointestinal Disease: Physiology, Diagnosis, Management, 6th edition. China: People's Medical Publishing House; 2018.

8. A 10-year-old girl visited the outpatient department with complaints of abdominal pain and diarrhea for the last 3 months. There is history of passage of blood in stools intermittently for last 2 weeks. She has received two courses of antibiotics for her complaints. Now she has started feeling pain in her bilateral knee joints for the last 4 days. A provisional diagnosis of inflammatory bowel disease (IBD) has been made. Which one among the following statements regarding the arthropathy in IBD is *true*?

A. Arthropathy is the most common extraintestinal manifestation of IBD
B. Peripheral arthritis is asymmetric, deforming, and migratory polyarthritis
C. Exacerbations in pauciarticular disease do not correlate with bowel disease
D. Almost 20% of cases of IBD present with HLA-B27 positivity

EXPLANATION

Presence of chronic bloody diarrhea, abdominal pain/tenesmus, and weight loss with or without extra-intestinal manifestations is an indication to evaluate for the presence of IBD. 25–35% of patients with IBD have extraintestinal manifestations—arthropathy being the most common, present in 6% cases with pediatric ulcerative colitis (UC) and 7% cases with pediatric Crohn's disease. Presents as asymmetric, nondeforming, migratory polyarthritis involving one or more large joints, and the exacerbations in pauciarticular form (<5 joints involved) correlates well with the bowel disease. 1–4% cases present with axial arthropathy, sacroiliitis, or ankylosing spondylitis and it is associated with the HLA-B27 positivity.

Key: A

BOOST YOUR KNOWLEDGE

Manifestations such as fever, significant weight loss, anorexia, lethargy, and perianal disease (fissure, tag, etc.) are more common in cases with Crohn's disease in comparison to those with UC.

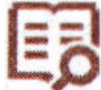

REFERENCES/SOURCES

- Croft N. Ulcerative and indeterminate colitis. In: Kleinman RE, Goulet OJ, Mieli-Vergani G, Sanderson IR, Sherman PM, Shneider BL (Eds). Walker's Pediatric Gastrointestinal Disease: Physiology, Diagnosis, Management, 6th edition. China: People's Medical Publishing House; 2018.
- Kliegman RM. Nelson Textbook of Pediatrics, 1st South Asia edition. Amsterdam, Netherlands: Elsevier; 2015.

9. Inflammatory bowel disease-ulcerative colitis (IBD-UC) is associated with the occurrence of multiple extra-intestinal manifestations involving the skin, eye, liver, and joints. According to the frequency of occurrence the correct order from most to least common extraintestinal manifestation is:

A. Skin, eye, liver, and joint manifestations
B. Joint, eye, liver, and skin manifestations
C. Joint, skin, eye, and liver manifestations
D. Skin, joint, liver, and eye manifestations

EXPLANATION

About 25–35% of patients with IBD-UC have extraintestinal manifestations. The order according to the frequency of involvement is arthropathy (6%), skin (erythema nodosum 3–8% and pyoderma gangrenosum 1–2%), eye (episcleritis and uveitis 1–3%), and liver (autoimmune hepatitis and primary sclerosing cholangitis 1%). Based on this explanation, the correct order of extraintestinal manifestations according to frequency is joint, skin, eye, and liver.

Key: C

BOOST YOUR KNOWLEDGE

Pediatric UC activity index is a tool which can help in making diagnosis or monitoring the response to treatment. It consists of the following items: Abdominal pain, rectal bleeding, stool consistency, number of stools per day, presence of nocturnal stools, and extent of limitation of activity.

REFERENCES/SOURCES

- Croft N. Ulcerative and indeterminate colitis. In: Kleinman RE, Goulet OJ, Mieli-Vergani G, Sanderson IR, Sherman PM, Shneider BL (Eds). Walker's Pediatric Gastrointestinal Disease: Physiology, Diagnosis, Management, 6th edition. China: People's Medical Publishing House; 2018.
- Kliegman RM. Nelson Textbook of Pediatrics, 1st South Asia edition. Amsterdam, Netherlands: Elsevier; 2015.

10. A 6-year-old girl presented with multiple episodes of nonbilious vomiting and abdominal pain since morning. On examination, the child appears pale and listless, she has tachycardia with tachypnea and severe dehydration, her systemic examination is normal. Results of all investigations are normal except for the presence of mild anemia. There is history of five similar episodes during last 6 months each requiring correction of dehydration, in between the episodes the child remains alright. There are no red flags on history and examination, family history is also not significant. What is the most preferred management in this case?

A. Correction of dehydration
B. Use of triptans
C. Use of sedative agents
D. Use of proton pump inhibitors

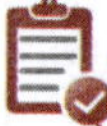

EXPLANATION

Based on history, this is a case of cyclical vomiting syndrome (CVS). Early and aggressive hydration in CVS corrects the volume deficit as well as shortens the episode. In cases with family history of migraine triptans can be started at the onset. Sedatives may reduce the severity or stop the episode. Proton pump inhibitors can be useful in some cases by reducing abdominal pain. Antiemetics like ondansetron can reduce nausea and emesis. In rare cases, general anesthesia may be used.

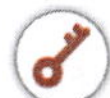

Key: A

BOOST YOUR KNOWLEDGE

Cyclical vomiting syndrome is a functional GI disorder. The Rome IV criteria for CVS are more than three episodes of intense nausea and paroxysmal vomiting lasting hours to days within a 6 months duration, return to baseline health in between the episodes separated by a gap of weeks to months, stereotypical pattern, and symptoms in the individual patient and not attributable to another disorder.

REFERENCES/SOURCES

- Kleinman RE, Goulet OJ, Mieli-Vergani G, Sanderson IR, Sherman PM, Shneider BL. Walker's Pediatric Gastrointestinal Disease: Physiology, Diagnosis, Management, 6th edition. China: People's Medical Publishing House; 2018.
- Kliegman RM. Nelson Textbook of Pediatrics, 1st South Asia edition. Amsterdam, Netherlands: Elsevier; 2015.

11. The presence of which of the following *does not* require further evaluation in child diagnosed as a case of chronic abdominal pain.

A. Deceleration of linear growth
B. Family history of celiac disease (CD)
C. Involuntary weight gain
D. Presence of perianal disease

EXPLANATION

Deceleration of linear growth, family history of CD, IBD or peptic ulcer disease, and presence of perianal disease—all are alarming signs and symptoms, presence of which requires further evaluation in a case of chronic abdominal pain. While involuntary weight gain is not an alarming sign.

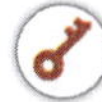

Key: C

BOOST YOUR KNOWLEDGE

According to Rome IV criteria, functional abdominal pain disorders consist of functional dyspepsia, pediatric irritable bowel syndrome, abdominal migraine, and functional abdominal pain not otherwise specified.

REFERENCES/SOURCES

- Kleinman RE, Goulet OJ, Mieli-Vergani G, Sanderson IR, Sherman PM, Shneider BL. Walker's Pediatric Gastrointestinal Disease: Physiology, Diagnosis, Management, 6th edition. China: People's Medical Publishing House; 2018.
- Kliegman RM. Nelson Textbook of Pediatrics, 1st South Asia edition. Amsterdam, Netherlands: Elsevier; 2015.

12. A 2-week-old baby boy presented with history of watery diarrhea since birth, passing 15–18 episodes per day. The baby had frequent episodes of dehydration requiring intravenous (IV) correction and he had not gained weight since birth. The diarrhea episodes persisted despite the baby being shifted on parenteral nutrition. On investigations, work-up for sepsis was negative, blood gas analysis revealed normal anion gap metabolic acidosis with serum sodium 130 mEq/L and potassium 2.8 mEq/L. Stool examination reveals fecal sodium concentrations between 100 and 130 mmol/L, normal alpha-1 antitrypsin clearance. Baby was born at term gestation to a second gravida mother with polyhydramnios. What is the most likely cause of diarrhea in this baby?

A. Microvillus inclusion disease (MVID)
B. Congenital tufting enteropathy
C. Syndromic diarrhea
D. Autoimmune enteropathy

EXPLANATION

Congenital diarrhea is a group of inherited disorders presenting as diarrhea with onset during early neonatal period. The first three conditions have an early onset compared to the autoimmune enteropathy which starts after 6 months of age.

	Microvillus inclusion disease	***Congenital tufting enteropathy***	***Syndromic diarrhea***	***Autoimmune enteropathy***
Age at onset	At birth	Within first few days to weeks	Within first 6 months	After 6 months
Severe dehydration	++	++	+	±
Failure to thrive	+	+	+	+
Metabolic acidosis	++	+	±	±
Impact of parenteral nutrition	–	–	±	+
Dysmorphism	–	– (present in syndromic type)	++	–
Polyhydramnios	++	±	±	–

Key: A

BOOST YOUR KNOWLEDGE

Microvillus inclusion disease is the most severe cause of congenital diarrhea. It is an autosomal recessive disorder which occurs due to the mutations of the *MYO5B* gene coding for a nonconventional motor protein, myosin Vb. This results in mislocalization of apical proteins and disrupted enterocyte polarization, leading to MVID. *t-SNARE syntaxin3 (STX3)* is another gene which has been described in patients with milder phenotype of MVID. Histopathological findings on light microscopy include diffuse thinning of the small bowel mucosa, with hypoplastic villus atrophy, no inflammatory infiltrate and periodic acid–Schiff (PAS) and CD10 positive intracellular inclusions.

REFERENCES/SOURCES

- Kleinman RE, Goulet OJ, Mieli-Vergani G, Sanderson IR, Sherman PM, Shneider BL. Walker's Pediatric Gastrointestinal Disease: Physiology, Diagnosis, Management, 6th edition. China: People's Medical Publishing House; 2018.
- Kliegman RM. Nelson Textbook of Pediatrics, 1st South Asia edition. Amsterdam, Netherlands: Elsevier; 2015.

13. A 3-year-old child was brought to the emergency with complaints of three episodes of bleeding per rectum over last 2 months. Child was apparently well 2 months back. During these episodes, the child had passed tarry red-colored stools, there is no history of abdominal pain, loose stools, rash, vomiting, headache, fever, joint pain, and on examination child is hemodynamically stable with no features of intestinal obstruction. What is the most likely cause of lower GI tract bleeding in the child?

A. Enterocolitis in Hirschsprung's disease
B. Henoch–Schönlein purpura
C. Ileoileal intussusception
D. Meckel's diverticulum

EXPLANATION

All of these conditions can present with acute onset lower GI bleeding, but we have to compare these on the basis of age at presentation, characteristics of bleeding, systemic symptoms, and signs, as discussed here.

	Enterocolitis in Hirschsprung's disease	*Henoch–Schönlein purpura*	*Ileoileal intussusception*	*Meckel's diverticulum*
Age at presentation	Can present at any age	Between 3 and 15 years	Usually under 3 years age	Usually Under 10 years age
Presentation	Acute onset over days	Onset over days to weeks	Acute onset	Insidious onset, present over weeks to months
Color of blood	Red to tarry stools	Red to tarry stools	Red currant jelly stools	Red to tarry stools
Volume of blood	Moderate	Moderate	Moderate with mucus	Moderate to Large
Consistency of Stools	Foul smelling, loose	Normal	Might be normal with mucus	Normal
Abdominal pain	+	++	++	–
Systemic symptoms (fever, headache, vomiting, rash, joint pain, etc.)	+	+	–	–
Hypovolemia	±	±	–	±
Intestinal obstruction	+	–	+	–

Key: D

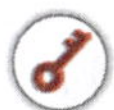

BOOST YOUR KNOWLEDGE

Lower gastrointestinal (LGI) bleeding is defined as bleeding with an origin distal to the ligament of Treitz. Anal fissure secondary to constipation, intussusception, Meckel's diverticulum, juvenile polyps, and IBD are the most common causes of LGI in the pediatric patient.

REFERENCES/SOURCES

- Kliegman RM. Nelson Textbook of Pediatrics, 1st South Asia edition. Amsterdam, Netherlands: Elsevier; 2015.
- Turck D, Michaud L. Lower gastrointestinal bleeding. In: Kleinman RE, Goulet OJ, Mieli-Vergani G, Sanderson IR, Sherman PM, Shneider BL (Eds). Walker's Pediatric Gastrointestinal Disease: Physiology, Diagnosis, Management, 6th edition. China: People's Medical Publishing House; 2018.

14. A 9-month-old male is brought with the complaints of infrequent passage of stools since birth. Child passes stool once in every 7–10 days, after application of enema. The baby was on exclusive breastfeeds till 6 months of age and thriving well. There is no history of any hospitalization in the past. On examination, child have some pallor and abdomen is grossly distended as shown in the given figure. On palpation there is no organomegaly, on percussion tympanic note is heard. What will be your next step as the attending pediatrician?

A. X-ray abdomen erect and supine
B. Barium enema
C. Ultrasound abdomen
D. Digital rectal examination (DRE)

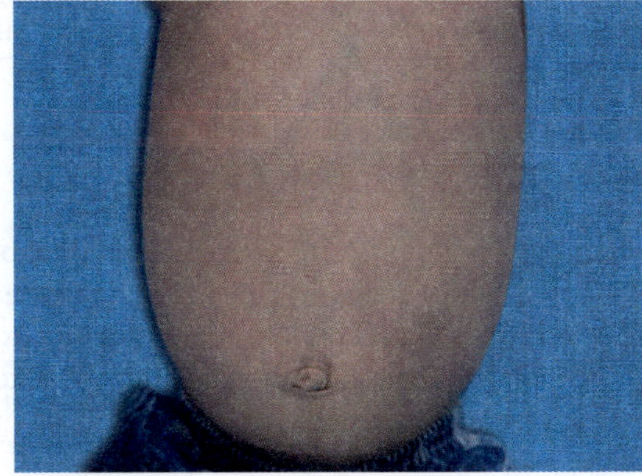

EXPLANATION

Based on history this is a case of chronic constipation. In chronic constipation before advising radiological investigations, a bedside DRE by the pediatrician/treating physician can help in differentiating Hirschsprung's disease from other causes of chronic constipation.

Key: D

BOOST YOUR KNOWLEDGE

In an approach to child with chronic constipation, detailed history and examination plays an important role. History includes the age at onset, progression, duration, time of passage of meconium, feeding history, growth and development, response to medications, pointers suggestive of hypothyroidism, and history suggestive of stool-withholding behavior and encopresis. On examination, abdomen is distended, tympanic, and fecal mass in left lower abdomen. On DRE, rectum is empty of feces, on removal of examining finger there is explosive discharge of feces and gas. Rectal biopsy is the gold standard for diagnosis, should be taken from a site at least 2 cm above the dentate line.

REFERENCES/SOURCES

- Gaiepy C, Ciciora SL. Hirschsprung disease. Kleinman RE, Goulet OJ, Mieli-Vergani G, Sanderson IR, Sherman PM, Shneider BL (Eds). Walker's Pediatric Gastrointestinal Disease: Physiology, Diagnosis, Management, 6th edition. China: People's Medical Publishing House; 2018.
- Kliegman RM. Congenital aganglionic megacolon. In: Kliegman RM (Ed). Nelson Textbook of Pediatrics, 1st South Asia edition. Amsterdam, Netherlands: Elsevier; 2015.

15. Regarding a child presenting with prolonged constipation and subsequently diagnosed as a case of Hirschsprung's disease, which of the following statements is true?

A. It is more common in premature babies
B. More common in females than males
C. Rectosigmoid region is most involved
D. Treatment includes temporary ostomy followed by corrective surgery

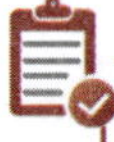

EXPLANATION

Hirschsprung's disease is the most common cause of lower intestinal obstruction in neonates, with an overall incidence of 1 in 5,000 live births. Males are affected more than the females. Hirschsprung's disease is uncommon in premature babies. Short aganglionic segment limited to rectosigmoid region is seen in 80% of cases. Definitive treatment is operative intervention in the form of excision/bypass of the aganglionic segment. Current guidelines recommend the 1 stage primary procedure in all cases of Hirschsprung's disease, except in cases having associated enterocolitis or other complications where decompressing ostomy is required.

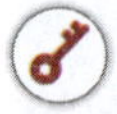

Key: C

BOOST YOUR KNOWLEDGE

Short-segment, long-segment, and total bowel aganglionosis is seen in 80%, 10–15%, and 5% cases, respectively. Ultra-short segment Hirschsprung's disease, i.e., aganglionic segment is limited to the internal anal sphincter only. It is also known as anal achalasia. In this, the ganglion cells are present in rectal suction biopsy, but internal anal sphincter fails to relax in response to rectal distension. Anal botulism injection or anorectal myectomy are the available treatment options.

REFERENCE/SOURCE

- Kliegman RM. Congenital aganglionic megacolon. In: Kliegman RM (Ed). Nelson Textbook of Pediatrics, 1st South Asia edition. Amsterdam, Netherlands: Elsevier; 2015.

16. A 3-year-old child was brought with history of persistent drooling, refusal to drink, and pain in abdomen since past 1 hour. On history, elder sibling mentioned that child has ingested a drain cleaner while playing 1 hour back. On examination, child is hemodynamically stable, has tachycardia, tachypnea, on local examination showed hyperemia over lips, tongue, and oropharynx. Rest of the systemic examination is normal. UGI endoscopy documented presence of hemorrhage exudate, blistering, and transmucosal injury along with scattered superficial ulceration. What will be the clinical outcome of this injury?

A. Temporary dysphagia, no long-term sequelae
B. Scarring, no long-term sequelae
C. Small risk of perforation, later stenosis
D. High risk of perforation, later stenosis

EXPLANATION

Classification of caustic injury describes it under 6 grades based on appearance on UGI endoscopy.

Grade	*Visible appearance*	*Clinical significance*
0	History of ingestion but no visible damage or symptoms	Able to take fluids immediately
1	Edema, loss of normal vascular pattern, hyperemia, no transmucosal injury	Temporary dysphagia, able to swallow within 0–2 days, no long-term sequelae
2a	Transmucosal injury with friability, hemorrhage, blistering, exudate, scattered superficial ulceration	Scarring, no circumferential damage (no stenosis), no long-term sequelae
2b	Grade 2a plus discrete ulceration and/or circumferential ulceration	Small risk of perforation, scarring that may result in later stenosis
3a	Scattered deep ulceration with necrosis of the tissue	Risk of perforation, high risk of later stenosis
3b	Extensive necrotic tissue	High risk of perforation and death, high risk of stenosis

Based on this classification of caustic injury, it is grade 2a injury. It will lead to scarring but no long-term sequelae.

Key: B

BOOST YOUR KNOWLEDGE

Liquid alkali substances are tasteless; thus, a larger amount is ingested compared to acids which are bitter. Children younger than 5 years of age account for half of the cases of caustic ingestions. Dilution by water or milk is recommended as acute treatment, but neutralization, induced emesis and gastric lavage are contraindicated.

REFERENCE/SOURCE

- Kliegman RM. Caustic ingestions. In: Kliegman RM (Ed). Nelson Textbook of Pediatrics, 1st South Asia edition. Amsterdam, Netherlands: Elsevier; 2015.

17. A single, term, 2.9 kg newborn was brought at 6 hours of life with recurrent bilious vomiting. There is a history of polyhydramnios in the mother. On examination, vitals were stable and abdomen is soft, nontender, and nondistended. X-ray abdomen is shown in given Figure. For the given condition, which of the following statement is true?

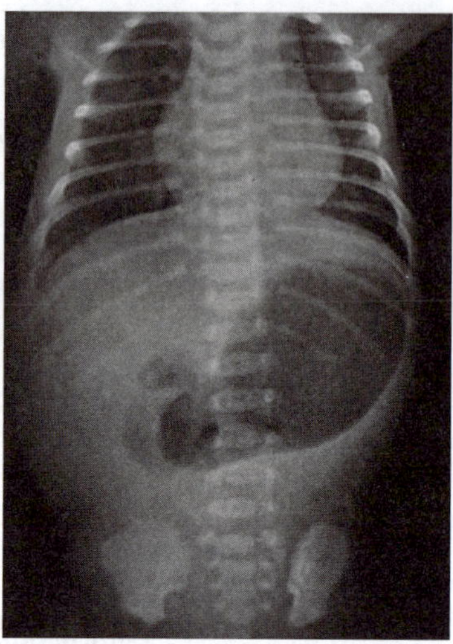

A. Majority of neonates born with this condition are term babies
B. This is result of failed vascularization of intestinal mesentery
C. Concomitant congenital anomalies are uncommon
D. Thin membranous type is the most common form

EXPLANATION

This is a case of intestinal obstruction as a newborn is presenting on first day of life with bilious vomiting, nondistended abdomen, and history of polyhydramnios during antenatal period. As X-ray abdomen is showing "double-bubble", this is case of duodenal atresia. Duodenal atresia is a result of failed recanalization of intestinal lumen during early gestation, in majority of cases there is a thin membrane near ampulla of Vater which occludes the lumen. Associated congenital anomalies are common in babies born with duodenal atresia and approximately 50% of neonates with DA born prematurely.

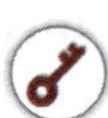

Key: D

BOOST YOUR KNOWLEDGE

Duodenal atresia accounts for 25–40% of intestinal atresia, it can present as thin membrane occluding lumen, fibrous cord connecting two blind duodenal pouches or as two nonconnecting ends of the duodenum. Congenital heart disease (30%), malrotation (20–30%), annular pancreas (30%), renal anomalies (5–15%), and skeletal malformations (5%) are the concomitant anomalies present in cases of duodenal atresia. Almost half of DA cases have chromosomal abnormalities—trisomy 21 being present in one-third cases.

REFERENCES/SOURCES

- Kliegman RM. Intestinal atresia and malrotation. Kliegman RM (Ed). Nelson Textbook of Pediatrics, 1st South Asia edition. Amsterdam, Netherlands: Elsevier; 2015.
- Lloyd D, Kenny SE, Wilkinson D. Congenital anomalies including hernias. In: Kleinman RE, Goulet OJ, Mieli-Vergani G, Sanderson IR, Sherman PM, Shneider BL (Eds). Walker's Pediatric Gastrointestinal Disease: Physiology, Diagnosis, Management, 6th edition. China: People's Medical Publishing House; 2018.

18. Which of the following statements regarding peptic ulcer disease in children is *incorrect*?

A. Esophagogastroduodenoscopy is the investigation of choice for diagnosis
B. Dyspepsia, epigastric pain is seen in older children
C. Feeding difficulty, vomiting, and crying seen in infants
D. In majority, epigastric pain is relieved after food intake

EXPLANATION

The symptoms of peptic ulcers in children vary with age. Infants and younger children usually present with feeding difficulty, vomiting, crying; while older children mainly have dyspepsia and epigastric pain or fullness. The classical history of epigastric pain alleviation after ingestion of food is present in few children only.

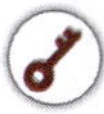

Key: D

BOOST YOUR KNOWLEDGE

Esophagogastroduodenoscopy is the investigation of choice for diagnosis of peptic ulcer disease. Biopsies taken from esophagus, stomach, and duodenum for histologic assessment as well as to screen for the presence of *Helicobacter pylori* infection. Both ^{13}C-urea breath tests and stool antigen tests are reliable as well as noninvasive methods for detecting *H. pylori* infection.

REFERENCE/SOURCE

- Kliegman RM. Nelson Textbook of Pediatrics, 1st South Asia edition. Amsterdam, Netherlands: Elsevier; 2015.

19. Celiac disease is an immune-mediated systemic disorder due to sensitization to gluten and related prolamins. Asymptomatic child detected to have histologic evidence of villous atrophy on UGI endoscopy is known as:

A. Latent CD case
B. Silent CD case
C. Potential CD case
D. Symptomatic CD case

EXPLANATION

Based on clinical spectrum, the cases of CD are classified as:

- *Symptomatic celiacs:* These children present with frank symptoms and signs of malabsorption and associated complications. Some also manifest extraintestinal symptoms and signs.
- *Silent celiacs:* These are asymptomatic children who are identified during serologic screening in at-risk groups (first-degree relatives, trisomy 21, and diabetes cases). UGI endoscopy shows histologic evidence of villous atrophy.
- *Latent celiacs:* These are children who have a normal intestinal histology, but at some other times have shown a gluten-dependent enteropathy.
- *Potential celiacs:* Children with positive celiac serology but without evidence of altered intestinal histology. These patients may or may not have symptoms and signs of disease and may or may not develop a gluten-dependent enteropathy later.

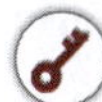

Key: B

BOOST YOUR KNOWLEDGE

The major predisposing genes for CD are the HLA-DQ2 and DQ8 genotypes, found in at least 95% of patients. Presence of family history of CD, autoimmune diseases, especially type 1 diabetes (T1D) and thyroiditis, immunoglobulin A (IgA) deficiency, and some genetic syndromes (particularly Down and Turner syndromes) are associated with increased incidence of CD.

REFERENCES/SOURCES

- Fasano A. Celiac disease. In: Kleinman RE, Goulet OJ, Mieli-Vergani G, Sanderson IR, Sherman PM, Shneider BL (Eds). Walker's Pediatric Gastrointestinal Disease: Physiology, Diagnosis, Management, 6th edition. China: People's Medical Publishing House; 2018.
- Kliegman RM. Nelson Textbook of Pediatrics, 1st South Asia edition. Amsterdam, Netherlands: Elsevier; 2015.

20. **A 3-year-old girl was brought with complaints of passage of pale, foul smelling, and bulky stools since birth. She also has complaint of poor physical growth despite adequate calorie intake. On examination, she has pallor, abdomen is distended, and her deep tendon reflexes are absent. Investigations reveal mild anemia and acanthocytes on peripheral smear, markedly low levels of cholesterol and triglycerides. What is the most likely diagnosis in this child?**

A. CD
B. Intestinal lymphangiectasia
C. Abetalipoproteinemia
D. Congenital microvillus atrophy

EXPLANATION

The key points in the clinical presentation are: (1) age at onset, (2) stool characteristics, (3) poor growth, (4) presence of pallor, and (5) absent deep tendon reflexes. Findings on investigations are: (1) anemia with acanthocytes on smear and (2) markedly low levels of cholesterol and triglycerides. Let us analyze these characteristics for each of the four options:

	Celiac disease	*Intestinal lymphangiectasia*	*Abetalipoproteinemia*	*Congenital microvillus atrophy*
Age at onset	Usually after 6 months	During first decade of life	Birth	Birth
Pale, foul-smelling bulky stools	±	+	++	Watery diarrhea
Poor growth	+	+	+	+
Pallor	+	+	+	–
Absent deep tendon reflexes	±	–	++	–
Acanthocytes on peripheral smear	–	–	++	–
Markedly low cholesterol and triglycerides	–	+	++	–

Key: C

BOOST YOUR KNOWLEDGE

Patients with abetalipoproteinemia have mutations of the *microsomal triglyceride transfer protein (MTTP)* gene. MTTP catalyzes the transfer of triglycerides to nascent ApoB particles in the endoplasmic reticulum (ER). There is no specific treatment of abetalipoproteinemia; supplementation of large doses of vitamin E arrests the neurological and retinal degeneration. Intake of medium chain triglycerides alleviates intestinal symptoms.

REFERENCES/SOURCES

- Cézard JP. Absorption and Digestion. In: Kleinman RE, Goulet OJ, Mieli-Vergani G, Sanderson IR, Sherman PM, Shneider BL (Eds). Walker's Pediatric Gastrointestinal Disease: Physiology, Diagnosis, Management, 6th edition. China: People's Medical Publishing House; 2018.
- Kliegman RM. Nelson Textbook of Pediatrics, 1st South Asia edition. Amsterdam, Netherlands: Elsevier; 2015.

CHAPTER

16.3

Vomiting: Causes, Approach, and Cyclical Vomiting

Ankit Agrawal, Moinak Sen Sarma

1. A 5-year-old boy with the history of accidental corrosive ingestion 4 weeks ago presents with symptoms of abdominal distension, postprandial, and stale food vomiting. During the abdomen examination, succussion splash is observed. What is the likely cause?

A. Esophageal stricture
B. Esophageal perforation
C. Pyloric stricture
D. Gastric ulcer

EXPLANATION

Given the provided symptoms and history, the most suitable answer would be pyloric stricture. Presence of the symptoms such as of abdominal distension, postprandial vomiting, stale food vomiting, and the finding of a succussion splash on examination suggests the gastric outlet obstruction caused by the pyloric stricture. Succussion splash is elicited by positioning the stethoscope over the upper abdomen and gently rocking the patient back and forth at the hips. If the gastric material retained in the stomach for >3 hours after a meal, it could produce a distinct splash sound.

Key: C

BOOST YOUR KNOWLEDGE

In children, the leading cause of upper gastrointestinal stricture is corrosive ingestion. Globally, children represent 80% of all corrosive substance ingestion cases. Accidental ingestions are common, particularly among children <5 years old, comprising 60–80% of incidents. Corrosives include both acidic and alkali substances. Esophagitis, necrosis, perforation, and stricture formation are the medical consequences of caustic ingestion. Esophageal stricture usually presents as dysphagia, while pyloric stricture as gastric outlet obstruction. Acids produce more gastric injury because of the less viscosity, however alkali are more viscous so they produce more esophageal injury. The complications are highlighted here.

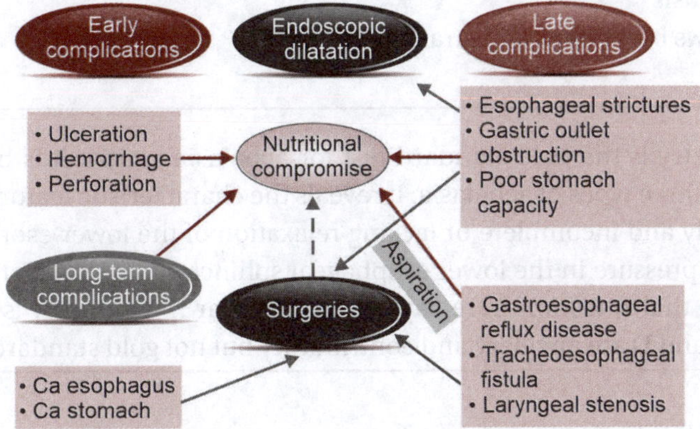

The management algorithm is given here.

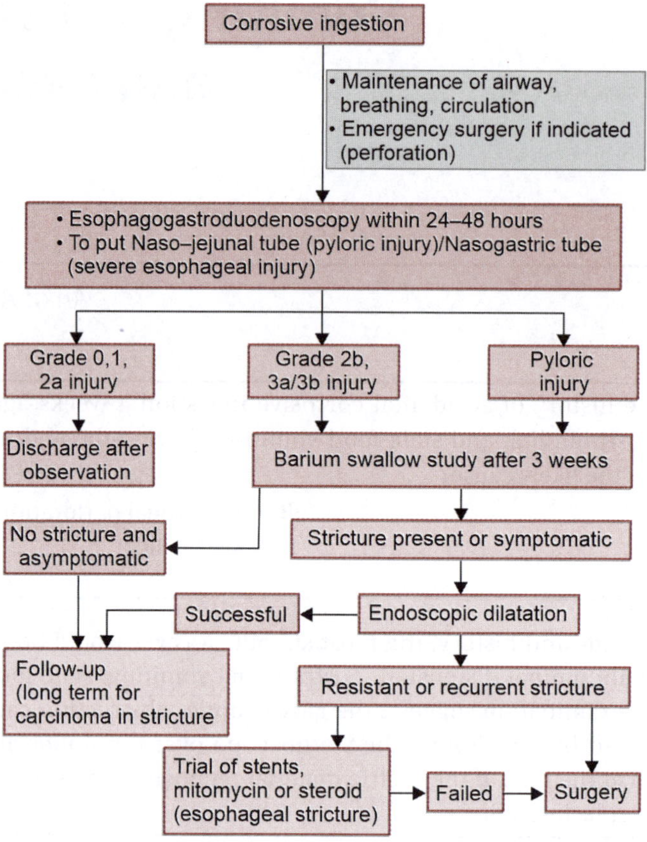

REFERENCES/SOURCES

- Ingestion. In: Kliegman RM, St Geme III JW, Blum NJ, Shah SS, Tasker RC, Wilson KM (Eds). Nelson Textbook of Pediatrics, 21st edition. Elsevier; 2019. p. 1943.
- Sarma MS, Tripathi PR, Arora S. Corrosive upper gastrointestinal strictures in children: difficulties and dilemmas. World J Clin Pediatr. 2021;10(6):124.

2. Which of the following is the gold standard investigation and finding for achalasia cardia?

A. Abnormal 24-hour pH monitoring
B. Complete absence of peristalsis in manometry and elevated resting pressure
C. Endoscopy showing stasis
D. Barium radiology shows bird's beak appearance

EXPLANATION

High-resolution manometry is the gold standard test for achalasia cardia. It is highly sensitive and helps to differentiate between the three types of achalasia. It reveals the characteristic features such as aperistalsis within the distal esophageal body and incomplete or lacking relaxation of the lower esophageal sphincter, frequently coupled with heightened pressure in the lower esophageal sphincter and diminished amplitude of esophageal body contractions. Note that question here says, "gold standard." Option A is valid for gastroesophageal reflux disease. Options C and D are ancillary and contributory but not gold standard for achalasia cardia.

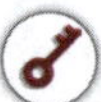

Key: B

BOOST YOUR KNOWLEDGE

Both solid and liquid dysphagia, regurgitation, and weight loss are the common manifestations. Classical achalasia in adults starts as dysphagia with liquid as it is a motor disorder, but in children, it may be dysphagia to solids or liquids. It can lead to undernutrition or chronic cough. Food retention in esophagus can lead to esophagitis. A chest radiograph may reveal an air-fluid level in a dilated esophagus. A barium esophagogram typically showed, bird's beak appearance (smooth tapering of the lower esophagus leading to the closed lower esophageal sphincter). Sigmoid esophagus is a rare complication of achalasia that occurs in advanced cases. Based on manometry, there are three types of achalasia.

Treatment options include pneumatic dilation and laparoscopic or surgical (Heller) myotomy. Pneumatic dilation is often preferred initially and does not preclude a future myotomy. Surgeons may combine myotomy with an anti-reflux procedure to address the potential gastroesophageal reflux disease. Peroral endoscopic myotomy (POEM) is possible alternative to the laparoscopic approach. Medications such as calcium channel blockers (such as nifedipine) and phosphodiesterase inhibitors can provide temporary relief. Botulinum toxin injection endoscopically into the lower esophageal sphincter can also be effective by inhibiting acetylcholine release, but it may require repeated injection. Botulinum toxin is effective in 50–65% of adult patients who are otherwise unfit for surgery or endoscopic dilatation. Eventually most require dilation or surgery.

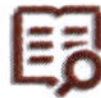

REFERENCE/SOURCE

- Khan S, Matta SKR. Dysmotility. In: Kliegman RM, St Geme III JW, Blum NJ, Shah SS, Tasker RC, Wilson KM (Eds). Nelson Textbook of Pediatrics, 21st edition. Elsevier; 2019. p. 1933.

3. A 2-month-old girl with Down syndrome presents with chronic nonbilious vomiting. X-ray of the abdomen revealed double bubble sign. What is the probable diagnosis?

A. Pyloric stenosis
B. Duodenal atresia
C. Antral web
D. Intussusception

EXPLANATION

The "double bubble sign" is classically seen in duodenal atresia or web and annular pancreas. Duodenal atresia affects approximately 1 in 10,000 live births and constitutes 25–40% of all intestinal atresia. During the 4th and 5th weeks of embryogenesis, there is rapid proliferation of epithelial cells in the duodenal mucosa. Persistence of these cells beyond 7th week of gestation results in occlusion of the lumen (atresia) in approximately 2/3rd of cases and narrowing (stenosis) in the 1/3rd. Duodenal atresia can be classified into three subtypes: Type I is membranous form, type II has atretic duodenal end, separated by some distance but attach by cord, type III has atretic duodenal end, separated by some distance but without any intervening tissue. The membranous form is most common and typically occurs near the ampulla of vater. In rare cases, the membrane may be distensible, referred to as a windsock web, causing obstruction several centimeters distal to the origin of the membrane. Around 50% of infants with duodenal atresia are born prematurely. Congenital heart disease (30%), malrotation (20–30%), annular pancreas (30%), renal anomalies (5–15%), esophageal atresia with or without tracheoesophageal fistula (5–10%), skeletal malformations (5%), and anorectal anomalies (5%) are the common concomitant congenital anomalies associated.

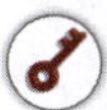

Key: B

BOOST YOUR KNOWLEDGE

Duodenal atresia, annular pancreas, tracheoesophageal fistula, Hirschsprung disease, and imperforate anus are the following gastrointestinal diseases associated with Down syndrome.

Intussusception occurs when a segment of the alimentary tract telescopes into an adjacent segment. It is the common cause of intestinal obstruction between 5 months and 3 years of age. In approximately 30% of cases, presence of pain, a palpable sausage-shaped abdominal mass, and bloody or currant jelly stool constitute the classical triad. When there is paroxysmal pain, vomiting, and a palpable abdominal mass, likelihood of the condition is over>90%, rising nearly to 100% when rectal bleeding is also present. Pyloric stenosis and antral web are obstructions at the gastric outlet.

REFERENCE/SOURCE

- Maqbool A, Bales C, Liacouras CA. Intestinal atresia, stenosis, and malrotation. In: Kliegman RM, St Geme III JW, Blum NJ, Shah SS, Tasker RC, Wilson KM (Eds). Nelson Textbook of Pediatrics, 21st edition. Elsevier; 2019. p. 1951.

4. Which of the following is the drug of choice for prophylaxis of cyclical vomiting syndrome (CVS) in a 4-year-old child?

A. Propranolol
B. Amitriptyline
C. Cyproheptadine
D. Sumatriptan

EXPLANATION

In patients <5 years, cyproheptadine is recommended for prophylaxis and for those >5 years old, amitriptyline is preferred. Propranolol can be considered as a secondary option for both the age groups.

Key: C

BOOST YOUR KNOWLEDGE

Therapy of Cyclical Vomiting Syndrome

Phase of illness	*Management*
Abortive management (at the onset of prodrome to prevent the acute attack)	• Dark quiet environment • Intravenous (IV) ondansetron • IV lorazepam • Sumatriptan intranasal (>12 year)
Acute attack	IV fluids: 10% dextrose with normal saline and potassium supplement. 1.5 times the requirement *Antiemetics*: • *Ondansetron:* 0.3–0.4 mg/kg/dose IV q 4–6 hours • *Diphenhydramine:* 1.0–1.25 mg/kg/dose IV q 6 hours • *Sedation:* Lorazepam 0.05–0.1 mg kg/dose IV q 6 hours
Prophylaxis	*Indications*: • Frequent episodes (>1–2 months) • Severe episodes (repeated hospitalization and school absences) *<5 years age*: • *First line:* Cyproheptadine 0.25–0.5 mg/kg/day • *Second line:* Propranolol 0.25–1 mg/kg/day *>5 years age*: • *First line:* Amitriptyline 0.25–0.5 mg/kg/day • *Second line:* Propranolol 0.25–1 mg/kg/day *Other drugs:* Topiramate and valproate *Supplements:* L-carnitine and coenzyme Q10 *If second-line therapy fails:* • Combination therapy using amitriptyline + any other drug • Add on supplements
General lifestyle changes	• Maintain "vomiting diary" • Avoid fasting—regular meals • Sleep hygiene • Avoid triggers/excitement (downplay big events) • Aerobics (avoid overexertion) • Supplement carbohydrates (fruit juices)—fasting, before exercise, and bedtime

REFERENCE/SOURCE

- In: Kliegman RM, St Geme III JW, Blum NJ, Shah SS, Tasker RC, Wilson KM (Eds). Nelson Textbook of Pediatrics, 21st edition. Elsevier; 2019. p. 2046-8.

5. A 1-year-old boy came to emergency department with history of recurrent bilious vomiting and abdominal distension. The abdomen is tympanic to percussion, and hyperactive bowel sound. A computed tomography (CT) scan of the abdomen is presented here. What is the likely diagnosis?

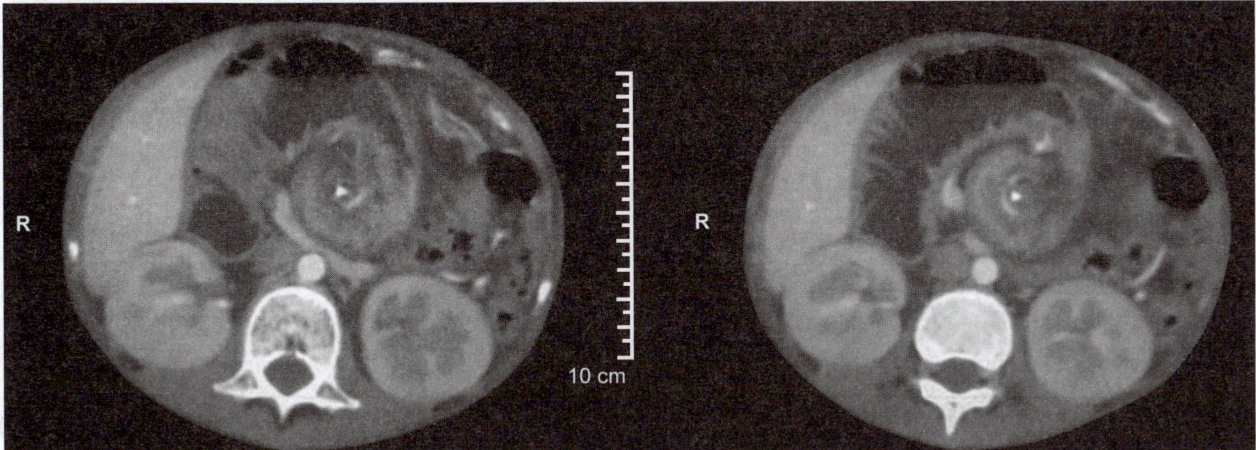

A. Malrotation
B. Intussusception
C. Meckel's diverticulum
D. Annular pancreas

EXPLANATION

The 'whirlpool sign' also known as whirl sign classically seen in malrotation or midgut volvulus on a CT abdomen. It represents the swirling appearance of mesentery and superior mesenteric vein around the superior mesenteric artery. The sensitivity and specificity of the "whirlpool sign" for midgut volvulus caused by malrotation are 92% and 100%, respectively. In cases of intussusception, diagnostic features on ultrasound or CT scans typically reveal a tubular mass in longitudinal views and a doughnut or target-like appearance in transverse images. Ultrasound is highly effective, with a sensitivity and specificity of around 98% in diagnosing intussusception.

Key: A

BOOST YOUR KNOWLEDGE

Malrotation refers to congenital anatomical anomaly that results from abnormal rotation of gut. It can be classified into various subtypes based on the stage of midgut development, including nonrotation, incomplete rotation, and reverse rotation. During the normal fetal development, gut initially begin to form as a straight tube extending from the stomach to the rectum. Intestinal rotation and attachment commence around the 5th week of gestation. Malrotation is estimated to affect approximately 1 in 500 infants. Around 75–85% of patients present within infancy, with over 50% presenting within the first month. Symptoms commonly include signs of acute or chronic obstruction. Vomiting, particularly bilious is the most predominant symptom in this age group, with infants frequently presenting in the first week of life along with acute bowel obstruction.

Meckel diverticulum is the common congenital anomaly of the gastrointestinal tract caused by incomplete obliteration of the vitelline duct during the 7th week of gestation. Symptoms typically manifest in the first or second year of life (average: 2.5 year) with painless intermittent rectal bleeding. Less commonly, it may lead to partial or complete bowel obstruction when the diverticulum acts as the lead point of an intussusception.

The "rule of 2" states that Meckel occur in 2% of population, usually 2 inches long, located in ileum around 2 feet from ileocecal valve, twice as common in males, and contain two types of ectopic tissue (gastric or pancreatic).

Intussusception occurs when a segment of the alimentary tract telescopes into an adjacent segment. It is the common cause of intestinal obstruction between 5 months and 3 years of age. In approximately 30% of cases, presence of pain, a palpable sausage-shaped abdominal mass, and bloody or currant jelly stool are the classical triad. When there is paroxysmal pain, vomiting, and a palpable abdominal mass, likelihood of the condition is over 90%, rising nearly 100% when rectal bleeding is also present. Pyloric stenosis and antral web are obstructions at the gastric outlet.

Annular pancreas results from incomplete rotation of ventral pancreatic bud, often associated with recessive mutations in the *IHH* or *SHH* genes. Patient typically presents with symptoms of complete or partial bowel obstruction either in infancy or later in the 4th or 5th decade. Maternal polyhydramnios is often noted in the medical history. Annular pancreas may be associated with various congenital anomalies, including Down syndrome, tracheoesophageal fistula, intestinal atresia, imperforate anus, malrotation, cardiorenal abnormalities, and pancreatitis. Some children may present with chronic vomiting, pancreatitis, or biliary colic. The preferred treatment is duodenojejunostomy.

REFERENCE/SOURCE

- Kliegman RM, St Geme III JW, Blum NJ, Shah SS, Tasker RC, Wilson KM. Nelson Textbook of Pediatrics, 21st edition. Elsevier; 2019. pp. 1954-55, 1966, 2031.

6. In which of the following gastrointestinal obstructive conditions, bilious vomiting and air-fluid level in X-ray of the abdomen may be absent?

A. Meconium ileus
B. Jejunoileal atresia
C. Hirschsprung disease
D. Midgut volvulus

EXPLANATION

Meconium ileus predominantly affects newborns with cystic fibrosis, a channelopathy marked by faulty chloride transport in exocrine glands, resulting in abnormally thick secretions. About 80–90% of infants with meconium ileus have cystic fibrosis, while only 10–15% of infants with cystic fibrosis present with meconium ileus. The absence of an air-fluid level is due to the viscosity of the secretions in the proximal bowel. Instead, a typical hazy or ground-glass appearance may be observed in the right lower quadrant. This haziness is caused by small bubbles of gas that become trapped in inspissated meconium in the terminal ileal region. If there is meconium peritonitis, patchy calcification may also be noted, particularly in the flanks. Plain films can reveal evidence of pneumoperitoneum due to intestinal perforation. Air may be seen in the subphrenic regions on the upright view and over the liver in the left lateral decubitus position.

Key: A

BOOST YOUR KNOWLEDGE

In patients with obstruction resulting from jejunoileal atresia or long-segment Hirschsprung disease, plain radiographs commonly reveal multiple air-fluid levels proximal to the obstruction in the upright or lateral decubitus position.

REFERENCE/SOURCE

- Maqbool A, Bales C, Liacouras CA. Intestinal Atresia, Stenosis, and Malrotation. In: Kliegman RM, St Geme III JW, Blum NJ, Shah SS, Tasker RC, Wilson KM (Eds). Nelson Textbook of Pediatrics, 21st edition. Elsevier; 2019. p. 1952.

7. Diaphragmatic breathing exercise is helpful in which of the following conditions?

A. Regurgitation
B. Rumination
C. CVS
D. Psychogenic vomiting

EXPLANATION

Rumination involves the repetitive regurgitation and rechewing or expulsion of food, typically commencing soon after a meal and occasionally during eating. This behavior is facilitated by a voluntary increase in abdominal pressure and does not occur during sleep.

Diagnostic criteria:

Criteria must include all the following:

- Repeated regurgitation and rechewing or expulsion of food that: (1) Begins soon after ingestion of a meal and (2) Does not occur during sleep.
- Not preceded by retching
- After appropriate evaluation, the symptoms cannot be fully explained by another medical condition. An eating disorder must be ruled out.

Diaphragmatic breathing exercise and postprandial gum chewing have been shown to be helpful in managing such patients.

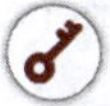

Key: B

BOOST YOUR KNOWLEDGE

Vomiting involves the forceful expulsion of stomach contents through the mouth, driven by contractions of the abdominal and chest wall muscles.

Regurgitation, on the other hand, is a passive process where food from the stomach flows back into the mouth without muscular activity from the abdomen or diaphragm.

Recurrent vomiting is characterized by experiencing at least three episodes of vomiting within a three-month period, which can be either chronic or cyclical.

Cyclical vomiting syndrome (CVS) is defined by recurrent, distinct episodes of vomiting that are self-limited. Diagnosis relies on symptoms, with laboratory, radiographic, and endoscopic tests typically yielding negative results.

Psychogenic vomiting occurs without an identifiable organic cause. It often persists chronically and is attributed to psychological or cortical factors. Stressful events can trigger these episodes, and some children may require hospitalization.

REFERENCES/SOURCES

- Gupta P, Agrawal M, Mathur GP, Mathur Sarla, Gupta Piyush. Piyush Gupta Textbook of Pediatrics, 2nd edition. New Delhi: CBS Publishers & Distributors; 2019. p. 1447.
- Maqbool A, Li BUK, Liacouras CA. Cyclic vomiting syndrome. Kliegman RM, St Geme III JW, Blum NJ, Shah SS, Tasker RC, Wilson KM (Eds). Nelson Textbook of Pediatrics, 21st edition. Elsevier; 2019. pp. 2046-8.

8. A 13-year-old boy is brought to the outpatient department by parents with the history of recurrent vomiting and not gaining weight. He also experiences food getting stuck in the throat. He has a history of eczema and asthma. Based on clinical presentation, what is the most likely underlying cause?

A. Pill esophagitis
B. Infective esophagitis
C. Eosinophilic esophagitis (EoE)
D. Gastroesophageal reflux disease

EXPLANATION

Given case scenario is pointing towards the possibility of eosinophilic esophagitis (EoE). It is characterized by esophageal dysfunction and infiltration of the esophageal epithelium by ≥15 eosinophils per hpf. In infants and toddlers, symptoms often include vomiting, feeding difficulties, and inadequate weight gain, while older children and adolescents typically experience solid food dysphagia with occasional food impaction or stricture.

Key: C

BOOST YOUR KNOWLEDGE

EoE is distinguished from gastroesophageal reflux disease by the presence of concurrent atopic diseases, the absence of erosive esophagitis, higher eosinophil levels, and normal esophageal pH-multichannel intraluminal impedance results.

Infective esophagitis can be caused by various fungal agents like *Candida albicans* and *Torulopsis glabrata*, viral agents including herpes simplex, cytomegalovirus, HIV, and varicella-zoster, and rarely bacterial infections such as diphtheria and tuberculosis, or parasites. Common symptoms include odynophagia, dysphagia, and chest pain. *Candida* is the most common cause of infective esophagitis in both immunocompetent and immunocompromised individuals. Diagnosis typically requires upper gastrointestinal endoscopy, which may reveal white plaques in the case of *Candida*, multiple superficial ulcers or volcano ulcers in herpes simplex virus, and single deep ulcers in cytomegalovirus.

Pill esophagitis is caused by medications such as tetracycline, doxycycline, potassium chloride, ferrous sulfate, nonsteroidal anti-inflammatory medications, cloxacillin, and alendronate. Progressive retrosternal pain, odynophagia, and dysphagia are the common symptoms. Endoscopic findings show a focal lesion localized to one of the anatomically narrowed regions of the esophagus.

Management algorithm for EoE is given here.

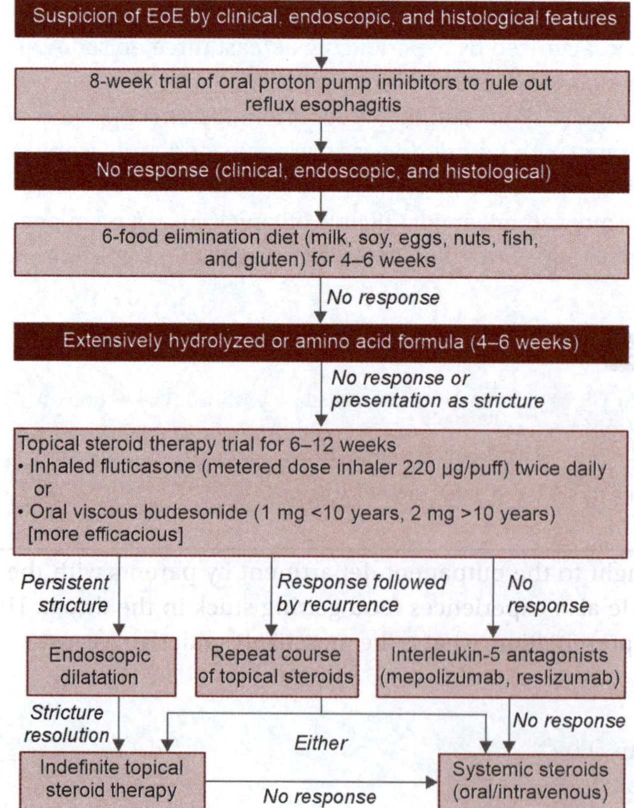

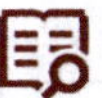

REFERENCE/SOURCE

- Kliegman RM, St Geme III JW, Blum NJ, Shah SS, Tasker RC, Wilson KM (Eds). Nelson Textbook of Pediatrics, 21st edition. Elsevier; 2019. pp. 1938-42.

9. A 6-week-old child presented with nonbilious projectile vomiting for the last 3 weeks. Blood test revealed unconjugated hyperbilirubinemia and abdominal radiograph suggested dilated gastric bubble. Which of the following is most likely diagnosis?

A. Pyloric stenosis
B. Meconium ileus
C. Duodenal atresia
D. Hirschsprung disease

EXPLANATION

Given case scenario is suggestive of pyloric stenosis with icteropyloric syndrome. Icteropyloric syndrome, due to hyperbilirubinemia (Primarily unconjugated) is the most common medical syndrome associated with pyloric stenosis. It often resolves following surgical correction of the pyloric stenosis in about 5% of affected infants. It is due to the decrease in glucuronyl transferase levels, and mutations in the bilirubin uridine diphosphate glucuronosyltransferase (*UGT1A1*) gene have also been implicated. The diagnosis is usually confirmed by abdominal ultrasonography in the majority of cases.

Key: A

BOOST YOUR KNOWLEDGE

Hypertrophic pyloric stenosis affects around 1–3/1,000 infants in the United States. It has a higher incidence in male affecting about 20% compared to 10% in females, whose mothers had the condition. Infants with B and O blood groups are at a higher risk. Vomiting typically starts after 3 weeks of age but can begin as early as the first week or as late as the 5th month. Persistent vomiting leads to electrolyte imbalance, resulting in hyperchloremic metabolic alkalosis. It is often diagnosed by abdominal ultrasonography, which is based on the following criteria: pyloric thickness of 3–4 mm, an overall pyloric length of 15–19 mm, and a pyloric diameter of 10–14 mm

Meconium ileus primarily affects newborns with cystic fibrosis, resulting in abnormally viscous secretions obstructing the intestines. Simple cases present with a collapsed distal ileum filled with pale stool pellets, while the proximal bowel is dilated and filled with thick, syrup-like meconium. Complicated cases may involve volvulus, intestinal ischemia, atresia, or perforation. Approximately 50% of patients with simple meconium ileus require laparotomy due to inadequate response to water-soluble enemas.

Hirschsprung disease is a developmental disorder (neurocristopathy), characterized by the absence of ganglion cells in the submucosal and myenteric plexus of enteric nervous system. It is typically diagnosed in the neonatal period secondary to a distended abdomen, failure to pass meconium, and/or bilious emesis or aspirates with feeding intolerance. A full thickness rectal biopsy is the "gold standard" for diagnosis, and surgery is the main stay of management with procedures such as Duhamel, Swenson, and Soave are commonly performed.

REFERENCE/SOURCE

- Pyloric stenosis and other congenital anomalies of the stomach. In: Kliegman RM, St Geme III JW, Blum NJ, Shah SS, Tasker RC, Wilson KM (Eds). Nelson Textbook of Pediatrics, 21st edition. Elsevier; 2019. p. 1947.

10. Pathological gastroesophageal reflux in infants presents with all, *except*:

A. Respiratory symptoms
B. Upper gastrointestinal bleeding
C. Bilious vomiting
D. Esophageal stricture

EXPLANATION

Gastroesophageal reflux in infant is of two types: Physiological and pathological. In the first few months of life, physiological infant reflux typically becomes noticeable, reaching its peak around 4 months, and often resolves in up to 88% of cases by 1 year, with nearly all cases resolving by 2 years. The vast majority of healthy infants present with daily regurgitation or vomiting with no failure to thrive referred to as "happy spitters." Gastroesophageal reflux disease in infants may manifest as obstructive apnea or as stridor or lower airway disease in which reflux complicates primary airway disease such as laryngomalacia or bronchopulmonary dysplasia. Bilious vomiting suggests small bowel obstruction.

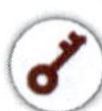

Key: C

BOOST YOUR KNOWLEDGE

Symptoms and signs of gastroesophageal reflux in infants and older children encompass recurrent regurgitation with or without vomiting, inadequate weight gain or weight loss, irritability (especially in infants), rumination behavior, heartburn or chest pain, blood in vomitus (hematemesis), difficulty swallowing (dysphagia), painful swallowing (odynophagia), wheezing, stridor, coughing, and hoarseness. Signs may include esophagitis, narrowing of the esophagus (esophageal stricture), Barrett's esophagus, recurrent lung infections (pneumonia), anemia, erosion of dental enamel, refusal to eat, and abnormal neck movements (Sandifer syndrome).

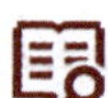

REFERENCES/SOURCES

- Khan S, Matta SKR. Gastroesophageal reflux disease. In: Kliegman RM, St Geme III JW, Blum NJ, Shah SS, Tasker RC, Wilson KM (Eds). Nelson Textbook of Pediatrics, 21st edition. Elsevier; 2019. pp. 1935-7.
- Rosen R, Vandenplas Y, Singendonk M, Cabana M, DiLorenzo C, Gottrand F, et al. Pediatric Gastroesophageal Reflux Clinical Practice Guidelines: Joint Recommendations of the North American Society for Pediatric Gastroenterology, Hepatology, and Nutrition and the European Society for Pediatric Gastroenterology, Hepatology, and Nutrition. J Pediatr Gastroenterol Nutr. 2018; 66(3):516-54.

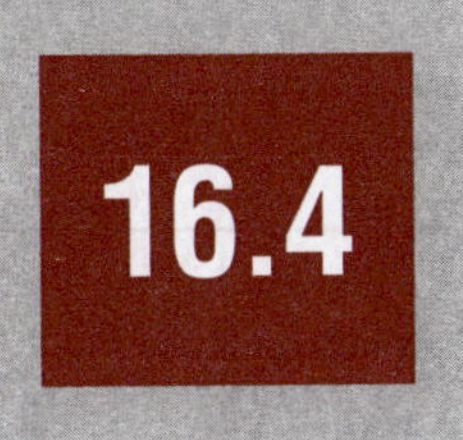

Gastroesophageal Reflux and Gastroesophageal Reflux Disease

Amrit Gopan

1. A 4-month-old infant is brought with the complaint of immediate postfeeding regurgitation of feeds for the past 2 months. The child is exclusively breastfed. The amount is a fraction of what is ingested; there are no nocturnal episodes, excess irritability, and skin or respiratory complaints. The baby had an uneventful neonatal period, and no surgical history. The child is thriving well and has started vocalizing for the past 1 month and is able to roll over. Examination does not reveal any significant abdominal findings and other systems are clinically normal. Which of the following would best describe the condition and management approach?

A. The baby has a narrowing in the esophagus and the next best step would be to proceed for a contrast esophagogram and involve the surgeon

B. The baby is suffering from gastroesophageal reflux disease (GRED) and requires an upper gastrointestinal (GI) endoscopy to confirm the same

C. The baby has a benign condition called gastroesophageal reflux and the caregiver needs to be counseled and reassured that it will likely improve with time

D. The baby is suffering from milk protein allergy and should be subjected to a proctosigmoidoscopy and rectal biopsies and switch to soy-based formula feeds

EXPLANATION

The key clinical information here are current age (4 months), age at onset (2 months), amount of regurgitation being a fraction of what is ingested, and the absence of any red flags. Analyzing this information in the background of a well-thriving child with normal developmental milestones leads us to think of a benign, nonsurgical condition with absence of extraintestinal manifestations.

There are four conditions which have been listed and we can compare them for ease of understanding:

Option	*Condition*	*Pointers for*	*Pointers against*
A	Esophageal stricture/atresia	Immediate postfeed regurgitation	• Onset is delayed (2 month) • No nocturnal episodes/salivary drooling • No surgical events • No positive history to support any caustic ingestion • Thriving well
B	GERD	Immediate postfeed regurgitation	No irritability, arching of back, and failure to thrive
C	Gastroesophageal reflux	• Immediate postfeed regurgitation • Well thriving • Achieved milestones • No other system involvement	
D	Cow milk protein allergy	Immediate postfeed regurgitation	• No irritability/fussiness • Exclusively breastfed • No skin changes/family history of atopy or allergy mentioned

Tip: Information not provided (for instance family history of atopy/allergy, in this case) is to be considered absent unless mentioned.

 **Key: C**

 **BOOST YOUR KNOWLEDGE**

Infant reflux becomes evident in the first few months of life, peaks at 4 months, and resolves in up to 88% by 12 months and in nearly all by 2 years of age.

Signs of esophagitis in infants are irritability, arching, choking, gagging, and feeding aversion.

Milk protein allergy when severe and presenting when baby is on exclusive breastfeeding is most often immunoglobulin E (IgE) mediated, has a strong atopic background, and is due to antigen passed from mother's milk due to ingestion of milk or milk products by the mother. This is treated by asking the mother to follow a strict milk/milk product free diet herself and continue to breastfeed.

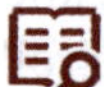 **REFERENCE/SOURCE**

- Khan S, Matta SKR. Gastroesophageal reflux disease. Kliegman RM, St Geme JW (Eds). Nelson Textbook of Pediatrics, 21st edition. Amsterdam, Netherlands: Elsevier; 2019.

2. **A 6-month-old child has wringing neck movements, noted for past one and half month. The child has sudden arching movements of neck, back, and head, with no abnormal movements of extremities. This appears predominantly postfeeding, and the child is conscious and responsive to physical and auditory stimuli during the event. These are not noticed during sleep. The neonatal and developmental history is uneventful; no other hospital visits were evident. Physical examination is essentially normal. What best describes the condition and what is the next best step in management?**

A. Possibility of seizures; involve pediatric neurologist and consider electroencephalogram (EEG) and neuroimaging
B. Torticollis; to refer for physical therapy
C. *Sandifer syndrome:* Counsel regarding natural history of GERD and consider nonpharmacological measures followed by proton pump inhibitor (PPI)
D. *Metabolic disorder:* Involve geneticist and consider urine and blood metabolic screening

 **EXPLANATION**

Identify the key words: Current age: 6 months; age of onset: 4.5 months; abnormal movements of back and neck without involving extremities, and a normal sensorium; all episodes postfeeding. Background history of gastroesophageal reflux.

Let's look at each option individually:

A. Seizures with a normal sensorium, involving only the upper trunk, and without any background risk factor, and appearing only postfeeds is a rare possibility. The fact that the child has not had any neurological sequelae, has been developmentally well and without any other systemic illness, and a normal neurological examination also precludes seizures as the first differential diagnosis. The presence of these paroxysms in sleep would have supported the possibility of seizures, but absence (as in this case) though supportive, does not confirm the non-neurological basis.
B. Congenital muscular torticollis is a true torticollis and has muscular shortening of the sternocleidomastoid. There is no worsening specifically postfeeds as described in this child. True torticollis responds to physical therapy.

C. Sandifer syndrome refers to the dystonic movements of back and neck associated in infants or young children with GERD, usually postfeeds at the time of reflux. These are possibly learned or adaptive behaviors secondary to, and to relieve abdominal discomfort and esophageal motility in those with GERD. It is important to note that these movements subside dramatically once GERD is alleviated, unlike seizures or extrapyramidal causes for dystonia which would not abate. Peak of GERD occurs at about 4 months, which is when the symptoms have started in this case.

D. Metabolic disorders could be suspected in the presence of lethargy, vomiting, and episodes of unresponsiveness. Seizures may be a part of metabolic disorders. There may be other pointers too, such as poor feeding, poor developmental milestones, and hospital admission for "periods of sickness". This option would figure lower in the list of possibilities.

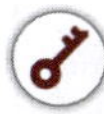

Key: C

BOOST YOUR KNOWLEDGE

Sandifer syndrome should be kept as a differential diagnosis for nonepileptic paroxysmal dystonic events and abnormal posturing. One of the key features of Sandifer syndrome is exacerbation of the abnormal posturing immediately after eating and improvement between feeds. When the clinical picture is not clear for Sandifer syndrome, in certain cases, EEG can provide valuable clinical information to rule in or out seizure disorders. Failure of nonpharmacological and pharmacological measures to treat Sandifer syndrome should prompt evaluation for an associated hiatal hernia, in which case a surgical consult should be sought.

REFERENCE/SOURCE

- Patil S, Tas V. Sandifer syndrome. Treasure Island (FL): StatPearls Publishing; 2024.

3. Which statement is correct regarding contrast esophagogram in GERD?

A. It has a high sensitivity but poor specificity for GERD
B. It correlates with severity of disease in GERD
C. It can differentiate physiological gastroesophageal reflux (GER) from GERD
D. It has poor accuracy in assessing mucosal involvement in GERD

EXPLANATION

Contrast esophagogram (barium or nonionic water-soluble contrast) studies have a limited value in diagnostics in GERD. It has *both poor sensitivity and specificity* (option A is incorrect) in diagnosing or discriminating GERD from GER (option C is incorrect). It is limited by its duration of assessment of the esophageal mucosa and has poor accuracy in mucosal inflammation assessment (option D is correct) or severity of disease (option B is incorrect).

It may be useful in assessing the presence of esophageal strictures, especially peptic strictures in lower esophagus and as an initial investigation before upper GI endoscopy to have a road map of the esophagus in patients with dysphagia.

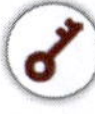

Key: D

BOOST YOUR KNOWLEDGE

Barium swallow is very useful in demonstrating Schatzki's ring, webs, and minimally narrowed peptic strictures, which may be missed by endoscopy.

REFERENCE/SOURCE

- Richter JE, Vaezi MF. Gastroesophageal reflux disease. In: Feldman M, Friedman LS, Brandt LJ (Eds). Sleisenger and Fordtran's Gastrointestinal and Liver Disease, 11th edition. Amsterdam, Netherlands: Elsevier; 2020. pp. 675.

4. Which of the following constitutes the postepithelial tissue resistance in the three-tiered esophageal defense system?

A. Mucous layer
B. Lumen to surface pH gradient
C. Intercellular buffers
D. Continuous mucosal blood flow

EXPLANATION

The three-tiered esophageal defense against gastric acid reflux is:

Anti-reflux barrier	***Esophageal acid clearance***	***Tissue resistance***
1. Intrinsic lower esophageal sphincter (LES)	1. *Volume/bolus clearance:* Primary and secondary peristalsis and gravity	1. *Pre-epithelial:* • Mucous layer/mucin • Lumen to surface pH gradient • Prostaglandin E2 (PGE2)
2. Diaphragmatic crura	2. *Acid clearance:* Salivary and esophageal gland secretions	2. *Epithelial:* • Cell membrane • Intercellular junctional complexes • Intercellular buffers • Ion transporters
3. Intra-abdominal location of LES		3. *Postepithelial: Continuous mucosal blood flow*
4. Phrenoesophageal ligaments		
5. Acute angle of His		

Tissue resistance is one among the three-tiered esophageal defense mechanisms (other two being antireflux barrier and esophageal acid clearance). This is further categorized as pre-, intra-, and postepithelial.

One of the most important factors in tissue resistance is the *pre-epithelial mucin layer* which constitutes the *first line of defense.* Mucin secretion of the esophageal squamous epithelium can be demonstrated by using *a periodic acid–Schiff stain*, which stains the esophageal mucins with *a light-blue color*.

The second epithelial barrier is composed of the *multilayered stratified nonkeratinized squamous epithelium.*

Postepithelial factors like adequate vascular perfusion with a *continuous mucosal blood flow* ensure that epithelial damage does not progress to necrosis of deeper layers of the mucosa.

Tip: When question in any part of the gastrointestinal tract (GIT) pertains toward "postmucosal", think of either lymphatic vessels/lacteals or blood vessels.

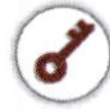

Key: D

BOOST YOUR KNOWLEDGE

Gastroesophageal reflux disease-related esophagitis is due to an imbalance between "aggressive factors" and "defensive factors". Defensive factors are antireflux barrier, esophageal acid clearance, and tissue resistance. *Aggressive factors* include gastric acid, pepsin, pancreatic enzymes, and bile acids.

REFERENCE/SOURCE

- Richter JE, Vaezi MF. Gastroesophageal reflux disease. In: Feldman M, Friedman LS, Brandt LJ (Eds). Sleisenger and Fordtran's Gastrointestinal and Liver Disease, 11th edition. Amsterdam, Netherlands: Elsevier; 2020. p. 675.

5. Which of the following is true regarding the role of esophageal pH monitoring in the diagnosis and management of GERD?

A. Dual pH probes involve adding a distal pH probe to the standard proximal esophageal pH probe and are confirmatory for diagnosing typical GERD
B. Most important indication is in assessing efficacy of acid suppression on treatment and for evaluating atypical symptoms of GERD
C. Esophageal pH monitoring documents acidic reflux episodes with poor sensitivity, but high specificity
D. Normal values of distal esophageal acid exposure (pH <4) are generally established as <20% of the total monitored time

EXPLANATION

Dual pH probes involve addition of a proximal pH probe in addition to the standard distal pH probe which is pre-existent. This helps in evaluating atypical symptoms of GERD such as chronic cough, stridor, and asthma. The cut-off of 1% of total monitored time is used for proximal esophageal acid exposure time for it to be considered as pathological.

Use of extended esophageal pH monitoring is used mainly for assessing efficacy of acid suppression during treatment, evaluating apneic episodes, and for evaluating atypical GERD presentations. pH-metry documents acid exposure time quantitatively and with high sensitivity.

The normal value established for distal esophageal acid exposure in a healthy individual is <5–8% of total measured time.

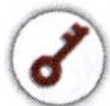

Key: B

BOOST YOUR KNOWLEDGE

- A standard pH-metry catheter has *two* pH sensors/probes, *one* for distal esophagus and the other *one* at the tip for gastric pH measurement.
- A dual pH probe means adding *another* pH sensor/probe in the standard catheter so that now the catheter has *three* pH probes, *two* esophageal and *one* gastric.

REFERENCE/SOURCE

- Khan S, Matta SKR. Gastroesophageal reflux disease. Kliegman RM, St Geme JW (Eds). Nelson Textbook of Pediatrics, 21st edition. Amsterdam, Netherlands: Elsevier; 2019.

6. Which of the following accurately describes diagnostics in GERD?

A. Endoscopy has both diagnostic and therapeutic roles in patients with GERD
B. Multichannel intraluminal impedance (MII) is not useful in atypical GERD with respiratory symptoms
C. Esophageal manometry has a key role in identifying gastroesophageal reflux
D. Amylase in tracheal fluid is a marker of reflux-associated aspiration of gastric contents

EXPLANATION

- Endoscopy is useful in diagnosing erosive esophagitis and also in taking biopsies to diagnose histologic reflux esophagitis in absence of erosions while simultaneously eliminating allergic and infectious etiologies. It can be useful for dilating esophageal strictures formed because of acid exposure to lower esophagus.
- MII is an important tool in those with respiratory symptoms, particularly for the determination of nonacid reflux. It helps in understanding bolus flow, volume clearance, and motor patterns in GERD.

- Esophageal manometry has no role in identifying reflux episodes directly. However, it can help identify pressure patterns like transient lower esophageal sphincter relaxation (tLESr).
- Detection of pepsin in tracheal fluid obtained while performing laryngo-tracheo-bronchoscopy can permit diagnosis of silent aspirations, while swallowing or during episodes of reflux. It is a marker of reflux-associated aspiration of gastric contents. Subsequent quantification of lipid-laden macrophages in airway secretions can be performed on the obtained fluid.

Key: A

BOOST YOUR KNOWLEDGE

Upper GI endoscopy is the first line investigation in the following situations:

1. Presence of warning signs like upper gastrointestinal bleeding, dysphagia, and significant weight loss
2. Failure of first-line therapy
3. Older patients (>50 years)

The classification system used in case of erosive esophagitis is the *Los Angeles classification*, which has four grades:

Grade	*Description*
Grade A	Esophageal mucosal breaks no longer than 5 mm
Grade B	At least one mucosal break longer than 5 mm, confined to the mucosal fold but not continuous between twofold
Grade C	Mucosal breaks that are continuous between the tops of mucosal folds but not circumferential
Grade D	Extensive mucosal breaks that involve at least 75% of the esophageal circumference

Lyon consensus on GERD diagnosis defined grade C and D esophagitis as strong evidence for GERD while grade A was considered insufficient for diagnosis of GERD.

In adults, presence of *peptic stricture and Barrett's esophagus >1 cm* is considered indicative of pathological GERD.

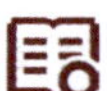
REFERENCES/SOURCES

- Khan S, Matta SKR. Gastroesophageal reflux disease. Kliegman RM, St Geme JW (Eds). Nelson Textbook of Pediatrics, 21st edition. Amsterdam, Netherlands: Elsevier; 2019.
- Shaheen NJ, Weinberg DS, Denberg TD, Chou R, Qaseem A, Shekelle P. Upper endoscopy for gastroesophageal reflux disease: best practice advice from the clinical guidelines committee of the American College of Physicians. Ann Intern Med. 2012;157(11):808-16.

7. Which of the following is *incorrect* regarding management of GERD in infants?

A. Feed thickening with rice-based feed thickeners is hypothesized to be associated with arsenic exposure in children
B. Feed thickening with xanthan gum-based commercial thickeners is associated with necrotizing enterocolitis
C. Rice or oat cereal as thickeners provides only a low caloric density in the feeds, affecting weight gain
D. Trial of hypoallergenic diet can be tried prior to starting any pharmacologic therapy in infants with GERD

EXPLANATION

Thickening of feeds or use of commercially available pre-thickened formulas decreases the percentage of infants with regurgitation, frequency of emesis, and promotes weight gain in infants. Studies have demonstrated increased risk of arsenic exposure in children with rice and rice product consumption used as feed thickeners. Xanthan-based thickeners have a possible association with necrotizing enterocolitis in preterm infants.

Rice and oat-based thickeners provide a high caloric density (30 cal/oz) and not a low-calorie density. They are also helpful in decreasing the total crying time.

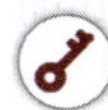

Key: C

BOOST YOUR KNOWLEDGE

A combination of modified feeding volumes, hydrolyzed infant formulas, proper positioning techniques, and avoidance of smoke exposure satisfactorily improve GERD symptoms in up to 50% of infants with GERD.

REFERENCE/SOURCE

- Khan S, Matta SKR. Gastroesophageal reflux disease. Kliegman RM, St Geme JW (Eds). Nelson Textbook of Pediatrics, 21st edition. Amsterdam, Netherlands: Elsevier; 2019.

8. Which of the following best qualifies for the definition of refractory GERD in children?

A. GERD not responding to optimal treatment after 12 weeks
B. GERD not responding to optimal treatment after 8 weeks
C. Gastroesophageal reflux leading to troublesome symptoms affecting daily functioning
D. Gastroesophageal reflux leading to troublesome symptoms leading to complications

EXPLANATION

Joint recommendations of the North American Society for Pediatric Gastroenterology, Hepatology, and Nutrition (NASPGHAN) and the European Society for Pediatric Gastroenterology, Hepatology, and Nutrition (ESPGHAN):

GER: Passage of gastric contents into the esophagus with or without regurgitation and vomiting.

GERD: When GER leads to troublesome symptoms that affect daily functioning and/or complications.

Refractory GERD: GERD, not responding to optimal treatment after 8 weeks.

Optimal therapy: Maximum pharmacologic and/or nonpharmacologic therapy based on available healthcare facilities in the region of practice.

Rumination: Effortless regurgitation of recently ingested food into the mouth with subsequent mastication and reswallowing.

Rumination syndrome: A distinct clinical entity wherein rumination follows minutes after ingestion of a meal, does not occur during sleep, and does not respond to standard treatment for GER. In infant rumination syndrome there are repetitive contractions of the abdominal wall muscles, diaphragm, and tongue.

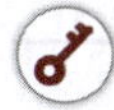

Key: B

BOOST YOUR KNOWLEDGE

Refractory GERD should prompt further investigations including esophageal biopsies for ruling out *eosinophilic esophagitis*.

REFERENCE/SOURCE

- Rosen R, Vandenplas Y, Singendonk M, Cabana M, DiLorenzo C, Gottrand F, et al. Pediatric Gastroesophageal Reflux Clinical Practice Guidelines: Joint Recommendations of the North American Society for Pediatric Gastroenterology, Hepatology, and Nutrition and the European Society for Pediatric Gastroenterology, Hepatology, and Nutrition. J Pediatr Gastroenterol Nutr. 2018;66:516-54.

9. A 14-year-old boy has complained of retrosternal burning sensation for past 3 months. You advised him for empirical PPI therapy for 4 weeks, but he returns with same complaints. You plan an upper GI endoscopy and pH-metry following which you establish a diagnosis of functional heartburn. Which of the following best describes the term functional heartburn?

A. Absence of erosions on upper GI endoscopy, pH-metry showing abnormal acid exposure
B. Absence of erosions on upper GI endoscopy, pH-metry showing normal acid exposure and positive correlation with reflux episodes
C. Absence of erosions on upper GI endoscopy, pH-metry showing normal acid exposure and negative correlation with reflux episodes
D. pH-metry showing normal acid exposure and positive correlation of symptoms with reflux episodes irrespective of upper GI endoscopy findings

EXPLANATION

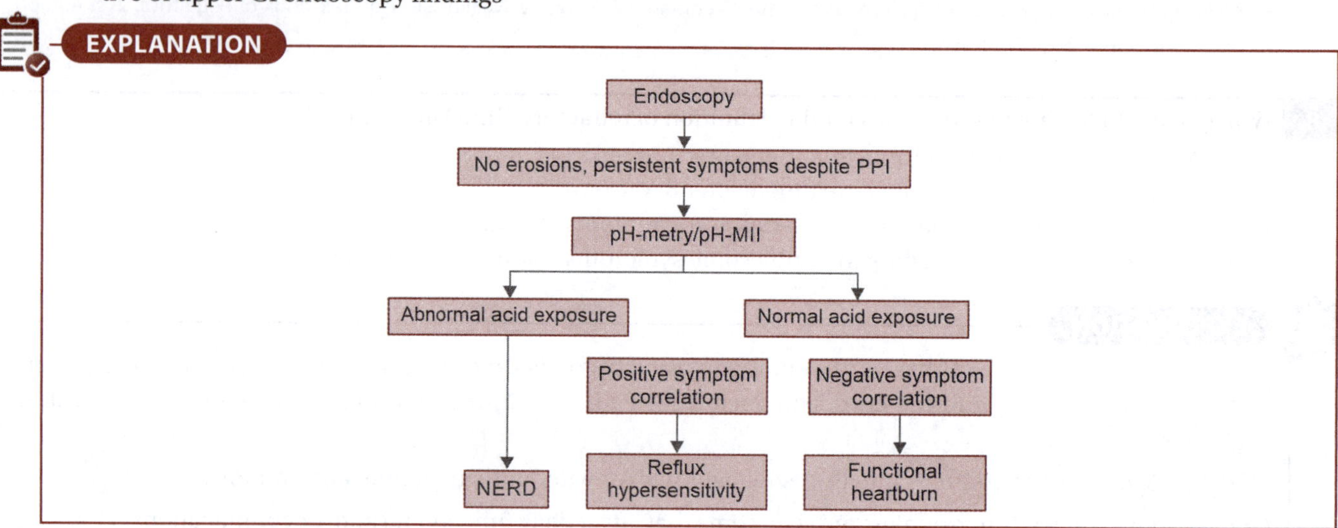

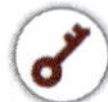

Key: C

BOOST YOUR KNOWLEDGE

Nonerosive reflux disease (NERD) responds to PPI therapy. Reflux hypersensitivity and functional heartburn patients are less likely to respond to PPI.

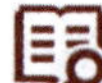

REFERENCE/SOURCE

- Richter JE, Vaezi MF. Gastroesophageal reflux disease. In: Feldman M, Friedman LS, Brandt LJ (Eds). Sleisenger and Fordtran's Gastrointestinal and Liver Disease, 11th edition. Amsterdam, Netherlands: Elsevier; 2020. p. 684.

10. Which of the following is correct regarding PPI use for diagnosis in GERD in pediatric age group?

A. A short trial of PPI therapy can be given in infants with suspected GERD
B. Greatest symptomatic improvement occurs in the first 2–4 weeks of PPI administration
C. Data supports the use of diagnostic trial of PPI for extraesophageal symptoms in GERD
D. Older children and adolescents can be given a diagnostic trial of PPI for 2–4 weeks

EXPLANATION

Short PPI trials are not advocated *in infants* (option A is false) with suspected GERD. Randomized control trials in older children support the hypothesis that *maximum symptomatic improvement* occurs in children in the *first 2–4 weeks* of PPI administration (option B is true). However, since these studies were not powered to arrive to this conclusion, the NASPGHAN working group suggests *a 4–8 weeks trial of PPIs for typical symptoms (heartburn, retrosternal, or epigastric pain) in children as a diagnostic test for GERD* (option D is false).

No data conclusively supports the use of PPIs in the diagnosis of extraesophageal symptoms in the pediatric literature. Only one randomized trial by Holbrook et al. addressed the use of PPI in asthma and did not find any improvement in interval analysis.

A 2-week randomized controlled trial (RCT) of lansoprazole was powered to assess improvement in GERD symptoms but found no benefit of lansoprazole compared with placebo for extraesophageal symptoms, but again this study was not powered for these outcomes. *Hence insufficient evidence exists to support a short trial of PPIs as a diagnostic test for extraesophageal reflux symptoms* (option C is false).

 **Key: B**

 **BOOST YOUR KNOWLEDGE**

- Jejunal feeding/transpyloric feeding trials for *diagnosis* of GERD are not recommended in both infants and children. However, transpyloric feeding has been used in cases of refractory GERD as a *therapeutic* measure.
- Gastric scintigraphy is not recommended as a diagnostic test for GERD in infants and children.

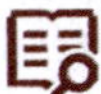 **REFERENCE/SOURCE**

- Rosen R, Vandenplas Y, Singendonk M, Cabana M, DiLorenzo C, Gottrand F, et al. Pediatric Gastroesophageal Reflux Clinical Practice Guidelines: Joint Recommendations of the North American Society for Pediatric Gastroenterology, Hepatology, and Nutrition and the European Society for Pediatric Gastroenterology, Hepatology, and Nutrition. J Pediatr Gastroenterol Nutr. 2018;66:516-54.

11. Which of the following is *true* regarding drug therapy for GERD in children?

A. Baclofen can be considered prior to surgery in children in whom other pharmacological treatments have failed
B. Metoclopramide is superior to domperidone in infants with GERD in reducing visible regurgitation/vomiting
C. Omeprazole reduces visible distress in infants with GERD compared to H_2 receptor antagonists (H_2RA) or antacid therapy
D. Use of an H_2RA improves histology/macroscopy in infants and children with GERD compared with antacids/alginates

 **EXPLANATION**

- Baclofen can be considered prior to surgery in children in whom other pharmacological treatments have failed. Baclofen *reduces* the frequency of tLESRs, reduces acid reflux, and *accelerates* gastric emptying, but it has not been evaluated in controlled trials for treatment of GERD in children. Based on adult studies, baclofen may be useful for treatment of GERD patients, but *should not be regarded as first-choice therapy* in view of adverse effects such as dyspeptic symptoms, drowsiness, dizziness, fatigue, and lowered threshold for seizures (option A is true).
- A study compared domperidone and metoclopramide in infants and children with a clinical diagnosis of GER and found significant improvement in the percentage of patients vomiting at the end of treatment in the group treated with domperidone. However, there is no sufficient evidence to recommend any one drug over the other (option B is false). Dysrhythmia, respiratory distress/arrest, neuroleptic malignant syndrome, and tardive dyskinesia are rarely associated with metoclopramide use and its therapeutic and toxic dose profile show a very narrow safe dosing range. Most serious adverse effect with domperidone is prolongation of QT interval.
- It is uncertain whether the use of omeprazole reduces crying/distress or chest pain as signs and symptoms of GERD in infants and children with GERD compared with H_2RA/antacids (option C is false). Rates of healing of erosive or histologic esophagitis are higher after 12 weeks of therapy with a PPI in contrast to H_2RA. Therefore, based upon evidence from adult literature and expert opinion, the NASPGHAN-ESPGHAN working group recommends PPIs as first line treatment and H_2RA as second-line treatment if first-line therapy is not available.
- H_2RA does not result in a significantly higher histological recovery in comparison with antacids/alginates.

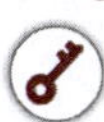 **Key: A**

BOOST YOUR KNOWLEDGE

- Rapid PPI metabolism is seen with *CYP2C19 polymorphism*. 30–40% Asians are rapid metabolizers. *Rabeprazole and esomeprazole* are least affected by this and hence may achieve better acid suppression.
- *Nocturnal acid secretion* is driven by *histamine* and less responsive to PPI therapy and better responsive to H_2RA. H_2RA has a useful role in "as-needed" medication over and above PPI in those with nocturnal symptoms when on PPI.

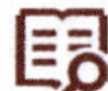

REFERENCES/SOURCES

- Richter JE, Vaezi MF. Gastroesophageal reflux disease. In: Feldman M, Friedman LS, Brandt LJ (Eds). Sleisenger and Fordtran's Gastrointestinal and Liver Disease, 11th edition. Amsterdam, Netherlands: Elsevier; 2020. p. 687.
- Rosen R, Vandenplas Y, Singendonk M, Cabana M, DiLorenzo C, Gottrand F, et al. Pediatric Gastroesophageal Reflux Clinical Practice Guidelines: Joint Recommendations of the North American Society for Pediatric Gastroenterology, Hepatology, and Nutrition and the European Society for Pediatric Gastroenterology, Hepatology, and Nutrition. J Pediatr Gastroenterol Nutr. 2018;66:516-54.

12. Which of the following is correct regarding Barrett's esophagus?

A. Replacement of nonkeratinized stratified squamous epithelium with stratified squamous epithelium in lower esophagus
B. Most common etiology is smoking and tobacco chewing in adults and GERD in children
C. The condition is associated with increased risk of adenocarcinoma of the esophagus
D. Medical therapy is superior to surgical fundoplication to prevent malignant transformation

EXPLANATION

Barrett's esophagus is replacement of nonkeratinized stratified squamous epithelium with intestinal epithelium (nonciliated columnar with goblet cells); (option A is not correct). Most common cause in both adults and children is long standing GERD (option B is not correct). There is an increased risk of adenocarcinoma of lower esophagus with above (option C is correct). There are studies which suggest that surgical fundoplication may prevent progression of Barrett's esophagus to esophageal cancer, compared to medical therapy.

The risk of developing Barrett's esophagus is very low in childhood. Three studies have looked at long-term outcomes in pediatric GERD with esophagitis on endoscopy and none of them found Barrett's esophagus over a follow-up of 12 months to 5 years. A large multicenter prospective study of 840 consecutive children who underwent elective endoscopies reported a 25.7% prevalence for reflux esophagitis, and a mere 0.12% for Barrett's esophagus in children without neurologic disorders or tracheoesophageal anomalies.

Key: C

BOOST YOUR KNOWLEDGE

Malignancy	*Esophagus part*	*Predisposing/risk factors*	*Remark*
Adenocarcinoma	Lower 1/3rd	Chronic GERD, obesity, tobacco smoking, Barrett's esophagus	More common in North America
Squamous cell carcinoma	Upper 2/3rd	Alcohol, liquids, smoking, caustic ingestion, achalasia cardia	More common in rest of the world

REFERENCES/SOURCES

- Khan S, Matta SKR. Gastroesophageal reflux disease. Kliegman RM, St Geme JW (Eds). Nelson Textbook of Pediatrics, 21st edition. Amsterdam, Netherlands: Elsevier; 2019.
- Rosen R, Vandenplas Y, Singendonk M, Cabana M, DiLorenzo C, Gottrand F, et al. Pediatric Gastroesophageal Reflux Clinical Practice Guidelines: Joint Recommendations of the North American Society for Pediatric Gastroenterology, Hepatology, and Nutrition and the European Society for Pediatric Gastroenterology, Hepatology, and Nutrition. J Pediatr Gastroenterol Nutr. 2018;66:516-54.

13. **Which of the following is hypothesized to influence long-term outcomes of pediatric GERD?**

A. Number of visits to primary physician for GERD
B. Age of onset of symptoms <5 years
C. Male gender
D. Family history of GERD

EXPLANATION

Age of onset of GERD symptoms <5 years (option B is correct) and use of acid-suppression at time of initial diagnosis may result in less favorable outcome in GERD in children. Drawing firm conclusions based on the above are, however, limited by the poor quality of the studies. No evidence exists showing an association between gender (option C is incorrect), ethnicity, and/or family history of GERD (option D is incorrect) or number of visits to the primary care physician (option A is incorrect) with poor outcomes in GERD in childhood.

Key: B

BOOST YOUR KNOWLEDGE

Family history of GERD does not predict outcome of GERD in children. However genetic linkage is indicated by the strong evidence of GERD in studies with monozygotic twins. A pediatric autosomal dominant form with otolaryngologic and respiratory manifestations has been located to chromosome 13q14, known as GERD1 locus.

REFERENCES/SOURCES

- El-Serag HB, Gilger M, Carter J, Genta RM, Rabeneck L. Childhood GERD is a risk factor for GERD in adolescents and young adults. Am J Gastroenterol. 2004;99:806-12.
- Ruigomez A, Lundborg P, Johansson S, Wallander M-A, Rodríguez LAG. Follow-up of a cohort of children and adolescents with gastro-esophageal reflux disease who were free of reflux esophagitis at initial diagnosis. Scand J Gastroenterol. 2010;45:814-21.

14. **Which of the following is the most common finding in oral cavity involvement in GERD in children?**

A. Geographic tongue
B. Dental erosions
C. Aphthous ulcers
D. Glossitis

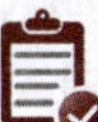

EXPLANATION

- Most common oral cavity lesions in GERD in children are dental erosions. Such lesions are seen on the lingual surface of teeth. Severity *correlates with* presence of symptoms of reflex and amount of acid in oral cavity and proximal esophagus.
- Acid suppressive therapy is useful in countering the damage to teeth lining.
- Similar lesions in oral cavity are seen in bulimia nervosa and excessive juice consumption.

Key: B

BOOST YOUR KNOWLEDGE

Posterior one-third of the vocal cord and interarytenoid areas are most common location for laryngitis secondary to GERD.

REFERENCE/SOURCE

- Khan S, Matta SKR. Gastroesophageal reflux disease. Kliegman RM, St Geme JW (Eds). Nelson Textbook of Pediatrics, 21st edition. Amsterdam, Netherlands: Elsevier; 2019.

15. The role of pH-MII is accurately described by which of the following statements with respect to diagnostics in GERD?

A. It can be used as the single best agent to diagnose GERD in infants and children
B. It is recommended to differentiate NERD in patients with normal endoscopy
C. It is a poor modality to assess treatment response following acid suppression
D. It is useful for only acid reflux symptoms in postprandial period

EXPLANATION

The pH-MII cannot be used as a diagnostic technique for GERD alone.

The advantage of pH-MII above the isolated monitoring of the esophageal pH lies in its ability to accurately detect:

- Refluxate with pH <4 and >4
- Full esophageal column reflux
- Liquid versus gas reflux
- Decreases in esophageal pH due to reflux versus swallow-related drops in pH

pH-MII testing is recommended for the following indications:

1. Correlate persistent troublesome symptoms with acid and nonacid gastroesophageal reflux events
2. Clarify the role of acid and nonacid reflux in the etiology of esophagitis and other signs and symptoms suggestive for GERD
3. Determine the efficacy of acid suppression therapy
4. Differentiate NERD, hypersensitive esophagus, and functional heartburn in patients with normal endoscopy

Key: B

BOOST YOUR KNOWLEDGE

The pH-MII had a *high sensitivity* compared to pH-metry for the detection of reflux episodes, particularly when *nonacid reflux* was prevalent, for instance those on acid suppression and in infants who are frequently fed. This has been very useful in understanding the *role of reflux with pH >4.*

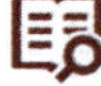

REFERENCE/SOURCE

- Rosen R, Vandenplas Y, Singendonk M, Cabana M, DiLorenzo C, Gottrand F, et al. Pediatric Gastroesophageal Reflux Clinical Practice Guidelines: Joint Recommendations of the North American Society for Pediatric Gastroenterology, Hepatology, and Nutrition and the European Society for Pediatric Gastroenterology, Hepatology, and Nutrition. J Pediatr Gastroenterol Nutr. 2018;66:516-54.

16. Which of the following is true regarding biomarkers for GERD?

A. Salivary pepsin has been studied as an extraesophageal biomarker for GERD
B. Pepsin from bronchoalveolar lavage (BAL) and middle ear fluid acts as a sensitive biomarker
C. Lipid laden macrophage index in BAL fluid is a marker for GERD
D. Bilirubin monitoring using fiber-optic measurements in esophagus is reliable biomarker for GERD

EXPLANATION

Pepsin: Studies have measured the diagnostic value of salivary pepsin (option A is true) by comparing it to results from pH-MII testing found it to be of limited sensitivity with results depending on concentration cut-off used. Apart from saliva, pepsin has also been measured in BAL and middle ear fluid. Findings of these studies also suggest a lack of sensitivity (57–84%) of the biomarker (option B is false).

Lipid-laden macrophage index: Studies comparing the lipid-laden macrophage index in BAL fluid to impedance and endoscopy did not show any relationship suggesting that it is not a biomarker for gastroesophageal reflux diagnosis (option C is false).

Bilirubin: Continuous monitoring of bilirubin using fiber-optic measurements in the esophagus is limited by the mandatory dietary restrictions during testing, thereby limiting its reliability and sensitivity (option D is false) and utility in children, hence not recommended for use in clinical practice at present.

Key: A

BOOST YOUR KNOWLEDGE

Based on expert opinion, the NASPGHAN-ESPGHAN working group *suggests against* the use of currently available extraesophageal biomarkers for the diagnosis of GERD in infants and children.

REFERENCE/SOURCE

- Rosen R, Vandenplas Y, Singendonk M, Cabana M, DiLorenzo C, Gottrand F, et al. Pediatric Gastroesophageal Reflux Clinical Practice Guidelines: Joint Recommendations of the North American Society for Pediatric Gastroenterology, Hepatology, and Nutrition and the European Society for Pediatric Gastroenterology, Hepatology, and Nutrition. J Pediatr Gastroenterol Nutr. 2018;66:516-54.

17. Wireless pH recording has been proposed as an alternative to the routine pH probe monitoring. It has certain limitations and some advantages. Which of the following statements can be considered as an advantage with respect to this technique?

A. Upper GI endoscopy is required to clip the device to the lower esophagus
B. It can be used in patients with developmental delay/autism
C. Wireless pH recording results are comparable to the pH probe
D. The device records pH changes for a minimum of 48 hours

EXPLANATION

Wireless pH monitoring is an alternative to the wired pH probe. It has to be affixed in the esophagus using upper GI endoscopy and is not a home-based alternative when it comes to initial attachment (option A is not an advantage).

A key advantage of the device is that the patient does not have a catheter in the nose, so for children with developmental delay or autism or in those with cystic fibrosis and chronic cough, the wireless device is preferable (option B is an advantage). Also, patients with exercise induced GERD symptoms find the device more comfortable when exercising including swimming.

Studies in children have shown that wireless pH recording results are comparable to the pH probe in patients that underwent both simultaneously (option C is a fact, but not an advantage over the standard probe).

The device records data for a minimum of 48 hours and up to 5 days according to some studies (option D is a fact, but not an advantage over the standard probe).

Key: B

BOOST YOUR KNOWLEDGE

Wireless pH recording is a minimally invasive diagnostic procedure used to evaluate the pH levels in the esophagus, which helps in diagnosing and assessing the severity of GERD. The test involves attaching a small capsule, about the size of a pencil eraser, to the lower part of the esophagus using an endoscope. The capsule measures the acid levels in the esophagus over a period of 48 hours and transmits the data to a recording device worn by the patient. This data is then analyzed by a doctor to determine the extent of acid reflux.

Advantages of Wireless pH Recording for GERD:

- *Accuracy:* Wireless pH recording is a highly accurate method for diagnosing GERD. It is more accurate than traditional 24-hour esophageal pH monitoring, as it provides a continuous record of pH levels over a longer period.
- Wireless pH recording for GERD

- *Minimally invasive:* The procedure is minimally invasive and does not require any incisions. The capsule is naturally eliminated through the digestive system.
- *Comfortable:* The capsule is small and lightweight, and most patients do not experience any discomfort during the test.
- *Convenient:* The patient can go about their normal activities during the test.

Risks of wireless pH recording:

The risks of wireless pH recording are minimal. Some patients may experience mild discomfort or throat soreness after the procedure. There is also a very small risk of the capsule becoming dislodged and causing esophageal obstruction.

Overall, wireless pH recording is a safe, accurate, and convenient method for diagnosing and assessing GERD.

REFERENCE/SOURCE

- Rosen R, Vandenplas Y, Singendonk M, Cabana M, DiLorenzo C, Gottrand F, et al. Pediatric Gastroesophageal Reflux Clinical Practice Guidelines: Joint Recommendations of the North American Society for Pediatric Gastroenterology, Hepatology, and Nutrition and the European Society for Pediatric Gastroenterology, Hepatology, and Nutrition. J Pediatr Gastroenterol Nutr. 2018;66:516-54.

18. Which of the following is correct regarding nonpharmacological measures for GERD in pediatric population?

A. Positioning therapy with head end elevation can be used to treat GERD in sleeping infants
B. Maternal massage therapy is recommended in fussy infants with GERD
C. *Lactobacillus reuteri* drops have shown improvement in GERD in infants
D. Weight loss is shown to improve GERD symptoms in children

EXPLANATION

Positioning therapy with head-end elevation/lateral position is not recommended for sleeping infants in view of increased risk of sudden infant death syndrome (option A is incorrect). Since elevating the head of an infant's crib while supine may result in the infant rolling to the foot of the crib into a position that may compromise respiration, elevating the head end of the crib is not recommended by the American Academy of Pediatrics.

There is a single trial on massage therapy versus sham therapy and it did not show any advantage of massage therapy after 6 weeks of intervention (option B is incorrect), hence the NASPGHAN group recommends against using any massage therapy for infants with GERD.

A preventive study used probiotics (*L. reuteri*) given as drops daily for 90 days in 589 term newborns (age <1 week) in the prevention of colic, regurgitation, and functional constipation. It showed significantly lower reflux episodes in the *L. reuteri* group compared to placebo (option C is correct). However, this is insufficient to be recommended as a standard of care.

There is an association between obesity and mild increase in GERD symptoms in children. No pediatric studies determine if weight reduction changes GERD symptoms (option D is incorrect). No pediatric studies have shown a relationship between obesity and reflux events by pH-metry. There are adult studies which show that weight loss may be useful in decreasing symptoms of GERD.

Key: C

BOOST YOUR KNOWLEDGE

Passive tobacco/alcohol exposure (maternal intake in breastfeeding infants) is implicated in GER symptoms in infants. Limiting the above exposure may be a reasonable trial before proceeding to more expensive therapies.

REFERENCE/SOURCE

- Indrio F, Di Mauro A, Riezzo G, Civardi E, Intini C, Corvaglia L, et al. Prophylactic use of a probiotic in the prevention of colic, regurgitation, and functional constipation: a randomized clinical trial. JAMA Pediatr. 2014;168:228-33.

19. Which of the following is true regarding fundoplication in GERD management in children?

A. Increases the LES baseline pressure and decreases the number of transient LES relaxations
B. Leads to an increase in the length of the intra-abdominal esophagus, accentuating the angle of His
C. Laparoscopic Nissen fundoplication is the gold standard for surgical treatment of severe GERD
D. All of the above

EXPLANATION

- Fundoplication decreases reflux by increasing the LES baseline pressure, decreasing the number of tLESRs and hence the nadir pressure during swallow induced relaxation, increasing the length of the intra-abdominal esophagus, accentuating the angle of His, and reducing a hiatal hernia if present (options A and B are true).
- Laparoscopic Nissen fundoplication is now considered the gold standard for surgical management of severe GERD and has largely replaced open Nissen fundoplication as the preferred antireflux surgery due to lower morbidity, shorter hospital stays, and lesser perioperative problems (option C is true).
- Robot-assisted Nissen fundoplication is a safe alternative to conventional laparoscopic surgery in children but does not provide any significant clinical advantage over conventional procedure.

Key: D

BOOST YOUR KNOWLEDGE

- Anti-reflux surgery may be superior in preventing esophageal adenocarcinoma compared with medical therapy in adults with Barrett's esophagus.
- Total esophagogastric disconnection (TED, *Bianchi procedure*) is an alternative surgical procedure in *resistant GERD in adults.*
- *Stretta procedure* refers to a form of radiofrequency ablation of the LES and is an *endoscopic therapy* for GERD.

REFERENCE/SOURCE

- Auyang ED, Patrice Carter, Thomas Rauth, Robert D Fanelli; SAGES Guidelines Committee. SAGES clinical spotlight review: endoluminal treatments for gastroesophageal reflux disease (GERD). Surg Endosc. 2013;27:2658-72.

20. Which of the following is true with respect to GERD?

A. Montreal consensus statement is used for defining GER in adults
B. *Helicobacter pylori* has a causal association with GERD
C. Delayed gastric emptying is a significant contributor to GERD in children
D. Bile salts are more noxious than acid and pepsin of the gastric reflux in GERD

EXPLANATION

Montreal consensus statements are used for defining GER in adults and the NASPGHAN-ESPGHAN consensus borrows the definition for pediatric population *(option A is true)*. GER is defined as the passage of gastric contents into the esophagus with or without regurgitation and/or vomiting. The association of *H. pylori* with GERD is controversial.

As a tip remember: One of the hypotheses with respect to variable association between *H. pylori* infection and GERD is gastric antral infection with *H. pylori* leads to hypergastrinemia and when *H. pylori* is treated, it improves GER symptoms. On the other hand, gastric body infection with *H. pylori* leads to atrophic gastritis and decreased acid production, and when *H. pylori* is treated, it may worsen GER symptoms *(option B is false)*.

Importance of delayed gastric emptying is controversial with earlier studies showing rates as high as up to 50%; however, recent studies show a prevalence of delayed gastric emptying in only 10–15% in adults *(option C is false)*. Data in children is further limited.

Gastric acid and pepsin are more noxious than bile acids in leading to mucosal injury in GERD *(option D is false)*:
- Deconjugated bile acids and pancreatic enzymes get inactivated in acidic pH of stomach.
- Bile acids do not reach cytotoxic concentration in refluxate
- Typical signs of bile acid injury usually missing

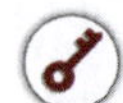

Key: A

BOOST YOUR KNOWLEDGE

- Nocturnal GERD has an association with obstructive sleep apnea.
- Progressive dysphagia due to peptic stricture formation *decreases* heartburn symptoms as there is a mechanical barrier for reflux.

REFERENCE/SOURCE

- Vakil N, van Zanten SV, Kahrilas P, Dent J, Jones R; Global Consensus Group. The Montreal definition and classification of gastroesophageal reflux disease: a global evidence-based consensus. Am J Gastroenterol. 2006;101:1900-20.

CHAPTER 16.5

Functional Abdominal Pain Disorders

Srinivas Srinidhi Vadlapudi, Moinak Sen Sarma

1. A 6-year-old child has presented with periumbilical pain abdomen for last 1 year. Pain occurs only during daytime, lasts for 1–2 hours, and occurs almost every alternate day. Father is a known case of Crohn's disease on treatment for the last 10 years. There is no history of growth failure in this child. Which of the following in history is a red flag sign which helps us to differentiate between functional and organic etiology?

A. Duration of pain of 1 year

B. Periumbilical pain abdomen

C. Pain occurring at daytime

D. Family history of Crohn's disease

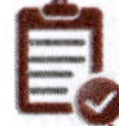

EXPLANATION

Family history of inflammatory bowel disease, celiac disease, and peptic ulcer disease is a red flag sign. Duration, frequency, and intensity of pain cannot differentiate between functional and organic etiology. Midline pain favors functional abdominal pain while pain in the right upper or lower quadrants requires work-up for organic etiology. Pain which awakens the child is a red flag and not daytime pain.

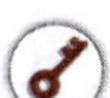

Key: D

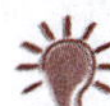

BOOST YOUR KNOWLEDGE

Alarm symptoms in a child with chronic abdominal pain which require further investigations include:

- Pain that wakes a child from sleep
- Persistent right upper or lower quadrant pain
- Significant vomiting
- Unexplained fever
- Genitourinary symptoms
- Dysphagia or odynophagia
- Chronic severe diarrhea or nocturnal diarrhea
- Gastrointestinal blood loss
- Involuntary weight loss
- Deceleration of linear growth
- Delayed puberty
- Family history of inflammatory bowel disease, celiac disease, or peptic ulcer disease

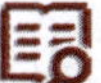

REFERENCES/SOURCES

- Hyams JS, Di Lorenzo C, Saps M, Shulman RJ, Staiano A, Van Tilburg M. Childhood functional gastrointestinal disorders: child/adolescent. Gastroenterol. 2016;150(6):1456-68.
- Maqbool A, Liacouras CA. Functional gastrointestinal disorders (Table 368.10). In: Kliegman RM, St Geme III JW, Blum NJ, Shah SS, Tasker RC, Wilson KM (Eds). Nelson Textbook of Pediatrics, 21st edition. Elsevier; 2019. p. 2044.

2. A 10-year-old child presented with periumbilical pain abdomen for 1 month duration. Pain occurs daily only during daytime, lasts for 30 minutes and does not affect general well-being. Elder sibling is a known case of celiac disease. On examination, there is no growth failure, anemia, jaundice, pedal edema, abdominal tenderness, or organomegaly. Due to which feature in this child, a diagnosis of functional abdominal pain cannot be established?

A. Abdominal pain occurring daily
B. Duration of pain of 1 month only
C. Family history of celiac disease
D. Periumbilical pain abdomen

EXPLANATION

For the diagnosis of functional abdominal pain disorders, the criteria must be fulfilled for at least 2 months duration. Frequency of pain (at least 4 days in a month) and presence of midline pain cannot differentiate from organic or functional etiology. Family history of celiac disease will require further investigation for the child but does not stop him from being diagnosed as functional abdominal pain.

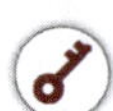

Key: B

BOOST YOUR KNOWLEDGE

Functional dyspepsia (FD), irritable bowel syndrome (IBS), functional abdominal pain not otherwise specified (FAP-NOS), and abdominal migraine constitute functional abdominal pain disorders. The criteria for FD, IBS, and FAP-NOS need to be fulfilled for ≥4 days/month for ≥2 months. For abdominal migraine, the criteria need to be satisfied for at least 6 months before the diagnosis.

REFERENCES/SOURCES

- Hyams JS, Di Lorenzo C, Saps M, Shulman RJ, Staiano A, Van Tilburg M. Childhood functional gastrointestinal disorders: child/adolescent. Gastroenterol. 2016;150(6):1456-68.
- Maqbool A, Liacouras CA. Functional gastrointestinal disorders. In: Kliegman RM, St Geme III JW, Blum NJ, Shah SS, Tasker RC, Wilson KM (Eds). Nelson Textbook of Pediatrics, 21st edition. Elsevier; 2019. pp. 2041-5.

3. A 14-year-old boy presented with upper abdominal discomfort and early satiety for 3 months. Symptoms are present for at least 20 days in each month. There were no red flag signs on history or examination. Upper gastrointestinal endoscopy and ultrasonography of the abdomen were found to be normal. Which of the following is the most likely diagnosis in this child?

A. Irritable bowel syndrome
B. Rumination syndrome
C. Peptic ulcer disease
D. Functional dyspepsia

EXPLANATION

Functional dyspepsia is characterized by postprandial fullness, early satiety, epigastric pain, or burning sensation not associated with defecation. These symptoms should not be explained by any other condition and the criteria should be fulfilled for at least 2 months. IBS is characterized by abdominal pain and change in bowel habits. Rumination is associated with effortless regurgitation of food. As endoscopy did not reveal any ulcer, it is unlikely to be peptic ulcer disease.

Key: D

BOOST YOUR KNOWLEDGE

Functional dyspepsia is diagnosed when one or more of the following is/are present for ≥4 days/month for ≥2 months:

- Postprandial fullness
- Early satiation
- Epigastric pain or burning not associated with defecation
- After appropriate evaluation, symptoms cannot be explained as another medical condition.

Within FD, the following subtypes are now adopted:

- Postprandial distress syndrome includes bothersome postprandial fullness or early satiation that prevents finishing a regular meal. Supportive features include upper abdominal bloating, postprandial nausea, or excessive belching.
- *Epigastric pain syndrome includes all of the following:* Bothersome (severe enough to interfere with normal activities) pain or burning localized to the epigastrium. The pain is not generalized or localized to other abdominal or chest regions and is not relieved by defecation or passage of flatus. Supportive criteria can include: (1) Burning quality of the pain but without a retrosternal component and (2) the pain commonly induced or relieved by ingestion of a meal but may occur while fasting.

REFERENCES/SOURCES

- Hyams JS, Di Lorenzo C, Saps M, Shulman RJ, Staiano A, Van Tilburg M. Childhood functional gastrointestinal disorders: child/adolescent. Gastroenterol. 2016;150(6):1456-68.
- Maqbool A, Liacouras CA. Functional gastrointestinal disorders (Table 368.9). In: Kliegman RM, St Geme III JW, Blum NJ, Shah SS, Tasker RC, Wilson KM (Eds). Nelson Textbook of Pediatrics, 21st edition. Elsevier; 2019. p. 2044.

4. Irritable bowel syndrome is further subclassified on the basis of:

A. Stool pattern
B. Pain duration
C. Location of pain
D. Associated extraintestinal symptoms

EXPLANATION

Irritable bowel syndrome is further classified into the following four subtypes based on the predominant stool pattern:

1. IBS with constipation
2. IBS with diarrhea
3. IBS with constipation and diarrhea
4. Unspecified IBS

Key: A

BOOST YOUR KNOWLEDGE

Irritable bowel syndrome patients are classified into the earlier mentioned four subtypes based on stool pattern. The stool pattern is assessed by *Bristol Stool Form Scale* depicted in the picture.

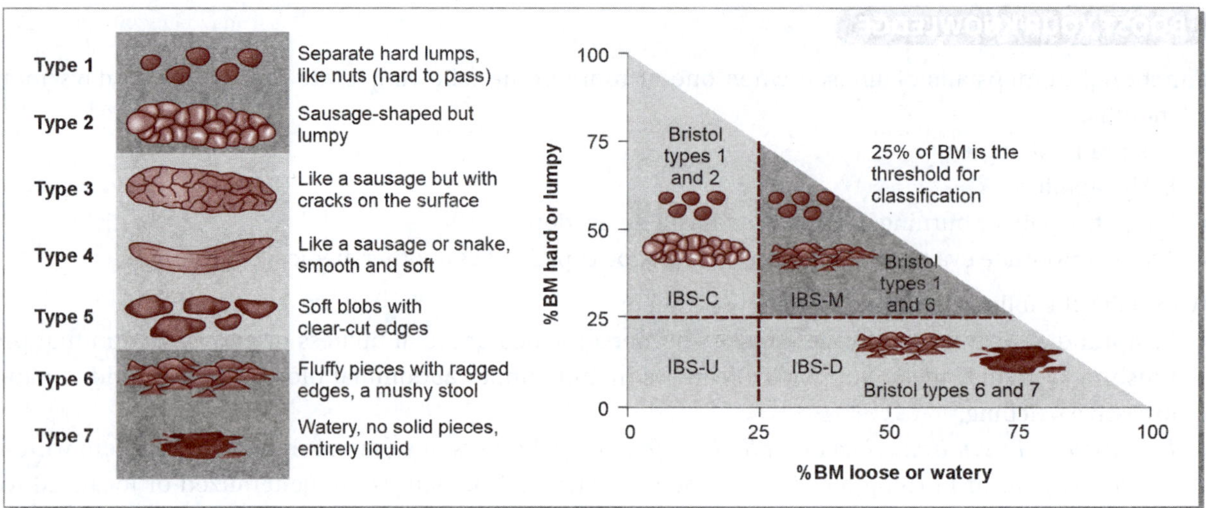

The Bristol Stool Form Scale and classification of subtypes of IBS.
(BM: bowel movement; C: constipation; D: diarrhea; M: mixed; U: unsubtyped)
Source: Adapted from Lacy BE, Mearin F, Chang L, Chey WD, Lembo AJ, Simren M, et al. Bowel disorders. Gastroenterol. 2016; 150(6):1393-407.e5.

REFERENCES/SOURCES

- Ford AC, Talley NJ. Irritable bowel syndrome. In: Feldman M, Friedman LS, Brandt LJ (Eds). Sleisenger and Fordtran's Gastrointestinal and Liver Disease, 11th edition. Elsevier; 2020. pp. 2008-22.
- Hyams JS, Di Lorenzo C, Saps M, Shulman RJ, Staiano A, Van Tilburg M. Childhood functional gastrointestinal disorders: child/adolescent. Gastroenterol. 2016;150(6):1456-68.
- Maqbool A, Liacouras CA. Functional gastrointestinal disorders (Table 368.9). In: Kliegman RM, St Geme III JW, Blum NJ, Shah SS, Tasker RC, Wilson KM (Eds). Nelson Textbook of Pediatrics, 21st edition. Elsevier; 2019. p. 2044.

5. **Which of the following dietary modifications is approved for the treatment of IBS?**

A. Low residue diet
B. Low FODMAP (fermentable oligosaccharide, disaccharide, monosaccharide, and polyol) diet
C. Six-food elimination diet
D. Exclusive enteral nutrition

EXPLANATION

Low FODMAP diet has been used for the treatment of IBS. Low residue diet is low in fiber and considered for patients with partial bowel obstruction. Exclusive enteral nutrition is used for induction of remission in mild-to-moderate Crohn's disease patients. Six-food elimination diet is used for the treatment of eosinophilic gastrointestinal disorders.

Key: B

BOOST YOUR KNOWLEDGE

Low FODMAP diet was introduced by Gibson and Shepherd in 2005. It was identified that there is exacerbation of symptoms in some patients of IBS while on FODMAP diet. The hypothesis for the use of low FODMAP diet is that poorly absorbed carbohydrates reach the colon, where they undergo fermentation by the colonic flora, resulting in higher osmolality and gas production. This results in the development of symptoms. Patients are advised to exclude FODMAPs in a top-down approach. It includes three phases: (1) Exclusion, (2) reintroduction, and (3) maintenance phases.

Foods rich in FODMAPs include the following:

- *Vegetables:* Beetroot, onion, garlic, pumpkin, broccoli, asparagus, cabbage, capsicum, and cauliflower
- *Cereals:* Corn, wheat, and rye
- *Fruits:* Banana, blueberry, cranberry, pomegranate, watermelon, and custard apple
- *Nuts:* Almonds, cashew, and pistachio
- *Legumes:* Chickpea, soybean, red bean, and lentils
- Lactose, sweeteners and fructose, honey, jams, and jelly.

Low FODMAP diet is recommended by the American College of Gastroenterology as the second-line therapy for adults with IBS.

The evidence regarding the effectiveness of the low FODMAP diet in the treatment of FGID in children is currently insufficient to guide clinical practice.

REFERENCES/SOURCES

- Ford AC, Talley NJ. Irritable bowel syndrome. In: Feldman M, Friedman LS, Brandt LJ (Eds). Sleisenger and Fordtran's Gastrointestinal and Liver Disease, 11th edition. Elsevier; 2020. pp. 2008-22.
- Maqbool A, Liacouras CA. Functional gastrointestinal disorders (Table 368.9). In: Kliegman RM, St Geme III JW, Blum NJ, Shah SS, Tasker RC, Wilson KM (Eds). Nelson Textbook of Pediatrics, 21st edition. Elsevier; 2019. p. 2044.
- Thomassen RA, Luque V, Assa A, Borrelli O, Broekaert I, Dolinsek J, et al. An ESPGHAN position paper on the use of low-FODMAP diet in pediatric gastroenterology. J Pediatr Gastroenterol Nutr. 2022;75(3):356-68.

6. An 8-year-old boy presented with complaints of abdominal pain and constipation for 6 months. There are no red flag signs on history and examination of the child. For constipation, the child was started on polyethylene glycol following which his symptoms completely subsided. What is his most likely diagnosis?

A. Abdominal migraine
B. Functional dyspepsia
C. Functional constipation
D. Functional abdominal pain—not otherwise specified

EXPLANATION

As abdominal pain subsided after treatment of constipation, this is likely functional constipation. In IBS with constipation, abdominal pain persists even after resolution of constipation. In FD, abdominal pain is not associated with change in bowel habits. Functional abdominal pain not otherwise specified is a diagnosis of exclusion.

Key: C

BOOST YOUR KNOWLEDGE

As many as 75% of children with constipation report pain, and studies have shown that IBS patients often receive a diagnosis of functional constipation. The committee recommends that patients with constipation and abdominal pain initially be treated for constipation only. If abdominal pain resolves with constipation treatment, the patient has functional constipation. If pain does not resolve with appropriate constipation treatment alone, the patient likely has IBS with constipation.

REFERENCES/SOURCES

- Hyams JS, Di Lorenzo C, Saps M, Shulman RJ, Staiano A, Van Tilburg M. Childhood functional gastrointestinal disorders: child/adolescent. Gastroenterol. 2016;150(6):1456-68.
- Maqbool A, Liacouras CA. Functional gastrointestinal disorders (Table 368.9). In: Kliegman RM, St Geme III JW, Blum NJ, Shah SS, Tasker RC, Wilson KM (Eds). Nelson Textbook of Pediatrics, 21st edition. Elsevier; 2019. p. 2044.

7. A 7-year-old child presented with intense periumbilical pain in the abdomen lasting for 1–2 hours, interfering with day-to-day activities occurring in a similar manner once every 2 months for the last 1 year. These episodes of abdominal pain are associated with nausea, photophobia, and nonbilious vomiting. Work-up for metabolic disorders and imaging of the abdomen were unyielding. What is the likely diagnosis?

A. Abdominal migraine
B. Rumination syndrome
C. Acute recurrent pancreatitis
D. Acid peptic disease

EXPLANATION

Abdominal migraine is a functional abdominal pain syndrome characterized by stereotypical symptoms in an episodic manner like that in the question. *Rumination syndrome* is an effortless regurgitation of stomach contents which is not associated with nausea. Episodes of *acute pancreatitis* are associated with epigastric and not periumbilical pain in the abdomen. Urea cycle defect is unlikely as basic screening for metabolic disorders would identify some abnormality.

Key: A

BOOST YOUR KNOWLEDGE

Diagnostic criteria for abdominal migraine include all of the following occurring at least twice:

- Paroxysmal episodes of intense, acute periumbilical, midline, or diffuse abdominal pain lasting 1 hour or more (should be the most severe and distressing symptom).
- Episodes are separated by weeks to months.
- The pain is incapacitating and interferes with normal activities.
- Stereotypical pattern and symptoms in the individual patient.
- The pain is associated with two or more of the following:
  - Anorexia
  - Nausea
  - Vomiting
  - Headache
  - Photophobia
  - Pallor
- After appropriate evaluation, the symptoms cannot be fully explained by another medical condition.

REFERENCES/SOURCES

- Hyams JS, Di Lorenzo C, Saps M, Shulman RJ, Staiano A, Van Tilburg M. Childhood functional gastrointestinal disorders: child/adolescent. Gastroenterol. 2016;150(6):1456-68.
- Maqbool A, Liacouras CA. Functional gastrointestinal disorders (Table 368.14). In: Kliegman RM, St Geme III JW, Blum NJ, Shah SS, Tasker RC, Wilson KM (Eds). Nelson Textbook of Pediatrics, 21st edition. Elsevier; 2019. p. 2045.

8. Which of the following drugs is used to treat abdominal migraine?

A. Fiber
B. Rifaximin
C. Amitriptyline
D. Loperamide

EXPLANATION

Amitriptyline is an effective agent for abdominal migraine. Fiber is used for treatment of IBS. Rifaximin is helpful in a subset of IBS with diarrhea patients. Loperamide is helpful in patients with IBS with diarrhea.

Key: C

BOOST YOUR KNOWLEDGE

Exposure to known triggers such as any stressful events will help prevent attacks. Cyproheptadine, propranolol, and amitriptyline can be used as prophylactic agents to prevent attacks. Pizotifen (antiserotonin and antihistamine) is also useful. Triptans may be used to abort an episode. Abdominal migraine has many overlaps with cyclical vomiting syndrome and migraine headaches. Abdominal migraine may evolve into migraine headaches in adulthood.

REFERENCES/SOURCES

- Hyams JS, Di Lorenzo C, Saps M, Shulman RJ, Staiano A, Van Tilburg M. Childhood functional gastrointestinal disorders: child/adolescent. Gastroenterol. 2016;150(6):1456-68.
- Maqbool A, Liacouras CA. Functional gastrointestinal disorders. In: Kliegman RM, St Geme III JW, Blum NJ, Shah SS, Tasker RC, Wilson KM (Eds). Nelson Textbook of Pediatrics, 21st edition. Elsevier; 2019. pp. 2041-5.

9. **Which of the following drugs may be helpful in patients of IBS with constipation?**

A. Fiber
B. Rifaximin
C. Eluxadoline
D. Loperamide

EXPLANATION

Soluble fiber is used for treatment of IBS. Rifaximin is helpful in a subset of IBS with diarrhea patients. Eluxadoline is a μ- and κ-opioid receptor agonist and δ-opioid receptor antagonist, which reduces visceral hypersensitivity and intestinal motility. Loperamide (μ receptor agonist) is helpful for patients with IBS with diarrhea.

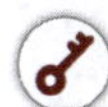

Key: A

BOOST YOUR KNOWLEDGE

For the treatment of IBS dietary modifications like low FODMAP diet may be helpful for patients with mild symptoms. Antispasmodics may be helpful for abdominal pain and postprandial symptoms. Antidepressants can improve abdominal pain and global symptoms. They may be useful for patients with moderate-to-severe symptoms. Fiber may relieve mild symptoms and constipation. Polyethylene glycol relieves constipation, but pain does not improve. Lubiprostone and linaclotide can be tried in patients who have not responded to polyethylene glycol. Loperamide reduces postprandial urgency and stool frequency but does not improve global symptoms. Rifaximin and eluxadoline (μ- and κ-opioid receptor agonist and δ-opioid receptor antagonist) are more effective than a placebo in patients of IBS with diarrhea. Alosetron (5-HT_3 antagonist) is reserved for women with severe unresponsive IBS with diarrhea.

REFERENCES/SOURCES

- Hyams JS, Di Lorenzo C, Saps M, Shulman RJ, Staiano A, Van Tilburg M. Childhood functional gastrointestinal disorders: child/adolescent. Gastroenterol. 2016;150(6):1456-68.
- Maqbool A, Liacouras CA. Functional gastrointestinal disorders (Table 368.13). In: Kliegman RM, St Geme III JW, Blum NJ, Shah SS, Tasker RC, Wilson KM (Eds). Nelson Textbook of Pediatrics, 21st edition. Elsevier; 2019. p. 2045.

10. **A 10-year-old boy presented with abdominal pain in periumbilical and hypogastric regions, which relieves with defecation for the last 6 months. The child passes hard stools once every day or alternate day (Bristol stool form 2). There are no red flag signs on history and physical examination. The child has been taking laxatives like polyethylene glycol and lactulose intermittently. Abdominal pain continues to persist in spite of relief in constipation. What is the likely diagnosis?**

A. Functional dyspepsia
B. Abdominal migraine
C. Functional constipation
D. IBS with constipation

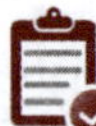

EXPLANATION

Irritable bowel syndrome with constipation (IBS-C) presents with abdominal pain, which relieves with passage of stools. In FD, functional constipation, and abdominal migraine, there is no relation of abdominal pain with defecation or change in stool form.

Key: D

BOOST YOUR KNOWLEDGE

Diagnostic criteria for IBS must include all the following:

- Abdominal pain at least 4 days per month is associated with one or more of the following:
  - Related to defecation
  - A change in frequency of stool
  - A change in form of stool
- In children with constipation, pain does not relieve with resolution of constipation.
- After appropriate evaluation, pain cannot be explained with any other medical condition.

REFERENCES/SOURCES

- Hyams JS, Di Lorenzo C, Saps M, Shulman RJ, Staiano A, Van Tilburg M. Childhood functional gastrointestinal disorders: child/adolescent. Gastroenterol. 2016;150(6):1456-68.
- Maqbool A, Liacouras CA. Functional gastrointestinal disorders (Table 368.12). In: Kliegman RM, St Geme III JW, Blum NJ, Shah SS, Tasker RC, Wilson KM (Eds). Nelson Textbook of Pediatrics, 21st edition. Elsevier; 2019. p. 2044.

11. A 10-year-old child presented with complaints of intermittent periumbilical pain in the abdomen for 1 year, which used to be relieved on passage of stool. There are no red flags on history or examination. For the abdominal pain, the child was prescribed a medication after which he started having difficulty in passing urine and constipation. Which drug was likely prescribed?

A. Paracetamol
B. Aceclofenac
C. Mefenamic acid
D. Hyoscine

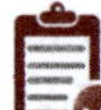

EXPLANATION

The child in question has developed acute retention of urine and constipation. This can be explained by the anticholinergic effect of hyoscine butylbromide. Paracetamol, aceclofenac, and mefenamic acid do not alter the gut motility.

Key: D

BOOST YOUR KNOWLEDGE

Gastrointestinal smooth muscle motility is affected by antimuscarinic agents, such as hyoscine. The tone and propulsive movements of the gut are diminished. The muscles of the gut wall are relaxed. Gastric emptying and intestinal transit are prolonged. However, intestinal "paralysis" induced by antimuscarinic drugs is temporary, local mechanisms within the enteric nervous system usually re-establish at least some peristalsis after 1–3 days of antimuscarinic drug therapy.

Smooth muscle of the bladder wall is also relaxed. Thus, voiding is delayed. It can precipitate urinary retention.

REFERENCE/SOURCE

- Katzung BG. Cholinoceptor-blocking drugs. In: Pappano AJ (Ed). Basic and Clinical Pharmacology, 14th edition. New York: McGraw-Hill Education; 2017.

CHAPTER 16.6

Acid-peptic Disease and *Helicobacter Pylori*

Parijat Ram Tripathi

1. Acid secretion in stomach is inhibited by which of the following hormone?

A. Acetylcholine
B. Somatostatin
C. Histamine
D. Gastrin

EXPLANATION

Acetylcholine is released from postganglionic enteric neurons. It stimulates parietal cells directly via M_3 receptor. Gastrin is secreted from G-cells and travels to parietal cells via circulation and activates cholecystokinin 2 (CCK-2) receptors on parietal cells. Histamine is released from oxyntic enterochromaffin-like cells, diffuses to parietal cells, and activates histamine subtype 2 receptors. All these three pathways are neural, hormonal, and paracrine pathways to stimulate acid secretion.

On other hand, somatostatin is released from oxyntic D-cells and diffuses to parietal cells in paracrine fashion, stimulate somatostatin subtype-2 receptors, and inhibit acid secretion.

Key: B

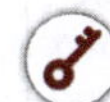

BOOST YOUR KNOWLEDGE

The stomach contains two types of glands: Oxyntic and pyloric glands. Hallmark of oxyntic glands is parietal cells while pyloric glands have G or gastrin cells predominantly. D-cells, containing somatostatin, are present predominantly in the pyloric gland area.

REFERENCE/SOURCE

- Feldman M, Friedman LS, Brandt LJ. Sleisenger and Fordtran's Gastrointestinal and Liver Disease, 10th edition. Saunders; 2015. Chapter 50.

2. Which of the following is *not* caused by *Helicobacter pylori* (*H. pylori*)?

A. Chronic gastritis
B. Duodenal ulcer
C. Enteropathy-associated T-cell lymphoma (EATL)
D. Mucosa-associated lymphoid tissue (MALT) lymphoma

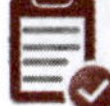

EXPLANATION

Children with colonization of *H. pylori* usually have chronic gastritis. Despite the presence of chronic gastritis, majority of patients remain asymptomatic. *H. pylori* is found in the antral mucosa of almost 90% of children with duodenal ulcer disease. Eradication of *H. pylori* from the gastric mucosa leads to long-term healing of duodenal ulcer disease. *H. pylori* is an etiologic factor in mucosa-associated lymphoid tissue (MALT) lymphomas of the stomach. Normal gastric mucosa is devoid of organized lymphoid tissue. For lymphoma to develop, the gastric wall must first acquire organized lymphoid tissue, which occurs as a reaction to infection with *H. pylori*.

 **Key: C**

 **BOOST YOUR KNOWLEDGE**

Enteropathy-associated T-cell lymphoma is associated with celiac disease. EATL is a rare type of non-Hodgkin lymphoma in general population, but it can develop in more than half of the patients of refractory celiac disease type 2. It is further very rare in pediatric population.

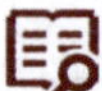 **REFERENCE/SOURCE**

- Walker WA, Goulet OJ, Kleinman RE, Sherman PM, Shneider BL, Sanderson IR. Walker's Pediatric Gastrointestinal Diseases, 4th edition. BC Decker; 2004. Chapter 29.

3. Which of the following is *incorrect* about acid peptic disease?

A. Gastric acid and pepsinogen are major aggressive factors
B. Infant gastric acid level reaches to adult level by 24 weeks of age
C. Bicarbonate—mucous barrier protects mucosa from acidic injury
D. Acid secretion is an active process involving H^+/Na^+ ATPase

 **EXPLANATION**

The pathophysiology of acid-peptic disease involves imbalance of aggressive and protective factors. Gastric acid and pepsinogen are major aggressive factors while bicarbonate and mucous layer protects mucosa from acidic injury. Prostaglandins stimulate gastric epithelium to produce mucous and bicarbonate. These protective mechanisms are broken by infections, ischemia, or non-steroidal anti-inflammatory drugs (NSAIDs). In term neonates, acidification of gastric mucosa starts soon after birth and reaches adult level by 24 weeks. Gastric acid is secreted by parietal cells through H^+/K^+ ATPase, not by H^+/Na^+ ATPase.

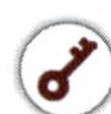 **Key: D**

 **BOOST YOUR KNOWLEDGE**

H^+/K^+ ATPase is present in parietal cells. They pump hydrogen ions against concentration gradient. Acid secretion is increased by activation of intracellular cAMP- and calcium-dependent signaling pathways that activate protein kinases, finally leading to fusion and activation of H^+/K^+ ATPase. In the resting state, H^+/K^+ ATPase is sequestered within cytoplasmic tubulovesicles in inactive form. On stimulation, the tubulovesicles move to and fuse with the apical membrane. Translocation of H^+/K^+ ATPase into the canalicular membrane and presence of luminal K^+ activate the enzyme.

 **REFERENCE/SOURCE**

- Pillai RBV. Chapter 36.11: Acid peptic disease. In: Gupta P, Menon PSN, Ramji S, Lodha R (Eds). PG Textbook of Pediatrics, 3rd edition. New Delhi: Jaypee Brothers Medical Publishers; 2022.

4. Which of the following is *true* about peptic ulcer disease?

A. Primary peptic ulcers are commonly present in the stomach
B. *H. pylori* is one of the most common causes of secondary peptic ulcer
C. Secondary peptic ulcers are usually chronic
D. Idiopathic primary peptic ulcers constitute 20% of all duodenal ulcers

EXPLANATION

Ulcers in children can be classified in two types. Primary peptic ulcers are chronic and more often duodenal. Secondary peptic ulcers are acute in onset and present in the stomach. Primary ulcers are most often associated with *H. pylori* infection. In around 20% of peptic ulcers, no apparent cause is found, and they are usually situated in duodenum.

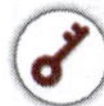

Key: D

BOOST YOUR KNOWLEDGE

The pathogenesis of peptic ulcer disease is multifactorial. Peptic ulcers are formed because of acid and pepsin on mucosal surface, which mucosal defense mechanism is not able to contain. Peptic ulcers are defined as deep mucosal lesions that disrupt the muscularis mucosa of the gastric or duodenal wall. Gastric ulcers are generally located on the lesser curvature of the stomach, and 90% of duodenal ulcers are found in the duodenal bulb.

REFERENCE/SOURCE

- Kliegman R, Stanton B, St Geme JW, Schor NF, Behrman RE. Nelson Textbook of Pediatrics, 20th edition. Philadelphia: Elsevier; 2016. Chapter 335.

5. Which of the following is *not* a cause of peptic ulcer?

A. Watery diarrhea, hypokalemia, and achlorhydria (WDHA) syndrome
B. Zollinger–Ellison syndrome
C. Intracranial lesions
D. Sepsis

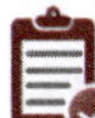

EXPLANATION

Zollinger–Ellison syndrome is due to gastrin secreting tumors which leads to refractory severe peptic ulcers. Intracranial pathologies lead to increased intracranial pressure and overstimulation of the vagus nerve. Increased secretion of gastric acid may occur which leads to gastroduodenal ulcer formation known as Cushing's ulcer. Patients with septic shock are at higher risk of peptic ulcer formation and bleeding.

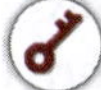

Key: A

BOOST YOUR KNOWLEDGE

Vasoactive intestinal peptide (VIP) is a neurotransmitter belonging to the secretin-glucagon family. It promotes vasodilation, glycogenolysis, lipolysis, and bone resorption. VIP-secreting tumors lead to watery diarrhea, hypokalemia, and achlorhydria (WDHA syndrome). Flushing and tetany can also be present. WDHA syndrome is also called VIPoma or Verner–Morrison syndrome.

REFERENCES/SOURCES

- Kemp WJ, Bashir A, Dababneh H, Cohen-Gadol AA. Cushing's ulcer: further reflections. Asian J Neurosurg. 2015;10(2):87-94.
- Kliegman R, Stanton B, St Geme JW, Schor NF, Behrman RE. Nelson Textbook of Pediatrics, 20th edition. Philadelphia: Elsevier; 2016. Chapter 335.

6. Which one is *true* about common symptoms of peptic ulcer in children?

A. Gastric perforation is not a feature of neonatal peptic ulcer
B. Hematemesis and melena are presenting symptoms in 20% of the patients
C. Young children usually present with epigastric pain
D. Older children usually present with dyspepsia, epigastric abdominal pain, or fullness

EXPLANATION

The presenting symptoms of peptic ulcer disease vary with the age of the patient. Hematemesis or melena is reported in up to half of the patients with peptic ulcer disease. School-age children and adolescents more commonly present with epigastric pain and nausea. Dyspepsia, epigastric abdominal pain, or fullness is seen in older children. Infants and younger children usually present with feeding difficulty, vomiting, crying episodes, hematemesis, or melena. In the neonatal period, gastric perforation can be the initial presentation. Although epigastric pain is a symptom of peptic ulcer disease, but it is not possible to localize the pain in infants.

Key: D

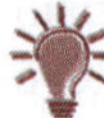

BOOST YOUR KNOWLEDGE

The predominant symptom of patients with uncomplicated peptic ulcer disease is epigastric pain. Pain typically is associated with hunger, occurs at night, and is often relieved by food and antacids. This typical pattern is usually present in adults and can be found in older children.

REFERENCE/SOURCE

- Kliegman R, Stanton B, St Geme JW, Schor NF, Behrman RE. Nelson Textbook of Pediatrics, 20th edition. Philadelphia: Elsevier; 2016. Chapter 335.

7. Which of the following is the right approach for management of *H. pylori* in children?

A. All children with pain abdomen should be actively investigated for *H. pylori*
B. Children with asymptomatic *H. pylori* infection should be treated
C. *H. pylori* can cause pain abdomen even without any inflammation or peptic ulcer disease
D. Test and treat strategy should be avoided

EXPLANATION

Diagnostic investigation for *H. pylori* in children is justified only in cases in which the expected benefits outweigh the costs and risks of testing and subsequent treatment. As per the recent evidence, *H. pylori* eradication treatment does not improve symptoms if they are not due to peptic ulcer disease. Therefore, if peptic lesions are not clinically suspected or identified by endoscopy, invasive diagnostic testing for the sole purpose of detecting *H. pylori* infection should not be undertaken. The goal of clinical investigation is to detect the cause of the child's symptoms. Since current evidence indicates that *H. pylori* infection does not cause symptoms in the absence of peptic ulcer disease (PUD), performing a noninvasive test to detect infection and treat if the test is positive is not warranted.

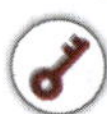

Key: D

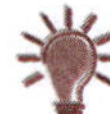

BOOST YOUR KNOWLEDGE

The primary aim of evaluation of a child with pain abdomen is to find underlying cause. Functional pain abdomen (FAP) is much more common than any other organic etiology. FAP is a diagnosis of exclusion but does not warrant extensive tests to rule out all possible causes. Investigations should be targeted and decided as per the detailed history and examination.

REFERENCE/SOURCE

- Jones NL, Koletzko S, Goodman K, Bontems P, Cadranel S, Casswall T, et al. Joint ESPGHAN/NASPGHAN Guidelines for the Management of *Helicobacter pylori* in Children and Adolescents (Update 2016). J Pediatr Gastroenterol Nutr. 2017;64(6): 991-1003.

8. Which of the following is the investigation of choice for diagnosis of *H. pylori* infection in a 6-year-old child?

A. Fecal *H. pylori* antigen
B. Anti *H. pylori* antibody
C. Urea hydrogen breath test
D. Gastric biopsy histology and culture

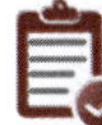

EXPLANATION

It is recommended that the initial diagnosis of *H. pylori* infection be performed using invasive gastric biopsy-based methods. The initial diagnosis of *H. pylori* infection should not be based on noninvasive tests. Urea hydrogen breath test and fecal antigen test can be utilized in follow-up to assess success of treatment. Antibody-based tests are not recommended either for diagnosis or follow-up in a clinical setting.

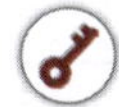

Key: D

BOOST YOUR KNOWLEDGE

The relief of symptoms is not an indicator of successful treatment of *H. pylori*. So, all children treated for *H. pylori* should be assessed for treatment success with a reliable test. Endoscopy and biopsy-based tests to confirm eradication are rarely needed in children with uncomplicated peptic ulcer disease. ^{13}C-urea breath test and fecal antigen testing can be utilized for assessment of success of therapy, but false-negative results can occur when medications are taken that decrease the bacterial load or suppress gastric acid. Therefore, testing for cure should be performed at least 4 weeks after completion of eradication therapy to avoid false negative results.

REFERENCE/SOURCE

- Jones NL, Koletzko S, Goodman K, Bontems P, Cadranel S, Casswall T, et al. Joint ESPGHAN/NASPGHAN Guidelines for the Management of *Helicobacter pylori* in Children and Adolescents (Update 2016). J Pediatr Gastroenterol Nutr. 2017;64(6):991-1003.

9. Which of the following grading systems is used for classification of peptic ulcer?

A. Los Angeles
B. Forrest
C. San Francisco
D. Rome

EXPLANATION

Forrest classification is used for classification of peptic ulcers as per the endoscopic finding. Los Angeles classification is used for extent of erosive reflux esophagitis. Rome criteria are for functional gastrointestinal disorders and not a grading system.

Forrest grade	*Endoscopic finding*
Ia Ib	• Active spurter • Active oozing
IIa IIb IIc	• Non-bleeding visible vessel • Adherent clot • Flat pigmented hematin on ulcer base
III	Clean-based ulcer

Key: B

BOOST YOUR KNOWLEDGE

Forrest classification of peptic ulcers is used as a tool to identify patients who are at an increased risk for bleeding, re-bleeding, and mortality. Grade I ulcers have higher chances of re-bleeding and mortality than grade II and III.

REFERENCE/SOURCE

- Feldman M, Friedman LS, Brandt LJ. Sleisenger and Fordtran's Gastrointestinal and Liver Disease, 10th edition. Saunders; 2015. Chapter 53.

10. Which of the following is true for *H. pylori* bacteria?

A. *H. pylori* can be cultured easily in an aerobic culture media
B. Rapid urease test is <60% sensitive and specific for *H. pylori*
C. Modified Giemsa and silver stains can be used for identification
D. *H. pylori* has multiple bipolar flagella

EXPLANATION

Helicobacter pylori are spiral bacteria with multiple unipolar flagella. They are difficult to culture as the organism is fastidious, slow growing and requires special media. Rapid urease test, which is performed from the biopsy sample, utilizes urease production from the bacteria. It has >90% sensitivity and specificity in detection for *H. pylori* from the gastric biopsy samples. Hematoxylin and eosin (H and E) stains can be utilized for identification of *H. pylori*, but modified Giemsa and silver stains improve detection rate significantly.

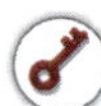

Key: C

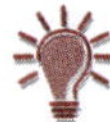

BOOST YOUR KNOWLEDGE

When culturing for *H. pylori*, tissue should be obtained before biopsy forceps become contaminated with formalin and then placed in a container with only a few drops of saline or appropriate media to preserve the specimen during transport. *H. pylori* is usually grown in jars with a standard microaerobic atmosphere, in CO_2 incubators or anaerobic chambers with a microaerobic atmosphere. Most studies with standardized atmospheres for culture of *H. pylori* use 2–5% O_2, 5–10% CO_2, and 0–10% H_2. *H. pylori* can grow on different solid media containing blood or blood products.

REFERENCES/SOURCES

- Andersen LP, Wadström T. Basic bacteriology and culture. In: Mobley HLT, Mendz GL, Hazell SL (Eds). *Helicobacter pylori*: physiology and Genetics. Washington (DC): ASM Press; 2001.
- Feldman M, Friedman LS, Brandt LJ. Sleisenger and Fordtran's Gastrointestinal and Liver Disease, 10th edition. Saunders; 2015. Chapter 51.

11. Which biopsy-based test is recommended for diagnosis of *H. pylori*?

A. Mandatory culture positivity
B. Rapid urease positivity
C. Histopathology showing *H. pylori*
D. Culture positivity or histopathology and urease positive

EXPLANATION

It is recommended that the initial diagnosis of *H. pylori* infection be performed using invasive gastric biopsy-based methods including the following:

- Positive bacterial culture OR
- *H. pylori* gastritis on histopathology with at least one other positive test such as rapid urease test, or molecular-based assays where available, including polymerase chain reaction, or fluorescent in situ hybridization.

The initial diagnosis of *H. pylori* infection should not be based on noninvasive tests (like urea breath test, *H. pylori* stool antigen test).

Culture positivity in isolation is enough for diagnosis but it is not mandatory and not easy to perform.

Key: D

BOOST YOUR KNOWLEDGE

Helicobacter pylori has a very high prevalence in the community. All noninvasive tests suggest presence or absence of *H. pylori* in the stomach with variable sensitivity and specificity. On the other hand, presence of *H. pylori* does not confirm causative association with the symptoms. Endoscopy and biopsy provide direct objective evidence of damage and inflammation in stomach and duodenal mucosa along with therapeutic utility in case of bleeding peptic ulcer.

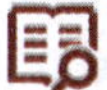

REFERENCE/SOURCE

- Jones NL, Koletzko S, Goodman K, Bontems P, Cadranel S, Casswall T, et al. Joint ESPGHAN/NASPGHAN Guidelines for the Management of *Helicobacter pylori* in Children and Adolescents (Update 2016). J Pediatr Gastroenterol Nutr. 2017;64(6): 991-1003.

12. An 8-year-old girl presented with history of pain abdomen for which she was given mefenamic acid. After 12 hours she had massive upper gastrointestinal (GI) bleed. Which of the following is an unlikely cause of upper GI bleed in this child?

A. Pancreatic rest of stomach
B. Peptic ulcer
C. Gastric varix
D. Dieulafoy lesion

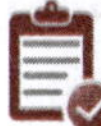

EXPLANATION

Peptic ulcer, gastric varix, and Dieulafoy lesion all can present with hematemesis and melena. NSAIDs (such as mefenamic acid) can increase chances of bleeding both in peptic ulcer disease and gastric varix. Dieulafoy lesion is an enlarged submucosal blood vessel that can lead to massive GI bleed even in absence of ulcer or erosion. Pancreatic rests are unlikely cause of GI bleed.

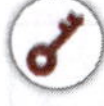

Key: A

BOOST YOUR KNOWLEDGE

Pancreatic rest is an ectopic pancreatic tissue which can present anywhere in GI tract but predominantly in stomach and proximal small bowel. It is an uncommon congenital anomaly defined as extrapancreatic tissue located far from the pancreas and without any connection via vascular or anatomical means. The pancreatic rests are usually asymptomatic.

REFERENCES/SOURCES

- Curfman K, Linders M, Poola A, O'Bryant L, Rashidi L. Pancreatic rest disguised as inflammatory bowel disease in young adult. J Surg Case Rep. 2022;2022(4):rjac153.
- Kliegman R, Stanton B, St Geme JW, Schor NF, Behrman RE. Nelson Textbook of Pediatrics, 20th edition. Philadelphia: Elsevier; 2016. Chapter 335.

13. Which of the following statements is *incorrect* about Zollinger–Ellison syndrome?

A. It can present like refractory peptic ulcer disease
B. Managed with 6–8 weeks of proton pump inhibitor (PPI) followed by tapering
C. Diarrhea can be a predominant symptom
D. More common in patients with multiple endocrine neoplasia

EXPLANATION

Zollinger–Ellison syndrome (ZES) is a rare syndrome characterized by refractory, severe peptic ulcer disease. There is gastric hypersecretion due to excessive production of gastrin by a neuroendocrine tumor, gastrinoma. It presents with peptic ulcer disease and diarrhea. The diagnosis is suspected by the presence of recurrent, multiple, or atypically located GI ulcers. ZES is commonly associated in patients with multiple endocrine neoplasia 1 and rarely with neurofibromatosis and tuberous sclerosis.

Proton pump inhibitors are an essential part of therapy and provide symptomatic relief. Patients with ZES may require long-term high dose of PPI until the tumor is removed surgically. Surgical intervention can be curative.

Key: B

BOOST YOUR KNOWLEDGE

First-line test to suspect ZES is fasting serum gastrin levels. Very high gastrin levels are suggestive of possible ZES. Other causes of hypergastrinemia are atrophic gastritis, proton pump inhibitors or H_2-receptor antagonist ingestion, *H. pylori* gastritis, chronic renal failure, and gastric outlet obstruction.

REFERENCE/SOURCE

- Kliegman R, Stanton B, St Geme JW, Schor NF, Behrman RE. Nelson Textbook of Pediatrics, 20th edition. Philadelphia: Elsevier; 2016. Chapter 335.

14. Which of the following is *incorrect* about *H. pylori* infection in children?

A. Prevalence of *H. pylori* in children can be >60% in developing countries
B. *H. pylori* is a common cause of recurrent pain abdomen in children
C. Treatment of *H. pylori* may require combination of multiple antibiotics in high doses
D. *H. pylori* is a Gram-negative, S-shaped rod that produces urease, catalase, and oxidase

EXPLANATION

Helicobacter pylori is a Gram-negative, S-shaped rod that produces urease, catalase, and oxidase. Prevalence of *H. pylori* is higher in developing countries as compared to developed nations. *H. pylori* can infect >80% of the population in developing countries and is acquired usually below 10 years of age. Treatment of *H. pylori* needs combination of antibiotics along with proton pump inhibitors. Combination of antibiotics and that too in high doses is required due to high antibiotic resistance.

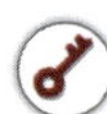

Key: B

BOOST YOUR KNOWLEDGE

Recurrent pain in abdomen in children is a very common condition in children and *H. pylori* should not be considered as the initial differential diagnosis. Although chronic gastritis is very common in children who harbor *H. pylori* but they usually remain asymptomatic.

REFERENCES/SOURCES

- Jones NL, Koletzko S, Goodman K, Bontems P, Cadranel S, Casswall T, et al. Joint ES-PGHAN/NASPGHAN Guidelines for the Management of *Helicobacter pylori* in Children and Adolescents (Update 2016). J Pediatr Gastroenterol Nutr. 2017;64(6):991-1003.
- Kliegman R, Stanton B, St Geme JW, Schor NF, Behrman RE. Nelson Textbook of Pediatrics, 20th edition. Philadelphia: Elsevier; 2016. Chapter 335.
- Poddar U, Yachha SK. *Helicobacter pylori* in children: an Indian perspective. Indian Pediatr. 2007;44(10):761-70.

15. Which of the following antibiotics is used for treatment of *H. pylori* in children?

A. Ciprofloxacin
B. Amoxicillin
C. Co-trimoxazole
D. Clindamycin

EXPLANATION

Amoxicillin, metronidazole, and clarithromycin are the primary antibiotics for treatment of *H. pylori*. Resistance to amoxicillin is very low while for metronidazole and clarithromycin it varies widely. Susceptibility testing is recommended before therapy. Resistance to amoxicillin is usually very low. There is high resistance to metronidazole and clarithromycin. If the strain is susceptible to clarithromycin and metronidazole both, triple therapy (PPI, amoxicillin, clarithromycin) for 14 days is the preferred choice. Antibiotics combination can be changed as per the regional resistance pattern.

Key: B

BOOST YOUR KNOWLEDGE

Standard dosing regimen for treatment of *H. pylori* in children is as follows:

Drug	*Body weight range*	*Morning dose (mg)*	*Evening dose (mg)*
PPI*	15–24 kg	20	20
	25–34 kg	30	30
	>35 kg	40	40
Amoxicillin	15–24 kg	500	500
	25–34 kg	750	750
	>35 kg	1000	1000
Clarithromycin	15–24 kg	250	250
	25–34 kg	500	250
	>35 kg	500	500
Metronidazole	15–24 kg	250	250
	25–34 kg	500	250[†]
	>35 kg	500	500
Bismuth[‡]	<10 years	262 QID	
	>10 years	524 QID	

*The doses of the different proton pump inhibitors are not equivalent. See comment on PPI in recommendation 14.
[†]If oral suspension of metronidazole is employed, the dose can be divided to be equal every 12 hours.
[‡]Bismuth in the United States and Canada comes as bismuth subsalicylate.
(PPI: proton pump inhibitor)

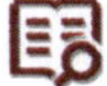

REFERENCE/SOURCE

- Jones NL, Koletzko S, Goodman K, Bontems P, Cadranel S, Casswall T, et al. Joint ESPGHAN/NASPGHAN Guidelines for the Management of *Helicobacter pylori* in Children and Adolescents (Update 2016). J Pediatr Gastroenterol Nutr. 2017;64(6):991-1003.

16. A 13-year-old boy presented with suspected peptic ulcer bleed. Which of the following is *true* about the management of this child?

A. Most acute peptic ulcer bleeds stop spontaneously
B. Proton pump inhibitors cannot control bleeding in most of the patients
C. Endoscopy should be performed immediately
D. Surgical intervention is required more frequently due to poor efficacy of medical management

EXPLANATION

The management of acute hemorrhage includes serial monitoring of pulse, blood pressure, and hematocrit to insure hemodynamic stability. Normal saline can be used to resuscitate a patient who has poor intravascular volume. Packed red blood cell transfusions may be required for significant anemia. A nasogastric tube should be placed to determine if the bleeding is continuing or has stopped. Most acute peptic ulcer bleeding stops spontaneously. All patients with suspected peptic ulcer bleed should be started on intravenous proton pump inhibitors. Intravenous proton pump inhibitors are very efficacious in controlling peptic ulcer bleed. With the availability of modern medical management, peptic ulcer disease requiring surgical treatment has become extremely rare.

Key: A

BOOST YOUR KNOWLEDGE

The indications for surgery are—uncontrolled bleeding, perforation, and obstruction. Surgical options are decided as per the indication. Surgical options for refractory peptic ulcers are vagotomy, antrectomy, and subtotal gastrectomy. Perforated peptic ulcer is managed with control of peritoneal contamination and closure of perforation. In the modern era of effective medical ulcer management, definitive ulcer surgery is rarely practiced.

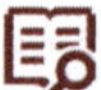

REFERENCE/SOURCE

- Kliegman R, Stanton B, St Geme JW, Schor NF, Behrman RE. Nelson Textbook of Pediatrics, 20th edition. Philadelphia: Elsevier; 2016. Chapter 335.

17. Which of the following contributes most to the mucosal defense of stomach?

A. Zinc
B. Histamine
C. Cyclic adenosine monophosphate (AMP)
D. Prostaglandin

EXPLANATION

The stomach has a high acidic milieu with pH of 1–2. A defense mechanism is required to avoid any damage to mucosa from the acidic contents. A continuous layer of mucous covers the stomach, which serves as a barrier to hydrogen ions and other chemicals. Mucus production and secretion are stimulated by prostaglandin E2. Underlying the mucous coat, the epithelium forms a second-line barrier, the characteristics of which are determined by the biology of the epithelial cells and their tight junctions. Secretion of bicarbonate into the mucous coat, which is regulated by prostaglandins, is important for neutralization of hydrogen ions.

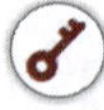

Key: D

BOOST YOUR KNOWLEDGE

A firmly adherent viscous mucus gel overlies the gastric surface. It is composed of 95% water and 5% extensively crosslinked mucin glycoproteins. Prostaglandin E2 (PGE2) analogs stimulate gastric bicarbonate secretion and blockade of endogenous PG synthesis reduces gastric bicarbonate secretion. Inhibition of PG synthesis is one of the important mechanisms through which NSAIDs cause peptic ulcers.

REFERENCE/SOURCE

- Kliegman R, Stanton B, St Geme JW, Schor NF, Behrman RE. Nelson Textbook of Pediatrics, 20th edition. Philadelphia: Elsevier; 2016. Chapter 335.

18. Which of the following is *true* about proton pump inhibitors (PPIs)?

A. Long-term use of proton pump inhibitors can cause pyridoxine deficiency
B. Half-life of PPIs is 30 minutes to 2 hours
C. PPIs work by temporarily binding and inhibiting H^+-K^+ ATPase enzyme complex
D. PPIs are strong bases

EXPLANATION

Proton pump inhibitors form a group of compounds called substituted benzimidazoles, which concentrate within the intracellular canaliculi of parietal cells. They irreversibly bind to the H^+-K^+ ATPase enzyme complex, and extensively inhibit acid production. PPIs are quickly absorbed (T_{max} = 1–3 hours), with variable bioavailability (omeprazole 35–65%, lansoprazole 80–91%, and pantoprazole 57–100%). They are rapidly metabolized (half-time = 0.6–2 hours). Chronic use of PPI can lead to osteopenia, chronic kidney disease and vitamin B_{12} deficiency. Although prolonged use of PPI in children is generally safe.

Key: B

BOOST YOUR KNOWLEDGE

Proton pump inhibitors are weak bases that concentrate in acidic spaces within the body that have a pH <4. Because of the same reason, concentration of PPIs in the secretory canaliculus is 100,000–1,000,000 times higher than in the blood.

The physiologic consequence of acid suppression by a PPI is hypergastrinemia. In the stomach, hypergastrinemia results in parietal and enterochromaffin cell hyperplasia, which persist for 2–3 months after stopping the PPI. And that may lead to rebound hypersecretion of acid.

REFERENCE/SOURCE

- Walker WA, Goulet OJ, Kleinman RE, Sherman PM, Shneider BL, Sanderson IR. Walker's Pediatric Gastrointestinal Diseases, 4th edition. BC Decker; 2004. Chapter 76.5.

19. An 11-year-old boy has a history of pain abdomen in epigastric region after eating food for last 3 days because of which oral intake has decreased. Before that child was normal. Which of the following is *unlikely* diagnosis?

A. Acute pancreatitis
B. Functional dyspepsia
C. Peptic ulcer disease
D. Acute gastritis

EXPLANATION

All the above etiologies can lead to epigastric pain after eating food. Acute pancreatitis, peptic ulcer disease, and acute gastritis all can present with short history. Functional dyspepsia is a diagnosis of exclusion and diagnosed when symptoms are present for a longer duration. If specific criteria are fulfilled and there are no other red flags, then diagnosis of functional dyspepsia can be made only on the basis of clinical history and examination. Pain or discomfort in functional dyspepsia is usually less severe and insidious in onset as compared to other organic etiologies.

Key: B

BOOST YOUR KNOWLEDGE

Diagnostic criteria for functional dyspepsia:

Must include one or more of the following bothersome symptoms at least 4 days per month:

- Postprandial fullness
- Early satiation
- Epigastric pain or burning not associated with defecation
- After appropriate evaluation, the symptoms cannot be fully explained by another medical condition.
- Criteria should be fulfilled for at least 2 months before diagnosis.

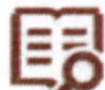

REFERENCE/SOURCE

- Hyams JS, Di Lorenzo C, Saps M, Shulman RJ, Staiano A, van Tilburg M. Functional disorders: children and adolescents. Gastroenterology. 2016:S0016-5085(16)00181-5.

CHAPTER

16.7 Acute and Persistent Diarrhea

Bishnupriya Sahoo

1. A 4-year-old male child presented to pediatric OPD with moderate-to-severe watery diarrhea along with pain abdomen for 2 days, associated with blood. On examination, he looked sick with features of severe dehydration. The child was diagnosed to have nephrotic syndrome 2 months back and is under treatment. Which of the following organisms is most likely to produce diarrhea in this child?

A. *Escherichia coli (E. coli)*
B. *Klebsiella*
C. *Clostridium difficile*
D. *Giardia lamblia*

EXPLANATION

Relevant information from mother is that her son had nephrotic syndrome and he is under treatment. This boy is probably on steroids for the last 2 months. Which indicates significant immune suppression. And the symptoms reveal he may be probably suffering from pseudomembranous colitis which is caused by *Clostridium difficile*. Though other organisms such as *E. coli*, *Klebsiella*, and *Giardia lamblia* may cause enteric infection in an immunocompromised host, but the given scenario would better fit with *Clostridium difficile*-associated pseudomembranous colitis.

Key: C

BOOST YOUR KNOWLEDGE

Pseudomembranous colitis is described as bloody diarrhea with accompanying fever, abdominal pain/cramps, nausea, and vomiting. The colonic mucosa contains 2–5 mm raised, yellowish plaques which can be visualized by sigmoidoscopy. Fatal cases are associated with toxic megacolon, systemic toxicity, and multisystemic involvement, sometime with organ failure, possibly related to systemic absorption of toxin. Symptoms of *Clostridium difficile* infection (CDI) generally begin <1 week after colonization and may develop during or weeks after antibiotic exposure. They are generally more severe in certain populations, including patients receiving chemotherapy prolong systemic steroid, patients with chronic gastrointestinal (GI) disease such as IBD (inflammatory bowel disease), and some patients with cystic fibrosis (CF). Other causes of pseudomembranous colitis include ischemia, verotoxin-producing *E. coli*, and drugs such as chlorpropamide, gold, linezolid, fluroquinolones, and nonsteroidal anti-inflammatory drugs (NSAIDs).

Treatment of severe/fulminant colitis: Vancomycin × 10 mg/kg/dose qid (maximum 500 mg qid) for 10 days PO or PR with or without Metronidazole × 10 mg/kg/dose (maximum 500 mg tid) tid for 10 days IV.

REFERENCES/SOURCES

- Ahmad OZ, Cohen MB. Chapter 239: *Clostridium difficile* infection (Table 239.1). In: Kliegman RM, St Geme III JW, Blum NJ, Shah SS, Tasker RC, Wilson KM (Eds). Nelson Textbook of Pediatrics, 21st edition. Elsevier; 2019. p. 6270.
- Kleinman RE, Goulet O-J, Mieli-Vergani G, Sanderson IR, Sherman PM, Shneider BL. Walker's Pediatric Gastrointestinal Disease: Physiology, Diagnosis, Management, 6th edition, Volume 1. USA: People's Medical Publishing House. Chapter 25.1: Drug induced bowel injury. pp. 2839-40.
- Kliegman RM, St Geme III JW. Nelson Textbook of Pediatrics, 21st edition. Elsevier; 2019. Chapter 366: Acute gastroenteritis in children. p. 2014.

2. Enteric infection caused by which of the following organism mimics appendicitis?

A. *Shigella sonnei*
B. Shiga toxin producing *E. coli* (*STEC*)
C. *Yersinia enterocolitica*
D. *Clostridium difficile*

EXPLANATION

Infections with *Yersinia* and sometimes with *Campylobacter* typically present with fever and abdominal pain. The abdominal pain is localized along with tenderness to the right lower quadrant of abdomen with or without diarrhea. It is called pseudoappendicitis; as there is no actual inflammation of the appendix (appendicitis), but mimics to it. Ultrasonogram and CT scan of abdomen may be helpful to distinguish between true appendicitis and pseudoappendicitis.

Key: C

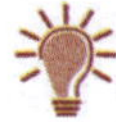

BOOST YOUR KNOWLEDGE

Clinical presentations suggestive of infectious diarrhea etiologies

Finding	***Likely pathogens***
Persistent or chronic diarrhea	*Cryptosporidium* spp., *Giardia lamblia, Cyclospora cayetanensis, Entamoeba histolytica (E. histolytica)*, nontyphoidal *Salmonella, Yersinia*, and *Campylobacter* spp.
Visible blood in stool	*STEC, Shigella, Salmonella, Campylobacter, Entamoeba histolytica*, noncholera *Vibrio parahaemolyticus, Yersinia, Balantidium coli*, and *Aeromonas*
Fever	Not highly discriminatory—viral, bacterial, and parasitic infections can cause fever. In general, higher temperatures are suggestive of bacterial etiology or *E. histolytica*. Patients infected with STEC usually are not febrile at time of presentation
Abdominal pain	STEC, *Salmonella, Shigella, Campylobacter, Yersinia*, noncholera *Vibrio* species, *Clostridium difficile*
Severe abdominal pain, often grossly bloody stools (occasionally non-bloody), and minimal or no fever	STEC, *Salmonella, Shigella, Campylobacter*, and *Yersinia enterocolitica*
Persistent abdominal pain and fever	*Y. enterocolitica and Y. pseudotuberculosis* may mimic appendicitis
Nausea and vomiting lasting ≤24 hours	Ingestion of *Staphylococcus aureus* enterotoxin or *Bacillus cereus* (short-incubation emetic syndrome)
Diarrhea and abdominal cramping lasting 1–2 days	Ingestion of *Clostridium perfringens* or *Bacillus cereus* (long-incubation emetic syndrome)
Vomiting and nonbloody diarrhea	Norovirus (low-grade fever usually present during the first 24 hours in 40% of infections); diarrhea usually lasts 2–3 days or less; other viral diarrheas (e.g., rotavirus, enteric adenovirus, sapovirus, astrovirus) usually last 3–8 days
Chronic watery diarrhea, often lasting a year or more	Brainerd diarrhea (epidemic secretory diarrhea, etiologic agent has not been identified); postinfectious irritable bowel syndrome

(STEC: Shiga toxin-producing *Escherichia coli*)

Source: Shane AL, Mody RK, Crump JA, Tarr PI, Steiner TS, Kotloff K, et al. 2017 Infectious Diseases Society for America clinical practice guidelines for the diagnosis and management of infectious diarrhea, Clin Infect Dis. 2017;65(12):e45-e80. (Table 3, p. e54).

REFERENCES/SOURCES

- Kliegman RM, St Geme III JW. Nelson Textbook of Pediatrics, 21st edition. Elsevier; 2019. Chapter 366: Acute gastroenteritis in children. p. 2026.
- Kotloff KL. Acute gastroenteritis in children (Table 366.10). In: Kliegman RM, St Geme III JW, Blum NJ, Shah SS, Tasker RC, Wilson KM (Eds). Nelson Textbook of Pediatrics, 21st edition. Elsevier; 2019. p. 8024.

3. Which of the following enteric virus infection usually causes prolonged diarrhea?

A. Rotavirus
B. Astrovirus
C. Norovirus
D. Adenovirus

EXPLANATION

In rotaviral diarrhea, the symptom resolution occurs by 7 days. Diarrheal illnesses caused by enteric adenovirus infections tend to be more prolonged than rotavirus (7–10 days), whereas astroviruses cause a shorter course ~5 days. For norovirus symptoms last for 1–3 days.

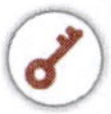

Key: D

BOOST YOUR KNOWLEDGE

Diarrhea can be classified into following categories on the basis of duration as:

- Acute diarrhea (remains for <7 days)
- Prolonged diarrhea (7–13 days)
- Persistent diarrhea (≥14 days)
- Chronic diarrhea (>4 weeks)

Most common viral etiology for acute diarrhea worldwide is Rotavirus. Due to extensive immunization coverage against Rotavirus, now Norovirus is emerging as the common cause of acute viral diarrhea in western countries.

Strains of Adenovirus that cause gastrointestinal manifestations are: 12, 18, 31, 40, 41, 52, 61. It spreads through feco-oral route and respiratory route. It is also known for nosocomial outbreaks.

REFERENCES/SOURCES

- Kotloff KL. Acute gastroenteritis in children (Chapter 366). In: Kliegman RM, St Geme III JW, Blum NJ, Shah SS, Tasker RC, Wilson KM (Eds). Nelson Textbook of Pediatrics, 21st edition. Elsevier; 2019. p. 8023.
- Weinberg JB, Williams JV. Adenoviruses (Chapter 289). In: Kliegman RM, St Geme III JW, Blum NJ, Shah SS, Tasker RC, Wilson KM (Eds). Nelson Textbook of Pediatrics, 21st edition. Elsevier; 2019. pp. 6997-7001.

4. A 6-year-old boy, otherwise healthy, presented with history of low-grade fever and watery stool and abdominal cramps for last 8 days. Mother also noticed blood and mucus in the stool. Clinical examination revealed no significant abnormality. There is no marked response after 3 days of oral cefixime. The stool routine examination showed the following finding. Identify the pathogen.

A. *Cryptosporidium*
B. *Cyclospora*
C. *E. histolytica*
D. *Giardia lamblia*

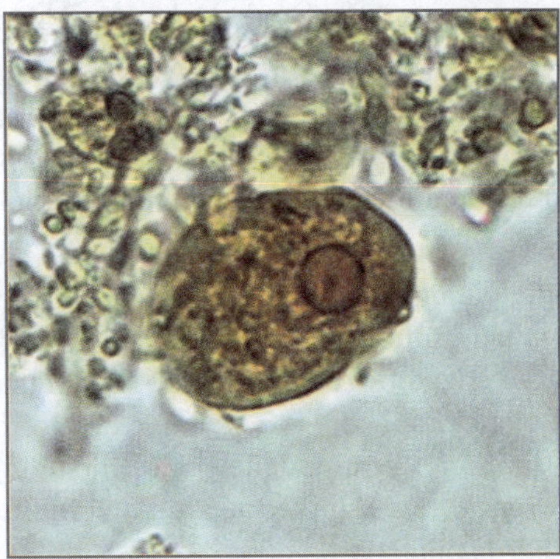

EXPLANATION

The above case explains a school-going child (6 years) where the degree of hygienic status might not be fully ensured. He is presented with prolong diarrhea (8 days). The stool is associated with blood and mucus, indicating dysentery. The child has no significant previous illness or immune deficient state. He is clinically fine. The illness has not improved with adequate antibiotics. The underlying pathogen is probably not a bacteria. As the stool contained blood, which indicates *Entamoeba histolytica* (*E. histolytica*) is the probable pathogen, as rest protozoa do not cause dysentery. Here, stool examination (wet mount stained) showed trophozoite state of *E. histolytica*.

Key: C

BOOST YOUR KNOWLEDGE

Entamoeba histolytica: Incubation period is 2–4 weeks. Gradual onset of cramps, watery diarrhea, and often dysentery but rarely fever. Duration of illness is variable with wax and wane; may be protracted (several weeks to several months). Chronic infection associated with weight loss. Infection with *Entamoeba* can cause severe ulcerating colitis, colonic dilation, and perforation.

The amebic liver abscess (ALA) is the most common extraintestinal manifestation of *Entamoeba histolytica* (*E. histolytica*) infection, more common in endemic areas. Amoebic trophozoites invade colonic mucosa and reach the liver through the portal circulation. Patients may not have an associated colitis. Fever, right upper quadrant pain, anorexia, and weight loss are often present. Laboratory evaluation typically reveals a leukocytosis without eosinophilia and increased alkaline phosphatase.

Ultrasonography or CT demonstrates the abscess. Most sensitive and specific among stool assays is polymerase chain reaction (PCR), followed by stool antigen detection, and least reliable is microscopy, because *E. histolytica* cannot easily be distinguished microscopically from its clinically benign relatives. Treatment involves 7–10 days of a nitroimidazole (most commonly metronidazole) to kill trophozoites, followed by 7 days of a luminal agent (such as paromomycin) to kill colonic cysts. Patients with large abscesses (≥5–7 cm in diameter) required percutaneous aspiration in addition to medical therapy.

Cryptosporidium: Cryptosporidium infection is associated with profuse, watery, nonbloody diarrhea that can be accompanied by diffuse crampy abdominal pain, nausea, vomiting, anorexia, and fever. Malabsorption, lactose intolerance, dehydration, weight loss, and malnutrition often occur in severe cases. Chronic diarrhea is common in individuals with immunodeficiency, such as congenital hypogammaglobulinemia or human immunodeficiency virus (HIV) infection.

Cyclospora: It infects both immunocompromised and immunocompetent individuals. Associated symptoms include anorexia; fatigue; abdominal bloating; abdominal cramps; nausea; muscle, joint, or body aches; low-grade fever; chills; headache, and weight loss. Vomiting may occur. Bloody stools are uncommon. Biliary disease has been reported. Travelers who harbor the organism almost always have diarrhea.

Infection is transmitted to humans through ingestion of fecally-contaminated food and water. Commonly seen in regions where there is poor sanitation and lack of access to clean water. After fecal excretion, the oocysts must sporulate outside the host to become infectious. This finding explains the lack of direct person-to-person transmission.

Giardia lamblia: Most symptomatic patients usually have acute diarrheal disease with or without low-grade fever, nausea, and anorexia. In a small proportion of cases may cause persistent or chronic diarrhea. It may cause more protracted course characterized by diarrhea, abdominal distention and cramps, bloating, malaise, flatulence, nausea, anorexia, and weight loss. There is no colonic involvement. It causes opportunistic infections in immunocompromised children (humoral immunodeficiencies, including common variable immunodeficiency selective immunoglobulin A deficiency and X-linked agammaglobulinemia), suggesting the importance of humoral immunity in controlling *Giardia* infection.

REFERENCES/SOURCES

- Flynn PM. *Cryptosporidium, Cystoisospora, Cyclospora,* and *Microsporidia* (Chapter 309). In: Kliegman RM, St Geme III JW, Blum NJ, Shah SS, Tasker RC, Wilson KM (Eds). Nelson Textbook of Pediatrics, 21st edition. Elsevier; 2019. pp. 7320-4.
- John CC. *Giardia duodenalis* (Chapter 308.1). In: Kliegman RM, St Geme III JW, Blum NJ, Shah SS, Tasker RC, Wilson KM (Eds). Nelson Textbook of Pediatrics, 21st edition. Elsevier; 2019. pp. 7309-16.
- Kotloff KL. Acute gastroenteritis in children (Chapter 366). In: Kliegman RM, St Geme III JW, Blum NJ, Shah SS, Tasker RC, Wilson KM (Eds). Nelson Textbook of Pediatrics, 21st edition. Elsevier; 2019. pp. 8002-3.

5. Which of the following is the best measure to assess the degree of dehydration in a child?

A. Urine output in last 24 hours
B. Skin turgidity
C. Percentage of body weight loss
D. Inspection of oral mucosa and tongue

EXPLANATION

Dehydration is the consequence of diarrhea, vomiting, and fever. It is a major risk for child health and the main reason for medical visit, hospitalization, and cause of death. Assessing dehydration in a reliable and rapid way is essential to prevent severe dehydration and its consequences and promptly start treatment.

In hospitalized children, although dehydration may also be considered, other parameters (such as respiratory distress, deep breathing, signs of shock, inability to drink, neurological signs, electrolyte abnormalities) may also be used as markers of severity.

However, the percentage of body weight lost is the best measure of dehydration. But in most circumstances, preillness weight is frequently not available to estimate weight loss during an episode of diarrhea. So, other clinically important parameters such as skin turgor, sunken eyes, general appearance, capillary refill time, and mucous membranes, urine output are included. But the reliability of the above signs may be reduced in malnourished children.

Key: C

BOOST YOUR KNOWLEDGE

Many guidelines divided patients into subgroups for mild (3–5%), moderate (6–9%), and severe (≥10%) dehydration basing on the percentage of body weight loss from the base line. However, it is difficult to distinguish between mild and moderate dehydration based on clinical signs alone. Therefore, most guidelines now combine mild and moderate dehydration and simply use none, some, and severe dehydration. The individual signs that best predict dehydration are prolonged capillary refill time >2 seconds, abnormal skin turgor, hyperpnea (deep, rapid breathing suggesting acidosis), dry mucous membranes, absent tears, and general appearance (including activity level and thirst). As the number of signs increases, so does the likelihood of dehydration. Tachycardia, altered level of consciousness, and cold extremities with or without hypotension suggest severe dehydration.

Clinical signs associated with dehydration

Symptom	*Minimal or no dehydration*	*Some dehydration*	*Severe dehydration*
Mental status	Well; alert	Normal, fatigued or restless, irritable	Apathetic, lethargic, unconscious
Thirst	Drinks normally; might refuse liquids	Thirsty; eager to drink	Drinks poorly; unable to drink severe cases
Quality of pulses	Normal	Normal to decreased	Weak, thready, or impalpable
Breathing	Normal	Normal; fast	Deep
Eyes	Normal	Slightly sunken	Deeply sunken
Tears	Present	Decreased	Absent

Contd...

Contd...

Symptom	*Minimal or no dehydration*	*Some dehydration*	*Severe dehydration*
Mouth and tongue	Moist	Dry	Parched
Skinfold	Instant recoil	Recoil in <2 seconds	Recoil in >2 seconds
Capillary refill	Normal	Prolonged	Prolonged; minimal
Extremities	Warm	Cool	Cold; mottled; cyanotic
Urine output	Normal to decreased	Decreased	Minimal

Sources:
- Modified from Duggan C, Santosham M, Glass RI. The management of acute diarrhea in children: oral rehydration, maintenance, and nutritional therapy. Centers for Disease Control and Prevention. MMWR Recomm Rep. 1992;41(RR-16):1-20.
- Modified from World Health Organization: The treatment of diarrhoea: a manual for physicians and other senior health workers, Geneva, 1995.
- Modified from World Health Organization; and Centers for Disease Control and Prevention: diagnosis and management of foodborne illnesses. MMWR 53(RR-4). 2004:1-33.

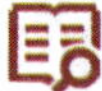

REFERENCES/SOURCES

- Guarino A, Lo Vecchio A, Dias JA, Berkley JA, Boey C, Bruzzese D, et al. Universal recommendations for the management of acute diarrhea in normal nourished children. J Pediatr Gastroenterol Nutr. 2018;67(5):586-93.
- Kotloff KL. Acute gastroenteritis in children (Chapter 366). In: Kliegman RM, St Geme III JW, Blum NJ, Shah SS, Tasker RC, Wilson KM (Eds). Nelson Textbook of Pediatrics, 21st edition. Elsevier; 2019. pp. 8022, 8031.

6. Which of the following findings in stool analysis is typical of secretory diarrhea?

A. Na^+ concentration is <70 mEq/L

B. Cl^- concentration is <35 mEq/L

C. Osmotic gap is <50 mOsm/kg

D. Stool pH is <5.5

EXPLANATION

Diarrhea can be categorized as osmotic or secretory depending on the underlying pathophysiological mechanism. It can be distinguished based on the stool electrolyte and osmolality analysis as follows:

Parameters	*Secretory*	*Osmotic*
Cl^- concentration	>40 mEq/L	<35 mEq/L
Na^+ concentration	>70 mEq/L	<70 mEq/L
Osmotic gap	<50 mOsm/kg	>135 mOsm/kg
pH	>6.0	<5.5
On fasting	No change in stool frequency	Stool frequency is decreased

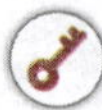

Key: C

BOOST YOUR KNOWLEDGE

Secretory diarrhea: It occurs when the intestinal epithelial cell solute transport system is in an active state of secretion. It is often caused by a secretagogue, such as cholera toxin, binding to a receptor on the surface epithelium of the bowel and thereby stimulating intracellular accumulation of cyclic adenosine monophosphate (c-AMP) or cyclic guanosine monophosphate (c-GMP). Some intraluminal fatty acids and bile salts cause the colonic mucosa to secrete through this mechanism. Diarrhea not associated with an exogenous secretagogue can also have a secretory component (congenital microvillus inclusion disease). Secretory diarrhea is usually of large volume and persists even with fasting. The stool osmolality is predominantly indicated by the electrolytes and the ion gap is <100 mOsm/kg.

Osmotic diarrhea: It occurs after ingestion of a poorly absorbed solute. The solute may be one that is normally not well absorbed (magnesium, phosphate, lactulose, or sorbitol) or one that is not well absorbed because of a disorder of the small bowel (lactose with lactase deficiency or glucose with rotavirus diarrhea). Unabsorbed carbohydrate is fermented in the colon, and short-chain fatty acids are produced. Although short chain fatty acids can be absorbed in the colon and used as an energy source, the net effect is an increase in the osmotic solute load. This form of diarrhea is usually of lesser volume than a secretory diarrhea and stops with fasting. The osmolality of the stool will not be explained by the electrolyte content, because another osmotic component is present and so the anion gap is >100 mOsm.

REFERENCE/SOURCE

- Kleinman RE, Goulet OJ, Mieli-Vergani G, Sanderson IR, Sherman PM, Shneider BL. Walker's Pediatric Gastrointestinal Disease: Physiology, Diagnosis, Management, 6th edition, Volume 1. USA: People's Medical Publishing House. Chapter 15(2b): Persistent and chronic diarrhea. p. 1106.

7. Which of the following statements is correct in context to acute inflammatory diarrhea?

A. Inflammatory diarrhea is due to enterotoxin or adherence/superficial invasion of pathogen
B. Most preferred site of involvement in inflammatory diarrhea is proximal small bowel
C. The nature of the stool is watery, profuse, and foul smelling
D. Stool analysis showed fecal polymorphonuclear leukocytes and increased lactoferrin

EXPLANATION

As per the etiopathological mechanism diarrhea can be classified as inflammatory, noninflammatory, and penetrating. Which can be followed as:

Pathophysiology	*Noninflammatory*	*Inflammatory*	*Penetrating*
Mechanism	Enterotoxin or adherence-mediated superficial invasion	Epithelial destruction (invasion, cytotoxin)	Penetrating
Location	Proximal small bowel	Colon	Distal small bowel
Illness	Watery diarrhea	Dysentery	Enteric fever
Stool examination	No fecal leukocytes, mild or no increase in lactoferrin	Fecal polymorphonuclear leukocytes ↑↑ lactoferrin	Fecal mononuclear leukocytes
Examples	• *Vibrio cholerae* • Enterotoxigenic *Escherichia coli (ETEC)* • *Clostridium perfringens* • *Bacillus cereus* • *Staphylococcus aureus* also *Giardia intestinalis* • Rotavirus Noroviruses • *Cryptosporidium* spp. • Enteropathogenic *Escherichia coli (EPEC)* • Enteroaggregative *Escherichia coli (EAEC)* • *Cyclospora*	• *Shigella* • *EIEC* • *STEC* • *NTS* • *Vibrio parahaemolyticus* • *Clostridium difficile* • *Campylobacter jejuni* • *Entamoeba histolytica*	• *Yersinia enterocolitica* • *Salmonella Typhi, Salmonella Paratyphi (S. Paratyphi)*, and occasionally *NTS, Campylobacter*, and *Yersinia*

Key: D

BOOST YOUR KNOWLEDGE

Special stool analysis and their implications:

Test	Normal values	Implication
α-1-antitripsin concentration	<0.9 mg/g	Increased intestinal permeability/protein loss
Steatocrit	• <2.5% (older than 2 years) • Fold increase over age-related values (below <2 years)	Fat malabsorption
Fecal reducing substances	Absent	Carbohydrate malabsorption
Elastase concentration	>200 µg/g	Pancreatic function
Chymotrypsin concentration	• >7.5 U/g • >375 U/24 hours	Pancreatic function
Fecal occult blood	Absent	Blood loss in the stools/inflammation
Fecal calprotectin concentration	<50 µg/g (older than 4 years)	Intestinal inflammation
Fecal leukocytes	<5/microscopic field	Colonic inflammation
Nitric oxide in rectal dialysate	<5 µM of NO_2^-/NO_3^-	Rectal inflammation

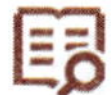

REFERENCES/SOURCES

- Kleinman RE, Goulet OJ, Mieli-Vergani G, Sanderson IR, Sherman PM, Shneider BL. Walker's Pediatric Gastrointestinal Disease: Physiology, Diagnosis, Management, 6th edition, Volume 1. USA: People's Medical Publishing House. Chapter 15(2b): Persistent and chronic diarrhea. p. 1103.
- Kotloff KL. Acute gastroenteritis in children (Chapter 366). In: Kliegman RM, St Geme III JW, Blum NJ, Shah SS, Tasker RC, Wilson KM (Eds). Nelson Textbook of Pediatrics, 21st edition. Elsevier; 2019. p. 8017.

8. A 4-year-old girl presented with complaints of fever and loose stool for 5 days. Initially stool was blood free but now associated with blood. She has vomiting and intermittent crampy abdominal pain and having puffy face with swollen limbs. On examination, the child looks sick, irritable, dehydrated, and pale. The abdominal examination was normal. Investigation showed leukocytosis with thrombocytopenia and deranged renal function. Identify the most important finding in peripheral smear in image below:

A. Acanthocytes
B. Schistocytes
C. Elliptocytes
D. Spherocytes

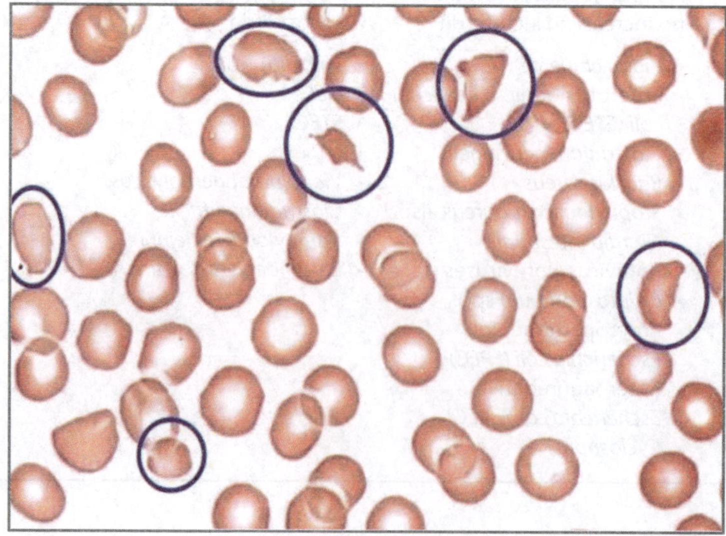

EXPLANATION

A 4-year-old female child presented with a short history of recent onset loose stool and vomiting. Suddenly, she developed bloody diarrhea along with generalized swelling and investigation showed deranged kidney function test, indicating renal involvement. This is pointing toward some complication resulting due to diarrhea which affects the kidney. Investigation also revealed leukocytosis which is told about the infective etiology probably of bacterial origin. The given image is a peripheral smear showing multiple fragmented red blood cells (RBCs) (blue circled) called schistocytes. If we combine all the above findings—it is a case of dysentery with complication, i.e., hemolytic uremic syndrome (HUS) which is a thrombotic microangiopathy (TMA) evidenced by thrombocytopenia and fragmented RBCs (schistocytes).

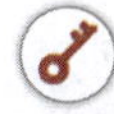

Key: B

BOOST YOUR KNOWLEDGE

Hemolytic uremic syndrome is the most dreaded complication of pediatric diarrhea and the leading cause of acquired renal failure in children, developing in 5–10% of patients infected with STEC. It is usually diagnosed 2–14 days after the onset of diarrhea. HUS is unlikely if there is no evidence of hemolysis. Risk factors include age 6 months–4 years, bloody diarrhea, fever, elevated leukocyte count, and treatment with antibiotics and antimotility agents. It is a common cause of community-acquired acute kidney injury in young children. It is the most common form of thrombotic microangiopathy (TMA) in children. Like all TMAs, HUS is characterized by the triad of microangiopathic hemolytic anemia, thrombocytopenia, and renal insufficiency. Mechanical injury to RBCs passing through the thrombotic microvasculature results in RBC breakdown and a severe nonimmune anemia with a negative direct Coombs test.

Diarrhea-associated HUS (D + HUS) mostly caused by Shiga toxin-producing *Escherichia coli* (STEC)—common in developed countries:

- STEC (*E. coli* O157:H7)
- STEC (*E. coli* 0121 and 0104:H4)

Non-STEC (*Shigella dysenteriae* type 1)—common in developing countries.

REFERENCES/SOURCES

- Kliegman RM, St Geme III JW. Nelson Textbook of Pediatrics, 21st edition. Elsevier; 2019. Chapter 366: Acute gastroenteritis in children.
- Kliegman RM, St Geme III JW. Nelson Textbook of Pediatrics, 21st edition. Elsevier; 2019. Chapter 538.5: Hemolytic-uremic syndrome.

9. A 7-month-old child was brought to pediatric OPD with history of 1 day of fever with vomiting one episode non-bilious not blood stained. It was followed by loose stools 4–5 episodes which were watery, greenish in color, and associated with mucus. On examination, he was alert and features of no dehydration. Which of the following is the most appropriate management.

A. Start oral rehydration therapy (ORT), oral antibiotics, zinc and send back to home
B. Start ORT, probiotics, zinc and send back to home
C. Start ORT, normal diet, zinc and send back home
D. Start ORT, probiotics, zinc and hospitalize for observation

EXPLANATION

The above case represents a case of acute gastroenteritis with no dehydration. It may be a case of rotaviral diarrhea as per the given clinical symptomatology. So, the appropriate management includes ORS and zinc as per the recommendations. As the infant has no features of dehydration, he can be sent back to home with proper explanation of the danger signs to the mother. Probiotics are not recommended routinely for acute diarrhea [World Health Organization (WHO)].

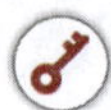

Key: C

BOOST YOUR KNOWLEDGE

Symptoms of rotavirus AGE usually begin with vomiting followed by frequent passage of watery nonbloody stools, associated with fever in about half the cases. The diarrhea lacks fecal leukocytes, but stools from 20% of cases contain mucus. Recovery with complete resolution of symptoms generally occurs within 7 days. Although disaccharide malabsorption is found in 10–20% of cases, it is rarely clinically significant. In routine, no investigations or treatment is required other than ORS and zinc.

REFERENCE/SOURCE

- Kliegman RM, St Geme III JW. Nelson Textbook of Pediatrics, 21st edition. Elsevier; 2019. Chapter 366: Acute gastroenteritis in children. pp. 2028-30.

10. An 18-month-old child with body weight of 12 kg was brought to emergency with complaints of loose stool for 3 weeks which was 4–5 times daily, stool volume was half to one cup per episode, not foul smelling, intermittently associated with blood. She had received oral antibiotics in OPD basis, but not relieved. On examination, she is thriving well and maintained hydration. But some pallor and perianal rash were noted. She is on predominant milk-based feeds. Stool analysis showed 8–10 RBCs and 5–7 pus cells and culture showed no growth of any organism. What is the first step of management?

A. Go for intravenous antibiotics
B. Stop all the milk and milk product from the diet
C. Go for low lactose or lactose free formula
D. Give albendazole and oral antibiotics

EXPLANATION

A well thriving 18 months old kid, who is predominantly on milk-based feeds, now having persistent diarrhea. It was associated with intermittent blood. Clinically, he had no dehydration but had pallor and perianal rash. Investigation showed RBCs and pus cells in the stool, but no organism was found in the stool culture. So, in the above case—first point, in spite of persistent diarrhea along with blood in the stool, the kid is not sick which indicate there might be some inflammatory condition which is not due to any infective pathology such as bacteria/protozoa or virus. Second point, the kid is on mostly milk-based diet. Third point, there was no response to antibiotics. So, considering the above points, the kid most probably has cow milk protein allergy (CMPA) or cow milk sensitive enteropathy (CMSE). Thus, for the diagnosis as well as for the treatment, we have to stop all the milk and milk products from his diet, as the first step in management.

For protozoal infestation, the kid does not have the features of malabsorption, undernutrition, and stool analysis does not show any cyst/ova/trophozoite.

Key: B

BOOST YOUR KNOWLEDGE

The best characterized syndrome is CMSE (cow milk sensitive enteropathy), classically presenting with chronic loose stools and failure to thrive. It begins with an episode of gastroenteritis in a formula-fed infant. Cow's milk β-lactoglobulin and casein are implicated in the development of CMSE.

Clinical features: Classic CMSE often demonstrates a period of good weight gain prior to the onset of symptoms, followed by abdominal distension, colic, gastroesophageal reflux, rectal bleeding, chronic loose stools, perianal erythema, or diaper rash (due to unabsorbed residual dietary carbohydrates), failure to thrive, eczema, and dermatographia. There may be evidence of micronutrient deficiency like iron and zinc.

Course: Classic CMSE is usually self-limiting, with most children tolerating reintroduction of milk or milk products at the age of 2–3 years. Some children may have persistent low-grade symptoms for a more prolonged period. A proportion of children (specifically IgE positive) manifests additional immediate reactions to food antigens, such as rash, urticaria, angioedema, or anaphylaxis. Others (non-IgE group) suffer enteropathy without immediate reactions, and it is important to recognize them, in the absence of systemic signs of food allergy. Here, skin prick tests and specific IgE are negative.

Overall, the prognosis of the child with CMSE appears good, and the great majority outgrow their sensitization by age 3 years, although other allergies subsequently develop in about half the cases. Up to 40% of infants with classic CMSE may later develop intolerance to soy.

REFERENCE/SOURCE

- Kleinman RE, Goulet OJ, Mieli-Vergani G, Sanderson IR, Sherman PM, Shneider BL. Walker's Pediatric Gastrointestinal Disease: Physiology, Diagnosis, Management, 6th edition, Volume 1. USA: People's Medical Publishing House. Chapter 16(2b): Food allergic enteropathy. pp. 509-17.

11. An 8-year-old male child is diagnosed as having acute lymphoblastic leukemia (ALL). He is undergoing chemotherapy for last 12 weeks. Now he developed fever, abdominal cramps, and loose stool for 1 week, associated with blood and mucus. On examination, he looks toxic and dehydrated. Stool PCR was positive for *Clostridium difficile*. What should be the treatment?

A. Starts IV ceftriaxone, amikacin, and metronidazole
B. Start oral vancomycin and metronidazole
C. Start IV vancomycin and metronidazole
D. Start IV fidaxomicin

EXPLANATION

An 8-year-old male child with background history of ALL on chemotherapy, all these points favor towards an immune-compromised state. He developed bloody and mucoid diarrhea with associated fever and abdominal cramps for 1 week. Physical examination revealed that he is very sick with dehydration and toxic look. So, all the above findings are well fitted to pseudomembranous colitis (severe form) which is evidenced by stool PCR positivity for *Clostridium difficile*. After hospitalization and all supportive measures the most preferred definitive therapy for this child is—first, hold the chemotherapy. Secondly, vancomycin PO 40 mg/kg/day divided qid × 10 days, maximum 500 mg/dose; OR, if ileus, give same dose PR as 500 mg/100 mL normal saline by retention enema with or without metronidazole IV 30 mg/kg/day divided tid × 10 days; maximum 500 mg/dose.

Fidaxomicin, a new antimicrobial agent which is recommended for adults, is yet to be approved for children.

Key: B

BOOST YOUR KNOWLEDGE

Clostridium difficile infections (CDI) are diagnosed by the detection of a *C. difficile* toxin in the stool of a symptomatic patient. Most patients present with a history of recent antibiotic use, but the absence of antibiotic exposure should not preclude this diagnosis in children. Conversely, high carriage rates without illness among infants should prompt careful consideration when testing and treating

Tests available for Clostridium difficile diagnosis:

- For toxin detection by enzyme immunoassay (EIA) both A and/or toxin B (most commonly done in laboratories)
- The real-time polymerase chain reaction (PCR) assay for toxin A/B (superior due to very high sensitivity)
- Nucleic acid amplification tests (NAATs) alone is not indicated to stamp the diagnosis.
- Culture for organism isolation is not specific because it does not differentiate between toxin-producing and nontoxin-producing strains (labor intensive, taking several days).

Recommendations for the treatment of *Clostridium difficile* infection in children

Clinical definition	*Recommended treatment*	*Pediatric dose*	*Maximum dose*	*Strength of recommendation/ quality of evidence*
Initial episode, nonsevere	Metronidazole × 10 days PO *or*	7.5 mg/kg/dose tid or qid	500 mg tid or qid	Weak/low
	Vancomycin × 10 days PO	10 mg/kg/dose qid	125 mg qid	Weak/low
Initial episode, severe/fulminant	Vancomycin × 10 days PO or PR *with or without*	10 mg/kg/dose qid	500 mg qid	Strong/moderate
	Metronidazole × 10 days IV*	10 mg/kg/dose tid	500 mg tid	Weak/low
First recurrence, nonsevere	Metronidazole × 10 days PO *or*	7.5 mg/kg/dose tid or qid	500 mg tid or qid	Weak/low
	Vancomycin × 10 days PO	10 mg/kg/dose qid	125 mg qid	Weak/low
Second or subsequent recurrence	Vancomycin in a tapered and pulsed regimen† *or*	10 mg/kg/dose qid	125 mg qid	Weak/low
	Vancomycin × 10 days, followed by rifaximin‡ × 20 days *or*	Vancomycin, 10 mg/kg/dose qid; rifaximin: no pediatric dosing	Vancomycin, 500 mg qid; rifaximin 400 mg tid	Weak/low
	Fecal microbiota transplantation			Weak/very low

*In cases of severe or fulminant *Clostridium difficile* infection associated with critical illness, consider addition of intravenous metronidazole to oral vancomycin.

†Tapered and pulsed regimen—vancomycin, 10 mg/kg with maximum of 125 mg 4 times daily for 10–14 days, then 10 mg/kg with maximum of 125 mg twice daily for 1 week, then 10 mg/kg with maximum of 125 mg once daily for 1 week, and then 10 mg/kg with maximum of 125 mg every 2 or 3 days for 2–8 weeks.

‡No pediatric dosing for rifaximin; not approved by the US Food and Drug Administration for use in children <12-year-old.

(IV: intravenously; PO: orally; PR: rectally; qid: four times daily; tid: three times daily)

Source: Adapted from McDonald LC, Gerding DN, Johnson S, Bakken JS, Carroll KC, Coffin SE, et al. Clinical practice guidelines for *Clostridium difficile* infection in adults and children 2017 update by the Infectious Diseases Society of America (IDSA) and Society for Healthcare Epidemiology of America (SHEA). Clin Infect Dis. 2018;66(7):e1-e48. (Table 2).

REFERENCE/SOURCE

- Kliegman RM, St Geme III JW. Nelson Textbook of Pediatrics, 21st edition. Elsevier; 2019. Chapter 366: Acute gastroenteritis in children (Table 366.14). p. 2031.

12. A 9-month-old male infant was brought to the emergency with complaints of excessive bilious vomiting along with bloody and mucoid scanty stools since evening. Mother was telling about the history of low-grade fever for 1 day along with loose stool 2 days back for which he was given some treatment from the local practitioner. On examination, the infant looked sick, dehydrated with abdominal distension. Urgent ultrasonography (USG) abdomen was carried out, which revealed the following (kindly refer the given image). What would be the next step of management?

A. Correct dehydration by oral or IV fluids, replace the ongoing loss, start IV antibiotics, and maintenance intravenous fluid (IVF)
B. Keep nil by mouth, start IVF and IV antibiotics, call for the pediatric surgeon
C. Keep nil by mouth, put a Ryle's tube, start IVF, and IV antibiotics, call for the pediatric surgeon
D. Call for the pediatric surgeon, urgently shift to OT for laparotomy

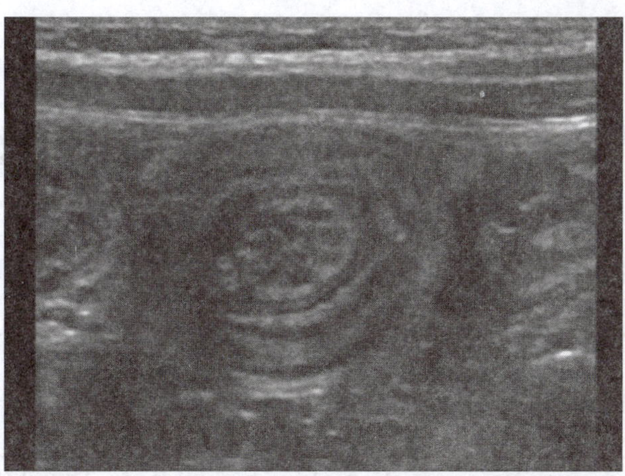

EXPLANATION

A 9-month-infant having an illness started as acute diarrhea and 2 days after it the kid was brought to emergency with excessive bilious vomiting and abdominal distension which may be suggestive of either paralytic ileus or small bowel obstruction. But the associated bloody and mucoid discharge per rectum, could not explain the paralytic ileus. Physical examination showed the kid was sick and dehydrated. USG revealed a transverse image of a target-shaped lesion in the abdomen which is multilayered and represents an intussusception. The bloody and mucoid discharge per rectum may be red currant jelly-like discharge which is seen in intussusception. So, the above case is an intussusception with intestinal obstruction. The appropriate management being keep nil by mouth, put a Ryle's tube, start IVF, and IV antibiotics, call for the pediatric surgeon. Initial management being the conservative step where enema reduction of the intussusception is done. If not resolved, then surgeon proceeds for laparotomy. Points to be noted that some surgical conditions can also present as acute diarrhea such as intussusception, acute appendicitis.

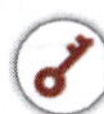

Key: C

BOOST YOUR KNOWLEDGE

Intussusception is one of the complications of enteric infection (viral AGE) that can be triggered by lymphoid hyperplasia of the gastrointestinal tract. A part of the intestine folds into the section next to it. Usually involves the small bowel and rarely the large bowel. It may be ileoileal or ileocolic. The part that prolapses into the other is called the intussusceptum. The part that receives it is called the intussuscipiens. Risk factors in children most often includes GI tract infections, cystic fibrosis, eosinophilic gastroenteritis, Meckel's diverticulum, and intestinal polyps.

Ultrasound is the test of choice for the diagnosis of intussusception. In the transverse image, the appearance of the target or doughnut sign, usually around 3 cm in diameter, confirms the diagnosis. In longitudinal imaging, intussusception may resemble a sandwich.

Intussusception requires rapid treatment. Treatment in children is typically by an enema (hydroreduction or pneumo-reduction) with barium, water-soluble, or an air-contrast enema, with success rate of 80%. If failed, then surgical reduction to be done.

REFERENCES/SOURCES

- Kleinman RE, Goulet OJ, Mieli-Vergani G, Sanderson IR, Sherman PM, Shneider BL. Walker's Pediatric Gastrointestinal Disease: Physiology, Diagnosis, Management, 6th edition, Volume 1. USA: People's Medical Publishing House. Chapter 15 (2a): Acute diarrhea. p. 1031.
- Kotloff KL. Acute gastroenteritis in children (Table 366.10). In: Kliegman RM, St Geme III JW, Blum NJ, Shah SS, Tasker RC, Wilson KM (Eds). Nelson Textbook of Pediatrics, 21st edition. Elsevier; 2019. p. 8024.

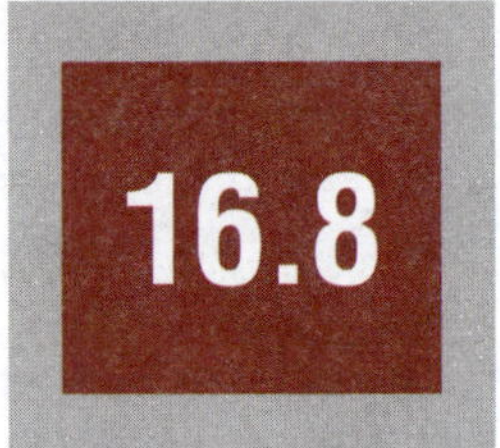

CHAPTER 16.8 Inflammatory Bowel Disease and Constipation

Shrish Bhatnagar

1. A 12-year-old boy is referred to you for evaluation of Crohn's disease. The child complained of fever, malaise, and easy fatigability and shows decreased growth velocity. Which of the following is most likely in this boy?

A. Puberty will be achieved on time
B. Final height will be achieved as per the genetic potential
C. There will be minimal extraintestinal symptoms such as oral aphthous ulcer, peripheral arthritis, and erythema nodosum
D. Perianal diseases, such as tag, fistula, and ulcer will be common

EXPLANATION

Systemic signs and symptoms are more common in Crohn's disease than in ulcerative colitis. Growth failure with delayed bone maturation with delayed sexual development is common in Crohn's disease as with ulcerative colitis. Sometimes growth failure is the only manifestation of Crohn's disease. Extraintestinal manifestations and perianal disease are seen in Crohn's disease.

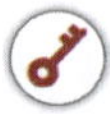

Key: D

BOOST YOUR KNOWLEDGE

Growth failure in Crohn's disease is caused by a variety of factors including insufficient calorie intake, inadequate absorption or overconsumption of nutrients, chronic inflammation of the bone system, alteration of appetite, and corticosteroid therapy. Perianal disease (tag, fistula, deep fissure, and abscess) is a common complication of Crohn's disease. Gastric involvement is also present with frequent vomiting and epigastric pain. Extraintestinal symptoms are more frequent in Crohn's disease including oral aphthous ulcers, peripheral arthritis, erythema nodosum, digital clubbing, episcleritis, kidney stones (uric acid and oxalate), and gallstones.

REFERENCE/SOURCE

- Stein RE, Baldassano RN. Inflammatory bowel disease. In: Kliegman RM, St Geme III JW, Blum NJ, Shah SS, Tasker RC, Wilson KM (Eds). Nelson Textbook of Pediatrics, 21st edition. Philadelphia: Elsevier Health Sciences; 2020. p. 1981.

2. A 14-year-old boy presents with the complaint of diarrhea, blood, mucus, and pus in the stools for the last 1 year. Double-contrast barium enema revealed small ulceration distributed uniformly about the colonic circumference and continuously from the rectum to the proximal transverse colon (as shown in given figure). Which of the following is true?

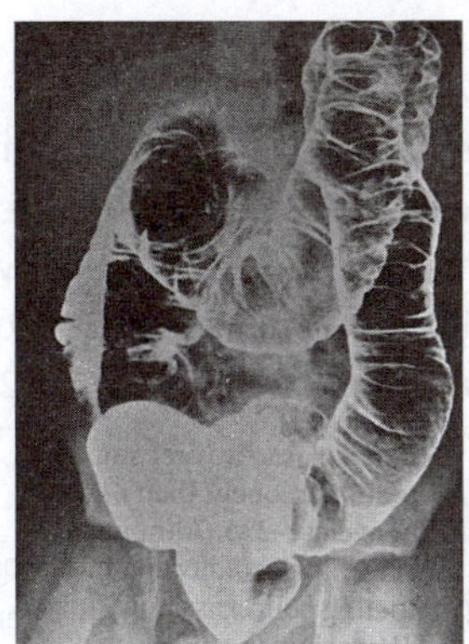

A. Strictures will be seen commonly
B. Discontinuous (skip) lesions will be seen
C. Toxic megacolon can be a complication
D. Transmural involvement will be seen

EXPLANATION

The child is having symptoms of ulcerative colitis in the form of colonic symptoms, supported by findings of double-contrast barium enema showing typical colon involvement with uniformly distributed small ulcerations. Strictures, discontinuous (skip) lesions, and transmural involvement are the classical features of Crohn's disease, while megacolon is a known complication of ulcerative colitis.

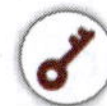

Key: C

BOOST YOUR KNOWLEDGE

Ulcerative colitis is an idiopathic chronic inflammatory disease. It is located in the colon and spares the upper gastrointestinal tract. Typical signs and symptoms include blood, mucus, and pus in the stool, as well as diarrhea. The important aspect of the diagnosis is the chronic nature of the disease. Symptoms that are >2–3 weeks old should be indicative of a differential of ulcerative colitis. The diagnosis must be confirmed through endoscopy and histology. Endoscopy shows the presence of micro ulcers. These micro ulcers give the impression of diffuse abnormality. Biopsy shows acute and chronic inflammation of the mucosa.

REFERENCE/SOURCE

- Stein RE, Baldassano RN. Inflammatory bowel disease. In: Kliegman RM, St Geme III JW, Blum NJ, Shah SS, Tasker RC, Wilson KM (Eds). Nelson Textbook of Pediatrics, 21st edition. Philadelphia: Elsevier Health Sciences; 2020. p. 1976.

3. A teenage boy is diagnosed with mild ulcerative colitis as per Montreal classification. He needs to be started on drug therapy. Which of the following is true regarding the drug therapy in this patient?

A. Aminosalicylate is the first drug class to be used in this child
B. Medication should be discontinued once the disorder is in remission
C. The dose of sulfasalazine is 10–20 mg/kg/24 hours given once a day
D. Sulfasalazine is a very well-tolerated drug with no side effects

EXPLANATION

Aminosalicylate is the first class of drug to be used in mild-to-moderate colitis. The dose of sulfasalazine is 30–100 mg/kg/24 hours (divided into 2–4 doses). Hypersensitivity to the sulfa component is the major side effect of sulfasalazine and occurs in 10–20% of patients. It is recommended that the medication be continued even when the disorder is in remission.

Key: A

BOOST YOUR KNOWLEDGE

Aminosalicylate is the first drug to be used in mild-to-moderate ulcerative colitis. Sulfasalazine is composed of a sulfur moiety linked to the active ingredient 5-aminosalicylic acid (5-ASA). This linkage prevents the premature absorption of the medication in the upper gastrointestinal tract, where the two components are separated by the bacterial cleavage. Because of the poor tolerance, sulfasalazine is used less commonly than other, better-tolerated 5-ASA preparations (mesalamine 50–100 mg/kg/day; balsalazide 2.25–6.75 g/day).

REFERENCE/SOURCE

- Stein RE, Baldassano RN. Inflammatory bowel disease. In: Kliegman RM, St Geme III JW, Blum NJ, Shah SS, Tasker RC, Wilson KM (Eds). Nelson Textbook of Pediatrics, 21st edition. Philadelphia: Elsevier Health Sciences; 2020. p. 1979.

4. A 15-year-old known patient of ulcerative colitis presents with three stools per day containing blood. There is absence of systemic symptoms. Inflammatory markers are within normal limits. What is the severity of the disease in this patient as per the Montreal classification?

A. S0 (remission)
B. S1 (mild)
C. S2 (moderate)
D. S3 (severe)

EXPLANATION

Out of four types of severity (S0, S1, S2, and S3), this patient lies in S1 (mild) severity in which there are four or fewer stools per day (with or without blood), absence of systemic symptoms, and normal inflammatory markers.

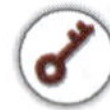

Key: B

BOOST YOUR KNOWLEDGE

Montreal classification of extent and severity of ulcerative colitis	
E1 (proctitis)	Inflammation limited to the rectum
E2 (left-sided; distal)	Inflammation limited to the splenic flexure
E3 (pancolitis)	Inflammation extends to the proximal splenic flexure
S0 (remission)	No symptoms
S1 (mild)	Four or less stools per day (with or without blood), absence of systemic symptoms, normal inflammatory markers
S2 (moderate)	Four stools per day, minimum signs of systemic symptoms
S3 (severe)	Six or more bloody stools per day, pulse rate of ≥90 beats/min, temperature ≥37.5°C (99.5°F), hemoglobin concentration <105 g/L, and erythrocyte sedimentation rate ≥30 mm/hour

(E: extent; S: severity)

REFERENCE/SOURCE

- Stein RE, Baldassano RN. Inflammatory bowel disease. In: Kliegman RM, St Geme III JW, Blum NJ, Shah SS, Tasker RC, Wilson KM (Eds). Nelson Textbook of Pediatrics, 21st edition. Philadelphia: Elsevier Health Sciences; 2020. p. 1976.

5. A 17-year-old girl is suffering from intractable ulcerative colitis and is unresponsive to medical management. She is planned for surgical management in the form of colectomy. What is true regarding this management?

A. Partial colectomy is the procedure of choice to preserve large bowel functions
B. The optimal approach is to combine colectomy with endorectal pull-through
C. Pouchitis is a rare complication (<5%) of colectomy with endorectal pull-through
D. No treatment is needed for pouchitis as it resolves spontaneously

EXPLANATION

Total colectomy is the surgical treatment for intractable or fulminant colitis. The optimal approach is to combine colectomy with an endorectal pull-through. The distal ileum is pulled down and sutured at the internal anus and a J-pouch is created. This procedure allows the child to maintain continence. The major complication of this operation is pouchitis, leading to bloody diarrhea, abdominal pain, and occasionally low-grade fever. Pouchitis is seen in 30–40% of patients with ulcerative colitis. It commonly responds to treatment with oral metronidazole or ciprofloxacin.

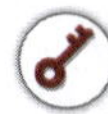

Key: B

BOOST YOUR KNOWLEDGE

A J-pouch is designed to maintain bowel continuity during a colectomy with an endorectal pull-through. A temporary ileostomy is typically performed to protect the small anastomosis between the pouch sleeve and the anus. This ileostomy is typically closed within a few months to restore bowel continuity.

REFERENCE/SOURCE

- Stein RE, Baldassano RN. Inflammatory bowel disease. In: Kliegman RM, St Geme III JW, Blum NJ, Shah SS, Tasker RC, Wilson KM (Eds). Nelson Textbook of Pediatrics, 21st edition. Philadelphia: Elsevier Health Sciences; 2020. p. 1980.

6. A child suffering from Crohn's disease is considered exclusive enteral nutrition therapy, as a primary mode of treatment. What is true regarding the enteral nutrition therapy in Crohn's disease?

A. Enteral nutrition therapy should be considered in those not responding to corticosteroids
B. Half of the calories should be given through formula, while half of the calories should be provided from daily food intake
C. These formulas are only given orally and they are well tolerated by the children
D. These formulas are relatively free of side effects and address nutritional rehabilitation

EXPLANATION

Exclusive enteral nutrition therapy is an effective primary as well as adjunctive treatment, whereby all of the patient's calories are delivered via formula. A novel approach is to give 80–90% of calories from formula, allowing children to have some food intake. These formulas are often administered via a nasogastric or gastrostomy infusion, usually overnight as these formulas are relatively unpalatable. These formulas are free of side effects, avoid problems associated with corticosteroid therapy, and simultaneously address nutritional rehabilitation.

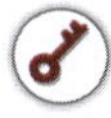

Key: D

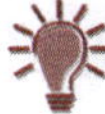

BOOST YOUR KNOWLEDGE

Although high-calorie oral supplements are effective, they are often not tolerated as they may cause premature hunger or worsen symptoms (such as abdominal pain, vomiting, or diarrhea). However, they should be given to children whose body weight gain is not optimal, even if they do not qualify for exclusive enteral nutrition therapy. Continuous oral nasogastric feeding for chronic malnourishment and growth failure has proven to be effective with much lower complication rates than parenterally hyperalimental feeding.

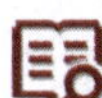

REFERENCE/SOURCE

- Stein RE, Baldassano RN. Inflammatory bowel disease. In: Kliegman RM, St Geme III JW, Blum NJ, Shah SS, Tasker RC, Wilson KM (Eds). Nelson Textbook of Pediatrics, 21st edition. Philadelphia: Elsevier Health Sciences; 2020. p. 1985.

7. A 5-year-old child is a known case of inflammatory bowel disease (IBD), having symptoms for the last 2 years, in the form of diarrhea, abdominal pain, vomiting, and growth failure. There is also a history of IBD in the elder brother of the child. What is the classification of the IBD as per the age of onset in this patient?

A. Pediatric onset
B. Early onset
C. Very early onset
D. Infant/toddler onset

EXPLANATION

Inflammatory bowel disease may be classified according to the age of onset: pediatric onset (<17 years), early onset (<10 years), very early onset (<6 years), infant/toddler onset (0–2 years), and neonatal-onset IBD (<28 days). This child is 5 years old with the age of onset of symptoms of 3 years, so the classification of the disease is very early onset (<6 years).

Key: C

BOOST YOUR KNOWLEDGE

Very early onset inflammatory bowel disease (VEO-IBD) makes up approximately 15% of all pediatric IBD and is estimated to affect 14 children out of 100,000 each year. Children with VEO-IBD have a higher chance of having a monogenic cause for their disease. VEO-IBD has a unique clinical phenotype with extensive colon involvement and a higher risk of a more aggressive disease course that is difficult to treat with conventional therapies. Most children with VEO-IBD will have isolated colorectal inflammation on ileocolonoscopy. However, this inflammation can be widespread and include the entire colon, making it difficult to distinguish between VEO-IBD and ulcerative colitis.

REFERENCE/SOURCE

- Stein RE, Baldassano RN. Inflammatory bowel disease. In: Kliegman RM, St Geme III JW, Blum NJ, Shah SS, Tasker RC, Wilson KM (Eds). Nelson Textbook of Pediatrics, 21st edition. Philadelphia: Elsevier Health Sciences; 2020. p. 1986.

8. A 15-year-old boy, with a known case of ulcerative colitis, presents with rectal bleeding, tenesmus, diarrhea, and abdominal cramping. There are no constitutional symptoms such as fatigue and fever. What is the extent of his disease as per the Montreal classification?

A. E0
B. E1
C. E2
D. E3

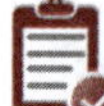

EXPLANATION

This patient lies in the E2 class of extent of the disease as per the Montreal classification. In E2 class, the inflammation is limited to splenic flexure. The symptoms are that of E1 class, such as rectal bleeding, urgency, tenesmus plus diarrhea, and abdominal cramping. There is no E0 class.

Montreal classification of extent and severity of ulcerative colitis	
E1 (proctitis)	Inflammation limited to the rectum
E2 (left-sided; distal)	Inflammation limited to the splenic flexure
E3 (pancolitis)	Inflammation extends to the proximal splenic flexure
S0 (remission)	No symptoms
S1 (mild)	Four or less stools per day (with or without blood), absence of systemic symptoms, normal inflammatory markers
S2 (moderate)	Four stools per day, minimum signs of systemic symptoms
S3 (severe)	Six or more bloody stools per day, pulse rate of ≥90 beats/min, temperature ≥37.5°C (99.5°F), hemoglobin concentration <105 g/L, and erythrocyte sedimentation rate ≥30 mm/h

(E: extent; S: severity)

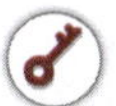

Key: C

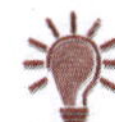

BOOST YOUR KNOWLEDGE

Montreal classification has three classes for the extent of the disease, i.e., E1, E2, and E3.

E1 (proctitis):

- 30–60% of patients
- Symptoms—rectal bleed, tenesmus, and urgency
- General treatment strategy—topical ± oral 5 ASA or steroid

E2 (left-sided colitis):

- 16–45% of patients
- Symptoms—E1 plus diarrhea and abdominal cramping
- General treatment strategy—oral ± topical 5-ASA or steroid, immunomodulators, biologics

E3 (extensive pan colitis):

- 15–35% of patients
- Symptoms—E2 plus constitutional symptoms (fatigue and fever)
- General treatment strategy—oral ± topical 5-ASA or steroid, immunomodulators, biologics

REFERENCE/SOURCE

- Stein RE, Baldassano RN. Inflammatory bowel disease. In: Kliegman RM, St Geme III JW, Blum NJ, Shah SS, Tasker RC, Wilson KM (Eds). Nelson Textbook of Pediatrics, 21st edition. Philadelphia: Elsevier Health Sciences; 2020. p. 1976.

9. The concerned parents want to know about the risk of their 2-year-old child having ulcerative colitis, as the father and 10 years old elder brother of the child suffer from ulcerative colitis. While evaluating the genes associated with the risk of IBDs, which of the following gene appears to be associated with ulcerative colitis rather than Crohn's disease?

A. Interleukin-2 (IL-2)
B. Interleukin-10 (IL-10)
C. Nucleotide-binding oligomerization domain-containing protein 2 (NOD2)
D. Immunity-related GTPase M (IRGM)

EXPLANATION

Interleukin-2 is associated with ulcerative colitis, while IL-10, NOD2, and IRGM are associated with Crohn's disease.

Genes associated with inflammatory bowel disease and the most associated physiological functions and pathway

	Gene name	*Associated disease*	*Gene function and associated pathways*	*Physiological function*
IL-2	Interleukin-2	Ulcerative colitis	Cytokine involved in immune cell activation	T-cell regulation
IL-10	Interleukin-10	Crohn's disease	Anti-inflammatory cytokine, NF-κB inhibition, JAK-STAT regulation	Immune tolerance
NOD2	Nucleotide-binding oligomerization domain-containing protein 2	Crohn's disease	Bacterial recognition and response, NF-κB activation, autophagy and apoptosis	Innate mucosal defense
IRGM	Immunity-related GTPase M	Crohn's disease	Autophagy and apoptosis in cells infected with bacteria	Autophagy

(JAK-STAT: Janus kinase-signal transducer and activator of transcription; NF-κB: nuclear factor kappa B)

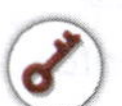

Key: A

BOOST YOUR KNOWLEDGE

Genetic factors play a significant role in the development of IBD as monozygotic twins will be affected more as compared to dizygotic. The concordance rate in twins is higher in Crohn's disease (36%) than in ulcerative colitis (16%). Genetic disorders that have been linked to IBD include Turner syndrome, Heřmanský–Pudlák syndrome, glycogen storage disease type Ib, and various immunodeficiency disorders.

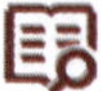

REFERENCE/SOURCE

- Stein RE, Baldassano RN. Inflammatory bowel disease. In: Kliegman RM, St Geme III JW, Blum NJ, Shah SS, Tasker RC, Wilson KM (Eds). Nelson Textbook of Pediatrics, 21st edition. Philadelphia: Elsevier Health Sciences; 2020. pp. 1973-4.

10. While evaluating a case of IBD clinically in a 14-year-old girl, which of the following symptoms will usually go against the diagnosis of Crohn's disease?

A. Perianal disease
B. Mouth ulceration
C. Abdominal mass
D. Pyoderma gangrenosum

EXPLANATION

Perianal disease, mouth ulceration, and abdominal mass are seen in Crohn's disease but pyoderma gangrenosum is a rare finding in Crohn's disease.

Key: D

BOOST YOUR KNOWLEDGE

Clinical, radiological, endoscopic, and histopathological difference between Crohn's disease and ulcerative colitis:

Feature	Crohn's disease	Ulcerative colitis
Rectal bleeding	Sometimes	Common
Diarrhea, mucus, and pus	Variable	Common
Abdominal pain	Common	Variable
Abdominal mass	Common	Not present
Growth failure	Common	Variable
Perianal disease	Common	Rare
Rectal involvement	Occasional	Universal
Pyoderma gangrenosum	Rare	Present
Erythema nodosum	Common	Less common
Mouth ulceration	Common	Rare
Thrombosis	Less common	Present
Colonic disease	50–70%	100%
Ileal disease	Common	None except backwash ileitis
Stomach: Esophageal disease	More common	Chronic gastritis can be seen
Strictures	Common	Rare
Fissures	Common	Rare
Fistulas	Common	Rare
Toxic megacolon	None	Present
Sclerosing cholangitis	Less common	Present
Risk for intestinal cancers	Increased	Greatly increased
Discontinuous (skip) lesions	Common	Not present

Contd...

Contd...

Feature	*Crohn's disease*	*Ulcerative colitis*
Transmural involvement	Common	Unusual
Crypt abscesses	Less common	Common
Granulomas	Common	None
Linear ulcerations	Uncommon	Common
Perinuclear antineutrophil cytoplasmic antibody—positive	<20%	70%

REFERENCE/SOURCE

- Stein RE, Baldassano RN. Inflammatory bowel disease. In: Kliegman RM, St Geme III JW, Blum NJ, Shah SS, Tasker RC, Wilson KM (Eds). Nelson Textbook of Pediatrics, 21st edition. Philadelphia: Elsevier Health Sciences; 2020. p. 1974.

11. A 4-year-old boy has been having complaints of difficulty in passing stools for the last 2 months with the frequency of two stools per week. Which of the following is the other criterion needed to diagnose constipation in this child?

A. Fecal incontinence ≥2 times per week after the acquisition of toileting skills
B. No significant finding per abdominal and digital rectal examination (DRE)
C. History of large-diameter stools but they are easily passed down the toilet
D. History of painful or hard bowel movements

EXPLANATION

Definition of constipation for use in Indian children:

- Duration of >4 weeks for all ages
- Presence of more than or equal to two of the following: (1) defecation frequency ≤2 times per week, (2) fecal incontinence ≥1 time per week after the acquisition of toileting skills, (3) history of excessive stool retention, (4) history of painful or hard bowel movements, (5) presence of a large mass in the rectum or on per abdomen examination, and (6) history of large-diameter stools that may obstruct the toilet (This may not be elicitable for the majority of Indian children who do not use the Western type of toilet).

In the above-given scenario, the child is having difficulty passing stools for >4 weeks. The defecation frequency is 2 per week. Out of the given options, a history of painful and hard bowel movements with the patient's complaint will define the presence of constipation in this patient.

Key: D

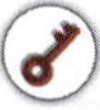

BOOST YOUR KNOWLEDGE

If inadequately treated, constipation can cause chronic abdominal pain, decreased appetite, and fecal incontinence. Additionally, it can lead to reduced self-esteem and social isolation.

REFERENCE/SOURCE

- Riyaz A, Matthai J. Gastrointestinal disorders. In: Gupta P, Menon PSN, Ramji S, Lodha R (Eds). PG Textbook of Pediatrics, 3rd edition. New Delhi: Jaypee Brothers Medical Publishers; 2022. p. 1321.
- Yachha SK, Srivastava A, Mohan N, Bharadia L, Sarma MS; Indian Society of Pediatric Gastroenterology, Hepatology and Nutrition Committee on Childhood Functional Constipation, and Pediatric Gastroenterology Subspecialty Chapter of Indian Academy of Pediatrics; et al. Management of Childhood Functional Constipation: Consensus Practice Guidelines of Indian Society of Pediatric Gastroenterology, Hepatology and Nutrition and Pediatric Gastroenterology Chapter of Indian Academy of Pediatrics. Indian Pediatr. 2018;55(10):885-92.

12. A 25-day-old newborn presents with the complaint of delayed passage of meconium (after 48 hours of birth), small-caliber stools, and failure to thrive. On examination, there is the presence of a palpable abdominal fecal mass; the anal sphincter is tight with an empty rectum on DRE. What should be the gold standard for the diagnosis in this child?

A. Contrast imaging
B. Rectal suction biopsy
C. Anorectal manometry
D. Colonic transit study

EXPLANATION

There is a history of delayed passage of meconium, small caliber stools, failure to thrive, and physical examination suggestive of per abdominal fecal mass and empty rectal. This is a case of Hirschsprung disease (HD). The rectal suction biopsy is the gold standard investigation of choice for this patient. The aganglionic segment is recognized by the absence of ganglion cells in the submucosa and the presence of hyperplastic nerve trunk.

Key: B

BOOST YOUR KNOWLEDGE

Imaging like X-ray should only be used in cases where the clinical examination is not reliable to exclude abdominal fecal impaction. In the cases of suspected HD, barium enema will show a transition zone that separates a dilated, stool-filled normally innervated ganglionic segment from an empty abnormal aganglionic bowel segment. Anorectal manometry helps in diagnosing abnormality of defecation by detecting the functional abnormality of the internal anal sphincter in diseases, such as HD, internal sphincter achalasia, and pelvic dyssynergia. In colonic transit study, radiopaque markers can be used to demonstrate dysfunctional (pan or segmental) colonic motility. It is a precise tool for the evaluation of colonic motor function and helps in differentiating myopathy from neuropathic causes.

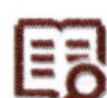

REFERENCE/SOURCE

- Riyaz A, Matthai J. Gastrointestinal disorders. In: Gupta P, Menon PSN, Ramji S, Lodha R (Eds). PG Textbook of Pediatrics, 3rd edition. New Delhi: Jaypee Brothers Medical Publishers; 2022. p. 1321.

13. While evaluating a case of functional constipation in a child of 12 months of age, faulty dietary practice appeared to be the factor leading to constipation. Which of the following history would indicate a faulty dietary practice leading to constipation?

A. Exclusive breastfeeding till 6 months of age
B. Vitamin D supplementation
C. Introduction of semisolid diet after 10 months of age
D. Combination of home-cooked semisolid food and breast milk

EXPLANATION

The introduction of a semisolid diet should not be delayed beyond 6 months. It should be readily available, culturally appropriate, affordable, hygienic, and home-cooked food of semisolid, porridge-like consistency. It should be given as complementary feed along with breast milk. Vitamin D supplementation does not lead to constipation.

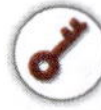

Key: C

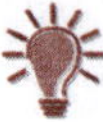

BOOST YOUR KNOWLEDGE

Exclusive and prolonged milk consumption with little or no solids in young babies is one of the primary causes of functional constipation. These babies are at a higher risk for iron deficiency anemia. During the assessment of a child with functional constipation, information such as consumption of fruits and vegetables, refined foods (such as bakery products), beverages in older children, the nature of the feeds (breast vs. top feeds), and the details of supplementary feeds in younger babies should be taken into consideration.

REFERENCE/SOURCE

- Yachha SK, Srivastava A, Mohan N, Bharadia L, Sarma MS; Indian Society of Pediatric Gastroenterology, Hepatology and Nutrition Committee on Childhood Functional Constipation, and Pediatric Gastroenterology Subspecialty Chapter of Indian Academy of Pediatrics; et al. Management of Childhood Functional Constipation: Consensus Practice Guidelines of Indian Society of Pediatric Gastroenterology, Hepatology and Nutrition and Pediatric Gastroenterology Chapter of Indian Academy of Pediatrics. Indian Pediatr. 2018;55(10):885-92.

14. While evaluating an 11-month-old child for constipation, some red flags signs, such as the history of delayed passage of stool, fever, recurrent pneumonia, and failure to thrive were seen. The patient had a history of hospital admissions due to severe pneumonia, three times in the past. Which of the following organic cause seems to be most appropriate according to the history provided?

A. Cystic fibrosis
B. Celiac disease
C. Cow milk protein intolerance
D. Hirschsprung disease

EXPLANATION

Cystic fibrosis patients have a history of delayed passage of stool, failure to thrive, fever, and recurrent pneumonia. Though fever and failure to thrive can be nonspecific, our patient had a significant history of repeated past hospitalization due to severe pneumonia which indicates the possibility of cystic fibrosis. Celiac disease will have chronic and recurrent diarrhea. Cow milk protein allergy will have diarrhea, failure to thrive, and occult blood positivity. The HD will have small caliber stools and no history of recurrent pneumonia.

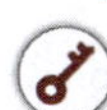

Key: A

BOOST YOUR KNOWLEDGE

Red flag signs indicating organic causes of constipation:

Clinical features	***Diseases***
Delayed passage of meconium (after 48 hours after birth), small-caliber stools, failure to thrive, tight anal sphincter, empty rectum with palpable abdominal fecal mass, gush of air, and liquid stool may follow withdrawal of the examining finger	Hirschsprung disease
Abdominal distension, bilious vomiting, and ileus	Pseudo-obstruction
• Decreased lower extremity tone and/or strength • Absence or delay in relaxation phase of lower extremity deep tendon reflexes, absence of anal wink and cremasteric reflex or presence of pilonidal dimple or hair tuft	Spinal cord abnormalities
Abnormal position or appearance of anus	Imperforate anus, anal stenosis, and anteriorly displaced anus
History of delayed passage of meconium, fatigue, cold intolerance, bradycardia, poor growth	Hypothyroidism
Polyuria and polydipsia	Diabetes insipidus
History of delayed passage of stool, failure to thrive, fever, and recurrent pneumonia	Cystic fibrosis
Chronic/recurrent diarrhea, pallor, and abdominal distension	Celiac disease
Diarrhea, failure to thrive, and occult blood positivity	Cow milk protein intolerance

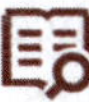

REFERENCE/SOURCE

- Riyaz A, Matthai J. Gastrointestinal disorders. In: Gupta P, Menon PSN, Ramji S, Lodha R (Eds). PG Textbook of Pediatrics, 3rd edition. New Delhi: Jaypee Brothers Medical Publishers; 2022. p. 1805.

15. A 10-year-old child is being treated with maintenance polyethylene glycol (PEG) for functional constipation. He needs to be evaluated for the response to the treatment. What is the cut-off duration after which you will label it as intractable constipation?

A. 1 month
B. 2 months
C. 3 months
D. 4 months

EXPLANATION

Constipation not responding to the optimal conventional management given for 3 months is called intractable constipation.

Key: C

BOOST YOUR KNOWLEDGE

Acute constipation: Constipation, which is of 4 weeks.

Chronic constipation: Constipation, which is of >4 weeks.

Fecal incontinence: It is defined as the involuntary passage of formed, semi-formed, or liquid stool in the child's underwear after achieving the age of continence. This may be a complication of chronic constipation. This is also called encopresis or soiling.

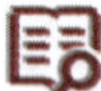

REFERENCE/SOURCE

- Riyaz A, Matthai J. Gastrointestinal disorders. In: Gupta P, Menon PSN, Ramji S, Lodha R (Eds). PG Textbook of Pediatrics, 3rd edition. New Delhi: Jaypee Brothers Medical Publishers; 2022. p. 1321.

16. You are prescribing oral laxatives for the treatment of constipation in a 9-year-old child; you wish to give osmotic laxatives as the first line of treatment. Which of the following is not an oral osmotic laxative?

A. Magnesium hydroxide
B. PEG 3350 with electrolytes
C. PEG 3350 without electrolytes
D. Sodium picosulfate

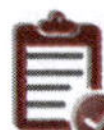

EXPLANATION

Sodium picosulfate is an oral stimulant laxative, while the rest of the others are osmotic laxatives. Lactulose is also an osmotic laxative, preferably given in acute constipation for a short duration.

Key: D

BOOST YOUR KNOWLEDGE

Osmotic laxatives are the mainstay of maintenance therapy in children. These laxatives draw water into the stool thereby making the stools softer and easy to pass. The two main osmotic laxatives are PEG and lactulose/lactitol. PEG is the first line of therapy and is more effective as compared to lactulose/lactitol. However, in children <1 year of age, the only drug recommended is lactulose/lactitol. In case of nonresponse or intolerance due to nonpalatability to PEG, the second line of treatment is lactulose/lactitol which is safe for all ages. Two osmotic agents such as PEG and lactulose/lactitol should not be given simultaneously. Combination therapy with two classes of laxatives is not recommended for children.

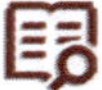

REFERENCE/SOURCE

- Yachha SK, Srivastava A, Mohan N, Bharadia L, Sarma MS; Indian Society of Pediatric Gastroenterology, Hepatology and Nutrition Committee on Childhood Functional Constipation, and Pediatric Gastroenterology Subspecialty Chapter of Indian Academy of Pediatrics; et al. Management of Childhood Functional Constipation: Consensus Practice Guidelines of Indian Society of Pediatric Gastroenterology, Hepatology and Nutrition and Pediatric Gastroenterology Chapter of Indian Academy of Pediatrics. Indian Pediatr. 2018;55(10):885-92.

17. An 18-month-old child is brought with the complaint of difficulty in passing stools for the last 2 months. A diagnosis of functional constipation was made after a detailed history and physical examination. History was suggestive of retentive posturing and toilet training from the age of 15 months. What should have been done to ensure proper toilet training and constipation?

A. Toilet training should not start before 24 months of age
B. Child should have been encouraged to go to the toilet whenever he had the urge to defecate
C. All family members should have contributed to the toilet training for a better response
D. Child should be allowed to sit whichever way they like to sit on the toilet

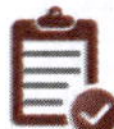

EXPLANATION

Toilet training should not be started before 24 months of age; however, there is a variation in recommended age of training between 3 and 4 years. This patient has a history of toilet training starting from 15 months which is too early and not recommended. Toilet training to be done by one person, one routine (5 minutes after each major meal), one place, one word, e.g., pooh/potty, etc. In a child with constipation, sit in a squatting position in the Indian toilet or with a footrest in the English toilet/potty seat to have appropriate angulation of knees and thighs to facilitate the expulsion of stools.

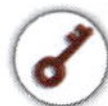

Key: A

BOOST YOUR KNOWLEDGE

In case of constipation in a child, (1) make the child sit in the toilet 2–3 times daily for a period of 5–10 minutes following a meal (within 30 minutes after eating); (2) provide painless defecation by treating any anal fissures that may be present; (3) have the child sit in a squatting position in an Indian toilet or with a footrest in an English toilet/potty seat so that the angulation of the knees and thighs is sufficient to facilitate the expulsion of stools; and (4) employ a positive reinforcement system to motivate the child and prevent parent-child conflict.

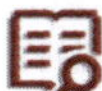

REFERENCE/SOURCE

- Yachha SK, Srivastava A, Mohan N, Bharadia L, Sarma MS; Indian Society of Pediatric Gastroenterology, Hepatology and Nutrition Committee on Childhood Functional Constipation, and Pediatric Gastroenterology Subspecialty Chapter of Indian Academy of Pediatrics; et al. Management of Childhood Functional Constipation: Consensus Practice Guidelines of Indian Society of Pediatric Gastroenterology, Hepatology and Nutrition and Pediatric Gastroenterology Chapter of Indian Academy of Pediatrics. Indian Pediatr. 2018;55(10):885-92.

18. A 12-year-old was evaluated for constipation. There were no red flag signs. History and physical examination were suggestive of functional constipation. Stool disimpaction was also needed with oral PEG. Maintenance PEG was started in adequate dose. There was no response to treatment despite compliance and with recurrence of impaction. What should be your next appropriate step in management?

A. Toilet training
B. Follow-up after 2 weeks
C. Increase the maintenance dose
D. Work-up for organic causes

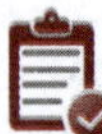

EXPLANATION

In this patient, stool disimpaction has been done and maintenance PEG which is the first-line treatment has been started in adequate doses. The patient has good compliance in follow-up. The next appropriate step of management should be the workup of organic causes and treatment accordingly.

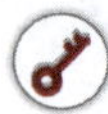

Key: D

BOOST YOUR KNOWLEDGE

Algorithm for evaluation of constipation:

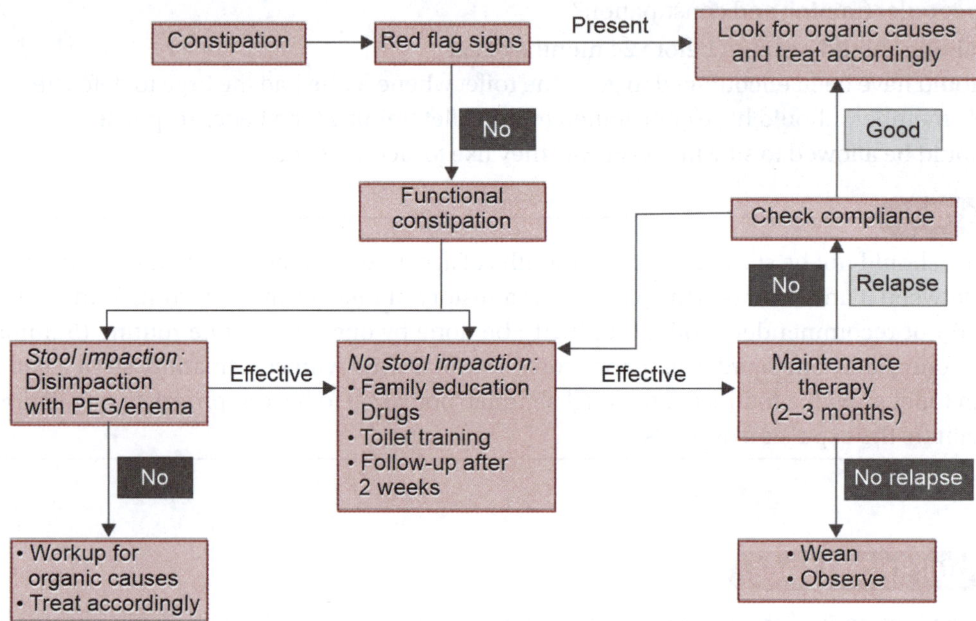

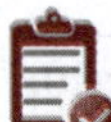

REFERENCE/SOURCE

- Riyaz A, Matthai J. Gastrointestinal disorders. In: Gupta P, Menon PSN, Ramji S, Lodha R (Eds). PG Textbook of Pediatrics, 3rd edition. New Delhi: Jaypee Brothers Medical Publishers; 2022. p. 1321.

19. While evaluating a 2-month-old, red flag signs such as a history of delayed passage of meconium and small caliber stools were noted. Physical examination is suggestive of fecal mass per abdomen. DRE revealed empty rectum and there was expulsion of stools after removal of the finger. What percentage of this disease contributes to the organic causes of constipation in young children?

A. 3% B. 6%
C. 9% D. 12%

EXPLANATION

Red flag signs such as the delayed passage of meconium, small caliber stools along with physical examination revealing fecal mass per abdomen and DRE indicating empty rectum suggest a clinical diagnosis of HD. It is the most common organic cause in young children accounting for 6% of all patients.

Key: B

BOOST YOUR KNOWLEDGE

Hirschsprung disease is the most common cause of lower intestinal obstruction in neonates, with an overall incidence of 1 in 5,000 live births. The male and female ratio for HD is 4:1 for short-segment disease and approximately 2:1 with total aganglionosis. The familial incidence of long-segment disease is higher.

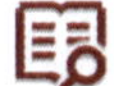

REFERENCES/SOURCES

- Kliegman RM, St Geme III JW, Blum NJ, Tasker RC, Wilson KM, Schuh AM, et al. Motility disorders and Hirschsprung disease. In: Kliegman RM, St Geme III JW, Blum NJ, Shah SS, Tasker RC, Wilson KM (Eds). Nelson Textbook of Pediatrics, 21st edition. Philadelphia: Elsevier Health Sciences; 2020. p. 1961.
- Riyaz A, Matthai J. Gastrointestinal disorders. In: Gupta P, Menon PSN, Ramji S, Lodha R (Eds). PG Textbook of Pediatrics, 3rd edition. New Delhi: Jaypee Brothers Medical Publishers; 2022. p. 1321.

20. An 8-month-old infant is being evaluated for constipation. There are no red flag signs and the patient is planned to be managed on the line of functional constipation in the form of parental counseling, dietary advice, and medical therapy. What medical maintenance therapy should be prescribed for this infant?

A. Polyethylene glycol
B. Lactulose/lactitol
C. A combination of PEG and lactulose/lactitol
D. A combination of PEG and sodium picosulfate

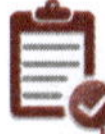

EXPLANATION

Polyethylene glycol is the first line of therapy and is more effective than lactulose/lactitol but in children <1 year of age, the only drug recommended is lactulose/lactitol. Two osmotic agents such as PEG and lactulose/lactitol should not be given in combination. Combination therapy with two classes of laxatives (osmotic—PEG and stimulant—sodium picosulfate) is not recommended for children. In case of nonresponse or intolerance due to nonpalatability to PEG, the second line of treatment is lactulose/lactitol which is safe for all ages.

Key: B

BOOST YOUR KNOWLEDGE

Stimulant laxatives are used only as rescue therapy (an acute or sudden episode of constipation while being on regular compliant maintenance therapy). Stimulants are given for a short duration of 2–3 days to overcome an acute episode of constipation and then stopped. Examples of stimulant laxatives are bisacodyl (oral and suppository), senna, and sodium picosulfate.

REFERENCES/SOURCES

- Riyaz A, Matthai J. Gastrointestinal disorders. In: Gupta P, Menon PSN, Ramji S, Lodha R (Eds). PG Textbook of Pediatrics, 3rd edition. New Delhi: Jaypee Brothers Medical Publishers; 2022. p. 1321.
- Yachha SK, Srivastava A, Mohan N, Bharadia L, Sarma MS; Indian Society of Pediatric Gastroenterology, Hepatology and Nutrition Committee on Childhood Functional Constipation, and Pediatric Gastroenterology Subspecialty Chapter of Indian Academy of Pediatrics; et al. Management of Childhood Functional Constipation: Consensus Practice Guidelines of Indian Society of Pediatric Gastroenterology, Hepatology and Nutrition and Pediatric Gastroenterology Chapter of Indian Academy of Pediatrics. Indian Pediatr. 2018;55(10):885-92.

CHAPTER

16.9 Celiac Disease

Rishi Bolia

1. A mother during an outpatient consultation for her 4-year-old child who was recently diagnosed with celiac disease (CeD) mentions that she is soon expecting another child. Is there anything that she can do differently to prevent the development of CeD in her next one. Which of the following is true?

A. Breastfeeding during gluten introduction reduces the risk of developing CeD
B. Early introduction (<4 months) of gluten sensitizes the body to it and reduces the overall likelihood of developing CeD
C. A normal vaginal delivery would reduce the risk of developing CeD
D. Infectious agents have been hypothesized to play a causative role

EXPLANATION

Neither breastfeeding during gluten introduction nor any breastfeeding has been shown to reduce the risk of CeD. The earlier introduction of gluten is associated with the earlier development of CeD autoimmunity (positive serology) and CeD, but the cumulative incidence of each in later childhood is not affected. It is advised to introduce gluten into the infant's diet anytime between 4 and 12 months of age. The mode of delivery, socioeconomic status, season of birth, and the use of drugs have been associated with the risk of developing CeD, but the evidence is contradictory. Infectious agents have been hypothesized to play a causative role as frequent rotavirus infections were shown to be associated with an increased risk of developing CeD. It is plausible that the contact with gliadin at a time when there is an ongoing intestinal inflammation alters intestinal permeability, and the enhanced antigen presentation can increase the risk of developing CeD.

Key: D

BOOST YOUR KNOWLEDGE

There are emerging data to suggest that the risk of developing celiac disease correlates with the amount of gluten intake in the early part of life. In a study it was found that the risk of developing CeD significantly increased if the child consumed >2 g/day of gluten at around 2 years of age. The source of gluten may also have a bearing on the risk of developing CeD.

REFERENCES/SOURCES

- Bolia R, Thapar N. Celiac disease in children: a 2023 update. Indian J Pediatr. 2024;91(5):481-9.
- Troncone R, Shamir R. Celiac disease. In: Kliegman RM, St Geme III JW, Blum NJ, Shah SS, Tasker RC, Wilson KM (Eds). Nelson Textbook of Pediatrics, 21st edition. Elsevier; 2019. pp. 1991-5.

2. A parent during a routine immunization appointment for their 6-week-old boy mentions that they have a strong family history of CeD and wonder if they should get some genetic testing done for their infant to ascertain whether he will go on to develop CeD or not. Which of the following statements is true?

A. The genes responsible for predisposing to CeD have not yet been conclusively identified
B. Most patients (~90–95%) carry a variant of human leukocyte antigen (HLA)-DQ8, whereas the remaining carry HLA-DQ2
C. A large proportion of patients who carry celiac genes will never develop CeD
D. There is no correlation between the risk of developing CeD and the number of copies of the *CeD* gene in an individual

EXPLANATION

Celiac disease occurs in genetically predisposed individuals who express certain specific HLAs [HLA-DQ2 (DQ2.5; DQA1*05/DQB1*02), and HLA-DQ8 (DQA1*03/DQB1*0302)] related to the DQ region. Most patients (~90–95%) carry a variant of HLA-DQ2, whereas the remaining carry HLA-DQ8. It is postulated that the "gene dose" has an effect on the clinical phenotype with those possessing a double dose of HLA-DQB1*02 more likely to have villous atrophy and classical manifestations of CeD. HLA-DQ2 or HLA-DQ8 is expressed in 30–35% of the populations, whereas CeD is prevalent with only ~2–5% of these carriers developing the disease. Thus, a large proportion of patients who carry these genes will never develop CeD.

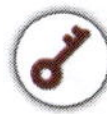

Key: C

BOOST YOUR KNOWLEDGE

Celiac disease has been found to have a 7.5% pooled prevalence among first-degree relatives. The risk varies in the first-degree relatives according to their relationship with the index patient with the highest prevalence reported in siblings.

REFERENCES/SOURCES

- Bolia R, Thapar N. Celiac disease in children: a 2023 update. Indian J Pediatr. 2024;91(5):481-9.
- Troncone R, Shamir R. Celiac disease. In: Kliegman RM, St Geme III JW, Blum NJ, Shah SS, Tasker RC, Wilson KM (Eds). Nelson Textbook of Pediatrics, 21st edition. Elsevier; 2019. pp. 1991-5.

3. A 10-year-old boy undergoing evaluation of chronic diarrhea is found to have elevated tissue transglutaminase (tTG) antibodies. He subsequently undergoes an upper endoscopy and duodenal biopsy which reveals normal intestinal histology. What is the term used to denote this finding?

A. Silent CeD
B. Potential CeD
C. Nonclassic CeD
D. Subclinical CeD

EXPLANATION

In 2013, a multidisciplinary task force of physicians proposed the "Oslo classification" of CeD providing uniform definitions for terms relating to CeD. Potential CeD refers to those with a normal small intestinal mucosa who are at increased risk of developing CeD as indicated by positive CeD serology. Potential CeD requires clinical and laboratory surveillance (serology, further biopsies) to monitor possible evolution to villous atrophy.

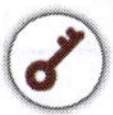

Key: B

BOOST YOUR KNOWLEDGE

When CeD presents without signs and symptoms of malabsorption it is called nonclassic CeD. In silent CeD, there is no apparent symptom in spite of histologic evidence of villous atrophy. Subclinical CeD is that which is below the threshold of clinical detection without signs or symptoms sufficient to trigger CeD testing in routine practice.

REFERENCES/SOURCES

- Bolia R, Thapar N. Celiac disease in children: a 2023 update. Indian J Pediatr. 2024;91(5):481-9.
- Troncone R, Shamir R. Celiac disease. In: Kliegman RM, St Geme III JW, Blum NJ, Shah SS, Tasker RC, Wilson KM (Eds). Nelson Textbook of Pediatrics, 21st edition. Elsevier; 2019. pp. 1991-5.

4. A pediatrician is evaluating a 7-year-old boy with diarrhea, loss of appetite, abdominal distention, and failure to thrive. He clinically suspects that the child may have CeD and decides to further evaluate for the same. What should be his first step?

A. Order antibody to tTG (IgA anti-tTG)
B. Order both IgA anti-tTG and total IgA levels
C. Order anti-endomysial IgA antibody (EMA)
D. Order both IgA anti-tTG and anti-EMA levels

EXPLANATION

Serological tests are the first screening tests performed when evaluating a patient for CeD. The preferred initial serologic test regardless of age for the detection of CeD is the IgA anti-tTG, which shows a sensitivity and specificity of around 97.7% and 70.2%, respectively. As the test is IgA based, children who are IgA deficient may have a false-negative tTG and so testing for total IgA levels should be done simultaneously.

Key: B

BOOST YOUR KNOWLEDGE

Endomysial IgA antibody has a higher specificity than tTG and is used as a confirmatory test in a second blood sample in cases where the tTG-IgA is ≥10 upper limit of normal (ULN).

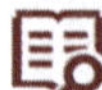

REFERENCES/SOURCES

- Bolia R, Thapar N. Celiac disease in children: a 2023 update. Indian J Pediatr. 2024;91(5):481-9.
- Troncone R, Shamir R. Celiac disease. In: Kliegman RM, St Geme III JW, Blum NJ, Shah SS, Tasker RC, Wilson KM (Eds). Nelson Textbook of Pediatrics, 21st edition. 2019. pp. 1991-5.

5. A pediatrician finds elevated tTG antibodies (tTG-IgA) in a 9-year-old boy with refractory constipation. The tTG-IgA level is 255 U/mL (normal <20 U/mL). The boy has normal growth parameters, and his complete blood count and iron studies are normal. What should be the next step of management?

A. CeD is unlikely and the child does not require any further testing
B. The anti-EMA should be checked
C. The child should be referred for an upper endoscopy and small bowel biopsies
D. Anti-deamidated gliadin peptide (DGP) IgA and IgG levels should be checked

EXPLANATION

Endomysial IgA antibody is used as a confirmatory test in a second blood sample in cases where the tTG-IgA is ≥10 ULN. Children who meet these criteria, i.e., a tTG-IgA of ≥10 ULN and a positive EMA, have a 99.75% positive predictive value (PPV) for CeD diagnosis and can be diagnosed without the need for duodenal biopsies.

Key: B

BOOST YOUR KNOWLEDGE

High values of tTG-IgA correlate with a greater degree of villous atrophy and a cut-off of ≥10 ULN has a >97% PPV for CeD diagnosis. However, a positive anti-tTG serology alone does not confirm the diagnosis of CeD as false-positive serologic tests may occur in several conditions including chronic liver disease, rheumatoid arthritis, inflammatory bowel disease, and other autoimmune diseases.

The addition of EMA to the algorithm decreases the probability of a false-positive diagnosis of CeD.

REFERENCES/SOURCES

- Bolia R, Thapar N. Celiac disease in children: a 2023 update. Indian J Pediatr. 2024;91(5):481-9.
- Troncone R, Shamir R. Celiac disease. In: Kliegman R, St Geme (III) JW. Nelson Textbook of Pediatrics, 21st edition. Elsevier; 2019. pp. 1991-5.

6. An 11-year-old girl with refractory iron deficiency anemia undergoes an upper endoscopy and small bowel biopsy for evaluation for suspected CeD. Which of the following findings on histopathology would suggest CeD?

A. Decrease in intraepithelial lymphocytes (IELs) and a villous to crypt ratio of >2

B. Decrease in IELs and a villous to crypt ratio of <2

C. Increased IELs and a villous to crypt ratio of >2

D. Increased IELs and a villous to crypt ratio of <2

EXPLANATION

The reading of biopsies should be performed on properly orientated biopsies using the modified Marsh-Oberhuber classification of villous abnormalities, which grades severity of villous atrophy based on two parameters, i.e., increase in IELs and reduced villous height to crypt depth ratio. A correctly orientated biopsy showing >25 IELs/100 epithelial cells and a villous to crypt ratio of <2 (Marsh Grade 2–3) indicates significant mucosal lesions.

Key: D

BOOST YOUR KNOWLEDGE

At least four biopsies from the distal duodenum and at least one from the duodenal bulb should be taken for histology assessment during a gluten-containing diet. In a meta-analysis of 11 pediatric studies, it was found that the addition of a duodenal bulb biopsy increased the diagnostic yield by 8%.

REFERENCES/SOURCES

- Bolia R, Thapar N. Celiac disease in children: a 2023 update. Indian J Pediatr. 2024;91(5):481-9.
- Troncone R, Shamir R. Celiac disease. In: Kliegman RM, St Geme III JW, Blum NJ, Shah SS, Tasker RC, Wilson KM (Eds). Nelson Textbook of Pediatrics, 21st edition. Elsevier; 2019. pp. 1991-5.

7. A physician is counseling a family with a child with newly diagnosed CeD. Which of the following statements is true?

A. Gluten is found in wheat, barley, maize, and rye

B. Oats are safe and can be consumed

C. A product is considered gluten-free if the gluten content is <200 parts per million

D. Continued exposure to even small amounts of gluten leads to persistence of the disease

EXPLANATION

Lifelong complete dietary avoidance of gluten is the cornerstone of the management of CeD. Gluten is found in wheat, barley, and rye. Oats do not contain gluten but often gets contaminated during milling. Patients and families need to be educated about sources of accidental contamination of gluten. Continued exposure to even small amounts of gluten leads to persistence of the disease.

All patients and their families should be encouraged to check labels of packaged foods, and only those labeled as "gluten-free" should be consumed. A product is considered gluten-free if the gluten content is <20 parts per million.

Key: D

BOOST YOUR KNOWLEDGE

IgA-TGA using the same assay as at diagnosis acts as a surrogate marker for healing of the small bowel mucosa and should be performed every 6 months until normalization and then every 12–24 months thereafter.

REFERENCES/SOURCES

- Bolia R, Thapar N. Celiac disease in children: a 2023 update. Indian J Pediatr. 2024;91(5):481-9.
- Troncone R, Shamir R. Celiac disease. In: Kliegman RM, St Geme III JW, Blum NJ, Shah SS, Tasker RC, Wilson KM (Eds). Nelson Textbook of Pediatrics, 21st edition. Elsevier; 2019. pp. 1991-5.

8. A 6-year-old girl is being evaluated for short stature. She is found to have elevated celiac antibodies [tTG-IgA -27 U/mL (normal <7 U/mL)]. What should be the next step?

A. This test confirms the diagnosis of CeD and she should be started on a gluten-free diet (GFD)
B. This mild elevation in tTG-IgA can be ignored and should be retested in 12 months
C. The child should undergo a gastroscopy and small bowel biopsies
D. The anti-EMA should be checked

EXPLANATION

All children who do not meet the serological diagnostic criteria for CeD (a tTG-IgA of ≥10 ULN and a positive EMA) should undergo a duodenal biopsy irrespective of the titers of the tTG antibodies.

Key: C

BOOST YOUR KNOWLEDGE

In recent times, it has been found that many patients of CeD present with nonclassical manifestations such as anemia unresponsive to oral iron therapy, osteoporosis, increase in transaminases, infertility, short stature, irritability, chronic fatigue, neuropathy, unexplained infertility, etc., and one should consider evaluating for CeD in all such situations.

REFERENCES/SOURCES

- Bolia R, Thapar N. Celiac disease in children: a 2023 update. Indian J Pediatr. 2024;91(5):481-9.
- Troncone R, Shamir R. Celiac disease. In: Kliegman RM, St Geme III JW, Blum NJ, Shah SS, Tasker RC, Wilson KM (Eds). Nelson Textbook of Pediatrics, 21st edition. Elsevier; 2019. pp. 1991-5.

9. A 6-year-old boy with type 1 diabetes is found to have elevated celiac antibodies on routine screening. The tTG-IgA level is 255 U/mL (normal <20 U/mL). The boy has normal growth parameters, and his complete blood count and iron studies are normal. What should be the next step?

A. Celiac disease is confirmed, and the child does not require any further testing
B. The anti-EMA should be checked
C. The child should be referred for an upper endoscopy and small bowel biopsies
D. Anti-DGP IgA and IgG levels should be checked

EXPLANATION

The "no-biopsy" criteria of CeD are not validated for children with type 1 diabetes mellitus (T1DM). Duodenal biopsies should be performed in all as a part of the diagnostic work-up. The only other condition where the no-biopsy approach is not validated is the cohort with IgA deficiency.

Key: C

BOOST YOUR KNOWLEDGE

Children with T1DM are at high risk for developing CeD. Other conditions which have a high risk include autoimmune conditions (such as thyroid diseases) or genetic disorders such as IgA deficiency, Down syndrome, Turner syndrome, and Williams-Beuren syndrome.

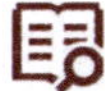

REFERENCES/SOURCES

- Bolia R, Thapar N. Celiac disease in children: a 2023 update. Indian J Pediatr. 2024;91(5):481-9.
- Troncone R, Shamir R. Celiac disease. In: Kliegman RM, St Geme III JW, Blum NJ, Shah SS, Tasker RC, Wilson KM (Eds). Nelson Textbook of Pediatrics, 21st edition. Elsevier; 2019. pp. 1991-5.

10. A 14-year-old boy with CeD is seen in clinic around 3 years after his initial diagnosis which was based on elevated celiac serology and duodenal biopsy demonstrating unequivocal subtotal villous atrophy. He currently has ongoing abdominal pain and diarrhea. He says he has been following his GFD strictly. On examination, his growth parameters are normal and abdominal examination is unremarkable. Blood test, including tTG antibodies, complete blood count, and iron studies, is normal. What should be the next step?

A. Referral to dietetics as the symptoms would likely be a result of ongoing noncompliance to GFD
B. The initial diagnosis was likely erroneous and needs to be revisited
C. An upper endoscopy and duodenal biopsies
D. Anti-EMA

EXPLANATION

The symptoms, signs, and laboratory abnormalities of CeD should resolve within 6–12 months of initiation of a GFD. Serologic titers fall soon after initiating a GFD. In those with persisting symptoms and/or lack of decreasing tTG levels 6–12 months after GFD initiation, the most common cause is ongoing advertent/inadvertent gluten exposure.

Causes of ongoing symptoms in those with normal tTG serology include irritable bowel syndrome, lactose intolerance, microscopic colitis, pancreatic insufficiency, and bacterial overgrowth. A small subset of CeD patients are refractory to a GFD with persistent malabsorption and intestinal villous atrophy, which is called refractory celiac disease (RCD). While tTG antibodies are usually positive at the initial diagnosis of CeD, most patients have negative antibodies at the time of RCD diagnosis reflecting strict adherence to GFD. A small bowel biopsy is indicated to differentiate between RCD and other causes of ongoing symptoms in a child with a normal tTG.

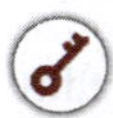

Key: C

BOOST YOUR KNOWLEDGE

Even though the above child was compliant to GFD, compliance is an issue and is the most common cause of ongoing symptoms with studies showing that up to 25% of the celiac patients are likely to transgress from their diet. Adherence is lower in those who were initially asymptomatic or diagnosed at an older age.

REFERENCE/SOURCE

- Troncone R, Shamir R. Celiac disease. In: Kliegman RM, St Geme III JW, Blum NJ, Shah SS, Tasker RC, Wilson KM (Eds). Nelson Textbook of Pediatrics, 21st edition. Elsevier; 2019. pp. 1991-5.

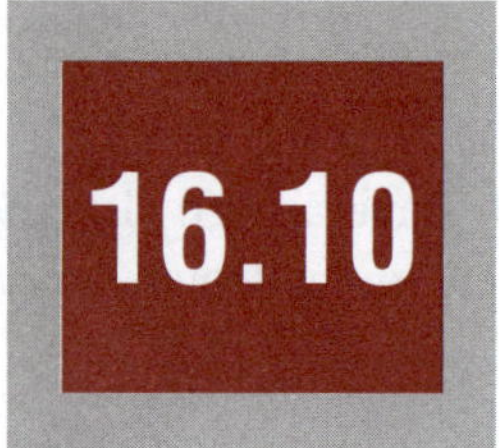

Chapter 16.10 Malabsorption Disorders

Aathira Ravindranath

1. A 12-year-old known case of chronic pancreatitis presented with bulky, foul smelling, difficult to flush, and greasy stools. Which of the following tests would you order?

A. Fecal calprotectin
B. Fecal elastase
C. Fecal occult blood
D. Fecal tryptase

EXPLANATION

The clue in the question is the background of chronic pancreatitis. Description of the stools is suggestive of steatorrhea which indicates pancreatic exocrine insufficiency. Hence, the test needs to determine either fat malabsorption or pancreatic insufficiency.

A. *Fecal calprotectin* is elevated in inflammatory conditions of the intestine like inflammatory bowel disease. Calprotectin is mainly found in neutrophils and elevated fecal calprotectin is a consequence of neutrophil migration into the gastrointestinal tract.
B. *Fecal elastase* is a protease produced by the pancreatic acinar cells. It is stable and unaffected by pancreatic enzyme supplementation.
C. *Fecal occult blood* test is performed to assess microscopic blood loss in stools in those with iron deficiency anemia.
D. *Tryptase* is produced by activated mast cells and can be elevated in allergic conditions.

Key: B

BOOST YOUR KNOWLEDGE

- *Other tests to detect fat malabsorption are* 72-hour fecal fat estimation, acid steatocrit, and stools for fat globules.
- *Other tests for pancreatic exocrine insufficiency:* Fecal chymotrypsin and C^{14}/C^{13} triolein breath test after ingestion of triglyceride.

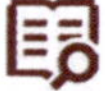

REFERENCE/SOURCE

- Feldman M, Friedman LS, Brandt LJ. Sleisenger and Fordtran's Gastrointestinal and Liver Disease, 10th edition. Philadelphia, PA: Elsevier Health Sciences; 2015. pp. 1804-5.

2. A 5-year-old child presented with loose stools for 4 months and increasing anasarca for 1 month. Investigations showed total protein—4g/dL, serum albumin—1.5 g/dL. Endoscopy showed "snow-flake" appearance of duodenal mucosa. What do you expect to see in the histopathology?

A. Absence of plasma cells
B. Dilated lacteals
C. Granulomatous duodenitis
D. Crypt hyperplasia

EXPLANATION

Loose stools with anasarca are a pointer toward either severe malabsorption or protein losing enteropathy. Investigation showing low total protein and albumin are clues to protein losing enteropathy. "Snow-flake" lesion in endoscopy is seen in intestinal lymphangiectasia. The classical histological finding is dilated lacteals.

- Granulomas in duodenum in the background of diarrhea are seen in Crohn's disease.
- Absence of plasma cells is in immunodeficient states like common variable immunodeficiency.
- Crypt hyperplasia is a finding in Marsh grade I of celiac disease, but the endoscopic finding would be that of scalloping of duodenal folds.

Key: B

BOOST YOUR KNOWLEDGE

Children with lymphangiectasia can also have calcium and vitamin D deficiency.

Treatment: Provide a diet low in long-chain triglyceride and high in medium-chain triglyceride (MTC). The diet should also be protein rich with calcium and vitamin supplements.

Medications: Subcutaneous octreotide and tranexamic acid.

Secondary causes of intestinal lymphangiectasia include lymphoma, tuberculosis, and retroperitoneal fibrosis.

REFERENCE/SOURCE

- Von der Weid PY. Lymphatic disorders. In: Kleinman RE, Goulet OJ, Mieli-Vergani G, Sanderson IR, Sherman PM, Shneider BL. Walker's Pediatric Gastrointestinal Disease: Physiology, Diagnosis, Management, 6th edition. USA: People's Medical Publishing House; 2018.

3. **A 3-year-old girl presented with small bowel diarrhea for 8 months, weight loss, and anemia. Initial possibility of celiac disease was considered. Which of these serological markers would you order for?**

A. Antitissue transglutaminase immunoglobulin M (IgM)
B. Antigliadin IgG
C. Antiendomysial antibody (anti-EMA) IgG
D. Antitissue transglutaminase IgA (anti-tTG IgA)

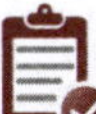

EXPLANATION

Antitissue transglutaminase IgA is the serological marker usually elevated >10 ULN in celiac disease. Anti-EMA IgA is also positive in celiac disease. Antigliadin antibodies have poor sensitivity in diagnosing celiac disease. In those with IgA deficiency IgG tTG or EMA can be used.

Key: D

BOOST YOUR KNOWLEDGE

In celiac disease, a typical duodenal biopsy would show villous atrophy, crypt hyperplasia and increase in intraepithelial lymphocytes (>20/hpf). HLA-DQ2/DQ8 will be positive in 95% of cases.

REFERENCE/SOURCE

- ESPGHAN. (2020). ESPGHAN guidelines 2020. [online] Available from https://espghan.info/ [Last accessed June, 2024].

4. **A 12-year-old girl presented with abdominal bloating, intermittent loose stools, and macrocytic anemia. Breath hydrogen test after oral lactulose was prescribed. What is the underlying condition suspected?**

A. Strongyloidiasis
B. Small intestinal bacterial overgrowth
C. Microscopic colitis
D. Functional dyspepsia

EXPLANATION

Breath hydrogen test after lactulose measures the increase in hydrogen in the exhaled breath after giving oral lactulose. Anaerobic organisms ferment unabsorbed sugar to produce hydrogen. Hydrogen produced by bacteria is absorbed through the intestinal wall and eventually reaches the lungs where it is exhaled. Increase in small bowel bacterial load would produce an early peak of hydrogen. Fermentation of carbohydrates would produce excessive gas resulting in bloating. Macrocytic anemia develops due to vitamin B_{12} deficiency which gets consumed by the bacteria. However, folate levels may be elevated as bacteria produce folic acid.

Key: B

BOOST YOUR KNOWLEDGE

- Strongyloidiasis is an opportunistic infestation in immunocompromised children caused by *Strongyloides stercoralis*. It can cause diarrhea and malabsorption.
- Microscopic colitis presents like chronic diarrhea. Colonoscopy would be normal; however, histopathology would show either lymphocytic colitis or collagenous colitis.
- Functional dyspepsia with postprandial distress syndrome variant can have bloating as a symptom but loose stools and macrocytic anemia are not explainable.

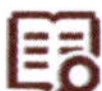

REFERENCE/SOURCE

- Feldman M, Friedman LS, Brandt LJ. Sleisenger and Fordtran's Gastrointestinal and Liver Disease, 10th edition. Philadelphia, PA: Elsevier Health Sciences; 2015. pp. 1824-30.

5. An 8-year-old child was admitted with pneumonia. He was put on intravenous antibiotics. After 10 days, he developed watery diarrhea. Which test you would order next?

A. Stool for *Clostridium difficile* culture
B. Stool for *C. difficile* gram staining
C. Stool for *C. difficile* toxin assay by polymerase chain reaction (PCR)
D. Stool for *C. difficile* antigen

EXPLANATION

The clinical scenario presented here represents that of antibiotic associated diarrhea and the options have different modalities to test for *C. difficile*. Only the toxigenic strains of *C. difficile* are responsible for antibiotic associated diarrhea.

Clostridium difficile culture alone is not sufficient because all organisms are not toxin producing. Gram staining and antigen test for *C. difficile* in stools has very poor sensitivity. Toxin A and B assay by nucleic acid amplification has good sensitivity and specificity.

Key: C

BOOST YOUR KNOWLEDGE

Clostridium difficile colonization is very common in infancy up to 84%. Hence, in the setting of diarrhea in an infant, testing for alternate cause is recommended. The risk factors for developing *C. difficile* diarrhea are exposure to antibiotics and exposure to the organism. Glutamate dehydrogenase is produced in large quantities compared to toxin A and B. Hence, it can be used as a screening test and if found to be positive further confirmation by nucleic acid amplification assay for toxin A and B can be done. Treatment includes stoppage of antibiotics, oral metronidazole, oral vancomycin, and in cases of recurrent *C. difficile* infection, fecal microbiota transplantation.

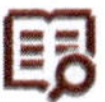

REFERENCE/SOURCE

- ACG Clinical Guidelines: Prevention, Diagnosis, and Treatment of Clostridioides difficile Infections. Am J Gastroenterol. 2021; 116(6):1124-47.

6. A 2-month-old boy presented with intractable watery diarrhea and weight loss. He also had extensive eczema. Duodenoscopy showed duodenal scalloping and biopsy was suggestive of villous atrophy. Mutation in which of these genes can cause this condition?

A. *SPINK*
B. *FOXP3*
C. *BSEP*
D. *NOTCH*

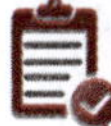

EXPLANATION

The clues in the question are: male child, small bowel diarrhea, eczema, duodenal scalloping and villous atrophy. These point to an underlying diagnosis of IPEX (immune dysregulation, polyendocrinopathy, enteropathy, X-linked). These patients can develop other autoimmune manifestations like diabetes mellitus type 1, autoimmune thyroiditis, hemolytic anemia, etc. The genetic mutation in IPEX is in *FOXP3* gene.

SPINK gene is mutated in those with recurrent acute pancreatitis, bile salt export pump (BSEP) in progressive familial intrahepatic cholestasis (PFIC) type 2 and NOTCH is mutated in those with Alagille syndrome (other gene is *JAGGED*).

Key: B

BOOST YOUR KNOWLEDGE

Autoimmune enteropathy can occur in the context of other autoimmune conditions like APECED (autoimmune phenomena, polyendocrinopathy, candidiasis, ectodermal dysplasia) which has a mutated autoimmune regulator (*AIRE*) gene. Patients with autoimmune enteropathy can have villous atrophy with apoptotic bodies in duodenal biopsies and they may be positive for antienterocyte antibodies.

REFERENCE/SOURCE

- Ruemmele FM, Brousse N, Goulet O. Autoimmune enteropathy and IPEX syndrome. In: Kleinman RE, Goulet OJ, Mieli-Vergani G, Sanderson IR, Sherman PM, Shneider BL (Eds). Walker's Pediatric Gastrointestinal Disease: Physiology, Diagnosis, Management, 6th edition. USA: People's Medical Publishing House; 2018.

7. A 15-year-old boy presented with large volume diarrhea for 3 years associated with anorexia and weight loss. Examination revealed pandigital clubbing and weight below the 3rd centile. Endoscopy showed nodular hypertrophied folds in the duodenum. Colonoscopy showed ulcerated edematous ileocecal valve. Biopsies showed atypical lymphocytic infiltrations in duodenum and ileum. What is the most likely diagnosis?

A. Celiac disease
B. Immunoproliferative small intestinal disease (IPSID)
C. Tropical sprue
D. Crohn's disease

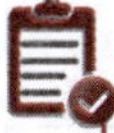

EXPLANATION

The given patient has long-standing small bowel type of diarrhea associated with weight loss and clubbing. All the given options can present with small bowel diarrhea. Options A, B, and D can have clubbing. Endoscopy in celiac disease and tropical would show scalloping of duodenal folds because of villous atrophy. Crohn's disease would show ulcers and erythema. Hypertrophied folds with nodularity along with ulceration can be seen in IPSID. Atypical lymphocytes on biopsy are also suggestive of IPSID.

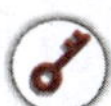

Key: B

BOOST YOUR KNOWLEDGE

Immunoproliferative small intestinal disease presents with chronic diarrhea, malabsorption, weight loss, and clubbing. Prolonged antigenic stimulation due to repeated intestinal infections would lead to proliferation of enteric lymphoplasmacytic cells which would initially be benign but can later progress to malignancy. Immunoelectrophoresis can detect alpha heavy chain (devoid of light chain) in the serum. Chronic infection with *Helicobacter pylori* and *Campylobacter jejuni* is known to trigger IPSID.

REFERENCE/SOURCE

- Fine KD, Stone MJ. Alpha-heavy chain disease, Mediterranean lymphoma, and immunoproliferative small intestinal disease: a review of clinicopathological features, pathogenesis, and differential diagnosis. Am J Gastroenterol. 1999;94(5):1139-52.

8. Which of the following would help to differentiate between tropical sprue and celiac disease?

A. Villous atrophy
B. Anemia
C. Response to antibiotics
D. Response to lactose-free diet

EXPLANATION

Tropical sprue presents with chronic diarrhea and is characterized by malabsorption of two or more unrelated nutrient groups. Villous atrophy is noted in duodenal biopsies. Malabsorption of nutrients absorbed in the proximal and distal intestine will occur. Secondary lactose intolerance can be associated with any condition causing villous atrophy. Pathogenesis is related to chronic infections seen in tropical countries due to poor hygiene. Treatment is by administering prolonged antibiotics like tetracycline.

Key: C

BOOST YOUR KNOWLEDGE

Carbohydrate, fat, vitamin B_{12}, folate, and iron malabsorption occur in tropical sprue. Tropical sprue may be associated with small intestinal bacterial overgrowth.

REFERENCE/SOURCE

- Feldman M, Friedman LS, Brandt LJ. Sleisenger and Fordtran's Gastrointestinal and Liver Disease, 10th edition. Philadelphia, PA: Elsevier Health Sciences; 2015. pp. 1873-86.

9. In a child with suspected celiac disease, tTG IgA was 10 ULN and EMA was negative. What would be the next step?

A. Send HLA-DQ2/DQ8
B. Take duodenal biopsies
C. Send tTG IgG
D. Start on gluten-free diet

EXPLANATION

If tTG IgA is <10 ULN with negative EMA, the next step is to perform duodenal biopsy and establish villous atrophy, crypt hyperplasia, and increase in intraepithelial lymphocytes. HLA-DQ2/DQ8 shows the genetic predisposition to celiac disease and is not confirmatory. Gluten-free diet should be started only after confirming celiac disease.

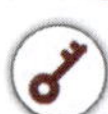

Key: B

 **BOOST YOUR KNOWLEDGE**

Histopathology in celiac disease is described as per Marsh grading. Marsh 0—normal, Marsh 1—increase in intraepithelial lymphocytes, Marsh 2—crypt hyperplasia, Marsh 3—villous atrophy, and Marsh 4—hypoplastic mucosa.

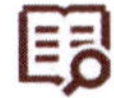 **REFERENCE/SOURCE**

- ESPGHAN. (2020). ESPGHAN guidelines 2020. [online] Available from https://espghan.info/ [Last accessed June, 2024].

10. Which of the following tests is recommended in diagnosis of Cow's milk protein allergy (CMPA)?

A. Atopy patch test
B. Endoscopic biopsy
C. Serum IgE level
D. Milk elimination and rechallenge

 **EXPLANATION**

Atopy patch test and IgE levels are not recommended to diagnose CMPA due to subjective nature of test and poor sensitivity respectively. Endoscopic biopsy showing eosinophilic infiltrates is not specific for CMPA. Diagnostic elimination of milk followed by improvement of symptoms and reappearance of symptoms upon reintroduction is the diagnostic test for CMPA.

 **Key: D**

 **BOOST YOUR KNOWLEDGE**

Treatment of CMPA is by elimination of milk and milk products from the diet for 6 months or up to 9–12 months of age. In case of severe IgE-mediated allergy elimination is recommended up to 12–18 months of age. About 15% babies with CMPA would have cross-reaction to soy protein also.

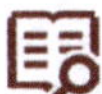 **REFERENCE/SOURCE**

- ESPGHAN. (2020). ESPGHAN guidelines 2020. [online] Available from https://espghan.info/ [Last accessed June, 2024].

11. Which of the following is not used in the maintenance treatment of Crohn's disease?

A. Azathioprine
B. Steroids
C. Infliximab
D. Methotrexate

 **EXPLANATION**

In the management of Crohn's disease, there is an initial induction phase and a maintenance phase. Steroids, exclusive enteral nutrition, and biologicals such as infliximab and adalimumab are used in inducing remission. Maintenance of remission is by azathioprine, methotrexate, sulfasalazine (in mild colonic Crohn's disease) and biologicals. Steroids are not used for maintaining remission.

 **Key: B**

 **BOOST YOUR KNOWLEDGE**

For perianal Crohn's disease, stricturing and penetrating disease and panenteric disease biologicals can be considered upfront.

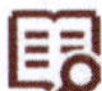 **REFERENCE/SOURCE**

- The Medical Management of Paediatric Crohn's Disease: an ECCO-ESPGHAN Guideline Update. J Crohns Colitis. 2021;15:171-94.

12. A 10-year-old girl with history of steatorrhea presented with ataxia. Her plasma cholesterol and triglyceride were undetectable. She was treated with high dose vitamin E. What is the likely diagnosis?

A. Pancreatic insufficiency
B. Tropical sprue
C. Abetalipoproteinemia
D. Celiac disease

EXPLANATION

From the presentation, it is apparent that the child has fat malabsorption with deficiency of fat-soluble vitamins which can be seen in pancreatic insufficiency, tropical sprue, and abetalipoproteinemia. The clue that is specific is undetectable cholesterol and triglycerides in blood which is seen in abetalipoproteinemia. Abetalipoproteinemia is characterized by absent plasma apoB-containing lipoproteins that results from MTP mutations.

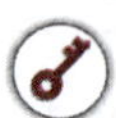

Key: C

BOOST YOUR KNOWLEDGE

Abetalipoproteinemia is otherwise known as Bassen–Kornzweig syndrome. Other manifestations of abetalipoproteinemia are retinitis pigmentosa, hepatic steatosis, ataxia, and peripheral neuropathy due to vitamin E deficiency.

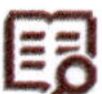

REFERENCE/SOURCE

- Wetterau JR, Gregg RE. Abetalipoproteinemia. Encycloped Endocr Dis. 2004;6-8.

13. Which of the following congenital diarrhea gets exacerbated with oral rehydration solution administration?

A. Congenital glucose-galactose malabsorption
B. Congenital chloride diarrhea
C. Congenital sucrase-isomaltase deficiency
D. Congenital sodium diarrhea

EXPLANATION

In congenital glucose-galactose malabsorption, mutations in *SLC5A1* gene encoding sodium-glucose cotransporter 1 (SGLT1) causes severe osmotic diarrhea upon introduction of glucose and galactose, hence it gets exacerbated with oral glucose containing solutions. Congenital chloride diarrhea is caused by mutations in SLC26A3 encoding Cl/HCO_3 transporter and causes severe dehydrating secretory diarrhea. Congenital sucrase-isomaltase deficiency becomes symptomatic after introduction of sucrose and starch in the diet. Congenital sodium diarrhea is a group of disorders associated with mutations in different genes like *GUCY2C* (associated with infantile inflammatory bowel disease), *SLC9A3*, and *SPINT2* (tufting enteropathy).

Key: A

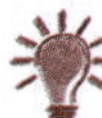

BOOST YOUR KNOWLEDGE

Absorption of fructose by GLUT5 is unaffected in congenital glucose-galactose malabsorption and hence it is treated with fructose-based formula.

REFERENCE/SOURCE

- Terrin G, Tomaiuolo R, Passariello A, Elce A, Amato F, Di Costanzo M, et al. Congenital diarrheal disorders: an updated diagnostic approach. Int J Mol Sci. 2012;13:4168-85.

14. A 9-year-old child developed ileal perforation following abdominal trauma and underwent resection of terminal ileum and ileotransverse anastomosis. Which of the following nutrient deficiencies is likely to occur in her on follow-up?

A. Iron
B. Folic acid
C. Vitamin C
D. Vitamin B_{12}

EXPLANATION

Iron, folic acid, and vitamin C are absorbed in the proximal small intestine. Vitamin B_{12} is absorbed in terminal ileum. Major forms of cobalamin are methylcobalamin, deoxyadenosylcobalamin, and hydroxycobalamin. Cobalamin is released from the food proteins in the stomach in the presence of acidic medium and pepsin. It then binds to R protein or haptocorrin secreted by salivary glands. On reaching the duodenum pancreatic proteases cleave the R protein from cobalamin and transfer it to intrinsic factor secreted by gastric parietal cells. Cobalamin-intrinsic factor complex reach the terminal ileum and bind to the cubilin-amnionless complex called the cubam receptors from where cobalamin is internalized and transferred after binding to transcobalamin II.

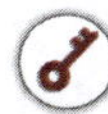

Key: D

BOOST YOUR KNOWLEDGE

Imerslund–Gräsbeck syndrome–selective vitamin B_{12} malabsorption with proteinuria occurs due to mutation in cubilin (*CUBN*) gene and amnionless (*AMN*) gene affecting the terminal ileal receptor for cobalamin absorption. Cubam has a role in renal protein reabsorption too.

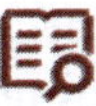

REFERENCE/SOURCE

- Feldman M, Friedman LS, Brandt LJ. Sleisenger and Fordtran's Gastrointestinal and Liver Disease, 10th edition. Philadelphia, PA: Elsevier Health Sciences; 2015. pp. 1770-1.

15. All of the following disorders can present with chronic diarrhea as well as intestinal obstruction *except:*

A. Tuberculosis
B. Eosinophilic gastroenteritis
C. Autoimmune enteropathy
D. Crohn's disease

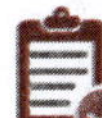

EXPLANATION

A. Tuberculosis can have ulcerative or hyperplastic (stricturing) involvement in the intestine. Ulcerative variety can present with diarrhea and the stricturing variety can present like subacute intestinal obstruction.
B. Manifestations in eosinophilic gastroenteritis would depend on the layer of involvement. Mucosal disease will present like diarrhea, and muscular involvement can present like subacute intestinal obstruction and serosal form can present with eosinophil predominant ascites.
C. Autoimmune enteropathy is a mucosal disease which presents with chronic diarrhea.
D. Crohn's disease can present with watery or bloody diarrhea. They can develop strictures due to the transmural nature of the disease.

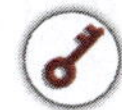

Key: C

BOOST YOUR KNOWLEDGE

Eosinophilic esophagitis can present like gastroesophageal reflux, food bolus impaction, and sometimes like achalasia. Typical endoscopic appearance is with multiple ring-like appearances in the esophageal mucosa called trachealization or felinization. Esophageal biopsies would demonstrate >20 eosinophils/hpf. It can be treated with six allergenic food elimination, proton pump inhibitors, and steroids.

REFERENCE/SOURCE

- Feldman M, Friedman LS, Brandt LJ. Sleisenger and Fordtran's Gastrointestinal and Liver Disease, 10th edition. Philadelphia, PA: Elsevier Health Sciences; 2015. pp. 1788-823.

16. Which of the following may not be the underlying cause in a child with steatorrhea?

A. Chronic pancreatitis
B. Bile acid synthetic defect
C. Ileal Crohn's disease
D. Hypolactasia

EXPLANATION

Fat absorption requires luminal hydrolysis aided by pancreatic lipase and colipase, formation of micelles with the help of bile acids, absorption into the enterocytes, and formation of chylomicrons and lymphatic transport of the chylomicrons. Chronic pancreatitis patients can develop exocrine insufficiency resulting in steatorrhea due to absence of lipase and colipase. Bile acid synthetic defects can impair micelle formation. Any condition affecting terminal ileum will interfere with enterohepatic circulation of bile acids thereby reducing the total bile acid pool.

Hypolactasia results from deficiency of the lactase enzyme at the tips of the villi. These patients would develop osmotic diarrhea on consumption of lactose.

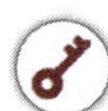

Key: D

BOOST YOUR KNOWLEDGE

Other conditions that can result in fat malabsorption are small intestinal bacterial overgrowth as the bacteria in the small bowel would deconjugate the bile acids affecting micelle formation; Zollinger–Ellison syndrome because of low luminal pH; generalized mucosal diseases like celiac disease and lymphangiectasia.

REFERENCE/SOURCE

- Feldman M, Friedman LS, Brandt LJ. Sleisenger and Fordtran's Gastrointestinal and Liver Disease, 10th edition. Philadelphia, PA: Elsevier Health Sciences; 2015. p. 1791.

17. In which of the following conditions, histopathology of duodenal mucosa is diagnostic of the specific disease?

A. Lymphangiectasia
B. Celiac disease
C. Tropical sprue
D. Food protein allergy

EXPLANATION

Celiac disease and tropical sprue can both have villous atrophy with lymphocytic infiltrates and many other conditions can also have similar histopathology; hence, they are not specific findings. Food protein allergy would show eosinophilic infiltrates; however, this finding is also nonspecific as it can be seen in worm infestations, Crohn's disease, and eosinophilic gastrointestinal disorders. Lymphangiectasia would have dilated lacteals on histopathology which is specific.

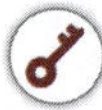

Key: A

BOOST YOUR KNOWLEDGE

Other conditions that have a diagnostic specific histopathology of the small bowel are abetalipoproteinemia, Whipple's disease, *Mycobacterium avium* complex infection, collagenous sprue, amyloidosis, and mastocytosis.

REFERENCE/SOURCE

- Feldman M, Friedman LS, Brandt LJ. Sleisenger and Fordtran's Gastrointestinal and Liver Disease, 10th edition. Philadelphia, PA: Elsevier Health Sciences; 2015. pp. 1800-1.

18. Which of the following conditions can present with chronic diarrhea, malabsorption, and cholestatic liver disease?

A. Tufting enteropathy
B. Microvillous inclusion disease (MVID)
C. Enterokinase deficiency
D. Shwachman–Diamond syndrome

EXPLANATION

A. *Tufting enteropathy* is characterized by disorganized surface enterocytes and crowded tips of villi caused due to mutations in EpCAM affecting tight junction protein.

B. In MVID, there is atrophy of the microvilli and intracellular accumulation of periodic acid–Schiff positive granules containing typical inclusion bodies. Mutations in *MYO5B* gene cause MVID and bile acid transport defect also called progressive familial intrahepatic cholestasis type 5. Hence, these patients may present only with diarrhea, only with cholestasis, or with a combination of diarrhea and cholestasis.

C. In *enterokinase deficiency*, there is defective activation of pancreatic enzymes resulting in diarrhea, hypoproteinemia, and edema.

D. Shwachman–Diamond syndrome is characterized by mutations in the SBDS protein, and these patients can have pancreatic insufficiency, bone marrow failure, and skeletal abnormalities.

Key: B

BOOST YOUR KNOWLEDGE

Trichohepatoenteric syndrome (phenotypic diarrhea of infancy) presents with secretory diarrhea, dysmorphism, and may develop liver fibrosis and even cirrhosis. Mutation in *TTC37* gene causes THES1 and mutation in SKIV2L results in THES-2. Mutated *TTC37* gene causes defective trafficking of apical transport proteins.

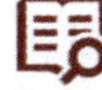

REFERENCE/SOURCE

- Ye Z, Huang Y, Zheng C, Wang Y, Lu J, Wang H, et al. Clinical and genetic spectrum of children with congenital diarrhea and enteropathy in China. Genet Med. 2019;21(10):2224-30.

19. If the stool osmotic gap was found to be <50 mOsm/kg, which of the following could possibly be the etiology?

A. Hypolactasia
B. Lactulose overdose
C. Magnesium ingestion
D. Verner–Morrison syndrome

EXPLANATION

Stool osmotic gap is calculated as 290 mOsm/kg – 2 × (Stool Na + Stool K) and normal is between 50 and 100 mOsm/kg. In secretory diarrhea, sodium and potassium ions make up for a large percent of stool osmolarity and hence, osmotic gap will be <50 mOsm/kg. In osmotic diarrhea, stool osmotic gap will be >100 mOsm/kg as other unabsorbed molecules contribute to the osmolarity of stools. Lactulose and magnesium are poorly absorbed and when ingested in large quantities can cause osmotic diarrhea. In hypolactasia, there is deficiency of lactase enzyme and unabsorbed lactose would contribute to stool osmolarity. In Verner–Morrison syndrome, there is excessive secretion of vasoactive intestinal peptide (VIP) which leads to activation of adenyl cyclase and cyclic adenosine monophosphate (cAMP) production. This will in turn lead to excessive luminal secretion of sodium, potassium, chloride, and water.

Key: D

BOOST YOUR KNOWLEDGE

Features suggesting osmotic diarrhea are improvement with fasting, low stool pH, reducing substance positive in stools, explosive stools, perianal rash whereas in secretory diarrhea there will be no improvement with fasting. Secretory diarrhea is caused by exogenous or endogenous secretagogues, absence of ion transporter, loss of intestinal surface area, and rapid intestinal transit. Osmotic diarrhea is caused by reduced nutrient transport such as lactase deficiency and ingestion of poorly absorbed agent. FODMAPs (fermentable oligosaccharides, disaccharides, monosaccharides, and polyols) can also cause osmotic diarrhea.

REFERENCE/SOURCE

- Feldman M, Friedman LS, Brandt LJ. Sleisenger and Fordtran's Gastrointestinal and Liver Disease, 10th edition. Philadelphia, PA: Elsevier Health Sciences; 2015. pp. 221-3.

20. Which of the following statements is *true*?

A. Micelle formation is mandatory for absorption of MTCs
B. Fructose absorption into the enterocytes requires GLUT5
C. Ferrous form gets converted to ferric form of iron for absorption into enterocyte
D. Rate of absorption of amino acids is faster than peptides

EXPLANATION

A. Medium-chain triglycerides can be directly absorbed into the portal circulation without formation of micelles. Hence, MCT is supplemented in cases with cholestasis where micelle formation gets affected by lack of bile acids in the intestinal lumen.
B. Fructose is absorbed into enterocyte by GLUT5 and transported across the basolateral membrane by GLUT2.
C. Dietary iron mostly contains ferric form which needs to be converted to ferrous form to be transported into the enterocytes by the divalent metal transporter (DMT). This conversion is aided by the presence of ascorbic acid.
D. Protein absorption is more efficient in the form of peptides than amino acids with the help of peptide transporters in the enterocytes. After absorption, peptidases convert them into amino acids.

Key: B

BOOST YOUR KNOWLEDGE

Sodium-glucose cotransporter 1 binds to two sodium ions and one glucose molecule and transports it into the enterocyte. For every glucose molecule absorbed, two sodium ions, two accompanying anions, and 1,100 water molecules are absorbed to maintain iso-osmolarity. This is the rationale behind the use of oral rehydration solution for diarrhea.

REFERENCE/SOURCE

- Feldman M, Friedman LS, Brandt LJ. Sleisenger and Fordtran's Gastrointestinal and Liver Disease, 10th edition. Philadelphia, PA: Elsevier Health Sciences; 2015. pp. 1736-87.

CHAPTER 16.11

Pancreatitis

Srinivas Srinidhi Vadlapudi, Moinak Sen Sarma

1. Which of the following is a criterion for the diagnosis of acute pancreatitis?

A. Serum amylase two times upper limit of normal
B. Periumbilical pain abdomen
C. Imaging of the abdomen revealing a dilated pancreatic duct with parenchymal and ductal calcification
D. Serum lipase ≥3 times the upper limit of normal

EXPLANATION

Diagnosis of acute pancreatitis is established by the presence of two of the following three criteria:

1. Pain abdomen compatible with acute pancreatitis
2. Elevation of serum amylase and/or lipase ≥3 times the upper limit normal (ULN)
3. Imaging findings consistent with acute pancreatitis

Pain abdomen of acute pancreatitis is typically epigastric pain, radiating to the back and worsens with food intake. Dilated pancreatic duct and ductal calcifications are imaging findings of chronic pancreatitis.

Key: D

BOOST YOUR KNOWLEDGE

Serum amylase and lipase are measured to diagnose acute pancreatitis. Serum lipase is more specific than amylase to make a diagnosis of acute pancreatitis. Amylase producing tumors, salpingitis, and macroamylasemia are conditions where estimation of serum lipase especially helps. It is normal in conditions such as amylase producing tumors, salpingitis, and macroamylasemia which have elevated serum amylase levels. Mild elevations of serum amylase are noted in renal insufficiency and gastrointestinal ischemia. Serum lipase rises by 4–8 hours, peaks at 24–48 hours, and remains elevated for 8–14 days. Typically, serum amylase stays elevated for 4 days. Serum amylase levels may be normal in case of mild attack, fatal pancreatitis, during recovery or when there is superimposed chronic pancreatitis (as pancreas has little superimposed pancreatic tissue). Serum amylase may be normal in hypertriglyceridemia associated pancreatitis because an amylase inhibitor may be associated with triglyceride elevations. Hyperamylasemia due to other condition are generally not more than three times the ULN.

REFERENCES/SOURCES

- Abu-El-Haija M, Kumar S, Quiros JA, Balakrishnan K, Barth B, Bitton S, et al. Management of Acute Pancreatitis in the Pediatric Population: A Clinical Report From the North American Society for Pediatric Gastroenterology, Hepatology and Nutrition Pancreas Committee. J Pediatr Gastroenterol Nutr. 2018;66(1):159-76.
- Werlin SL, Wilschanski M. Pancreatitis (Chapter 378). In: Kliegman RM, St Geme III JW, Blum NJ, Shah SS, Tasker RC, Wilson KM (Eds). Nelson Textbook of Pediatrics, 21st edition. Philadelphia: Elsevier Health Sciences; 2020. p. 2074.

2. Which type of intravenous fluid must be administered for the management of acute pancreatitis?

A. 10% dextrose
B. 0.9% normal saline (NS)
C. 5% albumin
D. Isolyte P

EXPLANATION

Recommended fluid for the management of acute pancreatitis is 0.9% NS or Ringer lactate (RL). Crystalloids are the fluids of choice to maintain the intravascular volume. Isolyte P (23 mEq/L of Na^+) and 10% dextrose do not maintain the intravascular volume as well as 0.9% NS or RL. Colloids are recommended only when hematocrit is <25% or serum albumin is <2 g/dL.

Key: B

BOOST YOUR KNOWLEDGE

Early in the course of disease, inflammation causes extravasation of fluid resulting in a capillary leak syndrome. End result is hemoconcentration, elevation of blood urea nitrogen (BUN) and decreased tissue perfusion. The decreased perfusion pressure into the pancreas results in pancreatic necrosis. Factors predicting the development of acute necrotizing pancreatitis include hematocrit at admission >44 or nonreduction of the hematocrit after 24 hours of admission. Rising BUN is a marker of increased mortality. As hematocrit and BUN are predictors of increased severity, measures to reduce the same by early vigorous intravenous volume repletion will improve the outcomes. Thus, the intravascular volume needs to be repleted adequately to decrease the hematocrit and BUN, thereby increasing pancreatic perfusion.

As of now, the recommendation is to use lactated ringers or 0.9% NS at a rate of 150–200% the maintenance IV fluid rate with monitoring of urine output for aggressive fluid resuscitation.

REFERENCES/SOURCES

- Abu-El-Haija M, Kumar S, Quiros JA, Balakrishnan K, Barth B, Bitton S, et al. Management of Acute Pancreatitis in the Pediatric Population: A Clinical Report From the North American Society for Pediatric Gastroenterology, Hepatology and Nutrition Pancreas Committee. J Pediatr Gastroenterol Nutr. 2018;66(1):159-76.
- Riyaz A, Govindaraj GM. Pancreatitis and pancreatic tumors (Chapter 36.12) In: Gupta P, Menon PSN, Ramji S, Lodha R (Eds). PG Textbook of Pediatrics, 2nd edition. New Delhi: Jaypee Brothers Medical Publishers; 2018.

3. Severity of acute pancreatitis is established on which of the following criteria?

A. Duration of hospital stay
B. Duration and intensity of pain abdomen
C. Elevation of hematocrit and neutrophilic leukocytosis
D. Presence of local complications like acute fluid collection or organ dysfunction

EXPLANATION

Pancreatitis is classified as mild, moderate, and severe as per the presence of local or systemic complications or organ dysfunction. Duration, intensity of pain, hematocrit, leukocytosis, and duration of hospital stay are not considered for classifying into mild, moderately severe, or severe acute pancreatitis.

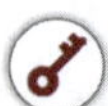

Key: D

BOOST YOUR KNOWLEDGE

Pediatric mild acute pancreatitis: It is the most common form of acute pancreatitis. It is characterized by absence of organ failure, local, or systemic complications. It generally resolves within a week of presentation.

Pediatric moderately severe acute pancreatitis: Acute pancreatitis accompanied by transient organ failure (<48 hours)/dysfunction or local or systemic complications is defined as moderately severe acute pancreatitis.

Pediatric severe acute pancreatitis: Acute pancreatitis accompanied by organ dysfunction lasting >48 hours. One or more organs may be affected and may be involved even 48 hours after presentation.

Local complications: These include pancreatic and peripancreatic necrosis, peripancreatic fluid collections, necrotic fluid collection, pseudocysts, or walled off necrosis (may be sterile or infected).

Systemic complications: These include exacerbation of comorbid disorders priorly diagnosed such as lung or kidney disease.

Criteria for organ dysfunction:

Cardiovascular dysfunction	*Respiratory dysfunction*	*Renal dysfunction*
≥1 of the following despite fluid bolus ≥40 mL/kg in 1 hour 1. Hypotension, i.e., blood pressure (BP) <5th centile for age or systolic blood pressure <2 standard deviation (SD) for age 2. Requirement of vasoactive drugs to maintain normal BP (dopamine >5 µg/kg/min or dobutamine, epinephrine, or norepinephrine at any dose) 3. Two of the following: a. Unexplained metabolic acidosis (base deficit >5.0 mEq/L) b. Increased arterial lactate >2 ULN c. Urine output <0.5 mL/kg/hour d. Core to peripheral temperature gap >3° Celsius e. Prolonged capillary refill >5 s	≥1 of the following in absence of preexisting lung disease or cyanotic heart disease: I. PaO_2/FIO_2 <300 in the absence of cyanotic heart disease or preexisting lung disease II. $PaCO_2$ >65 torr or 20 mm Hg over baseline $PaCO_2$ III. Need for >50% FIO_2 to maintain saturation ≥92 IV. Mechanical ventilation (nonelective)	Serum creatinine ≥2 times upper limit of normal for age or two-fold increase in baseline creatinine

REFERENCES/SOURCES

- Abu-El-Haija M, Kumar S, Szabo F, Werlin S, Conwell D, Banks P, et al. Classification of Acute Pancreatitis in the Pediatric Population: Clinical Report From the NASPGHAN Pancreas Committee. J Pediatr Gastroenterol Nutr. 2017;64(6):984-90.
- Werlin SL, Wilschanski M. Pancreatitis (Chapter 378). In: Kliegman RM, St Geme III JW, Blum NJ, Shah SS, Tasker RC, Wilson KM (Eds). Nelson Textbook of Pediatrics, 21st edition. Philadelphia: Elsevier Health Sciences; 2020. p. 2074.

4. When should enteral nutrition be started in patients with acute pancreatitis?

A. Within 48–72 hours if there are no gut-related contraindications
B. Start only after pain has subsided completely
C. After normalization of serum amylase and lipase
D. Immediately after hemodynamic stabilization

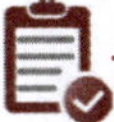

EXPLANATION

Enteral nutrition should be established as soon as possible once contraindications like ileus, shock requiring multiple inotropes are safely ruled out. It is recommended to start enteral nutrition within 48–72 hours. At presentation, keeping the patient nil per oral is necessary to provide pain relief and to rule out conditions such as ileus or phlegmonous collections which may present as intestinal obstruction.

Key: A

BOOST YOUR KNOWLEDGE

Keeping the patient of acute pancreatitis fasting adversely affects the gut mucosal barrier and facilitates translocation of bacteria from the lumen of the gut to extraluminal tissues including the inflamed pancreas. This increases the morbidity and mortality. By starting enteral feeding early, the complication rate and length of hospital stay can be reduced. Enteral feeding by mouth, nasogastric or nasojejunal tube feeding should be initiated in 48–72 hours of the attack.

REFERENCES/SOURCES

- Abu-El-Haija M, Kumar S, Quiros JA, Balakrishnan K, Barth B, Bitton S, et al. Management of Acute Pancreatitis in the Pediatric Population: A Clinical Report From the North American Society for Pediatric Gastroenterology, Hepatology and Nutrition Pancreas Committee. J Pediatr Gastroenterol Nutr. 2018;66(1):159-76.
- Werlin SL, Wilschanski M. Pancreatitis (Chapter 378). In: Kliegman RM, St Geme III JW, Blum NJ, Shah SS, Tasker RC, Wilson KM (Eds). Nelson Textbook of Pediatrics, 21st edition. Philadelphia: Elsevier Health Sciences; 2020. p. 2074.

5. Acute recurrent pancreatitis is defined as:

A. Two episodes of acute pancreatitis separated by a pain-free interval of 4 weeks
B. Two episodes of acute pancreatitis with any pain-free interval
C. Three or more episodes of acute pancreatitis occurring in a year
D. Three or more episodes of acute pancreatitis occurring in any time frame

EXPLANATION

Pediatric acute recurrent pancreatitis is defined as occurrence of two distinct episodes of acute pancreatitis with intervening 1 month symptom-free interval or two distinct episodes of acute pancreatitis with complete normalization of serum amylase and lipase in the intervening period with no symptoms.

Key: A

BOOST YOUR KNOWLEDGE

The INSPPIRE (International Study Group of Pediatric Pancreatitis: In Search for a Cure) consortium recommends systematic evaluation of anatomical, metabolic, and genetic causes for patients with acute recurrent pancreatitis including a sweat chloride test or CFTR genetic testing (even if newborn screening for CF was negative), PRSS1, CTRC, and SPINK1 genetic testing and for screening for celiac disease. Testing for exocrine pancreatic insufficiency and related vitamin and nutritional deficiencies, diabetes, and complications should also be evaluated annually.

REFERENCE/SOURCE

- Werlin SL, Wilschanski M. Pancreatitis (Chapter 378). In: Kliegman RM, St Geme III JW, Blum NJ, Shah SS, Tasker RC, Wilson KM (Eds). Nelson Textbook of Pediatrics, 21st edition. Philadelphia: Elsevier Health Sciences; 2020. p. 2080.

6. Which of the following commonly used antiepileptic is a known cause for drug-induced pancreatitis?

A. Midazolam
B. Levetiracetam
C. Phenytoin
D. Sodium valproate

EXPLANATION

Sodium valproate is a known cause of drug-induced pancreatitis. It falls under class 1A of drug-induced pancreatitis. Midazolam, phenytoin, and levetiracetam are relatively safe and are not commonly considered to cause pancreatitis.

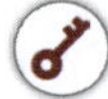

Key: D

BOOST YOUR KNOWLEDGE

Classification of drug-induced pancreatitis is as follows:

Class 1A: At least one case report with positive rechallenge, excluding all other causes, such as alcohol, hypertriglyceridemia, gallstones, and other drugs.

Class 1B: At least one case report with positive rechallenge; however, other causes, such as alcohol, hypertriglyceridemia, gallstones, and other drugs were not ruled out.

Class 2: At least four cases in the literature. Consistent latency (75% of cases).

Class 3: At least two cases in the literature. Latency not consistency established. No report of a rechallenge.

Class 4: Drugs that do not fit into the previous classes, single case report in literature without a rechallenge.

Common drugs causing pancreatitis:

Class 1A	*Class 1B*	*Class 2*	*Class 3*	*Class 4*
• Alpha-methyldopa • Carbimazole • Dapsone • Enalapril • Furosemide • Isoniazid • Mesalamine • Metronidazole • Valproic acid	• All-trans-retinoic acid • Amiodarone • Azathioprine • Dexamethasone • Lamivudine • Methimazole • Omeprazole • Trimethoprim-sulfamethazine	• Acetaminophen • Chlorothiazide • Erythromycin • L-asparaginase • Propofol	• Atorvastatin • Carbamazepine • Ceftriaxone • Cyclosporine • Hydrochlorothiazide • Indomethacin • Naproxen • Prednisolone	• Ampicillin • Cyclophosphamide • Cyproheptadine • Doxorubicin • Nitrofurantoin • Ranitidine • Rifampicin • Tacrolimus • Lamotrigine • Vincristine

REFERENCES/SOURCES

- Badalov N, Baradarian R, Iswara K, Li J, Steinberg W, Tenner S. Drug-induced acute pancreatitis: an evidence-based review. Clin Gastroenterol Hepatol. 2007;5(6):648-61; quiz 644.
- Werlin SL, Wilschanski M. Pancreatitis (Chapter 378). In: Kliegman RM, St Geme III JW, Blum NJ, Shah SS, Tasker RC, Wilson KM (Eds). Nelson Textbook of Pediatrics, 21st edition. Philadelphia: Elsevier Health Sciences; 2020. p. 2074.

7. A 12-year-old boy was diagnosed as a case of acute pancreatitis (typical pancreatic pain, serum amylase, and lipase ≥3 normal value and ultrasonography showing diffusely enlarged and bulky pancreas) and managed conservatively. Five weeks after the episode of pancreatitis, he started noticing a lump in epigastric region and had features of early satiety. A contrast-enhanced computed tomography (CECT) of the abdomen revealed a well encapsulated, homogeneous fluid collection with no necrosis in the peripancreatic region compressing the antrum of the stomach. Which of the following is likely?

A. Acute peripancreatic fluid collection
B. Pancreatic pseudocyst
C. Acute necrotic collection
D. Walled-off necrosis

EXPLANATION

Well-encapsulated collection occurring 4 weeks after the onset of pancreatitis is pancreatic pseudocyst. Acute peripancreatic fluid collection and acute necrotic collection occur within 4 weeks of the onset of pancreatitis and are differentiated based on the presence of necrosis. Acute necrotic collection matures into walled off necrosis (>4 weeks of illness).

Key: B

BOOST YOUR KNOWLEDGE

Acute pancreatitis may be interstitial edematous pancreatitis or necrotizing pancreatitis. Majority of the patients have interstitial edematous pancreatitis characterized by diffuse enlargement of the pancreas with CECT of the abdomen showing homogeneous enhancement of the pancreas with inflammatory changes of the peripancreatic fat with or without peripancreatic fluid collections. Necrotizing pancreatitis is seen in 5–10% of the patients of acute pancreatitis and is characterized by necrosis of pancreatic parenchyma and peripancreatic tissue and may have associated collections.

Acute peripancreatic fluid collection: Occurs in patients of interstitial edematous pancreatitis in the first 4 weeks of illness. On CECT, it is characterized by homogeneous nature, lack of mature wall encapsulating the collection, confined by normal peripancreatic fascial planes, and is adjacent to the pancreas without any intrapancreatic extension.

Acute necrotic collection: It occurs in patients of necrotizing pancreatitis in the first 4 weeks of illness. Necrosis of the pancreas and peripancreatic tissues takes place. On CECT, it is characterized by heterogeneous and nonliquid density of varying degrees in different locations (some appear homogeneous early in their course) without any definable wall encapsulating the collection and may be intrapancreatic and/or extrapancreatic.

Pancreatic pseudocyst: It is an encapsulated fluid collection with a well-formed inflammatory wall outside the pancreas with no or minimal necrosis. It occurs 4 weeks after the onset of interstitial edematous pancreatitis. On CECT, it appears as a well-circumscribed collection of homogeneous fluid density with no nonliquid component and a well-encapsulated wall.

Walled-off necrosis: It is a mature, encapsulated collection of pancreatic and/or peripancreatic necrosis surrounded by a well-defined inflammatory wall. It occurs after 4 weeks of the onset of necrotizing pancreatitis. On CECT, it is characterized by heterogeneous liquid and nonliquid density with varying degrees of loculations (some may appear homogeneous) surrounded by a well-defined encapsulated wall, located in intrapancreatic and/or peripancreatic region. Maturation usually requires at least 4 weeks from the onset of acute necrotizing pancreatitis.

REFERENCES/SOURCES

- Banks PA, Bollen TL, Dervenis C, Gooszen HG, Johnson CD, Sarr MG, et al. Classification of acute pancreatitis—2012: revision of the Atlanta Classification and Definitions by International Consensus. Gut. 2013;62(1):102-11.
- Wilschanski M, Werlin SL. Pancreatic fluid collections (Chapter 379). In: Kliegman RM, St Geme III JW, Blum NJ, Shah SS, Tasker RC, Wilson KM (Eds). Nelson Textbook of Pediatrics, 21st edition. Philadelphia: Elsevier Health Sciences; 2020. p. 2074.

8. Which of the following characterizes chronic pancreatitis?

A. Abdominal pain suggestive of pancreatitis lasting for >1 month
B. Steatorrhea present for >1 month
C. Abdominal pain suggestive of pancreatitis for >3 months
D. Endocrine pancreatic insufficiency and suggestive pancreatic imaging

EXPLANATION

A diagnosis of chronic pancreatitis is made if any one of the following is satisfied:

- Abdominal pain consistent with pancreatic origin and imaging findings suggestive of chronic pancreatic damage
- Evidence of exocrine pancreatic insufficiency and suggestive pancreatic imaging findings
- Evidence of endocrine pancreatic insufficiency and suggestive pancreatic imaging findings

Duration of symptoms is not considered while making a diagnosis of chronic pancreatitis. Steatorrhea or diabetes mellitus alone without imaging findings of pancreatitis cannot be labeled as chronic pancreatitis.

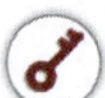

Key: D

BOOST YOUR KNOWLEDGE

Computed tomography, magnetic resonance cholangiopancreatography, or endoscopic retrograde cholangio-pancreatography (ERCP) are the imaging modalities to diagnose chronic pancreatitis. Findings that are suggestive of chronic pancreatitis include ductal changes (irregular contour of the main pancreatic duct or its radicles, strictures or dilatation of the ducts or intraductal calculi) and parenchymal changes (generalized or focal enlargement, accentuation of lobular architecture, heterogeneous echotexture, cavities, or calcifications).

Exocrine pancreatic insufficiency is diagnosed by fecal elastase-1 monoclonal assay or 72 hours fecal fat collection. Fecal elastase must be <100 mg/g stool on two separate occasions done at least 1 month apart. When a 72-hour fecal collection is done, coefficient of dietary fat absorption must be <90%. Neither test should be performed during an acute pancreatitis episode because the results may be temporarily low. Children with classic cystic fibrosis, exhibiting early-onset pancreatic insufficiency without earlier evidence of any meaningful pancreas sufficiency, typically should not be diagnosed as having chronic pancreatitis. They do not have chronic abdominal pain and pancreatic imaging findings described in the chronic pancreatitis criteria.

The diagnosis of endocrine pancreatic insufficiency is by the 2006 World Health Organization criteria for diagnosis of diabetes mellitus [fasting blood glucose >7.0 mmol/L (126 mg/dL) or plasma glucose >11.1 mmol/L (200 mg/dL)] 2 hours after a glucose load of 1.75 g/kg in children (maximum 75-g glucose load).

REFERENCE/SOURCE

- Morinville VD, Husain SZ, Bai H, Barth B, Alhosh R, Durie PR, et al. Definitions of pediatric pancreatitis and survey of present clinical practices. J Pediatr Gastroenterol Nutr. 2012;55(3):261-5.

9. Which of the following tests is used for determining exocrine pancreatic insufficiency?

A. Glycosylated hemoglobin (HbA1c)
B. Fecal α1-antitrypsin
C. Fecal calprotectin
D. Fecal elastase

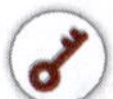

EXPLANATION

Fecal elastase is used to determine exocrine insufficiency of pancreas. HbA1c is for diagnosis and follow up of diabetes mellitus. Fecal α1-antitrypsin is a screening test for protein losing enteropathy. Fecal calprotectin is a marker of bowel inflammation.

Key: D

BOOST YOUR KNOWLEDGE

Fecal elastase-1 levels <200 µg/g of stool are considered abnormal and suggestive of exocrine pancreatic insufficiency. Levels <100 µg/g of stool are considered evidence of exocrine pancreatic insufficiency. Elastase is a stable endopeptidase secreted by the pancreas. The sensitivity and specificity of fecal elastase is >90%. A value >100 µg/g of stool has a 99% predictive value in ruling out pancreatic insufficiency. Falsely abnormal levels occur in other enteropathies and in the setting of diarrhea.

Pancreatic function testing can broadly be classified into direct and indirect tests. Direct tests include measurement of bicarbonate concentration and levels of enzymes trypsin, chymotrypsin, lipase, and amylase after secretin or cholecystokinin stimulation. As it is invasive and cumbersome it is rarely used.

Indirect tests include measurement of fecal fat, stool examination for fat globules, and measurement of fecal elastase and chymotrypsin.

Fecal fat estimation requires stool collection for 72 hours. During this time, a proper dietary record should be maintained so that fat intake can be calculated accordingly. A plastic container that is priorly weighed and can be sealed is used for stool collection. This must be refrigerated once stool collection begins. Freezing will preserve the sample and reduce odor. In the case of infants, diapers must be used with the plastic side facing the skin so that the entire sample can be emptied into the plastic container. Normal fat absorption is >93% of intake.

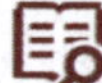

REFERENCES/SOURCES

- Riyaz A, Govindaraj GM. Pancreatitis and pancreatic tumors (Chapter 36.12). In: Gupta P, Menon PSN, Ramji S, Lodha R (Eds). PG Textbook of Pediatrics, 2nd edition. New Delhi: Jaypee Brothers Medical Publishers; 2018.
- Wilschanski M, Werlin SL. Pancreatic function test (Chapter 375). In: Kliegman RM, St Geme III JW, Blum NJ, Shah SS, Tasker RC, Wilson KM (Eds). Nelson Textbook of Pediatrics, 21st edition. Philadelphia: Elsevier Health Sciences; 2020.

10. Which of the following parasite is implicated for developing acute pancreatitis?

A. *Ascaris lumbricoides*
B. *Taenia solium*
C. *Enterobius vermicularis*
D. *Trichuris trichiura*

EXPLANATION

Ascaris lumbricoides or roundworm generally inhabits the jejunum. Proximal migration of the worm is known to occur when the worm load is huge. Upon proximal migration, the worm tends to explore orifices like the papilla thus causing cholangitis or pancreatitis. *T. solium, E. vermicularis,* and *T. trichiura* are not known to cause pancreatitis.

Key: A

BOOST YOUR KNOWLEDGE

Hepatobiliary and pancreatic ascariasis (HPA) is prevalent in Kashmir and eastern parts of India. Ascaris normally resides in the jejunum. Whenever there is a heavy worm load, the worm migrates proximally to the duodenum. As the nature of the worm is to explore orifices, the worm tends to move in and out of the ampulla of Vater. During this invasion of the ampulla of Vater, it obstructs the bile duct or the pancreatic duct and causes HPA. It can also cause marked sphincter spasm and dysmotility. On many occasions, the worms get trapped inside the bile ducts, die, and become a nidus for formation of choledocholithiasis. Ascarides in the bile ducts lead to impaired drainage, stasis, and formation of biliary sludge and stones. HPA can present in the following six ways: (1) Biliary colic, (2) acute cholangitis, (3) acalculous cholecystitis, (4) hepatic abscess, (5) acute pancreatitis, and (6) recurrent pyogenic cholangitis.

Hepatobiliary and pancreatic ascariasis occurs more commonly in females (female: male ratio 3:1). HPA is seen more so in pregnant women due to relaxation of the papilla caused by the hormones. Other risk factors for HPA include prior biliary surgeries and interventions such as cholecystectomy, choledocholithotomy, sphincterotomy, and so on. Ascariasis is more prevalent in childhood but HPA occurs more in adults. This is likely due to the smaller size of the papilla and absence of the above risk factors in children.

Diagnosis of HPA can be made by ultrasonography with the worm appearing as a linear echogenicity or by direct visualization of the worm on endoscopy or ERCP. Anthelmintic drugs that are effective include pyrantel pamoate, mebendazole, albendazole, and ivermectin. ERCP and retrieval of worms from the bile or pancreatic ducts is needed in case of severe symptoms or when the worms are dead within the ducts.

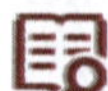

REFERENCE/SOURCE

- Khuroo MS, Rather AA, Khuroo NS, Khuroo MS. Hepatobiliary and pancreatic ascariasis. World J Gastroenterol. 2016;22(33): 7507-17.

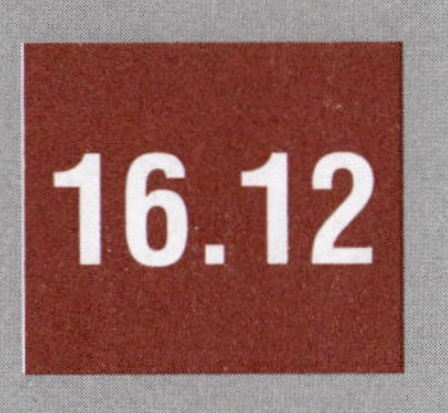

CHAPTER 16.12

Ascites, Abdominal Tuberculosis, and Appendicitis

Arghya Samanta, Moinak Sen Sarma

1. Which of the following is *not* a feature of chylous ascites?

A. Milky white appearance
B. Ascitic fluid triglyceride level >200 mg/dL
C. Serum ascites albumin gradient (SAAG) falsely high
D. Treatment is long-chain triglyceride (LCT)-based diet

EXPLANATION

Chylous ascites is defined as a milky appearing, triglyceride-rich peritoneal fluid in the abdominal cavity. It is characterized by the accumulation of true chyle from thoracic or intestinal lymph. Etiology of chylous ascites can be due to rupture of obstructed or distorted abdominal lymphatics as occurs in congenital lymphangiectasia or other acquired conditions such as trauma, malignancy, and tuberculosis. Chylous ascites is suspected when ascites appears milky. A triglyceride level in the ascitic fluid should be obtained, and a concentration >200 mg/dL supports the diagnosis. Fat globules and leukocytes with a predominance of lymphocytes is seen. Ascitic fluid total protein is high as ascitic fluid contains high concentration of chyle. However, SAAG is falsely high instead of being low as lipid interferes with estimation of albumin. The teaching point of this case is to recognize the milky appearance of chylous ascites and to order a triglyceride level to confirm the diagnosis. A special diet is recommended for treatment that is low in LCT and high in medium-chain triglyceride (MCT), and high in protein. MCTs spare the lymphatic system through absorption by enterocytes and being transported directly into the liver as free fatty acids and glycerol. When these dietary changes are insufficient, bowel rest, and total parenteral nutrition (TPN), octreotide should be considered.

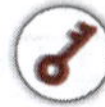

Key: D

BOOST YOUR KNOWLEDGE

Constituent of chyle: Protein, lymphocytes, immunoglobulin, and chylomicrons which contains LCTs. More than 50% of total body lymph originates in the gut and liver. Thoracic duct lymph flow averages 1 mL/kg/hour but may increase to 200 mL/kg/hour after ingestion of a fatty meal.

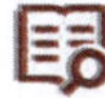

REFERENCES/SOURCES

- Chylous ascites. In: Kliegman RM, Stanton BF, St Geme JW III, Schor NF (Eds). Nelson Textbook of Pediatrics, 20th edition. Amsterdam, Netherlands: Elsevier; 2016.
- Sathiyasekaran M, Ganesh R. Ascites. In: Gupta P, Menon PSN, Ramji S, Lodha R (Eds). PG Textbook of Pediatrics, 3rd edition. New Delhi: Jaypee Brothers Medical Publishers; 2022.

2. Chylous ascites is associated with all of the following conditions *except*:

A. Edward syndrome
B. Turner syndrome
C. Yellow nail syndrome
D. Klippel–Trénaunay syndrome

EXPLANATION

Abdominal malignancy, cirrhosis, and tuberculosis are the most common causes of chylous ascites in adults, whereas congenital abnormalities of the lymphatic system and trauma are most common in children. Primary lymphatic hypoplasia is a condition seen most commonly in children and presents with lymphedema, chylothorax, chylous ascites, or combination. The Klippel–Trénaunay syndrome is an autosomal dominant inherited disorder characterized by venous and lymphatic hypoplastic malformations which can manifest as lower limb lymphedema and it is often associated with chylous ascites. The yellow nail syndrome is a childhood disorder of unknown etiology. The patients have hypoplastic or aplastic lymphatics leading to the characteristic features of lower limb lymphedema, pleural effusion, and/or chylous ascites and a yellow discoloration with dystrophy of the nails. Turner syndrome can present with severe lymphedema and chylous ascites. But Edward syndrome has not been reported to be associated with chylous ascites.

Key: A

BOOST YOUR KNOWLEDGE

Etiology of chylous ascites	
Primary (common in children)	***Secondary (common in adults)***
• Primary lymphatic hypoplasia • Primary lymphangiectasia • Lymphangioma • *Syndromic association:* Turner syndrome, Noonan syndrome, Klippel–Trénaunay syndrome, and Yellow nail syndrome	• *Neoplastic:* Lymphoma, lymphangiomyomatosis, and neuroendocrine tumor • *Infection:* Tuberculosis and filariasis • *Inflammation:* Pericarditis, radiation, retroperitoneal fibrosis, and acute pancreatitis • Trauma and abdominal surgery • Cirrhosis

REFERENCES/SOURCES

- Chylous ascites. In: Kliegman RM, Stanton BF, St Geme JW III, Schor NF (Eds). Nelson Textbook of Pediatrics, 20th edition. Amsterdam, Netherlands: Elsevier; 2016.
- Sathiyasekaran M, Ganesh R. Ascites. In: Gupta P, Menon PSN, Ramji S, Lodha R (Eds). PG Textbook of Pediatrics, 3rd edition. New Delhi: Jaypee Brothers Medical Publishers; 2022.

3. All are associated with high SAAG ascites *except*:

A. Nephrotic syndrome
B. Congestive cardiac failure
C. Cirrhosis
D. Portal vein thrombosis

EXPLANATION

Serum ascites albumin gradient is calculated by subtracting the value of ascitic fluid albumin from the serum albumin estimated concurrently. SAAG is classified as high gradient ascites (>1.1) and low gradient ascites (<1.1). High gradient ascites is seen in portal hypertension with a diagnostic accuracy of 97%. Acute liver failure hypothyroidism and cardiac conditions also lead to high gradient ascites.

Key: A

BOOST YOUR KNOWLEDGE

Etiological classification of ascites according to serum ascites albumin gradient	
High SAAG ascites: • Portal hypertension • Cardiac causes • Acute liver failure • Hypothyroidism	*Low SAAG ascites:* • Nephrotic syndrome • Biliary ascites • Pancreatic ascites • Tubercular ascites • Chylous ascites • Secondary bacterial peritonitis • Serositis • Malignant ascites
Falsely high SAAG ascites: • Chylous ascites (lipid interferes with albumin estimation)	*Falsely low SAAG ascites:* • Serum albumin <1.1 g/dL • Hypergammaglobulinemia

Note: Corrected SAAG = uncorrected SAAG × 0.16 × (serum globulin + 2.5)

REFERENCES/SOURCES

- Ascites. In: Kliegman RM, Stanton BF, St Geme JW III, Schor NF (Eds). Nelson Textbook of Pediatrics, 20th edition. Amsterdam, Netherlands: Elsevier; 2016.
- Sathiyasekaran M, Ganesh R. Ascites. In: Gupta P, Menon PSN, Ramji S, Lodha R (Eds). PG Textbook of Pediatrics, 3rd edition. New Delhi: Jaypee Brothers Medical Publishers; 2022.

4. Which of the following is not a feature of secondary bacterial peritonitis?

A. Ascitic fluid glucose low
B. Ascitic fluid lactate dehydrogenase (LDH)/serum LDH >0.5
C. Ascitic fluid protein <1 g/dL
D. Ascitic fluid cultures showing growth of multiple microorganisms

EXPLANATION

Secondary bacterial peritonitis describes peritoneal infections secondary to intraabdominal lesions, such as perforation of the hollow viscus, bowel necrosis, nonbacterial peritonitis, or penetrating infectious processes.

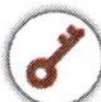

Key: C

BOOST YOUR KNOWLEDGE

Ascitic fluid analysis in secondary bacterial peritonitis:

- Absolute polymorphonuclear leukocyte (PMN) count ≥250 cells/mm^3
- Multiple organisms on gram stain and culture
- *Runyon's Criteria (at least two of the following findings):*
  - Total protein >1 g/dL
  - Glucose <50 mg/dL (2.8 mmol/L)
  - LDH greater than the upper limit of normal for serum

REFERENCE/SOURCE

- Peritonitis. In: Kliegman RM, Stanton BF, St Geme JW III, Schor NF (Eds). Nelson Textbook of Pediatrics, 20th edition. Amsterdam, Netherlands: Elsevier; 2016.

5. A patient with cirrhosis was found to have shifting dullness on examination. What should be the appropriate management?

A. Only salt restriction
B. Only diuretics
C. Salt restriction and diuretics
D. Paracentesis

EXPLANATION

Mild ascites usually responds to salt restriction only (80–120 mmol/day of sodium, corresponding to 4.6–6.9 g of salt daily). Moderate ascites is treated with diuretics along with salt restriction. Tense ascites requires paracentesis, followed by diuretic and salt restriction.

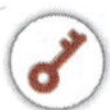

Key: C

BOOST YOUR KNOWLEDGE

The mainstay of ascites formation is renal sodium retention due to the activation of sodium retaining systems, such as the renin-angiotensin-aldosterone system (RAAS) and sympathetic nervous system. The resulting positive fluid balance ultimately leads to extracellular fluid volume expansion. Reduced effective volume secondary to splanchnic arterial vasodilation is a main determinant of these alterations.

Ascites is graded according to the International Club of Ascites as Grade 0 if there is no clinically demonstrable ascites, Grade 1 if mild ascites detected only by ultrasound, Grade 2 if moderate ascites without fluid thrill, and Grade 3 if large/tense ascites with marked distension of abdomen and fluid thrill.

REFERENCES/SOURCES

- Chylous ascites. In: Kliegman RM, Stanton BF, St Geme JW III, Schor NF (Eds). Nelson Textbook of Pediatrics, 20th edition. Amsterdam, Netherlands: Elsevier; 2016.
- Sathiyasekaran M, Ganesh R. Ascites. In: Gupta P, Menon PSN, Ramji S, Lodha R (Eds). PG Textbook of Pediatrics, 3rd edition. New Delhi: Jaypee Brothers Medical Publishers; 2022.

6. A 7-year-old boy had history of abdominal trauma 4 days back and now presented with diffuse abdominal distension and abdominal pain for past 2 days. Physical examination revealed shifting dullness. Ascitic tap was done and found to be hemorrhagic. Ultrasound abdomen showed laceration in mid body of pancreas. Which of the following features is *likely* in this scenario?

A. Normal ascitic fluid amylase
B. Ascitic fluid showing leukopenia
C. Normal serum amylase
D. Low SAAG

EXPLANATION

Pancreatic ascites refers to the accumulation of peritoneal fluid in the presence of pancreatic disease and is usually secondary to pancreatic pseudocysts or pancreatic duct disruption. Pancreatic ascites is an exudative ascites characterized by high amylase concentration in ascitic fluid (usually over 1000 IU/L) and protein concentration over 3 g/dL and low SAAG (<1.1) that differentiates it from ascites secondary to cirrhosis (SAAG >1.1). Serum amylase level is also elevated due to the release of pancreatic enzymes from damaged pancreatic tissue. The clinical presentation includes mild abdominal pain, weight loss, and progressive ascites. Peritoneal reaction due to seepage of pancreatic juice causes elevated total leukocyte count of ascitic fluid. Treatment can be medical (nasojejunal feeding and octreotide) or interventional (endoscopic retrograde cholangiopancreatography or surgical).

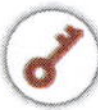

Key: D

BOOST YOUR KNOWLEDGE

Formation of pancreatic ascites:
- *Breach in main pancreatic duct:* Anterior pancreatic duct → pancreatic ascites; posterior pancreatic duct → pleural effusion (pancreaticopleural fistula)
- Leakage of peripancreatic fluid collection

Types of ascites in the setting of acute pancreatitis:
- Reactionary peritonitis
- Pancreatic duct disruption
- Hypoalbuminemia-related ascites
- Chylous ascites (pancreatic fluid collection causing lymphatic obstruction)
- Splenic vein/portal vein thrombosis

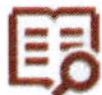

REFERENCE/SOURCE

- Kanneganti K, Srikakarlapudi S, Acharya B, Sindhaghatta V, Chilimuri S. Successful Management of Pancreatic Ascites with both Conservative Management and Pancreatic Duct Stenting. Gastroenterology Res. 2009;2(4):245-7.

7. All of the following are causes of pseudoascites (PA) *except*:

A. Mesenteric cyst
B. Retroperitoneal lymphangioma
C. Biliary ascites
D. Omental cyst

EXPLANATION

Pseudoascites is an uncommon cause of abdominal distention mimicking ascites. When PA is caused by large abdominal cysts, it is difficult to distinguish from simple ascites because of the presence of an ultra-thin wall and large liquid collection. It can present both in adult and pediatric patients. Its etiology comprises mostly benign conditions. The most common entities are cystic lymphangiomas, mesenteric and omental cysts, renal cysts, cystadenomas and ovarian cysts, mesothelial cysts, enteric cysts, mature cystic teratomas, and pancreatic or traumatic cysts. Sometimes a PA can be secondary to an infection, as for example of hydatid cyst. Because the diagnosis of a PA is usually not evoked primarily, and because a positive diagnosis is difficult, most PA patients experience a significant delay in the identification of their condition. Another radiological sign is the way the fluid is distributed while it accumulates in the peritoneal cavity. A free ascites occupies any disposable space (firstly the Morison's pouch and the Douglas space, then the upper abdominal quadrants and the whole cavity) separating progressively any organ from the abdominal wall. There are however some specific areas, i.e., the space between the diaphragm and the liver—where a free ascites is found and which distinguishes the latter from a large abdominal cyst—that usually does not extend in that space. Biliary ascites is ascites caused by rupture of bile duct and leakage of its content in peritoneal cavity. Here, bile floats freely in liver, hence its true ascites.

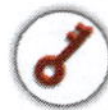

Key: C

BOOST YOUR KNOWLEDGE

Etiology of pseudoascites in children:
- Omental cyst
- Mesenteric cyst
- Ovarian cyst
- Filariasis
- Cerebrospinal fluid (CSF)—cyst in vicinity of ventriculoperitoneal shunt
- Cystic mesothelioma

REFERENCE/SOURCE

- Sathiyasekaran M, Ganesh R. Ascites. In: Gupta P, Menon PSN, Ramji S, Lodha R (Eds). PG Textbook of Pediatrics, 3rd edition. New Delhi: Jaypee Brothers Medical Publishers; 2022.

8. Hemorrhagic ascites is *not* seen in which of the following conditions?

A. Budd–Chiari syndrome (BCS)
B. Malignant ascites
C. Acute pancreatitis
D. Abdominal trauma

EXPLANATION

Acute pancreatitis can cause hemorrhagic ascites by rupture of pseudoaneurysm, necrosis while malignancy causes hemorrhagic ascites by involvement of blood vessels. Abdominal trauma causes hemorrhagic ascites by rupture of major vessels. BCS causes ascites due to postsinusoidal portal hypertension. Ascitic fluid in BCS is clear fluid.

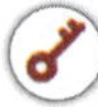

Key: A

BOOST YOUR KNOWLEDGE

Budd–Chiari syndrome is a vascular disorder of liver, characterized by obstruction of the hepatic venous outflow. The obstruction may be thrombotic or nonthrombotic anywhere along the venous course from hepatic vein to junction of inferior vena cava to right atrium. Hepatic veno-occlusive disease and structural cardiac disorders are excluded from this definition. BCS is considered primary or secondary depending on the origin of the obstructive lesion. If obstruction is the result of endoluminal venous lesion-like thrombosis, primary BCS is considered. In secondary BCS, the cause originates from neighboring structures like extrinsic compression or tumor invasion. BCS usually present with reaccumulating ascites with prominent abdominal vein, organomegaly, or gastrointestinal (GI) bleeding. Fulminant presentation with abdominal pain and liver failure is uncommon. It is rare but a potentially treatable cause of portal hypertension with favorable prognosis with various radiological interventions.

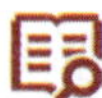

REFERENCE/SOURCE

- Sathiyasekaran M, Ganesh R. Ascites. In: Gupta P, Menon PSN, Ramji S, Lodha R (Eds). PG Textbook of Pediatrics, 3rd edition. New Delhi: Jaypee Brothers Medical Publishers; 2022.

9. A child presented with fever, anorexia, and weight loss for past 4 months. Examination revealed ascites and an enlarged axillary lymph node. Which of the following is typically expected in the ascitic fluid analysis?

A. SAAG of 0.9
B. Low LDH elevated
C. Positive mycobacterial culture of ascitic fluid
D. Adenosine deaminase (ADA) (20 U/L)

EXPLANATION

Ascitic fluid analysis shows turbid appearance grossly and on standing for some time, forms a cobweb coagulum. Total leukocyte count of ascitic fluid is mostly elevated with a predominance of lymphocytic cells. Ascitic fluid total protein is >3 g/dL with SAAG is <1.1 g/dL in peritoneal tuberculosis. Ascitic fluid ADA >39 U/L and elevated LDH can be used as adjunct test in diagnosis. Ascitic fluid acid-fast bacillus (AFB) stain positivity is seen in <3% cases. Ascitic fluid mycobacterial culture (after centrifugation) is positive in only 20% of cases. Laparoscopy with histology and culture of peritoneal biopsies has better sensitivity. Gastric lavage for AFB and positive Mantoux test are useful supportive investigations. Serological tests and nucleic acid amplification [e.g., polymerase chain reaction (PCR)] are not useful.

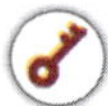

Key: A

BOOST YOUR KNOWLEDGE

Abdominal tuberculosis consists of tuberculosis of intestine, peritoneum/omentum, mesentery, lymph node, and other solid organs such as liver, spleen, and pancreas. Peritoneal tuberculosis (TB) can be wet type (with ascites/loculated ascites) or dry type (adhesion and abdominal cocoon) or fibrotic type with omental caking. Ascitic fluid analysis can provide many diagnostic clues—Cobweb formation, lymphocytic predominance, elevated ADA level, and positive mycobacterial culture. Yield of GeneXpert testing of ascitic fluid is very low, hence not routinely recommended.

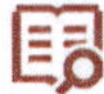

REFERENCES/SOURCES

- Lodha R, Kabra SK, Seth V. Essential of Tuberculosis in Children, 5th edition. New Delhi: Jaypee Brothers Medical Publishers; 2022.
- Meena RK, Ray S. Abdominal tuberculosis. In: Gupta P, Menon PSN, Ramji S, Lodha R (Eds). PG Textbook of Pediatrics, 3rd edition. New Delhi: Jaypee Brothers Medical Publishers; 2022.

10. Which of the following solid organ/system is most commonly involved in abdominal tuberculosis?

A. Genitourinary system
B. Hepatobiliary system
C. Spleen
D. Pancreas

EXPLANATION

The tubercle bacillus reaches the GI system by hematogenous spread from the primary lung focus, ingestion of bacilli from the sputum from an active pulmonary focus, direct spread from adjacent organs, or through lymph channels from infected abdominal nodes. Ileocecal region is commonly involved. Mesenteric and peritoneal tuberculosis are seen in approximately one-third of patients. The initial infection is localized to the Peyer's patches leading to local ulcers followed by mesenteric lymphadenitis and peritonitis. Intestinal tuberculosis is commonly classified as ulcerative, ulcerohyperplastic, and hyperplastic forms. Isolated involvement of abdominal solid organs is relatively uncommon and occurs in 15–20% of all patients with abdominal tuberculosis. The genitourinary system is the most involved followed by liver, spleen, and pancreas. Solid organs get involved by the tubercle bacillus leading to formation of tuberculoma. Esophageal tuberculosis is rare (0.2% of all cases). It occurs mainly by extension of disease from adjacent intrathoracic lymph nodes. Duodenal tuberculosis is also rare (1% of abdominal tuberculosis cases), presenting as stricture. Abdominal tuberculosis can also present as malabsorption. Involvement of colon, rectum and anal canal in tuberculosis is rare.

Key: A

BOOST YOUR KNOWLEDGE

Spectrum of abdominal tuberculosis			
Intestinal tuberculosis	***Peritoneal tuberculosis***	***Lymph nodal tuberculosis***	***Solid organs***
Ulcerative (mostly in malnourished children)	Wet type (ascites)	Mesenteric	Liver
Hypertrophic (in healthy children)	Dry plastic type (adhesion)	Peripancreatic and periportal	Spleen
Ulcerohypertrophic	Fibrotic type (omental caking)	Retroperitoneal	Pancreas

REFERENCES/SOURCES

- Lodha R, Kabra SK, Seth V. Essential of Tuberculosis in Children, 5th edition. New Delhi: Jaypee Brothers Medical Publishers; 2022.
- Meena RK, Ray S. Abdominal tuberculosis. In: Gupta P, Menon PSN, Ramji S, Lodha R (Eds). PG Textbook of Pediatrics, 3rd edition. New Delhi: Jaypee Brothers Medical Publishers; 2022.

11. In congenital tuberculosis, most commonly involved organ is:

A. Liver
B. Ileocecal region
C. Lungs
D. Peritoneum

EXPLANATION

Congenital tuberculosis is rare. Congenital infection depends on the presence and intensity of hematogenous dissemination of *Mycobacterium tuberculosis* during pregnancy, resulting in infection of the placenta or maternal genital tract. Transmission to the fetus occurs by hematogenous spread from the placenta or aspiration or ingestion of amniotic fluid. In hematogenous congenital tuberculosis, *M. tuberculosis* reaches the fetus via the umbilical vein and disseminates widely. If bacilli infect the liver, a primary focus develops, with involvement of periportal lymph nodes. Hematogenous primary focus in the fetal lung usually remains dormant until after birth, when oxygenation and circulation increase significantly. Congenital infection of the infant also occurs via aspiration or ingestion of infected amniotic fluid. The most common manifestations are respiratory distress, fever, hepatosplenomegaly, poor feeding, lethargy or irritability, lymphadenopathy, abdominal distention, ear drainage, and skin lesions.

Key: A

BOOST YOUR KNOWLEDGE

Cantwell et al. proposed diagnosis of congenital tuberculosis in the presence of proven tuberculous disease and at least one of the following:

- Lesions in the newborn baby during the first week of life
- A primary hepatic complex or caseating hepatic granulomata
- Tuberculous infection of the placenta or the maternal genital tract
- Exclusion of the possibility of postnatal transmission by investigation of contacts, including hospital staff

REFERENCES/SOURCES

- Lodha R, Kabra SK, Seth V. Essential of Tuberculosis in Children, 5th edition. New Delhi: Jaypee Brothers Medical Publishers; 2022.
- Mittal H, Das S, Faridi MM. Management of newborn infant born to mother suffering from tuberculosis: current recommendations and gaps in knowledge. Indian J Med Res. 2014;140:32-9.

12. Which of the following is the most common type of ulcer in intestinal TB on colonoscopy?

A. Serpiginous ulcer
B. Linear ulcers
C. Aphthous ulcers
D. Circumferential ulcer

EXPLANATION

On colonoscopy, mucosal nodules of variable sizes and ulcers in segments of colon, ulcer between nodules, and deformed, edematous and wide gaping of ileocecal valve, are characteristic. Ulcers in intestinal tuberculosis are usually transversely oriented/circumferential contrast to Crohn's disease where there is linear and serpiginous ulcers. Linear ulcers can rarely be seen in intestinal tuberculosis (<10%); however, aphthous ulcer has not been reported. Biopsies should be taken from the edge of the ulcers. The characteristic caseous granulomas are seen only in about one-third of cases. While AFB staining has a variable yield, cultures are rarely positive. Culture positivity is seen in 40% cases. Combination of histology and culture improves diagnostic yield to 60%. GeneXpert testing of colonic tissue from ulcer site is recommended.

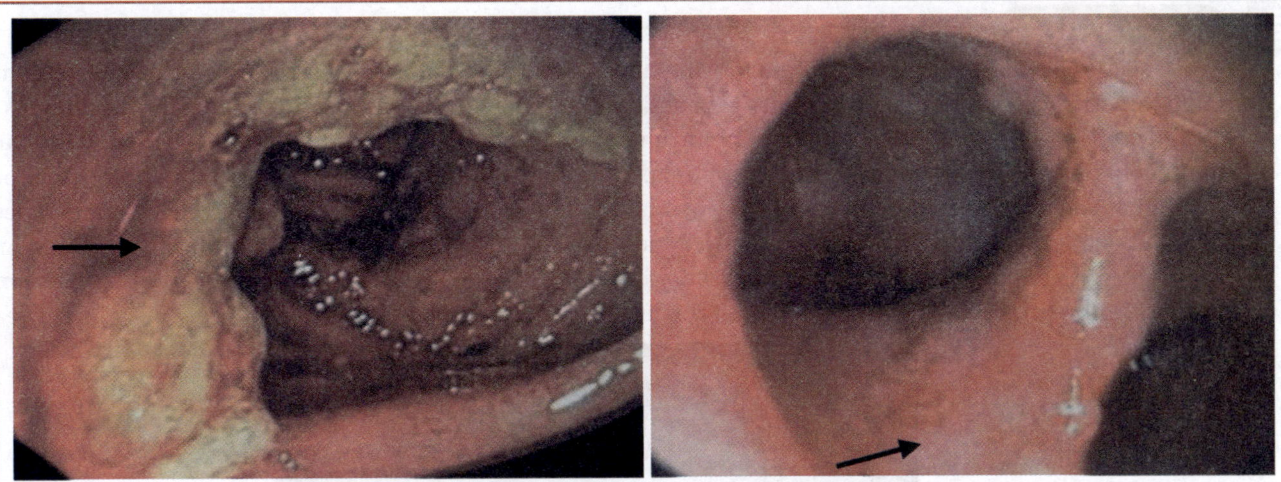

Courtesy: Dr Arghya Samanta, Department of Pediatric Gastroenterology, Sanjay Gandhi Postgraduate Institute of Medical Sciences, Lucknow, Uttar Pradesh, India

Key: D

BOOST YOUR KNOWLEDGE

In intestinal tuberculosis, there is submucosal expansion of tubercles → endarteritis → subsequent denudation → deep ulcer. Superficial ulcers are uncommon which are mostly seen in ulcerative colitis.

Endoscopic features of intestinal tuberculosis and Crohn's disease

Intestinal tuberculosis	*Crohn's disease*
Deep and circumferential ulcers	Deep serpiginous and linear ulcers
Occasionally linear ulcer	Stellate/bear-claw ulcers
Pseudopolyps	Pseudopolyps
Cobblestoning uncommon	Cobblestoning common
Ileocecal involvement common	Can be seen
Aphthous ulcer extremely rare	More common
Internal fistula can be seen	More common
Skip lesion can be seen	More common
Perianal sinus, fistula, and abscess less common	More common

REFERENCE/SOURCE

- Lodha R, Kabra SK, Seth V. Essential of Tuberculosis in Children, 5th edition. New Delhi: Jaypee Brothers Medical Publishers; 2022.

13. Which of the following is the most common feature of abdominal tuberculosis in CT scan?

A. Involvement of retropharyngeal lymph nodes
B. Homogeneous enhancement
C. Comb sign
D. Omental caking

EXPLANATION

Cross-sectional imaging is useful in diagnosing abdominal tuberculosis. Mesenteric and periportal lymph nodes are involved more often in patients with abdominal tuberculous, while retroperitoneal lymph nodes are more with lymphoma. While peripheral enhancement is seen more often in tuberculous lymphadenopathy, homogeneous enhancement suggests lymphoma. Smooth and uniform thickening with nodularity of peritoneum as well as loculated ascites is seen. The omentum is often smudged and nodular, giving appearance of omental caking. Space-occupying lesions in liver and spleen are also a characteristic feature seen in CT abdomen in patients of abdominal tuberculosis. Mesentery is often thickened with conglomerated and necrotic lymph nodes. Comb sign is a radiological sign due to congestion of mesenteric vessels which is seen in Crohn's disease.

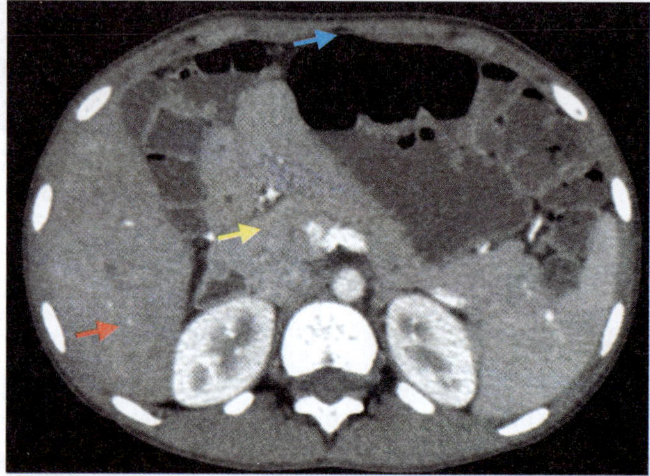

Courtesy: Dr Arghya Samanta, Department of Pediatric Gastroenterology, Sanjay Gandhi Postgraduate Institute of Medical Sciences, Lucknow, Uttar Pradesh, India

- Peritoneum *(blue arrow)*—smooth and uniform thickening
- Omentum—smudged and omental caking
- Necrotic lymph node (*yellow arrow*)
- Space-occupying lesion in liver (*red arrow*)

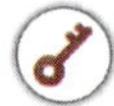

Key: D

BOOST YOUR KNOWLEDGE

Radiological difference between abdominal tuberculosis and Crohn's disease

Abdominal tuberculosis	***Crohn's disease***
Ileocecal region most common site involved	Can involve any site of bowel
Mural thickening without stratification	Mural thickening with stratification
Short segment (<3 cm) stricture	Multifocal long segment (>3 cm) wall involvement with skip area
Concentric stricture	Eccentric stricture
Fibrofatty proliferation of mesentery rare	Fibrofatty proliferation of mesentery common
Mesenteric inflammation but no vascular engorgement	Hypervascular mesentery (comb sign)
Large and hypodense lymph node with peripheral enhancement	Small, isodense, and nonenhancing lymph node
Loculated ascites	No ascites
Space-occupying lesion in liver and spleen	No space-occupying lesion in liver and spleen

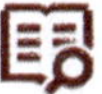

REFERENCES/SOURCES

- Lodha R, Kabra SK, Seth V. Essential of Tuberculosis in Children, 5th edition. New Delhi: Jaypee Brothers Medical Publishers; 2022.
- Meena RK, Ray S. Abdominal tuberculosis. In: Gupta P, Menon PSN, Ramji S, Lodha R (Eds). PG Textbook of Pediatrics, 3rd edition. New Delhi: Jaypee Brothers Medical Publishers; 2022.

14. Terminal ileum is the most involved area in intestinal tuberculosis. Which of the following is responsible for the same?

A. Maximum digestive activity
B. Paucity of lymphatic tissues
C. Increased permeability
D. Increased intestinal motility

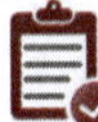

EXPLANATION

The most common site of GI tract involvement in abdominal tuberculosis is the ileocecal region. The terminal ileum is more commonly involved because of the various contributing factors such as:

- Increased physiological stasis due to ileal break (organisms get more time to stay in contact with intestinal mucosa and thus more time for invading mucosa)
- Presence of abundant lymphoid tissue (Peyer's patches which is the portal of entry for *Mycobacterium*)
- Increased rate of absorption at this site (intestinal permeability is maximum at this site, thus maximum chances of entry of *Mycobacterium* across intestinal mucosa)
- Minimal digestive activity (hence, mycobacteria survives the antimicrobial activity of digestive enzymes and can invades intestinal mucosa)

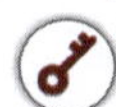

Key: C

BOOST YOUR KNOWLEDGE

Tubercular ulcers tend to be circumferential/transverse and surrounded by inflamed mucosa, with caseating granulomas. In early phases of the intestinal tuberculosis, there is circumferential thickening of the caecum and terminal ileum and a few regional nodes. Later the ileocecal valve and adjacent cecal wall are predominantly and asymmetrically thickened, producing a patulous/distorted ileocecal valve. In more advanced disease, gross wall thickening, adherent loops, large regional nodes, and mesenteric thickening can together form a soft-tissue mass centered around the ileocecal region.

REFERENCES/SOURCES

- Kapoor VK. Abdominal tuberculosis. Postgrad Med J. 1998;74(874):459-67.
- Lodha R, Kabra SK, Seth V. Essential of Tuberculosis in Children, 5th edition. New Delhi: Jaypee Brothers Medical Publishers; 2022.

15. Which of the following usually causes diarrhea in a patient with intestinal tuberculosis?

A. Enterohepatic fistula
B. Bacterial overgrowth in large bowel
C. Decreased bile acid deconjugation
D. Lymphatic obstruction

EXPLANATION

Intestinal tuberculosis is an uncommon cause of chronic diarrhea. Diarrhea occurs owing to malabsorption in intestinal tuberculosis which can be due to various reasons:

- Decreased small intestinal mucosal surface due to extensive ulceration
- Fistula formation between bowel loops
- Stricture formation leading to stagnation and small bowel bacterial overgrowth leading to increased bile acid deconjugation
- Decreased bile acid pool due to impaired active absorption in case of terminal ileum involvement
- Lymphatic obstruction by enlarged lymph nodes leading to secondary intestinal lymphangiectasia

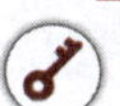

Key: D

BOOST YOUR KNOWLEDGE

Intestinal tuberculosis mostly present with subacute intestinal-like clinical picture. They can also present with bloody diarrhea (in case of colonic involvement), gastric outlet obstruction (duodenal tuberculosis), and bilious vomiting (secondary superior mesenteric artery syndrome due to loss of fat between aorta and superior mesenteric artery). Presentation as chronic small bowel type diarrhea or malabsorption is rare.

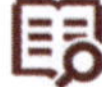

REFERENCES/SOURCES

- Lodha R, Kabra SK, Seth V. Essential of Tuberculosis in Children, 5th edition. New Delhi: Jaypee Brothers Medical Publishers; 2022.
- Thapa BR, Yachha SK, Mehta S. Abdominal tuberculosis. Indian Pediatr. 1991. 28(9):1093-100.

16. A 13-year-old boy was diagnosed as a case of ileocecal tuberculosis and was treated with antitubercular drugs for 6 months. Fever, anorexia, and non-colicky pain abdomen resolved within 4 weeks of starting antitubercular drugs. One year later, he complained of colicky abdominal pain, borborygmi, and ball rolling movements. Which is the most likely cause?

A. Inflammatory stricture
B. Fibrotic stricture
C. Fistula
D. Malrotation

EXPLANATION

Mycobacterium tuberculosis, upon penetration of the intestinal mucosa, initiates a local inflammatory reaction in the submucosal lymphoid tissue. This leads to lymphangitis, granuloma formation, caseation necrosis, mucosal ulceration, and scarring. Strictures in intestinal tuberculosis may be inflammatory or fibrotic, depending predominantly on the activity and duration of the disease. Response of the intestinal strictures to antitubercular therapy is varied as the inflammatory component may get resolved with treatment but also lead to healing and scarring with subsequent persistence of the fibrotic stricture and can present with intestinal obstruction like clinical feature without any constitutional features.

Key: B

BOOST YOUR KNOWLEDGE

Various complications due to intestinal tuberculosis:

- Fistula occurring at different sites (enteroenteric, enterocolic, and enterocutaneous)
- Stricture formation
- Intussusception
- Perforation
- Peritonitis
- Upper and lower GI bleeding
- Malabsorption
- Secondary lymphangiectasia (due to obstruction of lymphatics by enlarged lymph nodes, adhesion, and fibrosis)

REFERENCES/SOURCES

- Jena A, Mohindra R, Rana K, Neelam PB, Thakur DC, Singh H, et al. Frequency, outcomes, and need for intervention in stricturing gastrointestinal tuberculosis: a systematic review and meta-analysis. BMC Gastroenterol. 2023;23(1):46.
- Lodha R, Kabra SK, Seth V. Essential of Tuberculosis in Children, 5th edition. New Delhi: Jaypee Brothers Medical Publishers; 2022.

17. Which of the following is not an indication of surgery in a case of abdominal tuberculosis?

A. Loculated ascites
B. Perforation
C. Stricture leading to obstruction
D. Fistula formation

EXPLANATION

In a patient of abdominal tuberculosis, surgery is essentially reserved for those with acute surgical complications including free perforation, contained perforation with abscess or fistula, massive bleeding, complete obstruction, or obstruction not responding to medical management. Loculated ascites is not an indication for surgery in abdominal tuberculosis.

Key: A

BOOST YOUR KNOWLEDGE

Surgery in a case of abdominal tuberculosis is associated with high morbidity. Hence, abdominal tuberculosis should be managed conservatively unless there is absolute indication of surgery.

Postoperative complications in abdominal tuberculosis:

- Delayed wound healing
- Burst abdomen
- Fecal fistula
- Prolonged ileus
- Adrenal crisis
- Stress gastritis

REFERENCES/SOURCES

- Lodha R, Kabra SK, Seth V. Essential of Tuberculosis in Children, 5th edition. New Delhi: Jaypee Brothers Medical Publishers; 2022.
- Meena RK, Ray S. Abdominal tuberculosis. In: Gupta P, Menon PSN, Ramji S, Lodha R (Eds). PG Textbook of Pediatrics, 3rd edition. New Delhi: Jaypee Brothers Medical Publishers; 2022.

18. A patient with cirrhosis with Child-Turcotte-Pugh (CTP) score of 8, developed pulmonary tuberculosis. Which of the following antitubercular drug regimen will be most suitable for this patient?

A. Regimen with no potentially hepatotoxic drug
B. Regimen with one potentially hepatotoxic drug
C. Regimen with two potentially hepatotoxic drugs
D. Regimen with three potentially hepatotoxic drugs

EXPLANATION

Likelihood of drug-induced liver injury (DILI) is higher in patients of cirrhosis and the outcome of DILI in patients of cirrhosis may be serious, even fatal. The American Thoracic Society has given guidelines on use of antitubercular drugs in cirrhosis in 2016.

CTP score	*Liver disease status*	*Treatment*	*Antitubercular drug regimen and duration*
≤7, Class A	Stable	Regimen with two potentially hepatotoxic drug (rifampicin + isoniazid/pyrazinamide)	Rifampicin + isoniazid + ethambutol for 2 months followed by rifampicin + isoniazid for 7 months or rifampicin + pyrazinamide + ethambutol for 6 months
8–11, Class B	Advanced	Regimen with only one potentially hepatotoxic drug (rifampicin or isoniazid)	Rifampicin or isoniazid + ethambutol + streptomycin + quinolone or cycloserine for 12–18 months
>11, Class C	Very advanced	Regimen with no potentially hepatotoxic drug	Ethambutol + streptomycin + quinolone or cycloserine for ≥18 months

Key: B

BOOST YOUR KNOWLEDGE

Potentially hepatotoxic antitubercular drugs	
First-line drugs	***Second-line drugs***
• Isoniazid • Rifampicin • Pyrazinamide	• Ethionamide • Para-amino salicylic acid (PAS)

REFERENCES/SOURCES

- Kumar N, Kedarisetty CK, Kumar SK, Khillan V, Sarin SK, et al. Antitubercular therapy in patients with cirrhosis: challenges and options. World J Gastroenterol. 2014;20:5760-72.
- Nahid P, Dorman SE, Alipanah N, Barry PM, Brozek JL, Cattamanchi A, et al. Official American Thoracic Society/Centers for Disease Control and Prevention/Infectious Diseases Society America Clinical Practice Guidelines: Treatment of Drug-Susceptible Tuberculosis. Clin Infect Dis. 2016;63(7):e147-95.

19. Which of the following is true for tuberculosis in chronic liver disease?

A. ADA for diagnosis of tuberculosis in cirrhosis with ascites has high sensitivity
B. Tuberculin skin testing is sensitive for the diagnosis of tuberculosis in cirrhotic patients
C. Likelihood of antitubercular drug-induced hepatotoxicity is higher in preexisting liver disease patients
D. Isoniazid-induced hepatotoxicity is more common in fast acetylators

EXPLANATION

Cirrhotic patients demonstrate impaired delayed-type hypersensitivity; hence, there is a higher likelihood of false-negative tuberculin test results. Although ADA level is generally helpful in the detection of tubercular peritonitis, the presence of cirrhosis may reduce its sensitivity to 30%.

In the setting of preexisting liver disease, the likelihood of developing drug-induced hepatitis may be higher. Also, the outcome of drug-induced hepatitis in patients with compromised liver function may be poor. Monitoring of drug-induced hepatitis may be confounded in the presence of underlying liver disease due to fluctuating liver function tests related to the preexisting liver disease.

Fast acetylators clear acetyl hydrazine more rapidly compared to slow acetylators and thus have lesser risk of drug-induced hepatic injury.

Key: C

BOOST YOUR KNOWLEDGE

Isoniazid metabolism: In the metabolism in isoniazid in liver, two enzymes are most important, i.e., amidase and N-acetyltransferase 2. Among these two enzymes, N-acetyltransferase 2 has genetic polymorphism in the general population—fast acetylators and slow acetylators. In persons with fast acetylator, >90% of drug is excreted as acetyl isoniazid which is nontoxic while only 67% is excreted as acetyl isoniazid. Fast acetylators clear acetyl hydrazine (which is toxic) more rapidly compared to slow acetylators. Thus, slow acetylators are at higher risk of developing isoniazid-induced hepatotoxicity.

REFERENCES/SOURCES

- Kumar N, Kedarisetty CK, Kumar SK, Khillan V, Sarin SK, et al. Antitubercular therapy in patients with cirrhosis: challenges and options. World J Gastroenterol. 2014;20:5760-72.
- National Tuberculosis Elimination Programme. Pediatric TB Management Guideline 2022. New Delhi: National Tuberculosis Elimination Programme, Ministry of Health and Family Welfare; 2022.

20. A child presents with history of right iliac fossa pain and vomiting for last 5 days. 3 days later, he develops fever, a lump in the right iliac fossa, and localized abdominal tenderness. What would be the most appropriate next line of management?

A. Emergency appendicectomy
B. Intravenous antibiotics followed by interval appendicectomy
C. Intravenous antibiotics for 7 days and conservative management
D. Exploratory laparotomy

EXPLANATION

Appendicitis remains the most common acute surgical condition of the abdomen in children. Luminal obstruction due to fecalith remains the most common cause of acute appendicitis. Salient clinical features of acute appendicitis are right iliac fossa pain, nausea and vomiting, fever associated with tachycardia, and elevated leukocyte count. The gold standard treatment for appendicitis is laparoscopic appendicectomy. The gold standard treatment for appendicitis is prompt surgery. Majority of the appendicitis today are operated by laparoscopic methods. If not treated in time acute appendicitis may lead to complications such as perforation and peritonitis.

Once the diagnosis of appendicitis is confirmed or highly suspected, the standard treatment for acute appendicitis is most often prompt appendectomy. In patients in whom perforated appendicitis is identified at the time of diagnosis, the operation is even less urgent and proper preoperative management is more critical. Based on the patient's status, findings on CT scan, and availability of experienced radiologists, the initial plan may be percutaneous drainage of fluid collections by interventional radiology and continued fluid resuscitation and antibiotics. An inflammatory mass (phlegmon) without an identifiable fluid component might initially respond to nonoperative management with fluids and antibiotics. Placement of one or more drainage catheters under imaging (CT or ultrasound) guidance has been successful in >80% of patients. Most pediatric surgeons recommend delayed appendectomy (during the same hospitalization) or interval appendectomy (4–6 weeks after the initial presentation).

Key: B

BOOST YOUR KNOWLEDGE

Diagnostic laparoscopy and laparoscopic appendectomy (minimally invasive technique) for both simple and perforated appendicitis are the preferred approaches in most pediatric centers; the open surgery is still performed but in selected cases. Laparoscopic appendectomy has significant advantages in administrative factors (cost, resource utilization, and length of stay), and slight improvement in clinical outcome measures (wound infection rate, intra-abdominal abscess, analgesic requirements, and return to full activity).

REFERENCES/SOURCES

- Acute appendicitis. In: Kliegman RM, Stanton BF, St Geme JW III, Schor NF (Eds). Nelson Textbook of Pediatrics, 20th edition. Amsterdam, Netherlands: Elsevier; 2016.
- Agarwal P. Appendicitis. In: Gupta P, Menon PSN, Ramji S, Lodha R (Eds). PG Textbook of Pediatrics, 3rd edition. New Delhi: Jaypee Brothers Medical Publishers; 2022.

21. Which of the following is a characteristic radiological feature of acute appendicitis on ultrasonography?

A. A compressible open-ended tube
B. Outer diameter of appendix >10 mm
C. Hypoechoic appendicolith
D. Loss of submucosal echogenicity

EXPLANATION

Acute appendicitis is an acute inflammation of the vermiform appendix. Ultrasonography is the initial imaging modality while CT abdomen is the most sensitive modality to detect appendicitis. In a case of acute appendicitis, we find an inflamed appendix which looks like a noncompressible blind ending tube. Edema of the walls of appendix leads to thickened wall diameter (>3 mm for a single wall or >6 mL for both wall/outer diameter of appendix). Because of inflammation and edema, there is loss of submucosal echogenicity of appendix.

Key: D

BOOST YOUR KNOWLEDGE

Radiological findings supportive of the diagnosis of appendicitis include:

- A peristaltic, noncompressible, and dilated appendix (>6 mm outer diameter)
- Hyperechoic appendicolith with posterior acoustic shadowing
- *Distinct appendiceal wall layers:*
  - Implies non-necrotic (catarrhal or phlegmon) stage
  - Loss of wall stratification with necrotic (gangrenous) stages
- Loss of submucosal echogenicity
- Echogenic prominent pericecal and periappendiceal fat
- *Periappendiceal hyperechoic structure:* Amorphous hyperechoic structure (usually >10 mm) seen surrounding a noncompressible appendix with a diameter >6 mm
- Periappendiceal fluid collection
- Target sign
- Periappendiceal reactive nodal prominence/enlargement
- Single wall thickening (3 mm or above)

REFERENCES/SOURCES

- Acute appendicitis. In: Kliegman RM, Stanton BF, St Geme JW III, Schor NF (Eds). Nelson Textbook of Pediatrics, 20th edition. Amsterdam, Netherlands: Elsevier; 2016.
- Agarwal P. Appendicitis. In: Gupta P, Menon PSN, Ramji S, Lodha R (Eds). PG Textbook of Pediatrics, 3rd edition. New Delhi: Jaypee Brothers Medical Publishers; 2022.

SECTION 17

Hepatology

Section Editor: *Moinak Sen Sarma*

Hepatobiliary System

Vipul Gautam, Moinak Sen Sarma

1. The hepatobiliary system develops from the cells of ventral foregut endoderm. This part of the endoderm acquires competence to receive signals arising from the:

A. Cardiac mesoderm
B. Neural crest cells
C. Ectoderm
D. Metanephros

EXPLANATION

Ventral foregut endoderm gives rise to the lung, liver, and ventral pancreatic diverticula. Ventral wall of foregut endoderm is positioned adjacent to developing heart. Signals from heart (cardiac mesoderm) induce underlying endoderm to initiate its development toward hepatic fate.

Key: A

BOOST YOUR KNOWLEDGE

During the early embryonic process of gastrulation, the three embryonic germ layers (endoderm, mesoderm, and ectoderm) are formed. The liver and biliary system arises from cells of the ventral foregut endoderm (3.5 weeks); their development can be divided into three distinct processes. First, the ventral foregut endoderm acquires competence to receive signals arising from the cardiac mesoderm as shown in the given Figure. These mesodermal signals lead to specification of cells that have the potential to form the liver and activate liver-specific genes. Newly specified cells then delaminate from the ventral foregut endoderm and migrate in a cranial ventral direction into the septum transversum in the fourth week of human gestation to initiate liver morphogenesis. The given Table summarizes the timeline of liver development.

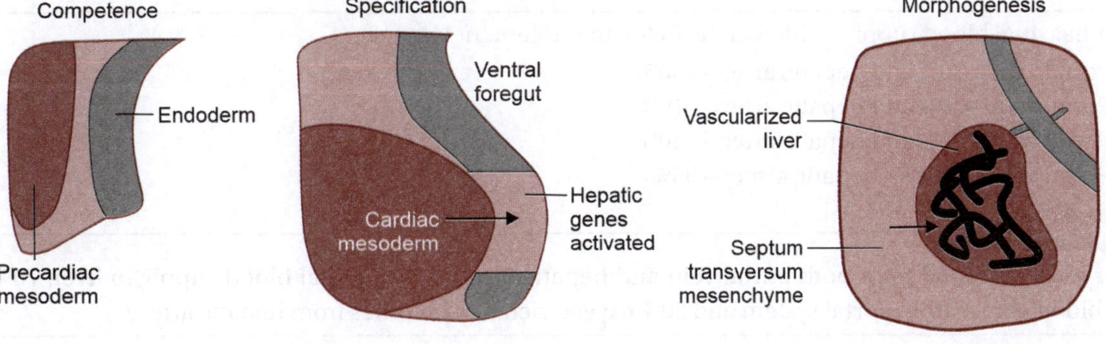

Developmental age (weeks)	*Characteristic*
3–4	Hepatic diverticulum appears as an evagination of the foregut
5	Umbilical veins connect with the developing hepatic sinusoids. Ductal plate begins to form
6	Hematopoiesis begins
7	Definitive venous pattern established within the liver
9	Liver accounts for 10% of fetal weight
12	Remodeling of the ductal plate. Bile formation begins
16	Major bile ducts formed at porta hepatis
36	Hematopoiesis reduced to small widely spaced *islands*

REFERENCES/SOURCES

- Gupta P, Menon PSN, Ramji S, Lodha R. PG Textbook of Pediatrics, 3rd edition. New Delhi: Jaypee Brothers Medical Publishers; 2022. p. 1861.
- Kliegman RM, Stanton BF, St Geme JW III, Schor NF. Nelson Textbook of Pediatrics, 20th edition. Amsterdam, Netherlands: Elsevier; 2016. pp. 1918-9.

2. Which of the following is the fixed macrophage found in liver?

A. Stellate cells
B. Kupffer cells
C. Sinusoidal endothelial cells
D. Cholangiocyte

EXPLANATION

Kupffer cells constitute almost 90% of the total fixed macrophages in the body and 20% of the nonparenchymal cells in the liver.

Key: B

BOOST YOUR KNOWLEDGE

Kupffer cells are ameboid-shaped and are attached to the sinusoidal endothelial cells. These cells are derived from circulating monocytes and reside in the periportal area in the sinusoids of liver. They function to clear endotoxins from the passing blood and to phagocytose debris, microorganisms, and apoptotic hepatocytes.

REFERENCE/SOURCE

- Chaudhry S, Emond J, Griesemer A. Immune Cell Trafficking to the Liver. Transplantation. 2019;103(7):1323-37.

3. Liver has dual blood supply. Which of the following statement is true?

A. Portal vein—70% and hepatic artery—30%
B. Portal vein—30% and hepatic artery—70%
C. Portal vein—50% and hepatic artery—50%
D. Portal vein—5% and hepatic artery—95%

EXPLANATION

Liver receives blood from both portal vein and hepatic artery. Of the total blood supply to liver, 70% nutrient rich blood comes from portal system and 30% oxygen rich blood comes from hepatic artery.

Key: A

BOOST YOUR KNOWLEDGE

A portal system is one, which begins and ends with capillaries. Portal vein is a large vein which collects blood from abdominal part of gut, gallbladder, pancreas, spleen, and conveys it to the liver. Splenic vein and superior mesenteric vein combine to form portal vein. After entering the liver, each branch of portal vein divides and redivides along with the hepatic artery to end ultimately in the hepatic sinusoids, where the portal venous blood mixes with the hepatic arterial blood.

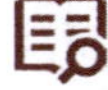

REFERENCES/SOURCES

- Chaurasia BD. BD Chaurasia's Human Anatomy, 8th edition. New Delhi: CBS Publishers and Distributors (P) Ltd; 2021. p. 331.
- Gupta P, Menon PSN, Ramji S, Lodha R. PG Textbook of Pediatrics, 3rd edition. New Delhi: Jaypee Brothers Medical Publishers; 2022. p. 1861.

4. Ductal plate malformation in the liver histology is seen in which of the following?

A. Bile acid synthetic defect
B. Congenital hepatic fibrosis
C. Progressive familial intrahepatic cholestasis (PFIC)
D. Alagille syndrome

EXPLANATION

Ductal plate malformation is a histological feature of a variety of liver diseases, such as congenital hepatic fibrosis, Caroli disease, and biliary atresia.

Key: B

BOOST YOUR KNOWLEDGE

Around the eighth week of gestation, starting at the hilum of the liver, primitive hepatoblasts adjacent to the mesenchyme around the portal vein branches form a cylindrical sleeve, termed the ductal plate. From 12 weeks of gestation onward, a "remodeling" of the ductal plate occurs, with some segments of the ductal plate undergoing tubular dilation and excess ductal plate cells gradually disappearing. The ramification of the biliary tree continues throughout human fetal life and at the time of birth the most peripheral branches of the portal veins are still surrounded by ductal plates; these require 4 more weeks to develop into definitive portal ducts. Lack of remodeling of the ductal plate results in persistence of primitive ductal plate configurations, an abnormality called ductal plate malformation.

REFERENCE/SOURCE

- Kliegman RM, Stanton BF, St Geme JW III, Schor NF. Nelson Textbook of Pediatrics, 20th edition. Amsterdam, Netherlands: Elsevier; 2016. pp. 1918-9.

5. Liver is the main site of protein synthesis. Which of the following statements is true?

A. Albumin level is high in a neonate reaching adult levels after several months
B. Infantile levels of ceruloplasmin and complement factors decrease slowly to adult values
C. Serum α-fetoprotein is high in the early infantile period
D. Synthesis of albumin is proportionate to that of α-fetoprotein

EXPLANATION

Synthesis of albumin appears at approximately the 7th–8th week in the human fetus and increases in inverse proportion to that of α-fetoprotein, which is the dominant fetal protein. Albumin concentrations are low in a neonate (~2.5 g/dL), reaching adult levels (~3.5 g/dL) after several months. Levels of ceruloplasmin and complement factors increase slowly to adult values in the first year.

Key: C

BOOST YOUR KNOWLEDGE

The postnatal patterns of protein synthesis vary with the class of protein. Lipoproteins of each class rise abruptly in the first week after birth to reach levels that vary little until puberty. Transferrin levels at birth are similar to those of an adult, decline for 3–5 months, and rise thereafter to achieve their final concentrations. Low levels of activity of specific proteins have implications for the nutrition of an infant. A low level of cystathionine γ-lyase (cystathionase) activity impairs the trans-sulfuration pathway by which dietary methionine is converted to cysteine. Consequently, the latter must be supplied in the diet. Similar dietary requirements might exist for other sulfur-containing amino acids, such as taurine.

REFERENCE/SOURCE

- Kliegman RM, Stanton BF, St Geme JW III, Schor NF. Nelson Textbook of Pediatrics, 20th edition. Amsterdam, Netherlands: Elsevier; 2016. pp. 1919-20.

6. Which of the following is correct for the given Figure?

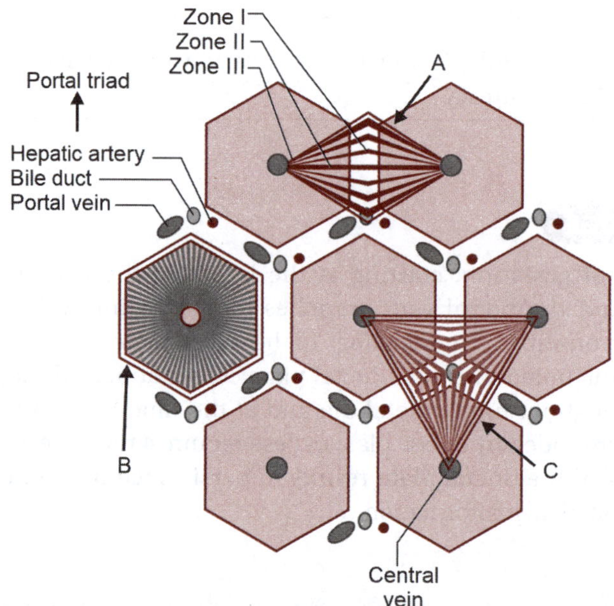

A. A—portal acinus, B—hepatic lobule, and C—portal lobule
B. A—portal lobule, B—hepatic lobule, and C—portal acinus
C. A—hepatic lobule, B—portal acinus, and C—portal lobule
D. A—portal lobule, B—portal acinus, and C—hepatic lobule

EXPLANATION

The parenchyma of liver is composed of several hepatic lobules. Each hepatic lobule is a hexagonal structural unit with hepatocytes arranged in the form of sheets or cords radiating outward from a central vein like the spokes of a wheel. Another way of considering the function is a triangular or biliary unit known as portal lobule, the corners of which are formed of three central veins. The third unit of structure function is the portal acinus. Each acinus is a diamond-shaped unit connecting the two adjacent hepatic lobules.

Key: A

BOOST YOUR KNOWLEDGE

Each hepatic/portal acinus is divided into three zones. There is an oxygen gradient (from high to low) between zones I, II, and III. The cells of the zone III, being least oxygenated, are the first to undergo necrosis due to ischemia or drug reaction. After a meal, glycogen will be stored first in the zone I, later in the zone II, and finally in the zone III. The reverse is true when glucose is needed: Zone III is depleted of its glycogen first, followed by zones II and I.

REFERENCE/SOURCE

- Gupta P, Menon PSN, Ramji S, Lodha R. PG Textbook of Pediatrics, 3rd edition. New Delhi: Jaypee Brothers Medical Publishers; 2022. pp. 1757-8.

7. Cholesterol is excreted from the body via:

A. Urine
B. Sweat
C. Bile
D. Lungs

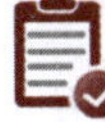

EXPLANATION

Bile is also the only route by which the body can dispose of cholesterol—either in its native form, or after conversion into bile acids.

Key: C

BOOST YOUR KNOWLEDGE

Some of the components of the bile, especially the bile acids and bile salts, are reabsorbed in the intestine and then excreted again by the liver (enterohepatic circulation). It is estimated that bile acids may be recycled up to 20 times before finally being excreted. Bile serves as a critical excretory fluid by which the body disposes of lipid-soluble end products of metabolism as well as lipid-soluble xenobiotics (compounds that are foreign to an organism or are not part of nutrition, e.g., drugs and food additives).

REFERENCE/SOURCE

- Gupta P, Menon PSN, Ramji S, Lodha R. PG Textbook of Pediatrics, 3rd edition. New Delhi: Jaypee Brothers Medical Publishers; 2022. pp. 1758-9.

8. Which of the following genes are involved in the embryological development of biliary system?

A. *HNF-1β* and *HNF-6*
B. *ABCB11* and *MYO5B*
C. *ABCB4* and *NR1H4*
D. *ATP8B1* and *TJP2*

EXPLANATION

The development of the intrahepatic biliary tree begins between the 5th and 9th week postfertilization. Biliary epithelium is believed to arise from precursor bipotential hepatoblasts that can differentiate into either hepatocytes or biliary epithelial cells. *HNF-1β* and *HNF-6* genes or gene products regularize this process. The Notch pathway is also involved in bile duct development; the Jagged1/Notch2 interaction may be critical for induction of biliary differentiation and repression of hepatocytic differentiations.

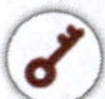

Key: A

BOOST YOUR KNOWLEDGE

Secretion of factors such as bone morphogenic protein (BMP) by the mesenchymal cells of the septum transversum and of fibroblast growth factors (FGFs) by the precardiac mesoderm appear to play an important role in the induction of hepatogenesis.

REFERENCE/SOURCE

- Gupta P, Menon PSN, Ramji S, Lodha R. PG Textbook of Pediatrics, 3rd edition. New Delhi: Jaypee Brothers Medical Publishers; 2022. p. 1861.

9. Which is the most preferred classification of functional liver anatomy?

A. Hailey
B. Bismuth
C. Couinaud
D. Brisbane

EXPLANATION

Liver is divided into eight segments by Claude Couinaud on basis of distribution of portal and hepatic vein as shown in the given Figure. Couinaud lobes were numbered in clockwise fashion from 1 to 8 starting from caudate lobe being segment 1. Segments 1–4 form left lobe and segments 5–8 form the right lobe. Segment anatomy is helpful during surgery, especially tumor resection or for taking graft for liver transplant.

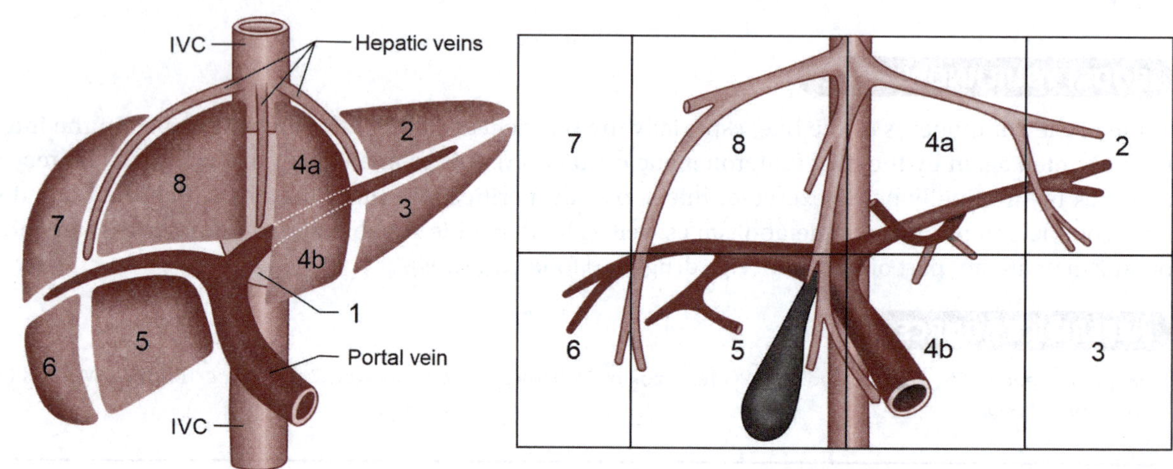

Key: C

BOOST YOUR KNOWLEDGE

The true right and left lobes of the liver are roughly equal size and are not divided by the falciform ligament, but by a plane passing though the bed of gallbladder and the notch of the inferior vena cava (IVC), which is known as Cantlie's line.

REFERENCES/SOURCES

- Gupta P, Menon PSN, Ramji S, Lodha R. PG Textbook of Pediatrics, 3rd edition. New Delhi: Jaypee Brothers Medical Publishers; 2022. p. 1861.
- van Gulik TM, van den Esschert JW. James Cantlie's early messages for hepatic surgeons: how the concept of preoperative portal vein occlusion was defined. HPB (Oxford). 2010;12(2):81-3.

10. Which organ plays the most important role in glycogen storage?

A. Brain
B. Spleen
C. Liver
D. Pancreas

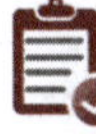

EXPLANATION

Glucose homeostasis is monitored by gut–brain–liver axis. Glucose levels are maintained mainly by the liver. Glucose when in excess gets stored as glycogen in hepatocytes and glycogen gets degraded to glucose during fasting stage.

Key: C

BOOST YOUR KNOWLEDGE

In fetal life, glycogen synthesis starts around 9 weeks of gestation, which increases before birth. After birth, this glycogen is metabolized to glucose preventing hypoglycemia in full-term neonate.

REFERENCE/SOURCE

- Gupta P, Menon PSN, Ramji S, Lodha R. PG Textbook of Pediatrics, 3rd edition. New Delhi: Jaypee Brothers Medical Publishers; 2022. p. 1863.

11. Somatostatins are secreted by which pancreatic cells?

A. Alpha-cells
B. Beta-cells
C. Delta-cells
D. Pancreatic polypeptide (PP) cells

EXPLANATION

Islets of Langerhans are found in abundance near the tail end of the pancreas. Four types of cells constitute the islets, i.e., (1) alpha-cells secreting glucagon, (2) beta-cells secreting insulin, (3) delta-cells secreting somatostatin, and (4) PP-cells secreting pancreatic peptide.

Key: C

BOOST YOUR KNOWLEDGE

Pancreas performs two distinct functions. The exocrine part secretes digestive enzymes and the endocrine part secretes hormones such as insulin and glucagon. The pancreatic juice is alkaline and has high HCO_3 content, which plays an important role in neutralizing the acidity of the chyme emptied from the stomach into the duodenum. The pancreatic enzymes are responsible for the digestion of all three forms of food—carbohydrate, protein, and fat.

REFERENCE/SOURCE

- Gupta P, Menon PSN, Ramji S, Lodha R. PG Textbook of Pediatrics, 3rd edition. New Delhi: Jaypee Brothers Medical Publishers; 2022. p. 1758.

12. Which of the following genes play role in hepatobiliary transport?

A. *ATP8B1*
B. *JAGGED1*
C. *SMN1*
D. *DDR1*

EXPLANATION

Progressive familial intrahepatic cholestasis is an autosomal recessive genetic disease [low to normal γ-glutamyl transpeptidase (GGT) cholestasis]. PFIC is characterized by the defect in the hepatocyte biliary transporters. PFIC type 1 is related to *ATP8B1* gene, PFIC type 2 to *ABCB11*, and PFIC type 3 to *ABCB4*.

Key: A

BOOST YOUR KNOWLEDGE

Progressive familial intrahepatic cholestasis accounts for 3–13% cases of neonatal cholestasis syndrome and accounts for 10–15% of children requiring liver transplantation. PFIC type 2 is the most common subtype.

To summarize:

ATP8B1 gene → FIC1 protein → PFIC type 1 (Byler disease)
ABCB11 gene → BSEP protein → PFIC type 2
ABCB4 gene → MDR3 protein → PFIC type 3 (high GGT PFIC)
TJP2 gene → TJP2 protein → PFIC type 4
NR1H4 gene → FXR protein → PFIC type 5
Myo5B gene → Myosin 5B → PFIC type 6
(BSEP: bile salt export pump; FIC1: familial intrahepatic cholestasis protein 1; FXR: farnesoid X receptor; MDR3: multidrug resistance protein 3; Myo5B: myosin 5B; TJP2: tight junction protein 2)

Summarizing:

Progressive familial intrahepatic cholestasis

	PFIC 1	*PFIC 2*	*PFIC 3*
Inheritance	Autosomal recessive	Autosomal recessive	Autosomal recessive
Mutated protein	FIC1 deficiency	BSEP deficiency	MDR3 deficiency
Gene	*ATP8B1*	*ABCB11*	*ABCB4*
Function	Translocation of aminophospholipids from outer to inner leaflet of lipid bilayer (flippase)	Bile salt transport	Translocation of phosphatidylcholine from inner to outer leaflet of lipid bilayer (floppase)
GGT	Normal	Normal	High
Extrahepatic features	++ (diarrhea, pancreatitis, deafness, and respiratory distress)	–	–
Histology	Bland cholestasis, coarse granular canalicular bile on electron microscopy	Giant cell transformation	Bile ductular proliferation and cholangiolytic changes
Treatment	Biliary diversion, liver transplantation (postliver transplant diarrhea, steatorrhea, and fatty liver)	Biliary diversion and liver transplantation	Ursodeoxycholic acid therapy and liver transplantation

REFERENCES/SOURCES

- Khanna R, Gautam V. Progressive Familial Intrahepatic Cholestasis. Ann Pediatr Gastroenterol Hepatol. 2020;2(2):1-20.
- Kliegman RM, Stanton BF, St Geme JW III, Schor NF. Nelson Textbook of Pediatrics, 20th edition. Amsterdam, Netherlands: Elsevier; 2016. p. 1931.

13. How many portal tracts should be present in an ideal liver biopsy tissue sample?

A. 2
B. 4
C. 5
D. 6

EXPLANATION

Minimum 6 g of liver tissue is considered as adequate and must contain at least six portal tracts. For enzyme analysis, 30 g tissue is required. For copper estimation, 1–2 g of liver tissue is sufficient.

Key: D

BOOST YOUR KNOWLEDGE

Usually, liver biopsy is done via percutaneous approach. In presence of coagulopathy or thrombocytopenia, transjugular approach is preferred. Transjugular biopsy specimen may be small and fragmented, especially in patients with cirrhosis, but are usually adequate for histological diagnosis.

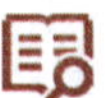

REFERENCE/SOURCE

- Gupta P, Menon PSN, Ramji S, Lodha R. PG Textbook of Pediatrics, 3rd edition. New Delhi: Jaypee Brothers Medical Publishers; 2022. p. 1863.

14. 1 g of hemoglobin produces how much bilirubin?

A. 10 mg
B. 24 mg
C. 34 mg
D. 62 mg

EXPLANATION

Hemoglobin from senescent RBCs is broken down to heme and protein. Heme is then converted into bilirubin, which is unconjugated and in insoluble form. 1 g of hemoglobin produces 34 mg of bilirubin.

Key: C

BOOST YOUR KNOWLEDGE

Unconjugated bilirubin, insoluble form, is taken up by hepatocytes, gets converted by enzyme uridine-5'-diphosphate (UDP) glucuronyl transferase enzyme to soluble form, bilirubin mono- or diglucuronide conjugates which is excreted into canaliculi by canalicular protein multiple drug-resistant protein 2 (MRP 2) against concentration gradient (energy dependent). From canaliculi, conjugated bilirubin is excreted into intestine via bile duct system. In intestine, bilirubin is broken down to stercobilirubin which is excreted into feces and urobilinogen which is reabsorbed by intestine. This reabsorbed urobilinogen either gets excreted into urine or recycled by the liver.

Mutation in MRP2 leads to Dubin-Johnson syndrome.

REFERENCES/SOURCES

- Gupta P, Menon PSN, Ramji S, Lodha R. PG Textbook of Pediatrics, 3rd edition. New Delhi: Jaypee Brothers Medical Publishers; 2022. p. 1863.
- Keitel V, Nies AT, Brom M, Hummel-Eisenbeiss J, Spring H, Keppler D. A common Dubin-Johnson syndrome mutation impairs protein maturation and transport activity of MRP2 (ABCC2). Am J Physiol Gastrointest Liver Physiol. 2003;284(1): G165-74.

15. Normal histology of a portal tract is shown in the given Figure. Identify the correct labels.

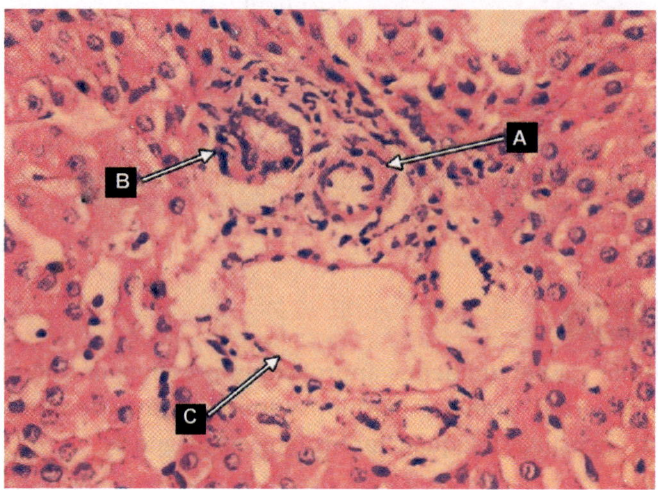

A. A—bile duct, B—portal vein, and C—central vein
B. A—hepatic arteriole, B—bile duct, and C—portal vein branch
C. A—central vein, B—bile duct, and C—portal vein branch
D. A—portal vein branch, B—arteriole, and C—bile duct

EXPLANATION

Portal triad consists of hepatic arteriole, bile duct, and branch of portal vein. Hepatic artery—lined by endothelium and a thin muscular layer, approximately the same diameter as a bile duct. Portal vein—lined by endothelium. Bile duct—lined by cuboidal epithelium, approximately the same diameter as a hepatic artery.

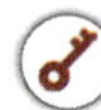

Key: B

BOOST YOUR KNOWLEDGE

Blood from both portal venules and arterioles pass through the sinusoidal system to reach efferent hepatic venules (central vein). From these, the blood drains into successively larger veins to reach the IVC. Bile is secreted into bile canaliculi, which flows toward canals of Hering and to the bile ductules and hence to interlobular bile ducts, further from the smallest ducts into larger ducts, to reach the small intestine by the way of common bile duct.

REFERENCES/SOURCES

- Gupta P, Menon PSN, Ramji S, Lodha R. PG Textbook of Pediatrics, 3rd edition. New Delhi: Jaypee Brothers Medical Publishers; 2022. p. 1862.
- Leonard N, Evason KJ. Histology. [online] Available from https://www.pathologyoutlines.com/topic/livernormalhistology.html. [Last accessed June, 2024].

16. Portal vein is formed by the union of which two veins?

A. Superior mesenteric vein and inferior mesenteric vein
B. Superior mesenteric vein and umbilical vein
C. Splenic vein and superior mesenteric vein
D. Splenic vein and inferior mesenteric vein

EXPLANATION

Splenic vein and superior mesenteric vein unite to form portal vein. Inferior mesenteric vein merges with splenic vein before the formation of portal vein.

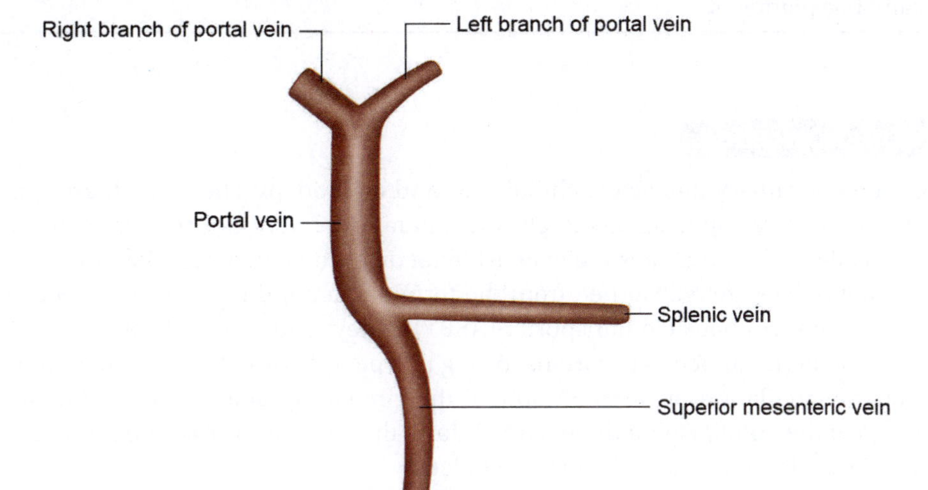

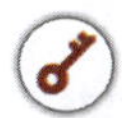

Key: C

BOOST YOUR KNOWLEDGE

Portal vein divides into two branches in the liver. The left branch is longer and narrower than the right branch. Just before entering the left lobe of the liver, it receives paraumbilical veins and ligamentum venosum. The right branch of portal vein is shorter and wider than the left branch, receives cystic vein.

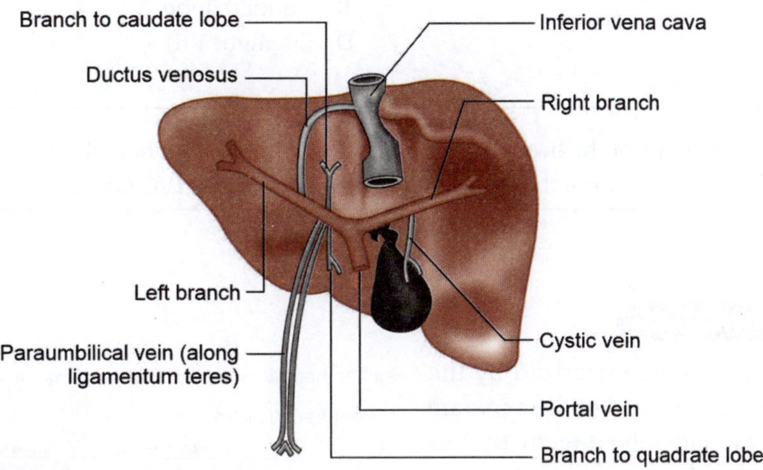

REFERENCE/SOURCE

- Chaurasia BD. BD Chaurasia's Human Anatomy, 8th edition. New Delhi: CBS Publishers and Distributors (P) Ltd; 2021. p. 330.

17. Bile is composed of:

A. Bilirubin, bile acids, and phospholipids
B. Ammonia and urea
C. Alpha-fetoprotein and albumin
D. Albumin and globulin

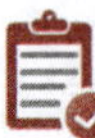

EXPLANATION

Bile is a complex and lipid-rich micellar solution that is isosmotic with plasma and composed primarily of water, inorganic electrolytes, and organic solutes such as bile acids, phospholipids (mostly phosphatidylcholine), cholesterol, and bile pigments.

Key: A

BOOST YOUR KNOWLEDGE

In humans, the two primary bile acids, cholic acid and chenodeoxycholic acid, are synthesized in the liver. Before excretion, they are conjugated with glycine and taurine. In response to a meal, contraction of the gallbladder delivers bile acids to the intestine to assist in fat digestion and absorption. After mediating fat digestion, the bile acids themselves are reabsorbed from the terminal ileum through specific active transport processes [apical sodium-dependent bile acid transporter (ASBT)]. They return to the liver via portal blood, are taken up by liver cells [via sodium taurocholate cotransporting polypeptide (NTCP)] and are excreted in bile. In an adult, this enterohepatic circulation involves 90–95% of the circulating bile acid pool. Bile acids that escape ileal reabsorption reach the colon, where the bacterial flora, through dehydroxylation and deconjugation, produce the secondary bile acids, deoxycholate, and lithocholate.

REFERENCES/SOURCES

- Kliegman RM, Stanton BF, St Geme JW III, Schor NF. Nelson Textbook of Pediatrics, 20th edition. Amsterdam, Netherlands: Elsevier; 2016. p. 1921.
- Podgórski P, Przybyłkowski A, Nehring P. Bile Composition—which Components Can Have Clinical Significance? A Review of the Literature. J Gastrointest Liver Dis. 2023;32:110-7.

18. Which of the following is *not* drained by hepatic veins?

A. Quadrate lobe
B. Caudate lobe
C. Riedel's lobe
D. Segment VIII

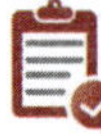

EXPLANATION

Majority of the venous drainage of the liver is accomplished by three major hepatic veins, i.e., (1) right, (2) middle, and (3) left drains into the IVC, except that the caudate lobe drains into IVC directly.

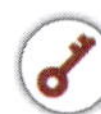

Key: B

BOOST YOUR KNOWLEDGE

Budd-Chiari syndrome is characterized by the blockage of hepatic veins. Provided the separate venous drainage of caudate lobe directly to IVC, caudate lobe hypertrophy is observed in the patients of Budd-Chiari syndrome or hepatic venous outflow tract obstruction.

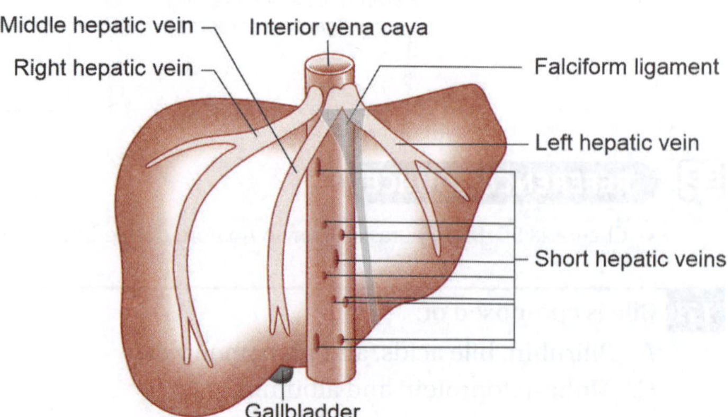

REFERENCES/SOURCES

- Chaurasia BD. BD Chaurasia's Human Anatomy, 9th edition. New Delhi: CBS Publishers and Distributors (P) Ltd; 2022.
- Desser TS, Sze DY, Jeffrey RB. Imaging and intervention in the hepatic veins. Am J Roentgenol. 2003;180(6):1583-91.

19. Hepatic artery is a branch of:

A. Phrenic artery
B. Subclavian artery
C. Celiac trunk
D. Superior mesenteric artery

EXPLANATION

Celiac trunk is 1.25 cm long and it ends by dividing into the left gastric, common hepatic, and splenic arteries.

Key: C

BOOST YOUR KNOWLEDGE

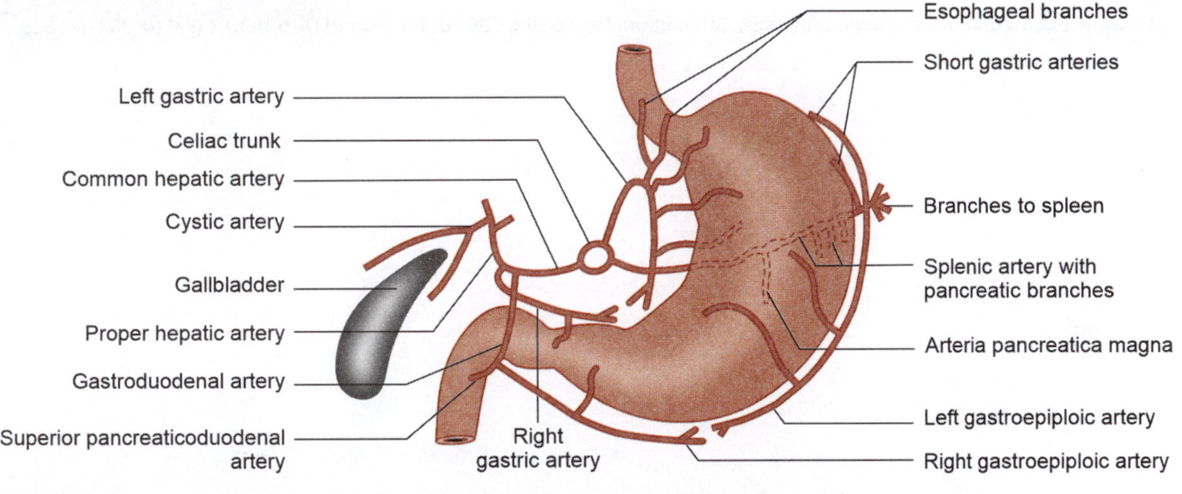

Arteries arising from the branches of the celiac trunk

REFERENCES/SOURCES

- Chaurasia BD. BD Chaurasia's Human Anatomy, 8th edition. New Delhi: CBS Publishers and Distributors (P) Ltd; 2021. p. 324.
- Gupta P, Menon PSN, Ramji S, Lodha R. PG Textbook of Pediatrics, 3rd edition. New Delhi: Jaypee Brothers Medical Publishers; 2022. p. 1861.

20. Spiral valve of Heister is related to:

A. Common hepatic duct
B. Common bile duct
C. Gallbladder
D. Cystic duct

EXPLANATION

The mucous membrane of the cystic duct forms a series of 5–12 crescentic folds, arranged spirally to form the so-called spiral valve of Heister. This is not a true valve.

Key: D

BOOST YOUR KNOWLEDGE

Cystic duct is about 3–4 cm long. It begins at the neck of the gallbladder, runs downward, backward, and to the left, and ends by joining the common hepatic duct at an acute angle to form the bile duct.

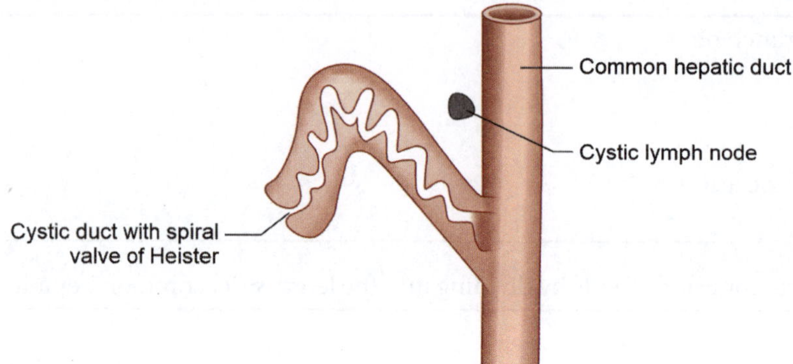

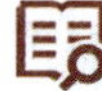

REFERENCE/SOURCE

- Chaurasia BD. BD Chaurasia's Human Anatomy, 8th edition. New Delhi: CBS Publishers and Distributors (P) Ltd; 2021. p. 338.

Liver Function Tests

Arti Pawaria, Vikrant Sood

1. A 4-week-old playful, normally nourished infant presented with suspected neonatal cholestasis with total bilirubin of 10 mg/dL. Which of the following combination would be the first line of evaluation for this child?

A. Liver function test (LFT), ultrasound (US) abdomen, and liver biopsy
B. Stool color, LFT, prothrombin time-international normalized ratio (PT-INR), and US abdomen
C. LFT, liver biopsy, blood tandem mass spectrometry (TMS), and urine gas chromatography mass spectrometry (GCMS)
D. Liver biopsy and magnetic resonance cholangiopancreatography (MRCP)

EXPLANATION

Neonatal cholestasis demands clinical, laboratory, and radiological investigation, as early diagnosis of surgically treatable conditions leads to favorable outcomes. The role of radiology in the work-up of conjugated hyperbilirubinemia is to make a distinction between obstructive cholestasis due to structural biliary anomalies and nonobstructive conditions such as genetic, metabolic, endocrine, or infective disorders, in which imaging investigations are often normal at presentation. The value of visual stool color (acholic or pale stools in obstructive conditions like biliary atresia) inspection is very important as early pointers to etiology. Nonsick and playful child favors obstructive pathology over metabolic/infectious.

The first-line investigations should include basic complete LFT with gamma-glutamyl transferase (GGT), PT-INR, and ultrasonography abdomen is the imaging modality of choice in the screening of these patients and provides the radiologist with a noninvasive and nonionizing tool. The US approach to these patients needs to be systematic, with thorough examination of the liver parenchyma, gallbladder, bile ducts, portal venous system, spleen, and pancreas. In particular, the examiner should concentrate on the intra- and extrahepatic bile ducts, to detect dilatation. The common bile duct (CBD) should not exceed a caliber of 1 mm in neonates, 2 mm in infants up to 1 year of age, 4 mm in older children, and 7 mm in adolescents. The gallbladder needs to be evaluated in its length (normal range between 1.5 and 3 cm) and shape and for the presence of gallstones, inspissated bile and irregular, thickened walls. Evaluation of portal vein patency and direction of flow, presence of collaterals as well as splenic length and ascites is needed to assess signs of portal hypertension.

Initial US can detect coarse nodular liver parenchyma, retrograde flow in the portal vein, ascites, varices, and splenomegaly. In biliary atresia, hepatic scintigraphy will show normal uptake of radiotracer in the liver but failure of biliary excretion after 24 hours; however, neonatal hepatitis could also show absent bowel activity due to poor hepatocellular function.

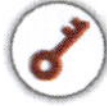

Key: B

BOOST YOUR KNOWLEDGE

- *Specific findings on US abdomen in cases of neonatal cholestasis:*
    - *Biliary atresia:*
        - Small gallbladder <15 mm (or absent)
        - Triangular cord sign—a band-like periportal echogenicity [echogenic anterior wall of the right portal vein (EARPV)] ≥4 mm in thickness, which represents a proximal biliary remnant
        - No/poor contraction of gallbladder (post-feed)
        - Increased hepatic artery diameter and subcapsular flow
    - *Choledochal cyst:*
        - Dilated CBD with or without dilated intrahepatic biliary radicles

REFERENCE/SOURCE

- Guandalini S, Dhawan A. Textbook of Pediatric Gastroenterology, Hepatology and Nutrition, 2nd edition. New York: Springer Cham; 2022. p. 743.

2. Which of the following best defines cholestasis?

A. Conjugated/direct hyperbilirubinemia >1 mg/dL if total serum bilirubin is at or below 5 mg/dL or direct bilirubin fraction >20% of total bilirubin when the total is higher than 5 mg/dL
B. Conjugated/direct hyperbilirubinemia >2 mg/dL if total serum bilirubin is at or below 5 mg/dL or direct bilirubin fraction >20% of total bilirubin when the total is higher than 5 mg/dL
C. Cholestasis can be opined only on liver biopsy, not by biochemical assessment of LFTs
D. It is defined only the presence of bile pigments in urine

EXPLANATION

Clinical jaundice in the first 2 weeks after birth is a common finding, occurring in 2.4–15% of newborns. Often benign, it resolves spontaneously by 2 weeks of age but may persist as long as 3 weeks in a breastfed but otherwise healthy infant. Any jaundice beyond 2 weeks is considered abnormal and requires evaluation with a fractionated serum bilirubin level. Cholestasis, defined as a decrease in bile formation or flow secondary to hepatocellular or obstructive cholestasis, respectively, stems from a variety of etiologies including genetic, metabolic, infectious, and toxin-mediated causes. Hepatocellular cholestasis is secondary to reduced bile formation, such as due to sepsis or toxins. Obstructive cholestasis is due to either intra- or extrahepatic obstruction, a product of either anatomic or functional obstruction of the biliary system such as with biliary atresia and Alagille syndrome. Cholestasis is defined as a conjugated/direct hyperbilirubinemia >1 mg/dL if total serum bilirubin is at or below 5 mg/dL or direct bilirubin fraction >20% of total bilirubin when the total is >5 mg/dL. Histologically, bile pigment is present in hepatocytes and bile ducts. Physiologically, the accumulation of substances normally excreted in bile is present in blood and extrahepatic tissues. But the definition of cholestasis is based solely on the total bilirubin and conjugated bilirubin fraction as mentioned earlier.

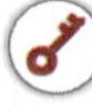

Key: A

BOOST YOUR KNOWLEDGE

- Any infant noted to be jaundiced after 2 weeks of age should be evaluated for cholestasis with measurement of total and direct serum bilirubin, and that an elevated serum direct bilirubin level (direct bilirubin levels >1.0 mg/dL or >17 μmol/L) warrants timely referral to a pediatric gastroenterologist or hepatologist.
- The most common causes of early onset infantile cholestasis are biliary atresia (25–40%) and genetic cholestatic disorders (25%).

REFERENCES/SOURCES

- Fawaz R, Baumann U, Ekong U, Fischler B, Hadzic N, Mack CL, et al. Guideline for the Evaluation of Cholestatic Jaundice in Infants: Joint Recommendations of the North American Society for Pediatric Gastroenterology, Hepatology, and Nutrition and the European Society for Pediatric Gastroenterology, Hepatology, and Nutrition. J Pediatr Gastroenterol Nutr. 2017;64(1):154-68.
- Guandalini S, Dhawan A. Textbook of Pediatric Gastroenterology, Hepatology and Nutrition, 2nd edition. New York: Springer Cham; 2022. p. 765.

3. **Tests that detect impaired bile flow or cholestasis are based on measurement of which of the following?**

A. Alkaline phosphatase (ALP), GGT, and 5′-nucleotidase (5′-NT)
B. Alanine aminotransferase (ALT), aspartate aminotransferase (AST), and lactic acid dehydrogenase (LDH)
C. Albumin, INR, PT, and partial thromboplastin time (PTT)
D. ALP, GGT, ALT, and AST

EXPLANATION

Alkaline phosphatase is a group of isoenzymes originating in different tissues in the body that hydrolyze organic phosphate esters at alkaline pH, generating inorganic phosphate and an organic radical. The ALPs are true isoenzymes because they all catalyze this reaction, with differences in physicochemical properties. ALPs are found in several tissues, including the canalicular membrane of hepatocytes, bone osteoblasts, the brush border of enterocytes in the small intestine, proximal convoluted tubules of the kidney, the placenta, and white blood cells. While the bone ALP isoenzyme appears to be involved with calcification, the precise function of the liver ALP isoenzyme is not known, although some postulate that it may participate in transport processes. Normal growing children and rapidly growing adolescents have elevations of serum ALP of bone origin, with good correlation with the rate of bone growth that causes influx of enzymes from osteoid tissues. Therefore, an isolated increase in ALP may not indicate hepatic or biliary disease if other liver biochemical tests are normal. Initial management may involve repeating the test or confirming the hepatic origin with another liver chemistry test such as a GGT or 5′-NT.

Gamma-glutamyl transferase is a microsomal enzyme that catalyzes the transfer of γ-glutamyl groups from peptides such as glutathione to other amino acids. GGT is present in the cell membranes of multiple body organs, including the kidney, pancreas, liver, spleen, brain, breast, and the small intestine. Since the enzyme is found in so many tissues, including the biliary epithelium and hepatocytes, the usefulness of an elevated GGT level is limited by its lack of specificity. Because GGT does not increase in the serum of patients with bone disease or children with active bone growth, it is helpful in confirming the hepatic origin of an elevated ALP level in pediatrics. GGT is present in normal human serum.

5′-nucleotidase catalyzes the hydrolysis of nucleotides such as adenosine-5′-phosphate or inosine-5′-phosphate, which are unique for having the phosphate group attached to the 5′ position of a pentose sugar moiety. 5′-NT is found in the liver, intestine, brain, heart, blood vessels, and endocrine pancreas. Despite this widespread tissue distribution, marked serum elevations of 5′-NT levels are found almost exclusively in the setting of liver disease. In the liver, 5′-NT is located in both sinusoidal and canalicular membranes, but its precise physiologic purpose is not known.

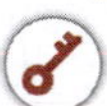

Key: A

BOOST YOUR KNOWLEDGE

- Serum GGT values can provide an early clue to the probable etiology of underlying cholestatic liver disease.
  - Normal or low levels are seen in progressive familial intrahepatic cholestasis (PFIC) type 1 (ATP8B1 deficiency) and 2 (ABCB11 deficiency), bile acid synthesis disorders (BASDs) and tight junction protein (TJP) type 2 deficiency.
  - High levels are seen in Alagille syndrome, PFIC3 (due to ABCB4 deficiency), and often, but not always, in biliary atresia.

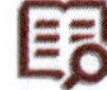

REFERENCES/SOURCES

- Fawaz R, Baumann U, Ekong U, Fischler B, Hadzic N, Mack CL, et al. Guideline for the Evaluation of Cholestatic Jaundice in Infants: Joint Recommendations of the North American Society for Pediatric Gastroenterology, Hepatology, and Nutrition and the European Society for Pediatric Gastroenterology, Hepatology, and Nutrition. J Pediatr Gastroenterol Nutr. 2017;64(1):154-68.
- Suchy FJ, Sokol RJ, Balistreri WF, Bezerra JA, Mack CL, Shneider BL. Liver Disease in Children, 5th edition. Cambridge, United Kingdom: Cambridge University Press; 2021. pp. 95-7.

4. An apparently healthy 4-year-old child's total and fractionated serum bilirubin, AST, ALT, and ALP were done as a part of routine health check-up offered by family health insurance. Serum ALP was more than two times upper limit of normal. Parents are worried. What is your next step?

A. Repeat the LFT from different laboratory
B. Send the child for US abdomen to rule out obstructive biliary pathology
C. Do serum GGT to confirm hepatic origin
D. Reassure the parents to go home

EXPLANATION

As stated, an isolated increase in ALP may not indicate hepatic or biliary disease if other liver biochemical tests are normal. Initial management involves confirming the hepatic origin with another liver chemistry test such as a GGT or 5′-NT. Interpretation of serum ALP levels in children is challenging due to extensive changes with growth and puberty leading to distinct sex- and age-specific dynamics. Recently developed percentile charts for ALP activity in girls and boys from birth to 18 years are available. As a rough guide serum ALP values more than three times the upper limit of normal of the adult reference values should be considered as significant for children. Differentiation about the origin of ALP will still be required with GGT.

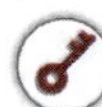

Key: C

BOOST YOUR KNOWLEDGE

A low serum ALP level may occur in patients with Wilson disease, especially those presenting with acute liver failure and hemolysis, possibly because of reduced activity of the enzyme owing to displacement of the cofactor zinc by copper. In such cases, ALP/bilirubin ratio is <4 (cf. other causes of acute liver failure with ratio >4).

REFERENCE/SOURCE

- Suchy FJ, Sokol RJ, Balistreri WF, Bezerra JA, Mack CL, Shneider BL. Liver Disease in Children, 5th edition. Cambridge, United Kingdom: Cambridge University Press; 2021. p. 96.

5. Serum AST and ALT levels are proportionately raised in which of the following clinical conditions?

A. Autoimmune hepatitis with associated intravascular hemolysis
B. Acute viral hepatitis A-related infection
C. Ischemic hepatic injury following prolonged hypotension
D. Viral infection-induced rhabdomyolysis

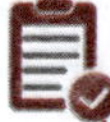

EXPLANATION

Pl, concentrations of liver enzymes in plasma are widely used as indicators of liver disease in children. The serum aminotransferases (also known as transaminases), AST and ALT, are the liver chemistry tests most commonly in use to assess injury to hepatocytes and to identify patients with liver disease.

- AST is an enzyme that catalyzes the reversible transfer of the amino group from aspartic acid to the α-keto group of α-ketoglutaric acid to form oxaloacetic acid plus glutamic acid [and hence AST's former name, serum glutamic oxaloacetic transaminase (SGOT)].

- Similarly, ALT is the enzyme that catalyzes the reversible α-amino group transfer from the amino acid alanine to the α-keto group of α-ketoglutaric acid to yield pyruvic acid plus glutamic acid [and hence ALT's former name, serum glutamic pyruvic transaminase (SGPT)].

Aspartate aminotransferase is present as both cytosolic and mitochondrial isoenzymes and found in high concentrations in many nonliver tissues, including heart muscle, skeletal muscle, kidney, brain, pancreas, lung, leukocytes, and red blood cells. ALT is a cytosolic enzyme that is present in highest concentrations in the liver, and to a lesser extent within skeletal muscle cells. Elevation of enzyme activities in serum results from damage to or destruction of tissues rich in the aminotransferases or to a change in cell membrane permeability allowing AST and/or ALT to leak from damaged cells into serum. However, because of the wide tissue distribution of AST, the hepatic origin of an isolated serum AST level elevation should be confirmed by simultaneously obtaining a serum ALT level. Acute viral hepatitis predominantly shows a proportionate increase in AST and ALT.

A disproportionately isolated increase in serum AST level should prompt a search for evidence of hemolysis, acute rhabdomyolysis (such as seen during a systemic viral illness); a myopathic process; myocardial disease (including undiagnosed cardiomyopathy); and recent vigorous physical activity (such as long-distance running or weightlifting). Serum haptoglobin, lactate dehydrogenase, creatine phosphokinase, or aldolase levels may verify hemolysis or myopathy/muscle disease as the underlying etiology of a disproportionately elevated AST level. Finally, spuriously high serum levels of AST can be due to the presence of a macro-AST, formed by the enzyme complexing with an immunoglobulin, usually immunoglobulin G, leading to decreased clearance, like the confusion that can occur in the case of macroamylasemia in the assessment of pancreatic diseases.

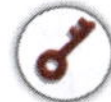
Key: B

BOOST YOUR KNOWLEDGE

- ALT is more specific for liver disease than AST. Half-life of AST (16–18 hours) is lower than that of ALT (40–48 hours); thus, in early stage of liver disease, AST rises before ALT but later levels come down and ALT levels go higher.
- If there is isolated rise in AST/ALT (and after exclusion of hepatic disorders), always exclude nonhepatic causes such as celiac disease, thyroid disease (hypo or hyper), muscle-related diseases, and strenuous exercise among others.

REFERENCE/SOURCE

- Suchy FJ, Sokol RJ, Balistreri WF, Bezerra JA, Mack CL, Shneider BL. Liver Disease in Children, 5th edition. Cambridge, United Kingdom: Cambridge University Press; 2021. p. 95.

6. Which of the following is *true* regarding hypoalbuminemia in the absence of other nonhepatic etiology?

A. Serum albumin has a long half-life in the serum of approximately 31 days, low serum levels are often taken as a sign of chronic liver disease rather than acute injury
B. Albumin synthesis is regulated only by changes in nutritional status and not by systemic inflammation and hormone levels
C. Serum albumin decreases only in decompensated chronic liver diseases
D. Albumin is synthesized in the rough endoplasmic reticulum of hepatocytes at a rate of 150 mg/kg/day under normal healthy condition

EXPLANATION

Albumin, the principal serum protein, is synthesized only in the liver. The serum albumin level at any point in time reflects the rate of synthesis, rate of degradation, and volume of distribution. Albumin is synthesized in the rough endoplasmic reticulum of hepatocytes at a rate of 150 mg/kg/day. Because serum albumin has a long half-life in the serum of approximately 21 days, low serum levels are often taken as a sign of chronic liver disease rather than acute injury. However, a patient with compensated chronic liver disease may demonstrate an abrupt decrease in serum albumin concentration during an acute illness, such as sepsis or even a flu-like minor illness. This is caused partly by an acute decrease in synthesis below that already present due to the parenchymal liver disease, possibly regulated by cytokines such as tumor necrosis factor and interleukin 1. Albumin synthesis is regulated by changes in nutritional status, osmotic pressure, systemic inflammation, and hormone levels. Traditionally, the biologic and therapeutic role of albumin in liver disease was attributed to its oncotic effects, but it is now understood that albumin has a wide range of other important physiologic functions such as immunomodulation, endothelial stabilization, antioxidant effects and binding multiple drugs, toxins, and other molecules. Hypoalbuminemia is not specific for liver disease because it also occurs in the setting of protein-losing enteropathy, chronic infection, and nephrotic syndrome. In the absence of other nonhepatic etiology, serum albumin levels can be useful in assaying hepatic synthetic function. Chronic inflammation, chronic liver disease, and protein malnutrition can inhibit albumin synthesis, whereas the presence of ascites causes an increased volume of distribution.

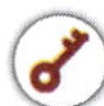

Key: D

BOOST YOUR KNOWLEDGE

- A normal serum albumin level does not exclude underlying advanced (or cirrhotic) liver disease since levels may be normal in early compensated disease stage.
- Being a negative acute phase reactant, serum albumin levels may decrease in presence of any significant acute hepatic insult (like acute severe hepatic infections or hepatitis); thus, low levels in these cases should not be attributed to underlying chronic (or cirrhotic liver disease).

REFERENCE/SOURCE

- Suchy FJ, Sokol RJ, Balistreri WF, Bezerra JA, Mack CL, Shneider BL. Liver Disease in Children, 5th edition. Cambridge, United Kingdom: Cambridge University Press; 2021. p. 98.

7. The liver is responsible for the synthesis of many of the procoagulant and anticoagulant proteins responsible for maintaining hemostasis. Which of the following derangements is true in liver disease?

A. Diminished hepatic synthesis of coagulation factors V, VII, IX, X, and XI, prothrombin, and fibrinogen
B. Only procoagulant production is decreased, hence liver diseases are always associated with increased risk of bleeding
C. Liver disease is associated with decreased fibrinolysis, due to increased synthesis of alpha2-plasmin inhibitor
D. All of the above are true

EXPLANATION

The liver is responsible for the synthesis of many of the procoagulant and anticoagulant proteins responsible for maintaining hemostasis. Abnormal hemostasis is a common complication of liver disease. Mechanisms resulting in these defects include: (1) diminished hepatic synthesis of coagulation factors V, VII, IX, X, and XI, prothrombin, and fibrinogen (reflected in prolongation of the PT); (2) dietary vitamin K deficiency due to inadequate intake or malabsorption (based on intrahepatic or extrahepatic cholestasis and intestinal malabsorption); (3) dysfibrinogenemia; (4) enhanced fibrinolysis, due to decreased synthesis of alpha2-plasmin inhibitor; (5) disseminated intravascular coagulation; and (6) thrombocytopenia due to hypersplenism. While liver dysfunction is often assumed to be associated with increased bleeding risk, other factors such as sepsis, hepatorenal syndrome, hypotension, and endothelial dysfunction also contribute to this bleeding tendency, rather than isolated liver disease or cirrhosis. Global tests of clot formation, such as rotational thromboelastometry and thromboelastography may eventually have a role in the evaluation of clotting in patients with advanced liver disease, but currently lack validated target levels, especially in pediatrics. As storage capacity of vitamin K in the liver is limited, depletion occurs quickly when absorption is impaired, and the PT and INR increases above normal ranges. The PT is the time (in seconds) it takes plasma to clot after addition of tissue factors. PT assesses how well the extrinsic and common pathways of the coagulation cascade work together. However, PT results will vary according to the type of analytical system and reagents employed by the laboratory. For this reason, INR is more frequently used instead of PT, since it is a calculated ratio and thus does not change no matter the testing method.

Key: A

BOOST YOUR KNOWLEDGE

- Although historically patients with cirrhosis were thought to have a hemostasis-related bleeding tendency, it is now widely accepted that the hemostatic system of patients with cirrhosis remains are in a state of rebalanced hemostasis as a result of simultaneous changes in pro- and antihemostatic systems. They can thus have either a bleeding or a thrombotic tendency based on the clinical situation and overall systemic homeostasis.
- Common hemostasis tests such as APTT and PT/INR do not predict bleeding risk (with controversial role of platelet count or fibrinogen levels). Thus, in liver disease patients, there is no role of artificial correction of PT/INR to prevent bleeding episodes. Viscoelastic tests such as thromboelastography, etc., may better reflect the true state of cirrhotic hemostasis.

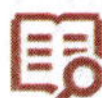

REFERENCE/SOURCE

- Suchy FJ, Sokol RJ, Balistreri WF, Bezerra JA, Mack CL, Shneider BL. Liver Disease in Children, 5th edition. Cambridge, United Kingdom: Cambridge University Press; 2021. p. 98.

8. A 6-month-old infant presents with conjugated jaundice, pruritus, and low serum GGT. Which of the following conditions could be a possible differential diagnosis?

A. Biliary atresia
B. Alagille syndrome
C. Choledochal cyst
D. PFIC type I

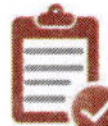

EXPLANATION

Serum GGT is most elevated in all children with biliary atresia, sclerosing cholangitis, paucity of intrahepatic bile ducts (Alagille syndrome), and cholestatic patients with α1-antitrypsin deficiency. The presence of increased serum GGT levels in both intrahepatic and extrahepatic cholestasis is variable and cannot be used to differentiate between them. Normal or decreased serum GGT levels in the clinical setting of persistent jaundice are utilized as a test to distinguish between the different subtypes of genetic cholestatic syndromes. PFIC is a general term encompassing a group of illnesses characterized by persistent and profound cholestasis without extrahepatic pathology typically presenting in the neonatal or infancy period, and with a progressive clinical course to cirrhosis.

Progressive familial intrahepatic cholestasis is often divided into two broad categories: "Low-GGT PFIC," in which serum activity of GGT is usually low (or normal), and "high-GGT PFIC," in which the activity is above normal. Occasional patients have intermediate levels and can be hard to categorize according to this criterion. While not typically correlated with genotype data, elevated serum levels of GGT are thought to distinguish PFIC type 3 [caused by mutations in *ABCB4*, the gene which encodes the multidrug resistance gene 3 (*MDR3*) protein] from the normal to low serum GGT levels more typical of PFIC type 1 (caused by mutations in *ATP8B1*, the gene which encodes the FIC1 protein) and PFIC type 2 [caused by mutations in *ABCB11*, the gene which encodes the bile salt export pump (BSEP) protein].

Recent scientific advances have helped clarify the molecular basis of many of these disorders. Low GGT familial intrahepatic cholestasis also occurs in infants with benign recurrent intrahepatic cholestasis (BRIC) with a good long-term prognosis. BRIC is an autosomal recessive liver disease characterized by intermittent attacks of cholestasis, which starts at any age and lasts for several weeks to months and shares a locus (chromosome 18q21) with PFIC type 1.

Low GGT cholestasis is also seen in children with defects in bile acid synthesis or conjugation, children with abnormalities of junctions (e.g., tight junctions) between liver cells, and children with abnormalities of cell organization manifest as arthrogryposis-renal dysfunction-cholestasis (ARC) syndrome.

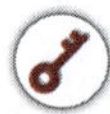

Key: D

BOOST YOUR KNOWLEDGE

- Genetic cholestatic disorders account for almost 25% of infantile cholestatic disorders.
- PFIC1 or ATP8B1 deficiency is characteristically associated with extrahepatic manifestations [cf. PFIC type 2 (ABCB11) and PFIC type 3 or ABCB4 defects] such as hearing loss, pancreatitis, or pancreatic exocrine insufficiency, and diarrhea (not attributable to fat malabsorption).

REFERENCE/SOURCE

- Suchy FJ, Sokol RJ, Balistreri WF, Bezerra JA, Mack CL, Shneider BL. Liver Disease in Children, 5th edition. Cambridge, United Kingdom: Cambridge University Press; 2021. p. 97.

9. A 9-month-old infant presents with conjugated jaundice and high serum GGT. Which of the following conditions is a possible differential diagnosis?

A. Bile acid synthetic defects
B. Alagille syndrome
C. BSEP (ABCB11) deficiency
D. PFIC type I

EXPLANATION

Please see Explanation for the Question 8. You should be able to answer on that basis only.

Key: B

BOOST YOUR KNOWLEDGE

Alagille syndrome is an autosomal dominant multisystem disorder characterized by cholestatic liver disease (with paucity of interlobular ducts on liver biopsy), characteristic facies (broad forehead and small pointy chin), posterior embryotoxon in the eye, butterfly vertebrae, renal disease, and cardiac defects (most commonly peripheral pulmonic stenosis). Diagnosis is usually made by the clinical findings, laboratory, and diagnostic evaluation, and confirmed by sequencing of *JAG1* and *NOTCH2* genes.

REFERENCES/SOURCES

- Fawaz R, Baumann U, Ekong U, Fischler B, Hadzic N, Mack CL, et al. Guideline for the Evaluation of Cholestatic Jaundice in Infants: Joint Recommendations of the North American Society for Pediatric Gastroenterology, Hepatology, and Nutrition and the European Society for Pediatric Gastroenterology, Hepatology, and Nutrition. J Pediatr Gastroenterol Nutr. 2017;64(1):154-68.
- Suchy FJ, Sokol RJ, Balistreri WF, Bezerra JA, Mack CL, Shneider BL. Liver Disease in Children, 5th edition. Cambridge, United Kingdom: Cambridge University Press; 2021. p. 97.

10. Conjugated hyperbilirubinemia is seen in which of the following conditions?

A. Congenital hypothyroidism
B. Crigler–Najjar syndrome type 1
C. Dubin–Johnson syndrome (DJS)
D. Gilbert syndrome

EXPLANATION

Bilirubin (from Latin, bilis, bile; rube, red) is formed from the degradation of heme-containing compounds. The largest source to produce bilirubin is hemoglobin. However, other heme-containing proteins are also degraded to bilirubin, including the cytochromes, catalases, tryptophan pyrrolase, and muscle myoglobin. The formation of bilirubin is initiated by cleaving the tetrapyrrole ring of protoheme (protoporphyrin IX), which results in a linear tetrapyrrole (biliverdin). The first enzyme system involved in the formation of bilirubin is microsomal heme oxygenase. Heme oxygenase reduces the porphyrin iron (Fe III to Fe II) and hydroxylates the α-methine = C-carbon. This carbon is then oxidatively excised from the tetrapyrrole ring, yielding carbon monoxide and opening the ring structure; this is associated with oxygenation of the two carbons adjacent to the site of cleavage. The cleaved α-carbon is excreted as carbon monoxide, which also functions as a neurotransmitter. The iron released by heme oxygenase can be reutilized by the body. The resultant linear tetrapyrrole is biliverdin IXα. The stereospecificity of the enzyme produces cleavage almost exclusively at the α-carbon of the tetrapyrrole.

Unconjugated hyperbilirubinemia may result from hemolysis or in genetic diseases such as Crigler–Najjar syndrome, a rare genetic disease that presents shortly after birth, characterized by a severe or total impairment of bilirubin conjugation by the liver due to a deficiency of bilirubin-uridine 5'-diphospho-glucuronosyltransferase (UGT). Diminished expression of the same enzyme is also the defect causing Gilbert syndrome, a benign, unconjugated hyperbilirubinemia occurring in up to 5% of the normal population. The term physiologic jaundice is used to describe the frequently observed jaundice in otherwise completely normal neonates, and the result of a few factors involving increased bilirubin production and decreased excretion. Congenital hypothyroidism is an important cause of prolonged unconjugated hyperbilirubinemia.

Key: C

BOOST YOUR KNOWLEDGE

Dubin–Johnson syndrome, first described in 1954, involves elevation of both the conjugated and unconjugated serum bilirubin fractions. More than half of the total serum bilirubin is conjugated, and total bilirubin levels usually range from 1.5 to 6 mg/dL, although they have been reported as high as 25 mg/dL during intercurrent illness. Patients with DJS sometimes report vague abdominal complaints although this is not believed to reflect serious pathology. Although hepatomegaly is sometimes seen, LFTs are otherwise normal, including bile acids, and there is no evidence of hemolysis. Although this syndrome occurs in both sexes, males predominate and present at an earlier age. It occurs in all races; however, Iranian and Moroccan Jews have an increased incidence. It is usually diagnosed after puberty, although cases have also been reported in neonates, at which time cholestasis can be significant. It is inherited as an autosomal recessive trait with heterozygotes manifesting normal serum bilirubin levels.

Dubin–Johnson syndrome is caused by defects in *ABCC2* gene which causes deficiency of canalicular MRP2 expression and impairs the transport of conjugated bilirubin into the bile duct system. The liver is grossly black in appearance and on light microscopy, the architecture of the liver is normal, but there is the accumulation of dark, coarsely granular pigment in the centrilobular hepatocytes. It is a benign disease and does not require any treatment.

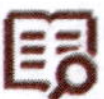

REFERENCE/SOURCE

- Suchy FJ, Sokol RJ, Balistreri WF, Bezerra JA, Mack CL, Shneider BL. Liver Disease in Children, 5th edition. Cambridge, United Kingdom: Cambridge University Press; 2021. p. 200.

11. Substantial prolongation of PT-INR disproportionate to degree of liver synthetic dysfunction in a nonencephalopathic child may point to which of the following disease condition of hepatic origin.

A. Fibrocystic liver diseases
B. Hepatitis E-related acute liver failure
C. Tyrosinemia type 1
D. Storage diseases of the liver

EXPLANATION

A persistently elevated INR time in a previously well child (with evidence of liver injury on clinical assessment or liver biochemical tests) can be the single laboratory test that draws attention to the possibility of the diagnosis of pediatric acute liver failure, and early communication with a pediatric liver transplant program is strongly recommended. In some inherited metabolic diseases in the newborn such as tyrosinemia, there may be profound elevations in INR out of proportion to other parameters of liver dysfunction. Most patients with extrahepatic obstruction respond promptly to parenterally administered vitamin K in early course of the disease. In patients with jaundice, the type of response to vitamin K is therefore of some value in differential diagnosis, especially because it can be summarized that parenchymal function is good if the PT or INR return to normal within 24 hours after a single parenteral injection of vitamin K.

Key: C

BOOST YOUR KNOWLEDGE

Tyrosinemia type I results from deficiency of the enzyme fumarylacetoacetate hydrolase (FAH). The diagnosis is made by increased succinylacetone concentration in the blood and urine and/or by the identification of pathogenic variants in *FAH* gene on genetic testing. It presents either in young infants with severe liver involvement or later in the first year with liver dysfunction and renal tubular dysfunction associated with growth failure and rickets. There may be repeated, often unrecognized, neurologic crises also. Management includes early initiation of nitisinone [2-(2-nitro-4-trifluoromethylbenzoyl)-1,3 cyclohexanedione (NTBC), which blocks parahydroxyphenylpyruvic acid dioxygenase (*p*-HPPD), the second step in the tyrosine degradation pathway], in combination with a low-tyrosine diet, with liver transplantation as definitive cure.

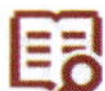

REFERENCE/SOURCE

- Suchy FJ, Sokol RJ, Balistreri WF, Bezerra JA, Mack CL, Shneider BL. Liver Disease in Children, 5th edition. Cambridge, United Kingdom: Cambridge University Press; 2021. p. 99.

12. Gamma-glutamyl transferase is an important biochemical marker of LFT because:

A. It helps differentiate bone origin of high ALP
B. It confirms the PFIC variants
C. It is a marker of synthetic function
D. It directly correlates with hepatic parenchymal regeneration

EXPLANATION

Gamma-glutamyl transferase is present in the cell membranes of multiple body organs, including the kidney, pancreas, liver, spleen, brain, breast, and the small intestine. Elevations in GGT have been described in adults with a wide range of clinical conditions including chronic alcoholism, exocrine pancreatic diseases, cardiovascular disease, heart failure, nonalcoholic fatty liver disease (NAFLD), renal failure, chronic obstructive pulmonary disease, and diabetes. Because GGT does not increase in the serum of patients with bone disease or children with active bone growth, it is helpful in confirming the hepatic origin of an elevated ALP level in pediatric population. GGT is present in normal human serum. The newborn may have very high levels of GGT, up to five to eight times the upper limit of normal for adults.

In premature infants, in the first few days of life the values of GGT may be even higher than in the full-term infant. Serum values then decline rapidly in both the full-term and premature infant and reach adult normal levels by 6–9 months of age. The highest levels of GGT are found in biliary obstruction. Serum GGT was most elevated in all children with biliary atresia, sclerosing cholangitis, paucity of intrahepatic bile ducts

(Alagille syndrome), and cholestatic patients with α1-antitrypsin deficiency. The presence of increased serum GGT levels in both intrahepatic and extrahepatic cholestasis is variable and cannot be used to differentiate between them.

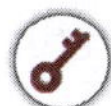

Key: A

BOOST YOUR KNOWLEDGE

GGTP levels may be elevated in patients taking antiepileptics (phenytoin, carbamazepine, valproic acid, and barbiturates), antiretroviral therapy (non-nucleoside reverse transcriptase inhibitors and the protease inhibitor abacavir), and also in alcoholics (thus, serum GGTP levels may be used for identifying unreported alcohol intake)

REFERENCE/SOURCE

- Suchy FJ, Sokol RJ, Balistreri WF, Bezerra JA, Mack CL, Shneider BL. Liver Disease in Children, 5th edition. Cambridge, United Kingdom: Cambridge University Press; 2021. p. 97.

13. Which of the following statements is true, while assessing serum AST and ALT levels?

A. There is a good correlation between serum elevations of aminotransferases and the extent of liver cell necrosis seen on liver biopsy

B. A rapid decline in aminotransferase levels, in association with coagulopathy carries a poor prognosis in acute liver failure

C. Levels of serum AST and serum ALT directly correlates with hepatic parenchymal regeneration

D. Impairment of functional hepatic blood flow leads to a resultant increase in hepatic sinusoidal uptake of AST in patients with cirrhosis

EXPLANATION

Some of the highest AST and ALT levels (elevations greater than 15 times normal) are seen following an acute episode of hypoxia or hypoperfusion (shock liver), and during the course of acute viral hepatitis, medication- or toxin-induced hepatotoxicity. Ischemic and hypoxic acute liver damage is more likely in patients with concomitant clinical conditions such as sepsis or low-flow hemodynamic states.

- There is a poor correlation between serum elevations of aminotransferases and the extent of liver cell necrosis seen on liver biopsy.
- A rapid decline in aminotransferase levels, reflecting massive destruction and loss of viable hepatocytes, in association with increasing bilirubin levels and a coagulopathy portends a poor prognosis in the setting of the child with acute liver failure.
- The value of an increased AST:ALT ratio is less relevant in pediatrics. Among adult alcoholic patients, often deficient in pyridoxal 5′-phosphate, the coenzyme needed for ALT synthesis, increased serum AST:ALT ratios reflect altered synthesis ratios in the liver.
- Physiologically, impairment of functional hepatic blood flow leads to a resultant decrease in hepatic sinusoidal uptake of AST in patients with cirrhosis.

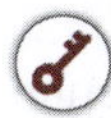

Key: B

BOOST YOUR KNOWLEDGE

- Pediatric experience with AST:ALT ratio is very limited; a retrospective review of 73 infants with chronic liver disease at one single center demonstrated an increase in AST:ALT ratio over a 13-month period of follow-up in those with a worse clinical outcome. An AST:ALT ratio of >4, in the appropriate clinical setting, is highly suggestive of fulminant Wilson disease.

- AST/ALT ratio >2.2 (along with ALP/total bilirubin ratio <4) has good sensitivity and specificity to differential fulminant Wilson disease from other causes of fulminant hepatic failure.
- As cirrhosis develops in a liver disease, AST/ALT ratio may exceed 1 (i.e., AST > ALT); the exact reason is still unknown (may be due to impaired functional hepatic blood flow, with a consequent decrease in hepatic sinusoidal uptake of AST)

REFERENCE/SOURCE

- Suchy FJ, Sokol RJ, Balistreri WF, Bezerra JA, Mack CL, Shneider BL. Liver Disease in Children, 5th edition. Cambridge, United Kingdom: Cambridge University Press; 2021. p. 97.

14. Which of the following statements is true about bilirubin metabolism?

A. Approximately 25% of total bilirubin produced comes from the heme moiety of hemoglobin released from senescent erythrocytes destroyed in the reticuloendothelial cells of the liver, spleen, and bone marrow

B. Unconjugated hyperbilirubinemia may result from hemolysis or in genetic diseases such as Crigler–Najjar syndrome, a rare genetic disease that presents shortly after birth

C. Bilirubin is a yellow hexapyrrole pigment produced from the breakdown of ferroprotoporphyrin IX (heme), an integral part of heme-containing proteins

D. Diminished expression UGT enzyme is also the defect causing Rotor's syndrome which is a benign, unconjugated hyperbilirubinemia occurring in up to 5% of the normal population

EXPLANATION

- Bilirubin is a yellow tetrapyrrole pigment produced from the breakdown of ferroprotoporphyrin IX (heme), an integral part of heme-containing proteins.
- Approximately 75% of total bilirubin produced comes from the heme moiety of hemoglobin released from senescent erythrocytes destroyed in the reticuloendothelial cells of the liver, spleen, and bone marrow. The remaining bilirubin is produced from the premature destruction of red blood cell precursors in the bone marrow (i.e., ineffective erythropoiesis) and from the turnover and catabolism of other heme-containing proteins such as cytochromes and peroxidases. Unconjugated hyperbilirubinemia may result from hemolysis or in genetic diseases such as Crigler–Najjar syndrome, a rare genetic disease that presents shortly after birth, characterized by a severe or total impairment of bilirubin conjugation by the liver due to a deficiency of bilirubin-UGT.
- Diminished expression of the same enzyme is also the defect causing Gilbert syndrome, a benign, unconjugated hyperbilirubinemia, occurring in up to 5% of the normal population.

Key: B

BOOST YOUR KNOWLEDGE

- First issue in a patient presenting with jaundice is to distinguish between conjugated and unconjugated jaundice.
- History of persistent dark urine in presence of jaundice points towards a conjugated jaundice, while presence of normal colored urine in the presence of jaundice is a strong indicator of unconjugated hyperbilirubinemia.
- Common causes of unconjugated jaundice are Gilbert syndrome, hemolytic anemia, megaloblastic anemia, and rarely, Crigler–Najjar syndrome. On the other hand, common causes of conjugated jaundice are hepatobiliary disorders and rarely, genetic syndromes such as Dubin–Johnson and Rotor syndrome.

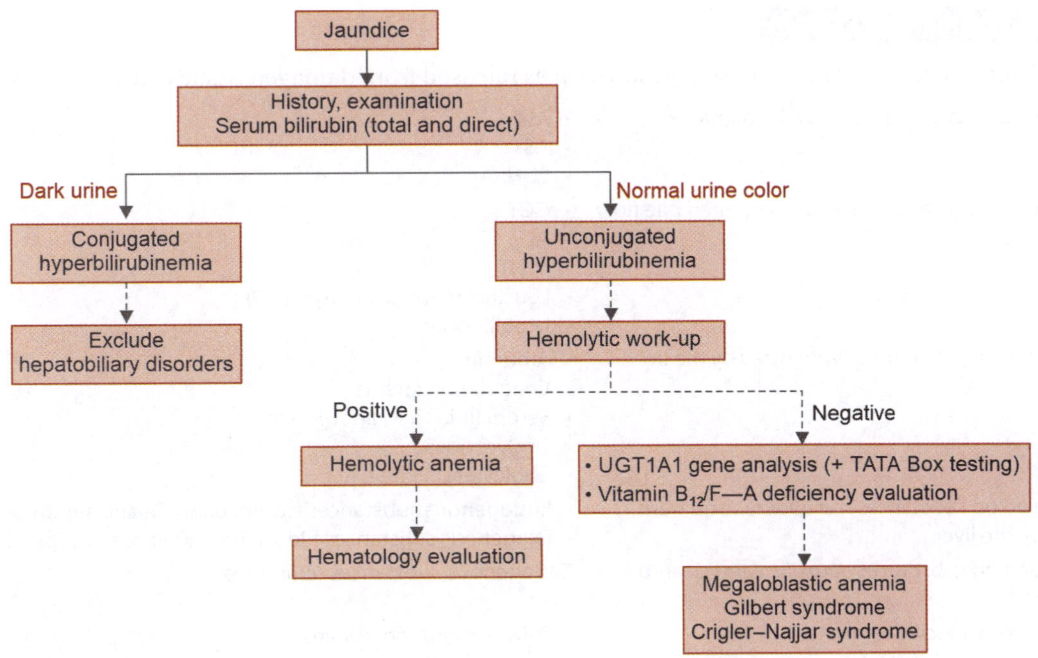

REFERENCE/SOURCE

- Suchy FJ, Sokol RJ, Balistreri WF, Bezerra JA, Mack CL, Shneider BL. Liver Disease in Children, 5th edition. Cambridge, United Kingdom: Cambridge University Press; 2021. p. 99.

15. Which of the following is *not* a marker of liver injury?

A. ALT B. AST
C. LDH D. ALP

EXPLANATION

Tests to evaluate liver disease can be divided into five categories, which are as follows:

1. Tests that detect liver injury are based on measurement of the serum level of endogenous substances released from damaged hepatocytes including ALT, AST, and LDH.
2. Tests that detect impaired damaged tissue such as ALP, GGT, and bile flow or cholestasis are based on measurement of the serum level of endogenous substances released from 5′-NT.
3. Tests of liver synthetic capacity include the serum levels of albumin, INR, PT and PTT, and individual clotting factors (such as factor VII and factor V). Triglyceride, cholesterol, lipid, and lipoprotein synthesis also occur in the liver.
4. Tests of hepatic excretory function are based on measurements of serum concentrations of substances metabolized and transported by the liver, including endogenously produced compounds such as bilirubin and serum bile acids, as well as the determination of the rate of clearance of exogenously administered dyes or drugs, such as indocyanine green, caffeine, lidocaine, and para-aminobenzoic acid (PABA).
5. Tests of hepatic metabolic function reflect the liver's central role in metabolic and regulatory pathways, including the detoxification and clearance of endogenous metabolites such as ammonia. Multiple metabolic abnormalities due to specific inherited deficiencies of enzymes which reside almost exclusively in the liver such as the urea cycle defects can have a primary or secondary effect on the liver.

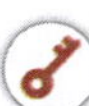 **Key: D**

BOOST YOUR KNOWLEDGE

Tests of liver function and injury based on substances released from damaged tissues are as follows:

Endogenous substances *released* by damaged hepatocytes	• ALT • AST • LDH
Endogenous substances *reflecting* impaired bile flow (cholestasis)	• GGT • ALP • 5'-NT • Leucine aminopeptidase (LAP) • Urobilinogen
Tests based on substances *synthesized* by the liver	• Albumin • Coagulation factors • Serum lipids and lipoproteins • Triglycerides • Cholesterol
Tests based on substances *metabolized* and transported by the liver	• Endogenous substances (serum bilirubin and serum bile acids) • Exogenous substances (lidocaine, caffeine, aminopyrine, and PABA)
Tests based on substances *detoxified* and cleared by the liver	Endogenous substances (ammonia)
Miscellaneous specific serum tests	• Serum immunoglobulins • Autoantibodies • Plasma and urine amino acids

Points to remember about LDH:

- Cytoplasmic enzymes present in many tissues
- Five isoenzymes of LDH
- Differential diagnosis of elevated serum LDH
- Skeletal or cardiac muscle injury, hemolysis, stroke, renal infarction, and acute and chronic liver disease

It is important to note that due to limited specificity, serum LDH levels rarely add information to that obtained from the aminotransferases alone. Uncommon clinical situations in which serum LDH levels may be diagnostically useful include the massive and transient elevation characteristic of ischemic hepatitis and the sustained elevation accompanying elevated ALP suggesting malignant infiltration of the liver.

REFERENCE/SOURCE

- Suchy FJ, Sokol RJ, Balistreri WF, Bezerra JA, Mack CL, Shneider BL. Liver Disease in Children, 5th edition. Cambridge, United Kingdom: Cambridge University Press; 2021. p. 94.

16. Which one of the following is *true* regarding utility of LFT?

A. LFT have no role in screening and documenting liver injury
B. LFT can help identify the type or pattern of liver disorder and the site of injury
C. These are not helpful in prognosis of children with chronic liver disease
D. These are not used to evaluate the response to treatment

EXPLANATION

Liver function tests have the following utilities: (1) Screen for and document liver injury; (2) identify the type or pattern of liver disorder and the site of injury; (3) prognosticate and follow-up children with chronic liver disease; and (4) serially monitor the course of liver disease, evaluate the response to treatment, and adjust a treatment regimen, when appropriate. After blunt abdominal trauma, parallel elevations in aminotransferase levels may provide an early clue to liver injury.

Key: B

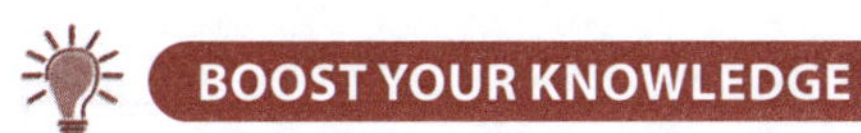

History
- Alcohol history/metabolic syndrome and BMI
- Drug history/risk factors for viral hepatitis
- Personal family history/comorbidities

Clinical pattern recognition

Hepatitic liver enzymes
↑ ALT or AST

Liver blood tests including AST, GGT and FBC
+
Ultrasound
+
Liver etiology screen
- Hepatitis B and C
- Autoantibodies and immunoglobulins
- Ferritin and transferrin saturation
- HbA1c

NAFLD
- T2DM
- BMI >25
- Dyslipidemia
- Hypertension

NAFLD fibrosis algorithm

- Normal USS
- Negative liver etiology screen
- No NAFLD risk-factors

ALT and AST remain abnormal

Refer for further diagnostic evaluation

Synthetic failure
Jaundice, low albumin, prolonged INR
OR
Suspected malignancy
- Weight loss
- Marked cholestasis

Urgent referral
Urgent ultrasound and/or
Consider urgent referral to secondary care or admission

Isolated raised bilirubin with otherwise normal liver blood tests

- Most commonly due to Gilbert's syndrome (unconjugated hyperbilirubinemia)
- Less commonly due to hemolysis (consider reticulocyte count, LDH, haptoglobin)

Repeat liver blood tests with split bilirubin and FBC
Consider: Reticulocyte and LDH if hemolysis

Gilbert's syndrome confirmed then inform patient and provide information

Isolated **cholestatic** liver enzymes
↑ ALP and GGT

Liver blood tests including GGT
+
Ultrasound
+
Liver etiology screen
- Autoantibodies and immunoglobulins
- Ferritin and transferrin saturation

Abnormal USS appearances and/or positive liver etiology screen

Normal USS and negative liver etiology screen

ALP and GGT remain abnormal

Refer for further specialist management/ investigation as defined by tests

Suspected alcohol risk
ARLD algorithm

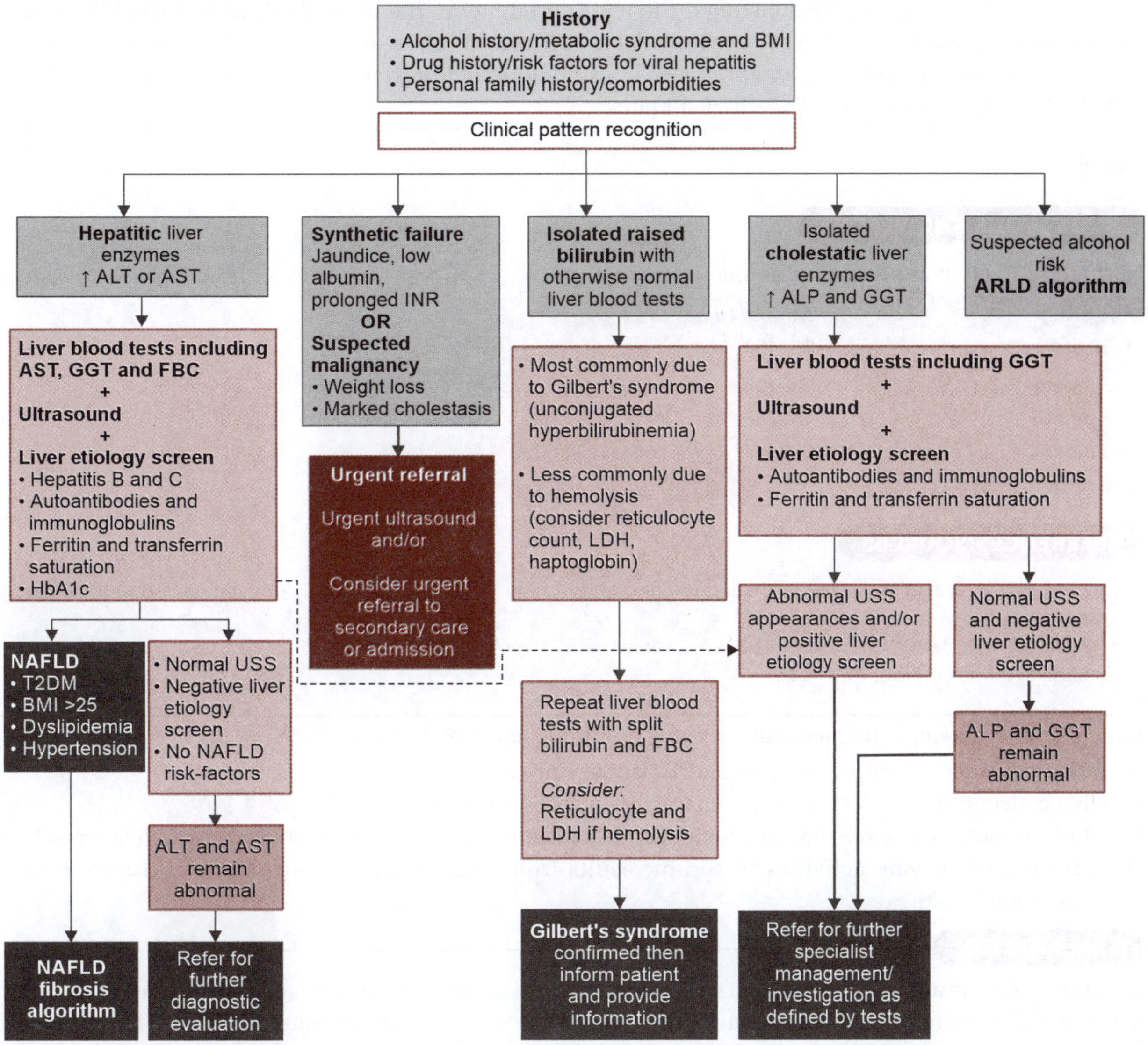

(ARLD: alcohol-related liver disease; BMI: body mass index; FBC: full blood count; USS: ultrasound scan)

REFERENCES/SOURCES

- Friedman SF, Martin P, Munoz JS. Hepatology: A Textbook of Liver Disease. Philadelphia: Saunders; 2003. pp. 661-709.
- Suchy FJ, Sokol RJ, Balistreri WF, Bezerra JA, Mack CL, Shneider BL. Liver Disease in Children, 5th edition. Cambridge, United Kingdom: Cambridge University Press; 2021. p. 94.

17. The SAFETY (Screening ALT for Elevation in Today's Youth) study recently demonstrated the wide variability in the upper limit of ALT used in acute care children's hospitals in the USA. What are the new proposed considerations of lowering the upper limit of normal threshold ALT for children?

A. ALT >15 IU/L for boys and ALT >12 IU/L for girls
B. ALT >25 IU/L for boys and ALT >22 IU/L for girls
C. ALT >45 IU/L for boys and ALT >42 IU/L for girls
D. ALT >65 IU/L for boys and ALT >62 IU/L for girls

EXPLANATION

The SAFETY study recently demonstrated the wide variability in the upper limit of ALT used in acute care children's hospitals in the USA. They concluded that ALT cut-off values are set too high for reliable detection of pediatric chronic liver diseases, and proposed consideration of lowering the upper limit of normal threshold to ALT >25 IU/L for boys and ALT >22 IU/L for girls.

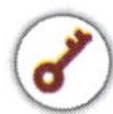

Key: B

BOOST YOUR KNOWLEDGE

Normal GGT values as per age are as follows:

Age group	*Normal values (U/L)*
1–30 day	16–450
1–3 month	16–267
3–5 month	16–267
5–8 month	8–84
9 months to 17 years	5–55

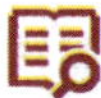

REFERENCES/SOURCES

- Hay W, Levin M, Deterding R, Sondheimer J. Current Diagnosis and Treatment: Pediatrics, 20th edition. New York: McGraw Hill Education; 2010.
- Suchy FJ, Sokol RJ, Balistreri WF, Bezerra JA, Mack CL, Shneider BL. Liver Disease in Children, 5th edition. Cambridge, United Kingdom: Cambridge University Press; 2021. p. 95.

18. Which of the following is *true* regarding serum aminotransferases?

A. AST is present primarily as a mitochondrial isoenzyme
B. High concentration of AST is unique characteristic of liver tissue
C. ALT is a cytosolic enzyme that is present in equal concentrations in the liver and within skeletal muscle cells
D. Elevation of enzyme activities in serum results from damage to or destruction of tissues rich in the aminotransferases

EXPLANATION

Aspartate aminotransferase is present as both cytosolic and mitochondrial isoenzymes and found in high concentrations in many nonliver tissues, including heart muscle, skeletal muscle, kidney, brain, pancreas, lung, leukocytes, and red blood cells. ALT is a cytosolic enzyme that is present in highest concentrations in the liver, and to a lesser extent within skeletal muscle cells. Elevation of enzyme activities in serum results from damage to or destruction of tissues rich in the aminotransferases or to a change in cell membrane permeability allowing AST and/or ALT to leak from damaged cells into serum. However, because of the wide tissue distribution of AST, the hepatic origin of an isolated serum AST level elevation should be confirmed by simultaneously obtaining a serum ALT level.

Key: D

BOOST YOUR KNOWLEDGE

Remember the following facts while analyzing AST and ALT:

- *AST:*
  - Origin from both mitochondria and cytoplasm of hepatocyte
  - True isoenzymes

- Less specific
- Early rise (t½ 16–18 hours)
- Clearance by reticuloendothelial system (RES) (primarily hepatic sinusoids)

- *ALT:*
  - Exclusively in cytosol
  - More specific
  - Longer t½ (40–48 hours)
  - Clearance by RES

REFERENCE/SOURCE

- Suchy FJ, Sokol RJ, Balistreri WF, Bezerra JA, Mack CL, Shneider BL. Liver Disease in Children, 5th edition. Cambridge, United Kingdom: Cambridge University Press; 2021. p. 95.

19. Asymptomatic elevation of serum ALT (and/or AST) levels is seen in which of the following disorders?

A. Celiac disease
B. Nephrotic syndrome
C. Severe acute malnutrition
D. Acute liver failure

EXPLANATION

The differential diagnosis of asymptomatic elevation of serum ALT (and/or AST) levels should consider underlying genetic diseases, including Wilson disease, alpha-1-antitrypsin deficiency, Alagille syndrome, hereditary fructose intolerance, glycogen storage disease and ornithine transcarbamylase deficiency, celiac disease, autoimmune hepatitis, drug-induced liver injury, and NAFLD. After blunt abdominal trauma, parallel elevations in aminotransferase levels may provide an early clue to liver injury. In the pediatric patient who has undergone liver transplantation, the differential diagnosis of elevated aminotransferase levels should include the different types of allograft rejection (hyperacute, acute cellular, or chronic), de novo autoimmune hepatitis, infection (hepatitis or intercurrent systemic), and biliary or vascular complications. Acute liver failure does not present as asymptomatic.

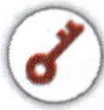

Key: A

BOOST YOUR KNOWLEDGE

Most accepted definition of acute liver failure (given by the Pediatric Acute Liver Failure study group) includes all the following:

- Acute onset of liver disease without evidence of chronic liver disease
- Biochemical evidence of severe liver injury
- Liver-based coagulopathy (not corrected by vitamin K) with PT >15 seconds or INR >1.5 with evidence of hepatic encephalopathy or PT >20 seconds or INR >2 with or without encephalopathy

REFERENCES/SOURCES

- Squires JE, Alonso EM, Ibrahim SH, Kasper V, Kehar M, Martinez M, et al. North American Society for Pediatric Gastroenterology, Hepatology, and Nutrition Position Paper on the Diagnosis and Management of Pediatric Acute Liver Failure. J Pediatr Gastroenterol Nutr. 2022;74(1):138-58.
- Suchy FJ, Sokol RJ, Balistreri WF, Bezerra JA, Mack CL, Shneider BL. Liver Disease in Children, 5th edition. Cambridge, United Kingdom: Cambridge University Press; 2021. p. 96.

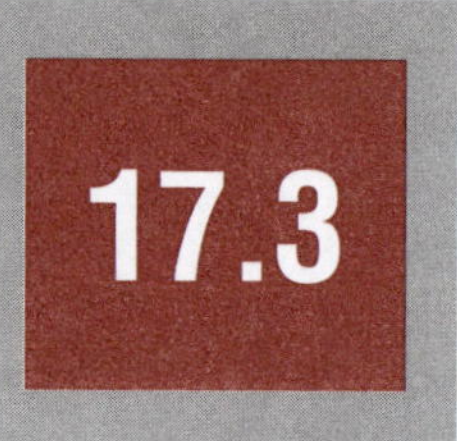

Acute Hepatitis and Hepatic Encephalopathy

Jayendra Seetharaman

1. Though blood-borne transmission is possible, what is the main reason behind feco-oral transmission being predominant mode of transmission of hepatitis A virus (HAV) in children?

A. Fecal contamination of the virus in the food is more common than blood product contamination
B. HAV predominantly grows in the small bowel epithelial cells
C. Fecal viral load is much higher and long lasting than the serum viral load
D. Children do not sanitize hands and do not follow hygiene practices well

EXPLANATION

The incubation period for hepatitis A is typically 2–6 weeks, averaging 28 days. Although HAV is present in serum, its concentration is several times lesser than in the feces. Hence, it is the high fecal viral load that results in feco-oral transmission. HAV grows predominantly in hepatocytes, so option B is wrong. Fecal contamination of the food and poor sanitation are secondary factors for feco-oral transmission but not the main factor.

Key: C

BOOST YOUR KNOWLEDGE

Fecal viral excretion may last up to 3 weeks. Children may excrete virus longer than adults. Virus replicates inside the hepatocytes and excreted with the bile in to the feces.

REFERENCE/SOURCE

- Suchy FJ, Sokol RJ, Balistreri WF. Liver Disease in Children, 4th edition. Cambridge: Cambridge University Press; 2014.

2. What is the reason behind the epidemiological shift of hepatitis A burden from younger children to adolescents and adults in India?

A. Increase in smoking and drinking in adolescents and adults
B. Compulsory childhood immunization with hepatitis A vaccine
C. Adults tend to travel more than the young children
D. Improvement in sanitation

EXPLANATION

In India, a rapid socioeconomic development has taken place in the recent decades. Many high endemicity areas for HAV infection made a transition to intermediate endemicity due to improvement in sanitation. Smoking and drinking do not have any relation with the transmission of virus, so option A is wrong. Hepatitis A vaccine in India is still an optional vaccine unlike countries like USA; hence, option B is also wrong. Adults travelling is not primary reason for the epidemiological shift.

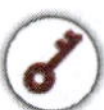

Key: D

BOOST YOUR KNOWLEDGE

Although feco-oral transmission is most common mode of transmission in hepatitis, sexual contact, contaminated needle for drug use, and intrauterine transmission also can result in transmission of the virus.

REFERENCE/SOURCE

- Advisory Committee on Vaccines and Immunization Practices. IAP Guidebook of Immunization 2018–2019, 3rd edition. New Delhi: Jaypee Brothers Medical Publishers; 2020.

3. A 2-year-old, well thriving girl present with vomiting, poor appetite, and fever for last 4 days. There was no history of jaundice, altered sensorium, or abdominal distention. There was no obvious history of drug intake. Paracetamol was given in therapeutic doses for fever. On examination, child had hepatomegaly. On evaluation her hemoglobin is 12.1 g/dL, total leukocyte count is 4,800 cells/mm^3, and platelet count is 2.3 lakh/mm^3. Her liver functions showed total bilirubin 0.4 mg/dL, alanine transaminase (ALT) 2,364 IU/L, aspartate aminotransferase (AST) 3,080 IU/L, serum albumin 4.4 g/dL, and international normalized ratio (INR) 1.12. Which of the following is the investigation of choice to confirm the diagnosis?

A. Serum ceruloplasmin
B. Paracetamol levels
C. Anti-HAV immunoglobulin M (IgM)
D. Ultrasonography (USG) abdomen

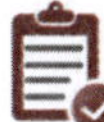

EXPLANATION

Initial clinical manifestations of HAV infection may present similar to a viral prodrome, with nonspecific symptoms such as nausea, vomiting, anorexia, fatigue, weight loss, low-grade fevers, myalgia, arthralgia, and headaches. Common signs of infection include hepatomegaly, and splenomegaly. In preschool children, acute HAV infection may be unapparent as they mostly remain anicteric. Jaundice is present only in 10% of the children with acute HAV infection under 6 years.

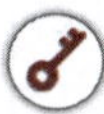

Key: C

BOOST YOUR KNOWLEDGE

Consider drug-induced liver injury and viral hepatitis when the transaminases are in thousands. Metabolic liver diseases like Wilson's disease rarely have very high transaminase levels.

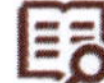

REFERENCE/SOURCE

- Suchy FJ, Sokol RJ, Balistreri WF. Liver Disease in Children, 4th edition. Cambridge: Cambridge University Press; 2014.

4. An 8-year-old boy presented with fever, vomiting, and abdominal pain for 5 days followed by jaundice and dark colored urine. There is no bleeding tendencies or encephalopathy. On examination, there is hepatomegaly. His IgM HAV was positive. His parents were reassured about the illness and the child was sent home. But 3 months later child again presented with persistent jaundice and recent onset itching. Which of the following medications is advised for this situation?

A. Cholestyramine
B. Lactulose
C. Ursodeoxycholic acid
D. Prednisolone

EXPLANATION

Prolonged jaundice for >3 months associated with pruritus, diarrhea, and weight loss with serum bilirubin levels >10 mg/dL is defined as cholestatic hepatitis, usually associated with HAV. Therapy with ursodeoxycholic acid is beneficial to reduce cholestasis. Lactulose and cholestyramine are not indicated. Corticosteroids can be beneficial but the data are sparse and currently not recommended due to risk of reactivation of virus.

Key: C

BOOST YOUR KNOWLEDGE

Relapsing hepatitis, bone marrow suppression, triggering autoimmune hepatitis, vasculitis, arthritis, pancreatitis, and hemophagocytic lymphohistiocytosis are other atypical manifestations of hepatitis A.

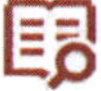

REFERENCE/SOURCE

- Suchy FJ, Sokol RJ, Balistreri WF. Liver Disease in Children, 4th edition. Cambridge: Cambridge University Press; 2014.

5. Which of the following is a significant difference between acute hepatitis caused by hepatitis A and hepatitis E viruses?

A. Mode of transmission
B. Incubation period
C. Protective antibody postinfection
D. Presence of cholestatic phase

EXPLANATION

Hepatitis E has similar presentation to hepatitis A with respect to prodromal illness which consists of fever, abdominal pain, anorexia, nausea, vomiting, etc. The mode of transmission for both acute hepatitis A and acute hepatitis E is predominantly feco-oral transmission. Posthepatitis A infection, IgG antibody provide protective immunity which is also similar in the case of acute hepatitis E postresolution. Hepatitis E is also known to have cholestatic phase like hepatitis A. The medical incubation period of hepatitis A is 28 days whereas the hepatitis E has longer incubation period, which is 45 days.

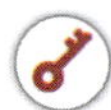

Key: B

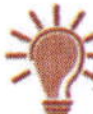

BOOST YOUR KNOWLEDGE

Longer incubation period, delayed age of presentation (15–40 years), fulminant manifestations in pregnancy, and risk of development of cirrhosis in immunosuppressed transplant recipients are specific for hepatitis E, and not a feature of hepatitis A.

REFERENCE/SOURCE

- Suchy FJ, Sokol RJ Balistreri WF. Liver Disease in Children, 4th edition. Cambridge: Cambridge University Press; 2014.

6. What is the current Indian Academy of Pediatrics (IAP) recommendation for HAV vaccine for adolescents in India?

A. Two doses of killed HAV vaccine should be given to all adolescents, irrespective of the past status of infection
B. One dose of live-attenuated HAV vaccine should be given to all adolescents
C. HAV vaccine should not be given for adolescents with cirrhosis
D. Hepatitis A IgG levels need to done before initiating hepatitis A vaccination

EXPLANATION

Multiple studies from India showed that the seropositivity of hepatitis A is over 50–75% in >15 years of age. Since the cost of screening to identify those susceptible to get hepatitis A infection is lower than the cost of vaccine, IAP Advisory Committee on Vaccines and Immunization Practices (ACVIP) recommends prevaccination screening for hepatitis A antibody in children >10 years of age. Hepatitis A in India is still an optional vaccine across all age group. Hepatitis A vaccine is to be considered in high-risk group, especially when there is underlying cirrhosis.

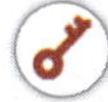

Key: D

BOOST YOUR KNOWLEDGE

High-risk groups where special emphasis should be given for vaccination are as follows: Patients with chronic liver disease (CLD), carriers of hepatitis B and hepatitis C, congenital or acquired immunodeficiency, transplant recipients, adolescents seronegative for HAV who are leaving home for residential school, travels to countries with high endemicity for hepatitis A, and household contacts of patients with acute HAV infection within 10 days of onset of illness in the index case are considered high-risk groups.

REFERENCE/SOURCE

- Advisory Committee on Vaccines and Immunization Practices. IAP Guidebook of Immunization 2018–2019, 3rd edition. New Delhi: Jaypee Brothers Medical Publishers; 2020.

7. An 8-year-old boy presented with nausea, abdominal pain and fever for 3 days, there after he developed jaundice. Within few days after he developed jaundice, he developed joint pain and skin rash in the legs and hands as shown in given Figure. There was no family history of jaundice or any drug intake in the past. But he had an ear piercing 6 months back in a local religious institution. What is the test required to confirm the etiology?

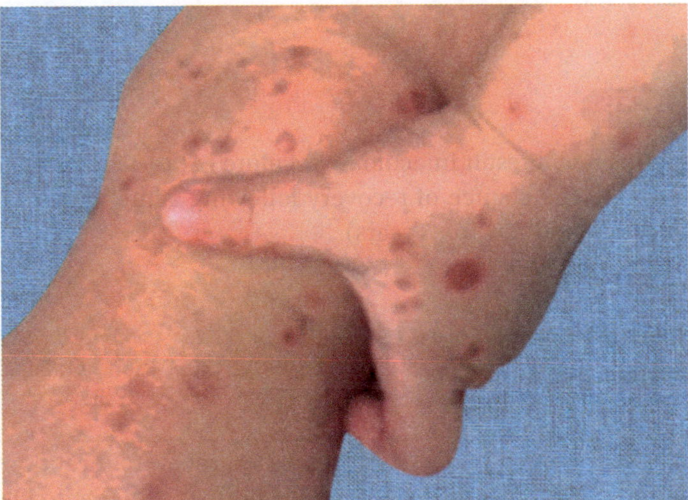

A. Leptospira serology
B. Antihepatitis A IgM
C. Antihepatitis B core (HBc) IgM
D. Antinuclear antibody (ANA) and anti-double-stranded deoxyribonucleic acid (dsDNA)

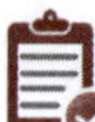

EXPLANATION

In the setting of acute hepatitis, which is a prodromal illness followed by jaundice, Acute viral hepatitis is to be considered. The ear piercing is the clue in the question that indicates likely possibility of transmission through contaminated needles, likely acute hepatitis B. Acute hepatitis B has associated extrahepatic manifestations. The picture depicts papular acrodermatitis which is called Gianotti–Crosti syndrome. To confirm the diagnosis, anti-HBc IgM needs to be done which is a marker of acute hepatitis B infection.

Key: C

BOOST YOUR KNOWLEDGE

Other extrahepatic conditions associated with HBV infections in children include polyarteritis nodosa, glomerulonephritis, and aplastic anemia.

REFERENCE/SOURCE

- Viral Hepatitis. In: Kliegman R, St Geme JW, Blum NJ, Shah SS, Tasker RC, Wilson KM (Eds). Nelson Textbook of Pediatrics, 21st edition. Amsterdam, Netherlands: Elsevier; 2019.

8. What is referred to as "window period" with respect to diagnosis of acute hepatitis B?

A. The period where transaminases resolve but hepatitis B surface antigen (HBsAg) is still present
B. The period when HBsAg has already resolved but anti-HBc IgM is still present
C. The period when HBV DNA titers have become negative but HBsAg is still positive
D. When there is jaundice but HBsAg has still not become positive

EXPLANATION

During recovery from acute infection, because HBsAg levels fall before symptoms wane, IgM antibody to hepatitis B core antigen (HBcAg) (anti-HBc IgM) might be the only marker of acute infection. Doing HBsAg at this point of time will fail to recognize acute hepatitis B. This is termed as window period. Anti-HBc IgM stays for many months till it is replaced by anti-HBc IgG.

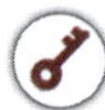

Key: B

BOOST YOUR KNOWLEDGE

About 1–5% of acute hepatitis B will result in acute liver failure (ALF). The mortality is as high as 30% without liver transplant in case of ALF. The chance of recovery following acute hepatitis B is more in older children (5% in neonate, 30% in 1–5 years, and 75% in >5 years).

REFERENCES/SOURCES

- Suchy FJ, Sokol RJ, Balistreri WF. Liver Disease in Children, 4th edition. Cambridge: Cambridge University Press; 2014.
- Viral Hepatitis. In: Kliegman R, St Geme JW, Blum NJ, Shah SS, Tasker RC, Wilson KM (Eds). Nelson Textbook of Pediatrics, 21st edition. Amsterdam, Netherlands: Elsevier; 2019.

9. Which of the following is *not* a routine Centers for Disease Control and Prevention (CDC) recommendation for the prevention of vertical transmission of the hepatitis B virus from the mother to the newborn?

A. HBsAg- and hepatitis B e antigen (HBeAg)-positive mothers should not breastfeed their infant
B. Antiviral should be started to mothers in the third trimester with high viral load
C. Hepatitis B vaccine along with hepatitis B immunoglobulin (HBIG) must be given within 12 hours of the birth of the infant
D. Postvaccination testing of HBsAg and anti-HBs should be done after 9 months of birth

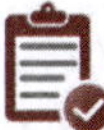

EXPLANATION

The HBsAg is inconsistently secreted in the breast milk, if there are no sore nipples or cracked nipple, mother can safely breastfeed their infant. Guidelines suggest that mothers with a HBV DNA viral load >200,000 IU/mL receive an antiviral such as telbivudine, lamivudine, or tenofovir during the third trimester. The children born to HBV mother must receive HBIG and the hepatitis B vaccine.

Key: A

BOOST YOUR KNOWLEDGE

Postvaccination testing must be done from 9 to 18 months or 1–2 months after the last dose of vaccine, if delayed. If HBsAg and anti-HBs are negative, will repeat all three doses of vaccine series. If HBsAg is negative and anti-HBs is positive, the child is adequately immunized. If HBsAg is positive, chronic hepatitis B infection is to be considered.

REFERENCES/SOURCES

- https://www.cdc.gov/hepatitis-b/hcp/prenatal-provider-overview/index.html.
- Viral Hepatitis. In: Kliegman R, St Geme JW, Blum NJ, Shah SS, Tasker RC, Wilson KM (Eds). Nelson Textbook of Pediatrics, 21st edition. Amsterdam, Netherlands: Elsevier; 2019.

10. A 12-year-old girl presented with fever and cough with expectoration for 3 weeks. She was sputum positive for acid-fast bacilli. She was started on four-drug antituberculosis therapy (ATT) (HRZE). 1 week later, she developed anorexia, vomiting, and jaundice. Her total bilirubin is 5.0 mg/dL and liver enzymes are AST 221 IU/L and ALT 206 IU/L. Considering ATT-induced liver injury, all the drugs were stopped. What is the next plan of action?

A. Start low dose of HRZ and continue ethambutol in usual dose
B. Wait for liver enzymes and bilirubin to normalize, then start ATT
C. Start each drug H, R, Z at low dose, one after another
D. Go for nonhepatotoxic ATT, as there is a risk of liver injury on restarting H, R, Z

EXPLANATION

In case of ATT-induced liver injury, once enzyme level improves, reintroduce remaining drugs, one at a time with the least hepatotoxic agents first, while monitoring liver function by testing enzymes every 3 days. Although there is difference of opinion, the schedule followed is to start R with 150 mg, repeat liver function test (LFT) after 3–5 days, if no increase and no symptoms, increase to 300 mg, repeat same as mentioned earlier and then full dose. For H and Z process is the similar. In most of the occasions, the hepatotoxicity would not recur when restarted slowly.

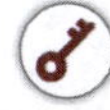

Key: B

BOOST YOUR KNOWLEDGE

Post-ATT, if there are any one of the following: (1) Presence of symptoms, (2) ALT/AST more than five times of upper limit of normal (ULN), and (3) total bilirubin >2 mg/dL, consider stopping all hepatotoxic drugs. If there are no symptoms, AST/ALT less than five times of ULN, total bilirubin <2 mg/dL, continue ATT with close monitoring of LFT and symptoms.

REFERENCE/SOURCE

- National Tuberculosis Elimination Programme. Pediatric TB Management Guideline 2022. [online] Available from https://tbcindia.gov.in/WriteReadData/l892s/9534339438Paediatric_TB_Mangement_Guideline_22082022_V1.pdf. [Last accessed June, 2024].

11. A 9-year-old child presented with progressively increasing jaundice for the past 3 weeks, there was cola-colored urine noticed for last 1 week associated with lethargy and confusion. He has diminished school performance noticed for last 1 year. The elder sibling also had developed jaundice at 10 years and died a year later. On examination, he was lethargic, pale, and deeply jaundiced. There was hepatosplenomegaly on abdominal examination. What is the probable diagnosis of ALF?

A. Hepatitis A
B. Autoimmune hepatitis
C. Hepatitis E
D. Wilson's disease

EXPLANATION

Child in this question had jaundice followed by encephalopathy which qualifies for ALF. Other clues in the history are cola-colored urine and anemia which signifies probable underlying intravascular hemolysis. Of the options, Wilson's disease can have Coombs-negative hemolytic anemia and autoimmune hepatitis can have associated autoimmune hemolytic anemia both presenting as intravascular hemolysis. Diminished school performance is much suggestive of neurological manifestation of Wilson's disease. As the Wilson's disease is autosomal recessive disorder, the possibilities of Wilson's disease in sibling are not uncommon.

Key: D

BOOST YOUR KNOWLEDGE

Wilson's disease is diagnosed by low ceruloplasmin levels (<20 mg/dL), presence of Kayser–Fleischer (KF) of ring and 24-hour urine copper (>100 µg/day in symptomatic cases). In ambiguous cases, liver biopsy needs to be done to look for dry weight of copper >250 µg/g with good sensitivity. Molecular studies also help to identify mutation in *ATP7B* gene to confirm Wilson's disease.

REFERENCES/SOURCES

- Suchy FJ, Sokol RJ, Balistreri WF. Liver Disease in Children, 4th edition. Cambridge: Cambridge University Press; 2014.
- Viral Hepatitis. In: Kliegman R, St Geme JW, Blum NJ, Shah SS, Tasker RC, Wilson KM (Eds). Nelson Textbook of Pediatrics, 21st edition. Amsterdam, Netherlands: Elsevier; 2019.

12. A 2-year-old child (10 kg) developed recurrent vomiting from 4 AM. Parents realized the child was playing with the Calpol syrup (5 mL/250 mg, volume 50 mL) at 9 PM and the bottle is empty now. The child was taken to pediatric emergency at 6 AM. There was no encephalopathy and he was treated for vomiting with intravenous (IV) fluids and antiemetics. Samples were reported at 7 AM showed paracetamol level 200 µg/mL, serum glutamic-oxaloacetic transaminase (SGOT) 781 IU/L and serum glutamic-pyruvic transaminase (SGPT) 344 IU/L. His INR is 1.2 and total bilirubin is <1 mg/dL. Currently the child is asymptomatic. What is the next line of management?

A. Child can be sent home safely from the emergency
B. Observe the child for 24–48 hours till liver enzymes improve
C. To start N-acetyl cysteine (NAC) and repeat paracetamol levels and liver enzymes after 24 hours
D. To refer to a transplant center for emergency liver transplantation

EXPLANATION

The paracetamol level at 9 hours (9 PM to 6 AM) of ingestion is 200 µg/mL which is the level of probable toxicity in Rumack–Matthew nomogram. Hence, the child needs to immediately started on NAC either oral or IV. 24 hours later paracetamol levels and liver enzymes need to be repeated. NAC needs to be continued till paracetamol levels are undetectable and liver enzymes are in down going trend.

Key: C

BOOST YOUR KNOWLEDGE

The King's College Criteria are applied to assess the need for liver transplant. Acidosis (pH < 7.3), INR > 6, creatinine > 3.4 mg/dL, lactate > 3 mmol/L, and grade III/IV hepatic encephalopathy (HE) predicts death without liver transplant with high sensitivity and specificity.

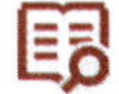

REFERENCE/SOURCE

- Poisoning. In: Kliegman R, St Geme JW, Blum NJ, Shah SS, Tasker RC, Wilson KM (Eds). Nelson Textbook of Pediatrics, 21st edition. Amsterdam, Netherlands: Elsevier; 2019.

13. In a child with multiple repeated supratherapeutic doses of paracetamol, which level of paracetamol in the blood needs monitoring and treatment?

A. 5 μg/mL
B. 10 μg/mL
C. 15 μg/mL
D. 20 μg/mL

EXPLANATION

Because the Rumack–Matthew nomogram is not helpful in repeated supratherapeutic ingestion of paracetamol, a conservative approach is taken. In the asymptomatic patient, if the SGOT is normal and the paracetamol level is <10 μg/mL, no therapy is required. If the paracetamol levels are above that NAC has to be started.

Key: B

BOOST YOUR KNOWLEDGE

If the SGOT is elevated, NAC needs to be started and LFT needs to be monitored to assess the need for liver transplantation. In case of symptoms such as abdominal pain and vomiting, NAC has to be started immediately till the drug levels are ready.

REFERENCE/SOURCE

- Poisoning. In: Kliegman R, St Geme JW, Blum NJ, Shah SS, Tasker RC, Wilson KM (Eds). Nelson Textbook of Pediatrics, 21st edition. Amsterdam, Netherlands: Elsevier; 2019.

14. Which of the following is the most appropriate biochemical marker that correlates with the stage of HE in cirrhosis?

A. Glutamine in cerebrospinal fluid (CSF)
B. Serum ammonia levels
C. Gamma-aminobutyric acid levels in serum
D. Serum tryptophan

EXPLANATION

In the setting of severe liver disease, blood from the intestine is shunted around the liver through collateral vessels or through the liver as the blood passes through the damaged or necrotic hepatocytes. Serum ammonia produced in the gut is converted to urea by urea cycle or glutamine by glutaminase in liver. In liver disease, the ammonia is shunted without conversion. But the ammonia levels do not correlate with stage of HE. Elevated ammonia, mercaptans, and aromatic amino acids such as tryptophan, octopamine, and GABA are all increased in HE. Out of all the markers, CSF levels of glutamine is said to correlate well with the stage of HE.

Key: A

 BOOST YOUR KNOWLEDGE

Glutaminase also is found in skeletal muscle and the brain. In individuals with CLD and skeletal muscle wasting, reduction of ammonia levels through synthesis of glutamine is diminished; hence, the risk of severe HE is high in malnourished cirrhotic patients.

 REFERENCE/SOURCE

- Suchy FJ, Sokol RJ, Balistreri WF. Liver Disease in Children, 4th edition. Cambridge: Cambridge University Press; 2014.

15. What is the most prominent difference between the HE in ALF and CLD?

A. Ammonia levels are much higher in ALF
B. False neurotransmitters play a major in CLD whereas ammonia plays a major role in ALF
C. Deposition of manganese in the basal ganglia is seen in CLD
D. Astrocyte swelling causing cerebral edema is more specific for ALF

 EXPLANATION

Ammonia levels increase in both ALF and CLD. False neurotransmitters are also responsible for HE in both ALF and CLD. Manganese deposition is seen in CLD, but it is also found in ALF. Production of glutamine inside the astrocytes causes absorption of water due to osmotic effect causing cerebral edema in ALF. This is not a prominent feature in CLD.

 **Key: D**

 BOOST YOUR KNOWLEDGE

In CLD, due to chronically increased ammonia levels, cerebral edema is less of a concern because of the activation of brain osmoregulatory mechanisms and the production of myoinositol to counter the osmotic effect of ammonia upon astrocytes.

 REFERENCE/SOURCE

- Suchy FJ, Sokol RJ, Balistreri WF. Liver Disease in Children, 4th edition. Cambridge: Cambridge University Press; 2014.

16. Which of the following is the clinical assessment method to identify minimal hepatic encephalopathy (MHE)?

A. Elicitation of asterixis
B. Hyperreflexia with extensor plantar reflex
C. Disoriented behavior
D. Psychometric hepatic encephalopathy score (PHES)

 EXPLANATION

Asterixis is flapping tremor seen in stage 2 of HE. Disorientation, stupor, and hyperreflexia are seen in late stages of HE. Neuropsychological testing with the PHES is a battery of tests evaluating memory and neuromotor function, has been used in studying MHE. Stroop test, portosystemic encephalopathy syndrome test, and critical flicker frequency are other tests to assess minimal HE.

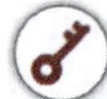 **Key: D**

 BOOST YOUR KNOWLEDGE

A battery of paper and pen tests contribute to PHES score. It consists of number connection tests, digit symbol tests, serial dotting tests, and line tracing tests. The tests are simple to perform and test multiple areas of cognition. However, the results depend on age, sex, level of education, and cultural background.

REFERENCES/SOURCES

- Suchy FJ, Sokol RJ, Balistreri WF. Liver Disease in Children, 4th edition. Cambridge: Cambridge University Press; 2014.
- Thanapirom K, Wongwandee M, Suksawatamnuay S, Thaimai P, Siripon N, Makhasen W, et al. Psychometric Hepatic Encephalopathy Score for the Diagnosis of Minimal Hepatic Encephalopathy in Thai Cirrhotic Patients. J Clin Med. 2023;12(2):519.
- Vilstrup H, Amodio P, Bajaj J, Cordoba J, Ferenci P, Mullen KD, et al. Hepatic encephalopathy in chronic liver disease: 2014 Practice Guideline by the American Association for the Study of Liver Diseases and the European Association for the Study of the Liver. Hepatology. 2014;60(2):715-35.

17. A 15-year-old boy who is a known cirrhotic, presented with hematemesis followed by melena. He has jaundice and diffuse abdominal distention along with fever after the vomiting episodes. On evaluation, his ascitic tap revealed spontaneous bacterial peritonitis, his hemoglobin is 7.5 g/dL, sodium is 132 mEq/L, potassium is 2.9 mEq/L, albumin is 2.4 g/dL, and calcium is 7.7 mg/dL. He was started on frusemide and spironolactone for ascites. One day later, he developed drowsiness, confusion, and disorientation. Which of the following *did not* contribute to his mental deterioration?

A. Spontaneous bacterial peritonitis
B. Hypokalemia
C. Diuretics
D. Anemia

EXPLANATION

Hepatic encephalopathy is initiated by a precipitating event, such as gastrointestinal (GI) hemorrhage, infection, the administration of sedatives, hypokalemia, hyponatremia, or high doses of diuretics. This child had spontaneous bacterial peritonitis which is known to precipitate HE. The child also had low sodium, potassium, and GI bleed that could have precipitated HE. Anemia is not a known factor to precipitate HE.

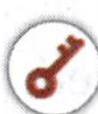

Key: D

BOOST YOUR KNOWLEDGE

Hypokalemia promotes ammoniagenesis in the renal tubules. High doses of diuretics precipitate HE by causing dehydration and hypokalemia. Sedatives, especially benzodiazepines, facilitate GABAergic neurons and worsen encephalopathy.

REFERENCE/SOURCE

- Suchy FJ, Sokol RJ, Balistreri WF. Liver Disease in Children, 4th edition. Cambridge: Cambridge University Press; 2014.

18. Which of the following is not a recommended drug for the treatment of HE?

A. Lactulose
B. Ampicillin
C. Neomycin
D. Branched chain amino acids

EXPLANATION

Lactulose is the first choice of drug for the treatment of overt HE. Rifaximin is an effective add-on for lactulose. In case of refractory cases of HE, oral branched chain amino acids and IV L-ornithine and L-asparagine are proven to be useful add-on for lactulose and rifaximin. Neomycin is an effective alternative drug to have beneficial effect in HE.

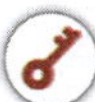

Key: B

BOOST YOUR KNOWLEDGE

Ammonia scavengers such as ornithine phenylacetate, glyceryl phenyl butyrate, probiotics, metronidazole, polyethylene glycol, and flumazenil are all studied and shown to have some benefit on HE apart from the drugs mentioned in the earlier section.

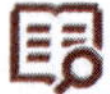

REFERENCE/SOURCE

- Vilstrup H, Amodio P, Bajaj J, Cordoba J, Ferenci P, Mullen KD, et al. Hepatic encephalopathy in chronic liver disease: 2014 Practice Guideline by the American Association for the Study of Liver Diseases and the European Association for the Study of the Liver. Hepatology. 2014;60(2):715-35.

19. A 4-year-old apparently normal child presented with jaundice for 2 weeks. 2 days before, he developed altered mentation in the form of confusion, irritability, and not recognizing his parents. He was admitted in intensive care for his altered mentation and started on midazolam infusion due to the irritability. He became stuporous after 24 hours that he has to be intubated to secure airway. He was started on IV meropenem and vancomycin empirically due to fever. He was started on IV proton pump inhibitor and intermittent mannitol boluses. Which of the following was *not* the appropriate management measure for this child?

A. Midazolam infusion
B. Initiation of antibiotics
C. Proton pump inhibitor
D. Mannitol

EXPLANATION

In case of HE, child has to be electively intubated especially in stage III/IV HE. Hypertonic saline and mannitol would help in reduction of cerebral edema. Isotonic fluids must be given for hypovolemia and inotropes to maintain blood pressure. Broad-spectrum antibiotics must be empirically started, especially in advanced HE (stage III/IV) as there is high chances of sepsis in these children. IV proton pump inhibitor is advised for prevention of GI bleed due to stress ulcers. Sedatives are avoided in early stages of HE as it may further worsen the sensorium and precipitate coma.

Key: A

BOOST YOUR KNOWLEDGE

Sedatives are avoided as far as possible and indicated only after the child is put on mechanical ventilation. Even when the sedatives are used benzodiazepines and opiates are better avoided.

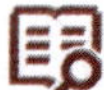

REFERENCE/SOURCE

- Acute hepatic failure. In: Kliegman R, St Geme JW, Blum NJ, Shah SS, Tasker RC, Wilson KM (Eds). Nelson Textbook of Pediatrics, 21st edition. Amsterdam, Netherlands: Elsevier; 2019.

20. Which of the following is the correct match with respect to the stages of HE as per the West Haven criteria?

A. Reversal of day-night sleep pattern—minimal HE
B. Q waves in electroencephalogram (EEG)—stage II
C. Asterixis—stage III
D. Coma not responding to noxious stimuli—stage IVa

EXPLANATION

Electroencephalogram would be normal in stage I, generalized background slowing, q waves are seen in stage II, triphasic waves in stage III, marked slowing, and d waves seen in stage IV. Asterixis is seen in stage II and stage III. Areflexia, flaccidity, and coma are seen in stage IV. Stage IVa is when there is response to noxious stimuli and Stage IVb is when there is no response to noxious stimuli. Minimal HE is when the child is clinically normal but able to elicit HE by neurophysiological and psychometric test.

Key: C

BOOST YOUR KNOWLEDGE

Spectrum of neurocognitive impairment in cirrhosis (SONIC) nomenclature is divided into unimpaired, covert HE, and overt HE. Unimpaired HE patients have no neuropsychometric abnormalities or clinical abnormalities. Covert HE comprises of minimal HE and stage I HE of West Haven criteria. Overt HE comprises stage II, III, and IV of West Haven criteria.

REFERENCES/SOURCES

- Acute hepatic failure. In: Kliegman R, St Geme JW, Blum NJ, Shah SS, Tasker RC, Wilson KM (Eds). Nelson Textbook of Pediatrics, 21st edition. Amsterdam, Netherlands: Elsevier; 2019.
- Other inherited metabolic disorders of the liver. In: Feldman M, Friedman LS, Brandt LJ (Eds). Sleisenger and Fordtran's Gastrointestinal and Liver Disease, 11th edition. Amsterdam, Netherlands: Elsevier; 2020.

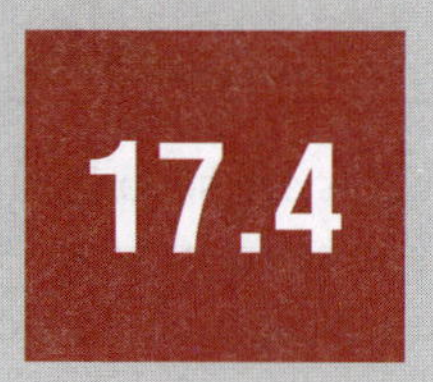

CHAPTER 17.4

Chronic Liver Disease

Moinak Sen Sarma

1. Chronicity of liver disease is best defined as presence of:

A. Liver dysfunction for at least 3 months
B. Features such as spider nevi and ascites
C. Firm hepatomegaly
D. Conjugated hyperbilirubinemia

EXPLANATION

Chronicity of liver disease is determined either by duration of liver disease (typically >6 months for viral diseases such as hepatitis B or C) or by evidence of chronic hepatic decompensation (hypoalbuminemia, coagulopathy, encephalopathy, and ascites) irrespective of duration or physical stigmata of chronic liver disease (CLD), described below. Firm hepatomegaly can be seen in acute viral hepatitis or CLD. Conjugated hyperbilirubinemia is not specific of CLD. It can be seen in many other conditions such as Dubin Johnson syndrome, Rotor syndrome, cholestasis, and acute hepatitis.

Key: B

BOOST YOUR KNOWLEDGE

Stigmata of CLD in children include spider nevi (typically over upper chest, back and face), paper money skin (skin telangiectasia), leukonychia (white nails), clubbing, palmar erythema (>2 years age). Parotitis and Dupuytren's contracture are typically seen in adults with alcoholic liver disease. Adolescents have delayed puberty. Typical features seen in adults such as breast and testicular atrophy are not seen in children. Early onset gynecomastia in boys can be attributed to CLD but not after the onset of adolescence. Gynecomastia (unilateral or bilateral) can be due to spironolactone therapy for controlling ascites in CLD.

REFERENCES/SOURCES

- Alam S, Khanna R. Chronic liver disease (Chapter 37.8). In: Gupta P, Menon PSN, Ramji S, Lodha R. PG Textbook of Pediatrics, 3rd edition. New Delhi: Jaypee Brothers Medical Publishers; 2022.
- Kliegman RM, St Geme III JW. Nelson Textbook of Pediatrics, 21st edition. Elsevier; 2019. Chapter 382: Manifestations of liver disease.
- Kliegman RM, St Geme III JW. Nelson Textbook of Pediatrics, 21st edition. Elsevier; 2019. Chapter 389: Autoimmune hepatitis.
- Yachha SK, Sarma MS. Portal hypertension (Chapter 37.4). In: Gupta P, Menon PSN, Ramji S, Lodha R. PG Textbook of Pediatrics, 3rd edition. New Delhi: Jaypee Brothers Medical Publishers; 2022.

2. Which of the combination of nail changes is present in chronic liver disease?

A. Clubbing and Terry nails
B. Muehrcke's lines and splinter hemorrhages
C. Half-and-half nail and Mees' lines
D. Melanonychia and Beau's lines

EXPLANATION

Various systemic disorders cause changes in the nails. Changes seen commonly in chronic liver diseases (CLD) are Terry nails, leukonychia, Muehrcke's lines, and clubbing. Additionally azure lunula is rarely seen in Wilson disease (WD).

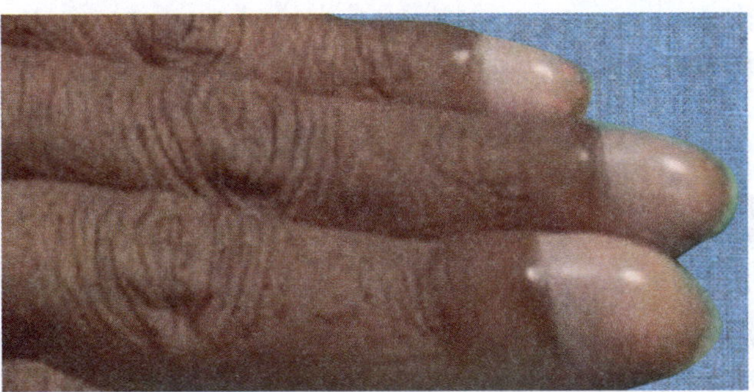

Key: A

BOOST YOUR KNOWLEDGE

Nail changes in systemic diseases occur as changes in nail shape (e.g., koilonychia, clubbing), surface (Beau's lines, longitudinal ridging), attachment (onycholysis), color (leukonychia, yellow nails), and abnormalities in lunula. Due to hypoalbuminemia, periods of edema, and poor nutrition, nail growth is affected in CLD, specifically affecting shape, surface, and color. Some of these changes may overlap with other systemic disorders. Clubbing in CLD occurs due to concomitant hepatopulmonary syndrome. Yellow nail syndrome is associated with conditions that have lymphedema.

The table here shows systemic disorders with specific nail changes:

Hematological	*Renal*	*Cardiac*	*Drugs and metals*	*Immunological*	*Respiratory*
• Koilonychia • Platynychia	• Half and half nail (Lindsay nails) • Mees' line • Muehrcke's lines	• Splinter hemorrhages (infective endocarditis) • Mees' lines	• Melanonychia • Mees' line	• Nail bed telangiectasia • Beau's lines	• Cyanosis • Clubbing • Yellow nails • Red lunula

REFERENCES/SOURCES

- Alam S, Khanna R. Chronic liver disease (Chapter 37.8). In: Gupta P, Menon PSN, Ramji S, Lodha R. PG Textbook of Pediatrics, 3rd edition. New Delhi: Jaypee Brothers Medical Publishers; 2022.
- Singal A, Arora R. Nail as a window of systemic diseases. Indian Dermatol Online J. 2015;6(2):67-74.
- Yachha SK, Sarma MS. Portal hypertension (Chapter 37.4). In: Gupta P, Menon PSN, Ramji S, Lodha R. PG Textbook of Pediatrics, 3rd edition. New Delhi: Jaypee Brothers Medical Publishers; 2022.

3. A 10-year-old boy was referred for an inguinal hernia surgery. In the presurgical screen, hepatitis B surface (HBs) antigen was found to be positive. On further workup, he was found to have normal liver functions, normal abdominal sonography, immunoglobulin M (IgM) anti-HBc (hepatitis B core) negative, HBe antigen positive, anti-HBe antibody negative, and hepatitis B virus deoxyribonucleic acid (HBV-DNA) 3×10^8 IU/mL. Which of the statements is true?

A. Child has an ongoing anicteric hepatitis
B. Child is not in an infective stage
C. Transmission is likely to have been vertical
D. Child is most likely having cirrhosis

EXPLANATION

Incidentally detected HBs antigen is a common scenario in children. Most children are infected vertically (i.e., mother-child transmission). 90% develop chronicity when infected during infancy. Chronic hepatitis B in this scenario is in an immune-tolerant phase with high infectivity. Here, the child remains anicteric with normal liver functions. In this scenario, the HBe antigen is positive, HBe antibody is negative, and HBV-DNA is many folds high (>10^6 IU/mL). IgM anti-HBc positivity with high liver enzymes is a marker of acute hepatitis.

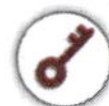

Key: C

BOOST YOUR KNOWLEDGE

Phases of chronic hepatitis B infection:

Characteristics	*Immune tolerance*	*Immune clearance*	*Inactive carrier*	*Reactivation*
New terminology	HBe antigen positive chronic infection	HBe antigen positive or negative chronic hepatitis	HBe antigen negative chronic infection	None
What does it mean?	Liver is quietly harboring the chronic infection, allowing viral replication	Liver is actively trying to clear the chronic infection	Liver has cleared the infection	Re-inflammation in an immunosuppressed individual with latent chronic infection; may progress to acute liver failure or fibrosis
Age (years)	Mostly in children	20–40	>35–40	>35–40
HBsAg	Positive for >6 months	Positive for >6 months	Positive for >6 months	Positive for >6 months
HBeAg	+	+ or –	–	+ or –
Anti-HBe	–	–	+	+
Liver enzymes	Normal	Elevated	Normal	Very high
HBV-DNA IU/mL	>10^6	>20,000 if HBeAg+ >2,000 if HBeAg-	<2000	>10^3
Necro-inflammation on liver biopsy	No/minimal	Moderate/severe	No/minimal	Moderate/severe
Progression to cirrhosis	Rare	2–4%/year	Rare	2–3%/year

REFERENCES/SOURCES

- Alam S, Khanna R. Chronic liver disease (Chapter 37.8). In: Gupta P, Menon PSN, Ramji S, Lodha R. PG Textbook of Pediatrics, 3rd edition. New Delhi: Jaypee Brothers Medical Publishers; 2022.
- Kliegman RM, St Geme III JW. Nelson Textbook of Pediatrics, 21st edition. Elsevier; 2019. Chapter 385: Viral hepatitis.

4. Which of the following is an approved therapy for chronic hepatitis B in children?

A. Interferon and nucleoside analogues
B. Infliximab and steroids
C. Directly acting antivirals
D. Ribavirin

EXPLANATION

Approved therapies for chronic hepatitis B are quite similar to adults. Therapy is usually recommended in patients who are in immune clearance or reactivation phases. This is a window of opportunity to boost up viral clearance with drugs in a liver which has already initiated the process. The drugs are interferon-alpha-2b [pegylated (PEG) or nonpegylated, plain] or nucleos(t)ide analogues (lamivudine, entecavir, adefovir, and tenofovir). Infliximab and steroids are used in inflammatory bowel disease, not chronic hepatitis B. Directly acting antivirals are used in chronic hepatitis C. Ribavirin has been discontinued as a therapy in chronic hepatitis C.

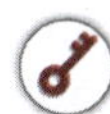 **Key: A**

BOOST YOUR KNOWLEDGE

Interferons (IFN) are immune modulators that encourage the host immune system to suppress replication, clear the virus, induce seroconversion and enhance loss of antigen positivity. IFN therapy has numerous systemic side effects and hence is no longer considered a first-line treatment of all patients. Nucleos(t)ide analogues (NAs), on the other hand, directly disrupt viral replication via DNA targets. Approved ages for initiating therapy are lamivudine (>3 years), entecavir (>2 years), adefovir (>12 years), tenofovir (>12 years). Lamivudine and adefovir were the first-generation NAs, blocking HBV reverse transcriptase, but do not affect intrahepatic covalently closed circular (ccc)-DNA, causing decreased HBsAg clearance. The second generation of NAs, entecavir and tenofovir, are now considered the first-line agents with PEG-IFN during the immune-active phase. The goals of treatment of HBV are to reduce the risk of transmission, infectivity, and complications, including cirrhosis and hepatocellular carcinoma and suppress HBV replication Treatment of children in the immune-tolerant phase has been tried with poor response and hence not currently indicated.

REFERENCES/SOURCES

- Indolfi G, Abdel-Hady M, Bansal S, Debray D, Smets F, Czubkowski P, et al. Management of hepatitis B virus infection and prevention of hepatitis B virus reactivation in children with acquired immunodeficiencies or undergoing immune suppressive, cytotoxic, or biological modifier therapies. J Pediatr Gastroenterol Nutr. 2020;70(4):527-38.
- Kliegman RM, St Geme III JW. Nelson Textbook of Pediatrics, 21st edition. Elsevier; 2019. Chapter 385: Viral hepatitis.
- Sokal EM, Paganelli M, Wirth S, Socha P, Vajro P, Lacaille F, et al. European Society of Pediatric Gastroenterology, Hepatology and Nutrition. Management of chronic hepatitis B in childhood: ESPGHAN clinical practice guidelines: consensus of an expert panel on behalf of the European Society of Pediatric Gastroenterology, Hepatology and Nutrition. J Hepatol. 2013;59(4): 814-29.

5. Which of the following is the most ideal endpoint of antiviral therapy in chronic hepatitis B?

A. Improvement in liver enzymes
B. Undetectable HBV-DNA titers
C. HBe antigen seroconversion
D. Loss of HBs antigen

EXPLANATION

Improvement of liver enzymes means liver inflammation has subsided and is the first step in antiviral therapy. As the inflammation improves, the HBV-DNA levels fall to the extent that it may be undetectable in serum. However, this does not mean that the disease is cured. Next step is occurrence of HBe antigen seroconversion which means development of anti-HBe antibody and loss of HBeAg. This is an achievable goal in those patients who are "e" antigen positive. In practice, antiviral drugs may be stopped at this point of time. However, a small proportion may have relapse of the disease. This step cannot be the goal of therapy in those cirrhotic patients who are already "e" antigen negative. Hence, the *most ideal* and durable endpoint is loss of HBs antigen which heralds the *cure* from the disease and almost eliminates any risk from hepatocellular carcinoma.

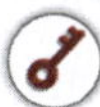 **Key: D**

BOOST YOUR KNOWLEDGE

Most treatments target the *immune active* phase of the disease, characterized by active inflammation, elevated liver enzymes and progressive fibrosis. Spontaneous HBeAg seroconversion, defined as the development of anti-HBe and loss of HBeAg, occurs in the immune-tolerant phase, albeit at low rates of 4–5% per year. It is more common in childhood acquired. HBV rather than in perinatally transmitted infections. Seroconversion can occur over many years, during which time significant damage to the liver may take place. There are no large studies that accurately assess the lifetime risks and morbidities of children with chronic HBV infection.

REFERENCES/SOURCES

- Indolfi G, Abdel-Hady M, Bansal S, Debray D, Smets F, Czubkowski P, et al. Management of hepatitis B virus infection and prevention of hepatitis B virus reactivation in children with acquired immunodeficiencies or undergoing immune suppressive, cytotoxic, or biological modifier therapies. J Pediatr Gastroenterol Nutr. 2020;70(4):527-38.
- Kliegman RM, St Geme III JW. Nelson Textbook of Pediatrics, 21st edition. Elsevier; 2019. Chapter 385: Viral hepatitis.
- Sokal EM, Paganelli M, Wirth S, Socha P, Vajro P, Lacaille F, et al. European Society of Pediatric Gastroenterology, Hepatology and Nutrition. Management of chronic hepatitis B in childhood: ESPGHAN clinical practice guidelines: consensus of an expert panel on behalf of the European Society of Pediatric Gastroenterology, Hepatology and Nutrition. J Hepatol. 2013;59(4):814-29.

6. A neonate is born to an incidentally detected anti-HCV antibody+ mother. Which of the following is used to test the neonate for presence of HCV infection?

A. Anti-HCV antibody in the first week of birth
B. HCV-RNA in the first week of birth
C. HCV-RNA and anti-HCV antibody at 3 months of age
D. Delay testing till 18 months of age

EXPLANATION

Maternal HCV antibodies cross the placenta, remain in circulation for a long time, and wane off by 12–24 months of age. Meanwhile the neonate's immune system is immature at birth and true self antibodies start peaking only by 18 months. Similarly, mother's HCV-RNA may be in the neonatal circulation for first 3 months. The neonate's HCV-RNA start appearing only from 3rd month onwards. HCV is a slow progressive disease in children, and most are asymptomatic. Therapy is approved only >3 years age. Hence, there is no urgency in testing or therapy. Testing of the infant is usually delayed till 18 months age. Only anti-HCV antibody is initially recommended. If positive, quantitative HCV-RNA is performed. Testing at an earlier age will lead to confusion as to whether baby is infected or not.

Key: D

BOOST YOUR KNOWLEDGE

American Academy of Pediatrics recommends all children born to HCV infected mothers should be screened. This screening will increase identification of HCV infections and halting future transmission. Anti-HCV antibodies are used for screening, with subsequent testing for HCV-RNA to distinguish current from previous infections. Children aged 18 months or younger have waning maternal antibodies, so screening is typically not conducted until that age. In select situations, screening-exposed infants at 2–6 months of age for HCV-RNA if needed, with confirmatory follow-up serologic testing at 18 months. Infected children are evaluated annually for progression of their disease. Untreated children are monitored with routine blood tests (e.g., liver function tests, complete blood count) and HCV-RNA levels. Annual abdominal ultrasonography is only indicated if there is a family history of early cirrhosis, hepatocellular carcinoma, or evidence of rapid disease progression.

REFERENCES/SOURCES

- American Association for the Study of Liver Diseases and the Infectious Diseases Society of America. (2021). HCV Guidance: Recommendations for Testing, Managing, and Treating Hepatitis C. [online] Available from https://www.hcvguidelines.org [Last accessed June, 2024].
- Sperry AB, Bennett A, Wen J. Hepatitis B and C in children. Clin Liver Dis. 2022;26(3):403-20.

7. In the natural history of untreated incidentally detected chronic HCV disease in children, which of the following statements is correct?

A. Jaundice ensues in all by adolescence
B. Cirrhosis may occur at fourth decade
C. Liver transplantation is required in most patients
D. Hepatocellular carcinoma is common complication

EXPLANATION

Chronic HCV in children has insidious progression. Hence, advanced liver disease is uncommon in the first two decades. Effective therapy reduces this risk even further. Cirrhosis develops in one-third at mean age of 33 years. Hepatocellular carcinoma ensues only after cirrhosis sets in.

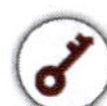

Key: B

BOOST YOUR KNOWLEDGE

Complications from chronic liver disease in children and adolescents are rare. Children often experience transaminase elevations, which do not correlate with histologic severity seen on biopsy. Cirrhosis develops in 1–2% of the population, but they rarely require transplantation. 30% may develop cirrhosis in the third-fourth decade. Development of hepatocellular carcinoma in the pediatric population has been reported but is exceedingly rare. This risk may be increased by comorbid conditions, including diabetes and obesity.

REFERENCES/SOURCES

- American Association for the Study of Liver Diseases and the Infectious Diseases Society of America. (2021). HCV Guidance: Recommendations for Testing, Managing, and Treating Hepatitis C. [online] Available from https://www.hcvguidelines.org [Last accessed June, 2024].
- Sperry AB, Bennett A, Wen J. Hepatitis B and C in Children. Clin Liver Dis. 2022;26(3):403-20.

8. Chronic HCV infection is *not* associated with:

A. Lichen planus
B. Inflammatory bowel disease
C. Membranoproliferative glomerulonephritis
D. Porphyria cutanea tarda

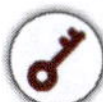

EXPLANATION

Chronic HCV infection can be associated with cutaneous vasculitis, porphyria cutanea tarda, lichen planus, membranoproliferative glomerulonephritis, and nephrotic syndrome. Inflammatory bowel disease is not associated.

Key: B

BOOST YOUR KNOWLEDGE

Chronic HCV is also associated small vessel vasculitis and is a common cause of essential mixed cryoglobulinemia. Adults may manifest also with sicca syndrome, peripheral neuropathy, cerebritis, polyarthritis. Antibodies to smooth muscle, antinuclear antibodies, and low thyroid hormone levels may also be present. A high prevalence of B-cell non-Hodgkin's lymphoma has also been noted with HCV.

REFERENCE/SOURCE

- Kliegman RM, St Geme III JW. Nelson Textbook of Pediatrics, 21st edition. Elsevier; 2019. Chapter 385: Viral hepatitis.

9. **A 12-year-old girl with chronic HCV infection (anti-HCV positive, HCV-RNA 100,000 IU/mL) is planned for therapy with directly acting antivirals. Which of the following statements is true?**

A. Genotype assessment is mandatory before initiating therapy in India
B. Ledipasvir and sofosbuvir are recommended across all genotypes
C. Recommended duration of therapy is 6 weeks
D. HCV-RNA should be checked 12 weeks after therapy completion

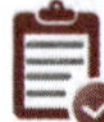

EXPLANATION

In India, the therapy has been simplified. There is no need to do genotype assessment before starting antivirals. Genotype 3 is the most common in India. Ledipasvir-sofosbuvir is recommended >3 years age for 12 weeks in genotype 1, 4, 5, and 6. Sofosbuvir-velpatasvir is recommended >3 years age for 12 weeks in all genotypes. The new glecaprevir-pibrentasvir can also be used >3 years in any genotype for 8 weeks. Sustained virological response (SVR) is an important landmark in chronic HCV therapy. It is the assessment of HCV-RNA levels at 12 weeks from end of therapy.

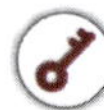

Key: D

BOOST YOUR KNOWLEDGE

Earlier therapy consisted of interferon and ribavirin. In the last 10 years, there is a paradigm shift in therapy. There are currently three types of directly acting antivirals (DAAs): Nonstructural protein 5A (NS5A) inhibitors, NS5B polymerase inhibitors, and NS3/4A protease inhibitors. Ledipasvir/sofosbuvir was the first DAA approved for use in the pediatric population. A once daily regimen for 12 weeks in children older than 12 years infected with genotypes 1, 4, 5, or 6 was the original indication, but approval has been extended to children aged 3 years and older. Sofosbuvir/ribavirin was initially approved for genotypes 2 and 3, as an option for those ineligibles for treatment with ledipasvir/sofosbuvir, but due to ribavirin side effects and the availability of newer pangenotypic DAAs, it is no longer recommended. Glecaprevir/pibrentasvir is approved for all six genotypes in children aged 3 years and older and is only 8 weeks of treatment for treatment-naive children with or without cirrhosis, but treatment is extended in treatment-experienced patients. Sofosbuvir/velpatasvir is another pangenotypic regimen approved for children aged 3 years and older. There are negligible side effects with DAAs. In types 1, 3, 4, 5, and 6 responses to therapy is approximately 92–100%, meaning complete cure from the disease is possible.

REFERENCES/SOURCES

- American Association for the Study of Liver Diseases and the Infectious Diseases Society of America. HCV Guidance: Recommendations for Testing, Managing and Treating Hepatitis C. [online] Available from: https://www.hcvguidelines.org/sites/default/files/fullguidance-pdf/AASLD-IDSA_HCVGuidance_October_05_2021.pdf.
- Kliegman RM, St Geme III JW. Nelson Textbook of Pediatrics, 21st edition. Elsevier; 2019. Chapter 385: Viral hepatitis.
- Sperry AB, Bennett A, Wen J. Hepatitis B and C in Children. Clin Liver Dis. 2022;26(3):403-20.

10. **A 13-year-old girl presents with recurrent jaundice and hepatosplenomegaly of 6 months duration. She had raised antinuclear and antismooth muscle antibodies. Which of the features in liver biopsy is consistent with autoimmune hepatitis?**

A. Rosetting and emperipolesis
B. Mallory-hyaline bodies
C. Orcein stain positivity
D. Ballooning degeneration of hepatocytes

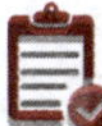

EXPLANATION

Interface hepatitis, lymphoplasmacytic infiltrates, rosetting of hepatocytes, and emperipolesis are characteristic features of autoimmune hepatitis. Mallory-hyaline bodies and orcein stain positivity (copper binding protein) are seen in Wilson disease. Ballooning degeneration of hepatocytes are nonspecific and mostly seen in viral hepatitis.

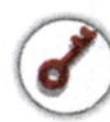

Key: A

BOOST YOUR KNOWLEDGE

Other histologic features that are not seen in autoimmune hepatitis—periodic acid-Schiff-positive, diastase-resistant granules (seen in α1-antitrypsin deficiency) and macrovascular and microvascular steatosis (seen in nonalcoholic steatohepatitis and Wilson disease).

Diagnosis of autoimmune hepatitis is based on simplified autoimmune criteria. Treatment can only be started if a score ≥6 is achieved.

Category	*Variable*	*Score*
Autoantibodies		
Anti-nuclear/smooth muscle	• 1:40 • ≥1:80	• +1 • +2
Anti liver kidney microsomal	≥1:40	+2
Anti soluble liver antigen	Positive	+2
Immunological level		
IgG	• >1 × ULN • >1.1 × ULN	• +1 • +2
Histologic findings		
Morphologic features	• Compatible with AIH • Typical of AIH	• +1 • +2
Viral diseases		
Absence of viral hepatitis	No viral markers	+2
Diagnosis		
Definite		≥7
Probable		6

REFERENCES/SOURCES

- Alam S, Khanna R. Chronic liver disease (Chapter 37.8). In: Gupta P, Menon PSN, Ramji S, Lodha R. PG Textbook of Pediatrics, 3rd edition. New Delhi: Jaypee Brothers Medical Publishers; 2022.
- Kliegman RM, St Geme III JW. Nelson Textbook of Pediatrics, 21st edition. Elsevier; 2019. Chapter 389: Autoimmune hepatitis.
- Yachha SK, Sarma MS. Portal hypertension (Chapter 37.4). In: Gupta P, Menon PSN, Ramji S, Lodha R. PG Textbook of Pediatrics, 3rd edition. New Delhi: Jaypee Brothers Medical Publishers; 2022.

11. Type II autoimmune hepatitis is diagnosed by which of the following antibodies?

A. Antismooth muscle
B. Antinuclear
C. Antiliver kidney microsomal
D. Antisoluble liver antigen

EXPLANATION

Antiliver kidney microsomal (LKM) antibodies are very specific of type II autoimmune hepatitis. Titers >1:40 is diagnostic. But lower titers up to 1:20 is acceptable in children. Antismooth muscle or antinuclear antibodies are specific for type I.

Key: C

BOOST YOUR KNOWLEDGE

A subgroup of female patients might demonstrate autoantibodies against a soluble liver antigen but not against nuclear or microsomal proteins. Antineutrophil cytoplasmic antibodies may be seen more commonly in autoimmune cholangiopathy. Autoantibodies are rare in healthy children, so that titers as low as 1:40 may be significant, although nonspecific elevation in autoantibodies can be observed in a variety of liver diseases. Up to 20% of patients with apparent autoimmune hepatitis might not have autoantibodies at presentation but have histological features and clinical course consistent with the disorder. They are called seronegative autoimmune hepatitis.

Table to differentiate autoimmune hepatitis type I and II is given here:

	Type I (80–90%)	***Type II (10–15%)***
Age of onset	Peripubertal	Younger age
Presentation	Mostly chronic	Mostly acute
Antibody	ANA/SMA	LKM
Overlap with sclerosing cholangitis	Yes	Rare
Cirrhosis at diagnosis	One-third	Rare
Progression	Slower	Rapid
Stopping of drug	Possible	Almost never

REFERENCES/SOURCES

- Alam S, Khanna R. Chronic liver disease (Chapter 37.8). In: Gupta P, Menon PSN, Ramji S, Lodha R. PG Textbook of Pediatrics, 3rd edition. New Delhi: Jaypee Brothers Medical Publishers; 2022.
- Kliegman RM, St Geme III JW. Nelson Textbook of Pediatrics, 21st edition. Elsevier; 2019. Chapter 389: Autoimmune hepatitis.

12. Which of the following skin conditions is *not* associated with autoimmune hepatitis?

A. Acne
B. Vitiligo
C. Psoriasis
D. Nevus

EXPLANATION

Autoimmune hepatitis is associated with autoimmunity of skin. Manifestations are acne, vitiligo, psoriasis, alopecia areata, and pyoderma gangrenosum. Nevus is a collection of melanocytes in dermis or epidermis not caused due to autoimmune process. Other chronic liver diseases with skin conditions are lichen planus in hepatitis C and papular acrodermatitis (Gianotti–Crosti syndrome) in hepatitis B.

Key: D

BOOST YOUR KNOWLEDGE

Extrahepatic features of autoimmune hepatitis (AIH) include arthritis, vasculitis, nephritis, thyroiditis, adrenalitis, Coombs positive anemia, and celiac disease. AIH can also be associated to autoimmune regulatory (*AIRE)* mutations which cause autoimmune polyendocrinopathy-candidiasis-ectodermal dystrophy. An important association of AIH is with primary sclerosing cholangitis (PSC). PSC can be large duct disease (involving extrahepatic common bile duct) or small duct disease (intrahepatic bile ducts). Large duct disease is diagnosed by presence of high gamma-glutamyl transpeptidase (GGT) and abnormal cholangiogram (on magnetic resonance cholangiography or endoscopic retrograde cholangiography). Small duct disease is diagnosed on histology with features of ductopenia, ductular proliferation or "onion-skin appearance" of bile ducts. AIH with PSC is also called as *overlap syndrome*. Overlap syndrome is strongly associated with inflammatory bowel disease, mostly ulcerative colitis.

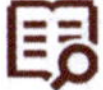

REFERENCE/SOURCE

- Kliegman RM, St Geme III JW. Nelson Textbook of Pediatrics, 21st edition. Elsevier; 2019. Chapter 389: Autoimmune hepatitis.

13. A 14-year-old girl presenting with chronic hepatitis is diagnosed to have autoimmune hepatitis type I and is being started on therapy. Which of the following is *not* correct about the protocol for therapy?

A. Start with azathioprine followed by a course of steroids

B. Measurement of thiopurine methyltransferase activity is ideal before azathioprine

C. In those with overlap syndrome, ursodeoxycholic acid should be tried

D. Cyclosporine should be reserved as a second-line agent

EXPLANATION

Steroids (prednisolone) are the induction drugs that suppress inflammation. Azathioprine is started after 2 weeks of starting steroids. Thiopurine methyltransferase activity is ideally tested before starting azathioprine. Cyclosporine, tacrolimus, mycophenolate mofetil, and sirolimus are second-line agents.

Key: A

BOOST YOUR KNOWLEDGE

Steroids (prednisolone) are the induction drugs that suppress inflammation. Initially it is given at 1–2 mg/kg/day and tapered off over 2–4 months. In those with chronic hepatitis and compensated cirrhosis, azathioprine is started after 2 weeks of starting induction. Azathioprine is not given in those without decompensated cirrhosis and acute severe hepatitis. Thiopurine methyltransferase activity is ideally tested before starting azathioprine. Patients with low activity (10% prevalence) or absent activity (prevalence 0.3%) are at risk for developing severe drug-induced myelotoxicity from the accumulation of the unmetabolized drug. Measurement of the drug metabolites, 6-thioguanine nucleotide and 6-methylmercaptopurine, is useful in determining as to why a patient is not responding to a standard dose of a thiopurine drug. This may help in avoiding myelosuppression and hepatotoxicity. Cyclosporine, tacrolimus, mycophenolate mofetil, and sirolimus have been used in the management of cases refractory to standard therapy. In those with overlap syndrome, ursodeoxycholic acid can be tried. There is a potential role for budesonide combined with azathioprine in treatment of noncirrhotic adult patients. Budesonide is a corticosteroid with high first-pass clearance by the liver and fewer systemic side effects including suppression of hypothalamic-pituitary axis. However, budesonide therapy is not popular in children.

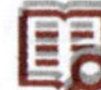

REFERENCES/SOURCES

- Kliegman RM, St Geme III JW. Nelson Textbook of Pediatrics, 21st edition. Elsevier; 2019. Chapter 389: Autoimmune hepatitis.
- Mack CL, Adams D, Assis DN, Kerkar N, Manns MP, Mayo MJ, et al. Diagnosis and management of autoimmune hepatitis in adults and children: 2019 practice guidance and guidelines from the American Association for the Study of Liver Diseases. Hepatology. 2020;72(2):671-22.

14. A 10-year-old girl with autoimmune hepatitis type II, on immunosuppression has been in remission for 2 years. Which of the following statements is correct?

A. Drug withdrawal is seldom possible in type II disease due to high chances of relapse
B. Drug withdrawal can be attempted without a repeat liver biopsy in children
C. Biochemical remission signifies histological remission
D. Relapses should be treated with second-line agents

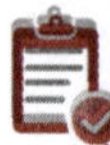

EXPLANATION

Those who have normalized liver enzymes, immunoglobulins and become seronegative for at least 2 years may be considered for drug withdrawal. Biochemical remission is not parallel to histological remission and hence, a repeat liver biopsy is mandatory in children, not in adults. Relapses after drug withdrawal are common and should be promptly treated with the original immunosuppression. Type II disease is more aggressive than type I. Drug withdrawal is seldom possible in type II autoimmune hepatitis as relapses are inevitable.

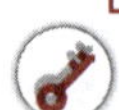

Key: A

BOOST YOUR KNOWLEDGE

The initial response to therapy in autoimmune hepatitis is generally prompt, with a >75% rate of remission. Transaminases and bilirubin fall to near-normal levels, often in the first 1–3 months. When present, abnormalities in serum albumin and prothrombin time respond over a longer period (3–9 months). Intermittent flares of hepatitis can occur and can necessitate recycling of prednisone therapy. In patients meeting the criteria for tapering and then withdrawal of treatment (25–40% of children), 50% are weaned from all medication; in the other 50%, relapse occurs after a variable period. Relapse usually responds to retreatment. Many children will not meet the criteria for an attempt at discontinuation of immunosuppression and should be maintained on the smallest dose of prednisolone that minimizes biochemical activity of the disease. Histologic progress does not necessarily need to be assessed by sequential liver biopsies, although biochemical remission does not ensure histologic resolution. Follow-up liver biopsy is an important consideration in patients for whom consideration is given to discontinuing corticosteroid therapy. In patients with disappearance of symptoms and biochemical abnormalities and resolution of the necroinflammatory process on biopsy, an attempt at gradual discontinuation of medication is justified. There is a high rate of relapse after discontinuation of therapy. Relapses require reinstitution of induction dosing of immunosuppression.

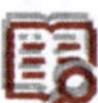

REFERENCES/SOURCES

- Kliegman RM, St Geme III JW. Nelson Textbook of Pediatrics, 21st edition. Elsevier; 2019. Chapter 389: Autoimmune hepatitis.
- Mack CL, Adams D, Assis DN, Kerkar N, Manns MP, Mayo MJ, et al. Diagnosis and Management of Autoimmune Hepatitis in Adults and Children: 2019 Practice Guidance and Guidelines from the American Association for the Study of Liver Diseases. Hepatology. 2020;72(2):671-722.

15. Which one of the following statements is *correct* for diagnosis of Wilson disease with hepatic manifestation?

A. Children with neurologic manifestations are much younger than those with primary hepatic manifestation
B. Kayser–Fleischer ring is seen in 50% of patients with neurological diseases
C. Cholelithiasis can be a manifestation due to chronic hemolysis
D. Mutation analysis is mandatory for diagnosis

EXPLANATION

Age-phenotypic effect is a feature seen in Wilson disease (WD) where children with primary hepatic manifestation are much younger than those with primary neurological manifestation. Approximately 10–12% present with both neurological and hepatic features. Kayser-Fleischer ring is seen in 40–60% of hepatic and 97% of neurological patients. Due to a concomitant chronic hemolytic process, cholelithiasis can be seen. There are more than 600 mutations in WD and genotyping can be a cumbersome process. Detection of a homozygous mutation of ATP7B is confirmatory but not mandatory.

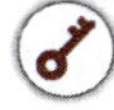

Key: C

BOOST YOUR KNOWLEDGE

The following figures describe the myriads of presentations in WD and a simplified diagnostic approach.

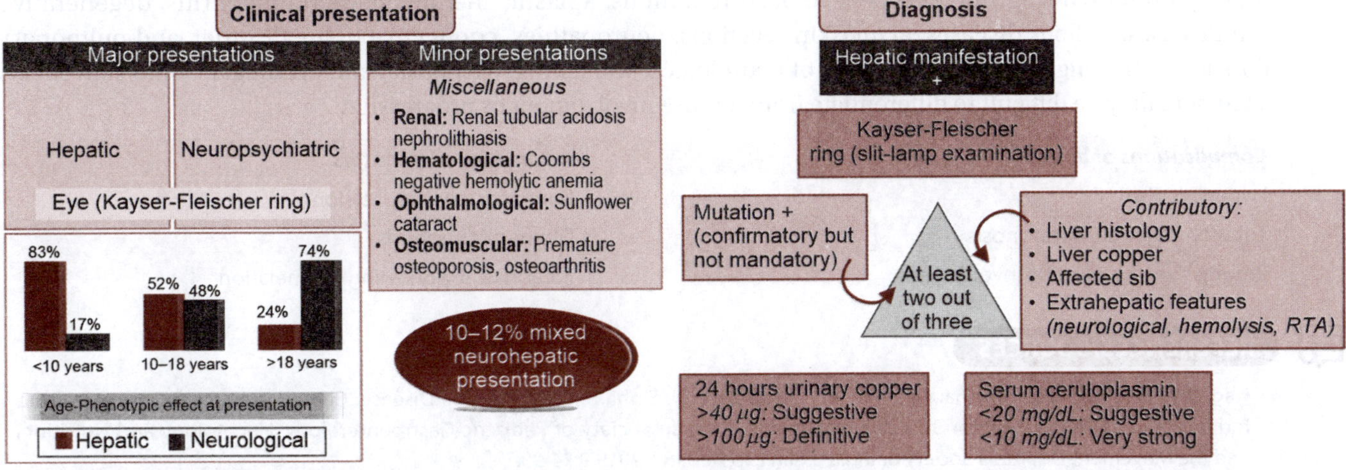

Source: Walshe JM, Yealland M. Wilson's disease: the problem of delayed diagnosis. J Neurol Neurosurg Psychiatry. 1992;55(8):692-6.

REFERENCES/SOURCES

- Nagral A, Sen Sarma M, Matthai J, Kukkle PL, Devarbhavi H, Sinha S, et al. Wilson's Disease: Clinical Practice Guidelines of the Indian National Association for Study of the Liver, the Indian Society of Pediatric Gastroenterology, Hepatology and Nutrition, and the Movement Disorders Society of India. J Clin Exp Hepatol. 2019;9:74-98.
- Peters AL, Balistreri WF. Wilson disease (Chapter 384.2). In: Kliegman RM, St Geme III JW, Blum NJ, Shah SS, Tasker RC, Wilson KM (Eds). Nelson Textbook of Pediatrics, 21st edition. Elsevier; 2019.

16. A 10-year-old girl with chronic hepatitis is diagnosed to have Wilson disease. Which of following statements is correct regarding her further management.

A. Zinc is the drug of choice for induction
B. Trientine is contraindicated in this situation
C. D-penicillamine is associated with glomerular proteinuria
D. Liver transplantation is the only option

EXPLANATION

Drug of choice for hepatic manifestation of Wilson disease (WD) is D-penicillamine or trientine which have systemic chelating ability. D-penicillamine is started in most cases as it is a stronger chelator as compared to trientine. Trientine is also expensive presently in India and is, hence, reserved as second-line agent in those who have D-penicillamine toxicity or intolerance. D-penicillamine has a higher adversity profile as compared to trientine, one of the majors being glomerulonephritis. Zinc is not a true chelator. It competitively displaces copper in the gut lumen and prevents the absorption of dietary copper. Hence, it is not very efficacious in those with symptomatic liver disease who already have a high copper overburden. Zinc is used presymptomatic siblings of WD (on screening) to delay onset of disease, for maintenance (in those who are well controlled and wish to switch back from a systemic chelator) and in those with severe neurological illness intolerant to systemic chelators. Liver transplantation is indicated in those with advanced disease or liver failure not responding to chelation.

Key: C

BOOST YOUR KNOWLEDGE

D-penicillamine is known to have side effects in up to 20% of patients. Absolute contraindications to rechallenge of drug if the following side effects have occurred: lupus, aplastic anemia, glomerulonephritis, degenerative skin diseases, bullous diseases, acute skin reactions, neuropathies, connective tissue disorder, and pulmonary fibrosis. Rechallenge is possible in cases of neurological worsening, dyspepsia, and arthralgia. Some side effects listed here may be difficult to differentiate from disease involvement or progression.

Complications of disease		*Adversities of chelators*
Hypersplenism	vs.	Bone marrow suppression
Tubulopathy/nephrocalcinosis	vs.	Glomerulonephritis
Progressive neurological involvement	vs.	Paradoxical worsening on chelation

REFERENCES/SOURCES

- Nagral A, Sen Sarma M, Matthai J, Kukkle PL, Devarbhavi H, Sinha S, et al. Wilson's Disease: Clinical Practice Guidelines of the Indian National Association for Study of the Liver, the Indian Society of Pediatric Gastroenterology, Hepatology and Nutrition, and the Movement Disorders Society of India. J Clin Exp Hepatol. 2019;9:74-98.
- Peters AL, Balistreri WF. Wilson disease (Chapter 384.2). In: Kliegman RM, St Geme III JW, Blum NJ, Shah SS, Tasker RC, Wilson KM (Eds). Nelson Textbook of Pediatrics, 21st edition. Elsevier; 2019.

17. An anicteric 7-year-old boy has massive ascites, hepatomegaly, and dilated tortuous veins over abdomen and back. Which of the following statements is the likely to be correct?

A. Doppler abdomen will show a block in extrahepatic part of inferior vena cava
B. Liver function tests will be markedly deranged
C. Ascites will rapidly reaccumulate once paracentesis is performed
D. Portal vein has undergone a cavernomatous change

EXPLANATION

The features above are most consistent with the diagnosis of chronic Budd-Chiari syndrome (BCS). The back veins are the best clue which suggests an inferior vena cava block in the intrahepatic part. Cirrhosis is close differential. The presentation is not consistent with extrahepatic portal hypertension (EHPVO, portal cavernoma). Dilated veins over the abdomen occur over the abdomen due to the patent umbilical veins that communicate between the left branch of portal vein and superior/inferior epigastric veins. In EHPVO, the left branch of portal vein is blocked and hence, dilated abdominal veins do not appear. In BCS, liver function test is near normal. Ascites is intractable in BCS and difficult to manage due to a tendency of rapid refilling after each large volume paracentesis.

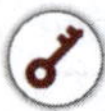

Key: D

BOOST YOUR KNOWLEDGE

Chronic Budd–Chiari syndrome is an important differential diagnosis in a cirrhotic patient. All three hepatic veins and (or) inferior vena cava (IVC) is blocked. Most often the etiology is idiopathic in children. Since this a postsinusoidal disease, the liver functions are usually preserved till late stages. Intractable ascites is the most common presentation. Some patients present with variceal bleeding. Doppler findings include absent hepatic veins, IVC thrombus or web, intrahepatic collaterals, and caudate lobe hypertrophy. Treatment is hepatic vein and (or) IVC angioplasty and stenting to restore the hepatic venous outflow.

REFERENCES/SOURCES

- Alam S, Khanna R. Chronic liver disease (Chapter 37.8). In: Gupta P, Menon PSN, Ramji S, Lodha R. PG Textbook of Pediatrics, 3rd edition. New Delhi: Jaypee Brothers Medical Publishers; 2022.
- Yachha SK, Sarma MS. Portal hypertension (Chapter 37.4). In: Gupta P, Menon PSN, Ramji S, Lodha R. PG Textbook of Pediatrics, 3rd edition. New Delhi: Jaypee Brothers Medical Publishers; 2022.

18. Ascites can be primary manifestation in all of the following *except*:

A. Autoimmune hepatitis
B. Wilson disease
C. Hepatitis B infection
D. Extrahepatic portal venous obstruction

EXPLANATION

Note that the question says, "primary manifestation". In other words, the question is asking which of the diseases can present as decompensated cirrhosis as a presenting feature. The meaning of decompensation is development of ascites, hepatic encephalopathy and (or) uncorrectable coagulopathy. Autoimmune hepatitis, Wilson disease, and hepatitis B have intrinsic pathologies in the parenchyma of liver. When there is a destruction of parenchyma, ascites is likely. Chronic Budd–Chiari syndrome is a postsinusoidal block where ascites occurs frequently due to liver congestion and ooze from the hepatic lymph. Extrahepatic portal venous obstruction (EHPVO) is a prehepatic lesion which does not destroy the hepatic parenchyma till terminal stage. Hence, it does not present with ascites as a primary manifestation. Rarely transient ascites can be seen due to severe hypoalbuminemia after a bout of massive variceal bleeding in EHPVO. Hence, the farther the lesion is from the portal vein, the higher the chances of developing ascites.

Key: D

BOOST YOUR KNOWLEDGE

Table shows the common conditions that may appear as cirrhosis and the features that distinguish the same.

Differential diagnosis of cirrhosis: Clinical features and investigations

	Cirrhosis	*Chronic Budd–Chiari syndrome*	*Congenital hepatic fibrosis*	*Extrahepatic portal venous obstruction*
GI bleed	Rarely (20%)	± (35%)	± (40–50%)	Mostly (85%)
Jaundice	Recurrent or persistent (36%)	Absent (unless end stage)	Absent	Absent (unless complicated)
Encephalopathy	± (30%) Recurrent	Absent (unless end stage)	Absent	Absent

Contd...

Contd...

	Cirrhosis	*Chronic Budd–Chiari syndrome*	*Congenital hepatic fibrosis*	*Extrahepatic portal venous obstruction*
Ascites	± (21%) Recurrent	Massive rapidly reaccumulating	Absent	Absent (occasionally postbleed)
Liver	Shrunken or enlarged irregular, nodular	Enlarged irregular, nodular	Left lobe > right lobe hard liver	Normal span
Spleen	Enlarged	Enlarged	Enlarged	Enlarged
Dilated veins	Anterior abdominal wall caput medusae	• Abdominal wall • Back veins in IVC block	May or may not be	None
Liver function tests	Abnormal	Near normal (unless end stage)	Normal except high alkaline phosphatase	Normal (unless complicated)
Doppler ultrasonography	• Irregular liver outline, liver nodularity • Dilated portal vein	Hepatic veins ± IVC block	Irregular liver outline left lobe enlarged	Portal cavernoma or block
Varices	Varices (esophageal and gastric) are seen in all four conditions			

REFERENCES/SOURCES

- Alam S, Khanna R. Chronic liver disease (Chapter 37.8). In: Gupta P, Menon PSN, Ramji S, Lodha R. PG Textbook of Pediatrics, 3rd edition. New Delhi: Jaypee Brothers Medical Publishers; 2022.
- Yachha SK, Sarma MS. Portal hypertension (Chapter 37.4). In: Gupta P, Menon PSN, Ramji S, Lodha R. PG Textbook of Pediatrics, 3rd edition. New Delhi: Jaypee Brothers Medical Publishers; 2022.

19. Which of the following is an important modality of management of cirrhotic ascites?

A. Restriction of dietary sodium to 5 mEq/kg/day
B. Water restriction if serum sodium >125 mEq/L
C. Administration of furosemide: spironolactone in ratio 2:1
D. Albumin infusion

EXPLANATION

In infants and children, sodium is restricted to a maximum of 1–2 mEq/kg/day and 1–2 g/day (44–88 mEq) in adolescents. Water restriction is necessary only if serum sodium is <125 mEq/L. Furosemide: spironolactone ratio 2:5 have the best synergistic action. Albumin infusion especially during large volume paracentesis restores the oncotic pressure.

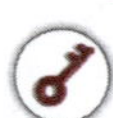

Key: D

BOOST YOUR KNOWLEDGE

Ascites occurs in 44% of children with cirrhosis. Progressive deterioration of liver functions, portal hypertension, splanchnic arterial vasodilatation, and reduced plasma oncotic pressure due to low serum albumin all contribute to development of ascites. Inappropriate sequestration of fluid in splanchnic vascular bed leading to renin-angiotensin stimulation (underfilling theory) or primary inappropriate renal retention of sodium and water in the absence of volume depletion (overflow theory) are the other postulated mechanisms. Large volume paracentesis (LVP) in severe ascites (defined as tense ascites with fluid thrill, respiratory distress and/or difficulties in ambulation) may result in postparacentesis circulatory dysfunction and hyponatremia that in turn predisposes to early mortality. In single time LVP, it is recommended to drain the ascitic fluid preferably under albumin cover (0.5–1 g/kg) and limit drainage volume <200 mL/kg to prevent the above effects. In the absence of albumin cover (limited resource setting), the fluid drainage rate must be limited to <680 mL/hour.

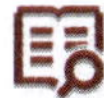

REFERENCE/SOURCE

- Yachha SK, Sarma MS. Portal hypertension (Chapter 37.4). In: Gupta P, Menon PSN, Ramji S, Lodha R. PG Textbook of Pediatrics, 3rd edition. New Delhi: Jaypee Brothers Medical Publishers; 2022.

20. A 12-year-old girl with cirrhosis and ascites develops fever and diarrhea. Ascitic fluid shows total leukocytes count 850 cells/cu mm, neutrophils 60%, lymphocytes 40%. Ascitic fluid culture shows *Escherichia coli.* Which of the following statements is correct?

A. This condition is called monomicrobial non-neutrocytic bacterial ascites
B. *Escherichia coli* is a normal commensal in the ascitic fluid
C. Third-generation cephalosporins is the antibiotic of choice
D. Prophylactic antibiotics are not required

EXPLANATION

The peritoneal cavity and ascites are usually sterile. Development of fever, diarrhea, and abdominal pain in a setting of ascites is the hallmark of spontaneous bacterial peritonitis (SBP). There are three different variants of the same.

Variants of spontaneous bacterial peritonitis

Nomenclature	*Ascitic fluid absolute neutrophil count/mm^3*	*Ascitic fluid culture*	*Antibiotic treatment*
Spontaneous bacterial peritonitis (SBP) (monomicrobial neutrocytic)	>250	Positive for single organism	Yes
Culture negative neutrocytic ascites (CNNA)	>250	Negative	Yes
Monomicrobial non-neutrocytic bacterascites (MNB)	<250	Positive	• Yes, if symptomatic • No, if asymptomatic

The ascitic fluid neutrophil count in this case is 510 and the culture is positive. Hence, the condition is SBP. Antibiotic of choice is intravenous cefotaxime 50 mg/kg/dose every 8 hours for 5 days. This covers 95% of flora and is effective in 85% of cases. Prophylactic antibiotics are required to prevent further episodes of SBP in those patients with cirrhosis who have already developed an episode of SBP in the past. Recurrent SBP leads to hepatic encephalopathy and renal failure.

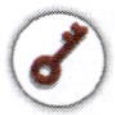

Key: C

BOOST YOUR KNOWLEDGE

Spontaneous bacterial peritonitis (SBP) is the most common complication of ascites occurring in 10–30% due to translocation of bacteria from the gut into peritoneal cavity. *Escherichia coli* (*E. coli*), *Klebsiella,* and *Staphylococcus aureus* (*S. aureus*) are the most frequently isolated organisms. In a setting of ascites, presence of unexplained fever, abdominal pain, increased frequency of stools, or worsening of encephalopathy in a cirrhotic should raise a suspicion for SBP. Frequently, SBP may be asymptomatic and incidentally detected on ascitic fluid analysis. Treatment should be started empirically if SBP is suspected clinically, regardless of the availability of laboratory results. Antibiotic of choice is intravenous cefotaxime 50 mg/kg/dose every 8 hours for 5 days. This covers 95% of flora and is effective in 85% of cases. However, increasing bacterial resistance is observed in tertiary care centers. Repeat ascitic tap is advocated after 48 hours to see the leukocyte response in selected cases.

Upgrading to carbapenems is considered if fever persists >48 hours, rising ascitic fluid counts, nosocomial setting, previous exposure of beta-lactams, and patients already on SBP prophylaxis. Secondary antibiotic prophylaxis refers to prevention of further episodes of SBP in a patient who has already had one episode in the past. Primary antibiotic prophylaxis refers to prevention of SBP in those patients who have low total protein content (<1 g/dL) in ascitic fluid without prior episode of SBP. Risk factors for development of SBP are ascitic fluid protein concentration <1 g/dL, variceal hemorrhage, and prior episode of SBP. Long-term administration of oral norfloxacin 5–7.5 mg/kg once a day in cirrhotic patients with ascitic fluid protein content of <1 g/dL or prior episode of SBP is recommended for prevention of SBP.

REFERENCE/SOURCE

- Yachha SK, Sarma MS. Portal hypertension (Chapter 37.4). In: Gupta P, Menon PSN, Ramji S, Lodha R. PG Textbook of Pediatrics, 3rd edition. New Delhi: Jaypee Brothers Medical Publishers; 2022.

CHAPTER 17.5

Portal Hypertension and Gastrointestinal Bleed

Nishant Wadhwa

1. Which pathological change depicted in the image here is responsible for portal hypertension in cirrhosis?

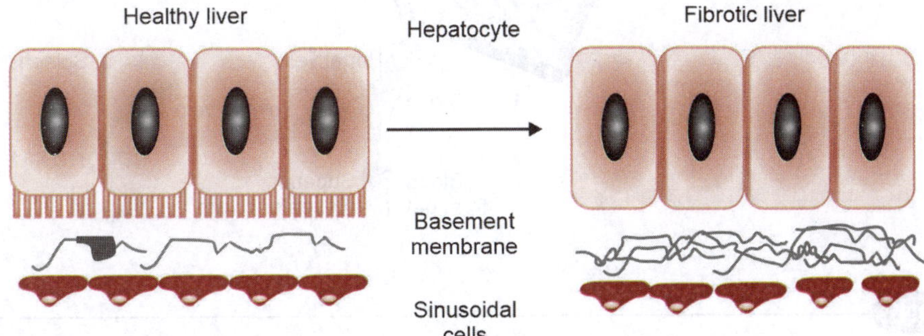

A. Capillarization of sinusoids
B. Microvascular thrombus
C. Parenchymal loss
D. Hepatocyte atrophy

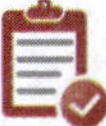

EXPLANATION

The figure depicts the laying of fibrous collagen in the basement membrane of sinusoidal cells. This deposition leads to transformation of a porous sinusoidal barrier to a nonporous barrier termed capillarization of sinusoids. The other options, microvascular thrombi and hepatocyte atrophy, also contribute to portal hypertension; however, they are secondary causes and not depicted in the figure.

Key: A

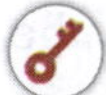

BOOST YOUR KNOWLEDGE

Portal hypertension occurs because of resistance to portal flow followed by an increase in portal venous inflow. The resistance to blood flow increases as fibrosis in liver biopsy increases. Fibrosis can be semiquantitatively classified according to the Ishak stage or METAVIR stage, wherein bridging fibrosis and above are considered advanced fibrosis stages.

REFERENCES/SOURCES

- Iwakiri Y, Trebicka J. Portal hypertension in cirrhosis: Pathophysiological mechanisms and therapy. JHEP Rep. 2021;3(4): 100316.
- Natarajan V, Harris EN, Kidambi S. SECs (sinusoidal endothelial cells), microenvironment, and fibrosis. Biomed Res Int. 2017; 2017:4097205.

2. Correctly identify the sites of obstruction in portal hypertension.

A. 4-Extrahepatic portal vein obstruction
B. 3-Veno-occlusive disease
C. 5-Cirrhosis
D. 1-Budd–Chiari syndrome

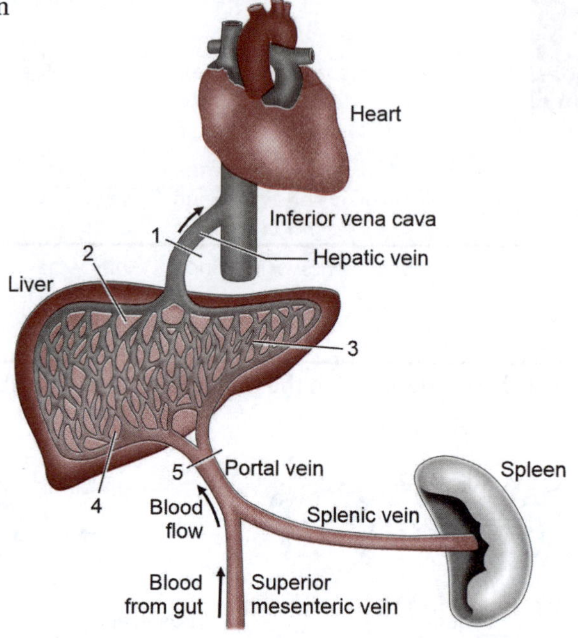

EXPLANATION

Option D is correctly matched. Budd–Chiari syndrome occurs due to obstruction of hepatic vein outflow tract and is correctly matched. Regarding the other options, the site of extrahepatic portal vein obstruction is depicted by number 5, veno-occlusive disease by number 2, and cirrhosis by number 3.

Key: D

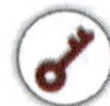

BOOST YOUR KNOWLEDGE

Portal hypertension can be classified according to the site of increased resistance to portal vein flow into three categories: (1) Prehepatic—site of resistance prior to entry into liver; (2) intrahepatic—resistance within the liver; and (3) posthepatic—resistance after blood exists in the liver. Intrahepatic portal hypertension is further subdivided into presinusoidal, sinusoidal, and postsinusoidal. In India, the most common cause of hematemesis in children is prehepatic obstruction due to extrahepatic portal vein obstruction. In cirrhosis, the site of obstruction is intrahepatic sinusoidal.

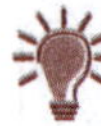

REFERENCES/SOURCES

- Berzigotti A, Seijo S, Reverter E, Bosch J. Assessing portal hypertension in liver diseases. Expert Rev Gastroenterol Hepatol. 2013;7(2):141-55.
- Khanna R, Sarin SK. Noncirrhotic portal hypertension: current and emerging perspectives. Clin Liver Dis. 2019;23(4):781-807.

3. A 4-year-old boy presents with blood in vomitus, single episode 2 days back. On examination, his heart rate (HR) is 98 beats/min, respiratory rate (RR) is 14 breaths/min, blood pressure (BP) is 98/62 mm Hg. He does not have any petechial rash, ecchymosis, or lymphadenopathy. His spleen is enlarged, 3 cm below costal; however liver is not palpable. What is the next investigation to establish the diagnosis?

A. Bone marrow
B. Peripheral smear to look for blasts
C. Ultrasonography (USG) of abdomen with Doppler
D. Noncontrast computed tomography (CT)

EXPLANATION

The question describes the typical scenario of a child with extrahepatic portal vein obstruction presenting with first hematemesis episode. These children present around 5 years of age with growth failure, splenomegaly, and hematemesis. They have evidence of hypersplenism, decrease in two or more blood cell lines, in hemogram report. USG abdomen with Doppler is 95% sensitive in establishing the diagnosis. As these children have splenomegaly with decreased cell lines, initial evaluation by a hematologist with bone marrow (option A) and peripheral smear (option B) is not uncommon, before a final diagnosis is established.

Key: C

BOOST YOUR KNOWLEDGE

Ultrasonography findings in extrahepatic portal vein obstruction include nonvisualization of portal vein, with multiple collaterals, leading to the formation of a portal cavernoma. Pericholecystic, pericholedochal collaterals, and spontaneous portosystemic shunts like lienorenal shunts may also be seen.

REFERENCE/SOURCE

- Pargewar SS, Desai SN, Rajesh S, Singh VP, Arora A, Mukund A. Imaging and radiological interventions in extra-hepatic portal vein obstruction. World J Radiol. 2016;8(6):556-70.

4. A 4-year-old boy presents with history of large amount blood in vomitus 2 hours back. On examination, his HR is 120 beats/min, respiratory rate is 28 breaths/min, BP is 69/38 mm Hg, and peripheries are cold. Per abdomen examination reveals splenomegaly 2 cm below costal margin, no hepatomegaly. What is the next step?

A. Secure 2 peripheral lines, fluid resuscitation, and packed red blood cell (PRBC) transfusion with target Hb 7–9 g/dL
B. Immediately shift for endoscopy as stoppage of bleeding is the primary determinant of outcome
C. Start propranolol immediately via nasogastric tube as nonselective beta-blockers (NSBBs) are best modality to stop bleed
D. Start octreotide and give PRBC transfusion to target Hb 10–11 g/dL

EXPLANATION

This child has presented with large volume hematemesis and is in shock. The first step would be to stabilize the patient by securing intravenous (IV) access, restoring perfusion and correcting anemia. Target Hb is 7–9 g/dL as overtransfusion can overload the venous system, precipitating further bleed. Option B is incorrect as this patient requires immediate resuscitation, prior to endoscopy. Immediate mortality is due to reduced organ perfusion. There is no role of propranolol in acute hematemesis, hence option C is incorrect. Option D is incorrect as target Hb is on the higher side, which can cause further bleeding.

Key: A

BOOST YOUR KNOWLEDGE

Octreotide is a somatostatin analog and inhibits glucagon-like peptide 1 (GLP-1) action, causing splanchnic vasoconstriction and reducing portal vein blood flow. Continuous octreotide infusion has been found to be beneficial in emergency control of bleeding.

REFERENCES/SOURCES

- Kaplan DE, Ripoll C, Thiele M, Fortune BE, Simonetto DA, Garcia-Tsao G, et al. AASLD practice guidance on risk stratification and management of portal hypertension and varices in cirrhosis. Hepatology. 2024;79(5):1180-211.
- Koul PB, Totapally BR, Raszynski A. Continuous octreotide infusion for treatment of upper gastrointestinal bleeding due to portal hypertension in children: an observational study from pediatric intensive care unit. J Pediatr Intensive Care. 2012;1(2):99-103.

5. A 5-year-old girl, case of biliary atresia post-Kasai portoenterostomy, presents with blood in vomitus. On examination, she has HR 98 beats/min, RR 23 breaths/min, and BP 105/74 mm Hg. What is the next step?

A. Injection octreotide infusion and upper gastrointestinal endoscopy
B. Injection octreotide followed by propranolol
C. Pantoprazole infusion followed by upper gastrointestinal endoscopy
D. Immediate upper gastrointestinal endoscopy

EXPLANATION

This child has presented with hematemesis; however, her vitals are stable, and she does not require immediate resuscitation. In all these children, after securing IV access, IV octreotide infusion should be initiated followed by upper gastrointestinal endoscopy. The door to needle time to initiate octreotide should be ideally less than 2 hours, and the door to endoscopy time, less than 12 hours. Option B is incorrect as all children with hematemesis merit an endoscopy. Option C is incorrect as octreotide infusion is missing in that option. Option D is incorrect as octreotide infusion should be started prior to endoscopy.

Key: A

BOOST YOUR KNOWLEDGE

Nonselective beta-blockers like propranolol reduce portal pressure by reducing cardiac output via beta-1 blockage and splanchnic arterial vasoconstricts by beta-2 blockage. Carvedilol with additional alpha-1 blockage further reduces portal pressure by decreasing intrahepatic portal resistance, however, has not yet been studied for this indication in children less than 12 years.

REFERENCE/SOURCE

- de Franchis R; Baveno VI Faculty. Expanding Consensus in Portal Hypertension—Report of the Baveno VI Consensus Workshop: stratifying risk and individualizing care for portal hypertension. J Hepatol. 2015;63(3):743-52.

6. A 7-year-old boy, known case of biliary atresia, with history of Kasai portoenterostomy at 65 days of life presents for a routine checkup. His blood investigations show Hb 12 g/dL, total leukocyte count (TLC) 11,000/mm^3, platelet count 2.1 lakh/mm^3, total bilirubin 0.6 mg/dL. Liver is palpable at 2 cm below costal margin, and spleen is palpable at 1 cm below costal margin. A screening upper GI endoscopy shows grade 1 varices without any red color signs. What should be the next step?

A. Endoscopic sclerotherapy to eradicate the varices
B. Endoscopic band ligation
C. Start propranolol prophylaxis
D. Advice urgent liver transplant in view of variceal development

EXPLANATION

This child has normal bilirubin, suggesting a successful Kasai portoenterostomy. His hemogram report does not suggest hypersplenism. Endoscopy shows grade 1 varices, which have a low risk of bleeding.

Primary prophylaxis of varices to prevent hematemesis is recommended in adults; however, no studies exist in the pediatric age group. In adults, NSBBs are preferred to endoscopic therapy due to additional mortality benefit of starting NSBBs. Liver transplantation is not recommended in case of successful Kasai portoenterostomy with low-risk varices, hence option D is incorrect.

Key: C

BOOST YOUR KNOWLEDGE

Varices are graded according to their size and presence of red color signs. Small varices (<5 mm) without red color signs are unlikely to bleed and are classified as low risk of bleeding varices. Large varices (>5 mm) or even small varices with red color signs are classified as high risk of bleeding varices. Bleeding risk also depends on underlying liver status. Small size varices, but with underlying advanced disease with Child-Turcotte-Pugh Score B or C, are also considered high risk of bleeding varices.

REFERENCE/SOURCE

- Abby Philips C, Sahney A. Oesophageal and gastric varices: historical aspects, classification and grading: everything in one place. Gastroenterol Rep (Oxf). 2016;4(3):186-95.

7. A 5-year-old girl, known case of biliary atresia, history of Kasai portoenterostomy at 98 days of life, lost to follow-up for past 2 years, now presents with history of jaundice and increasing abdominal distention. On examination, she is icteric with moderate ascites, firm enlarged liver 4 cm below costal margin with irregular outline, and splenomegaly 4 cm below costal margin. *Investigations:* Hb 6.9 g/dL, TLC 1,690/mm^3, and platelet 60,000/mm^3. Total bilirubin 5.2 mg/dL, direct bilirubin 3.2 mg/dL, protein 4.5 g/dL, albumin 2.9 g/dL, international normalized ratio (INR) 2.5, urea 34 mg/dL, and creatinine 0.7 mg/dL. On Day 2 of admission, she develops hematemesis. She is started on octreotide infusion and taken for endoscopy.

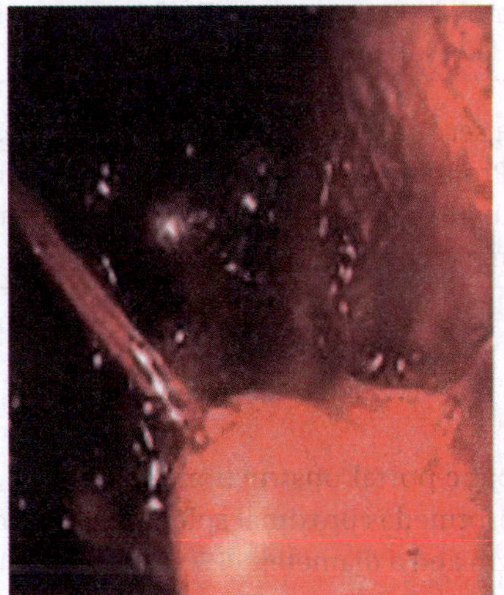

Endoscopy shows active variceal spurter. Despite endotherapy, she again has hematemesis 36 hours after the procedure. Repeat endotherapy session is also unsuccessful in controlling the bleed. What is the next step?

A. Give fresh-frozen plasma
B. Rescue transjugular intrahepatic portosystemic shunt (TIPS) and list for liver transplant
C. Self-expanding metal stent
D. Propranolol at 5 mg/kg/day

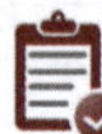

EXPLANATION

This case describes a child with failed Kasai portoenterostomy with decompensated chronic liver disease along with portal hypertension with hematemesis. As after an initial endotherapy has failed to control the bleed and the child also has underlying cirrhosis, there is high probability of failure of repeat endotherapy sessions. Such children should be taken for TIPS to decompress the portal system and be listed for liver transplant. Fresh-frozen plasma is not recommended in case of variceal bleed as coagulopathy is not the cause of bleed in such patients, hence option A is incorrect. Self-expanding metal stent can temporarily control bleed in such patients, however, is available only for patients 16 years or older, hence option C is incorrect. Propranolol has no role in acute hematemesis.

Key: B

BOOST YOUR KNOWLEDGE

Transjugular intrahepatic portosystemic shunt done for repeat hematemesis is called rescue TIPS. TIPS can also be done preemptively in patients with Child-Turcotte-Pugh score B with active bleeding and patients with Child-Turcotte-Pugh score C. In such cases, early TIPS have been found to reduce mortality due to hemorrhage. However, all such evidence comes from adult studies.

REFERENCE/SOURCE

- Edelson J, Basso JE, Rockey DC. Updated strategies in the management of acute variceal haemorrhage. Curr Opin Gastroenterol. 2021;37(3):167-72.

8. A 3-year-old boy presents with hematemesis. He is diagnosed as a case of extrahepatic portal vein obstruction. What current plan should be adopted to prevent further bleeds?

A. Starting on propranolol alone
B. Repeated endotherapy sessions alone
C. Endotherapy along with propranolol
D. Liver transplant

EXPLANATION

Secondary prophylaxis to prevent a second episode of bleeding includes both endoscopic variceal eradications along with beta-blocker therapy. Propranolol alone (option A) or endotherapy sessions alone (option B) are not the standard of care. Liver transplant (option D) is not recommended after a single episode of bleed in extrahepatic portal vein obstruction patients.

Key: C

BOOST YOUR KNOWLEDGE

Surgical management of extrahepatic portal obstruction is the most effective treatment for reducing hematemesis. Most common surgery performed is proximal splenorenal shunt (PSRS) with splenectomy. This surgery requires adequate splenic vein length and a diameter >6.5 mm and is usually done around 6–8 years of age.

REFERENCE/SOURCE

- Sarin SK, Khanna R. Non-cirrhotic portal hypertension. Clin Liver Dis. 2014;18(2):451-76.

9. In management of extrahepatic hepatic portal vein obstruction, which of the following surgeries restores physiological portovenous flow?

A. Proximal splenorenal shunt
B. Distal splenorenal shunt
C. Meso-Rex bypass
D. Distal splenogonadal shunt

EXPLANATION

Meso-Rex bypass surgery creates a flow conduit from superior mesenteric vein to left branch of portal vein (Rex vein). This surgery is feasible in those patients of extrahepatic portal vein obstruction who still have a patent left branch of portal vein. This procedure restores portal vein flow to the liver, by bypassing the portal vein obstruction site. Other options do not restore portal flow to liver, rather create a portosystemic shunt to decompress the portal system.

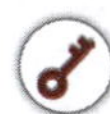

Key: C

BOOST YOUR KNOWLEDGE

Meso-Rex bypass requires a patency of superior mesenteric vein and left branch of portal vein with a minimum diameter of 2 mm. Rex vein patency decreases as age progresses, hence this surgery is generally only feasible in early age group patients.

REFERENCE/SOURCE

- Zhang J, Li L. Rex shunt for extra-hepatic portal venous obstruction in children. Children (Basel). 2022;9(2):297.

10. A 17-year-old girl with autoimmune hepatitis (on maintenance azathioprine) presents to OPD. Her per abdomen examination shows liver 2 cm below costal margin and spleen 4 cm below costal margin. Her liver function test (LFT) is total bilirubin/direct bilirubin/AST/ALT/ALP/GGT/total protein/albumin 0.9/0.3/45/43/114/37/6.4/3.8, INR 1.2, and CBC—Hb/TLC/platelet 10.5 g/dL/3,100/mm^3/90,000/mm^3. Her liver stiffness measurement by transient elastography (FibroScan) is 30 kPa. What is the next step?

A. Start carvedilol
B. Upper gastrointestinal endoscopy is necessary to assess for varices
C. No further intervention required as LFT is normal
D. Increase azathioprine dose

EXPLANATION

FibroScan value more than 25 kPa is a noninvasive marker for clinically significant portal hypertension (CSPH). In patients with chronic liver disease with FibroScan >25 kPa, NSBB therapy has shown to reduce risk of decompensation. Option B is incorrect as NSBB may be started without a prior endoscopy to assess variceal status. This is based on Baveno VII recommendations. Option C is incorrect as despite having normal LFT, patients may still have portal hypertension, which may gradually decrease as the underlying disease resolves.

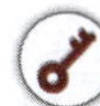

Key: A

BOOST YOUR KNOWLEDGE

Clinically significant portal hypertension is defined as hepatic venous pressure gradient (HVPG) >10 mm Hg. Such patients are at increased risk of variceal hemorrhage and ascites, thus benefit from measures to reduce portal pressure. HVPG is an invasive test and is not suitable for children as it requires cooperation of the patient, and sedation can alter hemodynamics, leading to erroneous values. Other markers of CSPH include the presence of varices on endoscopy, portosystemic collaterals on imaging. Liver stiffness measurement by transient elastography (FibroScan) has been found to correlate with HVPG in adult cirrhotics and is used as a guide to start nonselective beta-blocker therapy.

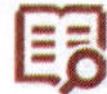

REFERENCE/SOURCE

- de Franchis R, Bosch J, Garcia-Tsao G, Reiberger T, Ripoll C; Baveno VII Faculty. Baveno VII—renewing consensus in portal hypertension. J Hepatol. 2022;76(4):959-74.

11. A 9-year-old child with Wilson disease presents with hematemesis. He is started on octreotide infusion, and upper gastrointestinal endoscopy is done which shows large high-risk varices. Endoscopic band ligation is done, and bleeding is controlled. What should be the next step?

A. Repeat endoscopy should be done every 6 months, and patient should be maintained on propranolol
B. Repeat endoscopy should be done every 4 weeks till variceal eradication is achieved alongside propranolol maintenance therapy
C. Propranolol maintenance therapy is required for a long duration. There is no need of repeating endoscopy, if there is no further hematemesis
D. Propranolol maintenance therapy should be given along with yearly endoscopy

EXPLANATION

Secondary prophylaxis of variceal hemorrhage entails repeated endotherapy till variceal eradication along with beta blocker maintenance therapy. Repeat endoscopy should be done every 4 weeks. Once varices have been eradicated, the frequency of endoscopy can be decreased to once every 1–2 years. Thus, option B is the only correct option.

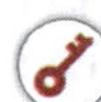

Key: B

BOOST YOUR KNOWLEDGE

Repeat endoscopy done at 2 weekly intervals has been shown to have increased ulcer formation. 4-week interval between endoscopies gives time for postbanding ulcers to heal.

REFERENCE/SOURCE

- Kaplan DE, Ripoll C, Thiele M, Fortune BE, Simonetto DA, Garcia-Tsao G, et al. AASLD Practice Guidance on Risk Stratification and Management of Portal Hypertension and Varices in Cirrhosis. Hepatology. 2024;79(5):1180-211.

12. An 18-year-old boy, case of biliary atresia postsuccessful Kasai portoenterostomy, currently asymptomatic, comes for a routine checkup. He has splenomegaly with investigations showing thrombocytopenia (platelet count 120,000/mm^3), Model for End-Stage Liver Disease (MELD) Na 5, and FibroScan of 22 kPa. He also has moderately persistent asthma. What is the next step to manage his portal hypertension?

A. Start propranolol as he has high FibroScan with thrombocytopenia
B. Upper gastrointestinal endoscopy with band ligation
C. No need for any therapy as MELD Na is low
D. Liver transplant

EXPLANATION

The FibroScan and platelet count of this patient suggest the presence of CSPH. Patients with CSPH benefit with NSBBs as risk of variceal bleeding is reduced. However, this patient has asthma, which is a contraindication to NSBB. In such cases, endoscopy with band ligation and eradication of varices is recommended. Patient should then undergo yearly screening endoscopies. Option D is incorrect as currently MELD Na is low, and patient is otherwise asymptomatic.

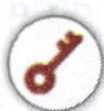

Key: B

BOOST YOUR KNOWLEDGE

According to Baveno VII guidelines, noninvasive markers of CSPH include: (1) FibroScan >25 kPA; (2) FibroScan between 20 and 24.9 kPa with platelet <150,000/mm^3; and (3) FibroScan between 15 and 19.9 kPa with platelet count <110,000/mm^3. These recommendations are mostly based on adults with viral hepatitis-associated cirrhosis.

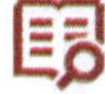

REFERENCE/SOURCE

- de Franchis R, Bosch J, Garcia-Tsao G, Reiberger T, Ripoll C; Baveno VII Faculty. Baveno VII—renewing consensus in portal hypertension. J Hepatol. 2022;76(4):959-74.

13. All of the following are sequelae of advanced portal hypertension in patients of biliary atresia, *except*:

A. Increasing hepatic artery resistive index (HARI)
B. Hepatorenal syndrome–acute kidney injury (HRS-AKI)
C. Hepatopulmonary syndrome (HPS)
D. Cholangitis with increasing bilirubin

EXPLANATION

Cholangitis in biliary atresia patients is not a sequelae of portal hypertension, but a cause. Repeated cholangitis can lead to increased fibrosis and accelerate portal hypertension in such patients. All other options develop due to portal hypertension.

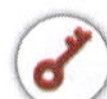

Key: D

BOOST YOUR KNOWLEDGE

Hepatic artery resistive index calculated on Doppler sonography has good correlation with portal hypertension in biliary atresia patients. According to one study, with every 0.1 increase in HARI, there is 5.2 mm Hg increase in portal pressure. HARI >0.8 is associated with poor outcome in biliary atresia patients.

REFERENCE/SOURCE

- Mittal D, Bhatnagar V, Agarwala S, Srinivas M, Jana M, Gupta AK, et al. Preoperative hepatic artery resistive index is a non-invasive predictive indicator of prognosis in biliary atresia. J Indian Assoc Pediatr Surg. 2017;22(4):237-41.

14. A 12-year-old known case of Wilson disease presents with hematemesis and melena. He is in hepatic encephalopathy grade II with compensated shock, with ongoing bleed. Which of the following is *not* recommended?

A. Prophylactic intubation prior to upper gastrointestinal endoscopy
B. Fresh-frozen plasma (FFP) transfusion to correct deranged INR
C. Prophylactic broad-spectrum antibiotic to prevent infection
D. Nasogastric tube should not be placed pre-endoscopy or prior to intubation

EXPLANATION

Fresh-frozen plasma or platelet transfusion based on INR and platelet values are not recommended in cases of variceal hemorrhage as these conventional markers of coagulopathy do not accurately predict bleeding in cirrhotics. FFP transfusion in such cases may increase variceal pressure exacerbating the bleed. Thus, option B is incorrect. In cases of ongoing hematemesis with altered mentation, prophylactic intubation is recommended to prevent aspiration pneumonia. Aspiration pneumonia is the most common infection posthematemesis, and all patients should be started on antibiotic prophylaxis. Nasogastric tube placement is not recommended as it may increase the risk of aspiration.

Key: D

BOOST YOUR KNOWLEDGE

In cirrhosis, both pro- and anticoagulant factors are reduced and exist in a state of delicate balance called "rebalanced hemostasis." Conventional coagulopathy markers such as INR and platelet count do not accurately predict bleeding in such cases. Viscoelastic tests like rotational thromboelastometry (ROTEM) and thromboelastogram (TEG), which measure blood coagulation in real time, are being increasingly studied in such patients to guide transfusion.

REFERENCES/SOURCES

- European Association for the Study of the Liver. EASL Clinical Practice Guidelines on prevention and management of bleeding and thrombosis in patients with cirrhosis. J Hepatol. 2022;76(5):1151-84.
- Maria A, Lal BB, Khanna R, Sood V, Mukund A, Bajpai M, et al. Rotational thromboelastometry-guided blood component use in cirrhotic children undergoing invasive procedures: randomized controlled trial. Liver Int. 2022;42(11):2492-500.

CHAPTER

17.6

Liver Abscess and Tumors

Jagadeesh Menon VR, Naresh Shanmugam

1. Which of the following *does not* form the clinical triad of liver abscess?

A. Fever
B. Right upper abdominal tenderness
C. Hepatomegaly
D. Jaundice

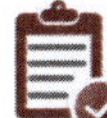

EXPLANATION

The classical triad of liver abscess—fever, hepatomegaly, and RUQ tenderness—is seen in up to 80% patients with liver abscess.

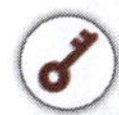

Key: D

BOOST YOUR KNOWLEDGE

Jaundice may also be seen in patients with liver abscess but does not form a part of triad. The possible mechanism is hepatic necrosis leading to damaged bile ducts and blood vessels, leading to a biliovascular fistula.

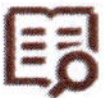

REFERENCES/SOURCES

- Lal SB, Venkatesh V, Kumar A, Anushree N, Seetharaman K, Aneja A, et al. Liver abscess in children-experience from a single tertiary care center of North India: etiology, clinical profile and predictors of complications. J Pediatr Infect Dis. 2021;40(5): e179-84.
- Longworth S, Han J. Pyogenic liver abscess. Clin Liver Dis (Hoboken). 2015;6:51-4.

2. Which of the following is the most common cause of liver abscess in children?

A. *Escherichia coli*
B. *Klebsiella*
C. *Staphylococcus aureus*
D. *Entamoeba histolytica*

EXPLANATION

As opposed to adults, in whom gram-negative bacilli predominate, *S. aureus* is the predominant etiologic agent in children. This may reflect the significant number of immunocompromised patients in pediatric series of pyogenic liver abscess.

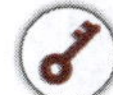

Key: C

BOOST YOUR KNOWLEDGE

Portal vein bacteria from intra-abdominal infectious processes (e.g., appendices abscess, abscess secondary to ingested foreign body, and inflammatory bowel disease) or umbilical vein catheterization can predispose to liver abscesses and could be multiple in these children.

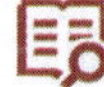 REFERENCE/SOURCE

- Suchy FJ (Ed). Liver Disease in Children, 5th edition. Cambridge University Press; 2021.

3. Which one of the following is *correct* for amoebic liver abscess?

A. It is the most common extraintestinal manifestation of amoebiasis
B. Up to 30% patients with intestinal amoebiasis develop liver abscess
C. Budd–Chiari syndrome is the most common complication
D. Percutaneous aspiration is always better than catheter drainage when the size is >5 cm, and the wall is thick

 EXPLANATION

Around 2–5% of patients with intestinal amoebiasis may end up with liver abscess. Catheter drainage is always better than aspiration. Budd–Chiari syndrome is rare after liver abscess.

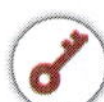 **Key: A**

 BOOST YOUR KNOWLEDGE

Metronidazole is the drug of choice in children with amoebic liver abscess, and this should be followed by treatment with paromomycin, which is a luminal amebicide to prevent transmission.

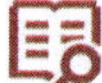 REFERENCE/SOURCE

- Arellano-Aguilar G, Marín-Santillán E, Castilla-Barajas JA, Bribiesca-Juárez MC, Domínguez-Carrillo LG. A brief history of amoebic liver abscess with an illustrative case. Rev Gastroenterol Mex. 2017;82:344-8.

4. Which of the following is *not* a characteristic of complicated liver abscess (rupture/vascular thrombosis)?

A. Elevated prothrombin time
B. Albumin <3 g/dL
C. Elevated alanine transaminase (ALT)
D. Elevated gamma-glutamyl transferase (GGT)

 EXPLANATION

In one the largest series of pediatric liver abscess, described from PGI Chandigarh India, these children were found to have a higher ALT, prolonged prothrombin time/international normalized ratio, low serum protein, and albumin levels. GGT was not affected.

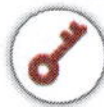 **Key: D**

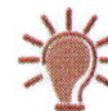 BOOST YOUR KNOWLEDGE

Rare complications of liver abscess include Budd–Chiari syndrome, pleural or pericardial fistulation, and acute pancreatitis.

 REFERENCE/SOURCE

- Lal SB, Venkatesh V, Kumar A, Anushree N, Seetharaman K, Aneja A, et al. Liver abscess in children-experience from a single tertiary care center of North India: etiology, clinical profile and predictors of complications. J Pediatr Infect Dis. 2021;40(5):e179-84.

5. A child with pyogenic liver abscess was noted to have palmoplantar hyperkeratosis. What is the probable diagnosis?

A. Gianotti–Crosti syndrome
B. Papillon–Lefèvre syndrome
C. Olmsted syndrome
D. Huriez syndrome

EXPLANATION

Papillon–Lefèvre syndrome is a rare autosomal recessive disorder caused by *cathepsin C* gene mutation, leading to the deficiency of cathepsin C enzymatic activity. The disease is characterized by palmoplantar hyperkeratosis, loss of deciduous and permanent teeth, and increased susceptibility to infections, especially liver abscess.

Key: B

BOOST YOUR KNOWLEDGE

Other primary immunodeficiency disorders associated with liver abscess include chronic granulomatous disease, other disorders of neutrophil dysfunction, and hyper-immunoglobulin E (IgE) syndrome.

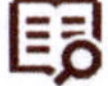

REFERENCE/SOURCE

- Ahmad M, Hassan I, Masood Q. Papillon-Lefevre syndrome. J Dermatol Case Rep. 2009;3(4):53-5.

6. Liver abscess in the post-transplant period happens in association with:

A. Hepatic artery thrombosis
B. Portal vein thrombosis
C. Hepatic vein thrombosis
D. Acute rejection

EXPLANATION

Hepatic abscess, a rare complication after liver transplantation, may be associated with hepatic artery thrombosis secondary to bilioma formation. This happens as the blood supply to the biliary system principally depends on the hepatic artery flow.

Key: A

BOOST YOUR KNOWLEDGE

Hepatic artery thrombosis is an important cause of graft loss and mortality in postliver transplant period. It is also an important indication of retransplantation.

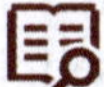

REFERENCE/SOURCE

- Ahmad M, Hassan I, Masood Q. Papillon-Lefevre syndrome. J Dermatol Case Rep. 2009;3(4):53-5.

7. Which of the following liver tumors can mimic a liver abscess in clinical presentation?

A. Hepatic adenoma
B. Teratoma
C. Mesenchymal hamartoma
D. Focal nodular hyperplasia (FNH)

EXPLANATION

Mesenchymal hamartoma may present with fever, pain, and hepatomegaly.

Key: C

BOOST YOUR KNOWLEDGE

Mesenchymal hamartoma usually presents as a large benign multicystic liver mass in a child <3 years. Treatment consists of complete resection. Malignant transformation to embryonal sarcoma is extremely uncommon.

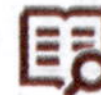

REFERENCE/SOURCE

- Suchy FJ (Ed). Liver Disease in Children, 5th edition. Cambridge University Press; 2021.

8. Which of the following organisms, responsible for liver abscess, is characterized by wheel within a wheel sign *or* Bull's eye sign on ultrasound imaging?

A. *Candida*
B. *Histoplasma*
C. *Coccidioides*
D. *Sporothrix schenckii*

EXPLANATION

Both are seen in *Candida* liver abscess. In wheel within a wheel sign, the wheely central hypoechoic area corresponds to necrosis/fungal debris; an inner hyperechoic ring of inflammatory cells; and a peripheral hypoechoic area representing fibrosis. The Bull's eye sign is similar to the above sign but lacks the central hypoechoic necrosis/fungal debris.

Key: A

BOOST YOUR KNOWLEDGE

Other Bull's eye signs (not confined to the liver) are seen in intussusception and cerebral toxoplasmosis.

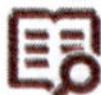

REFERENCE/SOURCE

- Cornely OA, Bangard C, Jaspers NI. Hepatosplenic candidiasis. Clin Liver Dis (Hoboken). 2015;6(2):47-50.

9. A 10-year-old child hailing from a rural area having thalassemia was diagnosed to have multiple liver abscess. An aspirate showed saprophytic gram-negative *Bacilli*. What is the most likely diagnosis?

A. Bartonellosis
B. Melioidosis
C. Tularemia
D. Septicemic plague

EXPLANATION

Melioidosis or *Whitmore disease* is an important but uncommon cause of liver abscess. The risk factors include diabetes and thalassemia and is more common in communities associated with farming. This is caused by gram-negative *Bacilli* named *Burkholderia pseudomallei*. Common presentations include pneumonia, liver and splenic abscess, septicemia, parotid abscess, and skin and soft tissue infections.

Key: B

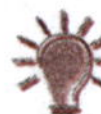

BOOST YOUR KNOWLEDGE

Abdominal CT scan findings of peripheral enhancement with "honeycomb" appearance increase the suspicion of melioidosis, especially in the presence of other affected intra-abdominal organs such as the spleen.

REFERENCE/SOURCE

- Martin PF, Teh CS, Casupang MA. Melioidosis: a rare cause of liver abscess. Case Reports Hepatol. 2016;2016(1):5910375.

10. A 3-year-old boy was diagnosed with multiple liver abscess. He was also noted to have hyperextensibility of joints. What is the probable underlying condition the child is suffering from?

A. Ehlers–Danlos syndrome
B. X-linked chronic granulomatous disease
C. Hyper-IgM syndrome
D. Hyper-IgE syndrome

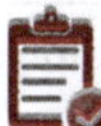

EXPLANATION

Hyper-IgE syndrome, also called Job's syndrome, is a primary immune deficiency state characterized by multisystemic manifestations apart from immunity-related issues. These include hyperextensibility of joints, coronary artery anomalies, fractures with trivial trauma, scoliosis, etc.

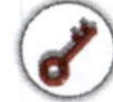

Key: D

BOOST YOUR KNOWLEDGE

An orthopantomogram can be helpful in diagnosing hyper-IgE syndrome, as these patients have persistent deciduous teeth along with noneruption of permanent teeth.

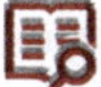

REFERENCE/SOURCE

- Saikia B. Clinical profile of hyper-IgE syndrome in India. Front Immunol. 2021;12:626593.

11. Which of the following gene mutations or chromosomal anomaly is *not* associated with hepatoblastoma in children?

A. Adenomatous polyposis coli (APC)-beta catenin
B. Insulin-like growth factor 2 (IGF-2)
C. *PTEN*
D. Trisomy 18

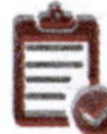

EXPLANATION

All the above-mentioned gene mutations/chromosomal anomaly are associated with hepatoblastoma, except the *PTEN* gene, which is associated with glioblastoma and prostatic cancer. *PTEN* gene mutation also causes hamartomas associated with Bannayan–Riley–Ruvalcaba syndrome and Proteus syndrome also with childhood autism.

Key: C

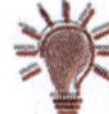

BOOST YOUR KNOWLEDGE

Adenomatous polyposis coli-beta catenin gene mutation is also seen in colorectal cancers and pancreatoblastomas.

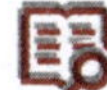

REFERENCE/SOURCE

- Zhu LR, Zheng W, Gao Q, Chen T, Pan ZB, Cui W, et al. Epigenetics and genetics of hepatoblastoma: linkage and treatment. Front Genet. 2022;13:1070971.

12. A 5-month-old infant, with a mass in the right lobe of the liver, had an alpha-fetoprotein (AFP) of 300 ng/dL. Biopsy showed a liver tumor with absent Integrase interactor 1 (INI1) expression. What is the most probable diagnosis?

A. Epithelial hepatoblastoma
B. Malignant teratoma
C. Inflammatory myofibroblastic tumor
D. Malignant rhabdoid tumor (MRT)

EXPLANATION

Malignant rhabdoid tumors are highly aggressive rare tumors that occur in early childhood. These are usually refractory to chemotherapy and radiation with high fatality. They typically have INI-1 negative expression.

Hepatoblastoma is the most common liver tumor in children, and it is basically divided into epithelial and mixed epithelial and mesenchymal types. The epithelial type, which is more common, includes various subtypes such as fetal, pleomorphic, embryonal, macrotrabecular, small cell undifferentiated (SCU), cholangioblastic, and mixed epithelial variants.

Inflammatory myofibroblastic tumor of the liver usually presents with persistent fever and elevated inflammatory markers like CRP and is treated with resection.

Malignant teratoma of the liver is an extragonadal germ cell tumor. This is a type of immature teratoma.

Key: D

BOOST YOUR KNOWLEDGE

Inflammatory myofibroblastic tumor expresses the rearrangements in *anaplastic lymphoma kinase* (*ALK*)-1 gene. It may also be associated with Epstein-Barr virus (EBV) infection.

REFERENCE/SOURCE

- Filips A, Maurer MH, Montani M, Beldi G, Lachenmayer A. Inflammatory myofibroblastic tumor of the liver: a case report and review of literature. World J Hepatol. 2020;12:170-83.

13. Which of the following disorders does *not* predispose to hepatoblastoma in children?

A. Classical galactosemia
B. Glycogen storage disorder (GSD)
C. Tyrosinemia type 1
D. Progressive familial intrahepatic cholestasis (PFIC)

EXPLANATION

Galactosemia does not predispose to developing hepatoblastoma in children, whereas the other disorders are reported to be associated with this tumor.

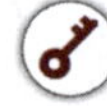

Key: A

BOOST YOUR KNOWLEDGE

Even though hepatocellular carcinoma (HCC) is more common in tyrosinemia, PFIC, and GSD, hepatoblastoma is also reported in the mentioned conditions.

14. Which of the following statements is *true* for hepatoblastomas?

A. Surgery is the only curative option
B. There is no correlation of birth weight with late developing hepatoblastoma
C. The presence of lung secondary is a contraindication to liver transplantation
D. Radiotherapy is the preferred treatment of choice

EXPLANATION

Patients that present with lung metastases are candidates for liver transplantation if their lung metastases resolve with chemotherapy or with resection.

Key: A

BOOST YOUR KNOWLEDGE

Those with extrahepatic disease that remains viable after full chemotherapy and not amenable to surgical resection represent the only absolute contraindication to orthotopic liver transplant (OLT) in patients with HB.

REFERENCE/SOURCE

- Khaderi S, Guiteau J, Cotton RT, O'Mahony C, Rana A, Goss JA. Role of liver transplantation in the management of hepatoblastoma in the pediatric population. World J Transplant. 2014;4:294-8.

15. Which of the following is correct regarding the SIOPEL IV classification of hepatoblastomas?

A. Pretext I tumor with rupture is very high-risk tumor
B. Pretext II tumors with low AFP are very high-risk tumors
C. Standard risk tumors need six cycles of chemotherapy followed by surgery
D. Pretext I tumor with portal vein involvement is a standard risk tumor

EXPLANATION

Irrespective of the pretext staging, patients with a low AFP are classified as very high-risk tumors as they are usually undifferentiated tumors and run an aggressive course. Pretext I tumor is a high-risk tumor (not a very high-risk tumor). Usually, four cycles of chemotherapy are provided before surgery following which a surgery is offered and then two more cycles are completed. Pretext tumor I with portal vein involvement is a high-risk tumor. So, options A, C, and D are incorrect.

Key: B

BOOST YOUR KNOWLEDGE

SIOPEL IV classification:

- *Standard risk*: Pretext I, II, and III, no metastasis, no extrahepatic extension, no tumor rupture, and AFP >100
- *High risk*: Pretext IV and/or extrahepatic abdominal disease or extension (vascular invasion) or tumor rupture
- *Very high risk*: Metastatic disease (usually lung) or AFP <100

REFERENCE/SOURCE

- Aronson DC, Czauderna P, Maibach R, Perilongo G, Morland B. The treatment of hepatoblastoma: its evolution and the current status as per the SIOPEL trials. J Indian Assoc Pediatr Surg. 2014;19:201-7.

16. Which of the following is *false* regarding pediatric HCC?

A. Fibrolamellar HCC has usually a normal AFP
B. Nitisinone should be started within 6 months of age to significantly reduce the risk of tyrosinemic children developing HCCs
C. Patients with Wilson disease on chelation rarely develop HCCs
D. Pediatric HCCs are more chemoresponsive than adult HCCs

EXPLANATION

NTBC or nitisinone must ideally be started within 4 weeks of age to significantly reduce the incidence of HCCs in TT-1.

Key: B

BOOST YOUR KNOWLEDGE

Fibrolamellar HCC is a type of HCC which usually occurs in adolescent age group, and only 10% of these patients have an elevated AFP (C/W 70–90% patients with HCC having an elevated AFP). Patients with Wilson disease on chelation usually do not develop HCC due to antineoplastic effect of these agents.

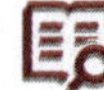

REFERENCE/SOURCE

- Suchy FJ (Ed). Liver Disease in Children, 5th edition. Cambridge University Press; 2021.

17. Hamartomas of the liver have all the features, *except*:

A. Marsupialization of the tumor is the treatment of choice
B. The presence of lymphatic channels
C. Diagnosed commonly in infancy
D. Malignant transformation is rare

EXPLANATION

The treatment of choice of mesenchymal hamartomas of the liver is complete surgical excision. Marsupialization is offered only if surgical excision cannot be done.

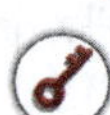

Key: A

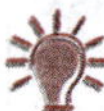

BOOST YOUR KNOWLEDGE

Mesenchymal hamartomas can grow as huge liver masses as they lack a capsule, and the majority have a stromal with cystic components.

REFERENCE/SOURCE

- Gupta R, Parelkar SV, Sanghvi B. Mesenchymal hamartoma of the liver. Indian J Med Paediatr Oncol. 2009;30:141-3.

18. Which of the following statements is *incorrect* regarding pediatric hepatic adenoma?

A. They have a central scar formation
B. *HNF-1 A* is a gene associated with this tumor
C. It is common in patients with GSD type 1
D. Malignant transformation to HCC can happen

EXPLANATION

Central scar formation is classical of FNH of the liver, and not hepatic adenomas.

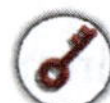

Key: A

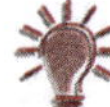

BOOST YOUR KNOWLEDGE

Glycogen storage disorder-1, the use of oral contraceptive pills (OCPs), HNF-1 mutation, the use of anabolic steroids, barbiturates, and obesity increase the risk to develop hepatic adenomas.

REFERENCE/SOURCE

- Beaufrère A, Paradis V. Hepatocellular adenomas: review of pathological and molecular features. Hum Pathol. 2021;112:128-37.

19. All are true for hepatic hemangiomas, *except*:

A. The most common benign liver tumor
B. Spontaneous regression is seen in many cases
C. The majority are asymptomatic
D. Can lead to hyperammonemia and encephalopathy

EXPLANATION

Hyperammonemia is caused by congenital extra- or intrahepatic portosystemic shunts and not vascular tumors of the liver. All other statements are true.

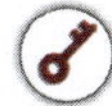

Key: D

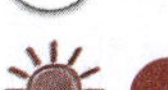

BOOST YOUR KNOWLEDGE

Patients with hemangiomas can have heart failure, hypothyroidism, and thrombocytopenia secondary to Kasabach-Merritt syndrome.

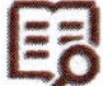

REFERENCE/SOURCE

- Aziz H, Brown ZJ, Baghdadi A, Kamel IR, Pawlik TM. A comprehensive review of hepatic hemangioma management. J Gastrointest Surg. 2022;26(9):1998-2007.

20. Which of the following is *correct* regarding Langerhans cell histiocytosis (LCH) of the liver?

A. Pseudotumor is the most common hepatic presentation
B. Biopsy shows positive CD1a in almost all the cases
C. Liver transplant is contraindicated in active multisystem LCH
D. Vinblastine therapy is not preferred in patients with synthetic liver failure

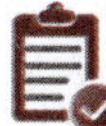

EXPLANATION

Vinblastine is contraindicated in liver cell failure as it worsens the liver failure, and the systemic toxicity of its metabolite increases to cause myelosuppression and peripheral neuropathy. The rest of the statements are false.

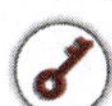

Key: D

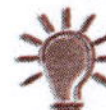

BOOST YOUR KNOWLEDGE

Langerhans cell histiocytosis is an important cause of secondary sclerosing cholangitis in children and is an important clinical presentation. Liver biopsy done during chronic phase may not show active cells as sclerosing cholangitis progresses even without active damage caused by the cancer cells. BRAF (V-Raf Murine Sarcoma Viral Oncogene Homolog B) inhibitors are a newer class of agents used to treat refractory LCH.

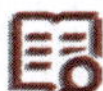

REFERENCE/SOURCE

- Menon J, Rammohan A, Vij M, Shanmugam N, Rela M. Current perspectives on the role of liver transplantation for Langerhans cell histiocytosis: a narrative review. World J Gastroenterol. 2022;28:4044-52.

SECTION 18

Hematology

Section Editor: Sidharth Totadri

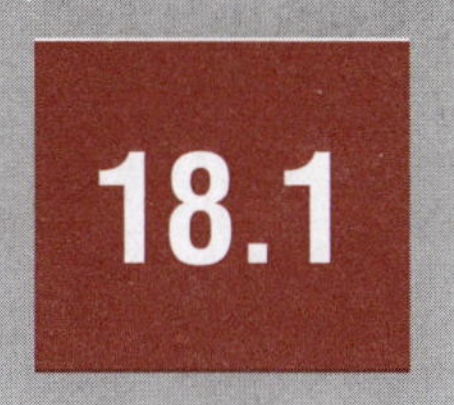

CHAPTER 18.1

Anemia, Etiology, Classification, and Approach to Diagnosis

Sanghamitra Ray

1. A male child of 5 months of age presented with severe anemia. The child had triphalangeal thumb, high-arched palate, and ventricular septal defect. Investigations showed macrocytic anemia, while other cell lines were preserved. High performance liquid chromatography (HPLC) showed high fetal hemoglobin (HbF), and erythrocyte adenosine deaminase (ADA) activity was increased. What is the most probable diagnosis?

A. Anemia of prematurity
B. Transient erythroblastopenia of childhood
C. Diamond–Blackfan anemia
D. Fanconi anemia

EXPLANATION

Pointers of diagnosis: (1) Age of onset; (2) Skeletal and cardiovascular deformity; (3) High HbF—very characteristic feature along with (4) increased red cell ADA level.

	Age of onset	*Other associated malformations*	*High HbF and High ADA*	*Macrocytosis*
Anemia of prematurity	3–6 weeks	–	–/–	±
Transient erythroblastopenia of childhood	Around 1 year	–	–/–	–
Diamond–Blackfan anemia	Before 1 year, median age 8 weeks	++	+/+	+
Fanconi anemia	Variable usually after 1 year	++	–/–	+

Key: C

BOOST YOUR KNOWLEDGE

Few hematological conditions with high HbF: Thalassemia major, hereditary persistence of fetal hemoglobin (HPFH), Diamond–Blackfan anemia, juvenile myelomonocytic leukemia, etc.

REFERENCE/SOURCE

- Thornburg CD. Congenital hypoplastic anemia (Diamond-Blackfan anemia). In: Kliegman RM, St Geme III JW, Blum NJ, Shah SS, Tasker RC, Wilson KM (Eds). Nelson Textbook of Pediatrics, 21st edition. Elsevier; 2019. pp. 2510-2.

2. Which among these is an acquired cause of hemolytic anemia?

A. Pyruvate kinase deficiency
B. Glucose-6-phosphate dehydrogenase (G6PD) deficiency
C. Paroxysmal nocturnal hemoglobinuria
D. Pyropoikilocytosis

EXPLANATION

Disease entity	*Inheritance*	*Diagnostic tests*
Pyruvate kinase deficiency	Hereditary	Pyruvate kinase assay—reduced level
G6PD deficiency	Hereditary	G6PD assay—reduced level
Paroxysmal nocturnal hemoglobinuria (PNH)	Acquired	Reduced white blood cell CD55 and CD59 or reduced red cell CD59 by flow cytometry
Pyropoikilocytosis	Hereditary	Extreme variability in red blood cell (RBC) size and shape. RBC shows thermal sensitivity—fragmentation occurs at 45°C for 15 minutes. Reduced level of decay accelerating factor

Key: C

BOOST YOUR KNOWLEDGE

Paroxysmal nocturnal hemoglobinuria is an acquired marrow disorder where there is complement-mediated lysis of RBCs. It can present with the expanded spectrum ranging from mild isolated cytopenia to pancytopenia. Most patients experience chronic hemolysis, thrombocytopenia, and leukopenia. Hemoglobinuria is rarely seen in children compared to adults. Thrombosis and thromboembolic phenomena are life-threatening complications.

REFERENCE/SOURCE

- Kliegman RM, St Geme III JW, Blum NJ, Shah SS, Tasker RC, Wilson KM (Eds). Nelson Textbook of Pediatrics, 21st edition. Elsevier; 2019. Chapters 484 to 491. pp. 2527-64.

3. A 3-year-old child is a known case of seizure disorder and is on syrup phenytoin for the last 2 years. The child presented to the outpatient department with complaints of weakness and increasing pallor. On examination, he was of normal nutritional status but pale with no organomegaly. He regularly consumed nonvegetarian food. Investigations showed Hb 5 g%, mean corpuscular volume (MCV) 110 fL, total leukocyte count (TLC) 3,000/mm^3, and platelet count 1.4 lacs/mm^3. Peripheral smear showed macrocytic red cells. What is the most probable cause of macrocytic anemia in this case?

A. Vitamin B_{12} deficiency
B. Folic acid deficiency
C. Iron deficiency
D. Copper deficiency

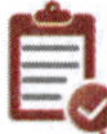

EXPLANATION

Chances of vitamin B_{12} deficiency are less as the child is of good nutritional status and on nonvegetarian diet. Iron deficiency does not cause macrocytic anemia. Phenytoin causes impaired folic acid absorption, leading to folate deficiency. Copper deficiency usually presents with microcytic anemia with neurological dysfunction in patients with malnutrition or in those who are on parenteral nutrition without copper supplementation.

Key: B

BOOST YOUR KNOWLEDGE

Hereditary folate malabsorption (HFM) is an autosomal recessive disorder. Loss-of-function mutations in the *SLC46A1* gene, which codes for the folate transporter, is behind its pathogenesis. There is inability to absorb folic acid, 5-tetrahydrofolate, 5-methyltetrahydrofolate, and folinic acid. Children present at 2–6 months of age with megaloblastic anemia, infections and diarrhea, and neurologic abnormalities including seizures, developmental delay, and subnormal IQ. Folate transport is impaired in the intestine and choroid plexus of the brain. Serum and cerebrospinal fluid (CSF) folate levels are very low, with a loss of the normal 3:1 ratio of CSF to serum folate.

REFERENCE/SOURCE

- Thornburg CD. Folic acid deficiency. In: Kliegman RM, St Geme III JW, Blum NJ, Shah SS, Tasker RC, Wilson KM (Eds). Nelson Textbook of Pediatrics, 21st edition. Elsevier; 2019. pp. 2518-9.

4. A child of 5 years of age presented with sudden onset pallor. He has history suggestive of upper respiratory tract infection 5 days back. On examination, no organomegaly was noted. On investigation, Hb was 2 g%, MCV 166 fL, TLC 11,000/mm^3, platelet count 1.7 lacs/mm^3, and reticulocyte count 12%. HPLC was normal and Direct *Coombs* test (DCT) was 3+ (IgM+/ C3d+). Peripheral smear finding is shown here.

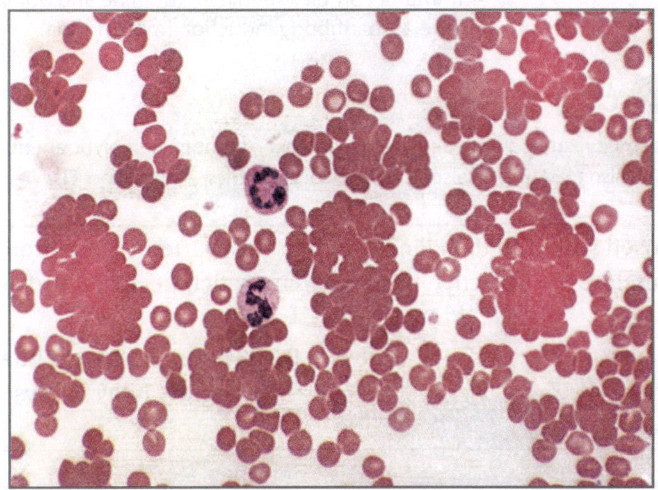

What is the most probable diagnosis?

A. Wilson disease
B. Warm antibody autoimmune hemolytic anemia (AIHA)
C. Cold agglutinin disease
D. Vitamin B_{12} deficiency

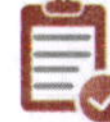

EXPLANATION

Wilson disease is generally a cause of DCT-negative hemolytic anemia, so it is ruled out. Warm antibody AIHA has immunoglobulin G (IgG) positive, and generally such high MCV is not seen. In megaloblastic anemia caused by vitamin B_{12} deficiency, MCV is not that high, and peripheral smear does not show any hypersegmented neutrophil typical of megaloblastic anemia. In cold agglutinin disease, there is often a preceding history of viral infection, MCV is very high, and peripheral smears typically show large clumps of RBCs.

Key: C

BOOST YOUR KNOWLEDGE

Causes of AIHA:

Disease entity	***Causes***
Warm antibody AIHA	• Primary (idiopathic) • *Secondary:* – Lymphoproliferative disorders – Connective tissue disorders – Nonlymphoid neoplasms (e.g., ovarian tumor) – Chronic inflammatory diseases (e.g., ulcerative colitis) – Immunodeficiency disorders
Cold antibody AIHA	• Primary cold agglutinin disease • Secondary cold agglutinin disease • Lymphoproliferative disorders • Infections (*Mycoplasma pneumoniae*) • Epstein-Barr virus) • Paroxysmal cold hemoglobinuria • Primary (idiopathic)
Drug-induced immune hemolytic anemia	• Hapten/drug adsorption (penicillin) • Immune complex mediated (quinine and quinidine) • True autoantibody induction (methyldopa)

REFERENCE/SOURCE

- Brandow AM. Hemolytic anemias resulting from extracellular factors—immune hemolytic anemias. In: Kliegman RM, St Geme III JW, Blum NJ, Shah SS, Tasker RC, Wilson KM (Eds). Nelson Textbook of Pediatrics, 21st edition. Elsevier; 2019. pp. 2562-64.

5. A 3-year-old child diagnosed with iron deficiency anemia was started on oral iron supplementation at a dose of 4 mg/kg/day. Average timeline of subjective improvement, reticulocytosis, and starting of hemoglobin rise are respectively:

A. 72 hours, 7 days, 14 days
B. 36 hours, 14 days, 21 days
C. 24 hours, 3 days, 7 days
D. 12 hours, 1 day, 7 days

EXPLANATION

Time after starting iron	***Response***
12–24 hours	Subjective improvement, increased appetite
36–48 hours	Erythroid hyperplasia
48–72 hours	Reticulocytosis, peaking at 5–7 days
4–30 days	Increase in hemoglobin level, increase in MCV, and increase in ferritin
1–3 months	Repletion of iron stores

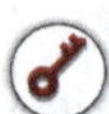

Key: C

BOOST YOUR KNOWLEDGE

The sequence of development of iron deficiency anemia is as follows:

- Tissue iron stores get depleted—marked by reduced serum ferritin (SF) (iron-storage protein).
- Serum iron levels decrease, the iron-binding capacity [serum transferrin (TF)] increases, and the TF saturation falls.

- Iron becomes scarce to bind with protoporphyrin to form heme. Free erythrocyte protoporphyrin accumulates.
- Hemoglobin synthesis is impaired.
- Iron deficiency progresses to iron-deficiency anemia.

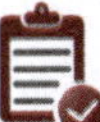

REFERENCE/SOURCE

- Rothman JA. Iron-deficiency anemia. In: Kliegman RM, St Geme III JW, Blum NJ, Shah SS, Tasker RC, Wilson KM (Eds). Nelson Textbook of Pediatrics, 21st edition. Elsevier; 2019. pp. 9923-8.

6. A 1-year-old boy presented with complaints of pain and swelling of digits of left hand. Initial laboratory investigations demonstrated hemoglobin of 4.5 g/dL, white cell count of 19,000/mm^3 (55% neutrophils and 45% lymphocytes), platelet count of 170,000/mm^3, and an erythrocyte sedimentation rate of 45 mm/hour. Peripheral blood smear showed sickling of RBC. Hb electrophoresis revealed that HbS was 80%, HbF 18%, and HbA2 2%, and the patient was diagnosed with sickle cell anemia. What will be the plan of treatment in this child in acute phase of dactylitis?

A. Antibiotic for 6–8 weeks, intravenous fluid and surgery
B. Blood transfusion only
C. Hydroxyurea and antibiotics
D. Intravenous fluid and pain relief measures

EXPLANATION

Dactylitis, also known as hand-foot syndrome, is often the first presentation of painful crisis in infants and young children with sickle cell anemia. It occurs in 50% of children aged <2 years. Dactylitis often manifests with symmetric or unilateral swelling of the hands and/or feet. Unilateral dactylitis is often confused with osteomyelitis. Detailed evaluation is needed to distinguish the two entities as treatment differs significantly. Dactylitis requires palliation with pain medications, including semisynthetic opioid derivatives—hydrocodone/oxycodone and maintaining proper hydration, whereas osteomyelitis requires minimum of intravenous antibiotic therapy for 6–8 weeks.

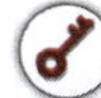

Key: D

BOOST YOUR KNOWLEDGE

Hydroxyurea, a myelosuppressive agent, is very effective in reducing the frequency of acute painful crisis. In adults with sickle cell anemia, hydroxyurea decreases the rate of hospitalization for painful episodes by 50% and blood transfusion by around 50%. It is well tolerated in children of more than 5 years of age. All children with sickle cell anemia should be on hydroxyurea from the age of 9 months. Hydroxyurea is started at the dose of 5–20 mg/kg once daily, with gradual increment, up to a maximum of 35 mg/kg per dose.

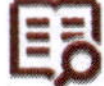

REFERENCE/SOURCE

- Smith-Whitley K, Kwiatkowski JL. Hemoglobinopathies. In: Kliegman RM, St Geme III JW, Blum NJ, Shah SS, Tasker RC, Wilson KM (Eds). Nelson Textbook of Pediatrics, 21st edition. Elsevier; 2019. pp. 2540-58.

7. A 5-year-old child presented to the pediatric outpatient department with bleeding from gums and fever for 4 days. On examination, the child was short statured with bifid thumb and multiple café-au-lait spots. There was no hepatosplenomegaly. Initial investigations showed pancytopenia (Hb 4 g%, TLC 2,000/mm^3, and platelet count 12,000/mm^3). Peripheral smear showed no atypical cells and reticulocyte count as 0.02%. What is the definitive treatment?

A. Antithymocyte globulin (ATG)
B. Cyclosporine
C. Allogenic bone marrow transplantation (BMT)
D. Androgens

EXPLANATION

The afore-mentioned entity is Fanconi anemia. Pancytopenia with café-au-lait spots, limb anomalies, and short stature favor the diagnosis of Fanconi anemia. The definitive treatment of Fanconi anemia is allogenic bone marrow transplantation. ATG with cyclosporine is used as the first-line treatment in aplastic anemia but is not effective in this entity. Androgens are used in Fanconi with a response rate of around 50% and has a high risk of relapse. Allogenic BMT is the only curative treatment option available.

Key: C

BOOST YOUR KNOWLEDGE

The diagnosis of Fanconi anemia is confirmed with lymphocyte chromosomal breakage study done with addition of crosslinking agents, such as diepoxybutane and mitomycin-C. Increased chromosome fragility is indicated by spontaneously occurring chromatid breaks, rearrangements, gaps, etc. in blood lymphocytes as well as in cultured skin fibroblasts. 10–15% of the patients can have somatic mosaicism and thus can have normal chromosomal fragility. Next-generation sequencing (NGS) is the new confirmatory test for this entity now.

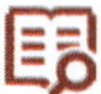

REFERENCE/SOURCE

- Dror Y, Cada M. Inherited bone marrow failure syndromes with pancytopenia. In: Kliegman RM, St Geme III JW, Blum NJ, Shah SS, Tasker RC, Wilson KM (Eds). Nelson Textbook of Pediatrics, 21st edition. Elsevier; 2019. pp. 2568-78.

8. Which of the following statements is *correct* regarding the management of thalassemia?

A. Iron chelation is to be started at 1 year of age irrespective of the ferritin level in transfusion-dependent thalassemia (TDT) children
B. Deferiprone is the only oral chelator drug available for pediatric population
C. Only indication of splenectomy in TDT is hypersplenism
D. Children with nontransfusion-dependent thalassemia (NTDT) are at higher risk of thromboembolism than TDT

EXPLANATION

Iron chelation is generally started after 1 year of transfusion therapy and/or when SF is >1,000 ng/mL. Iron chelation is not currently labeled for use in children <2 years. Three iron chelators available at present both for adults and children are deferoxamine, deferasirox, and deferiprone among which last two mentioned are administered orally. Indications of splenectomy in TDT are hypersplenism, rising red cell transfusion requirement, and mechanical discomfort due to massive enlargement of spleen. Causes of hypercoagulable state in NTDT are:

- Ineffective erythropoiesis
- Chronic hemolytic anemia leading to pathological RBCs
- Chronically activated platelets and enhanced platelet aggregation
- Increased platelet count and adhesiveness are a common finding in splenectomized patients and are a strong contributor to occlusive thrombus formation.

Key: D

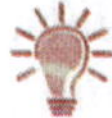

BOOST YOUR KNOWLEDGE

Iron chelation is initiated in NTDT patients ≥10 years of age if any of the below is present:

- Liver iron concentration ≥5 mg Fe/g dry weight (not done routinely)
- SF level ≥800 ng/mL
- SF level >300 to <800 ng/mL and other clinical or laboratory measures indicative of iron overload

Deferasirox therapy should be discontinued, if SF level 300 ng/mL and patients should continue to be monitored for iron overload. The use of other iron chelators other than deferasirox cannot be recommended as per the latest Thalassaemia International Federation (TIF) guideline for NTDT.

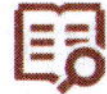

REFERENCES/SOURCES

- Hypercoagulablity and thrombotic disease. In: Taher A, Musallam K, Cappellini MD (Eds). Guidelines for the Management of Non-transfusion-dependent β-thalassemia, 3rd edition. Thalassaemia International Federation; 2023.
- Smith-Whitley Kim, Kwiatkowski JL. Hemoglobinopathies. In: Kliegman RM, St Geme III JW, Blum NJ, Shah SS, Tasker RC, Wilson KM (Eds). Nelson Textbook of Pediatrics, 21st edition. Elsevier; 2019. pp. 2540-58.

9. **A 5-year-old child with chronic renal disease was presented with anemia. After work-up, he was labeled as anemia of chronic disease. Which of the following laboratory parameters is *not* suggestive of anemia of chronic disease?**

A. Increased hepcidin
B. Normocytic normochromic anemia
C. Low serum iron
D. High serum TF

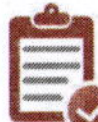

EXPLANATION

Anemia of chronic disease is usually associated with normocytic normochromic anemia although few patients can have hypochromia with microcytosis. Hepcidin level is increased because of inflammation-associated increased production. Serum iron is low but without an associated rise in iron-binding protein, TF, which is in contrast with iron-deficiency anemia. Low serum TF is a diagnostic feature of anemia of chronic disease.

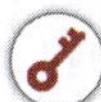

Key: D

BOOST YOUR KNOWLEDGE

Hepcidin is a key regulator of intestinal iron absorption and tissue distribution. It is predominantly synthesized in hepatocytes and in monocytes and macrophages. As it is excreted through the kidney, its level is also increased in patients with reduced glomerular filtration rate (GFR).

REFERENCE/SOURCE

- Anemia of chronic disease and renal disease. In: Kliegman RM, St Geme III JW, Blum NJ, Shah SS, Tasker RC, Wilson KM (Eds). Nelson Textbook of Pediatrics, 21st edition. Elsevier; 2019. pp. 2513-5.

10. **Which of the following is *incorrect* regarding physiological anemia of prematurity?**

A. Nadir is <10 g% most of the times
B. Anemia is due to suboptimal response of erythropoietin (EPO)
C. Nadir of anemia is never before 8 weeks
D. Premature infants' shortened RBC lifespan is one of the reasons

EXPLANATION

Premature infants develop a physiological anemia, which is called physiological anemia of prematurity. Hb decline is earlier than 8 weeks and is usually more severe than that of term infants. Shortened RBC lifespan of 40–60 days, suboptimal response of EPO to the degree of anemia along with increased metabolism of EPO, and repeated phlebotomies in these sick babies lead to severe anemia.

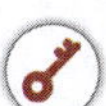

Key: C

BOOST YOUR KNOWLEDGE

During the intrauterine life, EPO synthesis occurs mainly in liver, which had oxygen sensors relatively insensitive to hypoxia compared to that of the kidney. The developmental switch from liver to kidney EPO production does not occur earlier in case of a premature birth. The preterm infant thus depends only on liver as the primary site for EPO generation, leading to diminished responsiveness to tissue hypoxia and anemia.

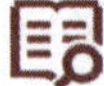

REFERENCE/SOURCE

- Thornburg CD. Physiologic anemia of infancy. In: Kliegman RM, St Geme III JW, Blum NJ, Shah SS, Tasker RC, Wilson KM (Eds). Nelson Textbook of Pediatrics, 21st edition. Elsevier; 2019. pp. 2516-7.

11. Which of the following is not a feature of hemolytic anemia?

A. Increased lactate dehydrogenase (LDH)
B. Increased serum haptoglobin
C. Increased urinary urobilinogen
D. Increased red cell distribution width (RDW)

EXPLANATION

Laboratory features of hemolytic anemia:

Laboratory features	***Cause***
Increased LDH	LDH (mainly iso-enzyme 1) is found intracellularly in RBCs. In hemolytic anemia, its level increases in blood secondary to increased red cell lysis
Reduced serum haptoglobin	Haptoglobin is primarily produced in liver, and its main function is to bind free hemoglobin from lysed RBCs in order to limit iron loss and renal damage due to free hemoglobin
Increased urinary urobilinogen	Hemolysis causes unconjugated hyperbilirubinemia. Unconjugated bilirubin not being hydrophilic is not excreted in urine. Bilirubin is deconjugated and converted to urobilinogen by bacteria in colon and is reabsorbed and excreted in urine
Increased RDW	The increased number of reticulocytes causes wide variation in RBC size causing increased RDW

Key: B

BOOST YOUR KNOWLEDGE

Haptoglobin is an acute phase reactant. Its level can also get elevated in infection and inflammation. It is also an antioxidant and has antibacterial activity.

REFERENCE/SOURCE

- Merguerian MD, Gallagher PG. Definitions and classification of hemolytic anemias. In: Kliegman RM, St Geme III JW, Blum NJ, Shah SS, Tasker RC, Wilson KM (Eds). Nelson Textbook of Pediatrics, 21st edition. Elsevier; 2019. pp. 2527-30.

12. Which of the following facts is *incorrect* regarding iron refractory iron deficiency anemia (IRIDA)?

A. Autosomal recessive disorder
B. Iron deficiency is because of impaired intestinal iron absorption
C. Reduced hepcidin level
D. SF is inappropriately low relative to the degree of iron deficiency

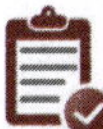

EXPLANATION

Serum ferritin is generally higher in comparison to the degree of iron deficiency in IRIDA. It is an autosomal recessive disorder caused by the loss of function mutation of the gene *TMPRSS6*, causing dysregulated production of hepcidin. As hepcidin regulates iron level of the body, its high-level causes impaired absorption of iron. Thus, patients are refractory to oral iron therapy.

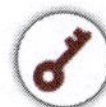

Key: D

BOOST YOUR KNOWLEDGE

The treatment of IRIDA requires parenteral iron therapy to correct anemia. Even with intravenous therapy, clinical response is usually slow and not correctable completely. Optimum dose and duration of therapy are not standardized till date due to rarity of the disease.

REFERENCE/SOURCE

- Finberg KE. Iron-refractory Iron-deficiency anemia. In: Kliegman RM, St Geme III JW, Blum NJ, Shah SS, Tasker RC, Wilson KM (Eds). Nelson Textbook of Pediatrics, 21st edition. Elsevier; 2019. p. 2525.

13. A 2-year-old male child born out of a nonconsanguineous marriage presented with pallor, icterus, and splenomegaly. The child had severe anemia with Hb of 4 g%. His peripheral smear examination showed significant amount of spherocytes (20–30 spherocytes per high power field) with features suggestive of hemolytic anemia. Investigations showed: MCV 84 fL, MCHC 36%, MCH 32 pg, RDW 15, reticulocyte count 10.2%. HPLC and DCT were negative. Osmotic fragility started at 0.92% of NaCl and ended at 0.38% of NaCl (markedly increased).

Which of the following tests will not aid in diagnosis in this index case?

A. Eosin-5-maleimide (EMA) binding test
B. Complement level
C. Acidified glycerol lysis test (AGLT)
D. Osmotic gradient ektacytometry

EXPLANATION

The diagnosis of the index case is hereditary spherocytosis. It can be established from a positive family history and the presence of typical clinical and laboratory features of the disease: Splenomegaly, spherocytes on the blood smear, reticulocytosis, and an elevated MCHC. If these are present, no additional testing is necessary to confirm the diagnosis clinically. If the diagnosis is less certain, additional testing can be performed. The binding of fluorescence labeled EMA to band 3 and other membrane proteins is decreased in HS erythrocytes. This flow cytometry-based test is easy. Other assays, such as the cryo-hemolysis test, the AGLT, and osmotic gradient ektacytometry, have been used for the diagnosis of HS. Complement level does have any role in diagnosis of the case. Study like exome sequencing offers accurate diagnosis.

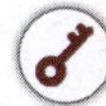

Key: B

BOOST YOUR KNOWLEDGE

Spherocytes can be found in many other conditions: Isoimmune hemolytic disease of the newborn, particularly in ABO incompatibility, thermal injury, hemolytic transfusion reaction, clostridial sepsis, severe hypophosphatemia, Wilson disease, congenital dyserythropoietic anemia type II, hereditary stomatocytosis, and snake, bee, or wasp envenomation, etc.

REFERENCE/SOURCE

- Merguerian MD, Gallagher PG. Hereditary spherocytosis. In: Kliegman RM, St Geme III JW, Blum NJ, Shah SS, Tasker RC, Wilson KM (Eds). Nelson Textbook of Pediatrics, 21st edition. Elsevier; 2019. pp. 2530-4.

14. All these diseases result in microcytic anemia, *except*:

A. Copper deficiency
B. Aceruloplasminemia
C. Atransferrinemia
D. Orotic aciduria

EXPLANATION

Disease entity	***Type of anemia***	***Cause***
Copper deficiency	Microcytic anemia	Copper is absorbed in the stomach and proximal duodenum. Deficiency is associated with malabsorption, severe malnutrition, and neurological dysfunction
Aceruloplasminemia	Microcytic anemia	• Defective transport of iron from macrophages to plasma to be available for RBC production • Iron accumulates in the brain and visceral organs • The diagnosis includes absent serum ceruloplasmin, low serum copper and iron, elevated ferritin, and raised liver iron concentration
Atransferrinemia	Microcytic anemia	Autosomal recessive disorder caused by mutations in the *TF* gene. Diagnosis is by low or absent serum TF and liver iron overload
Orotic aciduria	Macrocytic anemia	Autosomal recessive disorder. Appears in the first year of life: *Features:* Growth failure, developmental delay, megaloblastic anemia, and increased urinary orotic acid *Diagnosis:* Severe megaloblastic anemia with normal serum B12 and folate levels and no evidence of TC deficiency

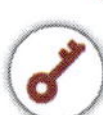

Key: D

BOOST YOUR KNOWLEDGE

Indicators of iron deficiency anemia:

Indicators	***Cut-off for iron deficiency anemia***
Hemoglobin	Hemoglobin (g/dL) <11.0 for non-Hispanic whites. Age (0.5–4) years
MCV (μm^3)	<70 for age 6–24 months
SF (μg/L)	*Age ≤5 years:* <12; children >5 years: <15 *All age groups in presence of infection:* <30–100
Reticulocyte hemoglobin content (CHr) (pg)	*Infants and young children:* <27.5; adults: ≤28.0
Serum transferrin receptor (sTfR)	Cutoff varies with assay and with patient's age and ethnic origin
Transferrin saturation	<16%
Erythrocyte zinc protoporphyrin (ZPP) (μmol/mol heme)	• *Age ≤5 years:* >70 • *Children >5 years:* >80 • *Children >5 years on washed red cells:* >40
Hepcidin	To be defined; usually ≤10 ng/mL

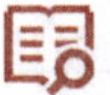

REFERENCES/SOURCES

- Rothman JA. Other microcystic anemias In: Kliegman RM, St Geme III JW, Blum NJ, Shah SS, Tasker RC, Wilson KM (Eds). Nelson Textbook of Pediatrics, 21st edition. Elsevier; 2019. p. 2526.
- Thomburg CD. Other rare megaloblastic anemias. In: Kliegman RM, St Geme III JW, Blum NJ, Shah SS, Tasker RC, Wilson KM (Eds). Nelson Textbook of Pediatrics, 21st edition. Elsevier; 2019. p. 2521.

15. Which of the following statements regarding iron deficiency anemia is *not true*?

A. Serum iron-binding capacity is low
B. Serum transferrin (TF) saturation is reduced in iron deficiency
C. Pica can lead to ingestion of lead-containing substances and result in plumbism along with iron deficiency anemia
D. Soluble transferrin receptor (sTfR) is a newer modality to diagnose iron deficiency, which is not affected by concomitant infection

EXPLANATION

- In term infants, anemia caused solely by inadequate dietary iron usually occurs at 9–24 months of age and is relatively uncommon after this age.
- As serum iron decreases, the iron-binding capacity of the serum transferrin (TF) increases, and the TF saturation reduces.
- Lead poisoning is also an important cause of microcytic anemia, which is often undiagnosed. Pica is a risk factor for developing plumbism in children.
- *Serum TF receptor:* This soluble receptor is upregulated in iron deficiency, and its level is increased in serum. It is also increased during enhanced erythropoiesis. sTfR is not substantially affected by the acute-phase response.

Key: A

BOOST YOUR KNOWLEDGE

The newborn infant has relatively higher hemoglobin content, which falls during the first 2–3 months of life, and this iron is mostly recycled. These iron stores are usually sufficient for blood formation in the initial 6–9 months in a term infant. Stores are depleted sooner in premature and low-birthweight infants, infants with perinatal blood loss as they have lesser iron stores. The excessive consumption of cow's milk increases iron deficiency due to its lesser iron content, lesser bioavailability of iron, and occult blood loss from milk protein colitis.

REFERENCE/SOURCE

- Rothman JA. Iron-deficiency anemia. In: Kliegman RM, St Geme III JW, Blum NJ, Shah SS, Tasker RC, Wilson KM (Eds). Nelson Textbook of Pediatrics, 21st edition. Elsevier; 2019. pp. 9920-8.

16. All the statements are true for congenital dyserythropoietic anemia (CDA) *except*:

A. Type I CDA has been associated with dysmorphic features
B. Type III CDA is also known as hereditary erythroblastic multinuclearity with a positive acidified serum (HEMPAS) test
C. Type I and type III CDA present with macrocytic anemia
D. Splenectomy is helpful in type II CDA and not in type I

EXPLANATION

Type of CDA	*Features*	*Diagnosis*
Type I CDA	Autosomal recessive, macrocytic anemia, associated with dysmorphic features in 4–14%, hepatosplenomegaly	Electron microscopy is the gold standard for diagnosis, revealing erythroblasts with a characteristic "Swiss cheese" heterochromatin
Type II CDA	Autosomal recessive, most common form, normocytic anemia, and hepatosplenomegaly	Known as HEMPAS test because it shows erythroblast multi-nuclearity and circulating RBCs that are sensitive to lysis by acidified normal serum. Diagnosis is done usually by SDS-PAGE
Type III CDA	Autosomal dominant, rare form, macrocytic anemia, and no splenomegaly	Bone marrow shows giant multinucleated erythroid precursors

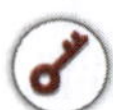

Key: B

BOOST YOUR KNOWLEDGE

- As HEMPAS test is technically difficult, the diagnosis is usually made by analyzing RBC membrane proteins with sodium dodecyl sulfate-polyacrylamide gel electrophoresis (SDS-PAGE). In type II CDA, there is a thinner band size and faster migration of erythrocyte anion transporter (EA1), or band 3, and band 4.5 proteins.
- Splenectomy is not recommended in type I CDA.
- Significant iron overload can occur in type I and type II CDA requiring iron chelation.

REFERENCE/SOURCE

- Thornburg CD. Congenital dyserythropoietic anemias. In: Kliegman RM, St Geme III JW, Blum NJ, Shah SS, Tasker RC, Wilson KM (Eds). Nelson Textbook of Pediatrics, 21st edition. Elsevier; 2019. pp. 2515-6.

17. Which of the following statements regarding HbF is *correct*?

A. At birth, neonate has 90–95% of HbF
B. It reduces to <2% by 4 years of age
C. Transfusion-dependent thalassemia patients have low HbF
D. At 6–8 weeks of gestation, HbF is the predominant hemoglobin

EXPLANATION

At 6–8 weeks, HbF becomes the predominant Hb in fetus. At 6 months of gestation, HbF constitutes 90% of total Hb, and it gradually reduces to 70–80% at birth. It further reduces to <2% by 6–12 months of postnatal life. HbF levels are elevated in hemoglobinopathies like TDT, HPFH, and bone marrow failure syndromes or may be associated with stress erythropoiesis.

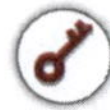

Key: D

BOOST YOUR KNOWLEDGE

Hereditary persistence of fetal hemoglobin is a benign genetic disorder caused by heterozygous deletions or nucleotide substitutions in β-globin locus, causing persistent pancellular HbF expression levels of approximately 30% of total hemoglobin. Individuals with HPFH do not exhibit significant anemia and mostly detected on routine screening.

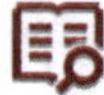

REFERENCE/SOURCE

- Chou ST. Development of the hematopoietic system. In: Kliegman RM, St Geme III JW, Blum NJ, Shah SS, Tasker RC, Wilson KM (Eds). Nelson Textbook of Pediatrics, 21st edition. Elsevier; 2019. pp. 2500-5.

18. A 10-year-old girl presented with pancytopenia. There was no history of fever. On initial investigation, Hb was 6 g%, TLC 2,000/mm^3, platelet count 90,000/mm^3, and MCV 112 fL. The child was on vegan diet and had no hepatosplenomegaly on examination. Which of the following is the first line of investigation?

A. Peripheral smear with reticulocyte count
B. Serum B12 and folate level
C. Flow cytometry
D. Iron studies

EXPLANATION

Pancytopenia with high MCV in a child with vegan diet indicates toward a nutritional cause—most likely megaloblastic anemia due to vitamin B_{12} deficiency, though the concomitant presence of iron deficiency due to inadequate dietary intake cannot be ruled out in such cases. So, it is better to document iron deficiency in such cases. Peripheral smear with reticulocyte count is the first investigation of choice. Peripheral smear findings in a case of megaloblastic anemia show large and oval RBCs with increased MCV. Neutrophils are hypersegmented, with many having >5 lobes. Reticulocyte count will depict the activity of the bone marrow. Serum B12 and folate are required to document the deficiency. Flow cytometry is not recommended as a first-line test unless there is strong suspicion of malignancy, and in that case, bone marrow examination will be done along with flow cytometry and other tests including cytogenetics as second-line investigations.

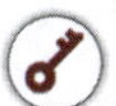

Key: A

BOOST YOUR KNOWLEDGE

In advanced cases of megaloblastic anemia, neutropenia and thrombocytopenia can occur, simulating aplastic anemia or leukemia. Serum concentrations of methylmalonic acid and homocysteine are elevated. Serum lactate dehydrogenase activity is markedly increased due to ineffective erythropoiesis. Serum bilirubin levels may be moderately increased (2–3 mg/dL). Excessive excretion of methylmalonic acid in the urine (normal: 0–3.5 mg/24 hour) is a reliable and sensitive index of vitamin B_{12} deficiency.

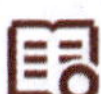

REFERENCE/SOURCE

- Thornburg CD. Megaloblastic anemia. In: Kliegman RM, St Geme III JW, Blum NJ, Shah SS, Tasker RC, Wilson KM (Eds). Nelson Textbook of Pediatrics, 21st edition. Elsevier; 2019.pp- 9910-16.

19. A 4-year-old child presented to pediatric outpatient department with severe pallor and moderate hepatosplenomegaly. Initial investigation showed microcytic anemia with hemoglobin level of 6 g%. Other cell lines were within normal limits. HPLC was suggestive of thalassemia. What of the following cannot be the cause of delayed presentation in this case of thalassemia?

A. Hereditary persistence of fetal hemoglobin
B. Coinheritance of alpha-thalassemia trait
C. Xmn polymorphism
D. Associated iron deficiency anemia

EXPLANATION

Nontransfusion-dependent thalassemia includes patients who are not chronically dependent on transfusion but may need transfusion sporadically. Coinheritance of α-thalassemia trait or polymorphisms of globin promoters such as BCL11 makes the disease less severe and results in NTDT. HbE β-thalassemia is a common cause of both TDT and NTDT. A single β-thalassemia mutation or autosomal dominant β-thalassemia trait has clinical features of NTDT. These patients with NTDT have increased iron load due to ineffective erythropoiesis, and iron deficiency is not seen in NTDT patients.

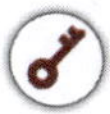

Key: D

BOOST YOUR KNOWLEDGE

Hydroxyurea, a DNA antimetabolite, increases HbF. It is used in children with NTDT. In general, there is a mean increase in Hb of 1 g/dL (0.1–2.5 g/dL). Hydroxyurea therapy in NTDT patients is associated with a reduced risk of leg ulcers, pulmonary hypertension, and extramedullary hematopoiesis. The initial starting dose for thalassemia intermedia is 10 mg/kg and may be escalated to 20 mg/kg/day.

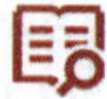

REFERENCE/SOURCE

- Smith-Whitley K, Kwiatkowski JL. Hemoglobinopathies. In: Kliegman RM, St Geme III JW, Blum NJ, Shah SS, Tasker RC, Wilson KM (Eds). Nelson Textbook of Pediatrics, 21st edition. Elsevier; 2019. pp. 2540-58.

CHAPTER 18.2

Nutritional Anemia (Iron, Folic Acid, and B_{12})

Shruti Kakkar

1. Regarding anemia in severe acute malnutrition (SAM), which of the following statements is *false*?

A. Anemia is observed in >75% of hospitalized children with SAM

B. Anemia in a child with SAM is associated with a higher risk of death and prolonged hospitalization

C. Iron supplementation should not be started in the first week of treatment

D. Hemoglobin (Hb) <6 g/dL will require red cell transfusion in a stable child

EXPLANATION

A. Anemia is observed in 73.5–90% of hospitalized children with SAM and 25% of hospitalized children with SAM require blood transfusion.

B. Anemia is associated with higher hazard ratio for death and prolonged hospitalization in children with SAM. Children with SAM have 1.36 times higher chances of recovery in absence of anemia.

C. Iron supplementation can increase the chances of infection, hence, should be done when the infections are controlled, usually after first week of starting therapy.

D. Packed red blood cell (PRBC) transfusion should be done at an Hb level of <4 g% if there is no cardiopulmonary compromise. PRBC transfusion should be done at an Hb level of 4–6 g% if there is cardiopulmonary compromise.

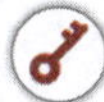

Key: D

BOOST YOUR KNOWLEDGE

- Iron supplementation should be done for 2 months for mild-to-moderate anemia as per World Health Organization (WHO) guidelines.
- For severe anemia, supplement iron for 3–6 months to replenish the store.
- Investigate for other nutritional deficiencies such as B_{12}, folate, and their prompt treatment can help improve prognosis.
- If repeat transfusion needed; should be done after 4 days.

REFERENCES/SOURCES

- Chandra J, Kumar P. Anemia in severe acute malnutrition: ten steps of management need to be fine-tuned. Indian J Pediatr. 2023;90:1061-4.
- World Health Organization. (2009). WHO Child Growth Standards and the Identification of Severe Acute Malnutrition in Infants and Children: Joint Statement by the World Health Organization and the United Nations Children's Fund. [online] Available from https://www.ncbi.nlm.nih.gov/books/NBK200775 [Last accessed June, 2024].

2. Which of the following phenomenon is a physiological adjustment to anemia?

A. Decreased cardiac output
B. Decreased arteriovenous oxygen difference
C. Increased concentration of 2,3-diphosphoglycerate
D. Shift of oxygen dissociation curve to the left

EXPLANATION

Physiologic adjustments to anemia include increased cardiac output, augmented oxygen extraction (increased arteriovenous oxygen difference), and a shunting of blood flow toward vital organs and tissues. In addition, the concentration of 2,3-diphosphoglycerate increases within the red blood cell (RBC). The resultant "shift to the right" of the oxygen dissociation curve reduces the affinity of hemoglobin for oxygen and results in more complete transfer of oxygen to the tissues. The same shift in the oxygen dissociation curve can also occur at high altitude.

Key: C

BOOST YOUR KNOWLEDGE

Higher levels of erythropoietin (EPO) and consequent increased RBC production by the bone marrow further assist the body to adapt.

Oxygen Hb dissociation curve:

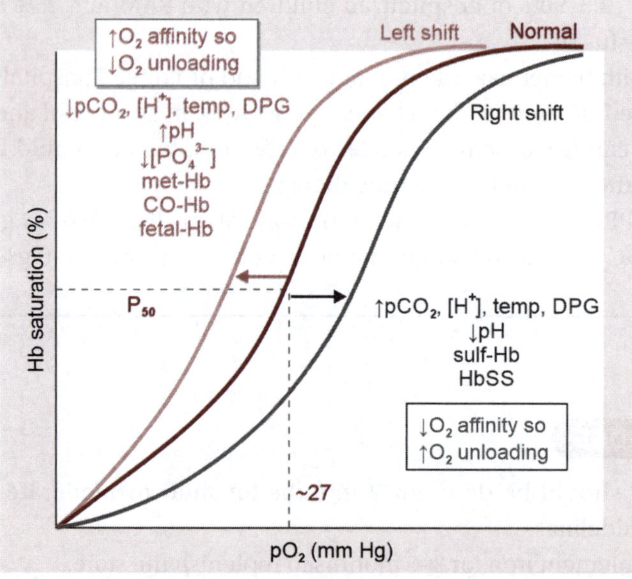

- Hemoglobin A (HbA) has lower affinity for O_2 as compared to hemoglobin F (HbF). Shift of HbF to HbA at birth results in better O_2 delivery to tissues, thus, resulting in reduced erythropoietin secretion.
- Hemoglobin F binds to 2,3 DPG (diphosphoglyceric acid) poorly and increased 2,3 DPG destabilizes spectrin-actin-protein 4.1 complex resulting in higher membrane instability and increased hemolysis in neonates with hereditary spherocytosis/elliptocytosis.
- In disorders of glycolytic pathway, the defective enzyme could be upstream (hexokinase deficiency) or downstream (pyruvate kinase deficiency) of 2,3 DPG. Levels of 2,3 DPG increase 2,3 folds in patients with pyruvate kinase deficiency leading to right shift of oxyhemoglobin (oxy Hb) dissociation curve and decrease in hexokinase deficiency shifts the curve to left.
- Hence, at same Hb levels patients with pyruvate kinase (PK) deficiency have greater exercise tolerance than one with hexokinase deficiency.

REFERENCES/SOURCES

- Kliegman RM, St Geme III JW. Nelson Textbook of Pediatrics, 21st edition. Amsterdam: Elsevier; 2019. Chapter 485. p. 2531.
- Orkin SH, Nathan DG, Ginsburg D, Look AT, Fisher DE, Lux S. Nathan and Oski's Hematology and Oncology of Infancy and Childhood, 8th edition. Philadelphia: Elsevier; 2014. Chapter 19, p. 648.
- Orkin SH, Nathan DG, Ginsburg D, Look AT, Fisher DE, Lux S. Nathan and Oski's Hematology and Oncology of Infancy and Childhood, 8th edition. Philadelphia: Elsevier; 2014. Chapter 2. p. 52.
- Orkin SH, Nathan DG, Ginsburg D, Look AT, Fisher DE, Lux S. Nathan and Oski's Hematology and Oncology of Infancy and Childhood, 8th edition. Philadelphia: Elsevier; 2014. Chapter 9, p. 293.

3. Which of the following can result in macrocytic anemia with high reticulocyte count?

A. Dyserythropoietic anemia type II
B. Active hemolysis
C. Pearson syndrome
D. Thiamine responsive anemia

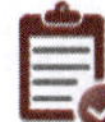

EXPLANATION

- Macrocytic anemia with low or normal reticulocyte counts includes congenital (Diamond-Blackfan and Fanconi syndromes) and acquired aplastic anemia and hypothyroidism.
- Patients with trisomy 21 have macrocytic cells, although an accompanying anemia is generally not present.
- High mean corpuscular volume (MCV) and reticulocytosis is seen in congenital dyserythropoietic anemia I and III and in active hemolysis results in reticulocytosis so that the mean MCV is abnormally high.
- Dyserythropoietic anemia type II—normocytic anemia with low reticulocyte count
- Active hemolysis—macrocytic anemia with high reticulocyte count
- Pearson syndrome and thiamine responsive anemia—macrocytic anemia with low reticulocyte count

Key: B

BOOST YOUR KNOWLEDGE

Pearson syndrome:
- Mitochondrial deoxyribonucleic acid deletion disorder
- Anemia, metabolic acidosis, and exocrine pancreatic insufficiency
- May present with nonimmune hydrops.
- Neutropenia and thrombocytopenia may occur.

Aase syndrome:
- Rare congenital hypoplastic anemia
- Abnormally digitalized thumbs ± growth failure ± bony abnormalities

Thiamine-responsive megaloblastic anemia:
- Autosomal recessive disorder
- Mutations in the *SLC19A2* gene encoding a thiamine transporter protein
- Megaloblastic anemia + diabetes mellitus + sensorineural hearing loss
- Responds to thiamine.

Congenital dyserythropoietic anemia:
- Inherited disorder of late erythropoiesis characterized by anemia, ineffective erythropoiesis, and secondary hemochromatosis.
- Three subtypes—based bone marrow morphology, clinical features, and genetic defects. Variants with GATA1 and KLF1 mutation described.

Comparison of the three major types of congenital dyserythropoietic anemia:

	CDA 1	CDA 2 or HEMPAS[#] (Hereditary erythroblastic multinuclearity with a positive acidified serum test)	CDA 3
Inheritance	AR	AR	AD
Defective gene	*CDAN 1*	*SEC23B*	*KIF23*
Gene product	Codanin 1	Cytoplasmic coat protein II	Mitotic kinesin-like protein
Age at presentation	Childhood/adolescence	Later in life	variable
Anemia	• Megaloblastic anemia • Reticulocyte count inadequate for the degree of anemia	• Normocytic anemia • Low reticulocyte count	Mild-to-moderate macrocytic anemia
EMH	+	+	–
Iron overload	+	+	–
Other features	Dysmorphism syndactyly, absence of toes, supernumerary toes	Patient's RBCs lyse in acidified serum due to an immunoglobulin M (IgM) antibody that recognizes an antigen present on RBCs	• Angioid streaks, macular degeneration • Intravascular hemolysis
Transfusion dependance	+	10% during childhood	–
BM	Incompletely divided cells with thin chromatin bridges between nuclei of pairs of erythrocytes	Binucleate late polychromatophils	Giant multinucleated erythroid precursors (up to 12 nuclei/cell)
Electron microscopy	Erythroblasts with "Swiss cheese" heterochromatin pattern.	Vesicles laden with endoplasmic reticulum proteins running beneath the plasma membrane	Clefts in heterochromatin, iron-laden macrophages, myelin figures in RBCs, autophagic vacuoles
Treatment	Human leukocyte antigen (HLA)-matched transplant Interferon may reduce transfusion requirement	HLA-matched transplant	Supportive, transplant may not be required
Splenectomy	Not recommended	May be beneficial	Not required

[#]Diagnosis is usually made by analyzing RBC membrane proteins with sodium dodecyl sulfate–polyacrylamide gel electrophoresis (SDS-PAGE).
In CDA II, there is a thinner band size and faster migration of erythrocyte anion transporter (EA1), or band 3, and band 4.5 proteins.

REFERENCES/SOURCES

- Kliegman RM, St Geme III JW. Nelson Textbook of Pediatrics, 21st edition. Amsterdam: Elsevier; 2019. Chapter 474. p. 2507.
- Kliegman RM, St Geme III JW. Nelson Textbook of Pediatrics, 21st edition. Amsterdam: Elsevier; 2019. Chapter 479. pp. 2515-6.
- Orkin SH, Nathan DG, Ginsburg D, Look AT, Fisher DE, Lux S. Nathan and Oski's Hematology and Oncology of Infancy and Childhood, 8th edition. Philadelphia: Elsevier; 2014. Chapter 7. p. 184.

4. Which of the following parameters is increased in iron deficiency anemia?

A. RBC count
B. Reticulocyte Hb concentration
C. Serum ferritin
D. Soluble transferrin receptor

EXPLANATION

Indices \ Clinical entity	IDA (iron deficiency anemia)	Thalassemia trait
RBC Count	↓ decrease	↑ increase
RDW (red cell distribution width)	↑ increase	Normal
Serum ferritin	↓ decrease	Normal
TIBC (total iron-binding capacity)	↑ increase	Normal
Free erythrocyte protoporphyrin	↑ increase	Normal
Soluble transferrin receptor	↑ increase	Normal
Reticulocyte Hb concentration	↓ decrease	Normal

Soluble transferrin receptor:

- Truncated form of the transferrin receptor that is cleaved from reticulocytes and erythroid cells.
- Circulates in plasma largely bound to transferrin
- Upregulated in IDA and enhanced erythropoiesis (hemolytic anemia or conditions that increase red cell mass)
- Not affected by the acute-phase response

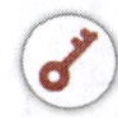

Key: D

BOOST YOUR KNOWLEDGE

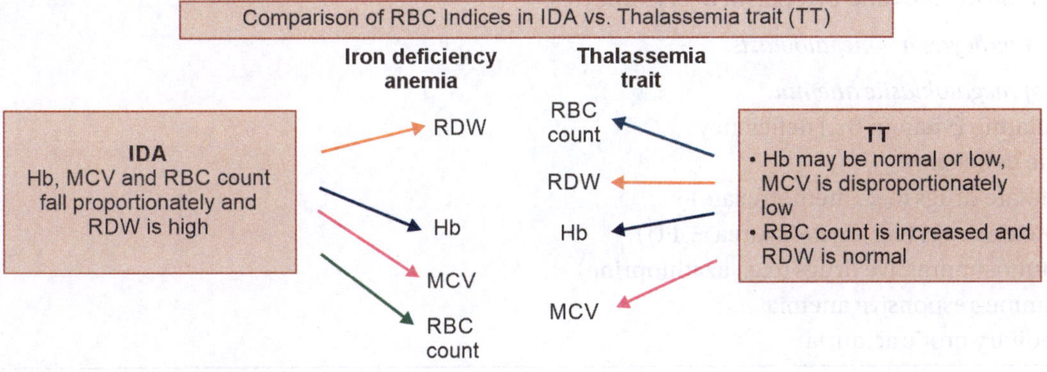

Free erythrocyte protoporphyrin:

- An accumulation of free erythrocyte porphyrin (FEP) occurs in the red cell precursors as iron deficiency limits the final step in heme synthesis.
- FEP is elevated in iron deficiency (FEP is >80 μg/dL for children >5 years of age and >70 μg/dL for children <5 years of age)
- Rapidly falls in response to treatment.
- Spuriously high levels of FEP can be seen in hyperbilirubinemia, thalassemia trait, and hemoglobin E disease

Zinc protoporphyrin:

- Can be measured directly on a drop of blood with a portable hematofluorometer.
- Useful screening test in field surveys, particularly in children
- Lead poisoning can increase zinc protoporphyrin (ZPP) values.

Reticulocyte hemoglobin:
- Falls within days of onset of iron-deficient erythropoiesis.
- Unaffected by inflammation
- Can recognize iron deficiency as well as IDA.
- False-normal values can be observed when MCV is increased and in thalassemia.

REFERENCES/SOURCES

- Chandra J, Dewan P, Kumar P, Mahajan A, Singh P, Dhingra B, et al. Diagnosis, Treatment and Prevention of Nutritional Anemia in Children: Recommendations of the Joint Committee of Pediatric Hematology-Oncology Chapter and Pediatric and Adolescent Nutrition Society of the Indian Academy of Pediatrics. Indian Pediatr. 2022;59(10):782-801.
- Kliegman RM, St Geme III JW. Nelson Textbook of Pediatrics, 21st edition. Amsterdam: Elsevier; 2019. Chapter 482. p. 2523.
- Orkin SH, Nathan DG, Ginsburg D, Look AT, Fisher DE, Lux S. Nathan and Oski's Hematology and Oncology of Infancy and Childhood, 8th edition. Philadelphia: Elsevier; 2014. Chapter 11. p. 362.

5. Which among the following causes megaloblastic anemia?

A. Hypothyroidism
B. Hereditary orotic aciduria
C. Blackfan-Diamond anemia
D. Methylenetetrahydrofolate reductase (MTHFR) deficiency

EXPLANATION

Megaloblastic anemia describes a group of disorders that are caused by impaired deoxyribonucleic acid (DNA) synthesis. RBCs are larger than normal at every developmental stage, and there is maturational asynchrony between the nucleus and cytoplasm of erythrocytes.

Not all macrocytes are megaloblasts.

Causes of megaloblastic anemia
- Cobalamin (vitamin B_{12}) deficiency
- Folate deficiency
- Antifolate drugs (e.g., methotrexate)
- Cytotoxic drugs (e.g., hydroxyurea, 5-FU)
- Immunosuppressive drugs (e.g., azathioprine)
- Thiamine-responsive anemia
- Hereditary orotic aciduria

Key: B

BOOST YOUR KNOWLEDGE

Hereditary orotic aciduria is a cause of megaloblastic anemia. Others are causes of macrocytic anemia but not megaloblastic anemia.

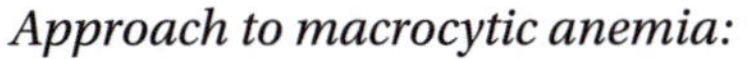

Approach to macrocytic anemia:

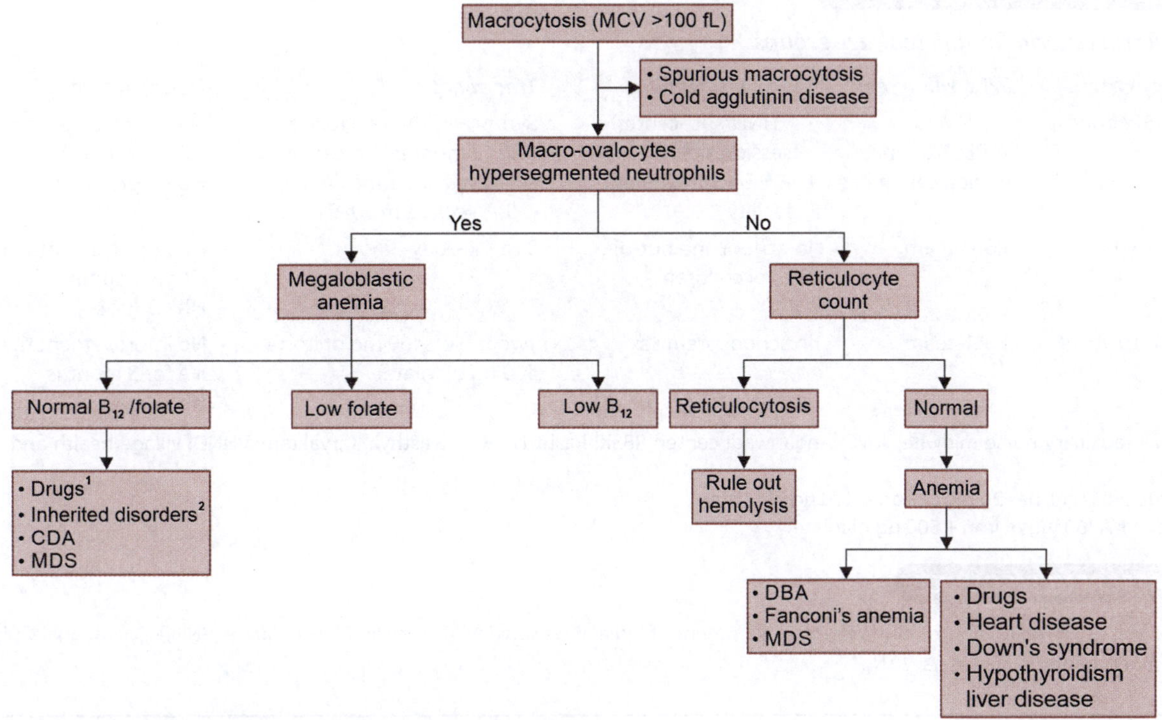

[1]*Drugs:* 6MP, Hydroxyurea, anticonvulsants, sulfa drugs, etc.
[2]*Inherited disorders:* Deficiency of IF, TC II, etc.
(CDA: congential dyserythropoietic anemia; MDS: myelodysplastic syndrome)

Although methylenetetrahydrofolate reductase (MTHFR) deficiency is the most common inborn error of folate metabolism, and severe cases can produce several neurologic and vascular complications, there is no associated megaloblastic anemia.

Hereditary orotic aciduria

- Inborn error of pyrimidine synthesis that leads to an excessive excretion of orotic acid in urine.
- Failure to thrive and intellectual disability.
- Anemia is refractory to vitamin B_{12} or folic acid but responds promptly to administration of uridine.

REFERENCES/SOURCES

- Kliegman RM, St Geme III JW. Nelson Textbook of Pediatrics, 21st edition. Amsterdam: Elsevier; 2019. Chapter 481. p. 2521.
- Orkin SH, Nathan DG, Ginsburg D, Look AT, Fisher DE, Lux S. Nathan and Oski's Hematology and Oncology of Infancy and Childhood, 8th edition. Philadelphia: Elsevier; 2014. Chapter 10. p. 341.
- Sobti PC. Pediatric Hematology Manual, PHO Chapter of IAP. Chandigarh, 2000.

6. Which among the following is an indication for referral in children of 5–9 years according to Anemia Mukt Bharat Guidelines?

A. Hb <10 g/dL
B. Hb <8 g/dL
C. Hb <7 g/dL
D. Hb <5 g/dL

EXPLANATION

Management of Hb <8 g/dL in children of 5–9 years is to be done by the medical officer at the first referral unit/district hospital based on investigations.

Key: B

BOOST YOUR KNOWLEDGE

Referral criteria for different age groups:

Age criteria	Who will screen	Place of screening	Treatment	Criteria for referral
6–59 months	• ANM • RBSK team medical officer	• VHND/sub-center/ session site • AWC/school health facility	Syrup IFA (iron and folic acid) • *6–12 months:* 1 mL daily • *1–3 years:* 1.5 mL daily • *3–5 years:* 2 mL daily	• No improvement to daily IFA for 2 months • Hb <7 g/dL
5–9 years	RBSK team	In-school and out-of-school children	3 mg/kg/day	• No improvement to daily IFA for 3 months • Hb <8 g/dL
10–19 years	RBSK team	In school premises	Two tablets (60 mg of iron + 500 µg of folate)	• No improvement to daily IFA for 3 months • Hb <8 g/dL

(ANM: auxiliary nurse midwife; AWC: Anganwadi center; RBSK: Rashtriya Bal Swasthya Karyakram; VHND: village health and nutrition day)
Syrup IFA (1 mL has 20 mg of iron + 100 µg of folate)
Tablet IFA (60 mg of iron + 500 µg of folate)

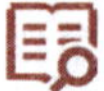

REFERENCE/SOURCE

- Ministry of Health and Family Welfare, Government of India. Intensified National Iron Plus Initiative (I-NIPI) Operational Guidelines for Programme Managers, 2018.

7. According to National Programme for Prevention and Control of Fluorosis (NPPCF), which of the following is *correct*?

A. High fluoride leads to destruction of gastrointestinal mucosa
B. Broad message of "*Kharaab Paani, Kamzor Paani*" signifies health and nutritional improvements through water
C. Dietary corrections include avoiding calcium magnesium and vitamin C
D. IFA supplementation is indicated through fluorosis control activities

EXPLANATION

A. High fluoride leads to destruction of gastrointestinal mucosa, thus reducing nutrient absorption including iron and folic acid.
B. One of the three key interventions include communicating a broad message of *"Accha Paani, Takatvar Paani"* signifies health and nutritional improvements through water.
C. Dietary corrections include *providing* calcium, magnesium vitamin C.
D. Iron and folic acid supplementation is not indicated through fluorosis control activities.

Key: A

BOOST YOUR KNOWLEDGE

Dental fluorosis:

- First indication of fluorosis—yellowish, brown, or black discoloration of the teeth (on the enamel surface away from the gums)
- Observed as spots or streaks, which are always horizontal in orientation.
- Commonly affected teeth are—central and lateral incisors, molars of permanent dentition.
- It affects permanent teeth because of hypomineralization of the enamel due to fluoride exposure during enamel mineralization.

Skeletal fluorosis:
- Neck, vertebral column, pelvic girdle, knee, and shoulder joints are affected maximally.
- Endemic, crippling skeletal fluorosis continuous exposure to very high levels of fluoride in drinking water for years.
- Malnutrition and/or renal dysfunction may aggravate skeletal fluorosis.

Phase	*Clinical manifestation*	*Radiological manifestation*
Preclinical phase	Asymptomatic	Increase bone mass
Phase I • Musculoskeletal fluorosis	Sporadic pain and stiffness of joints	Osteosclerosis of pelvis and spine
Phase II • Degenerative and destructive fluorosis	Chronic join pain and arthritic symptoms	• Calcification of ligaments • Osteoporosis of long bones
Phase III • Crippling fluorosis	• Muscle wasting • Neurological deficits • Crippling deformities of various joints	• Deformities joint/spinal cord • Spinal cord compression

REFERENCES/SOURCES

- Ministry of Health and Family Welfare, Government of India. Intensified National Iron Plus Initiative (I-NIPI) Operational Guidelines for Programme Managers. 2018. pp. 24-5.
- National Centre for Disease Control, Directorate General of Health Services, Government of India. Fluorosis CD Alert. 2022.

8. Which of the following is an *incorrect* specification for digital hemoglobinometers?

A. Should have a good diagnostic accuracy (at least 90% sensitivity)
B. Works on the principle of reflectance photometry
C. Testing time should be <1 minute
D. Range of measurement is from 4 g/dL to 16 g/dL

EXPLANATION

- Range of measurement is from 2 g/dL to 23 g/dL
- A screening test should be cheap, easy to perform, and results are available immediately.

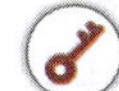

Key: D

BOOST YOUR KNOWLEDGE

Cyanmethemoglobin is the gold standard for estimation of Hb.

REFERENCE/SOURCE

- Ministry of Health and Family Welfare, Government of India. Intensified National Iron Plus Initiative (I-NIPI) Operational Guidelines for Programme Managers, 2018. p. 60

9. A 14-year-old boy with inflammatory bowel disease develops repeated episodes of diarrhea and takes zinc gluconate on a chronic basis. Parents have notices worsening fatigue, weakness, gait instability, and progressive weight loss. On examination, child has severe pallor and both weight and height are below 3rd centile. Complete blood count (CBC) shows Hb 5.1 g/dL with MCV 48 fL, TLC 3,300/mm^3 and platelet 3,92,000 with PBF showing ringed sideroblasts. Which of the following is responsible for child's anemia?

A. X-linked sideroblastic anemia
B. Cobalamin deficiency
C. Copper deficiency
D. Iron deficiency anemia

EXPLANATION

- Zinc and copper are competitively absorbed from the gastrointestinal (GI) tract, so zinc excess may inadvertently lead to copper deficiency.
- In copper deficiency, leukopenia (neutropenia) is common, however, thrombocytopenia is unusual. Bone marrow aspirates are hypocellular with relative erythroid hyperplasia and prominent vacuolization of erythroid precursors. Variable degrees of dyserythropoiesis/megaloblastoid changes with or without the presence of ringed sideroblasts can be seen.

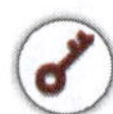

Key: C

BOOST YOUR KNOWLEDGE

- Copper deficiency is a rare cause of microcytic anemia and neurologic dysfunction.
- Copper is absorbed in the stomach and proximal duodenum.
- Deficiency is associated with malabsorption; severe malnutrition, often with feeding of milk alone; gastric surgery or feedings that bypass the stomach and duodenum; or parenteral nutrition with inadvertent omission of supplemental copper. Diagnosis is made by measuring a serum copper level and possibly a zinc level.
- Treatment includes either oral or parenteral supplementation, depending on the underlying cause.

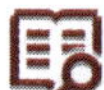

REFERENCES/SOURCES

- Kliegman RM, St Geme III JW. Nelson Textbook of Pediatrics, 21st edition. Amsterdam: Elsevier; 2019. Chapter 474. pp. 2526-7.
- Orkin SH, Nathan DG, Ginsburg D, Look AT, Fisher DE, Lux S. Nathan and Oski's Hematology and Oncology of Infancy and Childhood, 8th edition. Philadelphia: Elsevier; 2014. Chapter 11. p. 375.

10. Elevated HbA2 levels can be seen in which of the following condition?

A. Anti-retroviral therapy
B. δ-thalassemia
C. HPFH carriers
D. Capsite +1 (A > C) mutation

EXPLANATION

Borderline HbA_2 with near normal or reduced red cell indices in β-thalassemia heterozygotes is most often due to the Capsite +1 (A > C) mutation and the poly A (T > C) mutation.

Human immunodeficiency virus (HIV) positive patients on antiretroviral therapy (zidovudine and stavudine) and megaloblastic anemia (B_{12} and folate deficiency) may show elevated HbA_2 levels.

Delta-beta (δβ) thalassemia and hereditary persistence of fetal hemoglobin (HPFH) carriers have normal HbA2 (<3.5%) and high HbF (10–25%) with variable RBC indices.

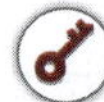

Key: A

BOOST YOUR KNOWLEDGE

Associated iron deficiency in a β-thalassemia carrier may reduce the level of HbA_2, however, it is not significant to bring it down to normal levels.

Algorithm for approach to thalassemia carrier/IDA:

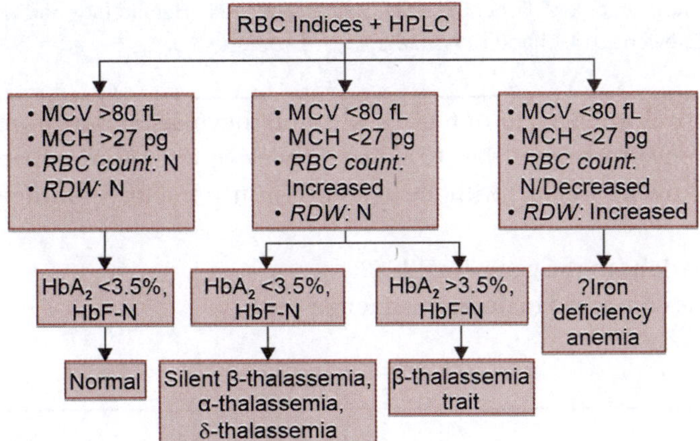

REFERENCES/SOURCES

- Colah R, Italia K, Gorakshakar A. Burden of thalassemia in India: The road map for control. Pediatr Hematol Oncol J. 2017;2(4):79-84.
- Kliegman RM, St Geme III JW. Nelson Textbook of Pediatrics, 21st edition. Amsterdam: Elsevier; 2019. Chapter 473. pp. 2505-6.

11. Which of the following is correct regarding oral iron therapy?

A. Ferrous form of iron has lower bioavailability compared with ferric form
B. Sulphate form has higher percentage of elemental iron than fumarate form
C. Enteric-coated tablets have better bioavailability
D. Addition of vitamin C in pharmaceutical form is not recommended

EXPLANATION

A. Iron is transported into the intestinal cell by DMT (di-metallic transporter). Ferric forms must be converted to ferrous form in the intestine; hence, ferrous forms are better absorbed.
B. The elemental iron content of common ferrous iron preparations viz., ferrous sulphate (FS), ferrous fumarate, and ferrous gluconate is 20% (anhydrous 30%), 33%, and 12% elemental iron, respectively.
C. Enteric-coated and delayed-release iron supplements release iron below the site of absorption, hence, iron is not absorbed as well as the standard preparations.
D. Randomized clinical trial in adults has shown no benefit of adding vitamin C to iron therapy. Hence, vitamin C is not recommended in pharmaceutical forms.

Key: D

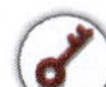

BOOST YOUR KNOWLEDGE

- Addition of citrus fruits to the diet just prior to medication enhances iron absorption.
- Consumption of tea, whole grains, cereals, soy, nuts, legumes, and phosphates should be restricted to increase iron absorption.
- Combined deficiency of B_{12} and iron is seen in 30% children of nutritional anemia.

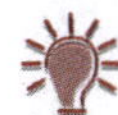

REFERENCES/SOURCES

- Chandra J, Dewan P, Kumar P, Mahajan A, Singh P, Dhingra B, et al. Diagnosis, Treatment and Prevention of Nutritional Anemia in Children: Recommendations of the Joint Committee of Pediatric Hematology-Oncology Chapter and Pediatric and Adolescent Nutrition Society of the Indian Academy of Pediatrics. Indian Pediatr. 2022;59(10):782-801.

- Kliegman RM, St Geme III JW. Nelson Textbook of Pediatrics, 21st edition. Amsterdam: Elsevier; 2019. Chapter 482. pp. 2522-5.
- Orkin SH, Nathan DG, Ginsburg D, Look AT, Fisher DE, Lux S. Nathan and Oski's Hematology and Oncology of Infancy and Childhood, 8th edition. Philadelphia: Elsevier; 2014. Chapter 11. p. 362.

12. A 2-year-old boy was found to have Hb of 6 g/dL with microcytosis, hypochromia, and raised RDW. He was started on oral iron therapy at 3 mg/kg/day. Child was reviewed after a month and repeat Hb was found to be 6.2 g/dL. Which of the following concurs with the diagnosis iron-refractory iron-deficiency anemia?

A. Very low ferritin
B. Loss-of-function mutations in the gene *TMPRSS2*
C. Decreased hepcidin as compared to degree of anemia
D. Transferrin saturation <5%

EXPLANATION

Iron refractory iron deficiency anemia (IRIDA) is a rare, autosomal recessive disorder characterized by defects in absorption and utilization of iron. Characterized by iron deficiency anemia refractory to oral iron therapy and partially responsive to parenteral iron administration.

Iron refractory iron deficiency anemia is characterized by:

- Anemia with variable degree of microcytic hypochromic indices
- Low-normal to normal serum ferritin
- Very low serum iron and transferrin saturation (TSAT)
- Inappropriately high serum hepcidin levels compared to degree of anemia
- Oral iron refractoriness as per standard criteria for evaluation of response to oral iron
- Presence of homozygous or compound heterozygous mutations in *TMPRSS6* gene

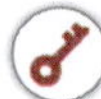

Key: D

BOOST YOUR KNOWLEDGE

Iron refractoriness: Defined as <1 g/dL Hb increase after 4 weeks of oral iron therapy, provided patient compliance is adequate and acquired forms of GI disorders have been ruled out.

Hepcidin:

- Master regulator of iron homeostasis
- Secreted by liver cells
- Acts on ferroportin channels at basal enterocytes in duodenum and on macrophages
- Blocks iron absorption into circulation and release from macrophages
- Causes of increased hepcidin—inflammatory cytokines and increased iron stores
- Causes of decreased hepcidin—iron deficiency, increased bone marrow erythropoietic states and hypoxia

REFERENCES/SOURCES

- Bhatia P, Jain R, Singh A. A structured approach to iron refractory iron deficiency anemia (IRIDA) diagnosis (SAID): the more is "SAID" about iron, the less it is. Pediatr Hematol Oncol J. 2017;2(2):48-53.
- Kliegman RM, St Geme III JW. Nelson Textbook of Pediatrics, 21st edition. Amsterdam: Elsevier; 2019. Chapter 474. p. 2525.

13. Which of the following is correct for anemia of prematurity?

A. Deficiency of vitamin E plays a role
B. Early transfusion increases risk of NEC and late transfusion is associated with IVH
C. Cord milking and delayed cord clamping do not reduce transfusions in anemia of prematurity
D. EPO synthesis is reduced as liver is the source in premature infants

EXPLANATION

In physiologic anemia of prematurity Hb drops to 7–9 g/dL at 3–6 weeks of age.

- Heightened anemia in prematurity is seen due to exaggeration of factors causing physiological anemia of infancy, increased phlebotomy losses, shortened RBC lifespan (40–60 days), low reserves of iron, and rapid growth.
- Vitamin E does not play a role in pathogenesis
- Early transfusion increases the risk of IVH
- Late transfusion increases the risk of NEC

Cord milking and delayed cord clamping reduce the need for transfusions. Delayed cord clamping (DCC) leads to 30% increase in neonatal blood volume.

- Erythropoietin (EPO) is synthesized in liver in utero and kidney becomes the main source after birth. The liver oxygen sensors are less sensitive than those in kidneys hence resulting in a lower EPO response to anemia.

Key: D

BOOST YOUR KNOWLEDGE

- Physiological nadir of anemia is exaggerated after fetal or neonatal transfusion.
- The degree of anemia depends upon the degree of prematurity, nutritional status and intake, chronologic age, and the type and severity of the underlying illness.
- *Treatment/prevention:* Iron supplementation at 1–2 mg/kg/day from 4 weeks to age of 1 year.

REFERENCES/SOURCES

- Kliegman RM, St Geme III JW. Nelson Textbook of Pediatrics, 21st edition. Amsterdam: Elsevier; 2019. Chapter 480. pp. 2516-17.
- Orkin SH, Nathan DG, Ginsburg D, Look AT, Fisher DE, Lux S. Nathan and Oski's Hematology and Oncology of Infancy and Childhood, 8th edition. Philadelphia: Elsevier; 2014. Chapter 2. p. 69.

14. **A 5-year-old boy presented with history of acute paleness for last 3 days. Also, his mother gives a history of cough, running nose, and watery eyes 7–10 days back. On examination, mild icterus is noted, there a palpable splenomegaly. Laboratory investigations reveal the following results:**

- *Hb:* 5.4 g/dL
- *MCV:* 152
- *Reticulocyte%:* 36%
- *LDH:* 3,508 IU/L

What is the possible diagnosis for the patient?

A. AIHA
B. CDA
C. B_{12} deficiency
D. Hypernatremia

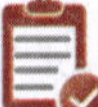

EXPLANATION

- All four options can cause macrocytosis. However, hypernatremia will not cause anemia, high lactate dehydrogenase (LDH), or high reticulocyte count.
- B_{12} deficiency can result in anemia, high LDH due to ineffective erythropoiesis however reticulocyte count is low.
- A MCV >150 fL is usually not seen in megaloblastic anemia and is indicative of a spuriously high MCV due to RBC agglutination secondary to cold agglutinin disease or rouleaux formation due to paraproteins.
- Congenital dyserythropoietic anemia does not have high LDH, reticulocytosis is seen in type I, III, and reticulocytopenia in type II.
- Autoimmune anemia can present with low Hb, high reticulocyte (marrow response), high LDH (increased red cell turnover), and high MCV as well.

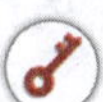

Key: A

BOOST YOUR KNOWLEDGE

Serologic findings in autoimmune hemolytic anemia:

Characteristic	***Warm reactive***	***Paroxysmal cold hemoglobinuria***	***Cold agglutinin disease***
Immunoglobulin	IgG	IgG	IgM
Thermal reactivity	37°C	4°C	4°C
Fixes complement	±	Yes	Yes
DAT 4°C 37°C	 Not performed IgG ± C_3	 IgG C_3	 C_3 C_3
Plasma titer	Low/absent	Moderate	High
Hemolysin	No	Yes	Variable
Antigenic specificity	Rh and others	P	I/i
Site of RBC destruction	Spleen	Intravascular	Intravascular

(DAT: direct antiglobulin test; IgG: immunoglobulin G; IgM: immunoglobulin M; RBC: red blood cell)

REFERENCES/SOURCES

- Kliegman RM, St Geme III JW. Nelson Textbook of Pediatrics, 21st edition. Amsterdam: Elsevier; 2019. Chapter 474. p. 2505.
- Kliegman RM, St Geme III JW. Nelson Textbook of Pediatrics, 21st edition. Amsterdam: Elsevier; 2019. Chapter 481.1. p. 2521.
- Orkin SH, Nathan DG, Ginsburg D, Look AT, Fisher DE, Lux S. Nathan and Oski's Hematology and Oncology of Infancy and Childhood, 8th edition. Philadelphia: Elsevier; 2014. Chapter 13. p. 416.

15. Which of the following is true regarding adverse effects of vitamin B_{12} administration?

A. Cyanocobalamin is more allergenic than hydroxocobalamin
B. Pre-medication with hydrocortisone is recommended before injecting B_{12}
C. Transient worsening of neurological symptoms may occur
D. Risk of hyperkalemia present especially in malnourished children

EXPLANATION

A. Injectable cobalamin is more allergenic than oral forms. Hydroxocobalamin is more allergenic than cyanocobalamin.
B. B_{12} is given intravenously over 45–60 minutes. IV administration results in rapid excretion of B_{12}. May be administered in patients with thrombocytopenia.
C. Hydrocortisone premedication should be given before injecting B_{12} only in those with previous history of sensitivity.
D. Monitor potassium levels in malnourished children with severe megaloblastic anemia in initial few days, because of risk of hypokalemia.

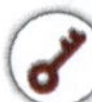

Key: B

BOOST YOUR KNOWLEDGE

- Parenteral vitamin B_{12} is preferably administered by intramuscular (IM) or deep subcutaneous (SC) injection as vitamin B_{12} is rapidly excreted after IV administration. Sublingual and intranasal routes of vitamin B_{12} administration have also been tried in children with vitamin B_{12} deficiency.

- Cyanocobalamin is contraindicated in optic nerve atrophy/Leber's hereditary neuropathy.
- Hydroxocobalamin is long acting and preferred in children requiring long-term supplementation, e.g., pernicious anemia.

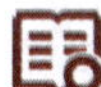

REFERENCES/SOURCES

- Chandra J, Dewan P, Kumar P, Mahajan A, Singh P, Dhingra B, et al. Diagnosis, Treatment and Prevention of Nutritional Anemia in Children: Recommendations of the Joint Committee of Pediatric Hematology-Oncology Chapter and Pediatric and Adolescent Nutrition Society of the Indian Academy of Pediatrics. Indian Pediatr. 2022;59(10):782-801.
- Kliegman RM, St Geme III JW. Nelson Textbook of Pediatrics, 21st edition. Amsterdam: Elsevier; 2019. Chapter 481.2. p. 2521.

16. Which of the following statements regarding folate replacement is false?

A. Supplement both B_{12} and folate if levels are not available

B. B_{12} supplementation alone may precipitate neurological symptoms if folate deficiency is also present

C. Folate doses >0.8 mg/day cause maximum reduction in homocysteine levels

D. In infants a dose of 50 µg/day suffices

EXPLANATION

A. Neurological manifestations of B_{12} deficiency may get precipitated if folic acid is supplemented alone.

B. Anemia due to dietary folic acid deficiency in children >1 year of age and adults should be treated using oral folic acid 1–5 mg daily.

C. Doses of 0.2 and 0.4 mg folate are associated with 60% and 90%, respectively, of the maximal effect (seen with 0.8 mg)

D. Vitamin B_{12} should be continued alongside in folate deficiency doses of at least 1–2 µg/day to prevent neurological deterioration.

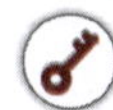

Key: B

BOOST YOUR KNOWLEDGE

- The British Society for Hematology Guidelines recommends 5 mg of FA to be given for 4 months to treat megaloblastic anemia due to dietary folic acid deficiency in adults. The duration of folic acid therapy is for 3–4 months to replenish the depleted stores. Vitamin B_{12} should be continued even if the levels are normal at a dose of 1–2 µg/day.
- Folinic acid is used for specific disorders of metabolism or chemotherapy toxicity.
- Cerebral folate deficiency has been linked with autism.

REFERENCES/SOURCES

- Chandra J, Dewan P, Kumar P, Mahajan A, Singh P, Dhingra B, et al. Diagnosis, Treatment and Prevention of Nutritional Anemia in Children: Recommendations of the Joint Committee of Pediatric Hematology-Oncology Chapter and Pediatric and Adolescent Nutrition Society of the Indian Academy of Pediatrics. Indian Pediatr. 2022;59(10):782-801.
- Devalia V, Hamilton MS, Molloy AM; British Committee for Standards in Haematology. Guidelines for the diagnosis and treatment of cobalamin and folate disorders. Br J Haematol. 2014;166(4):496-513.
- Kliegman RM, St Geme III JW. Nelson Textbook of Pediatrics, 21st edition. Amsterdam: Elsevier; 2019. Chapter 481.1. pp. 2518-9.

17. Which of the following is *correct* regarding red cell folate levels?

A. They reveal folate status over past 12 weeks

B. They are affected by transient fluctuations in folate consumption

C. They remain unaltered after reticulocyte stage

D. They can be falsely low in IDA

EXPLANATION

A. Red cell folate levels give information about folate status over 120 days (nearly 17 weeks).
B. Serum folate is affected by transient fluctuations in folate absorption much more than RBC folate.
C. Red cell folate levels are unaltered after reticulocyte stage.
D. It is falsely low in pernicious anemia.

Key: C

BOOST YOUR KNOWLEDGE

- False high levels occur in hemolysis (reticulocytes have higher folate content), IDA (which elevates RBC folate), and blood transfusion.
- False low levels occur in pernicious anemia.
- Red cell folate levels <100 ng/mL are suggestive of deficiency and have the advantage of depicting status of the last 120 days.
- These are recommended if there is a strong suspicion of folate deficiency, but serum folate levels reveal normal results.

REFERENCES/SOURCES

- Chandra J, Dewan P, Kumar P, Mahajan A, Singh P, Dhingra B, et al. Diagnosis, Treatment and Prevention of Nutritional Anemia in Children: Recommendations of the Joint Committee of Pediatric Hematology-Oncology Chapter and Pediatric and Adolescent Nutrition Society of the Indian Academy of Pediatrics. Indian Pediatr. 2022;59(10):782-801.
- Kliegman RM, St Geme III JW. Nelson Textbook of Pediatrics, 21st edition. Amsterdam: Elsevier; 2019. Chapter 481.1. p. 2518.
- Orkin SH, Nathan DG, Ginsburg D, Look AT, Fisher DE, Lux S. Nathan and Oski's Hematology and Oncology of Infancy and Childhood, 8th edition. Philadelphia: Elsevier; 2014. Chapter 10.

18. Which of the following statements is *false* regarding folate metabolism?

A. Increased folate losses occur in hyperthyroidism and in patients undergoing dialysis
B. Placenta has receptors for selective transport of folate to fetus
C. Folate-free diet can cause megaloblastic anemia in 2–3 weeks
D. Anticonvulsants can lead to frank megaloblastic anemia in rare cases

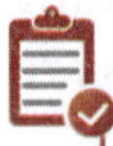

EXPLANATION

Increased folate losses occur in hyperthyroidism and in patients undergoing dialysis. Placenta has receptors for selective transport of folate to fetus, thus babies of mother's deficient in folate do not present with megaloblastic anemia at birth. Folate-free diet can cause megaloblastic anemia in 2–3 months.

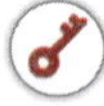

Key: C

BOOST YOUR KNOWLEDGE

- Diarrhea/IBD (inflammatory bowel disease) leads to decreased folate conjugase activity resulting in folate deficiency.
- Goat's milk is deficient in folate and can result in megaloblastic anemia. Folate content of food is reduced by cooking at high temperature.
- Anticonvulsants such as phenytoin, phenobarbitone, and primidone can present with megaloblastic anemia that responds rapidly to folic acid supplementation.
- Pancreatic replacement therapy may cause folic acid deficiency.

REFERENCE/SOURCE

- Kliegman RM, St Geme III JW. Nelson Textbook of Pediatrics, 21st edition. Amsterdam: Elsevier; 2019. Chapter 481.1. p. 2518.

19. Choose the correct match with respect to inherited disorders of folate metabolism.

Defective gene	*Disorder or its manifestation*
a. *DHFR*	1. No megaloblastic anemia
b. *MTHFR*	2. Hereditary folate malabsorption
c. *SCL46A1*	3. Megaloblastic anemia with neurological dysfunction
d. *FOLR1*	4. Cerebral folate deficiency syndrome

A. a-2, b-3, c-1, d-4
B. a-1, b-2, c-3, d-4
C. a-2, b-1, c-3, d-4
D. a-3, b-1, c-2, d-4

EXPLANATION

DHFR	Megaloblastic anemia with neurological dysfunction
MTHFR	No megaloblastic anemia
SCL46A1	Hereditary folate malabsorption
FOLR1	Cerebral folate deficiency syndrome

Key: D

BOOST YOUR KNOWLEDGE

Hereditary folate malabsorption is an autosomal recessive disorder caused by a mutation in the gene *SCL46A1*. Presents at 2–6 months with megaloblastic anemia. It may be precipitated following an infection or a diarrheal illness. The normal cerebrospinal fluid (CSF): serum folate ratio of 3:1 is lost. Central nervous system (CNS) manifestations include seizures, developmental delay, and intellectual disability. It may be associated with hypogammaglobinemia as well.

Methylenetetrahydrofolate reductase (MTFHR) deficiency is the most common inherited disorder of folate metabolism. It is associated with neurological and vascular disorders, however, there is no megaloblastic anemia. Elevated homocysteine (Hcy) levels and homocystinuria with decreased serum methionine level are seen in contrast to classic homocystinuria due to cystathionine β-synthase deficiency, both homocysteine and methionine levels are elevated.

Dihydrofolate reductase (DHFR) deficiency presents with both megaloblastic anemia and neurological dysfunction. Methotrexate binds to DHFR and blocks the conversion of dihydrofolate to tetrahydrofolate.

Functional methionine synthase deficiency results from mutations affecting the function of methionine synthase reductase or methionine synthase. Autosomal recessive (AR) inheritance. Clinical features include cerebral atrophy, nystagmus, blindness, and altered muscle tone in addition to megaloblastic anemia. Variable response to hydroxocobalamin plus betaine.

Cerebral folate deficiency syndrome: Isolated decreased cerebral methyl THF uptake and levels resulting in developmental delay or regression, hypotonia, seizures, visual disturbances, and autistic features. All other expected systemic features of folate deficiency are absent. Absence of megaloblastic anemia and normal plasma Hcy and serum and red cell folate levels are observed, and intestinal folate absorption is normal. The disorder is caused by decreased function of folate receptor-α at the choroid plexus. Treat with folinic acid (0.5–1 mg/kg), folic acid therapy is not useful.

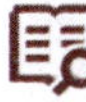

REFERENCES/SOURCES

- Kliegman RM, St Geme III JW. Nelson Textbook of Pediatrics, 21st edition. Amsterdam: Elsevier; 2019. Chapter 481.1. p. 2518.
- Orkin SH, Nathan DG, Ginsburg D, Look AT, Fisher DE, Lux S. Nathan and Oski's Hematology and Oncology of Infancy and Childhood, 8th edition. Philadelphia: Elsevier; 2014. Chapter 10.

20. **A 12-year-old girl child with progressive anemia comes to your clinic. Examination reveals mild icterus, sallow complexion, and hyperpigmented knuckles. The hemogram shows Hb 5.6 g/dL, TLC 2.9/mm^3, PLT 79,000/mm^3. Peripheral blood film has macrocytes and hypersegmented neutrophils. Which of the following statements is true?**

A. Bone marrow examination can help distinguish vitamin B_{12} deficiency from folate deficiency
B. If both methylmalonic acid (MMA) and homocysteine levels are elevated, folate deficiency is likely
C. If MMA is normal and homocysteine is raised, vitamin B_{12} deficiency is more likely
D. Testing for anti-parietal cell antibody is not recommended as a routine

EXPLANATION

- Bone marrow aspiration (BMA) is not needed in this patient to prove diagnosis as the clinical picture, CBC and peripheral blood smear (PBF) findings are diagnostic. BMA *cannot* help distinguishing vitamin B_{12} deficiency from folate deficiency.
- If both MMA and homocysteine levels are elevated, Vitamin B_{12} deficiency is likely.
- If MMA is normal and homocysteine is raised, folate deficiency is more likely.

Key: D

BOOST YOUR KNOWLEDGE

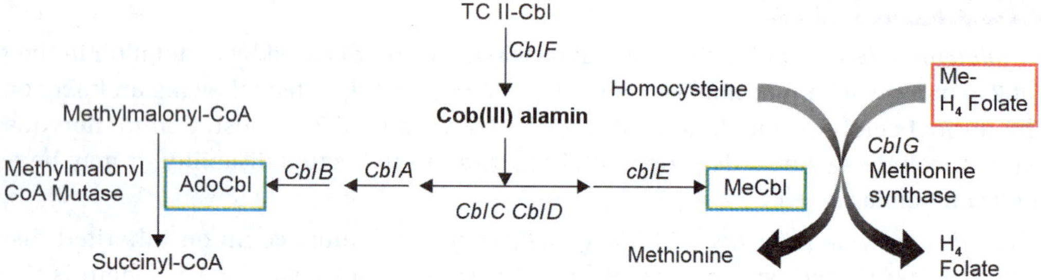

Folate is involved in conversion of homocysteine to methionine (red box), hence, resulting in high homocysteine levels in folate deficiency. Cobalamin is involved in both conversion of methylmalonic acid to succinyl CoA and homocysteine to methionine (green box), hence, both MMA and homocysteine levels are increased in cobalamin deficiency.

Cobalamin levels >300 pg/mL (>221 pmol/L) are considered normal and exclude significant vitamin B_{12} deficiency and levels between 200 and 300 pg/mL (148–221 pmol/L) are considered borderline. Levels <200 pg/mL (<148 pmol/L) are suggested to be used to define vitamin B_{12} deficiency.

The normal range of plasma MMA is 70–270 nmol/L and of homocysteine is 5–15 µmol/L. Plasma total homocysteine is more sensitive, but plasma MMA is more specific. The British Society of Hematology suggests MMA >750 nmol/L is indicative of vitamin B_{12} deficiency, and homocysteine above 15 mol/L could be indicative of folate deficiency.

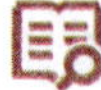

REFERENCES/SOURCES

- Chandra J, Dewan P, Kumar P, Mahajan A, Singh P, Dhingra B, et al. Diagnosis, Treatment and Prevention of Nutritional Anemia in Children: Recommendations of the Joint Committee of Pediatric Hematology-Oncology Chapter and Pediatric and Adolescent Nutrition Society of the Indian Academy of Pediatrics. Indian Pediatr. 2022;59(10):782-801.
- Devalia V, Hamilton MS, Molloy AM; British Committee for Standards in Haematology. Guidelines for the diagnosis and treatment of cobalamin and folate disorders. Br J Haematol. 2014;166(4):496-513.
- Kliegman RM, St Geme III JW. Nelson Textbook of Pediatrics, 21st edition. Amsterdam: Elsevier; 2019. Chapter 481.2.

CHAPTER 18.3

Bone Marrow Failure and Aplastic Anemia

Manas Kalra

1. A 12-year-old boy presents with a 1-month history of recurrent fevers and bruises. He has received blood transfusion and platelet transfusion multiple times. His first complete blood count (CBC) showed an hemoglobin (Hb) of 7 g/dL, white blood cell (WBC) count of 5,000/cu mm and a platelet of 24,000/cu mm. Differential count showed N-10%, L-85%, E-3%, B-2%, M-0%, and no blasts. What would be the most appropriate terminology for his cytopenia?

A. Bicytopenia
B. Pancytopenia
C. Aplastic anemia
D. Aleukemic leukemia

EXPLANATION

This child is suffering from pancytopenia as he has anemia, neutropenia, and thrombocytopenia. It is a common error to classify cytopenia based on only WBC count. The most important cell to fight bacterial infection is neutrophil and it is produced from bone marrow. Neutropenia may indicate a severe abnormality in the bone marrow. Definition of pancytopenia Hb <11.5 g/dL, WBC <4,000/cu mm, ANC <1,500/cu mm, and platelet <1.5 lakhs/cu mm.

Key: B

BOOST YOUR KNOWLEDGE

Causes of pancytopenia:

Hypocellular bone marrow	*Cellular bone marrow*	*Infiltrative bone marrow disorders*
• Acquired aplastic anemia • Inherited bone marrow failure syndrome (Fanconi's anemia, amegakaryocytic thrombocytopenia, dyskeratosis congenita (DC), and Shwachman–Diamond syndrome) • Paroxysmal nocturnal hemoglobinuria • Hypoplastic myelodysplastic syndrome • Virus-associated aplastic anemia	*Primary bone marrow disease:* • Myelodysplasia • Paroxysmal nocturnal hemoglobinuria *Secondary to systemic disease:* • Systemic lupus erythematosus, Sjögren's syndrome • Hypersplenism • Vitamin B_{12}, folate deficiency • Infection • Storage disease (Gaucher, Niemann–Pick) • Alcoholism • Sarcoidosis	• Acute myelogenous leukemia • Acute lymphoblastic leukemia • Hemophagocytic lymphohistiocytosis • Metastatic solid tumors • Osteopetrosis • Myelofibrosis

REFERENCE/SOURCE

- Orkin SH, Nathan DG, Ginsburg D, Look AT, Fisher DE, Lux S. Nathan and Oski's Hematology of Infancy and Childhood, 7th edition. Philadelphia, Pennsylvania: Saunders; 2008.

2. An 8-year-old is being evaluated for anemia. Due to underlying macrocytosis, she has received B_{12} and folic acid on multiple occasions. She is noted to have a progressive pigmentation of skin and short stature (below 10th centile). Following is the CBC trend. What is the most appropriate method to evaluate this child?

	20/1/2017	31/3/2019	3/2/2022
Hemoglobin (Hb)	9	8	7.5
RBC count	2.9	3.1	2.8
Hematocrit (HCT)	32	29	28
Mean corpuscular volume (MCV)	98	102	99
Mean corpuscular hemoglobin (MCH)	30	29	31
Mean cell hemoglobin concentration (MCHC)	34	31	32
Red cell distribution width (RDW)	13	14	14.5
WBC	5.1	4.5	3.2
Neutrophils	70	43	30
Lymphocytes	22	50	59
Monocytes	1	2	1
Eosinophils	4	3	8
Basophils	3	2	2
Platelet	1.6 L	92 K	1.2 L
Mean platelet volume (MPV)	9	7.8	8

A. Do chromosomal breakage study on peripheral blood
B. Give injectable B_{12} and folic acid
C. Do endoscopy to look for villous atrophy and scalloping in duodenum
D. Do endocrine work-up to rule out adrenal issues and growth hormone study

EXPLANATION

Note that the CBC shows macrocytic anemia. RDW is not elevated which points to non-nutritional cause. Failure of therapy also points toward an alternate diagnosis. She also has evolving cytopenia in other cell lines. Children with IBMFS have macrocytic anemia. FA is the most common cause. They are known to have failure to thrive and progressive darkening of skin. Most have other congenital anomalies as well. As age progresses, the chances of aplastic anemia and MDS increase. It is diagnosed by a positive chromosome breakage test.

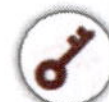

Key: A

BOOST YOUR KNOWLEDGE

Children or adults with B_{12} or folic acid deficiency have macrocytosis with low RBC count and high RDW. Their diet history is deficient, and it happens mostly in patients who are vegetarian or eat non-vegetarian diet occasionally. Peripheral smear shows large RBC or macro-ovalocytes with hypersegmented neutrophils. One may notice basophilic stippling, Cabot ring, and thrombocytopenia. Other causes of macrocytosis are hypothyroidism, marrow failure (inherited or acquired), Down syndrome, and liver disease.

REFERENCE/SOURCE

- Danewa A, Kalra M, Sachdeva A, Sachdeva P, Bansal D, Bhat S, et al. Diagnosis and management of acquired aplastic anemia: Consensus Statement of Indian Academy of Pediatrics. Indian Pediatr. 2022;59(6):467-75.

3. Complete blood count of a 4-year-old girl showed an Hb of 5 g/dL, PCV- 15, WBC count of 3,000/cu mm and a platelet of 70,000/cu mm. Differential count showed N-12%, L-83%, E-1%, B-2%, M-2%, no blasts. A reticulocyte count has been ordered which is reported as 1%. What is your comment on the retic count?

A. The retic count is adequate
B. Retic count cannot be interpreted as we do not have absolute retic number
C. It cannot be interpreted as we do not know the expected hematocrit
D. Reticulocyte count is based on bone marrow examination
E. Corrected reticulocyte count is low

EXPLANATION

The patient has pancytopenia. Evaluating reticulocyte count is important. In case of anemia, the retic count should normally increase to compensate for the degree of anemia. This can only happen if the bone marrow function is appropriate. If the bone marrow is hypo-functioning, then patient will not be able to mount a retic response. We need to check corrected reticulocyte count by the following formula: Retic count × patient hematocrit/expected hematocrit. The expected hematocrit can be approximately calculated by multiplying the expected Hb with 3. In this case, if we assume that the expected Hb is 12, the expected hematocrit is 36. So, corrected retic count is 1 × 15/36 = 0.4% which is lower than normal indicating erythrocyte hypoproduction.

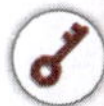

Key: E

BOOST YOUR KNOWLEDGE

Reticulocytes are the youngest form of erythrocytes that a bone marrow produces. They are larger than mature RBC. They are increased in hemolytic anemia especially those with extravascular hemolysis. Their rise post-administration of hematinic indicates a response to therapy. They are stained with supravital staining (brilliant cresyl blue, new methylene blue) and impart polychromatophilia in a peripheral smear.

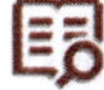

REFERENCE/SOURCE

- Parodi E, Romano F, Ramenghi U. How we use reticulocyte parameters in workup and management of pediatric hematologic diseases? Front Pediatr. 2020;8:588617.

4. A 5-year-old boy presented with history of gradually increasing pallor, petechiae all over the body from 1 month and fever from the past 15 days. CBC showed pancytopenia with severe reticulocytopenia. Which among the following is *not* an inherited cause of this situation?

A. Dyskeratosis congenita
B. Amegakaryocytic thrombocytopenia
C. Paroxysmal nocturnal hemoglobinuria
D. Fanconi anemia

EXPLANATION

Paroxysmal nocturnal hemoglobinuria is an acquired cause of aplastic anemia. The other three are forms of inherited bone marrow failure syndrome and have a genetic basis of inheritance with early presentation. However, diseases such as Fanconi have been identified in older patients as well. All children and young adults with aplastic anemia should undergo stress cytogenetics and preferably next generation sequencing too to identify an underlying inherited bone marrow failure syndrome (IBMFS).

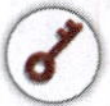

Key: C

BOOST YOUR KNOWLEDGE

Paroxysmal nocturnal hemoglobinuria (PNH) is an acquired complement-driven hemolytic anemia resulting from the clonal expansion of stem cells harboring a somatic phosphatidylinositol glycan biosynthesis class A protein (PIGA) mutation. The *PIGA* gene product is required for the biosynthesis of glycosylphosphatidylinositol (GPI) anchors, a glycolipid moiety that attaches numerous proteins to the cell surface. PNH blood cells have a deficiency of all GPI-anchored proteins. The absence of CD55 and CD59, both GPI-anchored complement regulators, leads to complement-driven erythrocyte lysis and a marked predisposition for venous and arterial thrombosis. The stem cell defect can also lead to aplastic anemia. It is not uncommon to identify a PNH clone in the work-up of a patient with aplastic anemia.

REFERENCE/SOURCE

- Brodsky RA. How I treat paroxysmal nocturnal hemoglobinuria. Blood. 2021;137(10):1304-9.

5. Which of the following drugs is a new addition to the anti-thymocyte globulin (ATG)-based immunosuppressive therapy for aplastic anemia?

A. Cyclosporin
B. Mycophenolate mofetil
C. Eltrombopag
D. Erythropoietin

EXPLANATION

Eltrombopag is an oral thrombopoietin-receptor agonist that is effective in both refractory and treatment-naive severe aplastic anemia. Currently, EPAG in combination with IST (ATG plus cyclosporin A) is approved by the United States Food and Drug Administration (US-FDA) for children aged ≥2 years as front-line treatment for severe aplastic anemia (SAA).

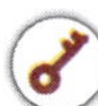

Key: C

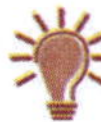

BOOST YOUR KNOWLEDGE

Eltrombopag is also used for chronic immune thrombocytopenia (ITP). Food or milk consumption should be avoided 2 hours before and after administration of this drug due to concerns of poor absorption with food intake. The dose is 25 mg for children <6 years and 50 mg for those >6 years. Common side effects are iron deficiency anemia and hepatotoxicity.

REFERENCE/SOURCE

- Barone A, Lucarelli A, Onofrillo D, Verzegnassi F, Bonanomi S, Cesaro S, et al. Diagnosis and management of acquired aplastic anemia in childhood. Guidelines from the Marrow Failure Study Group of the Pediatric Haemato-Oncology Italian Association (AIEOP). Blood Cells Mol Dis. 2015;55(1):40-7.

6. A 7-year-old child with severe aplastic anemia has three siblings. The family is offered human leukocyte antigen (HLA) typing of the index child and siblings. The family feels that transplant would be harmful for donor and recipient. What should be the doctor's advice?

A. Patient should be treated with cyclosporine and ATG as success rates similar
B. Transplant from a matched sibling donor carries the maximum chance of cure and has very minimal risks for the donor
C. Gene therapy should be tried if facilities are available as it has minimum risk
D. A trial of IV methylprednisolone can be given

EXPLANATION

Cure rates in excess of 90% can be achieved with a matched sibling donor transplant if it is performed before the patient develops life-threatening infections or bleeds. Risk to donor is minimal. Benefit of transplant outweighs its risk for the patient as this disease is uniformly fatal if untreated. Immunosuppressive therapy has a success rate of around 60–70% with higher chances of relapse and clonal evolution to secondary malignancy such as AML during follow-up.

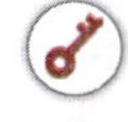

Key: B

BOOST YOUR KNOWLEDGE

Stem cells can be collected from the donor by a bone marrow harvest or peripheral stem cell harvest. Bone marrow harvest carries the risk of anesthesia as any surgical procedure. Peripheral blood stem cell harvest carries risk of complications of a central line insertion which is used to collect the apheresis after administration of granulocyte colony stimulating factor (GCSF) for 4 days. Patient can also have electrolyte abnormalities especially hypocalcemia during the procedure. Flu-like symptoms are common after administration of GCSF.

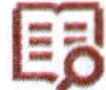

REFERENCE/SOURCE

- Danewa A, Kalra M, Sachdeva A, Sachdeva P, Bansal D, Bhat S, et al. Diagnosis and management of acquired aplastic anemia: Consensus Statement of Indian Academy of Pediatrics. Indian Pediatr. 2022;59(6):467-75.

7. A 24-year-old man with Fanconi anemia (FA) underwent a matched unrelated donor transplant at the age of 8 years for aplastic anemia. He has 100% donor chimerism. He developed severe acute graft-versus-host disease (GVHD) which improved with immunosuppressants. He later developed chronic GVHD of skin, oral mucosa, and eyes. He is on regular follow-up and his blood counts are normal. He presents with complaints of oral ulcer which has been troubling him for last 1 month. He has tried B complex vitamin and steroid application, but it has not improved. What is the next most appropriate step?

A. Try topical antifungal and oral fluconazole for a week
B. Increase immunosuppression to treat GVHD
C. Recurrent mucosal ulceration is part of disease process of Fanconi anemia and needs supportive care
D. He should undergo a biopsy to rule out oral cancer

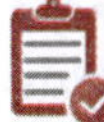

EXPLANATION

Children with FA have an increased risk of cancers. 11% develop some form of malignancy before 18 years of age. The most common cancer in younger patients is myelodysplastic syndrome (MDS) or acute myeloid leukemia. As they grow older, the chances of squamous cell carcinoma (SCC) in head and neck region increases. Children who develop GVHD have much higher chances of developing SCC. The ongoing inflammatory damage to skin and mucosa leads to further increase in risk of developing cancer.

Key: D

BOOST YOUR KNOWLEDGE

Stem cell transplant remains the treatment of choice for patients with FA who develop aplastic anemia or MDS. Their conditioning regimen differs from idiopathic aplastic anemia. The doses of chemotherapy and radiation are reduced to decrease the toxicity of treatment. Every precaution should be taken to avoid GVHD as this further aggravates risk of cancer. Human papillomavirus (HPV) vaccine is strongly recommended in FA patients to decrease the risk of SCC.

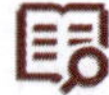

REFERENCE/SOURCE

- Kutler DI, Singh B, Satagopan J, Batish SD, Berwick M, Giampietro PF, et al. A 20-year perspective on the International Fanconi Anemia Registry (IFAR). Blood. 2003;101(4):1249-56.

8. A 16-year-old boy has severe aplastic anemia. He is awaiting a matched unrelated donor transplant from a German registry. He has been advised regular follow-up and neutropenic precautions. He presents for a weekly check-up to the pediatric hematologist. He has mild pallor and skin bruises. There is no mucosal bleeding, and he is afebrile. His CBC shows an Hb of 8.5 g/dL, TLC of 900/cu mm, and a platelet of 12,000/cu mm. Which of the following statements is true?

A. He needs urgent admission for platelet transfusion
B. He needs urgent admission for packed red blood cell and platelet transfusion
C. He needs IV antibiotics and packed red blood cells and platelet transfusion
D. He does not need any of the above

EXPLANATION

Children with aplastic anemia should not be unnecessarily transfused. Platelets should only be transfused if the child has mucosal bleeds or high-grade fever with severe thrombocytopenia. If a child is afebrile and does not have mucosal or any other life-threatening bleeds, he/she should not receive a platelet transfusion. Some physicians may transfuse if platelet count is <10,000/cu mm. Packed red blood cell should be given if a child has symptoms of anemia or the Hb falls <7 g/dL.

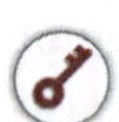

Key: D

BOOST YOUR KNOWLEDGE

Based on concerns with alloimmunization and iron overload, there should be a uniform approach to utilize as few transfusions as possible to keep the patient relatively asymptomatic. Unnecessary transfusion practice should be avoided in aplastic anemia.

A common problem in multi-transfused patients with aplastic anemia (AA) is that they may develop alloimmunization to leukocytes present in red cell and platelet transfusions by generating HLA or non-HLA (minor histocompatibility) antibodies. This can result in platelet refractoriness, as well as an increased risk of graft rejection and graft versus host disease after allogeneic BMT. Fever in neutropenic children warrants urgent admission and IV antibiotics. There is not much role of prophylactic antibiotics. Anti-mould prophylaxis (voriconazole or itraconazole) is used if ANC is <200.

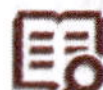

REFERENCE/SOURCE

- Danewa A, Kalra M, Sachdeva A, Sachdeva P, Bansal D, Bhat S, et al. Diagnosis and management of acquired aplastic anemia: Consensus Statement of Indian Academy of Pediatrics. Indian Pediatr. 2022;59(6):467-75.

9. A 3-year-old child presents with a history of recurrent fever. Each time he has fever, he also has oral ulcers which are painful. He is admitted to a hospital with severe respiratory distress and lower respiratory tract infection and a bad skin infection. CBC shows a hemoglobin of 9.5 g/dL. WBC count of 2,500/mm^3 and a platelet count of 1.8 lakh. The differential shows N 2%, L 95%, M 1%, E 1%, and B 1%. Bone marrow does not show any excess blasts. It shows maturation arrest in granulopoiesis. His records also show previous documented severe neutropenia. Which of the following statements is not true about this child?

A. Bone marrow report suggests the possibility of severe congenital neutropenia or cyclic neutropenia
B. Upfront treatment of choice for this condition is a stem cell transplant

C. There are high chances of evolution into acute myeloid leukemia or myelodysplastic syndrome

D. Blood counts should be performed once every 3 days for a period of 6 weeks to differentiate between severe congenital neutropenia and cyclic neutropenia

EXPLANATION

Children with severe congenital neutropenia can present with serious bacterial infections which can be life-threatening. Children with cyclic neutropenia develop neutropenia almost every 21 days. During the period of neutropenia, they can have mouth ulcers and bacterial infections. These infections can even turn fatal if not treated promptly. Most children respond very well to GCSF, and the dose may range from as low as 1 µg/kg per day to as high as 20 µg/kg per day. Children with severe congenital neutropenia who do not respond to GCSF need a stem cell transplant.

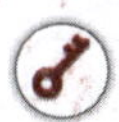

Key: B

BOOST YOUR KNOWLEDGE

The recognized subtypes of severe congenital neutropenia (SCN) are:

- SCN1 is the most common form of SCN, which accounts for 60–80% of SCN. This autosomal dominant form that arises from mutations of the *ELANE* (formerly *ELA2*) gene on chromosome 19p13.3, which encodes neutrophil elastase. Over a hundred ELANE mutations have been found in SCN1. This same gene is mutated in cyclic neutropenia.
- SCN2 is caused by heterozygous (autosomal dominant) mutation of the *GFI1* gene on chromosome 1p22.
- SCN3 is the "classical", autosomal recessive form of Kostmann disease which arises from homozygous mutations in the *HAX 1* gene on chromosome 1p22.1. About one-third of SCN3 individuals also have neurological changes including seizures, learning disabilities, or developmental delay.
- SCN4 is caused by autosomal recessive mutation of the *G6PC3* gene.

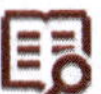

REFERENCE/SOURCE

- Orkin SH, Nathan DG, Ginsburg D, Look AT, Fisher DE, Lux S. Nathan and Oski's Hematology of Infancy and Childhood, 7th edition. Philadelphia, Pennsylvania: Saunders; 2008.

10. A 7.5-year-old child has severe aplastic anemia. He is admitted with fever for 7 days. His blood counts show an Hb 5 g/dL, platelet count of 5,000/mm^3, WBC count of 2,000/mm^3, and neutrophil of 3%. He has been receiving injection meropenem and polymyxin for the last 7 days, but the fever continues. What would be the most appropriate statement for the management of this child?

A. Invasive fungal infection should be presumed and treated

B. Do a CT chest and if it shows features of invasive fungal infection, treat. If not, voriconazole prophylaxis should be considered in this patient to prevent invasive fungal infection

C. Chest X-ray and galactomannan are highly sensitive to detect invasive fungal infection

D. Oral and rectal swab will help in detection of invasive candidiasis

EXPLANATION

Invasive candidiasis can be identified based on detection of *Candida* species in blood culture or ultrasound/CT scan of abdomen which can demonstrate lesions suggestive of hepato-splenic candidiasis. Beta D glucan is a serological assay to detect candidiasis. In patients with severe neutropenia, invasive aspergillosis is a frequent complication. High resolution computed tomography (HRCT) chest helps to detect aspergillosis in the lungs. It should be performed in any neutropenic child who is persistently febrile for >5 days.

Prolonged neutropenia, relapsed hematological malignancy, and steroid therapy are risk factors for invasive aspergillosis. The drug of choice for this condition is voriconazole.

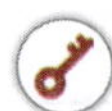

Key: B

BOOST YOUR KNOWLEDGE

Therapeutic drug monitoring is needed to optimize the dosage of voriconazole. The common side-effects of this drug are liver toxicity and visual toxicity. Amphotericin B is associated with renal toxicity, hypokalemia, and infusion reactions. Liposomal preparation has less chance of nephrotoxicity. Liposomal amphotericin B is used in patients with liver toxicity.

11. A 12-year-old boy presented with purpuric spots, fever, and oral ulcers. He had a history of jaundice 2 weeks back. At admission, his blood counts showed Hb 6.5 g/dL, TLC 2,200/cu mm, ANC 700/cu mm, and platelets of 35,000/cu mm. His serum glutamic oxaloacetic transaminase (SGOT) is 500 and serum glutamate pyruvate transaminase (SGPT) is 800 IU. Bone marrow aspiration showed hypocellular marrow. Bone marrow biopsy showed cellularity of 40%. What will be the next investigation in this case?

A. Serology for hepatitis A, B, C, E, reticulocyte count, stress cytogenetics, flowcytometry for PNH clone
B. HLA typing of patient and family members
C. Bone marrow cytogenetics
D. Next generation sequencing for inherited bone marrow failure syndrome

EXPLANATION

Hepatitis is a common cause of aplastic anemia. At least 10–15% of aplastic anemia patients have a history of jaundice and hepatitis. Hepatotropic viruses such as hepatitis A, B, C, E and even non-A, B, C, E viruses with their cytopathic effect cause failure of hematopoiesis in the marrow. The patient is suffering from post-hepatitis aplastic anemia. To ascertain the cause, we should go for viral serology.

Regarding options B, C, D—all the investigations paneled are done to find the etiology of aplastic anemia and decide further treatment. But if asked for the next appropriate investigation it would be serology for hepatotropic viruses.

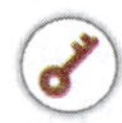

Key: A

BOOST YOUR KNOWLEDGE

Severe aplastic anemia is diagnosed if at least two of the following are fulfilled: (1) Granulocyte count <500/cu mm, (2) Platelet count <20,000/cu mm, and (3) Reticulocyte count $<20 \times 10^9$/cu mm.

The term "very severe aplastic anemia" is used when ANC <200/cu mm. Viral infections are known to cause aplastic anemia. Of the known viral infections, hepatitis viruses (A, B, C, E, and non-A, B, C, E), CMV, EBV, and Flaviviruses are well known to cause aplastic anemia.

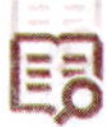

REFERENCES/SOURCES

- Bacigalupo A. How I treat acquired aplastic anemia. Blood. 2017;129(11):1428-36
- Orkin SH, Fisher DE, Ginsburg D, Look AT, Lux SE, Nathan DG. Nathan and Oski's Hematology and Oncology of Infancy and Childhood. 8th edition. Philadelphia, Pennsylvania: Saunders; 2015

12. **A 12-year-old boy whose height is 130 cm, and weight is 28 kg presented with oral lesions, abnormal skin pigmentation, and nail changes as shown in the figures.**

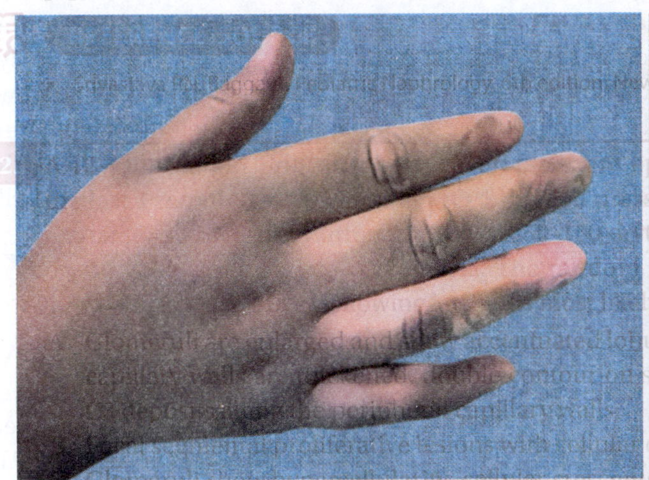
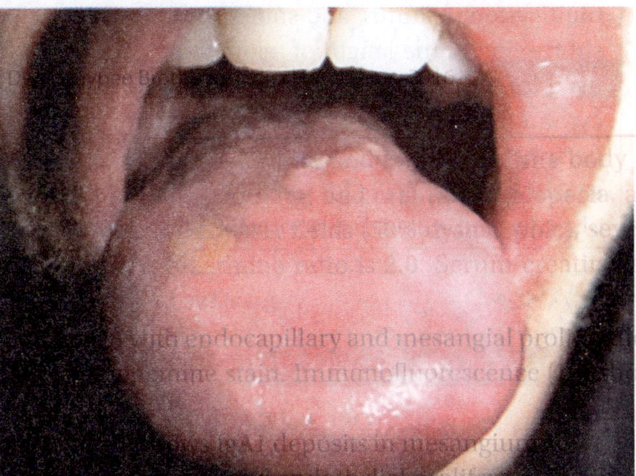
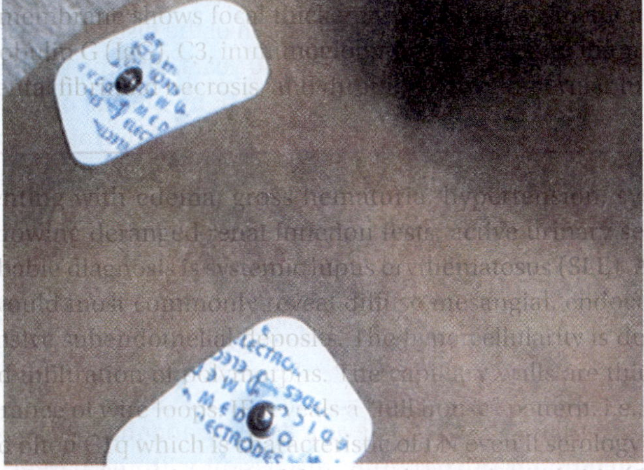

He has mild mental retardation. Complete blood count reveals Hb of 8.0 g/dL, TLC of 1,900/cu mm, and platelets of 52,000/cu mm. He has a history of pneumonia 3 months back. Which is *not* an appropriate investigation?

A. Fluorescence in situ hybridization (FISH) for telomere length assessment and flowcytometry for assessment of telomere length

B. Bone marrow aspiration and biopsy

C. Flowcytometry for PNH clone

D. Next generation sequencing and clinical exome sequencing for dyskeratosis congenita (DKC) and telomerase reverse transcriptase (TERT) mutations

EXPLANATION

The child is suffering from DKC. DKC is an IBMFS characterized by the classic triad of abnormal skin pigmentation, nail dystrophy, and oral leukoplakia. DKC is a disease of defective telomere maintenance and is heterogeneous at the genetic level. It can be inherited in X-linked, autosomal dominant, or autosomal recessive patterns. Mutations in at least 10 telomere- and telomerase-associated genes have been described in DKC. The clinical diagnosis of DKC is based on the presence of the four major features of the disease, which include the mucocutaneous triad and BMF, as well as the presence of multisystem features of the disease—epiphora, developmental delay or mental retardation, pulmonary disease, periodontal disease, esophageal stricture, premature hair greying or loss, hyperhidrosis, or development of malignant lesions. To make a correct clinical diagnosis of dyskeratosis congenita (DKC) requires at least two of four major features and at least two multisystem features, and sometimes it is difficult because of the disease heterogeneity. After demonstrating a shortening in the length of telomerase it is suitable to perform a genetic study. Three methods are commonly used for measuring telomere length, including Southern blot, real-time polymerase chain reaction, and flow cytometry and fluorescence in situ hybridization (Flow-FISH). Of these, measurement of telomere length in peripheral white blood cells by flow cytometry and fluorescence in situ hybridization was found to be both sensitive and specific for identifying patients with DKC. PNH on the other hand is an acquired clonal stem cell disorder and will not be positive in any inherited disorder.

Key: C

BOOST YOUR KNOWLEDGE

To date, ten genes (*DKC1, TERC, TERT, TINF2, NOP10, NHP2, TCAB1, C16orf57, RTEL1*) have been identified; nine of these are important in telomere maintenance. DKC can be inherited in one of three forms, X-linked, AD, or AR. De novo germline mutations are also relatively frequent in DKC, and to date, about 70% of DKC patients have an identifiable germline mutation. During the evolution of the disease, the abnormal skin pigmentation and nail changes usually appear first, often below the age of 10 years, and the patients usually develop BMF before the age of 20 years. Up to 80% of patients show signs of BMF by the age of 30 years. However, sometimes the manifestation of the disease is ambiguous, and BMF or another abnormality in another system could appear before the classic mucocutaneous features. This is being recognized in more cases with the advances in genetic diagnostic techniques.

REFERENCE/SOURCE

- Fernandez García MS, Teruya-Feldstein J. The diagnosis and treatment of dyskeratosis congenita: a review. J Blood Med. 2014;5: 157-67.

13. A 10-year-old girl was diagnosed as a case of severe aplastic anemia. There was no matched sibling donor (MSD) or matched unrelated donor (MUD). After discussion with the parents, immunosuppressive therapy was started with equine antithymocyte globulin (ATG) and cyclosporine. 3 weeks after starting treatment she developed pruritic erythematous maculopapular rash, high-grade fever, joint pains and joint swellings and severe muscle pains. Blood investigation revealed increased blood urea nitrogen (BUN) and creatinine. What will be next best step in management?

A. Start steroid with injection methyl prednisolone @2 mg/kg/day, assess response
B. Start non-steroidal anti-inflammatory drug (NSAID)
C. Start renal replacement therapy
D. Replace cyclosporine with tacrolimus and add antiallergics

EXPLANATION

Serum sickness is a common side effect of ATG. Serum sickness is characterized by fever, arthralgia, lymphadenopathy, and rash. Typically, serum sickness affects multiple large joints, occasionally joints involving the spine, or the temporal-mandibular joint. One important finding is that serum sickness presents as jaw pain along with polyarthralgia in all patients. Serum sickness can be treated with high dose steroids or plasmapheresis. NSAIDs may aid in bringing down inflammation but is contraindicated in this case owing to the high BUN and creatine values. Serum sickness is a self-limited entity that will usually resolve upon discontinuation of the offending agent, with or without additional treatment. Thus, treatment is generally aimed at reducing symptom severity and removing the agent. For mild or moderate presentations, symptomatic relief can be achieved with NSAIDs and/or antihistamines. The patient should be counseled that the rash and pruritis should stop progressing within 48 hours of initiation of these medications. For more severe symptoms, a 7–10-day course of 0.5–2 mg/kg of systemic glucocorticoids can be helpful.

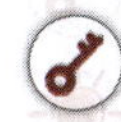

Key: A

BOOST YOUR KNOWLEDGE

Serum sickness is an immune-complex-mediated hypersensitivity reaction. It was first recognized as an entity in the early 1900s in patients who had received heterologous antisera, which was historically used to treat infectious diseases. The symptoms typically occur 1–2 weeks after exposure to an offending agent and resolve within several weeks of discontinuation. Certain patient populations are considered to be at a higher risk for developing serum sickness following rituximab infusion, including those with hypergammaglobulinemia and hepatitis C-related cryoglobulinemia vasculitis. When a patient is exposed to a foreign serum protein, it takes approximately 6–10 days for antibodies to develop and form antigen-antibody complexes and is considered a type III immune-mediated hypersensitivity reaction. If the macrophage activating system is not functioning properly, these complexes will become saturated in the circulation, leading to immune complex deposition, most commonly in parenchymal tissues, and synovial joint fluid. The deposition of immune complexes may also activate the classical complement pathway, leading to lower levels of circulating C3 and C4. These levels can be used to differentiate serum sickness from a serum sickness-like reaction, which will have normal complement levels. Also, the activation of the complement system will trigger histamine release and increase vascular permeability, which leads to an inflammatory response in the tissues and joints. It is the process of clearing these immune complexes and the subsequent inflammatory reaction that coincides with the onset of clinical symptoms. Note that in patients previously sensitized to the antigen, symptoms may develop within a few days of re-exposure to the causative agent.

REFERENCE/SOURCE

- Rixe N, Tavarez MM. Serum sickness. In: StatPearls. Treasure Island (FL): StatPearls Publishing; 2023.

14. A 6-month-old infant presents with failure to thrive and recurrent infections. On examination, the liver is enlarged. Fasting hypoglycemia is noted. A liver biopsy shows increased glycogen deposition. Molecular genetic testing reveals homozygous mutations in *SLC37A4*, the gene encoding the glucose-6-phosphate transporter and child gets diagnosed as GSD-1b. His CBC shows isolated neutropenia. What drugs have been recently approved for treatment of such a case?

A. Empagliflozin
B. Metformin
C. Celecoxib
D. Pioglitazone

EXPLANATION

For years, the mechanism behind neutropenia in glucose-6-phosphatase catalytic subunit 3 (G6PC3) deficiency and glycogen storage disease type Ib (GSDIB) was unclear, as the glucose-6-phosphatase (G6Pase) enzyme did not seem to directly affect neutrophils. The mystery was solved when 1,5-anhydroglucitol phosphate (1,5AG6P) was identified as a toxic metabolite that builds up when G6PC3 or the glucose-6-phosphate transporter (encoded by SLC37A4) are defective. 1,5AG6P inhibits neutrophil energy metabolism, causing dysfunction and death. This explained the neutropenia. Inhibitors of the sodium glucose cotransporter such as empagliflozin, used to treat diabetes, were then shown to reduce plasma 1,5AG and its toxic metabolite 1,5AG6P.

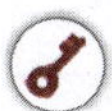

Key: A

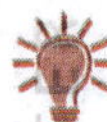
BOOST YOUR KNOWLEDGE

Empagliflozin normalized neutrophil counts in mouse models and humans with G6PC3 deficiency or GSDIB. These findings revealed the mechanism of neutropenia and opened up a targeted treatment approach using existing diabetes drugs.

15. A 7-year-old girl presents with a history of chronic diarrhea, recurrent pneumonia, and short stature. Physical examination is significant for short stature and diffuse bone pain. Laboratory findings reveal pancytopenia and low lipase level. Bone marrow biopsy shows hypocellularity with dysplastic changes. Karyotype shows monosomy 7. DNA sequencing identifies biallelic mutations in *SBDS* gene suggesting Shwachman–Diamond syndrome. Which of the following is the most accurate treatment for the pancytopenia in this patient?

A. GCSF therapy
B. Pancreatic enzyme therapy
C. Wait and watch
D. Allogeneic hematopoietic stem cell transplantation (HSCT)

EXPLANATION

The most accurate treatment for the pancytopenia in this 7-year-old girl with Shwachman–Diamond syndrome (SDS) is allogeneic HSCT. Specifically, the dysplastic changes in the patient's bone marrow indicate impaired hematopoiesis and increased risk of progression to myelodysplastic syndrome (MDS) or acute myeloid leukemia (AML). Additionally, the monosomy 7 identified on karyotyping portends a very poor prognosis. It is a common cytogenetic finding in MDS/AML arising from SDS.

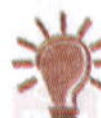
Key: D

BOOST YOUR KNOWLEDGE

Shwachman–Diamond syndrome is an IBMF due to AR defect in *SBDS* gene manifesting as neutropenia, pancreatic exocrine insufficiency, and metaphyseal chondrodysplasia.

G-CSF therapy: While G-CSF can help temporarily manage the neutropenia, it does not treat the underlying dysplastic bone marrow changes or high-risk monosomy 7 karyotype. Therefore, it is not an accurate long-term treatment.

Pancreatic enzyme therapy: This can help manage malabsorption from pancreatic insufficiency in SDS, but does not improve the hematologic manifestations or treat the dysplastic marrow or cytogenetic abnormalities.

16. A 9-month-old girl is brought to the pediatrician by her parents for evaluation of recurrent fevers and infections. The parents report that the child has had two episodes of otitis media: 1 episode of pneumonia and a urinary tract infection in the past month requiring antibiotic treatment. There is no family history of recurrent infections or immunodeficiency. On examination, the infant appears pale and irritable. Laboratory studies show hemoglobin 9.5 g/dL, platelet count 150,000/mm^3, and white blood cell count 3,200/mm^3 with an absolute neutrophil count of 200/mm^3. Peripheral blood smear shows decreased neutrophils with normal morphology and maturation. Which of the following is the most likely diagnosis?

A. Cyclic neutropenia
B. Severe congenital neutropenia
C. Shwachman–Diamond syndrome
D. Chronic benign neutropenia of childhood

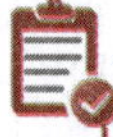
EXPLANATION

Severe congenital neutropenia (SCN) is a rare hematologic disorder characterized by an absolute neutrophil count (ANC) <500/mm^3 starting in infancy. The pathophysiology involves a maturation arrest of myeloid precursors in the bone marrow, leading to reduced neutrophil production and peripheral neutropenia.

The clinical features of SCN include:

- Onset of recurrent bacterial infections in the first few months of life—as seen in this infant with two ear infections and a UTI recently. Recurrent infections are the hallmark of SCN due to the lack of protective neutrophils.
- Persistent severe neutropenia on CBC—this infant has an ANC of only 200/mm^3, meeting the criteria for severe neutropenia.
- Normal neutrophil morphology and maturation on peripheral smear—this indicates an intrinsic defect in neutrophil production rather than an abnormality of the existing neutrophils.
- No identifiable secondary cause such as medications or autoimmune disease. The lack of family history makes this likely a de novo genetic mutation causing congenital neutropenia.
- Potential for progression to bone marrow failure over time.

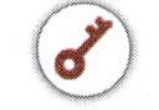

Key: B

BOOST YOUR KNOWLEDGE

The main alternative diagnosis is cyclic neutropenia, which is characterized by periodic oscillations in ANC over a 21-day cycle. This would not explain the persistent severe neutropenia in this infant. Other types of childhood neutropenia such as autoimmune neutropenia and chronic benign neutropenia also fail to account for the severe, unremitting neutropenia beginning in infancy in the absence of other causes. Cyclic neutropenia (100%) and 50–60% of *SCN* harbor *ELANE* gene mutation. Cyclic neutropenia is less severe and does not evolve into MDS/AML

17. A 7-year-old female child with dysmorphology was confirmed to have FA after genetic testing. She has no cytopenia at diagnosis and undergoes 3–6 monthly CBC monitoring. Which of the following is *incorrect* about malignancies in Fanconi patients?

A. Androgen therapy predisposes patients with FA to develop peliosis hepatis and hepatic adenomas
B. Patients with FA have a 30–40% cumulative risk of myeloid malignancies by age of 40 years
C. The head and neck cancers developing in a Fanconi patient are poorly responsive to conventional treatment
D. Girls with FA should ideally undergo breast and gynecological screening from the age of 5 years.

EXPLANATION

Patient with Fanconi on androgen therapy should undergo LFT and ultrasound abdomen monitoring every 3–6 monthly. Androgens predispose patients with FA to develop peliosis hepatis. Patients with FA have a 30–40% cumulative risk of myeloid malignancies by age of 40 years. Gain of chromosome 1q is the most common abnormality in FA; it can occur without MDS/AML. Conversely, monosomy 7/del(7q) is considered a marker of transformation, requiring urgent stem cell transplant. Other cytogenetic changes indicating a poor prognosis are gain of chromosome 3q, frequently preceding monosomy 7/del(7q), and *RUNX1* abnormalities. The head and neck cancers developing in a Fanconi patient are poorly responsive to conventional treatment. Girls should ideally undergo breast and gynecological screening from the age of 10 years.

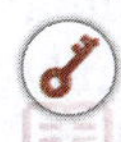

Key: D

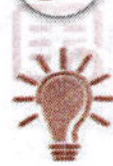

BOOST YOUR KNOWLEDGE

In addition to their well-known risk of AML, persons with FA have an extraordinary risk of developing a solid tumor. Compared to the general population, the risk is approximately 50-fold higher for all solid tumors combined, and several hundred- to several thousand-fold higher for cancers of the head and neck, esophagus, liver, vulva, and cervix.

18. Which of the following is *not true* about chromosomal breakage analysis?

A. It is performed on bone marrow sample.
B. DNA crosslinking agents (diepoxybutane or mitomycin C) are used
C. The test is gold standard for screening Fanconi anemia which can be confirmed by sequencing assay
D. Nijmegen breakage syndrome may have false positive chromosomal breakage

EXPLANATION

The test is performed on the peripheral blood samples because lymphocytes are needed to study chromosomal fragility. If the test fails in peripheral blood, it can be performed on skin fibroblasts.

Key: A

BOOST YOUR KNOWLEDGE

The test of chromosomal analysis is usually sent in a heparin vial and should reach the laboratory within 48 hours of its collection. Cell culture-based techniques utilize mitomycin or diepoxybutane (DEB). The reporting time is usually 12–20 days. The test does not pick carrier state. It is considered a gold standard for the diagnosis of FA and investigation of choice for sibling screening pretransplant donor selection. Causes of false +ve test—Nijmegen, Bloom, and cohesinopathies (Roberts syndrome, Warsaw breakage syndrome)

19. Which of the following is true about screening siblings of FA patients while selecting a suitable donor for stem cell transplant?

A. Clinical examination is enough to rule out Fanconi anemia
B. Chromosomal breakage should be ascertained as part of screening.
C. Sibling must undergo bone marrow evaluation prior to being a donor.
D. Male siblings should never be taken as donor as some cases of Fanconi are X-linked

EXPLANATION

Clinical examination is not enough, and siblings should be screened by chromosomal breakage testing. There is no indication of doing bone marrow for the donor. Though some cases of Fanconi may be X-linked, sibling screening clarifies donor selection and gender-based selections are not promoted.

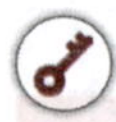

Key: B

BOOST YOUR KNOWLEDGE

It is critical that all potential siblings or other related donors undergo genetic testing or evaluation for chromosomal breakage, to ensure that they do not also have FA. This testing is necessary because family donors who are apparently asymptomatic and healthy may have FA, but lack classical findings due to mosaicism, incomplete penetrance of FA-associated abnormalities, or young age/late onset of disease manifestations. For potential-related donors who have non-hematologic features of FA, but in whom chromosomal breakage testing performed on a blood sample is normal. Chromosomal breakage testing should be performed on a fibroblast sample to exclude the possibility of testing a hematologic revertant. HSCT performed with a family donor who also turns out to have FA, even if mosaic/asymptomatic would carry a very high risk of graft failure. On the other hand, siblings who are only carriers of one heterozygous mutation in an autosomal recessive FA associated gene are eligible as donors.

REFERENCE/SOURCE

- Olson TS. Management of Fanconi anemia beyond childhood. Hematology Am Soc Hematol Educ Program. 2023;2023(1):556-62.

20. A 4-year-old patient diagnosed with FA is transfusion dependent. She showed poor response to Danazol. She underwent bone marrow screening a month back which showed clonal evolution and new translocations on karyotype. The parents are willing for HSCT at this stage and want 16-year-old sibling to be screened. Which is false regarding the HSCT?

A. This is the perfect time to do HSCT as bone marrow shows clonal evolution
B. Transplant outcomes are inferior in patients who are heavily pre-transfused
C. Pretransplant danazol/anabolic steroid therapy generally does not pose any additional challenge
D. Drug therapy is preferred over transplant in view of severe toxicity of transplant

EXPLANATION

The optimal time for HSCT is when cytopenia shifts from moderate to severe, prior to transfusion dependency, probably before androgen therapy, and before clonal evolution.

The androgens oxymetholone and danazol were shown to produce a transient hematologic response in two-thirds of patients, rendering this treatment a reasonable option in patients who cannot access HSCT at a given time, providing them a bridge until the possibility of a transplant occurs. Newer therapies for Fanconi include Eltrombopag, Quercetin, and metformin.

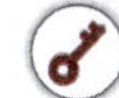

Key: D

BOOST YOUR KNOWLEDGE

Stem cell transplant for Fanconi provides a curative therapy for these patients. Other treatments mainly act as a bridge to transplant. Transplant performed before the onset of MDS/AML or complications of transfusion therapy such as iron overload and alloimmunization carries a better outcome.

REFERENCE/SOURCE

- Dufour C, Pierri F. Modern management of Fanconi anemia. Hematology. 2022;2022(1):649-57.

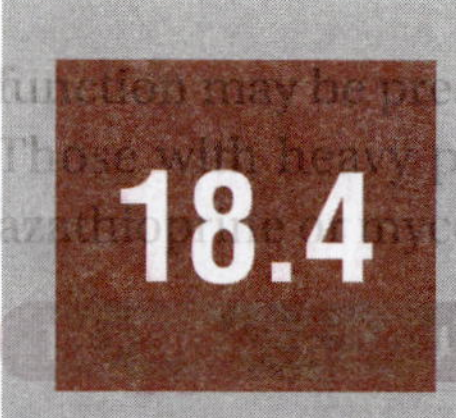

Thalassemia

Sidharth Totadri

1. A 9-month-old girl is brought with lethargy and a pale appearance for 2 months. She was transfused a week back for a low hemoglobin (Hb). She has hepatosplenomegaly on examination. The pretransfusion complete blood count shows Hb 5.4 g/dL, mean corpuscular volume (MCV) 65 fL, mean corpuscular hemoglobin (MCH) 18 pg, mean corpuscular hemoglobin concentration (MCHC) 29%, platelet count 1.52 lakhs/mm^3, and white blood cell (WBC) 35,200/mm^3. Pretransfusion smear picture is shown in given Figure. Which is the best way to confirm diagnosis now?

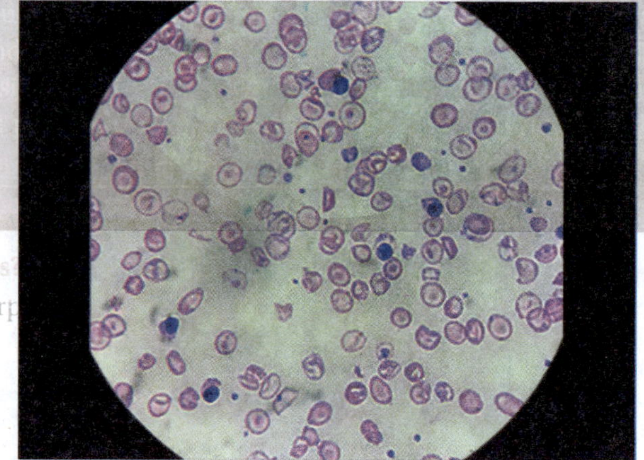

A. High-performance liquid chromatography (HPLC) and reverse dot blot test in the patient
B. HPLC and reverse dot blot test of parents
C. HPLC in parents and reverse dot blot test in the patient
D. HPLC in the patient and reverse dot blot test in parents

EXPLANATION

The child has presented in the second half of infancy with pallor and hepatosplenomegaly. The complete blood count shows microcytic hypochromic anemia and the smear shows target cells and nucleated red blood cells (NRBCs). The most likely clinical diagnosis would be thalassemia. A pretransfusion complete blood count and peripheral smear are crucial to the diagnosis of the etiology in children with anemia. Since red blood cells (RBCs) have a lifespan of 120 days, recent transfusion renders further functional or morphological testing in the blood unreliable. Hence, performing HPLC for Hb variant analysis should be avoided in this patient who has been transfused 1 week back. Since thalassemia is an autosomal recessive disease, both parents would be heterozygous carriers and an HPLC performed in them can identify their carrier state. Since mutational testing (reverse dot blot test) will not be affected by a transfusion 1 week back, it can be done in the patient.

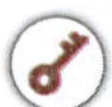

Key: C

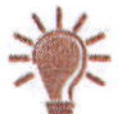

BOOST YOUR KNOWLEDGE

Beta-thalassemia major is a hemoglobinopathy with autosomal recessive inheritance. Approximately 3–4% of Indians are carriers of beta-thalassemia. Since fetal hemoglobin (HbF, $\alpha_2\gamma_2$) declines after birth and adult hemoglobin (HbA, $\alpha_2\beta_2$) emerges as the predominant Hb by 6 months age, beta-thalassemia manifests usually in the second 6 months of life. Microcytic hypochromic anemia with target cells and NRBCs on the peripheral smear characterizes the disorder. Notably, NRBC can cause spurious elevation of the WBC count [corrected WBC = reported WBC × {100/(100 + NRBC count per 100 WBC)}]. The diagnosis is confirmed by a quantification of Hb variants by HPLC or Hb electrophoresis which demonstrates high HbF levels in patients and >4% HbA2 ($\alpha_2\delta_2$) levels in carriers. Hb variant analysis can be affected by recent transfusions and an age of <6 months when HbF is physiologically high. Genetic confirmation of beta-thalassemia is done by demonstrating biallelic mutations by reverse dot-blot or amplification refractory mutation system-polymerase chain reaction (ARMS-PCR) technique which identifies the six common mutations prevalent in India.

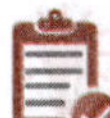

REFERENCE/SOURCE

- Ghosh K, Colah R, Manglani M, Choudhry VP, Verma I, Madan N, et al. Guidelines for screening, diagnosis and management of hemoglobinopathies. Indian J Hum Genet. 2014;20(2):101-19.

2. A 6-year-old boy from West Bengal is evaluated for anemia needing one to two transfusions per year since the age of 3 years and failure to thrive. Examination shows frontoparietal bossing and hepatosplenomegaly. The complete blood count shows Hb 6.4 g/dL, MCV 72 fL, MCH 28 pg, MCHC 32%, platelet count 1.505 lakhs/mm³, and WBC 15,200/mm³. HPLC showed HbA 6.8%, HbA2 41%, and HbF 52%. What is the most likely diagnosis?

A. Hemoglobin E (HbE)-beta-thalassemia, nontransfusion-dependent phenotype
B. Homozygous HbE, nontransfusion-dependent phenotype
C. Alpha-thalassemia, transfusion-dependent phenotype
D. HbE-alpha-thalassemia, nontransfusion-dependent phenotype

EXPLANATION

The contemporary phenotypic classification of thalassemia recognizes transfusion-dependent phenotype as patients needing regular blood transfusions without which they would have life-threatening complications and a limited lifespan. Patients with a nontransfusion-dependent phenotype seldom need or need intermittent or occasional transfusions. In Hb variant analysis, HbE elutes with HbA2, and therefore an unusually high level of HbA2 points to the presence of HbE. When there is also a high HbF and low HbA level, it suggests a HbE-beta-thalassemia syndrome.

Key: A

BOOST YOUR KNOWLEDGE

Hemoglobin E is a mildly unstable form of Hb that is predisposed to oxidant-induced hemolysis. HbE carrier state is common in the Eastern part of India. A heterozygous or homozygous state HbE does not manifest with significant anemia and only causes microcytic hypochromic RBC indices. However, in combination with another hemoglobinopathy, particularly a beta-globin chain defect it can present akin to beta-thalassemia. The spectrum of manifestations ranges from nontransfusion to transfusion-dependent thalassemia. The management is similar to beta-thalassemia.

REFERENCES/SOURCES

- Farmakis D, Porter J, Taher A, Domenica Cappellini M, Angastiniotis M, Eleftheriou A. 2021 Thalassaemia International Federation Guidelines for the Management of Transfusion-dependent Thalassemia. Hemasphere. 2022;6(8):e732.
- Fucharoen S, Weatherall DJ. The Hemoglobin E Thalassemias. Cold Spring Harb Perspect Med. 2012;2:a011734.

3. A 13-year-old boy weighing 35 kg with transfusion-dependent beta-thalassemia has a serum ferritin of 2,900 ng/mL and is receiving deferasirox 1,500 mg per day in a compliant manner. He undergoes a T2* MRI scan which shows a T2* value of 6 ms. For the last week, he is having exertional dyspnea. What is the most appropriate management strategy?

A. To continue the same chelation strategy
B. To increase the dose of deferasirox to 2,000 mg/day
C. To start desferrioxamine therapy
D. To start dexrazoxane therapy

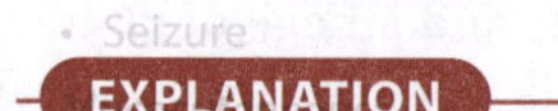

EXPLANATION

Monitoring and managing iron overload is a vital part of managing patients with thalassemia, particularly when they are transfusion-dependent. Serum ferritin is the most common measure used but is an indirect and nonspecific estimate of iron overload. It does not reflect the end-organ damage that has occurred due to the iron overload. T2* MRI scan can assess the iron content in myocardial septum and the T2* value is inversely related to the cardiac iron load. T2* <10 ms is associated with a high risk of cardiac failure. Of the three iron chelators that are available, namely, deferasirox, deferiprone, and desferrioxamine; the last one desferrioxamine has the best action on cardiac iron overload. Hence, in the index patient who has developed a critical cardiac iron overload despite a good dose of deferasirox, desferrioxamine therapy must be considered to reverse the risk of cardiac failure. Dexrazoxane is not used in thalassemia and is a drug that abrogates the cardiac toxicity of anthracyclines in patients with cancer.

Key: C

BOOST YOUR KNOWLEDGE

Transfusions with 1 mL of packed red blood cells (PRBCs) contributing 1.16 mg of iron and a hepcidin-suppressed state leading to increased gastrointestinal absorption of iron leads to iron overload in thalassemia. The cumulative iron overload predominantly affects the liver, heart, and endocrine organs. Serum ferritin is a cheap test to assess iron overload and can be repeated regularly to see the trend. A T2* MRI is a noninvasive test and gives an idea of cardiac iron overload. Invasive liver iron concentration (LIC) estimation by biopsy has fallen out of favor and contemporary MRI techniques are able to estimate the LIC in a noninvasive manner. A serum ferritin of <2,500 ng/mL, T2* of >20 ms, and LIC of <7 mg/g of dry weight of the liver indicate an optimal chelation strategy. The given Table summarizes the three available iron chelators. Deferasirox is the most popular drug due to its oral once-daily dose and better tolerance. Desferrioxamine is the only effective drug if there is heart failure.

Parameter	*Desferrioxamine*	*Deferiprone*	*Deferasirox*
Dose	20–50 mg/kg/day 5–7 days a week as infusion for 8–12 hours	75–100 mg/kg/day in three divided doses	20–40 mg/kg/day as a once-daily dose (30% lesser if film-coated tablets)
Route of administration	Subcutaneous/intravenous	Oral	Oral
Adverse events	Skeletal dysplasia, eye and ear toxicity, infection with *Yersinia/ Mucor*	Neutropenia/ agranulocytosis, arthralgia/ arthritis	Raised liver enzymes, increased creatinine, proteinuria
End organ effects	Only drug effective if established heart failure	Good cardiac chelation	Good whole-body effect

REFERENCES/SOURCES

- Farmakis D, Porter J, Taher A, Domenica Cappellini M, Angastiniotis M, Eleftheriou A. 2021 Thalassaemia International Federation Guidelines for the Management of Transfusion-dependent Thalassemia. Hemasphere. 2022;6(8):e732.
- Saliba AN, Harb AR, Taher AT. Iron chelation therapy in transfusion-dependent thalassemia patients: current strategies and future directions. J Blood Med. 2015;6:197-209.

4. A 5-year-old girl with beta-thalassemia was initially receiving monthly transfusions at a center that does extended phenotyping of RBCs and maintains a pretransfusion Hb of 8–9 g/dL. Since the last 6 months despite 2-weekly transfusions, the Hb is 5–6 g/dL. She has early satiety and is having poor weight gain. Her WBC count is 2,700/mm^3 and her platelet count is 50,000/mm^3. Which of the following strategies will benefit her?

A. Transfuse irradiated blood
B. Offer splenectomy
C. Test for alloimmunization and do direct Coombs test
D. Immunosuppression with steroids and rituximab

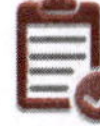

EXPLANATION

The recommended transfusion strategy for transfusion-dependent thalassemia is to transfuse PRBC every 2–5 weeks to maintain a pretransfusion Hb of above 9–10.5 g/dL. An extended red cell antigen typing including ABO, Rh, and Kell antigens, and issuing products compatible with all these antigens reduces the risk of alloimmunization with repeated transfusions. Although leukodepletion is recommended to reduce alloimmunization in thalassemia, irradiation of blood products is not necessary. Irradiation is relevant to reduce the risk of transfusion-associated graft-versus-host disease (GVHD) in immunocompromised patients and in the setting of a bone marrow transplant. The presence of early satiety and pancytopenia points to symptomatic splenomegaly and hypersplenism and this patient may benefit with splenectomy.

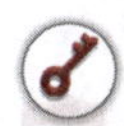

Key: B

BOOST YOUR KNOWLEDGE

An annual transfusion requirement of >200 mL/kg/year should alert the clinician. Alloimmunization and hypersplenism are two possible causes. Alloimmunization is avoided by leukodepletion of blood (can be done prestorage, pretransfusion, or during transfusion by the use of bedside leukocyte reduction filters). Symptomatic splenomegaly, hypersplenism, and increased blood requirements are indications to consider splenectomy. Postsplenectomy sepsis, pulmonary hypertension, and a prothrombotic state are adverse effects of splenectomy. Vaccination for pneumococcus, *Haemophilus influenzae*, and meningococcus must be administered 4–6 weeks before splenectomy and chemoprophylaxis with penicillin should be offered postprocedure.

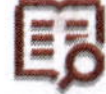

REFERENCE/SOURCE

- Farmakis D, Porter J, Taher A, Domenica Cappellini M, Angastiniotis M, Eleftheriou A. 2021 Thalassaemia International Federation Guidelines for the Management of Transfusion-dependent Thalassemia. Hemasphere. 2022;6(8):e732.

5. A 4-year-old boy who was planned for an elective surgical procedure and had no significant past medical history was referred for an abnormal complete blood count report to the hematologist. The complete blood count revealed Hb 9.4 g/dL, packed cell volume (PCV) 28.5, MCV 56 fL, MCH 18 pg, MCHC 32%, red cell distribution width (RDW) 16, platelet count 4.2 lakhs/mm^3, and WBC 11,200/mm^3. RBC count is 4.8 million/mm^3. The patient has been receiving regular iron supplementation for the last 2 months. Which of the following statements is correct?

A. The Mentzer index is <13 and the child is likely to be a thalassemia carrier
B. The Mentzer index is >13 and the child has iron refractory iron deficiency
C. The Mentzer index is >13 and the child is likely to be a thalassemia carrier
D. The Mentzer index is <13 and the child has iron deficiency

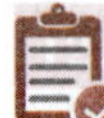

EXPLANATION

The Mentzer index is calculated by the formula MCV/RBC count. A value <13 favors the diagnosis of a thalassemia carrier status while a value >13 favors iron deficiency anemia. The distinction between the entities is important for management. Both present as microcytic hypochromic anemia. The other differentials for microcytic anemia include sideroblastic anemia and lead poisoning. The given table shows the differences between the two entities based on common parameters.

Differences between RBC indices and iron parameters in iron deficiency and thalassemia carrier state:

Parameter	*Iron deficiency anemia*	*Thalassemia minor*
Hemoglobin	Reduced	Normal to reduced (usually >9 g/dL)
RBC count	Reduced	Normal to increased
Mean corpuscular volume	Reduced	Reduced
RDW	Increased	Preserved*
Ferritin	Reduced	Normal
Total iron binding capacity	Increased	Normal
Peripheral smear	Microcytic hypochromic cells, pencil cells, and anisopoikilocytosis	Microcytic hypochromic cells, occasional target cells
HbA2 level in hemoglobin variant analysis	Normal	Increased >3.5%

*Note that RDW can be increased in patients with thalassemia disease (thalassemia major and intermedia) due to significant hemolysis and fragmented cells.

Key: A

BOOST YOUR KNOWLEDGE

Approximately 3.5% of the Indian population are thalassemia carriers. They are heterozygous for the thalassemia mutation and are clinically asymptomatic. They can be diagnosed based on the parameters given in the Table. A Hb <9 g/dL should prompt evaluation for deficiency of iron/folic acid/vitamin B_{12} which requires correction akin to the general population. A healthy carrier maintaining Hb >9 g/dL does not require any therapeutic intervention. It is also vital to counsel the family of a thalassemia carrier with regard to the inheritance of thalassemia and the 25% risk of disease in the offspring if two carriers marry. Rarely, mutations such as the Cap + 1 (A–C) and IVS-II-844 may lead to a "silent carrier" state with normal red cell indices. The NESTROFT (Naked Eye Single Tube Red Cell Osmotic Fragility Test) method is a screening test based on the relative resistance of thalassemic red cells to osmotic fragility in saline.

REFERENCE/SOURCE

- Choudhry VP. Thalassemia minor and major: current management. Indian J Pediatr. 2017;84(8):607-11.

6. A 14-month-old boy was found to be pale at the age of 2 months and was transfused for anemia twice till the age of 1 year. He had no organomegaly on examination. The complete blood count showed a Hb 5.8 g/dL, PCV is 19.2, MCV 71 fL, MCH 21.5 pg, MCHC 30.3%, RDW 21.2, platelet count 2.2 lakhs/mm^3, and WBC 6,500/mm^3. The peripheral smear showed microcytes, hypochromia, fine basophilic stippling, and nucleated red cells. Hb variant father: HbF 1.3%, HbA 85.7%, and HbA2 2.5%. Hb variant mother: HbF 0.4% HbA 97%, HbA2 3%. Identify the best test to confirm diagnosis.

A. ARMS-PCR for common beta-globin chain mutations
B. Sickle prep test
C. Lead levels in blood
D. Supravital staining of peripheral smear

EXPLANATION

This child has manifested with anemia in early infancy (before the HbF levels fall significantly) and his parents' Hb variant analyses do not show elevated HbA2. Hence, he is unlikely to have beta-thalassemia. Yet nucleated red cells with microcytic, hypochromic red cell indices point to thalassemia which can be alpha-thalassemia. Basophilic stippling in lead poisoning is coarse and the differential would be highly unusual in this baby who manifested so early in life. The parental Hb variant analyses also do not show evidence of sickle trait. A supravital staining of the smear will demonstrate the "golf-body" inclusions on red cell membranes that are typical of alpha-thalassemia.

Key: D

BOOST YOUR KNOWLEDGE

The alpha-globin chain of Hb is coded by two pairs of genes on chromosome 16. The deletion/mutation of 1, 2, 3, and all 4 genes respectively leads to asymptomatic carrier state, asymptomatic alpha-thalassemia minor, symptomatic hemoglobin H (HbH) disease, and life-threatening Hb Bart's hydrops fetalis. HbH and Bart's Hb are tetramers of beta- and gamma-globin chains, respectively, which are unstable and lead to membrane damage and hemolysis, HbH disease is more severe if the mutation is nondeletional than deletional. The clinical manifestations can range from mild anemia with an increased predisposition to oxidants to induced hemolysis to severe anemia requiring transfusions. The complete blood count and smear findings are similar to beta-thalassemia, but special staining with brilliant cresyl blue can show the HbH inclusions (giving the appearance of a golf ball). A Hb variant analysis can show the HbH as an early peak but can be missed in some techniques such as HPLC unless the instrument is set to detect. Gap-PCR is the test that is used to detect alpha-chain mutations. Management is similar to beta-thalassemia. However, HbF increasing strategies such as hydroxyurea will be less beneficial as alpha chains are not being produced.

REFERENCE/SOURCE

- Viprakasit V. Alpha-thalassemia syndromes: from clinical and molecular diagnosis to bedside management. Stockholm, Sweden: European Hematology Association; 2013. pp. 329-38.

7. An 18-year-old boy weighing 50 kg with transfusion-dependent thalassemia and a β^0/β^0 genotype was finding it increasingly difficult to obtain regular transfusions due to alloimmunization. Identify the *incorrect* statement from the options with regards to starting him on luspatercept.

A. The starting dose of the drug will be 50 mg
B. The β^0/β^0 genotype is a contraindication for the drug
C. He has to be administered the drug three weekly
D. The drug acts by enhancing erythropoiesis

EXPLANATION

Luspatercept is a transforming growth factor beta (TGF-β) superfamily ligand trap molecule that has been shown to enhance late erythropoiesis. It is administered at a starting dose of 1 mg/kg every 3 weeks and can be increased up to 1.25 mg/kg. β^0 genotype refers to an almost absent production of beta chains in comparison to a β^+ genotype where a reduced amount of beta chains are produced. Though the effect is lesser, luspatercept has been shown to benefit even the genotype with severe beta-chain deficiency.

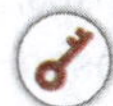

Key: B

BOOST YOUR KNOWLEDGE

Ligands belonging to the TGF-β super-family (e.g., activin) bind to their receptors and activate the Smad 2/3 pathway which in turn triggers hepcidin expression and ineffective erythropoiesis. Ineffective erythropoiesis is a unique feature of thalassemia that distinguishes it from other hemolytic anemias where the bone marrow is intact and hyperplastic in response to the anemia. The reticulocyte count as a result is less elevated in comparison to other hemolytic anemias such as membranopathies and enzymopathies. Activin ligand traps such as luspatercept prevent this downstream hepcidin activation and facilitate normal erythropoiesis to compensate for the hemolysis. The randomized phase 3 BELIEVE trial performed in adults with transfusion-dependent beta-thalassemia showed that the proportions of patients who had a >33% reduction (70% vs. 30%) and >50% reduction (40% vs. 6%) were greater in the luspatercept group in comparison to the placebo group. The drug was relatively well tolerated with musculoskeletal pain, hypertension, dizziness, and hyperuricemia noted as adverse events. The phase 2 BEYOND trial has shown a benefit in nontransfusion-dependent thalassemia too, with 77% showing an increased Hb of 1 g/dL. Trials in children are underway.

REFERENCE/SOURCE

- Cappellini MD, Viprakasit V, Taher AT, Georgiev P, Kuo KHM, Coates T, et al; BELIEVE Investigators: a phase 3 trial of luspatercept in patients with transfusion-dependent β-thalassemia. N Engl J Med. 2020;382(13):1219-31.

8. A 13-year-old girl with thalassemia major is brought by her parents to discuss the option of an allogeneic stem cell transplant. Her serum ferritin is 6,500 ng/mL and her liver is palpable 7 cm below the right costal margin. Her brother who is a full human leukocyte antigen (HLA)-match is a thalassemia carrier. Which of the following statements is correct?

A. The age and liver size will render her a very high-risk subset for transplant
B. The use of thiotepa in conditioning will reduce the risk of sinusoidal obstruction syndrome (SOS)
C. A liver biopsy must be performed before the transplant
D. The brother should not be used as the donor as he carries the thalassemia gene mutation

EXPLANATION

Allogeneic stem cell transplant remains the only curative therapy for thalassemia. Gene therapy is still not available outside clinical trials. The traditional Pesaro risk stratification for transplant in thalassemia used hepatomegaly >2 cm, history of inadequate chelation, and portal fibrosis in liver biopsy as three adverse factors to classify as class I (none present), class II (1 or 2 present), and class III (all 3 present). Performing a liver biopsy is cumbersome and is seldom performed in the current era of thalassemia management. The Vellore risk stratification identified the very-high risk subset with age >7 years and a liver span of >5 cm (the index case will thus be very high risk). The use of the drug treosulfan has been shown to reduce the risk of SOS in comparison to busulfan (though thiotepa is also used for conditioning, it is not related to the risk reduction of SOS). It is acceptable to use thalassemia carriers as donors as the recipient will also convert to a carrier phenotype post-successful transplant and will stop needing transfusions.

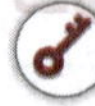

Key: A

BOOST YOUR KNOWLEDGE

Sinusoidal obstruction syndrome or veno-occlusive disease (VOD) of the liver is a life-threatening complication of transplant in thalassemia and is characterized by right upper quadrant pain, tender hepatomegaly, weight gain (>2–5% of baseline), jaundice, and ascites/pleural effusion occurring typically in the first 3 weeks of transplant. Refractory thrombocytopenia and multiorgan failure can ensue. In addition to fluid restriction and diuretics, defibrotide is the drug of choice for management when available. Patients with thalassemia are predisposed to this complication due to prior liver injury due to iron overload. Busulfan promotes VOD by depleting antioxidants. The use of treosulfan in place of busulfan has been shown to significantly reduce the risk of VOD posttransplant in thalassemia.

REFERENCE/SOURCE

- Mathews V, Balasubramanian P, Abraham A, George B, Srivastava A. Allogenic stem cell transplantation for thalassemia major in India. Pediatr Hematol Oncol. 2017;2(4):114-20.

9. An 8-year-old boy is brought for evaluation of poor height gain. He has received transfusions two times in the last 2 years. He has frontoparietal bossing, pallor, and hepatosplenomegaly. The height is 100 cm. The complete blood count showed a Hb of 7.2 g/dL, PCV is 22.2, MCV 56 fL, MCH 18.5 pg, MCHC 31%, RDW 19, platelet count 2.8 lakhs/mm^3, and WBC 5,500/mm^3. The peripheral smear showed target cells and nucleated red cells. The HPLC test showed HbA 22% and HbF 75%. Besides transfusion has not received any other medications. Identify the correct statement about his management.

A. Splenectomy should be performed upfront
B. A trial of hydroxyurea can be offered
C. He should be evaluated for iron overload and initiated on desferrioxamine infusion
D. He should be evaluated for hypogonadism and hormonal therapy

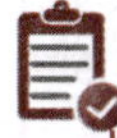

EXPLANATION

The phenotype of the patient is consistent with a nontransfusion-dependent beta-thalassemia (NTDT) or beta-thalassemia major as the patient has not required regular transfusions to sustain life. Splenectomy is currently not a favored approach in children with thalassemia. It is reserved for patients who have severe anemia affecting growth/development for whom transfusions or chelation are difficult, hypersplenism, symptomatic splenomegaly with pain or early satiety, and massive splenomegaly with a risk of splenic rupture. Hydroxyurea is a reasonable frontline approach for the management of a patient with newly diagnosed NTDT. Transfusional iron overload is contributed by an increased gastrointestinal absorption in patients with NTDT which in turn is a result of the ineffective erythropoiesis that increases erythropoietin and suppresses hepcidin. Serum ferritin assessment is recommended usually at the age of 10 years. A ferritin of >800 ng/mL should prompt the initiation of deferasirox at the dose of 10 mg/kg/day as the preferred iron chelator. Endocrinopathies due to iron overload usually manifest after the age of 10 years. Hypogonadism is suspected if puberty is delayed by 14 years in males/13 years in girls or absent testicular/breast development by the age of 16 years. Other complications of NTDT include osteoporosis, pulmonary hypertension, hypercoagulable state, leg ulcers, and extramedullary hematopoietic pseudotumors.

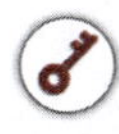

Key: B

BOOST YOUR KNOWLEDGE

Hydroxyurea is a HbF inducer that increases the gamma-chain production by enhancing the messenger ribonucleic acid (mRNA) expression for gamma-chain production and by inducing a stress erythropoiesis. It is started at a dose of 10 mg/kg/day and can be given up to 20 mg/kg/day and a rise in hemoglobin of >1 g/dL at 6 months of therapy is taken as response. Patients with the XmnI polymorphism have been shown to respond better to the drug. Complete blood count and hepatic and renal functions should be monitored during therapy.

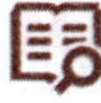

REFERENCE/SOURCE

- Taher A, Vichinsky E, Musallam K, Cappellini MD, Viprakasit V. Guidelines for the Management of Non Transfusion Dependent Thalassaemia (NTDT). Nicosia (Cyprus): Thalassaemia International Federation; 2013.

10. A 17-year-old girl with transfusion-dependent thalassemia is brought by her parents who wish to understand the option of gene therapy. Identify the correct sequence of events while performing gene therapy in thalassemia.

A. Infusion of a lentiviral vector containing the functional beta-globin gene to patient >myeloablation of the patient with chemotherapy >await count recovery
B. Mobilization of peripheral blood stem cells from the patient with filgrastim and plerixafor >transduction of cells with a lentiviral vector containing the functional beta-globin gene >myeloablation of the patient with chemotherapy >infusion of manipulated stem cells
C. Bone marrow harvest from the patient >transduction of cells with lentiviral vector containing the functional beta-globin gene >myeloablation of patient with chemotherapy >infusion of manipulated stem cells
D. Mobilization of stem cells from the patient with filgrastim and plerixafor >transduction with a lentiviral vector containing the functional beta-globin gene >reduced intensity conditioning to patient >infusion of manipulated stem cells

EXPLANATION

In gene therapy, the autologous hematopoietic stem cells from the patient are mobilized using granulocyte colony-stimulating factor (G-CSF) and plerixafor. A lentiviral vector integrates the normal beta-globin gene into the host genome as an ex vivo process. Similar to bone marrow transplant, myeloablation of the bone marrow using a busulfan-based or thiotepa/treosulfan-based conditioning regimen is done followed by reinfusion of the stem cells carrying the transduced gene back to the patient.

Key: B

BOOST YOUR KNOWLEDGE

Gene therapy offers potential cure to patients with thalassemia without the risk of a GVHD that threatens patients undergoing allogeneic transplant. Phase 1–2 clinical trials based in Europe and USA have evaluated the modality and found it to be safe and effective. High cost, toxicity of conditioning regimen, and the need for using G-CSF particularly in patients with splenomegaly are causes of concern in gene therapy. Besides the viral-vector-based addition of the functional beta-globin gene, other gene-based techniques in thalassemia include (1) gene correction or precision genome editing using nucleases that induce deoxyribonucleic acid (DNA) strand breaks at precise areas followed by repair (CRISPR-systems), (2) induction of gamma-chain production by targeting the *BCL11A* gene that suppresses gamma chains during the switch from HbF to HbA, and (3) suppression of alpha-chain production by short interfering RNAs.

REFERENCE/SOURCE

- Thompson AA, Walters MC, Kwiatkowski J, Rasko JEJ, Ribeil JA, Hongeng S, et al. Gene therapy in patients with transfusion-dependent β-thalassemia. N Engl J Med. 2018;378(16):1479-93.

11. A couple who are visiting the clinic with their first child who has beta-thalassemia major with a known mutation [homozygous for IVSI-5 (G>C)] say that the mother is now 10 weeks pregnant. They wish to know the thalassemia status of the fetus. What is the correct strategy?

A. Chorionic villus sampling followed by next-generation sequencing
B. Chorionic villus sampling followed by PCR
C. Amniocentesis followed by PCR
D. Cordocentesis followed by next-generation sequencing

EXPLANATION

Thalassemia is inherited in an autosomal recessive manner. If a child has thalassemia major or intermedia, it implies that both parents are thalassemia carriers and there is a 25% risk of thalassemia disease in each pregnancy. Therefore, it is essential to offer antenatal counseling and diagnosis to the parents after the diagnosis of thalassemia in a child. The options include chorionic villus sampling between 10 and 12 weeks, amniocentesis after 16 weeks of gestation, and cordocentesis at 18–20 weeks of gestation. Safe termination of pregnancy can be offered before 20 weeks of gestation. Since the genetic mutation is already known from the first child, there is no necessity for next-generation sequencing and a PCR-based method can identify the presence or absence of the mutation in the fetus.

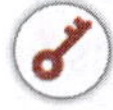

Key: B

BOOST YOUR KNOWLEDGE

About 90% of patients with beta-thalassemia in India have one of the five following mutations: IVSI-5 (G>C), IVSI-1 (G>T), 619-bp del, codon 41/42 (–TCTT), and codon 8/9 (+G). Since most patients have genetic mutations that are part of a known set of mutations, the most common techniques used for genetic diagnosis are reverse dot blot analysis or ARMS-PCR which will screen for and identify the most common mutations. In 10–15% of cases, if this does not identify the mutation, beta-globin chain DNA sequencing can be done. Next-generation sequencing is seldom needed if the clinical evaluation, complete blood count, peripheral smear, and Hb variant analysis all corroborate with the diagnosis of thalassemia.

REFERENCES/SOURCES

- Ministry of Health and Family Welfare. Prevention and Control of Hemoglobinopathies in India—Thalassemias, Sickle Cell Disease and Other Variant Hemoglobinopathies. New Delhi: Ministry of Health and Family Welfare, Government of India; 2016.
- Sinha S, Black ML, Agarwal S, Colah R, Das R, Ryan K, et al. Profiling β-thalassaemia mutations in India at state and regional levels: implications for genetic education, screening and counselling programmes. Hugo J. 2009;3(1-4):51-62.

12. A 5-year-old boy with NTDT is on regular follow-up. He has not been transfused till date. His Hb is maintained between 7 and 8 g/dL. He has a spleen that is palpable 3 cm below the costal margin. His height is 105 cm and his weight is 18 kg. He is active and attends school regularly. Select the correct statement with regard to blood transfusions.

A. He needs to be started on transfusions to maintain Hb 9–10.5 g/dL
B. He needs to be started on transfusions to address his growth
C. He needs to be started on transfusions as he has a significant splenectomy
D. He can be followed up further without transfusions

EXPLANATION

The target Hb of 9–10.5 g/dL is only for transfusion-dependent thalassemia who have life-threatening fall in Hb in the absence of periodic transfusions. However, in a nontransfusion-dependent thalassemia such as the index case, there is no particular target Hb in a clinically well child. Splenectomy is not indicated for palpable splenectomy. Rather, it is restricted to cases with symptomatic splenomegaly, hypersplenism, massive splenomegaly, or an increased transfusion requirement which is difficult to meet. A conservative strategy without transfusions is acceptable in a child with NTDT if he or she is growing well, the spleen is not progressively increasing in size with a relatively stable Hb, and the child is keeping up with peers at school.

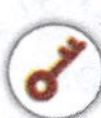

Key: D

BOOST YOUR KNOWLEDGE

As per the thalassemia international federation guidelines for NTDT, the indications for transfusion include the following: A fall in the Hb level accompanied by progressive enlargement of the spleen (at a rate of >3 cm/year in a growing child), falling height for age centiles, poor scholastic performance, reduced exercise tolerance, failure to develop secondary sexual characteristics in accordance with the bone age, significant musculoskeletal changes, and suboptimal quality of life. Occasionally, periods of stress, infection, and pregnancy may necessitate transfusion. Certain complications of NTDT such as a stroke, pulmonary hypertension (likely if tricuspid valve regurgitant jet velocity of >3.2 m/s or >2.5 m/s with symptoms/other echo findings; possible if only tricuspid regurgitation velocity (TRV) >2.5 m/s with no other symptoms/echo findings), extramedullary hematopoietic pseudotumors, and leg ulcers may benefit with transfusions for management and primary/secondary prevention. Alloimmunization is a very challenging complication to manage and the risk increases with increasing age of onset of transfusion. Hence, this risk must be balanced with the benefit of starting an older child with NTDT on transfusions.

REFERENCE/SOURCE

- Taher A, Vichinsky E, Musallam K, Cappellini MD, Viprakasit V. Guidelines for the Management of Non Transfusion Dependent Thalassaemia (NTDT). Nicosia (Cyprus): Thalassaemia International Federation; 2013.

13. An 18-year-old male with transfusion-dependent beta-thalassemia has presented with a fracture of the left femur after a trivial fall. He has been having bone pains for the last few months. A dual-energy X-ray absorptiometry was performed which showed a bone mineral density of T-score of –1.5. Serum vitamin D level is 18 nmol/L. Examination reveals delayed development of secondary sexual characteristics. Once the fracture is addressed, the most appropriate management will entail:

A. Hormonal replacement therapy, vitamin D and calcium supplementation, bisphosphonates
B. Hormonal replacement therapy, vitamin D, and calcium supplementation
C. Hormonal replacement therapy, bisphosphonates, avoid calcium/vitamin D with bisphosphonates
D. Calcium supplementation and hormonal replacement therapy

EXPLANATION

It is important to assess bone marrow density (BMD) annually in patients with transfusion-dependent and nontransfusion-dependent thalassemia after adolescence. A BMD of ≤2.5 is associated with osteoporosis and a high risk of fracture. Delayed puberty and hypogonadism can lead to overdiagnosis of osteoporosis. Hence, bone age must be used to interpret BMD rather than actual age. In the index case, the pathological fracture implies a definite osteoporotic state. Vitamin D level is low (<25 mmol/L) and needs supplementation too. The patient needs management of calcium/vitamin D status, hypogonadism, and severe osteoporosis with bisphosphonates.

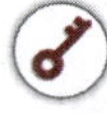

Key: A

BOOST YOUR KNOWLEDGE

Bone disease in thalassemia is multifactorial and contributed by the ineffective erythropoiesis/marrow expansion, iron overload-induced bone toxicity, hypogonadism, growth hormone/insulin-like growth factor 1 deficiency, and chelation-induced adverse events (desferrioxamine causes skeletal dysplasia and deferiprone causes arthralgia/arthropathy). Additional factors include nutritional deficiencies, hypoparathyroidism, diabetes mellitus, relative lack of physical activity, and liver disease. Regular transfusions to suppress marrow expansion, optimal iron chelation, encouragement of physical activity, encouraging adequate calcium/vitamin D intake, and monitoring/early management for endocrinopathies such as hypothyroidism and hypogonadism prevent bone loss.

Annual BMD measurement must be done from adolescence. Bisphosphonates (oral alendronate or intravenous zoledronate/pamidronate) are recommended to manage severe osteoporosis in thalassemia. It is important to supplement calcium and vitamin D with monitoring of urine calcium excretion to avoid hypercalciuria and nephrocalcinosis. Teriparatide, a recombinant parathyroid hormone analog; strontium ranelate, an anabolic agent; and denosumab, a RANKL antibody are novel agents in the management of bone disease in thalassemia.

REFERENCE/SOURCE

- Farmakis D, Porter J, Taher A, Domenica Cappellini M, Angastiniotis M, Eleftheriou A. 2021 Thalassaemia International Federation Guidelines for the Management of Transfusion-dependent Thalassemia. Hemasphere. 2022;6(8):e732.

14. A 9-year-old girl with transfusion-dependent thalassemia is on regular chelation with desferrioxamine at a dose of 20 mg/kg/day over 8 hours per day for 5 days a week with oral vitamin C 500 mg/day. On routine evaluation, her serum ferritin is 250 ng/mL. Her recent T2* MRI showed a cardiac T2* of 22 ms and an MRI estimated LIC of 2.8 mg/g. The correct action now is:

A. Continue the same management as the iron overload parameters are well within control
B. Stop vitamin C and continue desferrioxamine at the same dose
C. Stop desferrioxamine and do a hearing evaluation
D. Continue desferrioxamine at 3 days a week and reassess parameters after 1 month

EXPLANATION

Desferrioxamine has a narrow therapeutic index with a high risk of adverse events. The therapeutic index is calculated as daily dose (mg/kg) divided by serum ferritin (ng/mL). The index must be maintained at <0.025. In the index case, the value is 20/250 = 0.08 which is high, and therefore warrants discontinuation of the drug. Vitamin C is administered with desferrioxamine at a dose of 2–3 mg/kg/day to increase the availability of the chelatable iron and facilitate its iron secretion. Vitamin C is not started in the first few weeks of chelation.

Key: C

BOOST YOUR KNOWLEDGE

A serum ferritin level of A serum ferritin level of ≥2,500 ng/mL, LIC of >7 mg/g, and cardiac T2* MRI <20 ms are indications for intensifying chelation. Conversely a serum ferritin of <300 ng/mL and LIC of <3 mg/g are indications to stop chelation. Desferrioxamine, although efficacious in its effect on iron chelation, is less preferred for its parenteral route of administration and a high risk of toxicity. Adverse events with desferrioxamine include high-frequency sensorineural hearing loss, visual disturbances, growth retardation, skeletal dysplasia (sitting height is important to assess in patients as there can be a shortening of the vertebral bodies), infections with *Yersinia* and *Mucor* and rarely, hypersensitivity reactions.

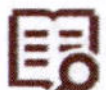

REFERENCE/SOURCE

- Taher AT, Bou-Fakhredin R, Kattamis A, Viprakasit V, Cappellini MD. Improving outcomes and quality of life for patients with transfusion-dependent β-thalassemia: recommendations for best clinical practice and the use of novel treatment strategies. Expert Rev Hematol. 2021;14(10):897-909.

15. A 19-year-old girl with transfusion-dependent thalassemia is requiring two weekly transfusions to maintain an Hb of 8–9 g/dL before transfusion. The family has heard about the use of thalidomide for reducing transfusion requirement and wishes to discuss the pros and cons. Which of the following is *not* a known toxicity of thalidomide?

A. Peripheral neuropathy
B. Teratogenicity
C. Hypercoagulable state
D. Arthropathy

EXPLANATION

In the absence of a curative therapy such as an allogeneic stem cell transplant or gene therapy which is still not within the reach of many patients with thalassemia, maintaining the ideal pretransfusion Hb is challenging. Several studies and a meta-analysis have shown that thalidomide use can benefit patients with thalassemia major and intermedia by increasing Hb. Transfusion independence has also been reported. However, it is not recognized as a standard of care treatment for thalassemia. The caveat is the risk of serious adverse events. While constipation, somnolence, elevated liver enzymes, and skin rash are mild and common; peripheral neurotoxicity, thrombosis, seizures, and teratogenicity are serious though infrequent. Arthropathy is not a known adverse event with thalidomide. Rather, it has been used in refractory, rheumatological conditions.

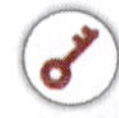

Key: D

BOOST YOUR KNOWLEDGE

Beta-thalassemia typically manifest after the first 6 months of life when the physiological switching from HbF ($\alpha2\gamma2$) to HbA ($\alpha2\beta2$) occurs. Suppression of the switch with continued production of HbF is an attractive target in thalassemia. Hydroxyurea is a time-tested drug, particularly in nontransfusion-dependent thalassemia. However, its effect is limited and seldom benefits patients with transfusion-dependent thalassemia. Thalidomide is a novel HbF inducer that induces γ-globin mRNA expression in a dose-dependent manner. Other mechanisms include enhancing erythroid transcription factors like GATA-1 and inhibiting inflammatory factors like tumor necrosis factor-alpha (TNF-alpha). A meta-analysis showed that thalidomide in doses of 50–200 mg improves the Hb, with a lower dose preferable to avoid side effects. Pomalidomide is an analogous drug with purportedly lesser side effects. Despite the promising effect, the pros and cons should be weighed particularly in children and young females in the reproductive age group. Serious side effects as mentioned earlier include peripheral neurotoxicity, thrombosis including central venous thrombosis, and teratogenicity.

REFERENCE/SOURCE

- Lu Y, Wei Z, Yang G, Lai Y, Liu R. Investigating the efficacy and safety of thalidomide for treating patients with β-thalassemia: a meta-analysis. Front Pharmacol. 2021;12:814302.

16. A 13-year-old boy with nontransfusion-dependent thalassemia required urgent transfusion during the management of malarial infection. At a peripheral healthcare facility, the father being the same blood group donor, donated blood for his transfusion. He recovered from the infection, but 2 weeks later presented with diarrhea and easy fatiguability. He had icterus and an erythematous maculopapular rash on the trunk. The complete blood count shows Hb 6.5 g/dL, WBC 2,100/mm^3, differential leukocyte count shows neutrophil of 12% and lymphocytes of 85%, the platelet count is 35,000/mm^3. Liver function test showed total bilirubin 6.5 mg/dL, conjugated bilirubin 6 mg/dL, serum glutamic oxaloacetic transaminase (SGOT) and serum glutamate pyruvate transaminase (SGPT) being 320 and 280, respectively. What is the most likely diagnosis?

A. Delayed hemolytic reaction
B. Cytomegalovirus (CMV) infection
C. Transfusion-associated GVHD
D. Acute viral hepatitis due to transfusion-transmitted hepatitis

EXPLANATION

Delayed transfusion reaction can occur after 12 weeks of transfusion, manifesting with a drop in Hb level with jaundice. The delayed reaction can be attributed to a hemolysis triggered by an alloantibody that has developed posttransfusion or was undetectable at the time of transfusion. In the index case, the skin rash, pancytopenia, and conjugated hyperbilirubinemia are not explained by this phenomenon.

Severe CMV infection can manifest with pneumonitis, hepatitis, and colitis. However, it would be unusual in this patient with NTDT who would otherwise be immunocompetent. Viral hepatitis such as hepatitis B virus (HBV) and hepatitis C virus (HCV) can occur following improperly screened blood products. The short duration between transfusion and symptoms, pancytopenia, and rash would be unusual with viral hepatitis. Hence, the most likely diagnosis is transfusion-associated GVHD (TA-GVHD) after transfusion from a close HLA-haploidentical relative.

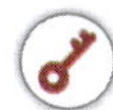
Key: C

BOOST YOUR KNOWLEDGE

Transfusion-associated GVHD is a deadly complication caused by the presence of viable donor lymphocytes in transfused blood products. The risk is high when the recipient is immunocompromised due to inherited or acquired defects in immunity following immunosuppressive therapy such as chemotherapy. Immunocompetent patients can also be affected when the donor is an HLA-haploidentical relative such as a parent or sibling. Following 1–4 weeks of transfusion the patient manifests with liver dysfunction, diarrhea, bone marrow aplasia, fever, and skin rash. Despite treatment with steroids, the outcome is often fatal. Hence, it is important to avoid blood from close relatives and use irradiation of blood products for all immunocompromised patients, such as in the setting of a hematopoietic stem cell transplantation (HSCT) for patients with thalassemia. Leukodepletion does not prevent this complication.

REFERENCE/SOURCE

- Goel R, Tobian AAR, Shaz BH. Noninfectious transfusion-associated adverse events and their mitigation strategies. Blood. 2019;133(17):1831-9.

17. A 3-year-old boy was evaluated for pallor noted by his mother. He had never been transfused before. His diet was predominantly cow milk based. He had no hepatosplenomegaly. His Hb was 7.5 g/dL with MCV 60 fL, MCH 22 pg, MCHC 30%, RDW of 20, WBC count was 5,600, and platelet count was 4.6 lakhs/mm^3 and peripheral smear showed anisopoikilocytosis and pencil cells. The HPLC analysis showed HbA1 70%, HbA2 1.7%, and HbF 28%. What is the most likely diagnosis?

A. Beta-thalassemia intermedia
B. Iron deficiency anemia
C. Iron deficiency anemia with beta-thalassemia trait
D. Iron deficiency with hereditary persistence of HbF

EXPLANATION

The case highlights the importance of a clinical evaluation before interpreting a Hb variant analysis report. The child has no clinical evidence of hemolysis and the cow's milk predominant diet at this age would certainly predispose to iron deficiency. The complete blood count shows a microcytic hypochromic anemia with high RDW and the smear with anisopoikilocytosis and pencil cells suggests iron deficiency. The HbA2 level of 1.7% makes beta-thalassemia trait unlikely as it would be expected to be >3.5%. The HbA level of 70% makes it very unlikely to be beta-thalassemia intermedia where one would expect a higher HbF and lower HbA level. The HbF elevation for the given age would be explained by the hereditary persistence of HbF.

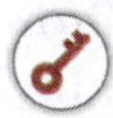
Key: D

BOOST YOUR KNOWLEDGE

Hereditary persistence of HbF is a benign hematological condition where mutations in gamma-globin promoter units or deletions in beta-globin subunit lead to inhibition of the switch that occurs after the first 6 months of life from fetal to HbA. HbF levels can vary from 10 to 40% in heterozygotes and up to 100% in homozygotes.

Mild erythrocytosis may be associated. Hereditary persistence of fetal hemoglobin (HPFH) can be pancellular or heterocellular. When coinherited with beta-thalassemia or sickle cell disease, the mutation can have a beneficial effect on phenotype.

REFERENCE/SOURCE

- Sharma DC, Singhal S, Woike P, Rai S, Yadav M, Gaur R. Hereditary persistence of fetal hemoglobin. Asian J Transfus Sci. 2020;14(2): 185-6.

18. A 3-year-old boy has transfusion-dependent beta-thalassemia. His genetic testing shows compound heterozygosity for the beta-globin chain mutations IVSI-1 (G>T) and 619-bp del with a coexisting heterozygosity for alpha-globin chain mutation $\alpha\alpha\alpha^{anti4.2}$. How will the alpha mutation contribute to the severity of the thalassemia?

A. Increase the severity of the thalassemia syndrome
B. Decrease the severity of the thalassemia syndrome
C. The mutation will have no effect
D. The mutation will lead to coexisting beta-thalassemia and HbH disease

EXPLANATION

Beta-thalassemia is characterized by the deficient production of beta-globin chains and the resulting imbalance between the alpha-beta chain ratio. Excess alpha chains contribute to peripheral hemolysis and premature erythrocyte precursor death and ineffective erythropoiesis. The index case is compound heterozygous for beta-thalassemia mutations. The alpha-chain mutation is notably a triplication which will increase the alpha-chain production. Thus, it will potentially increase the alpha/beta-chain imbalance and the severity of the disease. HbH disease needs deletional/nondeletional mutations involving three of the four genes coding for the alpha chain in the individual and will not occur in this child who has a heterozygous mutation for alpha triplication.

Key: A

BOOST YOUR KNOWLEDGE

Alpha triplication results from an unequal crossover during the recombination of the α1 and α2 Hb. $\alpha\alpha\alpha^{anti4.2}$ and $\alpha\alpha\alpha^{anti4.2}$ are the two mutations that result. Studies have shown up to 4% carrier rate in the Indian population for alpha triplication. The clinical syndrome of coexisting beta-thalassemia and alpha-triplication mutations can range from a thalassemia carrier status to a mild-to-moderate thalassemia intermedia status. Conversely, presence of alpha-chain mutations that lead to deficient alpha-chain production can ameliorate the severity of beta thalassemia by reducing the alpha-beta chain imbalance.

REFERENCE/SOURCE

- Sundaresan DD, Hira JK, Chhabra S, Trehan A, Khadwal AR, Malhotra P, et al. Hematological and genetic profiles of persons with co-inherited heterozygous β-thalassemia and supernumerary α-globin genes. Eur J Haematol. 2023;110(5):510-7.

19. A 6-year-old boy with transfusion-dependent beta-thalassemia weighing 15 kg is prescribed deferasirox dispersible tablet 500 mg per day. The mother finds it difficult to give the tablet in the morning on an empty stomach before he gets ready for school. Which of the following is a reasonable alternative?

A. To continue the same tablet with breakfast
B. To replace by film coated tablet deferasirox 360 mg strength
C. To replace by film coated tablet deferasirox 700 mg strength
D. To advise the same tablet just before going to bed

EXPLANATION

The original formulation of deferasirox is a dispersible tablet that is advised at a dose of 20–40 mg/kg/day as a suspension in water or in orange/apple juice. For best bioavailability, it is taken half an hour before a meal. It has to be taken in an upright position with a glass of water to avoid esophagitis and it is not recommended to lie down immediately after taking the drug. A recently introduced film-coated formulation has been shown to have better bioavailability and can be taken with a light meal at a dose that is 30% lesser than what is recommended for the dispersible form.

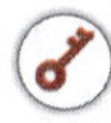

Key: B

BOOST YOUR KNOWLEDGE

The randomized ECLIPSE phase II study compared the safety of dispersible and film-coated tablets of deferasirox. There was better adherence and satisfaction with the film-coated tablets with a lesser frequency of adverse events. In India, the tablet is available as "Oleptiss" manufactured by Novartis. The starting dose is 14 mg/kg/day which can be increased to 28 mg/kg/day (0.7 times the dose used for the original dispersible form). Ensuring compliance with chelation is an important aspect of the management of thalassemia.

REFERENCE/SOURCE

- Taher AT, Origa R, Perrotta S, Kourakli A, Ruffo GB, Kattamis A, et al. New film-coated tablet formulation of deferasirox is well tolerated in patients with thalassemia or lower-risk MDS: results of the randomized, phase II ECLIPSE study. Am J Hematol. 2017; 92(5):420-8.

20. **An 8-year-old girl underwent a matched-sibling donor HSCT with her brother as the donor. At 30 days post-transplant, the donor chimerism is 95%, and at 120 days posttransplant, there is 80% donor chimerism. There is no GVHD. Her Hb is stable and she does not need transfusion. What is the most appropriate next step?**

A. Treat with rituximab
B. Treat with a course of systemic steroids
C. Taper immunosuppression and repeat chimerism
D. Counsel the family for a repeat transplant with an alternative donor

EXPLANATION

Chimerism testing ascertains the proportion of donor and recipient hematopoietic stem cells in the bone marrow after an allogeneic stem cell transplant using genetic tests based on unique tandem number repeats in the DNA sequences of individuals. Conventionally, >95% of donor cell is full donor chimerism; 5–95% is mixed chimerism, and <5% is absent donor chimerism. Compared to transplant for malignancies, where mixed chimerism portends relapse and aggressive treatment, it is more acceptable in benign diseases such as thalassemia as long as the donor cells are able to maintain transfusion-free hematopoiesis.

Key: C

BOOST YOUR KNOWLEDGE

Up to one-third of patients are reported to have mixed chimerism after transplant for hemoglobinopathy. Early mixed chimerism seen after 1 month of transplant has been associated with rejection. However, mixed chimerism at a later date with stable Hb can be tolerated with close follow-up. A reasonable approach to mixed chimerism is tapering the immunosuppression used for prophylaxis of GVHD. Donor lymphocyte infusions are also used, particularly when the chimerism drops with a drop in Hb. Immunosuppression with steroids or rituximab is not used in the management of mixed chimerism.

REFERENCES/SOURCES

- Fouzia NA, Edison ES, Lakshmi KM, Korula A, Velayudhan SR, Balasubramanian P, et al. Long-term outcome of mixed chimerism after stem cell transplantation for thalassemia major conditioned with busulfan and cyclophosphamide. Bone Marrow Transplant. 2018;53(2):169-74.
- Kharfan-Dabaja MA, Kumar A, Ayala E, Aljurf M, Nishihori T, Marsh R, et al. Standardizing Definitions of Hematopoietic Recovery, Graft Rejection, Graft Failure, Poor Graft Function, and Donor Chimerism in Allogeneic Hematopoietic Cell Transplantation: A Report on Behalf of the American Society for Transplantation and Cellular Therapy. Transplant Cell Ther. 2021;27(8):642-9.

CHAPTER

18.5

Hemoglobinopathies and Sickle Cell Disease

Arun Danewa

1. An 8-year-old boy presents to the clinic with complaints of fatigue, weakness, and occasional shortness of breath. On physical examination, he appears pale, and there is no hepatosplenomegaly. His complete blood count (CBC) reveals the following:

- *Hemoglobin:* 7.2 g/dL
- *Mean corpuscular volume (MCV):* 66 fL
- *Mean corpuscular hemoglobin (MCH):* 20 pg
- *Red blood cell (RBC) count:* 4.5 million/mm^3

Based on the provided information, calculate Mentzer index and it favoring which condition?

A. Mentzer index is 14.66 and favoring iron-deficiency anemia
B. Mentzer index is 14.66 and favoring thalassemia major (TM)
C. Mentzer index is 0.06 and favoring iron-deficiency anemia
D. Mentzer index is 3.3 and favoring iron-deficiency anemia

EXPLANATION

Various mathematical formulas have been made to help diagnose thalassemia trait when looking at a microcytic hypochromic anemia. However, it is important to know that none of these formulas are always perfectly accurate. Nonetheless, the Mentzer index is commonly used as an office screening test. It is ratio of MCV/RBC count (in million/mm^3). The RBC count is usually decreased in patients with iron deficiency while normal in thalassemia trait hence Mentzer index >13 in iron-deficiency anemia while <13 in thalassemia trait.

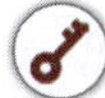

Key: A

BOOST YOUR KNOWLEDGE

Remember Mentzer index for differentiating between iron-deficiency anemia and thalassemia trait (not TM).

The ratio between microcytic (MCV <61 fL) and hypochromic [mean corpuscular hemoglobin concentration (MCHC) <28 g/dL] erythrocytes is a helpful parameter. A ratio >1.0 is highly suggestive of thalassemia trait, whereas a ratio <1.0 is mostly associated with iron deficiency.

	Thalassemia trait	*Iron deficiency*
Mentzer index: MCV/RBC	<13	>13
Shine and Lal index: (MCV)^2 × MCH	<1,530	>1,530

REFERENCE/SOURCE

- Look AT, Ginsburg D, Fisher DE, Nathan DG, Samuel L, Orkin SH. Nathan and Oski's Hematology and Oncology of Infancy and Childhood, 8th edition. Philadelphia: Saunders; 2014. pp. 751-2.

2. A 10-year-old girl is referred to you for the evaluation of an incidentally discovered anemia. Her mother noticed that her eyes occasionally turn yellow, mostly at time with cough and cold episodes. She has no history of recurring pain. Her growth and development parameter are normal. On examination, spleen is 2 cm below the costal margins. The following laboratory tests are available.

Hemoglobin (Hb)	10.2 g/dL
MCV	75 fL
MCHC	36.5 g/dL
Hematocrit (Hct)	31.6%
Reti count	1.5%
Platelet count	220,000/mm^3
Peripheral smear	Many target cells, polychromasia
High-performance liquid chromatography (HPLC)	Hb analysis shows >90% hemoglobin C (HbC) with slight increase in fetal hemoglobin (HbF)

What is this patient's most likely diagnosis?

A. Sickle-β$^+$-thalassemia
B. Sickle-Hgb C disease (Hgb SC)
C. β-thalassemia intermedia (TI)
D. Hemoglobin C disease (Hgb CC)

EXPLANATION

Hemoglobin C homozygosity, or HbC (HbCC) disease progresses in a similar way to sickle cell disease (SCD) but is less severe. Variable hemolytic anemia is the most dominant form.

Clinically mild-to-moderate splenomegaly is common. Laboratory evaluation shows Hb in the range of 10–11 g/dL with increased MCHC. Blood film shows an *abundance of target cells*, occasional microspherocytes. The MCHC may also be increased because of RBC dehydration.

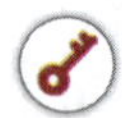

Key: D

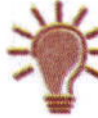

BOOST YOUR KNOWLEDGE

Hemoglobin C disease is mainly found in people with African heritage. It is not a type of SCD, even though it does not cause the same kind of "sickling" of RBCs. When someone has two copies of the *Hgb C* gene, it leads to mild and ongoing anemia. This anemia is usually not severe, but there might be times when the person has mild jaundice, giving their skin a yellowish tint.

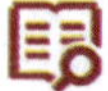

REFERENCE/SOURCE

- Gupta P, Menon PSN, Lodha R, Ramji S. PG Textbook of Pediatrics, 3rd edition. New Delhi: Jaypee Brothers Medical Publishers; 2022. p. 1857.

3. A 12-year-old child presents to the pediatric clinic for a routine check-up. On examination, there is no pallor, jaundice, or hepatosplenomegaly. The CBC shows a hemoglobin level of 9.5 g/dL, MCV is 68 fL, and the RBC is 5.27 million/mm^3. The physician decides to perform a hemoglobin electrophoresis using HPLC. Which of the following reports suggest thalassemia minor?

A. Elevated HbA2 >2.0%
B. Elevated HbA2 >2.5%
C. Elevated HbA2 >3.0%
D. Elevated HbA2 >3.5%

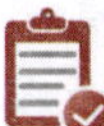

EXPLANATION

Children having thalassemia minor/carrier/trait are usually asymptomatic or may have mild anemia. Anemia in some cases may worsen during stress such as pregnancy and infection. It is inherited as heterozygous B-thalassemia. Hemoglobin levels may be normal or slightly reduced. Red cells have low MCV <78 fL and MCH <27 pg. RBC counts are higher for the hemoglobin level. HbA2, level is high, >3.5% is diagnostic.

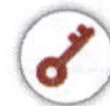

Key: D

BOOST YOUR KNOWLEDGE

In the following situations, the HbA2 level can be normal in individuals with thalassemia minor:

- Coexisting iron-deficiency anemia along with thalassemia trait
- Silent beta-thalassemia—mutations like 101 C-T
- Coinheritance of delta- and beta-thalassemia
- Alpha-globin chain triplication/quadruplication

REFERENCE/SOURCE

- Gupta P, Menon PSN, Lodha R, Ramji S. PG Textbook of Pediatrics, 3rd edition. New Delhi: Jaypee Brothers Medical Publishers; 2022. pp. 1871.

4. A 17-year-old boy with sickle cell trait presents with left-sided flank pain and gross hematuria. A CT scan of the abdomen shows an infiltrating mass of the left kidney that enhances with contrast. There is also retroperitoneal lymphadenopathy. Which of the following malignancies is associated with sickle cell trait?

A. Clear cell carcinoma
B. Renal medullary carcinoma
C. Rhabdoid tumor of the kidney
D. Wilms tumor

EXPLANATION

Sickle cell trait has been linked to the emergence of an uncommon and aggressive malignant kidney tumor known as renal medullary carcinoma. This form of cancer is particularly lethal, with a high fatality rate. In 1995, when the first 34 instances of renal medullary carcinoma were documented, the condition was referred to as the "seventh sickle cell nephropathy". Renal medullary carcinoma comprises a small fraction, <0.5%, of all cases of kidney carcinomas. It predominantly occurs in individuals with sickle cell trait, although cases have also been observed in individuals with sickle cell anemia, hemoglobin S with beta-thalassemia, and hemoglobin SC. However, this type of carcinoma does not manifest in hemoglobinopathies that do not induce sickling of RBCs.

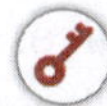

Key: B

BOOST YOUR KNOWLEDGE

Renal system complications in sickle cell: Sickle cell nephropathy includes papillary necrosis, nephrotic syndrome, renal infarction, hyposthenuria, pyelonephritis, and renal medullary carcinoma. The presentation of these entities could be hematuria (microscopic or gross), proteinuria, renal insufficiency, and urine concentrating detects.

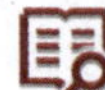

REFERENCES/SOURCES

- Gupta P, Menon PSN, Lodha R, Ramji S. PG Textbook of Pediatrics, 3rd edition. New Delhi: Jaypee Brothers Medical Publishers; 2022. p. 1865.
- Holland P, Merrimen J, Pringle C, Wood LA. Renal medullary carcinoma and its association with sickle cell trait: a case report and literature review. Curr Oncol. 2020;27(1):e53-6.
- Look AT, Ginsburg D, Fisher DE, Nathan DG, Samuel L, Orkin SH. Nathan and Oski's Hematology and Oncology of Infancy and Childhood, 8th edition. Philadelphia: Saunders; 2014. pp. 697-8.

5. You are seeing a 13-year-old girl with sickle cell anemia (Hb SS) for annual checkup. She is on hydroxyurea therapy. The neurological examination was normal. Screening transcranial Doppler (TCD) test using non-imaging technique shows elevated time average maximal mean velocity (TAMMV) of 207 cm/s in the left middle cerebral artery. What will be your strategy to prevent overt stroke in this scenario?

A. Increase hydroxyurea dose
B. Will start penicillin prophylaxis
C. Prophylactic anticonvulsant
D. Chronic transfusion therapy to maintain HbS <30%

EXPLANATION

An abnormal TCD velocity (200 cm/s by STOP trial criteria) confers a risk of overt stroke over the 3 years following the TCD examination of approximately 40%. Maintenance transfusion therapy to maintain "Hs" <30% can be considered in those children with time averaged blood velocity of >200 m/s. This results in 85% reduction in the rate of overt strokes.

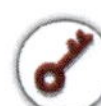

Key: D

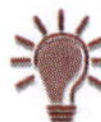

BOOST YOUR KNOWLEDGE

Indications of bone marrow transplant in SCD:

- Stroke or transient central nervous system (CNS) event
- Silent stroke with cognitive impairment
- MRI imaging changes of brain parenchymal damage
- MRI angiogram evidence of cerebrovascular disease
- Recurrent vaso-occlusive pain crises (>2 per year for the last 2 years), requiring hospitalizations
- Acute chest syndrome requiring recurrent hospitalizations
- Osteonecrosis of multiple joints
- Elevated TCD
- Red cell alloimmunization (>2 antibodies)

REFERENCES/SOURCES

- Gupta P, Menon PSN, Lodha R, Ramji S. PG Textbook of Pediatrics, 3rd edition. New Delhi: Jaypee Brothers Medical Publishers; 2022. p. 1866.
- Look AT, Ginsburg D, Fisher DE, Nathan DG, Samuel L, Orkin SH. Nathan and Oski's Hematology and Oncology of Infancy and Childhood, 8th edition. Philadelphia: Saunders; 2014. p. 708.

6. A 16-year-old boy from Assam presented with a history of mild fatigue and occasional episodes of jaundice. Examination did not reveal any pallor, jaundice, or hepatosplenomegaly. CBC reveals a hemoglobin level of 10.5 g/dL with normal white blood cell (WBC) and platelet count. Peripheral blood smear shows microcytic and hypochromic RBCs. Serum ferritin is 110 ng/mL. HPLC showed hemoglobin E (HbE) 93%, HbF 6.5, and HbA2 1.5%. Based on the clinical presentation and laboratory findings, what is the most likely diagnosis for this individual's condition?

A. HbE SCD
B. Beta-thalassemia minor (β-thalassemia minor)
C. HbE disease
D. HbE beta-thalassemia

EXPLANATION

Hemoglobin E disease is a hemoglobinopathy that results from the inheritance of two *HbE* genes. This combination leads to a mild form of anemia. Individuals with HbE disease may have microcytic and hypochromic RBCs, similar to beta-thalassemia minor.

The clinical presentation of mild fatigue, occasional jaundice, and patient belong to Northeastern part of India where HbE disease is prevalent favoring HbE disease. Option A is less likely given the absence of sickling and history. Option B is incorrect because beta-thalassemia minor would typically present with microcytic and hypochromic RBCs, but it is not characterized by the presence of HbE on HPLC. HbE-beta will have moderate anemia and HPLC will also show high HbF other than HbE.

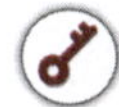

Key: C

BOOST YOUR KNOWLEDGE

Hemoglobin E disease is a genetic blood disorder that primarily affects people of Southeast Asian descent, particularly those from regions such as Thailand, Cambodia, and parts of India, especially Northeast region.

REFERENCE/SOURCE

- Gupta P, Menon PSN, Lodha R, Ramji S. PG Textbook of Pediatrics, 3rd edition. New Delhi: Jaypee Brothers Medical Publishers; 2022. p. 1858.

7. An adolescent boy diagnosed with sickle cell anemia (Hb SS) experiences recurrent painful episodes necessitating hospitalization. An initial treatment plan involves initiating hydroxyurea therapy at 15 mg/kg once daily. Subsequently, the dose is increased by 5 mg/kg every 2 months, reaching a dosage of 30 mg/kg for the past 3 months. However, there is no noticeable clinical improvement, and he continues to experience frequent painful episodes. Considering this, you decide to conduct blood tests, including a hemoglobin electrophoresis, to monitor his treatment response. What could be a possible reason for the lack of clinical improvement despite the escalated hydroxyurea dose?

Hb	6.9 g/dL
MCV	78 fL
MCHC	36.5 g/dL
WBC	15,600/mm^3
Platelet count	520,000/mm^3
Retics	4.5%
Peripheral smear	Severe normocytic anemia with polychromasia, many irreversibly sickled cells, and Howell–Jolly bodies

Hemoglobin electrophoresis: 97% Hgb S; Hgb F 1.5%; and 1.5% $HgbA_2$

A. Insufficient dosage of hydroxyurea
B. Limited duration of hydroxyurea therapy
C. The patient exhibits a biological nonresponder status to hydroxyurea
D. The patient's noncompliance with hydroxyurea treatment

EXPLANATION

Considering the appropriate dosage and duration of hydroxyurea therapy (as mentioned in options A and B), other potential factors contributing to nonresponse should be explored. While it is feasible to further increase the dose, it is prudent to initially investigate alternative explanations for the lack of response. While the possibility of this patient being a "nonresponder" to hydroxyurea (as indicated in option C) cannot be entirely ruled out, the most probable reason is the patient's inconsistency in adhering to the prescribed medication regimen. This assumption is reinforced by the absence of macrocytosis, along with the presence of both leukocytosis and thrombocytosis. In adults with sickle cell anemia, daily hydroxyurea at maximum tolerate doses leads to significant increases in percentage HbF, MCV, and Hb as well as decreases in WBC, neutrophils, and reticulocytes. Similar laboratory efficacy for hydroxyurea therapy is observed in children and adolescents. It is noteworthy that nonadherence to chronic medications poses a significant challenge in adolescent population, irrespective of the underlying medical condition.

Key: D

BOOST YOUR KNOWLEDGE

Deeper insights into the pathophysiology of SCD have led to the development of novel agents that target cellular adhesion, inflammation, oxidant injury, platelets and/or coagulation, vascular tone, and hemoglobin polymerization. Until 2017, hydroxyurea, which increases HbF and reduces RBC sickling, was the only disease-modifying therapy available for SCD and remains first-line therapy for most individuals with SCD. Three additional therapies, L-glutamine, crizanlizumab, and voxelotor, have been approved as adjunctive or second-line agents.

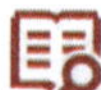

REFERENCE/SOURCE

- Ware RE. How I use hydroxyurea to treat young patients with sickle cell anemia. Blood. 2010;115(26):5300-11.

8. Which of the following mutational event is predominantly responsible for causing beta-thalassemia?

A. Chromosomal translocations
B. Large deletions
C. Inversions
D. Point mutations

EXPLANATION

Beta-thalassemia is primarily attributed to point mutations that lead to reduced or disrupted transcription or translation of beta-globin genes or transcripts. In contrast, alpha-thalassemia is more often linked to the deletion of complete alpha-globin genes. While deletional forms of beta-thalassemia and nondeletional forms of alpha-thalassemia do exist, they are less prevalent. Inversions, translocations, and uniparental disomy are not recognized as causal factors for thalassemia.

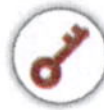

Key: D

BOOST YOUR KNOWLEDGE

The five common mutations, i.e., IVS 1-5 G → C, IVS 1-1 G → T, codon 41/42 (-TCTT), codon 8/9, and the 619 bp deletion account for over 90% of the mutations in β-thalassemia patients. IVS-I-5 (G → C) is the most common beta-thalassemia allele in the Indian population.

REFERENCE/SOURCE

- Look AT, Ginsburg D, Fisher DE, Nathan DG, Samuel L, Orkin SH. Nathan and Oski's Hematology and Oncology of Infancy and Childhood, 8th edition. Philadelphia: Saunders; 2014. p. 723.

9. You are called late at night for a 5-year-old boy with sickle cell anemia on hydroxyurea who presents to the emergency room of your hospital. The child is conscious, alert but pale and tachycardic. He has no history of ever. On abdominal examination, spleen is 4 cm below costal margin. Blood investigations are as follows:

Hb	5.6 g/dL
MCV	93 fL
WBC	17,600/mm^3
Platelet count	110,000/mm^3
Retics	11%
Peripheral smear	Severe normocytic anemia with polychromasia, many irreversibly sickled cells, and nucleated RBCs (NRBCs) 9/100 WBCs

Which of the following is the most plausible reason for the acute anemia in this child?

A. Recent aplastic crisis
B. Acute splenic sequestration
C. Acute chest syndrome
D. Hydroxyurea-related side effect

EXPLANATION

Among the given options, option B (acute splenic sequestration) is the most likely explanation for the child's sudden and severe anemia. Acute splenic sequestration crisis is a serious complication in individuals with SCD. It involves the rapid pooling of a large volume of blood within the spleen, leading to a sudden drop in hemoglobin levels and potentially life-threatening anemia. The spleen becomes enlarged, and the trapped blood can result in hypovolemic shock. Severe anemia, brisk reticulocytosis, and NRBCs in the peripheral circulation also favor this.

Option A: Aplastic crisis would give an anemia with reticulocytopenia.

Options C and D: There are no respiratory signs or symptoms to suggest acute chest syndrome. Hydroxyurea toxicity would cause low WBC and erythroid suppression and not reticulocytosis.

Key: B

BOOST YOUR KNOWLEDGE

Three major presentations of SCD:

1. Pain crisis
2. Splenic sequestration
3. Acute chest syndrome

The clinical characteristics of the transient aplastic crisis of SCD result from the abrupt cessation of erythropoiesis, most commonly, because of acute parvovirus infection. Patients usually have pallor and fatigue but are without jaundice and have laboratory evidence of severe anemia below baseline with associated severe reticulocytopenia. While in splenic sequestration, reticulocytosis occurs.

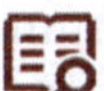

REFERENCE/SOURCE

- Look AT, Ginsburg D, Fisher DE, Nathan DG, Samuel L, Orkin SH. Nathan and Oski's Hematology and Oncology of Infancy and Childhood, 8th edition. Philadelphia: Saunders; 2014. pp. 687-93.

10. A 16-year-old boy was diagnosed with β-TM. He has been receiving RBC transfusions since the age of 1. Iron chelation therapy with deferoxamine (DFO) was started at age 2 but later became nonadherent, and transitioned to oral deferasirox. His ferritin is 3,540 ng/mL. What is the most probable cause of death if poor chelation practices continue?

A. *Yersinia enterocolitica* sepsis
B. Chronic liver disease
C. Hyperglycemia
D. Cardiovascular (CV) events like dysrhythmia

EXPLANATION

Inadequate iron chelation therapy in patients with β-TM who receive chronic blood transfusions can lead to iron overload and its complications. CV complications represent the leading cause of mortality in patients with thalassemia, including TM and TI. While other complications like sepsis (Option A) can occur, especially when on DFO.

Key: D

BOOST YOUR KNOWLEDGE

Exposure to *Yersinia enterocolitica* infection is a noteworthy hazard linked to the use of DFO therapy. This association underscores the significance of being vigilant about such infections, even though their diagnosis can be challenging. In circumstances where a substantial clinical suspicion of *Yersinia enterocolitica* infection arises (loose stool), it is recommended to temporarily halt the administration of DFO to the patient.

REFERENCE/SOURCE

- Farmakis D. Cardiovascular disease. In: Cappellini MD, Farmakis D, Porter J, Taher A (Eds). 2021 Guidelines for the Management of Transfusion Dependent Thalassemia (TDT), 4th edition. Cyprus: Thalassaemia International Federation; 2021. pp. 110-23.

11. A 2-year-old boy diagnosed with β-TM, has been receiving RBC transfusions every 3 weeks since the age of 9 months. When should you start iron chelation therapy?

A. It should start from beginning of chronic transfusion program
B. If serum iron >1,000 ng/mL
C. If any cardiac complications due to iron overload
D. If transfusion requirement is every 2 weeks

EXPLANATION

In TM, iron chelation should start before transfusions have deposited enough iron to cause tissue damage. This has not been formally determined, but current practice is to start after the first 10–20 transfusions, or when the ferritin level rises above 1,000 ng/mL. If chelation therapy begins before 3 years of age, particularly with DFO careful monitoring of growth and bone development is advised, along with reduced dosage.

Key: B

BOOST YOUR KNOWLEDGE

At low serum ferritin levels (<100 μg/L), the DFO dose needs to be reduced and DFO-related toxicities monitored particularly carefully. Dose reductions can be guided using the therapeutic index [mean daily dose (mg/kg)/serum ferritin μg/L] to keep this <0.025 (Porter index). This index is not a substitute for careful clinical monitoring. Liver iron concentration may be a more reliable alternative to serum ferritin in monitoring response.

REFERENCE/SOURCE

- Porter J. Iron chelation. In: Cappellini MD, Farmakis D, Porter J, Taher A (Eds). 2021 Guidelines for the Management of Transfusion Dependent Thalassemia (TDT), 4th edition. Cyprus: Thalassaemia International Federation; 2021. p. 76.

12. A 6-year-old boy, diagnosed with β-TM, has been on chronic transfusions since the age of 1 year. He is taking deferiprone (DFP) (Kelfer) as iron chelation therapy from last 2 months. He developed high-grade fever and CBC was done as part of fever workup which showed Hb 9.8, WBC 2,400, absolute neutrophil count (ANC) 240, and platelet 304,000/mm^3. What will be appropriate step regarding chelation therapy?

A. It should hold for till fever subsides and then restart at same dose
B. Can continue as this low WBC and low neutrophil count could be because of infection
C. It should hold for till fever subsides and then restart at 50% dose of previous dose
D. It should stop and switch to another iron chelation

EXPLANATION

Agranulocytosis (ANC <0.5×10^9/L) is a serious and potentially fatal adverse event. This may be preceded by neutropenia and is reported in approximately 1.7% of patients. Each patient's ANC should be estimated before starting deferiprone (DFP) therapy and every 1–2 weeks during treatment. DFP therapy should be interrupted, and the patient's neutrophil count closely monitored if an infection develops. It is not clear whether this effect is dose related. If severe neutropenia or agranulocytosis develops, the drug should be stopped and not reintroduced, and the use of granulocyte colony-stimulating factor (G-CSF) should be considered in the case of agranulocytosis.

Key: D

BOOST YOUR KNOWLEDGE

Other common side effect with DFP is joint pain. The frequency of arthropathy varies greatly between studies, from as low as 4.5% at 1 year to 15% after 4 years in a predominantly European patient group, and as high as 33–40% in studies of patients from India. Symptoms range from mild nonprogressive arthropathy, typically in the knees and controllable with nonsteroidal anti-inflammatory drugs to (more rarely) severe erosive arthropathy that may progress even after treatment is stopped.

REFERENCE/SOURCE

- Porter J. Iron chelation. In: Cappellini MD, Farmakis D, Porter J, Taher A (Eds). 2021 Guidelines for the Management of Transfusion Dependent Thalassemia (TDT), 4th edition. Cyprus: Thalassaemia International Federation; 2021. p. 94.

13. A 10-year-old boy from Punjab presents fever for 3 days. On examination, no pallor, no jaundice, and no hepatosplenomegaly. CBC reveals a hemoglobin level of 10.9 g/dL with normal WBC and platelet count. Peripheral blood smear shows normocytic normochromic with some microcytic and hypochromic RBCs. HPLC showed HbF 96%, HbA 2.5, and HbA2 1.5%. What is the most likely diagnosis?

A. Thalassemia trait
B. TM
C. Hereditary persistence of HbF
D. Sickle cell anemia

EXPLANATION

Hereditary persistence of fetal hemoglobin (HPFH) is a genetic condition characterized by the continued production of HbF into adulthood, instead of its normal decline shortly after birth; mutations are associated with a decrease in the production of either or both beta- and delta-globins. There is an imbalance in the nonsynthetic ratio characteristic of thalassemia.

Key: C

BOOST YOUR KNOWLEDGE

More than 20 variants of HPFH have been described. In the homozygous form, no manifestations of thalassemia are present. There is only HbF with very mild anemia and slight microcytosis. When inherited with other variant hemoglobins, HbF is elevated into the 20–30% range; when inherited with HbS, SCD is ameliorated, with fewer complications.

REFERENCE/SOURCE

- Kliegman RM, St Geme JW III, Blum NJ, Shah SS, Tasker RC, Wilson KM. Nelson Textbook of Pediatrics, 21st edition. Amsterdam: Elsevier; 2020. p. 2553.

14. A concerned couple rushes to your clinic with their 5-year-old son's blood test reports in hand. They explain that they had some routine blood tests done for their child, and the results have left them anxious. The CBC revealed mild anemia (hemoglobin 11.9 g/dL, RBC count 5.26 × 10^6/μL, MCV 78.9 fL, MCH 27.5 pg, and MCHC 34.9 g/dL). Peripheral smear revealed mildly microcytic red cells along with few target cells. HPLC analysis revealed something they did not understand: "HbD-Punjab."

Upon reviewing the HPLC results, you find the following information:

- Hemoglobin A (HbA0): 4.5%
- Hemoglobin A2 (HbA2): 1.6%
- Hemoglobin F (HbF): 0.3%
- HbD-Punjab: 89.4%

How will you counsel this family?

A. HbD-Punjab is a hemoglobin disorder which needs lifelong treatment
B. As child grows older, he can develop anemia
C. This child needs frequent follow-up with repeat blood tests for this condition
D. No active intervention is required

EXPLANATION

The substitution in HbD is a glutamic acid to glutamine at the 121st amino acid of the beta-globin chain (B121 Glu-GIn). HbD migrates with HbS on alkaline electrophoresis. HbD heterozygotes (HbAD) are asymptomatic, nonanemic, and have normal red cell indices.

Key: D

BOOST YOUR KNOWLEDGE

Homozygotes for HbD-Los Angeles (also known as HbD-Punjab) are asymptomatic and are hematologically normal with normal red cell indices. Blood films may show target cells. Osmotic fragility may be decreased. Compound heterozygotes for HbD-Los Angeles and a β-thalassemia mutation have mild microcytic anemia and show minimal hemolysis. Coinheritance of HbD-Los Angeles with HbS results in a severe SCD phenotype not different from homozygous HbS.

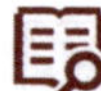

REFERENCE/SOURCE

- Gupta P, Menon PSN, Lodha R, Ramji S. PG Textbook of Pediatrics, 3rd edition. New Delhi: Jaypee Brothers Medical Publishers; 2022.

15. You are examining a 7-year-old child diagnosed with sickle cell anemia who presented with fever, coughing, headache, and vomiting. During the examination, the child appeared pale. Considering the child's medical history and presentation, which of the following infections is the *least probable* in this child?

A. *Pneumococcus* sepsis
B. *Haemophilus influenzae* meningitis
C. *Escherichia coli* urinary tract infection
D. Parvovirus B19 aplastic episode

EXPLANATION

In a child with sickle cell anemia, infections such as *Pneumococcus* sepsis (A), *Haemophilus influenzae* meningitis (B), and parvovirus infection (D) are more common and pose a greater risk to individuals with sickle cell anemia due to their compromised immune function. There is an increased incidence of urinary tract infection with bacteremia in young women with sickle cell anemia.

Key: C

BOOST YOUR KNOWLEDGE

All children with SCD should receive the complete routine immunization schedule that should include conjugated pneumococcal, conjugated *H. influenzae,* and hepatitis B vaccines. Additional vaccines including the 23-valent pneumococcal polysaccharide vaccine (Pneumovax; PPV23), seasonal influenza vaccine, and conjugated meningococcal vaccine (Menactra; MCV4) should be administered.

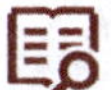

REFERENCE/SOURCE

- Look AT, Ginsburg D, Fisher DE, Nathan DG, Samuel L, Orkin SH. Nathan and Oski's Hematology and Oncology of Infancy and Childhood, 8th edition. Philadelphia: Saunders; 2014. pp. 694-6, 703.

16. A 10-year-old boy presented to the emergency department with profound cyanosis and diaphoresis, with a room air oxygen saturation of 89%. Despite use of a nonrebreathing face mask, the patient remained hypoxic, with oxygen saturations of around 88%. He was on Dapsone tablet for chronic immune thrombocytopenia (ITP). Chest X-ray, electrocardiogram (ECG), blood pressure (BP), and heart rate were normal. Arterial blood was noted to be chocolate brown in color, with a pH of 7.38, a PCO_2 of 37.2 mm Hg, a bicarbonate level of 24 mmol/L, and a PO_2 of 33.6 mm Hg. What is the most probable diagnosis?

A. Tetralogy of Fallot
B. Lobar pneumonia
C. Methemoglobinemia
D. Unstable hemoglobin

EXPLANATION

Portable co-oximetry can have identified a methemoglobin level. This class of Hb variants contains amino acid substitutions that alter the heme environment and stabilize the oxidized [ferric, Fe(III)] state over the reduced one [ferrous, Fe(II)]. Methylene blue is drug for this condition. Echo is normal so tetralogy of Fallot is unlikely in this condition. Chest X-ray is normal so lobar pneumonia is ruled out.

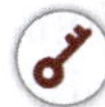

Key: C

BOOST YOUR KNOWLEDGE

Type of methemoglobinemia:

Disease	*Transmission*	*Cyanosis*	*Other symptoms*	*Gene*	*Meth Hb level*	*CYB5R activity*
Drug exposure	Acquired	Yes	–		Variable	Normal
Methemoglobinemia, type I	Autosomal recessive	Yes since birth	–	*CYB5R3*	20–30%	Decreased
Methemoglobinemia, type II	Autosomal recessive	Yes since birth	Neurological involvement	*CYB5R3*	8–40%	Decreased
Methemoglobinemia, type IV	Autosomal recessive	Yes	46,XY DSD ambiguous genitalia	*CYB5A*	12–19%	Normal

REFERENCE/SOURCE

- Iolascon A, Bianchi P, Andolfo I, Russo R, Barcellini W, Fermo E, et al. Recommendations for diagnosis and treatment of methemoglobinemia. Am J Hematol. 2021;96(12):1666-78.

17. A 3-month-old boy presented with dark urine, pallor, and mild jaundice. Moderate anemia (Hb 8.5 g/L) with reticulocytosis (13.4%) was detected in the peripheral blood. Biochemical analysis revealed elevated serum lactate dehydrogenase and hyperbilirubinemia. Coombs and autoantibody test results were negative. HPLC test results for thalassemia were normal. The patient was diagnosed with hemolytic anemia. Physical examination revealed generalized icterus accompanied by marked splenomegaly (3 cm below the costal margin). From then on, he was treated conservatively with multiple blood transfusions of an average of 2.5 units every month to maintain a Hb level of 9.0 g/L. He was re-evaluated at 2 years of age. Malnutrition or growth retardation was not observed. A blood smear examination revealed erythrocyte abnormalities with marked anisocytosis, poikilocytosis, and basophilic stippling. Specific enzyme activity assays for glucose-6-phosphate dehydrogenase (G6PD), phosphate isomerase, pyruvate kinase, and pyrimidine 5'-nucleotidase showed normal findings. HPLC was normal. Both heat stability and isopropanol tests showed positive results. What is the probable diagnosis?

A. Autoimmune hemolytic anemia (AIHA)
B. Thalassemia
C. G6PD disease
D. Unstable hemoglobin

EXPLANATION

- Direct Coombs test (DCT) test is negative so AIHA is unlikely.
- Normal HPLC rule out thalassemia.
- As G6PD can present in similar way but enzyme level normal rule out G6PD.

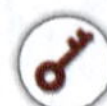

Key: D

BOOST YOUR KNOWLEDGE

In patients for whom standard evaluation does not identify the etiology of the hemolytic anemia, the possibility of a congenital unstable hemoglobinopathy should be considered. Among the more than 1,000 globin chain mutations described, several alpha- and beta-globin mutations are highly unstable, causing significant hemolysis. These children often present with hemolytic anemia, brisk reticulocytosis, jaundice, and splenomegaly, but can be difficult to diagnose. One of the challenges of correctly diagnosing unstable hemoglobin is the potentially misleading results from hemoglobin electrophoresis. Unstable hemoglobin variants undergo rapid denaturation, precipitation, and degradation within the erythrocyte. Analysis of the remaining hemoglobins may reveal a relatively normal hemoglobin electrophoresis pattern, particularly if the analysis is not performed quickly after collection. For some unstable beta-globin variants, the electrophoretic pattern may reveal increased hemoglobins A2 and F, suggesting the diagnosis of β-thalassemia trait. However, uncharacteristic severe hemolysis in this setting should prompt a more extensive evaluation including β-globin gene sequencing.

REFERENCE/SOURCE

- Yates AM, Mortier NA, Hyde KS, Hankins JS, Ware RE. The diagnostic dilemma of congenital unstable hemoglobinopathies. Pediatr Blood Cancer. 2010;55:1393-5.

18. Which of the following is *not* applicable for estimating iron overload in thalassemia patients?

A. Serum ferritin
B. SQUID
C. Liver biopsy
D. CT of liver

EXPLANATION

T2*MRI of liver is method of iron overload estimation not CT of liver. Rest all are method of iron overload estimation. Liver biopsy is considered as gold standard.

Key: D

BOOST YOUR KNOWLEDGE

- A unit processed from 420 mL of donor blood contains approximately 200 mg of iron, or 0.47 mg/mL of whole donor blood. For red cell preparations with variable Hct, the iron in mg/mL of blood can therefore be estimated from 1.16 × the Hct.
- Serum ferritin values exhibit variability, attributed in part to the impact of inflammation, which elevates serum ferritin levels. Additionally, the distribution of liver iron between macrophages (Kupffer cells) and hepatocytes significantly influences serum ferritin. A sudden surge in serum ferritin should prompt an investigation into potential causes such as hepatitis, other infections, or inflammatory conditions. It is important to note that a persistent elevation in serum ferritin despite chelation therapy does not conclusively establish the patient as a "nonresponder" to the chelation regimen.

REFERENCE/SOURCE

- Farmakis D. Cardiovascular disease. In: Cappellini MD, Farmakis D, Porter J, Taher A (Eds). 2021 Guidelines for the Management of Transfusion Dependent Thalassemia (TDT), 4th edition. Cyprus: Thalassaemia International Federation; 2021.

19. Severe thalassemia may not become clinically apparent until a child is several months old because:

A. Elevated HbA2 compensates for the missing β-globin genes.
B. The oxygen needs of a newborn are minimal. Overexpression of zeta-globin (zeta) compensates for the missing β-chain.
C. The gamma- to beta-globin switch is not complete until several months after birth.
D. The alpha-globin genes do not turn on until several months after birth.

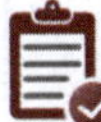

EXPLANATION

Severe thalassemia may not become clinically apparent until a child is several months old because fetal hemoglobin (HbF) production predominates during the initial months of life. As HbF declines and adult hemoglobin (HbA) synthesis increases, the imbalance in globin-chain production due to thalassemia becomes evident, leading to symptomatic anemia.

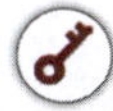

Key: C

BOOST YOUR KNOWLEDGE

The process of different hemoglobin species being produced and stopping production at certain periods of human development is known as "hemoglobin switching". In human, this switching starts before birth and complete by 1 year of life. Under normal conditions, the red cells of the adult human contain approximately 97–98% of HbA, 2–3% of HbA2, and traces of HbF.

REFERENCE/SOURCE

- Origa R. Genetic basis, pathophysiology and diagnosis of thalassaemias. In: Cappellini MD, Farmakis D, Porter J, Taher A (Eds). 2021 Guidelines for the Management of Transfusion Dependent Thalassemia (TDT), 4th edition. Cyprus: Thalassaemia International Federation; 2021. p. 20.

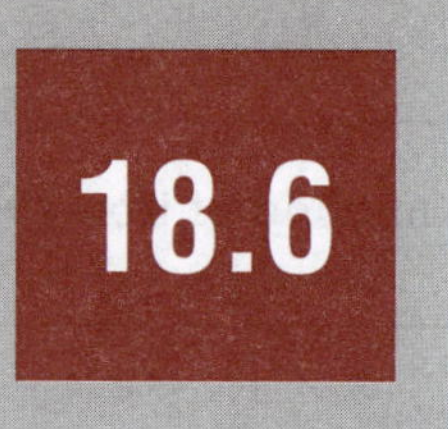

CHAPTER 18.6

Platelet Disorders

Swati Kanakia

1. A 14-year-old girl comes with a history of fatigue and overall tiredness. On clinical examination, the child looks pale and has hyperpigmentation of the knuckles. The peripheral smear showed hypersegmented neutrophils. Complete blood count (CBC) was as follows. Hb 4.1 g/dL, red blood cell (RBC) 1.2 million, packed cell volume (PCV) 12.6%, mean corpuscular volume (MCV) 105 fL, white blood cell (WBC) 2630, polymorphs 43%, lymphocytes 30%, monocytes 4%, eosinophils and basophils 0. Serum lactate dehydrogenase (LDH) was 5,600. What is the most likely diagnosis?

A. Megaloblastic anemia
B. Iron deficiency anemia
C. Immune thrombocytopenia
D. Aplastic anemia

EXPLANATION

Hyperpigmented knuckles are an important clinical finding. The important clues on CBC are, pancytopenia with macrocytosis, high red cell distribution width (RDW), with adequate neutrophils. A very high serum LDH along with the clinical setting points toward megaloblastic anemia.

It cannot be iron deficiency anemia because the RBCs in the given case are macrocytic and the characteristics of iron deficiency anemia are microcytosis and hypochromia. Immune thrombocytopenia is ruled out because there is a pancytopenia, and in immune thrombocytopenia (ITP), only the platelets are affected.

It is unlikely to be aplastic anemia because neutropenia and lymphocytosis are important features of aplastic anemia, which are absent in this child.

Also, a very high serum LDH is highly suggestive of megaloblastic anemia.

Key: A

BOOST YOUR KNOWLEDGE

A high serum LDH is a marker of ineffective erythropoiesis and often seen in megaloblastic anemia. It is a reliable and cost-effective marker for the diagnosis of megaloblastic anemia along with the CBC and peripheral smear. It can also be used to monitor therapy in megaloblastic anemia.

Another important diagnostic finding is hypersegmented neutrophils. Hypersegmented neutrophils are said to be present if there are more than five lobes in at least 5% of neutrophils or a single neutrophil shows six or more lobes. Macroovalocytes on peripheral smears are also indicative of megaloblastic anemia.

REFERENCE/SOURCE

- Dheendhayalan M, Abhilasha S, Gupta A. Standard Treatment Guidelines 2022, Megaloblastic Anemia. Indian Academy of Pediatrics; 2022.

2. A 22-month-old girl, preterm delivery, gaining adequate weight, breastfed, and bottle-fed, weaning not started as yet, comes to the pediatrician for routine immunization. On clinical examination, the child looks pale and has a just palpable spleen. Liver is not palpable and there are no significantly palpable lymph nodes. A complete blood count was carried out. The CBC report is as follows Hb 7.5%, RBC 4.0 million, MCV 64 fL, MCH 18.5 pg, RDW 22%, and platelet count 5.3 lakhs/cu mm. What is the most likely diagnosis?

A. Pure red cell aplasia
B. Iron deficiency anemia with thrombocytosis
C. Thalassemia minor
D. Thalassemia major

EXPLANATION

The most important clinical history is preterm delivery, inadequate weaning, and milk diet. The RBC indices, microcytosis hypochromia, and high RDW are diagnostic of iron deficiency anemia. Mild thrombocytosis often is seen in iron deficiency anemia.

Pure red cell aplasia is associated with microcytic anemia, generally tends to present earlier in life and thrombocytosis is not feature of this disorder.

It is unlikely to be thalassemia minor, because the RDW is high. It can be argued that thalassemia minor can coexist with iron deficiency anemia, but in this clinical context, iron deficiency anemia must be considered as the primary diagnosis.

Thalassemia major is ruled out due to absence of hepatosplenomegaly, and the peripheral smear findings which do not indicate presence of normoblasts. Also, thrombocytosis is not a feature of thalassemia major.

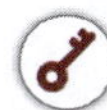

Key: B

BOOST YOUR KNOWLEDGE

Mild thrombocytosis is an important finding in iron deficiency anemia. The exact pathophysiology and implications are unknown. In adult studies, around 30% of patients with IDA had thrombocytosis. The counts revert in around 2/3 patients with replacement of iron. The dose is 3 mg/kg/day of elemental iron, once daily or in-between meals. It is advisable to continue iron for 2 months after the Hb normalizes.

REFERENCE/SOURCE

- Bansal D, Radhakrishna N, Prakash A. Standard Guidelines 2022, Iron Deficiency Anemia. Indian Academy of Pediatrics; 2022.

3. A 3-year-old boy comes with the complaints of severe leg pain, inability to bear weight, fever off and on, treated with multiple antibiotics for 1.5 months. On examination, the child looks pale, irritable, and has multiple ecchymotic spots. He has a hepatomegaly 3 cm below the costal margin, spleen 4 cm below the costal margin, and lymph nodes which are firm and palpable in the neck. In this child, what is the peripheral smear most likely to show?

A. Lymphoblasts with decreased platelets
B. Normoblasts with normal platelets
C. Normoblasts with decreased platelets
D. *Plasmodium vivax* (*P. vivax*) with decreased platelets

EXPLANATION

Lymphoblasts with decreased platelets. This child is likely to have acute lymphoblastic leukemia (ALL). The symptoms of fever, musculoskeletal complaints, and ecchymosis spots due to low platelet counts are highly suggestive of ALL.

Normoblasts or nucleated red blood cells are the cardinal feature of thalassemia major. A child with thalassemia major will have hepatosplenomegaly, but platelets will be normal, and the profound musculoskeletal symptoms would not be present. Also, the age of the child is not classical for thalassemia major.

Malaria also is unlikely because of the severity of the musculoskeletal symptoms.

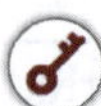 **Key: A**

 **BOOST YOUR KNOWLEDGE**

Bone pains in leukemia can be severe and are often accompanied by normal peripheral blood counts. This leads to delayed diagnosis or a misdiagnosis of juvenile rheumatoid arthritis (JRA), and steroids may be administered. Around 18–23% patients may present in this manner. JRA, has joint pain whereas ALL presents with bone pain. On a routine X-ray, leukemic lines may be seen, and magnetic resonance imaging (MRI) may show bone marrow changes, warranting a bone marrow aspirate, and further testing.

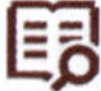 **REFERENCE/SOURCE**

- Pizzo PA, Poplack DG. Principles and Practice of Pediatric Oncology, 6th edition. Wolters Kluwer; 2011. pp. 539-40.

4. A playful active, 3.5-year-old female child, comes with the complaints of ecchymotic patches and petechiae all over the body. There is no history of any other symptoms. On examination, the child is otherwise fine, has multiple ecchymotic spots, and no stigmata of any syndrome. Systemic examination reveals no organomegaly/lymph nodes/pallor. What is the most likely diagnosis?

A. Acute leukemia
B. Persistent immune thrombocytopenia (ITP)
C. Newly diagnosed immune thrombocytopenia
D. Dengue hemorrhagic disease

 **EXPLANATION**

Newly diagnosed ITP as per the latest nomenclature. This child does not have any symptoms other than purpura. There are no constitutional symptoms such as weight loss, night sweats, fever, musculoskeletal symptoms, organomegaly, or lymph nodes. The child is playful and active. So, acute leukemia is ruled out.

By definition, persistent ITP is when the child has been diagnosed with ITP and the low platelet counts persist for >3 months and up to 12 months, after which the child is said to have chronic ITP.

It is not dengue hemorrhagic fever, because there is no fever and the child has no other symptoms.

Clinically, it is unlikely to be acute lymphoblastic leukemia because there is no lymphadenopathy, hepatosplenomegaly, or any other symptoms and a CBC would show solitary isolated thrombocytopenia in ITP.

 **Key: C**

 **BOOST YOUR KNOWLEDGE**

The recent nomenclature of ITP is as follows:

- A patient is called a newly diagnosed ITP or acute ITP if symptoms have lasted for <3 months. When symptoms are present from 3 months–1 year, then it is called persistent ITP. Beyond 12 months, the patient is said to have chronic ITP.
- The most important point here is not to give steroids without a detailed peripheral smear examination, to look for blasts and/or bone marrow examination, because acute leukemia remains a close differential and administration of steroids may mask the leukemia.

 **REFERENCE/SOURCE**

- Shah N, Kumar A, Rawat A. Standard Treatment Guidelines 2022, Immune Thrombocytopenic Purpura (ITP). Indian Academy of Pediatrics; 2022.

5. A 5-month-old male child is admitted to the hospital with the complaints of petechia all over the body. He has bloody diarrhea and anemia. The child has been having fever off and on. He has received antibiotics on numerous occasions and is an ill-looking child. Child had a history of rash on the scalp and cheeks after 1 month of life. He is born of a 2nd degree consanguineous marriage. There are two other siblings, both girls, both are fine. On examination, the child looks ill, has pallor, and petechiae all over the body. There are no physical stigmata suggestive of a syndrome. The child has achieved milestones for age. Systemic examination reveals a palpable liver and spleen. His CBC shows a pretransfusion Hb of 4.9 g% and indices suggestive of acute blood loss. Platelet count 31,000, mean platelet volume 5.4 fL, WBC 7,700, polymorphs 51%, lymphocytes 42%, eosinophils 5%, monocytes 2%. What is the primary or underlying diagnosis?

A. Disseminated intravascular coagulation (DIC)
B. Immune thrombocytopenia
C. Wiskott–Aldrich syndrome
D. Langerhans cell histiocytosis

EXPLANATION

The correct answer is Wiskott–Aldrich syndrome (WAS). The classic triad of eczema, thrombocytopenia with microplatelets, and recurrent infections, along with X-linked recessive inheritance, and two normal sisters nails the diagnosis. Langerhans cell histiocytosis can have skin rash, cytopenia in blood and hepatosplenomegaly. However, microplatelets and bloody diarrhea are not typically seen.

It is not immune thrombocytopenia, because the child is ill and there is anemia as well as thrombocytopenia. Of note, the MPV is very low. This is not generally the case in ITP where macroplatelets with a high MPV or IPF (immature platelet fraction) is seen.

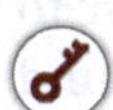

Key: C

BOOST YOUR KNOWLEDGE

Wiskott–Aldrich syndrome is an X-linked recessive disease. It is a primary immune deficiency, caused by a mutation in the gene that encodes for the WAS protein. This gene has been identified on the short arm of the X chromosome (Xp11.22-23). Gene mutation tests are now easily available for diagnosis as well as for antenatal genetic counselling. A popular mnemonic to remember features of WAS is WATER—Wiskott Aldrich, Thrombocytopenia, Eczema, Recurrent infections. Two additional symptoms include increased risk of malignancy and autoimmunity. It is imperative to diagnose these children early in life before complications set in. Also, hematopoietic stem cell transplant, the only potentially curative treatment, has best results when carried out early.

REFERENCE/SOURCE

- Hoffman R. Hematology: Basic Principles and Practice, 5th edition. Churchill-Livingstone; 1991. pp. 418-9.

6. A 9-year-old child presents to the pediatric oncology clinic with fatigue, pallor, and bruising. Complete blood count reveals leukocytosis, anemia, and thrombocytopenia. A bone marrow aspirate and biopsy confirms the diagnosis of acute myeloid leukemia (AML). Which of the following is the most appropriate initial management for this patient?

A. Immediate referral for bone marrow transplant
B. Induction chemotherapy with cytarabine and daunorubicin
C. Supportive care and observation without immediate intervention
D. Oral corticosteroids for symptom control

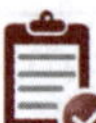

EXPLANATION

Acute myeloid leukemia in pediatric patients requires prompt initiation of chemotherapy. The standard initial treatment is induction chemotherapy, usually with a combination of cytarabine and daunorubicin. This aims to induce remission by reducing the number of leukemic cells in the bone marrow. Based on the gene mutations detected, other new agents can be added to the armamentarium, however cytarabine and daunorubicin are the backbone of chemotherapy to AML.

Key: B

BOOST YOUR KNOWLEDGE

While bone marrow transplant may be considered in the further management of AML, it is not the initial step. Induction chemotherapy is the primary treatment to achieve remission before considering transplantation.

Supportive care alone is not sufficient; induction chemotherapy is crucial to initiate the treatment and improve the chances of remission.

Corticosteroids are not the primary treatment for AML. Induction chemotherapy is the standard approach to address the underlying leukemia and achieve remission.

REFERENCE/SOURCE

- Pizzo PA, Poplack DG. Principles and Practice of Pediatric Oncology, 6th edition. Wolters Kluwer; 2011. pp. 576-81.

7. A 4-year-old boy was referred by the orthopedic surgeon for thrombocytopenia. The child had multiple limb abnormalities since birth which needed corrective surgery and thrombocytopenia. He went on to develop bloody diarrhea from 3 months of age until 1.5 years, after which the platelet counts were around 80,000–90,000. On examination, the child had bilateral upper limb abnormalities, with hypoplastic radii but thumbs were present. The child had achieved normal milestones. Based on the clinical history, what is the diagnosis?

A. Fanconi anemia
B. Thrombocytopenia with absent radius (TAR)
C. Congenital a megakaryocytic thrombocytopenia (CAMT)
D. VACTERL

EXPLANATION

The correct answer is thrombocytopenia with absent radius due to the limb abnormalities along with the thrombocytopenia. Fanconi anemia has pancytopenia with triphalangeal thumb or other thumb abnormalities. In this child, the thumb is normal. In children with CAMT, there is thrombocytopenia, which does not improve with age unlike in TAR. Patients with VACTERL (vertebral defects, anal atresia, cardiac defects, tracheoesophageal fistula, renal anomalies, and limb abnormalities) have congenital malformations including vertebral defects, anal atresia, cardiac defects, tracheoesophageal fistula, renal anomalies, and limb abnormalities. The thumb is usually absent in VACTERL.

Key: B

BOOST YOUR KNOWLEDGE

The correct answer is TAR or thrombocytopenia with absent radius. It is primarily a clinical diagnosis. The forearm is shortened with radius not palpable, and normal thumbs. Lower limb abnormalities are reported in 50% cases. Thrombocytopenia is severe until 2 years of age, and then improves, though it never normalizes.

The mainstay of treatment for thrombocytopenia is judicious single donor platelet transfusions for management of bleeding. Orthopedic interventions are needed to maximize limb function and they may be postponed until platelet counts improve. It is recommended to avoid cow's milk to reduce the severity of gastroenteritis and exacerbations of thrombocytopenia. Antenatal ultrasonography (USG) may pick up the skeletal abnormalities and amniocentesis with genetic testing is now available.

The genetic abnormality is a compound heterozygosity for a rare null mutation involving the *RBM8A* gene (605313) on chromosome 1q21 on 1 allele and 1 of 2 low-frequency noncoding single-nucleotide polymorphisms (SNPs) in RBM8A on the other.

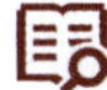

REFERENCE/SOURCE

- Hoffman R. Hematology: Basic Principles and Practice, 5th edition. Churchill-Livingstone; 1991. pp. 350-1.

8. **A 3-year-old girl was referred for multiple ecchymotic spots, and epistaxis, since 6 months of age. She was a full-term normal delivery born of a second-degree consanguineous marriage. The child was investigated on numerous occasions. A diagnosis of platelet function disorders was considered. Which of the following is a characteristic feature of platelet function disorders?**

A. Increased platelet count
B. Prolonged bleeding time
C. Elevated prothrombin time (PT)
D. Reduced von Willebrand factor levels

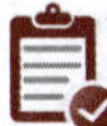

EXPLANATION

Platelet function disorders result in a prolonged bleeding time. This occurs because platelets play a crucial role in hemostasis by forming a plug at the site of vascular injury. In platelet function disorders, impaired aggregation, and adhesion lead to a delay in the formation of this plug, resulting in prolonged bleeding time.

The platelet count is not increased in platelet function disorders.

Prothrombin time assesses the extrinsic and common coagulation pathways, mainly involving factors in the liver-produced coagulation cascade. Platelet function disorders are more related to the platelet-mediated primary hemostasis.

Reduced von Willebrand factor levels are associated with von Willebrand disease, a distinct disorder.

Key: B

BOOST YOUR KNOWLEDGE

Platelet function disorders are characterized by qualitative defects in platelet function, not by an increase or decrease in platelet count. The total number of platelets may be normal, but their ability to aggregate and adhere is compromised.

A simple peripheral smear can point toward a platelet function defect especially macro platelets in case of Bernard–Soulier (BS) disease, or other macrothrombocytopenia. If a peripheral smear is prepared from a finger prick, it will show whether the platelets are clumping or not. An absence of clumping may point toward a platelet function defect such as Glanzmann's thrombasthenia (GT).

A platelet function assay will give further information on the functioning of the platelets. This helps to diagnose Glanzmann's thrombasthenia (absent aggregation with all mild agonists), Bernard–Soulier disease (absent aggregation to ristocetin, but normal aggregation with other agonists), and von Willebrand disease.

Receptor studies by flowcytometry will help to further consolidate the diagnosis. Typically, glycoprotein IIb/IIIA for Glanzmann's thrombasthenia and IB/IX for Bernard Soulier are studied.

Gene mutation analysis will seal the diagnosis of unclassified platelet abnormalities and help to characterize the exact mutation resulting in with GT or BS and may be done at a later stage after a diagnosis of the disorder is made.

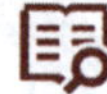

REFERENCE/SOURCE

- Hoffman R. Hematology: Basic Principles and Practice, 5th edition. Churchill-Livingstone; 1991. pp. 2133-44. Chapter: Disorders of platelet function.

9. A 15-year-old male child was referred for borderline low platelet counts on multiple occasions. He had a normal bone marrow, immature platelet fraction, and mean platelet volume. He was completely asymptomatic. Born of a non-consanguineous marriage there was no family history of bleeding. At our hospital, a CBC was repeated using Na citrate as an anticoagulant. The platelet count was now reported as 2.8 lakhs/cu mm. What is the diagnosis?

A. Chronic immune thrombocytopenia
B. Platelet satellitism resulting in pseudothrombocytopenia
C. Inherited bone marrow failure syndrome
D. May–Hegglin anomaly

EXPLANATION

Platelet satellitism resulting in pseudothrombocytopenia. The most important clue is that after changing the anticoagulant from ethylenediaminetetraacetic acid (EDTA) to trisodium citrate, the platelet count normalized. The cause for this phenomenon is that there is in vitro binding of platelets to neutrophils, thus resulting in a pseudothrombocytopenia. A peripheral sear examination is of utmost importance because it shows the platelets sticking to the neutrophils if done on the EDTA sample, and if a direct smear is prepared there are no platelet satellites. May–Hegglin anomaly or MYH9 group of platelet disorders is characterized by mild macrothrombocytopenia with or without additional features such as Döhle-like bodies in neutrophils, renal failure, hearing loss, and early onset cataracts.

It is not chronic ITP or inherited bone marrow failure because the count got corrected with a simple change in the anticoagulant, and also platelet satellitism was seen on the peripheral smear (PS).

Key: B

BOOST YOUR KNOWLEDGE

The pathophysiology of this phenomenon is not well understood. It is proposed that immunoglobin autoantibodies against the glycoprotein IIb/IIIa receptor complex and the neutrophil Fc-gamma (FcγRIII) receptor play a role.

Other hypotheses are:

- Ethylenediaminetetraacetic acid causes changes in platelet and neutrophil membranes resulting in bridge formation between the two.
- Ethylenediaminetetraacetic acid exposes cryptic epitopes on platelets or neutrophils.
- Autoantibodies recognize the same epitopes in the membrane of platelets and neutrophils.
- A non-immunologic mechanism has also been proposed.

REFERENCE/SOURCE

- Chakrabarti I. Platelet satellitism: a rare, interesting, in vitro phenomenon. J Hematol Blood Transfus. 2014;30(3):213-4.

10. A 6-year-old boy presents to the clinic with petechiae, easy bruising, and epistaxis over the past few weeks. On examination, he appears fine, playful active, afebrile, no organomegaly, or lymph nodes. The child has no history of recent infections or illnesses. The CBC is within normal limits except for a platelet count of 40,000/mm^3. What is the most likely diagnosis for this child's presentation?

A. Immune thrombocytopenic purpura (ITP)
B. Thrombotic thrombocytopenic purpura (TTP)
C. Hemolytic uremic syndrome (HUS)
D. von Willebrand disease

EXPLANATION

Immune thrombocytopenic purpura is characterized by isolated thrombocytopenia in the absence of other blood cell abnormalities. It often presents with petechiae, easy bruising, and mucosal bleeding. The absence of significant systemic symptoms and normal CBC except for thrombocytopenia are typical features of ITP in children.

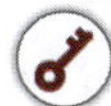

Key: A

BOOST YOUR KNOWLEDGE

- Thrombotic thrombocytopenic purpura is associated with microangiopathic hemolytic anemia and fever. This child does not exhibit those features.
- Hemolytic uremic syndrome typically presents with microangiopathic hemolytic anemia, thrombocytopenia, and acute kidney injury, which are not seen in this case.
- von Willebrand disease primarily affects platelet function rather than platelet count.

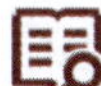

REFERENCE/SOURCE

- Neunert C, Lim W, Crowther M, Cohen A, Solberg L Jr, Crowther MA, et al. The American Society of Hematology 2011 Evidence-based Practice Guideline for Immune Thrombocytopenia. Blood. 2011;117(16):4190-207.

11. A 7-year-old girl is admitted to the ward with persistent fever, hepatosplenomegaly, and petechiae. CBC shows pancytopenia, with a platelet count of 20,000/mm^3, hemoglobin level of 6.0 g/dL, and a low absolute neutrophil count of 800/mm^3. The ferritin level is markedly elevated 45,00 ng/mL. The serum triglycerides are also elevated 290 mg/dL. What is the most likely diagnosis?

A. Immune thrombocytopenic purpura (ITP)
B. Hemophagocytic lymphohistiocytosis (HLH)
C. Thrombotic thrombocytopenic purpura (TTP)
D. Acute lymphoblastic leukemia (ALL)

EXPLANATION

Immune thrombocytopenic purpura typically presents with isolated thrombocytopenia without systemic symptoms such as hepatosplenomegaly and persistent fever.

Thrombotic thrombocytopenic purpura is characterized by microangiopathic hemolytic anemia and thrombocytopenia. ALL usually presents with symptoms related to bone marrow infiltration, such as anemia and thrombocytopenia, but it lacks the characteristic features of HLH.

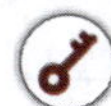

Key: B

BOOST YOUR KNOWLEDGE

Hemophagocytic lymphohistiocytosis is a hyperinflammatory syndrome characterized by persistent fever, cytopenia, coagulopathy, elevations in typical biomarkers, including ferritin and soluble interleukin-2 (IL-2) receptor (sIL-2R) splenomegaly, and hemophagocytosis in the bone marrow. Elevated ferritin levels and triglycerides are commonly seen and are useful simple tests to diagnose HLH. Patients may develop skin rash, hepatitis, and may progress to disseminated intravascular coagulation, acute liver failure, or central nervous system involvement, multiorgan failure, and other problems. The high mortality rate makes prompt recognition and treatment of this hyperinflammatory syndrome essential.

List of diagnostic criteria for hemophagocytic lymphohistiocytosis that were used in the Histiocyte Society HLH-2004 study:

(A) Genetic defect consistent with HLH or **(B) Five out of eight clinical and laboratory criteria fulfilled**
1. Fever
2. Splenomegaly
3. Cytopenia in >/=2 cell lineages Hemoglobin <9 g/dL, in neonates, 10 g/dL Platelet count <100 × 10^3/mL Neutrophil count <1 × 10^3/mL
4. Hypertriglyceridemia (>265 mg/dL) or hypofibrinogenemia (>150 mg/dL)
5. Hyperferritinemia (>500 ng/mL)
6. Soluble CD25 >2,400 U/mL (or elevated compared with laboratory defined normal ranges)
7. Hemophagocytosis in bone marrow, spleen, lymph nodes, or liver
8. Low or absent NK-cell cytotoxicity according to the revised diagnostic criteria guidelines

REFERENCES/SOURCES

- Canna SW, Marsh RA. Pediatric hemophagocytic lymphohistiocytosis. Blood. 2020;135(16):1332-43.
- Sachdeva A, Sachdeva D, Kalra M. Standard Treatment Guidelines 2022, Hemophagocytic Lymphohistiocytosis. Indian Academy of Pediatrics; 2022.

12. A 10-year-old girl is brought to the emergency department with complaints of fatigue, pallor, and easy bruising over the past few weeks. On examination, she appears lethargic. There is no hepatosplenomegaly or lymphadenopathy, and a CBC reveals pancytopenia with a markedly decreased absolute neutrophil count 150, hemoglobin level of 3.5 g/dL, and platelet count of 15,000/mm^3. The bone marrow aspirate shows hypocellular marrow with reduced cellularity. What is the most likely diagnosis?

A. Immune thrombocytopenic purpura (ITP)
B. Aplastic anemia
C. Hemolytic uremic syndrome (HUS)
D. Thalassemia

EXPLANATION

Aplastic anemia is characterized by pancytopenia and a hypocellular bone marrow. It presents with symptoms of fatigue, pallor, and easy bruising due to decreased production of blood cells.

Immune thrombocytopenic purpura primarily involves isolated thrombocytopenia without affecting other blood cell lines.

Hemolytic uremic syndrome typically presents with microangiopathic hemolytic anemia, thrombocytopenia, and acute kidney injury. Thalassemia is a hemoglobin disorder and does not present with pancytopenia.

Key: B

BOOST YOUR KNOWLEDGE

Aplastic anemia results in pancytopenia with a hypocellular bone marrow, without infiltration of the bone marrow with abnormal cells, dysplasia, or marrow fibrosis. In children, most cases are idiopathic and caused by T-lymphocyte-mediated destruction of hemopoietic stem and progenitor cells (HSPCs). It is mandatory to rule out inherited bone marrow failure syndromes (IBMFS). The modalities of treatment include hemopoietic stem cell transplantation (if a donor is available) and immunosuppressive therapy, with antithymocyte globulin and cyclosporin. Eltrombopag, the thrombopoietin receptor agonist, has also been used.

REFERENCE/SOURCE

- Danewa A, Kalra M, Sachdeva A, Sachdeva P, Bansal D, Bhat S, et al. Diagnosis and management of acquired aplastic anemia: Consensus Statement of Indian Academy of Pediatrics. Indian Pediatr. 2022;59(6):467-75.

13. A 5-year-old male presents to the pediatric emergency department with a 5-day history of persistent high-grade fever, conjunctival injection, strawberry tongue, and erythematous rash on his hands and feet. Physical examination reveals bilateral non-purulent conjunctivitis, cracked lips, and cervical lymphadenopathy. Investigations reveal elevated platelet count 12 lakhs, and a high C-reactive protein (CRP) and erythrocyte sedimentation rate (ESR). An echocardiogram shows coronary artery dilatation. What is the most likely diagnosis for this patient?

A. Scarlet fever
B. Measles
C. Kawasaki disease
D. Rocky Mountain spotted fever

EXPLANATION

- Kawasaki disease is an acute febrile illness that primarily affects children. It is characterized by systemic vasculitis, and common clinical features include fever, bilateral non-purulent conjunctivitis, erythematous rash, strawberry tongue, and cervical lymphadenopathy. Thrombocytosis is a common laboratory finding in Kawasaki disease.
- It is not Scarlet fever, because it is characterized by a sandpaper-like rash and is caused by Group A *Streptococcus*. The presentation in this case, including conjunctival injection, strawberry tongue, and cervical lymphadenopathy, is more suggestive of Kawasaki disease.
- Measles typically presents with a high fever, cough, and a characteristic maculopapular rash. It does not cause the specific findings seen in Kawasaki disease.
- Rocky Mountain spotted fever is a tick-borne illness characterized by fever and a rash that usually starts on the wrists and ankles. The symptoms and clinical features are not consistent with Kawasaki disease.

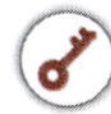

Key: C

BOOST YOUR KNOWLEDGE

Thrombocytosis is a normal reactive response to inflammation, and it is a common finding in inflammatory conditions, including Kawasaki disease. It is not indicative of a poor prognosis. The coronary artery complications can be prevented by administering intravenous immunoglobulin promptly, ideally within the first 10 days of illness. Without prompt treatment, Kawasaki disease can lead to the development of coronary artery aneurysms, which can have serious long-term consequences.

REFERENCE/SOURCE

- Kliegman RM, St Geme III JW. Nelson Textbook of Pediatrics, 21st edition. Elsevier; 2019. Chapter 191: Kawasaki disease.

14. A 4-year-old child has a sudden onset of ecchymotic spots all over the body. In addition, the child had headache for 1 week and confusion for the last few days. Investigations revealed severe thrombocytopenia, 26,000 with an Hb of 6.5 g%, total WBC count and differential were within the normal range for age. The peripheral blood smear showed schistocytes. The reticulocyte count was raised 11%, serum creatinine was raised 1.8 mg/dL so was the LDH, 1,600 units/liter. Thus, the child had a hemolytic anemia, and renal failure, with central nervous system (CNS) symptoms. What is the most likely diagnosis?

A. Hemolytic uremic syndrome (HUS)
B. Evans syndrome
C. Thrombotic thrombocytopenic purpura (TTP)
D. Disseminated intravascular coagulation (DIC)

EXPLANATION

Thrombotic thrombocytopenic purpura is a rare disorder caused by a deficiency in ADAMTS13 (a disintegrin and metalloproteinase with a thrombospondin type 1 motif, member 13), an enzyme responsible for cleaving von Willebrand factor. This disease is characterized by thrombocytopenia, microangiopathic hemolytic anemia, neurological symptoms, fever, and renal involvement. This is the classic pentad of TTP. However, all patients may not have all five features.

Hemolytic uremic syndrome is a disorder characterized by microangiopathic hemolytic anemia and thrombocytopenia, often associated with renal failure. However, HUS typically presents with gastrointestinal symptoms, such as bloody diarrhea, and is more commonly seen in the context of certain bacterial infections, particularly *Escherichia coli* O157:H7. The absence of significant gastrointestinal symptoms, and presence of neurological symptoms, makes HUS less likely in this case.

Evans syndrome is characterized by the simultaneous or sequential development of autoimmune hemolytic anemia and immune thrombocytopenic purpura. While it involves both red blood cells and platelets, the presentation does not typically include renal failure. Additionally, the presence of schistocytes on peripheral smear is not a prominent feature of Evans syndrome.

Disseminated intravascular coagulation is a complex disorder involving widespread activation of the clotting cascade, leading to both thrombosis and bleeding. While it can present with thrombocytopenia and hemolytic features, the combination of severe thrombocytopenia, schistocytes, and renal failure is more indicative of TTP. DIC is often secondary to underlying conditions such as sepsis, trauma, or malignancy.

It is crucial to differentiate between these disorders as their management and outcomes can vary significantly. In this case, the presence of schistocytes on the peripheral smear, along with the clinical presentation, points toward the diagnosis of TTP.

Key: C

BOOST YOUR KNOWLEDGE

Thrombotic thrombocytopenic purpura is characterized by the lack of ADAMTS13 leading to the formation of microthrombi in small blood vessels, causing microangiopathic hemolytic anemia, thrombocytopenia, and ischemic organ damage. The presence of schistocytes (fragmented red blood cells) on peripheral blood smear is a characteristic finding. The deficiency of ADAMTS-13 may be either acquired (associated anti-ADAMTS13 autoantibodies) or congenital (resulting from biallelic mutations of *ADAMTS13* gene). It is crucial to differentiate between these disorders as their management and outcomes can vary significantly. In this case, the presence of schistocytes on the peripheral smear, along with the clinical presentation, points toward the diagnosis of TTP. TTP is a medical emergency, and prompt diagnosis and treatment, with plasma exchange therapy are essential for a favorable outcome.

REFERENCE/SOURCE

- Joly BS. Pediatric thrombotic thrombocytopenic purpura. Eur J Haematol. 2018;101(4):425-34.

15. A 3-year-old child presents with easy bruising, petechiae, and mucosal bleeding. On examination, the child appears pale, and has significant hepatosplenomegaly. CBC reveals severe thrombocytopenia and low Hb. In addition, the child has a history of recurrent infections and developmental delay. A bone marrow aspirate carried out showed normal erythroid and myeloid maturation, and megakaryocytes. There were large clusters and aggregates of macrophages with eccentric nuclei, abundant blue-gray cytoplasm, and wrinkled tissue paper. What is the most likely diagnosis for this child's thrombocytopenia?

A. Immune thrombocytopenic purpura (ITP)
B. Gaucher disease
C. Thrombotic thrombocytopenic purpura (TTP)
D. Hemolytic uremic syndrome (HUS)

EXPLANATION

- Gaucher disease, an autosomal recessive lysosomal storage disorder, is characterized by a deficiency of glucocerebrosidase, leading to the accumulation of glucocerebroside in macrophages. This accumulation results in hepatosplenomegaly and hematologic abnormalities, including thrombocytopenia.
- It is not immune thrombocytopenic purpura. ITP is an immune-mediated disorder characterized by isolated thrombocytopenia without the hepatosplenomegaly and developmental delay seen in Gaucher disease.
- Thrombotic thrombocytopenic purpura is characterized by microangiopathic hemolytic anemia, thrombocytopenia, and organ involvement, typically without hepatosplenomegaly and developmental delay.
- Hemolytic uremic syndrome is characterized by microangiopathic hemolytic anemia and thrombocytopenia but is often associated with preceding gastrointestinal symptoms.

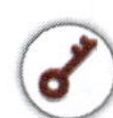

Key: B

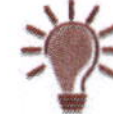

BOOST YOUR KNOWLEDGE

Gaucher's disease (GD) is diagnosed by the demonstration of characteristic "Gaucher cells" in the bone marrow. Pseudo-Gaucher cells have occasionally been described in various hematologic malignancies including multiple myeloma, myelodysplastic syndrome, lymphomas, chronic myelogenous leukemia, and thalassemia. Therefore, detection of reduced or absent β-glucosidase (glucocerebrosidase) enzyme activity is the gold standard for the diagnosis of all the variants of GD. However, molecular testing that involves single gene testing or a multigene panel is necessary for definitive diagnosis. Prenatal diagnosis is also possible. Enzyme replacement therapy is approved in pediatric patients.

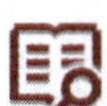

REFERENCE/SOURCE

- Weinreb NJ, Goker-Alpan O, Kishnani PS, Longo N, Burrow TA, Bernat JA, et al. The diagnosis and management of Gaucher disease in pediatric patients: Where do we go from here? Mol Genet Metab. 2022;136(1):4-21.

16. Which laboratory instrument is commonly used to measure immature platelet fraction (IPF)?

A. Automated hematology analyzer
B. Flow cytometer
C. Coagulation analyzer
D. Blood gas analyzer

EXPLANATION

- Immature platelet fraction is commonly measured using automated hematology analyzers from different companies. These analyzers use flow cytometry and fluorescent dyes to identify and quantify reticulated and other immature platelets, providing a comprehensive assessment of platelet maturation.
- It is not flow cytometer. While flow cytometers can be used for platelet analysis, automated hematology analyzers are more commonly employed in routine clinical settings for IPF measurement.
- Coagulation analyzers are primarily designed to assess blood clotting parameters, not platelet maturation. IPF is better assessed using hematology analyzers.
- Blood gas analyzers are used for measuring gases and electrolytes in blood, not for platelet analysis.

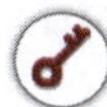

Key: A

BOOST YOUR KNOWLEDGE

The absolute number and percentage of reticulated platelets are a reflection of thrombopoiesis. Just like the reticulocyte count, reticulated platelets are useful for differentiating thrombocytopenia. However, it is difficult to reproduce the values when the test is carried out in different laboratories. The immature platelet fraction, on the other hand, is a reproducible and convenient parameter that is automatically measured by the hematology analyzers. A disproportionately high IPF is seen in patients with macrothrombocytopenia and may be useful to suspect this rare condition, which may be a mimic of chronic ITP.

REFERENCE/SOURCE

- Miyazaki K, Koike Y, Kunishima S, Ishii R, Danbara M, Horie R, et al. Immature platelet fraction measurement is influenced by platelet size and is a useful parameter for discrimination of macrothrombocytopenia. Hematology. 2015;20(10):587-92.

17. What does IPF measure in the peripheral blood?

A. Total platelet count
B. Proportion of newly formed platelets
C. Platelet aggregation capacity
D. Megakaryocytes in peripheral blood

EXPLANATION

Immature platelet fraction is a parameter that measures the percentage of circulating platelets that are newly formed and have not yet fully matured. It provides valuable information about platelet production and turnover. IPF is often used in conjunction with other platelet indices to assess bone marrow function and response in various clinical conditions.

Total platelet count represents the overall number of platelets in the blood and does not specifically measure the proportion of newly formed platelets. IPF provides additional information beyond the total platelet count.

Platelet aggregation is the ability of platelets to clump together in response to specific stimuli. IPF focuses on the immature fraction and does not directly assess platelet aggregation.

Key: B

BOOST YOUR KNOWLEDGE

It is important to determine the cause of thrombocytopenia because the treatment and management will be different. Most platelet parameters that are routinely analyzed in the diagnostic laboratory have not proven useful in identifying the etiology. The immature platelet fraction, indirectly provides a measure of bone marrow function, and response to thrombopoietin. The IPF percent is increased in cases of increased platelet consumption, pseudothrombocytopenia, idiopathic thrombocytopenic purpura, and hemorrhage. IPF helps in differentiating thrombocytopenia due to platelet consumption/destruction from bone marrow failure/suppression. It helps to predict platelet recovery in cases of dengue and chemotherapy, and unnecessary platelet transfusions and the associated risks can be prevented.

REFERENCE/SOURCE

- Ali I, Graham C, Dempsey-Hibbert NC. Immature platelet fraction as a useful marker in the etiological determination of thrombocytopenia. Exp Hematol. 2019;78:56-61.

18. Which of the following medications is commonly associated with drug-induced thrombocytopenia in pediatric patients?

A. Acetaminophen
B. Amoxicillin
C. Ibuprofen
D. Heparin

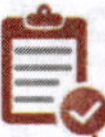

EXPLANATION

Heparin-induced thrombocytopenia (HIT) is a serious immune-mediated adverse reaction associated with the use of heparin. While HIT is more commonly observed in adults, it can also occur in pediatric patients. HIT is characterized by a rapid decrease in platelet count, usually occurring 5–14 days after exposure to heparin. The condition results from the formation of antibodies against the heparin-platelet factor 4 (PF4) complex, leading to platelet activation and consumption.

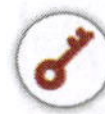

Key: D

BOOST YOUR KNOWLEDGE

- *Acetaminophen:* It is a widely used analgesic and antipyretic medication, but it is not known to cause thrombocytopenia. It does not have a significant impact on platelet function.
- *Amoxicillin:* Amoxicillin, a commonly prescribed antibiotic, is not typically associated with drug-induced thrombocytopenia. Thrombocytopenia is a rare adverse effect of beta-lactam antibiotics such as amoxicillin.
- *Ibuprofen:* It is a non-steroidal anti-inflammatory drug (NSAID) commonly used for pain relief and inflammation. It is not known to cause thrombocytopenia. NSAIDs primarily affect the coagulation system by inhibiting platelet function, rather than causing a decrease in platelet count.

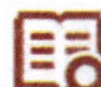

REFERENCE/SOURCE

- Greinacher A. Heparin-induced thrombocytopenia. N Engl J Med. 2015;373(3):252-61.

CHAPTER

18.7

Thrombosis, Disseminated Intravascular Coagulation, and Physiology of Hemostasis

Anusha Hegde

1. A 14-year-old girl presented with complaints of swelling in the right lower limb. There is no evidence of infection. Venous Doppler confirms thrombus in the femoral vein. On evaluation, hemoglobin was 9 g/dL, total count 5,600/mm, and platelets 125,000/mm^3; coagulation work-up showed prothrombin time (PT) 14 seconds (control 12) and activated partial thromboplastin time (APTT) 54 seconds (control 35 seconds). What is the most probable diagnosis?

A. Fibrinogen deficiency
B. Antiphospholipid antibody (APLA) syndrome
C. Protein C deficiency
D. Hyperhomocysteinemia

EXPLANATION

Here is an adolescent female presenting with spontaneous onset deep vein thrombosis (DVT) with mild anemia, thrombocytopenia, and prolonged APTT. Prolonged APTT in APLA syndrome is due to the presence of APLAs.

	Fibrinogen deficiency	*APLA*	*Protein C deficiency*	*Hyperhomocysteinemia*
Thrombosis		•	•	•
Bleeding	•	•		
Prolonged APTT	•	•		
Anemia and thrombocytopenia		•		

Key: **B**

BOOST YOUR KNOWLEDGE

Lupus anticoagulant:

- Antibody against phospholipids involved in phospholipid-based anticoagulation assay
- Prolonged APTT but predisposed to thrombus
- Mixing studies—patient plasma + normal plasma—APTT will not get corrected.

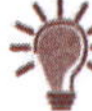

REFERENCE/SOURCE

- Raffini LJ, Scott JP. Thrombotic disorders in children. In: Kliegman RM, St Geme III JW, Blum NJ, Shah SS, Tasker RC, Wilson KM (Eds). Nelson Textbook of Pediatrics, 21st edition. Elsevier; 2019. pp. 2603-7.

2. Term neonate presented with history of (H/o) lethargy and seizures on the eighth day of life. Mother has difficulty in breastfeeding, and the baby has a weight loss of more than 20% of birth weight. What is the imaging modality of choice for evaluating this child?

A. Computed tomography (CT) of the brain
B. MR venogram
C. Ultrasound cranium
D. Lumbar puncture

EXPLANATION

In a neonate presenting with dehydration and central nervous system (CNS) symptoms, cerebral venous thrombosis should be suspected. MR venogram is the most sensitive modality in this setting.

Key: B

BOOST YOUR KNOWLEDGE

Site of thrombus	*Investigation of choice*
Thrombosis of the upper limb or lower limb	Ultrasound with Doppler flow
Pulmonary embolism	Spiral or helical CT chest
Cerebral venous thrombosis	MR venogram or diffusion-weighted imaging
Cardiac thrombus	Echocardiogram

REFERENCE/SOURCE

- Raffini LJ, Scott JP. Thrombotic disorders in children. In: Kliegman RM, St Geme III JW, Blum NJ, Shah SS, Tasker RC, Wilson KM (Eds). Nelson Textbook of Pediatrics, 21st edition. Elsevier; 2019. pp. 2603-7.

3. Identify the correct combination of anticoagulant agent and monitoring test.

A. Unfractionated heparin (UFH)—antifactor Xa, warfarin—D dimer, low-molecular-weight heparin (LMWH)—international normalized ratio (INR)
B. UFH—INR, LMWH—antifactor Xa, warfarin—D dimer
C. UFH—D-Dimer, LMWH—antifactor Xa, warfarin—partial thromboplastin time (PTT)
D. UFH—PTT, LMWH—antifactor Xa, warfarin—INR

EXPLANATION

Intravenous (IV) infusion of UFH is used to achieve PTT 1.5–2.5 the upper limit of normal. INR is maintained between 2 and 3 for most patients with venous thrombosis treated with warfarin. LMWH dose is adjusted according to antifactor Xa levels. The activity of recombinant tissue plasminogen activator is monitored using fibrin degradation product (FDP) or D-dimer levels.

Key: D

BOOST YOUR KNOWLEDGE

Low-molecular-weight heparin:

- Easy administration and less frequent monitoring
- Route of administration—subcutaneous and twice daily
- Monitoring—antifactor Xa
- Sample should be sent 4 hours after third dose.
- Target antifactor Xa levels between 0.5 and 1

REFERENCE/SOURCE

- Raffini LJ, Scott JP. Thrombotic disorders in children. In: Kliegman RM, St Geme III JW, Blum NJ, Shah SS, Tasker RC, Wilson KM (Eds). Nelson Textbook of Pediatrics, 21st edition. Elsevier; 2019. pp. 2603-7.

4. A 14-year-old girl with H/o joint pain and pallor was admitted for evaluation. No evidence of (E/o) bleeding was seen. On evaluation, hemoglobin was 7 g/dL, total count 6,200/mm^3, platelets 250,000/mm^3, PT 14 seconds (control 12 seconds), and APTT 60 seconds (control 35 seconds). What is the most appropriate test to be done next?

A. Mixing studies
B. Von Willebrand assay and Ristocetin cofactor (RCo)
C. Ferritin
D. Factor 13 assay

EXPLANATION

An adolescent girl with H/o joint pain and anemia is suggestive of evolving systemic lupus erythematosus (SLE). The prolongation of APTT in this setting is due to inhibitors. Von Willebrand disease will present with bleeding and prolonged PTT. Factor 13 deficiency would be associated with bleeding and normal PT/APTT. Either of these two will not cause anemia directly; however, immune-mediated cytopenias are possible in connective tissue disorders.

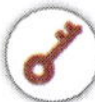

Key: A

BOOST YOUR KNOWLEDGE

Mixing study:
- A test is done to differentiate factor deficiency and circulating inhibitor.
- Patient's plasma is mixed with an equal amount of normal plasma
- Correction of APTT—factor deficiency
- Prolonged APTT—the presence of inhibitor

REFERENCE/SOURCE

- Gupta P, Menon PSN, Ramji S, Lodha R (Eds). PG Textbook of Pediatrics, 3rd edition. New Delhi: Jaypee Brothers Medical Publishers; 2022. Chapter 38.18.

5. A 9-month-old infant presented with H/o fever and decreased feeding and activity for 1 week. The child is admitted to the ICU in view of septic shock. On day 2 of admission, child was noticed with discoloration of the hand as shown here. What is the most appropriate immediate management?

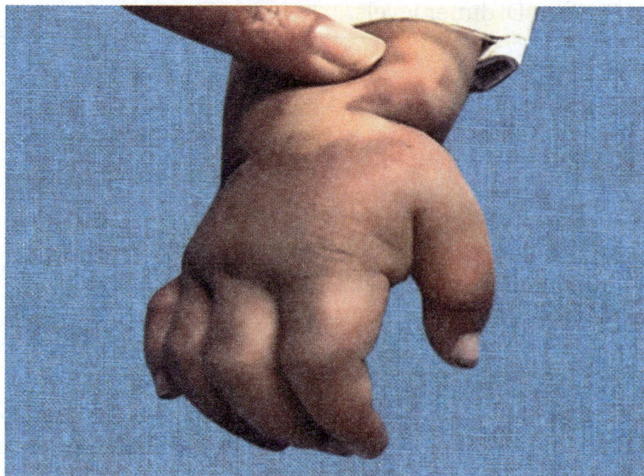

A. Platelet transfusion
B. Vitamin K administration
C. Fresh-frozen plasma (FFP) transfusion
D. Plasma exchange

EXPLANATION

Young infant presenting with septic shock and discoloration of skin is suggestive of sepsis-induced purpura fulminans. Skin discoloration is due to superficial thrombosis of the skin secondary to protein C deficiency. As FFP contains a considerable amount of protein C, it should be given immediately.

Key: C

BOOST YOUR KNOWLEDGE

Purpura fulminans:

- Neonatal period—homozygous or double heterozygous protein C/protein S deficiency
- Infants and older children—acquired deficiency of protein C secondary to sepsis

Treatment:

- FFP transfusion
- Infusion of protein C concentrate
- Liver transplant—in severe congenital deficiency of protein C

REFERENCE/SOURCE

- Inherited Disorders of Thrombosis and Fibrinolysis. In: Trenor CC, Bauer KA (Eds). Nathan and Oski's Hematology and Oncology of Infancy and Childhood, Elsevier; 8th edition, 2014.

6. A 16-year-old girl with a pelvic fracture following trauma developed deep vein thrombosis in her left leg. She was started on warfarin, and on Day 6 of warfarin, she developed skin discoloration and necrosis over her right thigh. What would have been done differently to prevent this complication?

A. To start with a high-loading dose of warfarin
B. To add antiplatelet agents along with warfarin
C. Bridge warfarin with LMWH
D. Add oral prednisolone along with warfarin

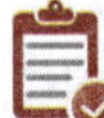

EXPLANATION

The patient discussed in the question is having warfarin-induced skin necrosis. Starting a high dose of warfarin is a risk factor for skin necrosis. Antiplatelet agents and steroids have no role.

Overlapping heparin and warfarin is known to reduce this complication.

Key: C

BOOST YOUR KNOWLEDGE

Warfarin-induced skin necrosis:

- Rapid depletion of anticoagulant factors like protein C and protein S following warfarin therapy creates a transient prothrombotic state, causing superficial vessel thrombosis.
- *Management:*
    - Immediately stop warfarin
    - FFP transfusion followed by adequate anticoagulation using heparin

REFERENCE/SOURCE

- Gupta P, Menon PSN, Ramji S, Lodha R (Eds). PG Textbook of Pediatrics, 3rd edition. New Delhi: Jaypee Brothers Medical Publishers; 2022. Chapter 38.22.

7. An 8-year-old child presented with ascites for the last 6 months. On examination, dilated veins over the abdomen and back were seen. Ultrasound Doppler showed absent flow in all branches of hepatic veins for the length of 2 cm. What is the treatment of choice?

A. Immediate thrombolysis
B. Aspirin
C. Angioplasty and stenting
D. Albumin infusion

EXPLANATION

Ascites, dilated veins over the abdomen and back, and absent hepatic flow are suggestive of chronic Budd–Chiari syndrome probably due to long segment thrombus in the hepatic vein. Thrombolysis and anticoagulation would be less likely to be beneficial as it is a chronic organized thrombus. Albumin infusion is not a definitive management in this setting.

Key: C

BOOST YOUR KNOWLEDGE

Treatment of Budd–Chiari Syndrome

Fulminant Budd–Chiari syndrome	*Acute Budd–Chiari syndrome*	*Chronic Budd–Chiari syndrome*
Liver transplantation	Thrombolysis	Angioplasty + stenting
	Stenting	Long-term anticoagulation to prevent restenosis

REFERENCES/SOURCES

- Gupta P, Menon PSN, Ramji S, Lodha R (Eds). PG Textbook of Pediatrics, 3rd edition. New Delhi: Jaypee Brothers Medical Publishers; 2022. Chapter 37.4.
- Shukla A, Shreshtha A, Mukund A, Bihari C, Eapen CE, Han G, et al. Budd-Chiari syndrome: consensus guidance of the Asian Pacific Association for the study of the liver (APASL). Hepatol Int. 2021;15(3):531-67.

8. An 8-year-old girl presented with progressive pallor and jaundice. On evaluation, hemoglobin was 6 g/dL, total count 1,800/mm^3, and platelets 64,000/mm^3. Total bilirubin was 5.2 g/dL and indirect bilirubin 4.3 g/dL. Ultrasound Doppler is showing portal vein thrombosis. Which of the following is the most likely investigation that would aid the diagnosis?

A. Increased osmotic fragility and decreased eosin-5'-maleimide (EMA) binding
B. Hemoglobin electrophoresis showing HbS peak
C. Reduced expression of CD55 and CD59 on peripheral blood flow cytometry
D. Bridging fibrosis in liver biopsy

EXPLANATION

The child has pancytopenia, indirect hyperbilirubinemia, and portal vein thrombosis.

Mostly due to paroxysmal nocturnal hemoglobinuria, in which case there will be reduced expression of CD55 and CD59 on flow cytometry.

Option A: Hereditary spherocytosis will have only anemia and indirect hyperbilirubinemia. Thrombosis risk increases postsplenectomy.

Option B: Sickle cell anemia will have anemia and indirect hyperbilirubinemia. Abdominal pain in sickle cell disease may be due to hemolytic crisis, sickle hepatopathy, or gut ischemia.

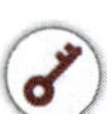

Key: C

BOOST YOUR KNOWLEDGE

Clinical presentation of paroxysmal nocturnal hemoglobinuria:

- Variable degree of pancytopenia due to marrow failure or mild anemia (intermittent or chronic)
- Intravascular hemolysis presenting as jaundice
- Thrombosis or thromboembolic phenomenon due to altered glycoproteins on platelets and release of procoagulants. It may present as Budd–Chiari syndrome, splenomegaly, or recurrent abdominal pain.

REFERENCE/SOURCE

- Merguerian MD, Gallagher PG. Paroxysmal nocturnal hemoglobinuria and acanthocytosis. In: Kliegman RM, St Geme III JW, Blum NJ, Shah SS, Tasker RC, Wilson KM (Eds). Nelson Textbook of Pediatrics, 21st edition. Elsevier; 2019. 2538-40.

9. Which of the following is not a risk factor for arterial ischemic stroke in children?

A. Hyperhomocysteinemia
B. Increased lipoprotein A
C. Protein C deficiency
D. Inhibitors to factor VIII

EXPLANATION

Options A, B, and C are procoagulant states that can contribute to arterial ischemic strokes or cerebral embolism of venous thrombus in case of congenital heart disease. Factor VIII inhibitors are seen after multiple exposures to factor VIII in children with hemophilia. These patients will have a high chance of bleeding.

Key: D

BOOST YOUR KNOWLEDGE

Causes of arterial ischemic stroke in children:

- Infections—CNS tuberculosis, human immunodeficiency virus (HIV), herpes simplex, and varicella zoster
- Hematological—sickle cell anemia
- Thrombophilia—protein C deficiency, elevated levels of lipoprotein, and hyperhomocysteinemia
- Other—neurofibromatosis type 1 and cranial irradiation for malignancies

REFERENCE/SOURCE

- Gupta P, Menon PSN, Ramji S, Lodha R (Eds). PG Textbook of Pediatrics, 3rd edition. New Delhi: Jaypee Brothers Medical Publishers; 2022. Chapter 38.22.

10. A 16-year-old child with fractured shaft femur following trauma was admitted to orthopedic ward. On Day 10 of hospital admission, the child develops sudden-onset chest pain, breathlessness, and hypoxia. What is the next line of management?

A. Chest X-ray and broad-spectrum antibiotics
B. CT angiography and tissue type plasminogen activator (tPA) infusion
C. Ultrasonography (USG) of chest and analgesics
D. CT chest and warfarin

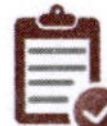

EXPLANATION

With sudden onset chest pain and breathlessness in a patient with prolonged immobilization, one should suspect pulmonary thromboembolism. CT angiography is the most sensitive investigation. As it is a life-threatening condition, immediate thrombolysis with tissue plasminogen activator is recommended.

Key: B

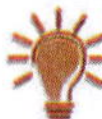

BOOST YOUR KNOWLEDGE

Tissue type plasminogen activator:

Intrinsic activator of the fibrinolytic system administered exogenously

Mechanism of action:

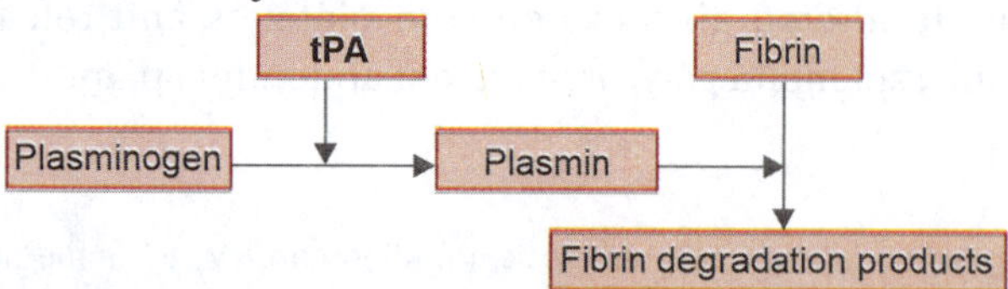

Indications:

- *Life-threatening thrombus:*
  - Massive pulmonary embolism with hemodynamic instability
  - Large arterial thrombus
  - Obstructive superior vena cava syndrome
  - Cerebral venous sinus thrombosis with worsening neurological status
  - Bilateral renal vein thrombus
- *Limb-threatening thrombus:*
  - Acute iliofemoral thrombus
  - Inferior vena cava (IVC) thrombus

REFERENCE/SOURCE

- Gupta P, Menon PSN, Ramji S, Lodha R (Eds). PG Textbook of Pediatrics, 3rd edition. New Delhi: Jaypee Brothers Medical Publishers; 2022. Chapter 38.22.

11. A term infant was admitted to the NICU with birth asphyxia and shock. On Day 3 of admission, the infant developed hematuria and flank mass suspected to have renal vein thrombosis (RVT). Which of the following is true?

A. Magnetic resonance imaging (MRI) abdomen should be done immediately to look for the size and echo structure of kidney
B. Mild thrombocytopenia is common in RVT
C. Thrombolysis is contraindicated in RVT
D. Long-term sequelae of RVT are negligible

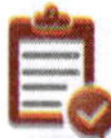

EXPLANATION

Renal vein thrombosis is one of the conditions where thrombocytopenia is seen along with major vessel thrombosis. The investigation of choice is USG renal Doppler to look for the extent of a renal vessel or IVC involvement. In the case of unilateral RVT with no renal vein involvement supportive care, radiological monitoring for the progression of thrombosis or anticoagulation with UFH/LMWH is indicated. Unilateral RVT with renal impairment warrants anticoagulation. Thrombolysis followed by anticoagulation is indicated in bilateral RVT with renal impairment, and significant sequelae like renal atrophy (70%), hypertension (20%), and chronic renal disease (3%) are seen.

Key: B

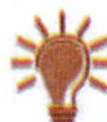

BOOST YOUR KNOWLEDGE

Predisposing factors for RVT in children:

- Maternal diabetes mellitus
- Shock

- Dehydration and perinatal asphyxia
- Polycythemia

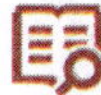

REFERENCES/SOURCES

- Blood coagulation. In: Orkin SH, Nathan DG, Ginsburg D, Look AT, Fisher DE, Lux S. Nathan and Oski's Hematology and Oncology of Infancy and Childhood, 8th edition. Elsevier; 2014.
- Gupta P, Menon PSN, Ramji S, Lodha R (Eds). PG Textbook of Pediatrics, 3rd edition. New Delhi: Jaypee Brothers Medical Publishers; 2022. Chapter 38.22.

12. Which of the following is false regarding warfarin use in children?

A. Dosing titration in infants is difficult as vitamin K-dependent factor levels are low
B. Green leafy vegetables and meat decrease the warfarin effect
C. Nonsteroidal anti-inflammatory drugs (NSAIDs) will increase the warfarin effect
D. Warfarin can cause thrombocytopenia

EXPLANATION

Warfarin is an oral anticoagulant that acts by inhibiting vitamin K, thus decreasing vitamin K-dependent coagulation factors. Foods containing high levels of vitamin K like meat, liver, and green leafy vegetables decrease the warfarin effect. Drugs like NSAIDs, sulfonamides, omeprazole, selective serotonin reuptake inhibitors (SSRIs), and fluconazole increase the warfarin effect. Barbiturates, oral contraceptive pills (OCPs), rifampicin, and vitamin C will decrease the effect. Thrombocytopenia is seen as a side-effect of heparin and not warfarin.

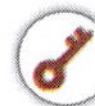

Key: D

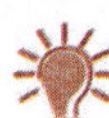

BOOST YOUR KNOWLEDGE

Side effects of warfarin:

- Bleeding
- Hair loss
- Reduced bone mineral density
- Fetal damage if used in pregnancy—nasal hypoplasia, skeletal deformities, and congenital heart defects

REFERENCE/SOURCE

- Gupta P, Menon PSN, Ramji S, Lodha R (Eds). PG Textbook of Pediatrics, 3rd edition. New Delhi: Jaypee Brothers Medical Publishers; 2022. Chapter 38.22.

13. Which of the following is not a procoagulant molecule?

A. Von Willebrand multimers
B. Fibrinogen
C. Adenosine diphosphate (ADP)
D. Nitric oxide

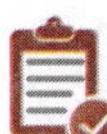

EXPLANATION

During endothelial injury, von Willebrand multimers are exposed on the endothelial surface which attracts platelets forming a primary plug. On activation of the coagulation cascade, fibrinogen converts into fibrin forming a stable clot. ADP helps in platelet aggregation. Nitric oxide causes vasodilation and acts as a natural anticoagulant.

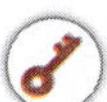

Key: D

BOOST YOUR KNOWLEDGE

Role of vascular endothelium in hemostasis		
Procoagulant	***Anticoagulant***	***Fibrinolytic***
Adhesive ligands—integrins and selectins	Platelet inhibition—nitric oxide and CD39 (ADPase)	tPA
Von Willebrand multimers	Tissue factor pathway inhibitor	Urokinase (uPA)-type plasminogen activator

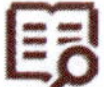

REFERENCE/SOURCE

- Gupta P, Menon PSN, Ramji S, Lodha R (Eds). PG Textbook of Pediatrics, 3rd edition. New Delhi: Jaypee Brothers Medical Publishers; 2022. Chapter 38.1.

14. Which of the following is not a vitamin K-dependent coagulation factor?

A. Factor II B. Fibrinogen
C. Protein C D. Factor X

EXPLANATION

Factors II, VII, IX, and X are vitamin K dependent for their activation. Protein C and protein S are the first to get affected by vitamin K deficiency. Fibrinogen is not dependent on vitamin K for its action.

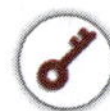

Key: B

BOOST YOUR KNOWLEDGE

Conditions associated with vitamin K-dependent factor deficiency:

- Malabsorption—celiac disease, biliary atresia, and cystic fibrosis
- Drugs—maternal intake of warfarin, valproate, carbamazepine, and antitubercular drugs
- Prolonged antibiotic use and dietary deficiency
- Liver diseases—cholestasis, acute hepatitis, Wilson disease, and Reye's syndrome
- Most common bleeding in vitamin K deficiency—intracranial bleed

	Early form	***Classic form***	***Late form***
Age of onset	<24 hours of birth	2–7 days of life	0.5–6 months
Cause	Medications during pregnancy	• Inadequate vitamin K intake • Breastfeeding	Malabsorption syndromes

REFERENCE/SOURCE

- Gupta P, Menon PSN, Ramji S, Lodha R (Eds). PG Textbook of Pediatrics, 3rd edition. New Delhi: Jaypee Brothers Medical Publishers; 2022. Chapter 38.18.

15. Which of the following coagulation markers is first to get affected in liver disease?

A. Fibrinogen B. Factor VII
C. Factor II D. Factor VIII

EXPLANATION

Clotting factors II, VII, IX, and X undergo vitamin K-dependent decarboxylation in the liver. Factor VII is the most sensitive and first to get affected by liver disease.

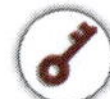

Key: D

BOOST YOUR KNOWLEDGE

- All clotting factors produced by the liver except Von Willebrand factor (VWF), factor VIII
- Factor VIII produced by sinusoidal endothelial cells
- VWF produced in endothelial cells and megakaryocytes
- Protein C and protein S also undergo decarboxylation in the liver.

REFERENCE/SOURCE

- Hemostasis in the newborn and infant. In: Orkin SH, Nathan DG, Ginsburg D, Look AT, Fisher DE, Lux S (Eds). Nathan and Oski's Hematology and Oncology of Infancy and Childhood, 8th edition. Elsevier; 2014.

16. What is the direct function of uPA?

A. Conversion of fibrin to FDPs
B. Conversion of plasmin to plasminogen
C. Conversion of zymogen plasminogen to active plasmin
D. Crosslinking of fibrin products to make a stable clot

EXPLANATION

Urokinase acts similarly as tissue plasminogen activator. Plasmin mediates the degradation of fibrin, leading to thrombolysis.

Key: B

BOOST YOUR KNOWLEDGE

Components of fibrinolytic system:

- Plasmin
- Tissue plasminogen activator
- uPA
- Accessary plasminogen activators—kallikrein, factor XIa, and factor XIIa

Inhibitor of fibrinolysis:

- Plasminogen activator inhibitors 1 and 2
- Alpha 2 antiplasmin

REFERENCE/SOURCE

- Molecular Basis of Fibrinolysis. In: Orkin SH, Nathan DG, Ginsburg D, Look AT, Fisher DE, Lux S (Eds). Nathan and Oski's Hematology and Oncology of Childhood, 8th edition. Elsevier; 2014.

17. Identify the correct pair. Coagulation factor—time to reach adult levels.

A. Protein C, Protein S—at birth
B. Antithrombin—at 1 year of age
C. Factor 8—around 6 months of age
D. VWF—at birth

EXPLANATION

Fibrinogen, factors V, VIII, and XIII, and anticoagulation factor levels are below normal adult range at birth and reach adult levels by 6 months of age. VWFs are high at birth and reach adult value at around 6 months of age.

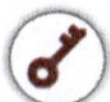

Key: C

BOOST YOUR KNOWLEDGE

Coagulation factors	Function
Factor XII and prekallikrein	Initiation of the intrinsic pathway
Factor VII and tissue factor	Initiator of the extrinsic pathway
Factors V and X	Common pathway activation

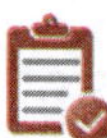

REFERENCE/SOURCE

- Hemostasis in the newborn and infant. In: Orkin SH, Nathan DG, Ginsburg D, Look AT, Fisher DE, Lux S (Eds). Nathan and Oski's Hematology and Oncology of Infancy and Childhood, 8th edition. Elsevier; 2014.

18. A 1-year-old male child, a diagnosed case of hemophilia B, had one episode of joint bleed. Parents have come for an opinion regarding the use of emicizumab for their child. What would be the most appropriate statement during counseling?

A. Emicizumab is highly effective in preventing bleeds in both hemophilia A and B
B. The child does not require emicizumab as child is not having the bleed currently
C. Emicizumab is not effective in hemophilia B
D. Emicizumab is used only in hemophilia with inhibitors

EXPLANATION

Emicizumab is a bispecific monoclonal antibody approved for use in hemophilia A. It can be used as prophylaxis as well as in hemophilia A with inhibitors. It has no role in hemophilia B.

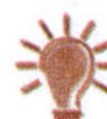

Key: C

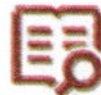

BOOST YOUR KNOWLEDGE

Emicizumab: It is a bispecific antibody that binds factor IXa and X, resulting in the activation of factor X. It is used as 2–3 weekly subcutaneous injection and licensed for primary prophylaxis as well as in patients with inhibitors in hemophilia A. It does not have benefit in hemophilia B as it needs factor IXa for binding and activation.

REFERENCE/SOURCE

- World Federation of Hemophilia. (2020). World Federation of Hemophilia Guidelines for the Management of Hemophilia. [online] Available from https://www1.wfh.org/publications/files/pdf-1863.pdf [Last accessed July, 2024].

19. Which among the following is most likely to present with disseminated intravascular coagulation (DIC)?

A. Hodgkin's lymphoma
B. Acute promyelocytic leukemia
C. Rhabdomyosarcoma
D. Localized Ewing's sarcoma

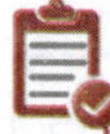

EXPLANATION

Hematological malignancies are more prone to DIC than solid tumors in children. In acute promyelocytic leukemia, high mortality at presentation is mainly due to DIC.

Key: B

BOOST YOUR KNOWLEDGE

Malignancies presenting as DIC:
- Acute promyelocytic leukemia
- Acute monoblastic leukemia

Hematological disorders presenting as DIC:
- Severe thrombotic thrombocytopenic purpura
- Giant hemangioma
- Antithrombin III deficiency
- Homozygous protein C/protein S deficiency
- Acute hemolytic transfusion reaction
- Heparin-induced thrombosis
- Infusion of prothrombin complex concentrates

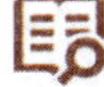

REFERENCE/SOURCE

- Scott JP, Raffini LJ. Disseminated intravascular coagulation. In: Kliegman RM, St Geme III JW, Blum NJ, Shah SS, Tasker RC, Wilson KM (Eds). Nelson Textbook of Pediatrics, 21st edition. Elsevier; 2019. pp. 2608-9.

20. A 5-month-old female child was admitted to pediatric intensive care unit with bronchopneumonia. On Day 3 of the hospital stay, she developed septic shock, needing ionotropic support; multiple ecchymosis noted along with prolonged bleeding at prick sites. What is the most likely combination of investigation results expected in this child?

A. Thrombocytosis, prolonged PT and APTT, and normal D dimer
B. Thrombocytopenia, prolonged PT and APTT, and increased D dimer
C. Decreased D dimer, thrombocytopenia, and normal PT and APTT
D. Normal platelets, increased PT and APTT, and normal D dimer

EXPLANATION

The child most probably has DIC secondary to sepsis. Due to the ongoing intravascular coagulation process, some factors (factors II, V, VIII, and fibrinogen) and platelets are consumed, leading to prolonged PT, prolonged APTT, and thrombocytopenia. At the same time, fibrinolytic mechanisms are also activated, and D dimers (fibrinogen degradation products) are increased in the blood.

Key: B

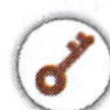

BOOST YOUR KNOWLEDGE

Isolated prolonged PT	*Isolated prolonged APTT*	*Prolonged PT and APTT*
• Congenital deficiency of factor VII • Drug-induced (warfarin) and mild liver disease	• Congenital deficiency of intrinsic pathway factors (factors VII, IX, XI, and XII) • Presence of circulating inhibitors • Von Willebrand disease	• Deficiency of common pathway factors (factors I, II, V, and X) • Combined deficiency of factors (factors V and VIII) • DIC, liver disease, and vitamin K deficiency

REFERENCES/SOURCES

- Gupta P, Menon PSN, Ramji S, Lodha R (Eds). PG Textbook of Pediatrics, 3rd edition. New Delhi: Jaypee Brothers Medical Publishers; 2022. Chapter 38.18.
- Scott JP, Raffini LJ. Disseminated intravascular coagulation. In: Kliegman RM, St Geme III JW, Blum NJ, Shah SS, Tasker RC, Wilson KM (Eds). Nelson Textbook of Pediatrics, 21st edition. Elsevier; 2019. pp. 2608-9.

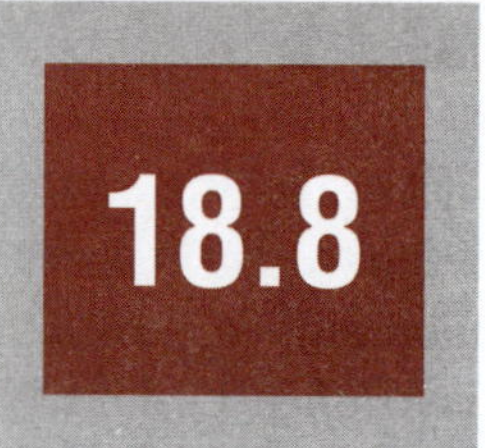

CHAPTER 18.8 Coagulation Disorders

Ritika Khurana, Purva Kanvinde, Sangeeta Mudaliar

1. A 2-year-old well child presented with recurrent epistaxis and easy bruisability since 7 months of age. His sibling at 3 years of age succumbed to massive hematemesis. Investigations revealed:

- Hemoglobin (Hb) 11 g/dL, white blood cell (WBC) count: 7,500/μL [absolute neutrophil count (ANC) 4,500 and absolute lymphocyte count (ALC) 3,500], platelet: 200 × 10^9/L
- *Platelet function studies:* Failure to aggregate with adenosine diphosphate (ADP) and epinephrine

How should we treat this condition?

A. Local measures for hemostasis and platelet transfusion may be required
B. Corticosteroids
C. Thrombopoietin (TPO) agonist like eltrombopag
D. Intravenous (IV) immunoglobulin

EXPLANATION

The child seems to be suffering from an inherited platelet type of disorder considering family history and early presentation of platelet type of bleeding (mucocutaneous).

Platelet function studies are suggestive of failure to aggregate in response to ADP, and epinephrine because they have a functional deficiency of platelet surface $\alpha IIb\beta_3$ receptors. This is diagnostic of Glanzmann's thrombasthenia.

The treatment recommended is local compression strategies, antifibrinolytic agents, and platelet transfusions as required.

Steroids, intravenous immunoglobulin (IVIG), TPO agonists, or other immunosuppressants have no role in this disorder.

Key: A

BOOST YOUR KNOWLEDGE

Glanzmann's thrombasthenia is a rare inherited autosomal recessive bleeding disorder due to a defect in the glycoprotein IIb/IIIa (Gp IIb-IIIa) platelet surface receptor. The hallmark of this is a failure of platelets to bind fibrinogen and aggregate after activation. Epistaxis and gastrointestinal bleeding are frequent issues in early childhood which often require intervention as well as iron supplementation.

Treatment options for mild bleeding are local compression strategies and antifibrinolytic agents. Moderate-to-severe bleeding requires platelet transfusion. Recombinant factor VIIa may be used in case of refractoriness to platelets.

REFERENCE/SOURCE

- Orkin SH, Nathan DG, Ginsburg D, Look AT, Fisher DE, Lux S. Nathan & Oski's Hematology and Oncology of Infancy and Childhood, 8th edition. Philadelphia: Saunders; 2014. pp. 1012-14.

2. A 5-year-old boy who is a known case of severe hemophilia A and is on regular prophylaxis is posted for appendicectomy. Choose the right preoperative plan for him.

A. Give appropriate factor VIII correction
B. Screen for inhibitors, if negative give appropriate factor correction preoperatively
C. 1 unit of cryoprecipitate per 10 kg body weight preoperatively
D. Must receive emicizumab 3 mg/kg preoperatively

EXPLANATION

Hemophilia patients on regular prophylaxis are prone to develop inhibitors post multiple exposures with factor therapy. They should be screened for the development of inhibitors by modified Bethesda assay before and after any surgery or invasive procedure. If negative for inhibitors, factor VIII should be given 80–100% preoperatively, followed by 60–80% postoperative Day 1–3; 40–60% Days 4–6, and 30–50% Days 7–14.

Cryoprecipitate is not the treatment of choice as it is not a specific treatment and is associated with the risk of viral transmitted infections. Emicizumab is used as prophylactic therapy and is not the choice of drug for surgery.

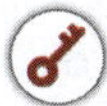

Key: B

BOOST YOUR KNOWLEDGE

The incidence of inhibitors is 33% in patients with severe hemophilia A, and 13% in mild-moderate hemophilia A.

Inhibitor screening is recommended by the modified Bethesda assay.

- Once every 5 exposure days till 20 exposure days, every 10 exposure days between 21 and 50 exposure days, at least two times a year till 150 exposure days, and later annually
- Before or after any surgery or invasive procedure
- Before or after a switch of products
- Bleeding episodes while on prophylaxis or suboptimal response to factor therapy during acute bleeding
- Low titer inhibitors have 0.6 to <5 Bethesda units (BU)/mL and high titer inhibitors have >5 BU/mL
- Low titer inhibitor will require higher doses of factor VIII. In the case of a high titer inhibitor, the treatment of choice is factor eight inhibitor bypassing agent (FEIBA) or recombinant factor VII or emicizumab.
- Emicizumab is a bispecific monoclonal antibody that binds factor IXa and X, resulting in the activation of factor X, thereby mimicking the actions of factor VIII.

REFERENCES/SOURCES

- Gupta P, Menon PSN, Lodha R, Ramji S. PG Textbook of Pediatrics, 3rd edition. New Delhi: Jaypee Brothers Medical Publishers; 2022. p. 1905.
- Rani S, Gupta V. (2022). IAP Hemophilia guidelines. [online] Available from https://iapindia.org/pdf/Ch-061-stg-hemophilia.pdf [Last accessed June, 2024].

3. A 13-day-old child presented with complaints of (c/o) lethargy, decreased oral intake, and bluish discoloration of the skin.

- *C-reactive protein (CRP):* 1, *procalcitonin:* 0.1
- *Prothrombin time (PT):* 22 seconds (normal 12)
- *Activated partial thromboplastin time (APTT):* 62 seconds (normal 35)
- *International normalized ratio (INR):* 1.8

What is the most likely diagnosis?

A. Purpura fulminans due to protein C/protein S deficiency
B. Severe sepsis
C. Hyperhomocysteinemia
D. Toxic shock syndrome

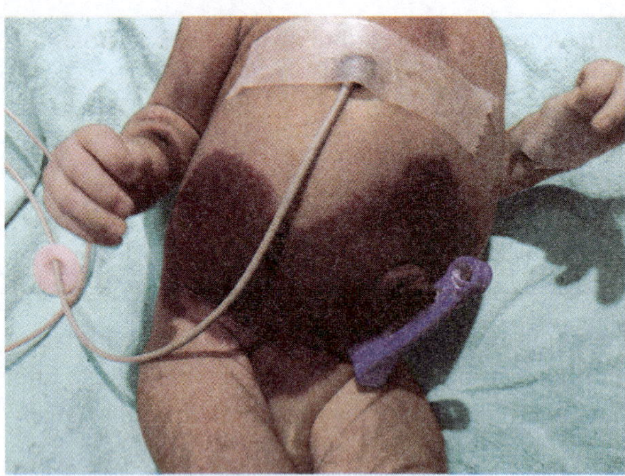
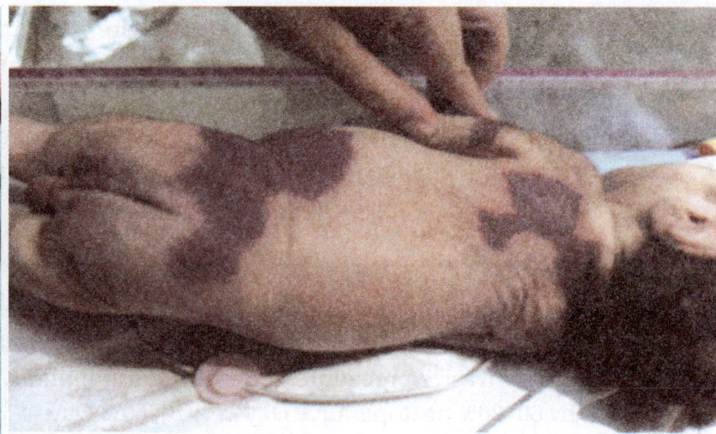

EXPLANATION

Here, it is a neonate presenting with extensive skin discoloration and deranged PT/APTT suggestive of purpura fulminans.

It is a clinical term to describe intravascular thrombosis with extensive skin necrosis. It occurs usually due to severe protein C or protein S deficiency.

Sepsis or toxic shock syndrome appears unlikely as with severe disseminated intravascular coagulation (DIC), usually, sepsis markers such as CRP and procalcitonin are deranged.

Hyperhomocysteinemia may predispose to thrombosis but does not present like purpura fulminans.

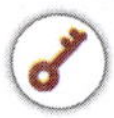

Key: A

BOOST YOUR KNOWLEDGE

Purpura fulminans is a rare but life-threatening clinical condition caused by homozygous or compound heterozygous deficiency of protein C or protein S. These neonates present shortly after birth with severe skin necrosis caused by thrombosis of small or medium-sized dermal vessels. It may progress to thromboembolic phenomena or DIC if not treated promptly. A pretreatment citrate sample of plasma must be sent for protein C and S activity and compared with age-specific reference ranges. Genetic testing is considered confirmatory.

Causes of Purpura Fulminans

Congenital/inherited states:

- Homozygous protein C deficiency
- Homozygous protein S deficiency

Acquired causes:

- *Increased consumption:*
  - Infection, e.g., group B *Streptococcus* infection
  - DIC
  - Acute venous thrombosis
  - Antiphospholipid antibodies
  - Cardiac bypass
- *Decreased synthesis:*
  - Severe hepatic dysfunction
  - Galactosemia
  - Severe congenital heart disease
  - Warfarin therapy

- *Initial treatment:*
  - *Fresh frozen plasma (FFP):* 10–20 mL/kg every 12 hourly
- *Definitive treatment:*
  - *Protein C concentrates (if available):* 100 units/kg followed by 50 units/kg every 6 hourly. The dose should be titrated to achieve protein C activity through levels of 50 units/dL. Low molecular weight heparin (LMWH) is also started.
- *Curative treatment:* Liver transplant

REFERENCES/SOURCES

- Bhat R, Monagle P. Anticoagulation in preterm and term neonates: Why are they special? Thromb Res. 2020;187:113-21.
- Orkin SH, Nathan DG, Ginsburg D, Look AT, Fisher DE, Lux S. Nathan & Oski's Hematology and Oncology of Infancy and Childhood, 8th edition. Philadelphia: Saunders; 2014. pp. 1064-66.
- Price VE, Ledingham DL, Krümpel A, Chan AK. Diagnosis and management of neonatal purpura fulminans. Semin Fetal Neonatal Med. 2011;16(6):318-22.

4. An 11-year-old female presented with acute onset of hematuria, severe headache, and confusion. She also developed a fever in the last few days.

Complete blood count (CBC):

- *Hb:* 9 g/dL
- *Mean corpuscular volume (MCV):* 75
- *WBC:* 4,500/mm^3
- *Platelets:* 11,000/μL

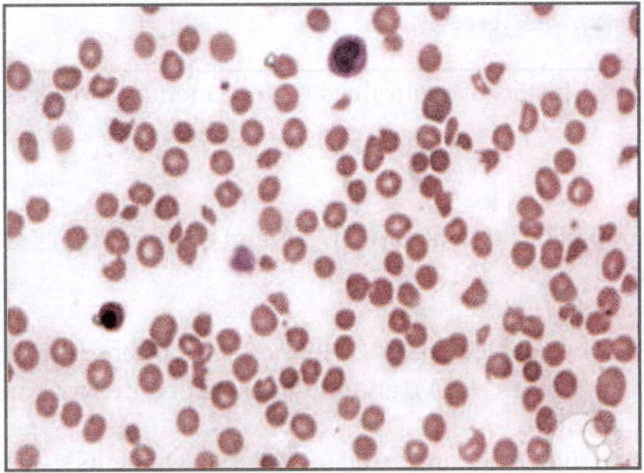

Peripheral smear picture

Pick up the most appropriate statement for this condition.

A. History and peripheral smear are suggestive of autoimmune hemolytic anemia, glucocorticoids are the treatment of choice

B. Thrombotic thrombocytopenia is the likely diagnosis, ADAMST13 activity should be checked, and plasma exchange initiated

C. Acute intravascular hemolysis in glucose-6-phosphate dehydrogenase (G6PD) deficiency

D. The main pathogenesis in TTP is persistently raised low molecular weight von Willebrand multimers

EXPLANATION

Acute onset bleeding manifestations with fever, neurological symptoms, thrombocytopenia, and evidence of microangiopathic anemia [schistocytes or fragmented red blood cells (RBCs)] are suggestive of thrombotic thrombocytopenic purpura (TTP). Autoimmune hemolytic anemia (AIHA) is an important differential, but it usually has very high MCV, and peripheral smear will have features of hemolysis, such as polychromasia and nucleated RBCs, and will show RBCs in clumps (in cold AIHA) or spherocytes (in warm AIHA). Thrombocytopenia and neurological symptoms are unusual in G6PD deficiency.

Key: B

BOOST YOUR KNOWLEDGE

Thrombotic thrombocytopenic purpura is a thrombotic microangiopathy caused by reduced activity of the vWF-cleaving protease ADAMTS13. TTP can be acquired, due to autoantibody inhibitors, or hereditary, due to homozygous or compound heterozygous ADAMTS13 mutations.

Plasma exchange is the treatment of choice to which 50–80% of patients respond.

Under conditions of sheer stress, ultra-large vWF (UL-vWF) multimers increase as they act more efficiently than other multimers. In a deficiency of ADAMTS13, cleaving of these UL multimers does not happen which leads to prothrombotic condition. Patients with Upshaw–Schulman syndrome, or congenital TTP have unusually large vWF multimers causing uncontrolled platelet aggregation and microvascular thrombosis.

REFERENCES/SOURCES

- Chiasakul T, Cuker A. Clinical and laboratory diagnosis of TTP: an integrated approach. Hematology Am Soc Hematol Educ Program. 2018;2018(1):530-8.
- Lazarchick J. https://imagebank.hematology.org/imageset/3/thrombotic-thrombocytopenic-purpura. ASH Image Bank; 2001.
- Orkin SH, Nathan DG, Ginsburg D, Look AT, Fisher DE, Lux S. Nathan & Oski's Hematology and Oncology of Infancy and Childhood, 8th edition. Philadelphia: Saunders; 2014. 1092-1094.

5. A 13-year-old well female with a history of menorrhagia since 2 months and occasional fatigue. No organomegaly/ lymphadenopathy.

- *CBC:*
  - *Hb:* 11 g/dL
  - *WBC:* 5,500/μL, neutrophil (N) 40, leukocyte (L) 56, and eosinophil (E) 4
  - *Platelet count:* 5 × 10^9/L
  - *Immature platelet fraction (IPF):* 22

Diagnosis of immune thrombocytopenic purpura (ITP) was made. Choose the right approach for this patient.

A. Screen for antinuclear antibodies (ANA), antidouble-stranded deoxyribonucleic acid (dsDNA), and viral markers and then initiate steroids

B. Bone marrow examination should be considered in adolescent patients suspected of ITP

C. There is no rationale for doing bone marrow or any blood investigations as it is suggestive of a typical ITP

D. The goal of treatment should be to achieve a platelet count of at least 50,000/L

EXPLANATION

Isolated thrombocytopenia in a well child, without any signs or symptoms of an underlying malignancy, etc., and a high IPF is suggestive of peripheral destruction due to ITP. ITP typically affects preschool toddlers aged 2–6 years.

In children <1 year of age, underlying immunodeficiency should be ruled out and autoimmune diseases, such as systemic lupus erythematosus (SLE) should be ruled out in adolescents; especially in females with additional symptoms, such as rash, photosensitivity, arthralgias, and fatigue.

Bone marrow examination is not mandatory if clinical signs and symptoms are typical of ITP and other cell lines are unaffected.

Key: A

BOOST YOUR KNOWLEDGE

Immune thrombocytopenic purpura now called immune Thrombocytopenia is an autoimmune disorder characterized by reduced peripheral blood platelet count due to a combination of premature platelet destruction and inadequate platelet production.

Patients with ITP have activated platelets, autoreactive B- and T-cells, and cytokine imbalance suggestive of peripheral intolerance.

Steroids or IVIG are the mainstay of treatment in acute ITP. TPO agonists (eltrombopag and romiplostim) are now widely used for persistent and chronic ITP with good results. Dapsone, rituximab, etc., are next-line drugs. Splenectomy is now rarely indicated.

The goal of treatment is to prevent life-threatening bleeding and to ensure a good quality of life, rather than chasing the platelet counts.

REFERENCES/SOURCES

- Gupta P, Menon PSN, Lodha R, Ramji S. PG Textbook of Pediatrics, 3rd edition. New Delhi: Jaypee Brothers Medical Publishers; 2022. 1916-8.
- Shah N, Kumar A, Rawat A. (2022). IAP standard treatment guidelines for Immune Thrombocytopenic purpura. [online] Available from https://iapindia.org/pdf/ch-072-immune-thrombocytopenic-purpura.pdf [Last access June, 2024].

6. A 10-year-old male child presented with fever since 3 days, pallor, and multiple ecchymotic patches. There has been hemiparesis and altered sensorium since morning.

- *CBC:*
    - *Hb:* 3 g/dL
    - *WBC:* 90,000/mm^3
    - *Platelets:* 4,000/μL
    - *PT:* 28(14)
    - *APTT:* 69(36)
    - *INR:* 2

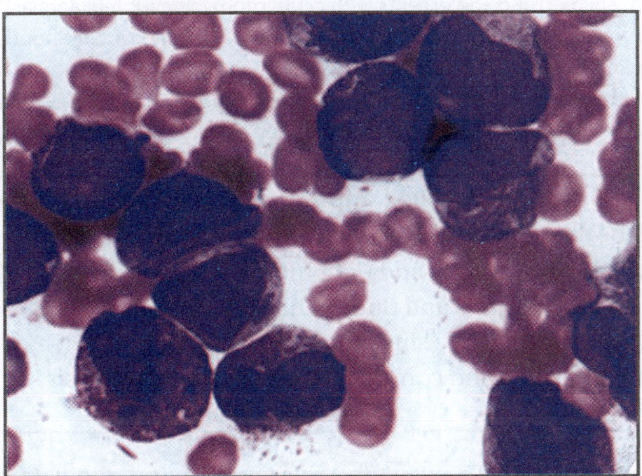

Peripheral blood smear

You are the registrar on call, what steps will you take?

A. Initiate unfractionated heparin (UFH) as soon as possible along with platelet and FFP transfusions
B. Give all-trans retinoic acid (ATRA) as soon as possible @45 mg/kg/day along with heparin
C. Give ATRA @25 mg/m^2/day and maintain platelets above 50,000 and fibrinogen >100
D. Plan bone marrow aspiration, depending on flow cytometry report start definitive treatment

EXPLANATION

Peripheral smear findings of leukemic promyelocytes with abundant, irregularly appearing primary azurophilic granules should raise suspicion of acute promyelocytic leukemia (APL). If APL is suspected, ATRA should be started immediately to rapidly ameliorate coagulopathy.

The International Consortium on Childhood APL (ICC APL-01) protocol (NCT01226303) recommends maintaining platelets >50 × 10^9/L and fibrinogen >1.5–2.0 g/L. Although heparin partially inhibits coagulation in DIC, a retrospective study comparing heparin with antifibrinolytic agents in the pre-ATRA era showed no benefit of heparin in APL-induced coagulopathy.

Complications such as pseudotumor cerebri and differentiation syndrome are more common in children, and many pediatric studies have shown that ATRA remains effective at 25 mg/m^2/day, with a lower incidence of side effects.

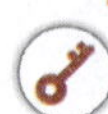

Key: C

BOOST YOUR KNOWLEDGE

Childhood APL is a medical emergency, and aggressive blood product support guided by frequent coagulation studies should commence promptly.

The presence of Auer rods and hypergranular promyelocyte blast cells is typical of APL. Frequently, the bone marrow classical morphology reveals promyelocytes with abundant Auer rods in multiple clusters (the so-called "faggot cells").

The classical hallmark of APL is the cytogenetic translocation t(15;17) (PML:RARA) present in 95–98% of cases, other translocations are also seen which may be resistant to ATRA.

All-trans retinoic acid acts as a differentiating agent for promyelocytic blasts whereas arsenic trioxide (ATO) induces apoptosis in blast cells. A combination of ATRA and ATO is now the preferred induction treatment in many centers, with the addition of anthracyclines in patients with WBC >10,000.

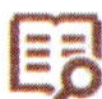

REFERENCES/SOURCES

- Abla O, Ribeiro RC. How I treat children and adolescents with acute promyelocytic leukaemia. Br J Haematol. 2014;164(1):24-38.
- De Botton S, Coiteux V, Chevret S, Rayon C, Vilmer E, Sanz M, et al. Outcome of childhood acute promyelocytic leukemia with all-trans-retinoic acid and chemotherapy. J Clin Oncol. 2004;22(8):1404-12.
- Tallman MS, Altman JK. How I treat acute promyelocytic leukemia. Blood. 2009;114(25):5126-35.
- Yilmaz M, Kantarjian H, Ravandi F. Acute promyelocytic leukemia current treatment algorithms. Blood Cancer J. 2021;11:123.

7. Direct oral anticoagulants (DOACs) have been approved for use in children with thrombosis in recent years. Which of the following will be the right candidate for putting on rivaroxaban?

A. A 5-year-old male with sickle cell disease and right middle cerebral artery (MCA) infarct
B. A 6-month-old female with cholestasis and Budd–Chiari syndrome
C. A 32-week neonate with cerebral venous sinus thrombosis
D. A 7-year-old child with Pott's spine and common femoral vein thrombosis

EXPLANATION

Two trials—EINSTEIN-Jr and DIVERSITY evaluated rivaroxaban and dabigatran for use in pediatric patients. They were found to be equally efficacious as LMWH and have an advantage of oral administration with the least side effects.

Till date, their use is approved for limited situations, restricting their use to venous thrombosis in children beyond 37 weeks of age, with normal liver and kidney function tests, following 4–5 days of unfractionated or LMWH. Budd–Chiari syndrome in the options given is associated with direct hyperbilirubinemia (cholestasis), hence not recommended.

Key: D

BOOST YOUR KNOWLEDGE

- DOACs exert their anticoagulant properties by affecting the common pathway in the coagulation cascade, with the two major oral medication classes being direct factor Xa inhibitors (DFXaI) and direct thrombin inhibitors (DTIs).
- An advantage of DOACs is their selective binding to their target factors (FXa for DFXaI and thrombin for DTIs) without the need for a cofactor.

Description of DOACs that have been studied in children

Drug	*Mechanism of action*	*Onset of action*	*Duration of action*	*Monitoring*	*Side effects*	*Available formulations in India*	*Reversal agent*	*Contra-indications*
Rivaroxaban	Direct factor Xa inhibitor	3–4 hours	24 hours	Requires no laboratory monitoring of PT or aPTT	Bleeding, dyspepsia, abdominal pain, pyrexia, fatigue, and headache	2.5, 10, 15, and 20 mg tabs	Andexanet alfa	Hepatic and renal impairment
Dabigatran	Reversibly blocks the catalytic site of thrombin	2 hours	24 hours	Though oral bioavailability is low, the anticoagulant effect is consistent, and no laboratory monitoring is required	Bleeding, dyspepsia, abdominal pain, pyrexia, fatigue, and headache	75, 110, and 150 mg caps	Idarucizumab	Renal impairment

Limitations for use of DOAC

- Due to the limited experience on DOACs long-term data on safety in children are lacking.
- DOACs need to be avoided in severe renal failure and rivaroxaban needs to be avoided in severe hepatic failure.
- DOACs have not been studied in neonates <37 weeks and birth weight <2.6 kg.
- In patients with arterial thrombus some studies have shown that warfarin is more beneficial. Hence the use in arterial thrombus is still not established.

REFERENCES/SOURCES

- Halton J, Brandão LR, Luciani M, Bomgaars L, Chalmers E, Mitchell LG, et al. DIVERSITY Trial Investigators. Dabigatran etexilate for the treatment of acute venous thromboembolism in children (DIVERSITY): a randomized, controlled, open-label, phase 2b/3, non-inferiority trial. Lancet Haematol. 2021;8(1):e22-33.
- Male C, Lensing AWA, Palumbo JS, Kumar R, Nurmeev I, Hege K, et al. EINSTEIN-Jr Phase 3 Investigators. Rivaroxaban compared with standard anticoagulants for the treatment of acute venous thromboembolism in children: a randomized, controlled, phase 3 trial. Lancet Haematol. 2020;7(1):e18-27.
- Whitworth H, Raffini L. Practical considerations for use of direct oral anticoagulants in children. Front Pediatr. 2022;10:860369.

8. A 3-month-old well boy, born of third-degree consanguinity presented with hematoma at the vaccine site. On investigation:

- *PT/APTT/INR:* 28/14, 95/42, *INR:* 2
- Fresh frozen plasma transfusion and vitamin K were given, after which the coagulation profile normalized. 10 days later child developed melena.

PT	26/14
APTT	65/40
INR	2
Protein induced by vitamin K absence (PIVKA)	40,000
Liver function tests	Normal

Which tests will clinch the diagnosis?

A. vWF assay
B. Coagulation factor levels, clinical exome
C. Coagulation factor levels and mixing studies
D. D dimer, fibrinogen, and thrombin time

EXPLANATION

Deranged PT/APTT/INR and increased PIVKAs are suggestive of vitamin K deficiency. It is commonly acquired but since this child is born of consanguinity and getting repeated symptoms. Congenital vitamin K deficiency should be ruled out.

Factor levels will show a reduced amount of vitamin K dependent factor II, VII, IX, and X. Clinical exome sequencing with clinch the diagnosis.

von Willebrand disease will not have such a grossly deranged coagulation profile and PIVKAs will not be high. Also unlikely to be hemophilia as both PT/APTT are deranged.

Key: B

BOOST YOUR KNOWLEDGE

Combined deficiency of vitamin K-dependent factors is usually acquired secondary to no administration of vitamin K at birth, liver disease, warfarin therapy, sepsis, etc.

Although rare, an inherited form of vitamin K deficiency also exists which leads to decreased levels of coagulation factors II, VII, IX, and X as well as natural anticoagulants protein C and protein S.

Vitamin K-dependent clotting factor deficiency (VKCFD) is an autosomal recessive disorder caused by mutations in the genes of either γ-glutamyl carboxylase or vitamin K2,3-epoxide reductase complex. VKCFD1, which is associated with point mutations in the γ-glutamyl carboxylase gene (*GGCX*), and *VKCFD2*, which results from point mutations in the vitamin K epoxide reductase gene (*VKOR*).

Bleeding manifestation ranges from mild to severe with onset in the neonatal period in severe cases.

Vitamin K administration is the mainstay of therapy in VKCFD; however, during surgery or severe bleeding episodes, FFP supplementation will be needed.

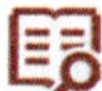

REFERENCES/SOURCES

- Bhattacharyya J, Dutta P, Mishra P, Dixit A, Srinivas U, K Meghanathan, et al. Congenital vitamin K-dependent coagulation factor deficiency: a case report. Blood Coagul Fibrinolysis. 2005;16(7):525-7.
- Napolitano M, Mariani G, Lapecorella M. Hereditary combined deficiency of the vitamin K-dependent clotting factors. Orphanet J Rare Dis. 2010;5:21.

9. A full-term baby born by normal vaginal delivery developed convulsion on Day 2 of life, a magnetic resonance imaging (MRI) brain was suggestive of intracranial hemorrhage.

- *CBC:*
    - *Hb:* 11 g/dL
    - *WBC:* 13,000
    - *Platelet count:* 12,000 and *PT/APTT/INR:* normal
    - *CRP:* Negative, *D-dimer:* negative, and *fibrinogen:* 250

Pick up the right diagnostic and management approach.

A. Neonatal alloimmune thrombocytopenia (NAIT) is the likely diagnosis. Screen for human platelet antigen (HPA)/human leukocyte antigen (HLA) antibody, administer platelet transfusion and IVIG
B. Child appears to be in DIC, administer FFP and platelet transfusion immediately
C. ITP is likely, to perform bone marrow studies and administer steroids
D. NAIT is likely, long-term monitoring and regular courses of IVIG are warranted

EXPLANATION

Neonatal alloimmune thrombocytopenia is caused by the placental transfer of maternal alloantibodies directed against paternally inherited antigens present on fetal platelets.

NAIT is suspected in patients with isolated thrombocytopenia in a term, otherwise, clinically well baby, in whom causes such as sepsis, are ruled out. ITP is extremely uncommon in this age group.

In all suspected cases of NAIT, HPA, and HLA antibody screening should be considered to confirm diagnosis as well as guide in subsequent pregnancies.

It is a transient disease, with resolution of thrombocytopenia by 2–3 weeks, when antibodies wean off.

Key: D

BOOST YOUR KNOWLEDGE

In Caucasians, the most commonly implicated alloantigen is HPA-1a, whereas in Asians HPA-4 is most common (80%). Antibodies to HLA class 1 antigen are also found as a cause of NAIT in a few patients. The degree of thrombocytopenia in neonates at risk for NAIT (mother immunized against HPA-1a) can be quite variable. The most serious complication of NAIT is intracranial hemorrhage, which occurs in 10–20% of symptomatic infants. Up to 80% of these bleeds occur prenatally. Flow cytometry using secondary probes specific for immunoglobulin G (IgG) and immunoglobulin M (IgM) immunoglobulin isotypes provides a rapid and sensitive means of detecting platelet reactive antibodies.

Irradiated maternal platelet transfusion is the treatment of choice in case of significant bleeding. If it is not feasible, then random donor platelets can be given. IVIG therapy should also be given at 1–2 g/kg/day for 2–4 days to deplete the formed antibodies.

REFERENCES/SOURCES

- Orkin SH, Nathan DG, Ginsburg D, Look AT, Fisher DE, Lux S. Nathan & Oski's Hematology and Oncology of Infancy and Childhood, 8th edition. Philadelphia: Saunders; 2014. pp. 1088-9.
- Peterson JA, McFarland JG, Curtis BR, Aster RH. Neonatal alloimmune thrombocytopenia: pathogenesis, diagnosis and management. Br J Haematol. 2013;161(1):3-14.

10. A 9-year-old boy with acute lymphoblastic leukemia (ALL) on induction chemotherapy, presented with induration and edema of the right upper limb. Ultrasonography (USG) Doppler is suggestive of right basilic vein thrombosis. He has a peripherally inserted central catheter (PICC) line in the same limb.

Choose the right statement for the management of line-associated thrombosis.

A. Port is associated with a higher risk of thrombosis compared to external devices like PICC line
B. Inherited thrombophilia work up is warranted in such situations
C. PICC line removal must be done and initiate enoxaparin
D. Initiate enoxaparin, and reassess after 6 weeks; the line can be salvaged in most situations

EXPLANATION

An internal device (port) has a lesser risk of thrombosis than an external tunneled device (Hickman or Broviac catheter). Amongst external devices, tunneled lines are less prone to thrombosis than PICC lines.

Since the child has conditions like malignancy, therapy involving steroids and L-asparaginase, and a line in-situ; all of which predispose to thrombosis, extensive thrombophilia workup is not warranted at this point.

If the line is necessary, is well positioned, and functioning well, needs not to be removed.

Enoxaparin in the dose of 1 mg/kg/dose 12 hourly is the treatment of choice. Reassessment scans should be done post 6 weeks of enoxaparin and if improving, it should be continued for another 6 weeks and then stopped. In case, the line is not required further or nonfunctional, it should be removed after 3–5 days of enoxaparin therapy to prevent embolization at the time of removal.

Key: D

BOOST YOUR KNOWLEDGE

Central venous access devices (CVADs) predispose patients to venous thrombosis because they impact each component of Virchow's triad: Stasis, hypercoagulability, and endothelial injury. CVAD insertion results in local vessel wall injury, activating coagulation and proinflammatory cascades.

Risk factors for thrombosis in cancer patients are listed in the given figure.

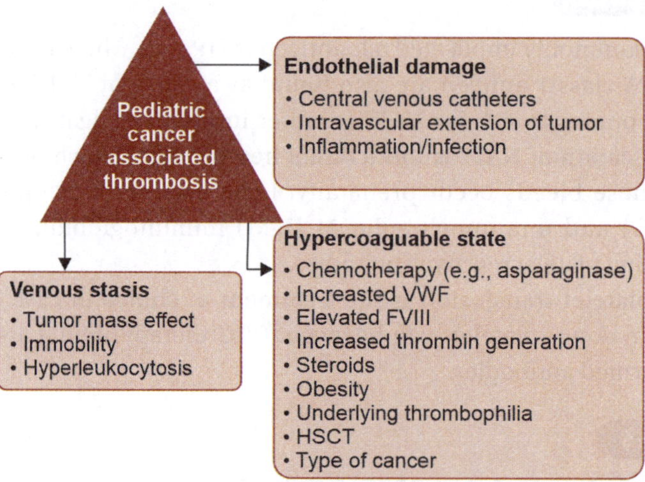

Cancer-associated thrombosis

Traditionally, UFH and LMWH have been the standard of care in pediatric oncology patients. Oral anticoagulants such as warfarin were typically avoided due to multiple food and drug interactions. However, with the EINSTEIN Jr and DIVERSITY trials demonstrating the safety and efficacy of DOACs such as rivaroxaban and dabigatran respectively; they are now extensively used.

For a child on chemotherapy, care should be taken to keep platelet count above 50,000 during anti-coagulation or reduce the dose of the drug when platelets are between 25,000 and 50,000 and withhold the drug when below 25,000.

REFERENCES/SOURCES

- Rajasekhar A, Streiff MB. How I treat central venous access device-related upper extremity deep vein thrombosis. Blood. 2017;129(20):2727-36.
- Samji N, Bhatt MD, Kulkarni K. Challenges in management of VTE in children with cancer: risk factors and treatment options. Front Pediatr. 2022;10:855162.

11. A 4-year-old girl was brought to the pediatric outpatient department (OPD) with a history of (H/O) easy bruisability noticed since the past 6 months. Bruises occurred episodically, usually observed a day after trivial trauma. On detailed history mother mentioned about similar episodes since early infancy. On examination, she had a large ecchymotic patch over the flank. No organomegaly/lymphadenopathy. History did not give any evidence of physical abuse.

Investigations:

- *Hb:* 10.8 g/dL
- *WBC count:* 6.4×10^9/L
- *Platelets:* 328×10^9/L
- *Peripheral smear:* Normal
- *Coagulation profile:* Normal
- *Platelet function tests:* Normal

What is the most likely diagnosis?

A. Factor XII deficiency
B. Factor V and VIII combined deficiency
C. Factor XIII deficiency
D. Factor X deficiency

EXPLANATION

History of episodic bruising with or without a history of umbilical cord bleeding with a normal coagulation profile and platelets are suggestive of factor XIII deficiency. Factor XII deficiency usually presents with incidentally found abnormal APTT in an asymptomatic child. Combined deficiency of factor V and VIII as well as factor X deficiency will have both PT and APTT deranged.

Key: C

BOOST YOUR KNOWLEDGE

Factor XIII is responsible for clot stability and crosslinking of fibrin polymer, protecting it from fibrinolysis, and hence factor 13 deficiency leads to delayed bleeding. Typically, the patient develops trauma, and a bruise or hematoma will be observed the next day. Other common symptoms are delayed umbilical cord hemorrhage, delayed umbilical cord separation, poor wound healing, or spontaneous abortion.

For a child with such bleeding manifestations and normal screening tests, factor XIII assay, and urea clot lysis test should be done.

12. A 7-year-old child with Marfan's syndrome undergoes cardiac surgery for severe aortic stenosis with valve replacement. He was initiated with UFH drip in the perioperative period. On the night of surgery, the child develops swelling and induration in the left upper limb near intravascular catheter insertion.

Investigations:

- *Hb:* 11 g/dL
- *WBC:* 9.3×10^9/L
- *Platelets:* 32×10^9/L
- *PT:* Normal and *APTT:* 62/34

You are the registrar on call that night, what are your thoughts on planning management of this patient?

A. Child has developed DIC, prompt FFP, and platelet transfusions should be initiated
B. Unlikely to be heparin-induced thrombocytopenia (HIT) as it occurs after 5 days of heparin infusion
C. Child has developed immune-mediated thrombocytopenia due to heparin, switch to LMWH
D. HIT is likely, stop heparin infusion and consider switching to lepirudin

EXPLANATION

Heparin-induced thrombocytopenia is an immune-mediated adverse drug reaction in which antibodies are generated against neoepitopes expressed when heparin binds to platelet factor-4 (PF4) and activate cellular FcγRIIA on platelets and monocytes to propagate a hypercoagulable state culminating in life-threatening thrombosis. It should be anticipated in children receiving heparin and presenting with thrombocytopenia with or without thrombosis and should be carefully differentiated from DIC as platelet transfusion may be detrimental. It usually occurs from Day 5 to 15 of heparin infusion, but rapid onset HIT can occur in children pre-exposed to heparin. Patients with HIT should be switched to direct thrombin inhibitors such as lepirudin and danaparoid and not LMWH which also has a risk of HIT.

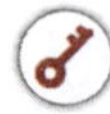

Key: D

BOOST YOUR KNOWLEDGE

Heparin-induced thrombocytopenia is an immune complication caused by antibodies directed to complexes containing heparin and an endogenous platelet protein, PF4.

The risk of children developing HIT is related to the extent of UFH exposure. Pediatric patients may receive UFH for various indications including prophylaxis and treatment of thromboembolic disorders, maintenance of indwelling arterial and venous cannulae, cardiac catheterization, cardiopulmonary bypass (CPB), extracorporeal membrane oxygenation (ECMO), dialysis, and perioperative anticoagulation or in cases of antiphospholipid and anticardiolipin antibodies or protein S deficiency.

Scoring system to estimate the pretest probability of HIT

Category	*2 points*	*1 point*	*0 point*
Thrombocytopenia	>50% fall, or nadir of 20–100 × 10^9/L	30–50% fall, or nadir of 10–19 × 10^9/L	30% fall or nadir <10 × 10^9/L
Timing of platelet count fall	Days 5–10, or ≤1 day if heparin exposure within the past 30 days	>Day 10 or unclear (but fits with HIT), or ≤1 day if heparin exposure within the past 30–100 days	≤1 day (no recent heparin)
Thrombosis or other sequelae	Proven thrombosis, skin necrosis, or, after heparin; bolus, acute systemic reaction	Progressive, recurrent, or silent thrombosis; erythematous skin lesions	None
Other cause of thrombocytopenia	None evident	Possible	Definite

Points assigned in each of the four categories are totaled, and the pretest probability of HIT by total points is as follows: 6–8 = high, 4–5 = intermediate; 0–3 = low.

Source: Adapted with permission from Warkentin TE, Aird WC, Rand JH. Platelet-endothelial interactions: sepsis, HIT, and antiphospholipid syndrome. Hematology Am Soc Hematol Educ Program. 2003:497-519.

The treatment of choice is DTIs, because DTIs act independently of antithrombin, they have an enhanced capacity to inhibit thrombin bound to fibrin, offering a unique advantage over heparins. Of the 33 pediatric HIT cases reported in the literature, lepirudin was used in 14 of them.

REFERENCES/SOURCES

- Arepally GM. Heparin-induced thrombocytopenia. Blood. 2017;129(21):2864-72.
- Vakil NH, Kanaan AO, Donovan JL. Heparin-induced thrombocytopenia in the pediatric population: a review of current literature. J Pediatr Pharmacol Ther. 2012;17(1):12-30.

13. A 13-day-old, breastfed female neonate, with a normal birth history, was brought to us with complaints of:
- Poor feeding and activities since 3 days
- Decreased urine output since 3 days
- One episode of convulsion
- One examination (O/E)—vitals stable
- Symptoms of (S/O) dehydration present (sunken eyes, skin pinch delayed, and depressed fontanelle)

Investigations: Na—190 mEq/L, K—5.1 mEq/L, blood urea nitrogen (BUN)—65 mg/dL, creatinine—1.6 mg/dL. MRI of the brain image is shown in the figure given here.

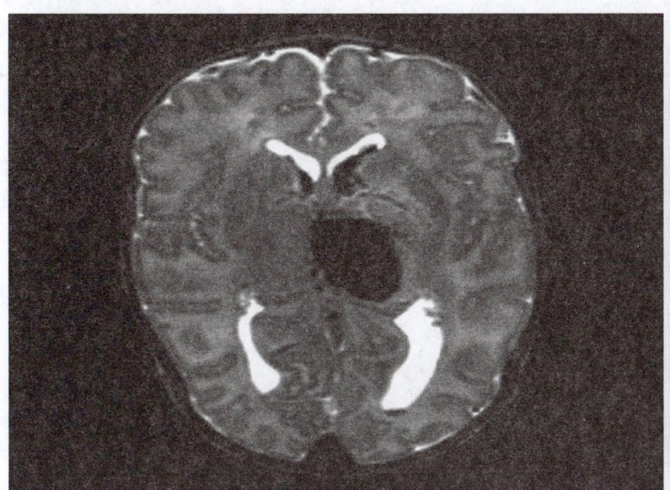
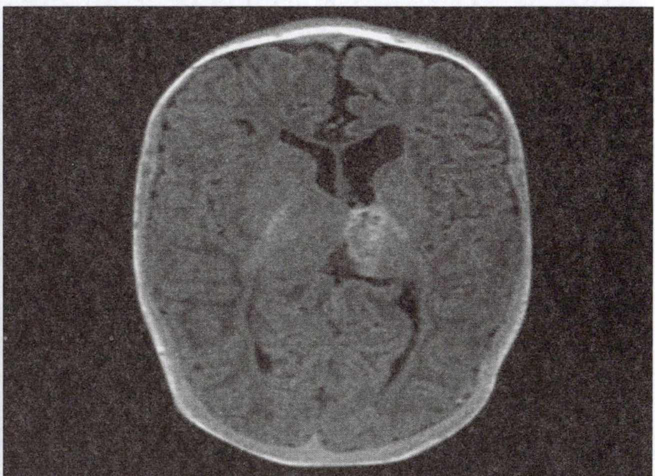

Which option seems to be least important at this point?

A. Correct hypernatremic dehydration and start antiepileptics
B. Start LMWH at 1.5 g/kg/dose twice daily
C. Thrombolysis with streptokinase should be initiated
D. Rule out underlying sepsis and initiate antibiotics

EXPLANATION

In neonates, common triggers for cerebral sinus venous thrombosis are asphyxia, septicemia, dehydration, and Maternal diabetes. The child should be treated for hypernatremic dehydration and acute renal failure with appropriate IV fluid and LMWH started at 1.5 mg/kg/dose BD and continued for at least 6 weeks.

Sepsis should be ruled out in all such neonates and empirical antibiotics should be given. Thrombolysis is not routinely performed in neonates with cerebral sinovenous thrombosis (CSVT).

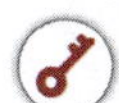

Key: C

BOOST YOUR KNOWLEDGE

Cerebral sinovenous thrombosis is an uncommon condition among pediatric patients involving major sinuses, with a preponderant occurrence in neonates. An early presentation (within the first 48 hours) may be accompanied by several comorbidities (respiratory distress, poor tone, fetal distress, and asphyxia), whereas a later presentation is more often associated with conventional neurological signs, such as seizures, lethargy, apnea, and poor feeding.

Magnetic resonance venography is the radiological investigation of choice. The two major goals of radiological diagnosis are imaging of the thrombus and the associated cerebral lesions such as hemorrhage due to venous infarction.

For neonates with CSVT without significant intracranial hemorrhage, the American Academy of Pediatrics (AAP) suggests anticoagulation with LMWH for a minimum of 6 weeks, and no longer than 3 months. In the case of significant intracranial hemorrhage associated with CSVT, radiological monitoring of the thrombosis at 5–7 days is suggested, and anticoagulation if thrombus propagation is noted.

REFERENCES/SOURCES

- Monagle P, Cambers E, Chan A, deVeber G, Kirkham F, Massicotte P, et al. Antithrombotic therapy in neonates and children: American College of Chest Physicians Evidence-Based Clinical Practice Guidelines (8th Edition). Chest. 2008;133(6 Suppl): 887S-968S.
- Ramenghi LA, Cardiello V, Rossi A. Neonatal cerebral sinovenous thrombosis. Handb Clin Neurol. 2019;162:267-80.

14. A 2-day-old infant born at home was brought to your center with the lesion shown in given figure.

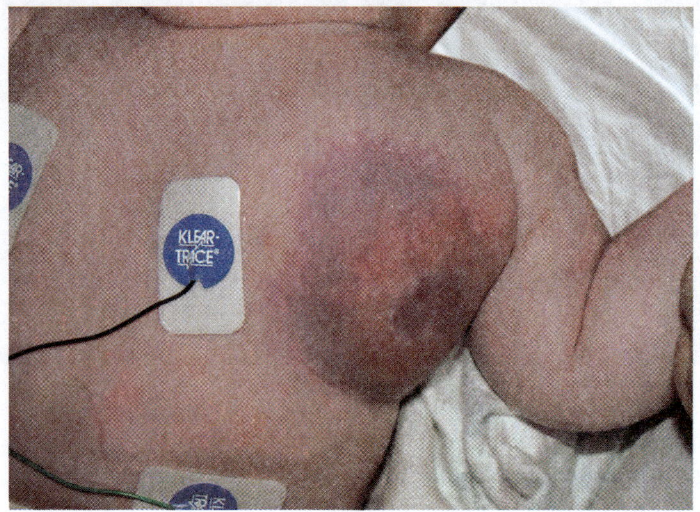

Investigation:
- *Hb:* 11 g/dL
- *WBC:* 7.2 × 10^9/L
- *Platelets:* 9 × 10^9/L
- *PT:* 19/12 and *APTT:* 110/34

Imaging revealed it to be a Kaposiform hemangioendothelioma (KHE). Pick up the right management strategy for this neonate.

A. It resolves spontaneously in most, hence consider observation
B. Child seems to be in consumptive coagulopathy, initiate steroids, and SOS sirolimus
C. Transfuse platelets and do surgical excision as early as possible
D. Most patients recover within a few days with mortality of <10%

EXPLANATION

Clinical presentation of a cutaneous hemangioma with signs of DIC, presenting in early infancy is suggestive of Kasabach-Merritt phenomenon (KMP) secondary to KHE. It is associated with a mortality of 30–50% due to the possibility of life-threatening bleeding. Treatment of choice is steroids, sirolimus, or vincristine may be considered in refractory cases. Platelet transfusion may be detrimental and surgical excision although definitive, is usually not feasible due to hemodynamic instability.

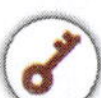

Key: B

BOOST YOUR KNOWLEDGE

Kasabach–Merritt phenomenon, first described in 1940, is a rare but life-threatening coagulopathy of infancy that presents with thrombocytopenia, microangiopathic hemolytic anemia, and consumptive coagulopathy in the setting of a rapidly enlarging vascular tumor-like KHE and tufted angioma (TA). KHE is locally aggressive and may involve multiple tissue planes; whereas, TA is benign and typically confined to a single tissue plane.

When identifying the underlying, cutaneous lesion, physical examination may be sufficient. If a visceral tumor is suspected, further imaging such as MRI may be useful.

While the thrombocytopenia of KMP may be profound, platelet transfusion is not recommended except in the cases of active bleeding. Transfused platelets may become trapped in the tumor and lead to further abnormal coagulation, worsening KMP.

Symptomatic anemia should be treated with red blood cell transfusion. In cases of bleeding or as preparation for surgery, cryoprecipitate may be administered apart from the therapies mentioned above.

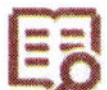

REFERENCES/SOURCES

- Drolet BA, Trenor CC, Brandão LR, Chiu YE, Chun RH, Dasgupta R, et al. Consensus-derived practice standards plan for complicated Kaposiform hemangioendothelioma. J Pediatr. 2013;163(1):285-91.
- Mahajan P, Margolin J, Iacobas I. Kasabach-Merritt Phenomenon: Classic Presentation and Management Options. Clin Med Insights Blood Disord. 2017;10:1179545X17699849.
- Schmid I, Klenk AK, Sparber-Sauer M, Koscielniak E, Maxwell R, Häberle B. Kaposiform hemangioendothelioma in children: a benign vascular tumor with multiple treatment options. World J Pediatr. 2018;14(4):322-29.

15. **A 4-year-old boy with intellectual disability, born to parents with third-degree consanguineous marriage, presents with sudden onset left-sided hemiparesis. There is no history of similar complaints in the past or any family member. On examination, the eyes showed an abnormality as shown in the below figure. There was decreased tone and power in the left upper limb and lower limb and associated right upper motor neuronal (UMN) facial nerve palsy. Rest systems normal.**

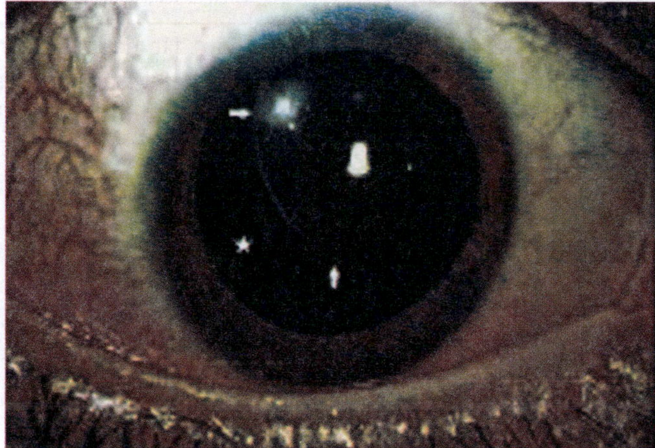

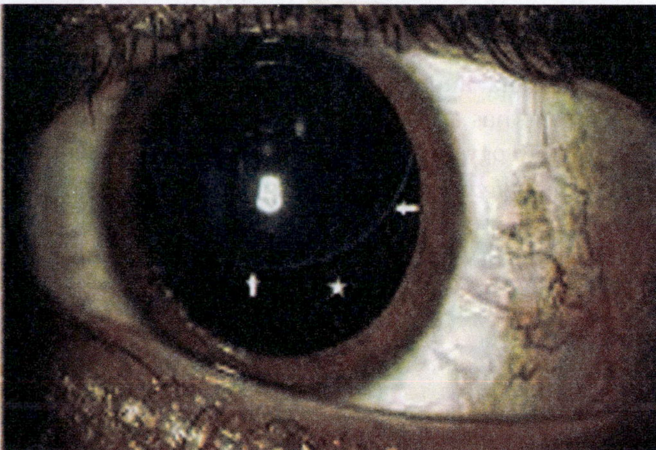

On baseline investigations, CBCs and coagulation profile were normal and sickling negative. Choose the diagnosis that is most likely in this case.

A. Adrenocortical leukodystrophy
B. Homocysteinemia due to folate deficiency
C. Factor V Leiden deficiency
D. Hyperhomocystinuria

EXPLANATION

Hyperhomocystinuria is a rare autosomal recessive disorder associated with the accumulation of homocysteine and hence homocystinuria. These patients are at increased risk of premature atherosclerosis leading to coronary artery disease, stroke, etc. They may also manifest mental retardation, ectopia lentis (mentioned in the above figure), and skeletal abnormalities. Homocysteinemia due to folate deficiency is the most common acquired cause of hyperhomocysteinemia but it is usually not associated with ectopia lentis or mental retardation. Heterozygosity of the factor V Leiden mutation is the most common inherited thrombophilia in the unselected White population (prevalence, approximately 1–5%) and is considered the most common inherited thrombophilia in individuals with venous thromboembolism, but considering the additional history in case, hyperhomocystinuria is more likely.

Adrenoleukodystrophy is a myelination disorder usually presenting with signs and symptoms of neurodegeneration and adrenal insufficiency.

Key: D

BOOST YOUR KNOWLEDGE

Hyperhomocystinuria is a rare autosomal recessive disorder due to a deficiency of cystathionine β-synthase. Due to impaired intracellular metabolism of homocysteine, increased amounts of amino acid accumulate in blood and are excreted in urine. In contrast to homocystinuria, a variant of methylenetetrahydrofolate reductase (MTFHR) can also lead to the prothrombotic condition.

Homocysteine levels are usually in the moderate (25–100 mmol/L) or severe (>100 mmol/L) range.

Folic acid, vitamin B_6, and vitamin B_{12} supplements help in reducing homocysteine levels.

REFERENCES/SOURCES

- Eldibany MM, Caprini JA. Hyperhomocysteinemia and thrombosis: an overview. Arch Pathol Lab Med. 2007;131(6):872-84.
- Hafidi Z, Berradi S, Handor H, Regragui A, Lezrek M, Daoudi R. Atypical presentation of ectopia lentis in homocystinuria. J Pediatr. 2015;166(4):1091.
- Orkin SH, Nathan DG, Ginsburg D, Look AT, Fisher DE, Lux S. Nathan & Oski's Hematology and Oncology of Infancy and Childhood, 8th edition. Philadelphia: Saunders; 2014. pp. 1069-70.

16. A 9-month-old boy presented with fever, productive cough, and increased respiratory activity. He had a history of neonatal intensive care unit (NICU) admission on Day 8 of life for melena and required platelet transfusions. He also has a history of recurrent otitis media which was managed on OPD basis. He is on follow-up with dermatology for generalized eczema which has responded partially to topical steroids.

On investigation:

- *Hb:* 8 × 10^9/L
- *WBC count:* 22.3 × 10^9/L, neutrophils: 17.1 × 10^9/L, and lymphocytes: 4.1 × 10^9/L
- *Platelets:* 25 × 10^9/L
- *Peripheral smear:* Small platelets noted
- *Direct Coombs test:* Positive
- *IgG:* Normal
- *Immunoglobulin A (IgA):* Increased
- *IgE:* Increased
- *IgM:* Reduced

What is the most likely diagnosis?

A. Wiskott–Aldrich syndrome (WAS)
B. Omenn syndrome
C. Hyper-IgE syndrome
D. IPEX (immune dysregulation, polyendocrinopathy, enteropathy, X-linked) syndrome

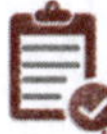

EXPLANATION

The clinical features of this child (sinopulmonary infections, thrombocytopenia, and eczema) are consistent with Wiskott–Aldrich syndrome. IPEX is due to forkhead box P3 *(FOXP3)* gene mutation presenting as eczema, autoimmune enteropathy, and endocrinopathy with high IgE, normal IgG, IgA, and IgM. Classical hyper-IgE syndrome is due to loss of function STAT 3 presenting with early onset eczema, recurrent cold abscesses, coarse facies, and skeletal defects with eosinophilia, IgE >2,000 IU/mL. Omenn's syndrome is an autosomal recessive disorder characterized by lymphocytic infiltration of the skin, gut, liver, and spleen, leading to erythroderma and protracted diarrhea with failure to thrive.

Key: A

BOOST YOUR KNOWLEDGE

Wiskott–Aldrich syndrome is an X-linked recessive disease characterized by eczema, immunodeficiency, and thrombocytopenia. Bloody diarrhea may be the initial feature. Recurrent otitis media and sinopulmonary infections occur frequently. Autoimmune manifestations including autoimmune hemolytic anemia, vasculitis, inflammatory bowel disease, and other autoimmune processes are frequently observed. The immune defects of Wiskott–Aldrich syndrome are variable, serum IgA and E are elevated, and IgM is low.

Aggressive treatment of all infections and irradiated blood products are recommended. The mainstay of treatment for WAS is HSCT.

REFERENCE/SOURCE

- Orkin SH, Nathan DG, Ginsburg D, Look AT, Fisher DE, Lux S. Nathan & Oski's Hematology and Oncology of Infancy and Childhood, 8th edition. Philadelphia: Saunders; 2014. pp. 898-9.

17. A 2-year-old female child presented with swelling of the knee joint (hemarthrosis). She had a history of easy bruisability since 6 months of age. Mother had a history of menorrhagia.

On investigation:

- *Hb:* 11
- *WBC:* 9.5×10^9/L, neutrophils: 5×10^9/L, and lymphocytes: 4.5×10^9/L
- *Platelet count:* 3.5×10^9/L
- *Peripheral smear:* Normal
- *PT:* 14/12
- *APTT:* 59/36
- *INR:* 1.2
- *Factor VIII levels:* <1%

Choose the most appropriate treatment.

A. Give appropriate correction for joint bleed with recombinant factor VIII
B. Send vWF antigen test and give appropriate factor VIII correction with intermediate purity factor VIII for joint bleed
C. Give FFP 10–15 mL/kg
D. Give Cryoprecipitate 1 unit/5 kg body weight

EXPLANATION

There is a history of mucocutaneous bleeding and now hemarthrosis in a girl child with a history of menorrhagia in the mother, pointing toward an autosomal disorder like von Willebrand disease rather than an X-linked disorder like hemophilia. For confirmation of diagnosis vWF antigen and activity are required. Intermediate purity factor VIII also contains vWF, so it should be preferred for the treatment of von Willebrand disease.

Key: B

BOOST YOUR KNOWLEDGE

von Willebrand disease is a disorder of vWF, a large multimeric glycoprotein that contributes to the adherence of platelets to damaged endothelium and serves as a carrier protein for plasma factor VIII. Deficiency of vWF results in mucocutaneous and posttraumatic or postsurgical bleeding, but if vWF is absent or severely reduced, the secondary reduction in plasma factor VIII may also result in joint or muscle bleeding.

Types of von Willebrand disease	
Type 1	Partial quantitative deficiency
Type 2	Qualitative defect
A	Absence of high-molecular-weight (HMW) multimers
B	Increased affinity for plt GPIb
M	Decreased platelet-dependent function but not caused by the absence of high-molecular-weight vWF multimers
N	Decreased affinity for factor VIII
Type 3	Complete deficiency—severe type

18. A 2.5-year-old boy was being evaluated for sensorineural hearing loss. No history of recent vaccinations or infections. His routine investigations revealed.

- *Hb:* 11.2 g/dL
- *WBC:* 7.5×10^9/L, *neutrophils*—4.5×10^9/L, and *lymphocytes*—3×10^9/L
- *Platelet count:* 60×10^9/L
- *MPV:* 25
- *PT:* 14/12
- *APTT:* 26/30
- *INR:* 1.1
- *Peripheral smear:* Below

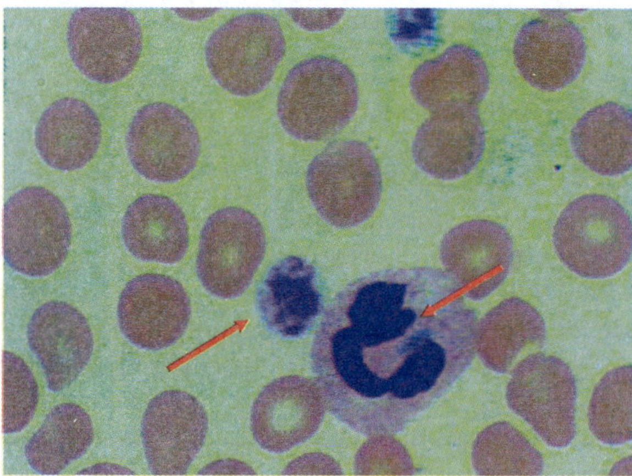

Peripheral smear

What is the likely diagnosis and marked peripheral smear finding?

A. May–Hegglin anomaly (MHA) showing giant platelet and Dohle bodies
B. X-linked anemia with severe thrombocytopenia showing giant platelet, Pseudo–Pelger–Huet anomaly
C. Gray platelet syndrome showing grey platelets, Dohle bodies
D. Chédiak–Higashi syndrome showing large platelets, intracytoplasmic granular deposits in neutrophils

EXPLANATION

In this figure, a neutrophil contains multiple prominent, light blue, round Dohle bodies, which are intracytoplasmic inclusions that consist of ribonucleic acid (RNA) and giant platelets with a history of sensorineural hearing loss which is seen with MHA.

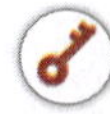

Key: A

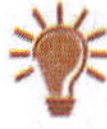

BOOST YOUR KNOWLEDGE

The MHA is a rare autosomal dominant disease due to *MYH9* gene mutation characterized by neutrophils with abnormal cytoplasmic inclusions, large platelets, and variable thrombocytopenia. It is part of the myosin heavy chain *(MHC)* single gene defect group that also includes Fechtner syndrome, Sebastian syndrome, and Epstein syndrome. All of these entities represent hereditary forms of macrothrombocytopenia associated with leukocyte inclusions (Dohle-like bodies), and variable clinical features of sensorineural hearing loss, presenile (early) cataracts, and renal failure. Most patients do not have clinically significant bleeding problems and are discovered incidentally. These patients require no specific treatment. In rare cases of severe bleeding, platelet transfusions may be necessary. Large platelets can also be seen in Bernard–Soulier syndrome, an inherited defect in the GPIb-IX-V membrane complex leading to platelet dysfunction.

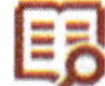

REFERENCES/SOURCES

- Hsia CC, Xenocostas A. Platelet and Megakaryocyte Disorders>Thrombocytopenia>Decreased Platelet Production. https://imagebank.hematology.org/image/12694/mayhegglin-anomaly. ASH Image Bank; 2014.
- Untanu RV, Vajpayee N. May-Hegglin anomaly. In: StatPearls [Internet]. Treasure Island (FL): StatPearls Publishing; 2024.

19. A 15-year-old girl is planned for appendicectomy. She had no history of previous bleeding episodes, menorrhagia, or family history of bleeding. She has a history of undergoing tooth extraction at 10 years of age with no excessive bleeding. On preoperative investigations:

- *Hb:* 12.5g/dL
- *White blood count:* 11.5 × 10^9/L, neutrophils: 8 × 10^9/L, and lymphocytes: 3.5 × 10^9/L
- *Platelet count:* 3.5 × 10^9/L
- *PT:* 14/12
- *APTT:* 85/34
- *INR:* 1.1
- *Postmixing studies APTT:* 26
- *Factor VIII:* 80%
- *Factor IX:* 75%

Which of the following is the most likely diagnosis?

A. Antiphospholipid antibody
B. Factor V deficiency
C. Factor XII deficiency
D. Plasminogen activator inhibitor 1 (PAI-1) deficiency

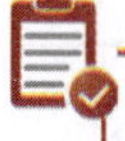

EXPLANATION

Incidentally found isolated APTT prolongation is seen with factor XII, prekallikrein, and high molecular weight kininogen deficiency. Antiphospholipid syndrome is associated with prolonged APTT which does not correct with mixing studies. Factor V deficiency is associated with deranged PT and APTT and mainly mucocutaneous bleeding. PAI-1 deficiency can be associated with bleeding postsurgery or trauma, but they are associated with normal PT, APTT, and TT.

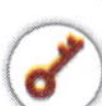

Key: C

BOOST YOUR KNOWLEDGE

Common etiologies of bleeding in children are classified based on the abnormal coagulation parameters

PT/APTT/INR	*With bleeding*	*Without bleeding*
Isolated PT abnormal	Factor VII deficiency, oral vitamin K antagonists, and early vitamin K deficiency	Oral vitamin K antagonist
Isolated APTT abnormal	• Factor VIII deficiency • Factor IX deficiency • Factor XI deficiency • Severe von Willebrand disease	Factor XII, prekallikrein, and high molecular weight kininogen deficiency
Both PT/APTT abnormal	• Factor V deficiency • Factor X deficiency • Fibrinogen deficiency • Combined factor deficiencies • Vitamin K deficiency • Liver disease	
Both PT/APTT normal	• Factor XIII deficiency • von Willebrand disease • Platelet function defects	

REFERENCES/SOURCES

- Gupta P, Menon PSN, Lodha R, Ramji S. PG Textbook of Pediatrics, 3rd edition. New Delhi: Jaypee Brothers Medical Publishers; 2022. p. 1896.
- Orkin SH, Nathan DG, Ginsburg D, Look AT, Fisher DE, Lux S. Nathan & Oski's Hematology and Oncology of Infancy and Childhood, 8th edition. Philadelphia: Saunders; 2014. p. 1060.

20. A 2.5-year-old boy presented with an abdominal mass palpated by his mother while bathing the child. On imaging, the child was diagnosed to be a case of Wilms tumor of the right kidney with lung metastasis. It was planned to start chemotherapy for 6 weeks preoperatively. On routine prechemotherapy investigations, he had a normal CBC. Coagulation screening revealed isolated APTT prolongation (patient value 35, for a control 25, mixing studies normal, factor VIII levels 25%, von Willebrand antigen levels 18%).

The child had undergone an uncomplicated circumcision at 6 months of age. There is no significant family history of bleeding. What is the correct statement regarding the management of a child?

A. Child will require factor VIII support during surgery and lifelong prophylaxis
B. Child will require factor VIII correction only during surgery and spinal anesthesia should be preferred
C. Child will not require factor VIII correction as we expect the coagulation profile to correct within 2–4 weeks of starting chemotherapy
D. Child will require factor VIII correction only during surgery and general anesthesia should be preferred

EXPLANATION

The diagnosis for the child is an acquired von Willebrand disease (AVWS) (uncomplicated surgery previously, no family history of bleeding, precipitating factor Wilms tumor). AVWS is seen in 4–8% of children with Wilms tumor. All children have had resolution of vWF abnormalities within 2–4 weeks of starting chemotherapy and do not require Factor support. In all patients with coagulation disorders neuraxial anesthesia is contraindicated.

Key: C

BOOST YOUR KNOWLEDGE

Acquired von Willebrand disease is characterized by structural or functional defects of vWF that are secondary to autoimmune, lymphoproliferative, or myeloproliferative, malignant, cardiovascular, or other disorders.

von Willebrand factor abnormalities in these disorders can result from:

- Antibody-mediated clearance or functional interference
- Adsorption to surfaces of transformed cells or platelets
- Increased shear stress and subsequent proteolysis

The treatment goals in AVWS are (1) to control acute bleeds, (2) to prevent bleeding in high-risk situations, and (3) to obtain long-term remission. Treatment should address the underlying disorder, thereby aiming to treat AVWS as well.

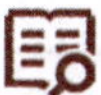

REFERENCES/SOURCES

- Callaghan MU, Wong TE, Federici AB. Treatment of acquired von Willebrand syndrome in childhood. Blood. 2013;122(12):2019-22.
- Tiede A, Rand JH, Budde U, Ganser A, Federici AB. How I treat the acquired von Willebrand syndrome? Blood. 2011;117(25):6777-85.

CHAPTER 18.9

Leukemia

Maharshi Trivedi

1. A 5-year-old girl presented with complaints of increasing pallor, bone pain, and skin bleeds. On examination, generalized lymphadenopathy, petechiae, and hepatosplenomegaly are present. There are no tachypnea, pedal edema, facial congestion, or abnormal chest findings. Her complete blood count (CBC) revealed hemoglobin (Hb)—5 g/dL, white blood cell (WBC)—175,700/mm^3, and platelets—9,000/mm^3. What is true for the management of this child?

A. Start prednisolone immediately
B. Start hyperhydration (2.5 L/m^2/day), allopurinol and monitor for tumor lysis syndrome
C. Give red blood cell transfusion at 10–15 mL/kg
D. Platelet transfusion can be avoided as there is no major active bleeding

EXPLANATION

The boy has presented with signs and symptoms of acute leukemia and has hyperleukocytosis with anemia and thrombocytopenia. Management of hyperleukocytosis includes hyperhydration at 2.5 L/m^2/day or twice the maintenance fluids depending upon cardiac status and the presence or absence of congestive heart failure due to anemia. Steroids should be started once all initial mandatory diagnostic samples are collected (i.e., peripheral smear, flow cytometry, cytogenetics, and molecular studies). In the case of hyperleukocytosis, red blood cell (RBC) transfusion should be avoided if there are no symptoms of congestive cardiac failure due to anemia. Platelets should be transfused as counts are below 9,000/mm^3 (most protocols consider cut-off of 20,000 in the absence of fever or hyperdynamic circulation) and signs of skin bleeds are present.

Key: B

BOOST YOUR KNOWLEDGE

Hyperleukocytosis is defined as a peripheral leukocyte count exceeding 100,000/mm^3 but clinically significant hyperleukocytosis typically occurs with WBC counts of greater than 200,000/mm^3 in AML, >300,000/mm^3 in acute lymphoblastic leukemia (ALL) and even higher in chronic myeloid leukemia (CML). Given the increased risk of tumor lysis with significant leukocytosis, therapies are often directed at preventing the metabolic derangements and hematologic complications associated with tumor lysis while aiming to decrease the WBC and risk of leukocytosis. IV hydration at two to four times maintenance and allopurinol or urate oxidase (rasburicase) should be started immediately. In the setting of hyperleukocytosis, a higher platelet count is desirable, with transfusions recommended if the count is <30,000–50,000/mm^3. Platelets do not add substantially to blood viscosity. In contrast, packed red cells increase viscosity. If a child is hemodynamically stable, packed red blood cell (PRBC) transfusion should be avoided until therapy for hyperleukocytosis is initiated. Coagulation abnormalities should be corrected. Exchange transfusion and leukapheresis are seldom advocated in the contemporary management of hyperleukocytosis. Expedited diagnosis with the early initiation of prednisolone/dexamethasone in ALL and cytarabine in AML is the key to establishing rapid cytoreduction. The procedures are invasive with the blast count rapidly increasing postprocedure in the absence of definitive therapy and are reserved for life-threatening situations with delay in diagnosis/ inadequate response to therapy.

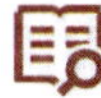

REFERENCES/SOURCES

- Jain R, Bansal D, Marwaha RK. Hyperleukocytosis: emergency management. Indian J Pediatr. 2013;80(2):144-8.
- Reingold S, Li A, Freedman JL. Oncological Emergencies. In: Blaney SM, Helman LJ, Adamson PC (Eds). Pizzo and Poplack's Pediatric Oncology, 8th edition. Philadelphia, USA: Lippincott Williams & Wilkins; 2020. pp. 918-20.

2. A 9-year-old boy presented with complaints of increasing pallor, facial congestion, and difficulty in breathing. On examination respiratory rate was 28 breaths/min, heart rate was 110 beats/min and saturation were 96% at room air. On general physical examination generalized lymphadenopathy, pallor, facial and pedal edema, and abdominal distension were present. There was decreased air entry on the left side with a dull note on percussion. Chest X-ray revealed mediastinal mass and left-sided pleural effusion. Choose the true sentence related to this condition:

A. Malignant mass is the second most common cause for superior vena cava syndrome second to the thrombotic complication related to implantable intravascular device
B. The child should be considered for urgent mediastinal mass biopsy for diagnosis
C. Steroids are the first line of empirical therapy when a child is in distress and diagnostic procedure cannot be performed
D. Radiotherapy is conventionally considered first-line empirical therapy

EXPLANATION

Malignant mass remains the most common cause of superior vena cava syndrome in children followed by thrombotic complications secondary to implantable intravascular devices. Common malignancies presenting with the superior mediastinal syndrome in children are ALL/lymphoma (particularly T-lymphoblastic lymphoma/leukemia), non-Hodgin lymphoma, germ cell tumor, rhabdomyosarcoma, neuroblastoma, and Ewing's sarcoma. The child should be evaluated for the least invasive diagnostic investigation first followed by mediastinal mass biopsy if other investigations are nondiagnostic. As most of the malignant mediastinal masses are responsive to steroids, and steroids are associated with less toxicities in comparison to chemotherapy and radiotherapy, steroids are considered first-line empirical therapy. For tumors unresponsive to steroids, emergent radiotherapy or broad-spectrum chemotherapy agents remain the alternatives.

Key: C

BOOST YOUR KNOWLEDGE

Superior vena cava syndrome refers to the signs and symptoms resulting from compression, obstruction, or thrombosis of the superior vena cava. The term superior mediastinal syndrome is used when tracheal compression also occurs. Initial evaluation includes chest X-ray and prone computed tomographic (CT) scan chest if the supine position aggravates the respiratory distress. The diagnostic investigation algorithm includes a least invasive procedure to start with, i.e., peripheral smear and peripheral blood flow cytometry, serum tumor markers [i.e., alpha-fetoprotein (AFP), beta-subunit of human chorionic gonadotropin (β-hCG)] bone marrow aspiration under local anesthesia, pleural or pericardial fluid aspiration, lymph node biopsy in this order and if these all remain nondiagnostic, mediastinal mass biopsy after evaluating for general anesthesia risk. When a child is in distress and a diagnostic procedure cannot be performed, steroids should be considered first-line empirical therapy. A diagnostic procedure/mediastinal mass biopsy should be performed as soon as the child's condition improves and allows for an invasive procedure.

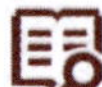

REFERENCES/SOURCES

- Biko DM, Lichtenberger JP 3rd, Rapp JB, Khwaja A, Huppmann AR, Chung EM. Mediastinal Masses in Children: Radiologic-Pathologic Correlation. Radiographics. 2021;41(4):1186-207.
- Reingold S, Li A, Freedman JL. Oncological Emergencies. In: Blaney SM, Helman LJ, Adamson PC (Eds). Pizzo and Poplack's Pediatric Oncology, 8th edition. Philadelphia, USA: Lippincott Williams & Wilkins; 2020. pp. 909-36.
- Verma S, Kalra K, Rastogi S, Sidhu HS. Clinical approach to childhood mediastinal tumors and management. Mediastinum. 2020; 4:21.

3. An 11-year-old boy presented with bone pain, increasing pallor, and abdominal distension. Physical examination showed pallor, petechiae, and moderately enlarged spleen. CBC revealed Hb—7 g/dL, WBC—120,000/mm^3, and platelets—30,000/mm^3. Bone marrow aspiration showed 79% blasts. Cytogenetic study revealed translocation t(9;22)(q34;q11) p190 variant. What is true about this condition?

A. This child is diagnosed with CML chronic phase
B. Treatment of this condition is tyrosine kinase inhibitor (TKIs) (i.e., imatinib) with chemotherapy
C. Hematopoietic stem cell transplant (HSCT) is considered a first-line treatment
D. Prognosis is excellent with 5-year overall survival of >95%

EXPLANATION

This child is having Philadelphia-positive ALL (Ph+ ALL). Bone marrow aspiration in the chronic phase of CML shows <10% blasts. CML is usually associated with p210 variant of t(9;22)(q34;q11). Previously HSCT was considered as a first-line therapy, however, after the advent of TKIs, chemotherapy with TKI is considered the initial therapy. HSCT is considered only in case of refractory [induction failure or postconsolidation minimal residual disease (MRD) positive] or relapsed Ph+ ALL. Prognosis is poor compared to Ph(-) ALL and with contemporary protocols, 5-year survival remains between 60 and 70%.

Key: B

BOOST YOUR KNOWLEDGE

Ph+ ALL is a distinctive biological group of ALL with t(9;22)(q34;q11) translocation where the *ABL1* kinase gene from chromosome 9 is translocated to the *BCR* gene on chromosome 22 forming *BCR-ABL1* fusion gene with tyrosine kinase activity. The P210 variant is associated with CML and <20% of cases of Ph+ ALL in children. P190 variant is associated with 80% ph+ ALL in children. Initial treatment consists of TKI (imatinib or dasatinib) added to ALL backbone chemotherapy. For CML chronic phase TKI alone is used without chemotherapy.

REFERENCES/SOURCES

- Ganguly S, Sasi A, Pushpam D, Bakhshi S. Philadelphia Chromosome Positive and Philadelphia-Like Acute Lymphoblastic Leukemia in Children and Adolescents: Current management, controversies and emerging concepts. Indian J Pediatr. 2024;91(1): 37-46.
- Gramatges M, O'Brien M, Rabin K. Acute lymphoblastic leukemia. In: Blaney SM, Helman LJ, Adamson PC (Eds). Pizzo and Poplack's Pediatric Oncology, 8th edition. Philadelphia, USA: Lippincott Williams & Wilkins (LWW); 2020. pp. 419-53.
- Slayton WB, Schultz KR, Silverman LB, Hunger SP. How we approach Philadelphia chromosome-positive acute lymphoblastic leukemia in children and young adults. Pediatr Blood Cancer. 2020;67(10):e28543.
- Tubergen D, Bleyer A, Ritchey AK, Friehling E. The leukemias. In: Kliegman RM, St Geme III JW (Eds). Nelson Textbook of Pediatrics, 21st edition. Philadelphia, USA: Elsevier; 2020. pp. 2020-651.

4. A 10-year-old boy was diagnosed with T-cell ALL (T-ALL). At presentation, the liver was 5 cm below the right costal margin and the spleen was 3 cm below the left costal margin. CBC revealed Hb—6 g/dL, WBC—212,300/mm^3, platelets—9,000/mm^3, and chest X-ray showed mediastinal mass. Initial cerebrospinal fluid (CSF) examination revealed blasts with 20 WBCs/mm^3. Treatment was started as per Associazione Italiana di Ematologia e Oncologia Pediatrica (AIEOP)-Berlin-Frankfurt-Muenster (BFM) 2009 protocol. On Day 8, CBC showed WBC—25,000/mm^3 and an absolute blast count of 500/mm^3. Postinduction and consolidation evaluation revealed MRD of 1 and 0.1%, respectively (positive MRD). Which of the following is the poor prognostic factor in this child?

A. Presence of mediastinal mass at presentation
B. Presence of blasts on Day 8
C. Anemia and thrombocytopenia at presentation
D. Positive MRD at the end of consolidation

EXPLANATION

The presence of mediastinal mass was considered a prognostic factor in the past; however, it is not considered of prognostic value in contemporary protocols. The BFM trials demonstrated that an absolute blast count of >1,000/mm^3 after a steroid prephase portended a poor prognosis in patients with ALL. Therefore, not only the presence of blasts but blast counts >1,000/mm^3 on Day 8 of treatment are considered as poor response to treatment and poor prognostic factor. Anemia and thrombocytopenia demonstrate the aggressive nature of the disease but are not considered prognostic. Positive MRD (>0.01%) at the end of consolidation is considered the most important prognostic factor.

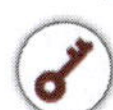

Key: D

BOOST YOUR KNOWLEDGE

High WBC at the time of presentation is considered a poor prognostic factor. However, there is a linear relation between the initial leukocyte count and outcome in B-ALL, with higher leukocyte counts associated with a poorer prognosis. This relationship is not observed in T-ALL. In early studies, male sex was a distinctly poor prognostic factor. However, contemporary trials do not show a significant survival difference in survival between males and females. While with immunophenotype in comparison with B-ALL which gives an opportunity for risk-stratified therapy, T-ALL requires a high-risk protocol and is more difficult to salvage on relapse. Poor prednisolone response (defined as the presence of ≥1,000 blasts/mm^3 after 7 days of steroids) is associated with poor prognosis. MRD assessed after induction and consolidation therapy (if still positive after induction) has emerged as the single most independent prognostic factor in patients with ALL. Generally, the earlier a patient is rendered MRD negative, the better the prognosis. MRD levels that are undetectable or at least $<10^{-4}$ at the end of a standard induction are associated with the best prognosis. In cases of TALL, a later achievement of MRD negativity (i.e., end of consolidation) may not significantly affect prognosis. Persistent or rising MRD at later time points after induction is associated with a poor outcome. MRD can be tested by flow cytometry (sensitivity up to 10^{-4}), polymerase chain reaction (PCR) (sensitivity up to 10^{-5}), and [next-generation sequencing (NGS)—sensitivity from 10^{-5} to 10^{-7}].

REFERENCES/SOURCES

- Gramatges M, O'Brien M, Rabin K. Acute lymphoblastic leukemia. In: Blaney SM, Helman LJ, Adamson PC (Eds). Pizzo and Poplack's Pediatric Oncology, 8th edition. Philadelphia, USA: Lippincott Williams & Wilkins; 2020. pp. 419-53.
- Lee JW, Cho B. Prognostic factors and treatment of pediatric acute lymphoblastic leukemia. Korean J Pediatr. 2017;60(5):129-37.
- Schrappe M, Valsecchi MG, Bartram CR, Schrauder A, Panzer-Grümayer R, Möricke A, et al. Late MRD response determines relapse risk overall and in subsets of childhood T-cell ALL: results of the AIEOP-BFM-ALL 2000 study. Blood. 2011;118(8):2077-84.
- Willemse MJ, Seriu T, Hettinger K, d'Aniello E, Hop WC, Panzer-Grümayer ER, et al. Detection of minimal residual disease identifies differences in treatment response between T-ALL and precursor B-ALL. Blood. 2002;99(12):4386-93.

5. A 5-year-old boy was diagnosed to have B ALL. His initial WBC counts were 12,000/mm^3. CSF studies did not show evidence of disease. He was started on the standard risk arm of the BFM 95 protocol. On Day 8, he showed a good prednisolone response. Results of cytogenetic studies sent at the time of diagnosis are available. Which of the following is true about cytogenetics and would be helpful for guiding further treatment and prognosis?

A. Trisomy 4, 10, and 17 are associated with poor prognosis
B. *KMT2A* rearrangement is commonly associated with infant leukemia and associated with a good prognosis
C. t(1;19) is a favorable aberration in ALL
D. t(17;19) is an indication for HSCT in first complete remission (CR1)

EXPLANATION

Trisomy 4, 10, and 17 (also known as triple trisomy) is associated with good prognosis. KMT2A (MLL) rearrangement is seen in infants with ALL and is associated with poor prognosis. Philadelphia chromosome t(9;22) (q34;q11) is seen in 3–5% of children with B ALL and portends a poor prognosis. t(8;21) and inv16 are favorable cytogenetic aberrations in acute myeloid leukemia. t(17;19) is a rare but high-risk mutation that is an indication for performing allogeneic HSCT in CR1. t(1;19) is not considered to alter the risk stratification in contemporary protocols for pediatric ALL.

Key: D

BOOST YOUR KNOWLEDGE

Chromosomal abnormalities are used to subclassify ALL into prognostic groups. Hyperdiploidy (>46 chromosomes) is the most common chromosomal abnormality in children with ALL (20%). Hyperdiploidy is associated with a good prognosis, while hypodiploidy seen in 2% of cases (<46 chromosomes) is associated with a poor prognosis. t(12;21) is the most common translocation (20%) in children with ALL and is associated with a good prognosis. Alterations of the *KMT2A* (formerly *MLL*) gene located at chromosome band 11q23 occur in 5% of pediatric ALL, in 70% of infant leukemia (both ALL and AML in patients <1 year of age), as well as in most therapy-related leukemias in patients who received topoisomerase II inhibitors and is associated with poor prognosis. Philadelphia chromosome is seen in approximately 3% of cases of pediatric ALL. t(1;19) is seen in approximately 3% of pediatric ALL and is associated with increased central nervous system (CNS) relapse in some studies but is no longer used to change risk stratification by most international groups. Intrachromosomal amplification of chromosome 21 is associated with poor prognosis and needs the high-risk arm of treatment.

REFERENCES/SOURCES

- Gramatges M, O'Brien M, Rabin K. Acute lymphoblastic leukemia. In: Blaney SM, Helman LJ, Adamson PC (Eds). Pizzo and Poplack's Pediatric Oncology, 8th edition. Philadelphia, USA: Lippincott Williams & Wilkins; 2020. pp. 419-53.
- Lee JW, Cho B. Prognostic factors and treatment of pediatric acute lymphoblastic leukemia. Korean J Pediatr. 2017;60(5):129-37.
- Peters C, Locatelli F, Bader P. Acute lymphoblastic leukemia in children and adolescents. In: Carreras E, Dufour C, Mohty M (Eds). The EBMT Handbook: Hematopoietic Stem Cell Transplantation and Cellular Therapies, 7th edition. Cham (CH): Springer; 2019.
- Tubergen D, Bleyer A, Ritchey AK, Friehling E. The leukemias. In: Kliegman RM, St Geme III JW (Eds). Nelson Textbook of Pediatrics, 21st edition. Philadelphia, USA: Elsevier; 2020. pp. 2020-651.

6. An 11-year-old boy presented with complaints of multiple large joint pain associated with swelling involving both knees and bilateral ankle of 2 months duration. There was a history of fever on-off for the last 1-month duration. On examination, there was cervical lymphadenopathy, and the liver was enlarged 4 cm below the right costal margin. Laboratory evaluation showed Hb—9 g/dL, WBC—20,000/mm^3, and platelets 125,000/mm^3. Erythrocyte sedimentation rate (ESR) was 55 mm/h. The rheumatoid factor was negative. What is true about this child and further management?

A. This child is diagnosed to have RF-negative systemic onset juvenile idiopathic arthritis (JIA)
B. Bone marrow studies should be done in the evaluation of systemic JIA before starting treatment in this child
C. This boy should be started on steroids along with methotrexate as disease-modifying antirheumatic drugs (DMARDs)
D. Improvement in symptoms after starting steroids will help in confirming the diagnosis of systemic JIA

EXPLANATION

This child has features suggestive of RF-negative systemic onset JIA (sJIA), however, sJIA is a clinical diagnosis and other differentials should be excluded before labeling sJIA. In this case, the hematological malignancy is a close differential, therefore bone marrow studies should be done before starting steroids. Treatment with steroids will also cause an improvement of leukemia-related symptoms, hence, improvement in symptoms should not be considered as supportive evidence for the diagnosis of sJIA.

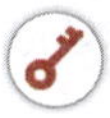

Key: B

BOOST YOUR KNOWLEDGE

Acute leukemia in children presents with variable symptoms. Fever is the most common presentation seen in 50–60% of children. On physical examination, hepatosplenomegaly is the most common finding 61–68%, followed by lymphadenopathy (41–50%), and bleeding (40–48%). Hyperleukocytosis (WBC >50,000) is seen in 15–20% of children. Severe anemia (<7 g/dL) is seen. Bone pain is seen in a quarter of children (20–26%). Children can also present with joint pain and swelling and association with fever can mimic sJIA. Severe pain with poor response to nonsteroidal anti-inflammatory drugs (NSAIDs), pain waking the child at night, and the presence of cytopenias in the blood must alert the physician to the possibility of leukemia.

REFERENCES/SOURCES

- Brix N, Rosthøj S, Glerup M, Hasle H, Herlin T. Identifying acute lymphoblastic leukemia mimicking juvenile idiopathic arthritis in children. PLoS One. 2020;15(8):e0237530.
- Clarke RT, Van den Bruel A, Bankhead C, Mitchell CD, Phillips B, Thompson MJ. Clinical presentation of childhood leukaemia: a systematic review and meta-analysis. Arch Dis Child. 2016;101(10):894-901.
- Gramatges M, O'Brien M, Rabin K. Acute lymphoblastic leukemia. In: Blaney SM, Helman LJ, Adamson PC (Eds). Pizzo and Poplack's Pediatric Oncology, 8th edition. Philadelphia, USA: Lippincott Williams & Wilkins; 2020. pp. 419-53.
- Tubergen D, Bleyer A, Ritchey AK, Friehling E. The leukemias. In: Kliegman RM, St Geme III JW (Eds). Nelson Textbook of Pediatrics, 21st edition. Philadelphia, USA: Elsevier; 2020. pp. 2020-651.

7. An 8-year-old child was diagnosed with T-ALL and was started on induction with four drugs of chemotherapy (vincristine, steroids, L-asparaginase, and daunorubicin). On Day 25 of induction, the child was presented with generalized tonic-clonic seizures. Which of the following drugs is not likely to be responsible for seizures?

A. Vincristine
B. Steroids
C. Daunorubicin
D. L-asparaginase

EXPLANATION

Children with ALL on induction can present with seizures because of various reasons. Vincristine can cause a syndrome of inappropriate antidiuretic hormone (SIADH). Sudden hyponatremia due to SIADH can precipitate seizures. Steroids can cause hypertension and posterior reversible encephalopathy syndrome (PRES). L-asparaginase is associated with coagulation abnormality, and hypercoagulability is more common than bleeding diathesis. The hypercoagulable state can cause cerebral sinus venous thrombosis. Rarely children can also present with intracranial bleeding secondary to coagulation abnormality and thrombocytopenia. Daunorubicin mainly causes myelosuppression, cardiac toxicity, and mucositis and does not directly contribute to neurotoxicity.

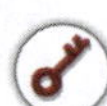 **Key: C**

 **BOOST YOUR KNOWLEDGE**

Vincristine, steroids (prednisolone, dexamethasone), L-asparaginase or pegylated asparaginase, and daunorubicin are commonly used drugs during induction. Common side effects of vincristine are neuropathy presenting as tingling, numbness, neuropathic pain, peripheral weakness, and loss of peripheral reflexes; can also cause central nerve abnormalities such as ptosis, hoarseness secondary to vocal cord palsy, autonomic neuropathy leading to constipation, and SIADH. Steroids can cause Cushing syndrome presenting as moon face, humpback, striae, pot belly, water retention; hyperglycemia; hypertension; avascular necrosis of bones, and proximal myopathy. Daunorubicin can cause myelosuppression (neutropenia, anemia, and thrombocytopenia), mucositis, acute heart failure, and rarely cardiac rhythm abnormality, and can cause cardiomyopathy as a long-term adverse effect.

Common adverse effects of L-asparaginase are hyperglycemia (including diabetic ketoacidosis), hypersensitivity, pancreatitis, coagulation abnormalities (hypercoagulability > bleeding), lipid abnormalities, and liver function abnormalities [rise in alanine aminotransferase (ALT) and aspartate aminotransferase (AST)].

 **REFERENCES/SOURCES**

- Anastasopoulou S, Heyman M, Eriksson MA, Niinimäki R, Taskinen M, Mikkel S, et al. Seizures during treatment of childhood acute lymphoblastic leukemia: a population-based cohort study. Eur J Paediatr Neurol. 2020;27:72-7.
- Rahiman EA, Rajendran A, Sankhyan N, Singh P, Muralidharan J, Bansal D, et al. Acute neurological complications during acute lymphoblastic leukemia therapy: a single-center experience over 10 years. Indian J Cancer. 2021;58(4):545-52.
- Reingold S, Li A, Freedman JL. Oncological Emergencies. In: Blaney SM, Helman LJ, Adamson PC (Eds). Pizzo and Poplack's Pediatric Oncology, 8th edition. Philadelphia, USA: Lippincott Williams & Wilkins; 2020. pp. 909-36.

8. A 12-year-old boy presented with bleeding and pallor for 1-week duration. On evaluation Hb—6 g/dL, WBC—12,000/mm^3, platelets—9,000/mm^3, prothrombin time (PT)—28.8, activated partial thromboplastin time (aPTT)—76.5, international normalized ratio (INR)—2.1, and fibrinogen 0.7 g/dL. Peripheral smear showed 28% strongly myeloperoxidase (MPO) positive blasts with an abundance of Auer rods. Bone marrow aspiration showed 79% blasts and flow cytometry revealed that blasts are positive for MPO, CD13, and CD33 and negative for CD34, CD11c, and CD14. Which is true for this condition?

A. t(8;21) is the most common cytogenetic abnormality associated with this subtype of AML
B. This child should be started on standard chemotherapy for AML with cytarabine and anthracycline
C. All transretinoic acid (ATRA) must be started immediately when the diagnosis is suspected
D. This leukemia is associated with poor prognosis because of coagulation abnormalities

 **EXPLANATION**

This child has been presented with bleeding diathesis and coagulopathy, and blasts are strong MPO positive and flowcytometry is suggestive of acute promyelocytic leukemia (APML). t(15:17) is the most common translocation associated with APML. Children with APML are conventionally treated with ATRA along with chemotherapy or ATRA and arsenic trioxide (ATO) depending on risk group and protocols. The standard chemotherapy regimen used for children with AML is not used for the treatment of children with APML. Children with APML have excellent prognoses with overall survival reaching >90% with contemporary protocols.

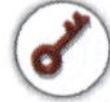 **Key: C**

 **BOOST YOUR KNOWLEDGE**

Acute promyelocytic leukemia is a distinct subtype of AML where children commonly present with abnormal coagulation and children are at high risk of bleeding complications. Previously included in the French-American-British (FAB) classification as M3, APML is considered a separate entity in the current

World Health Organization (WHO) classification as AML with t(15;17) translocation. Less commonly it is associated with other translocations such as t(11;17), t(5;17), and t(x;17). Children with APML are risk stratified based on initial WBC counts into standard risk (WBC <10,000/mm^3) and high-risk (WBC ≥10,000/mm^3). In contemporary protocols, children with standard-risk APML are treated with ATRA and ATO without chemotherapy. High-risk children are treated with either ATRA and chemotherapy or ATRA, ATO and chemotherapy. Components of the protocol where children are treated with ATRA and chemotherapy (without ATO) include induction, consolidation with ATRA, and chemotherapy followed by maintenance with ATRA, 6-mercaptopurine, and methotrexate for a total of 2 years duration. Maintenance chemotherapy is not required if children are treated with ATRA, ATO, or ATRA, ATO, and chemotherapy.

REFERENCES/SOURCES

- Abla O, Ribeiro RC. How I treat children and adolescents with acute promyelocytic leukaemia? Br J Haematol. 2014;164(1): 24-38.
- Aplenc R, Elgarten CW, Choi J, Meshinchi S. Acute myeloid leukemia and myelodysplastic syndrome. In: Blaney SM, Helman LJ, Adamson PC (Eds). Pizzo and Poplack's Pediatric Oncology, 8th edition. Philadelphia, USA: Lippincott Williams & Wilkins; 2020. pp. 454-95.
- Gurnari C, Voso MT, Girardi K, Mastronuzzi A, Strocchio L. Acute promyelocytic leukemia in children: a model of precision medicine and chemotherapy-free therapy. Int J Mol Sci. 2021;22(2):642.
- Sanz MA, Fenaux P, Tallman MS, Estey EH, Löwenberg B, Naoe T, et al. Management of acute promyelocytic leukemia: updated recommendations from an expert panel of the European LeukemiaNet. Blood. 2019;133(15):1630-43.
- Testi AM, Pession A, Diverio D, Grimwade D, Gibson B, de Azevedo AC, et al. Risk-adapted treatment of acute promyelocytic leukemia: results from the International Consortium for Childhood APL. Blood. 2018;132(4):405-12.
- Tubergen D, Bleyer A, Ritchey AK, Friehling E. The leukemias. In: Kliegman RM, St Geme III JW (Eds). Nelson Textbook of Pediatrics, 21st edition. Philadelphia, USA: Elsevier; 2020. pp. 2020-651.

9. An 11-year-old boy presented with pallor, bleeding, and hepatosplenomegaly and was diagnosed with AML. Cytogenetic and molecular studies were done at the time of diagnosis. Which of the following is not true about cytogenetic and molecular abnormality associated with AML?

A. t(8;21) is the most common cytogenetic abnormality associated with AML
B. Inv(16) alteration is sufficient to diagnose AML even if the bone marrow has <20% blasts
C. Children with FLT3-internal tandem duplication (ITD) mutation have a good prognosis
D. Children with monosomy 7 are risk stratified as poor-risk AML

EXPLANATION

t(8;21) and inv(16) are the most common cytogenetic abnormalities seen in 20% of children with AML. The presence of t(8;21) or inv(16) is sufficient to diagnose AML even if the bone marrow blasts are <20%. Children with FLT3-ITD and monosomy 7 have poor prognosis and are stratified to have high-risk AML.

Key: C

BOOST YOUR KNOWLEDGE

Children with AML are risk stratified into good, intermediate, and poor risk AML. The presence of t(8;21), inv(16), t(15;17), NPM1, and homozygous CEBPA (CCAAT enhancer binding protein alpha) mutation are considered as good risk. Children with monosomy 5, monosomy 7, inv(3), t(6;9), KMT2A rearrangement [t(4;11), t(6;11), t(10;11)], FLT3-ITD mutation, are included in poor risk group. Children who do not have any cytogenetic or molecular abnormality or who have t(8;21) along with c-kit mutation or who have FLT3-ITD mutation with NPM1 mutation are considered to have intermediate-risk disease.

REFERENCES/SOURCES

- Aplenc R, Elgarten CW, Choi J, Meshinchi S. Acute myeloid leukemia and myelodysplastic syndrome. In: Blaney SM, Helman LJ, Adamson PC (Eds). Pizzo and Poplack's Pediatric Oncology, 8th edition. Philadelphia, USA: Lippincott Williams & Wilkins; 2020. pp. 454-95.
- Conneely SE, Stevens AM. Acute myeloid leukemia in children: emerging paradigms in genetics and new approaches to therapy. Curr Oncol Rep. 2021;23(2):16.
- Rubnitz JE, Kaspers GJL. How I treat pediatric acute myeloid leukemia? Blood. 2021;138(12):1009-18.
- Tubergen D, Bleyer A, Ritchey AK, Friehling E. The leukemias. In: Kliegman RM, St Geme III JW (Eds). Nelson Textbook of Pediatrics, 21st edition. Philadelphia, USA: Elsevier; 2020. pp. 2020-651.

10. A 2-month-old infant presented with pallor and abdominal distension. On examination, features of Down's syndrome (DS) are present along with hepatosplenomegaly. Laboratory evaluation revealed Hb—7 g/dL, WBC—22,000/mm^3, and platelets—78,000/mm^3. Peripheral smear showed 2% blasts. Genetic studies showed the presence of *GATA1* mutation. The condition resolved spontaneously over the next 2 months. Which of the following is not true for children with Down's syndrome?

A. Children with DS have a 10- to 20-fold increased risk of leukemia compared to children who do not have DS

B. Approximately 20–30% of children with DS and transient abnormal myelopoiesis (TAM) develop AML later in life

C. Children with DS diagnosed with AML have a poor prognosis compared to other children with AML because of the increased risk of chemotherapy-related toxicity

D. Therapy with low-dose cytarabine should be considered in children with DS and TAM presenting with life-threatening symptoms or marked hepatomegaly

EXPLANATION

Children with DS have an increased risk of leukemia compared to children who do not have DS. The risk is asymmetric between ALL and AML with a 40-fold risk for ALL and a 150-fold risk for AML in children under 5 years; later in life, the respective incidence of ALL and AML in children is similar. Approximately 20–30% of children with TAM develop AML by the age of 4 years. AML blasts in children with trisomy 21 who are <4 years of age have increased sensitivity to cytarabine and remission rates of over 90% with OS of >80%. Therapeutic intervention with an exchange transfusion or low-dose cytarabine is necessary for infants with thrombotic microangiopathy (TMA) and life-threatening symptoms, as well as for those with marked hepatomegaly.

Key: C

BOOST YOUR KNOWLEDGE

Newborns with DS are also at risk for the transient myeloproliferative disorder (TMD) or TAM that occurs in approximately 10% of neonates with DS. Mutations of the *GATA1* transcription factor gene are nearly always found in DS-associated TMD. TAM presents with clinical signs and symptoms often indistinguishable from de novo AML. Although TAM usually undergoes spontaneous remission within 3 months from onset, some cases of TAM remit as late as 20 months. About 10–20% of patients have progressive hepatosplenomegaly, effusions, bleeding, liver dysfunction, and leukocytosis. In these infants, mortality is as high as 21%. Treatment with low-dose cytarabine has been reported to improve the 5-year event-free survival (EFS) of infants with severe TMD from 28 to 52%. Acute megakaryoblastic leukemia (AMKL) is the most common AML subtype in children with DS, and the diagnosis of AMKL in an infant prompts a consideration of an underlying DS mosaicism.

REFERENCES/SOURCES

- Aplenc R, Elgarten CW, Choi J, Meshinchi S. Acute myeloid leukemia and myelodysplastic syndrome. In: Blaney SM, Helman LJ, Adamson PC (Eds). Pizzo and Poplack's Pediatric Oncology, 8th edition. Philadelphia, USA: Lippincott Williams & Wilkins; 2020. pp. 454-95.
- Khan I, Malinge S, Crispino J. Myeloid leukemia in Down syndrome. Crit Rev Oncog. 2011;16(1-2):25-36.
- Roberts I. Leukemogenesis in infants and young children with trisomy 21. Hematology Am Soc Hematol Educ Program. 2022;2022(1):1-8.
- Taub JW, Berman JN, Hitzler JK, Sorrell AD, Lacayo NJ, Mast K, et al. Improved outcomes for myeloid leukemia of Down syndrome: a report from the Children's Oncology Group AAML0431 trial. Blood. 2017;129(25):3304-13.
- Tubergen D, Bleyer A, Ritchey AK, Friehling E. The leukemias. In: Kliegman RM, St Geme III JW (Eds). Nelson Textbook of Pediatrics, 21st edition. Philadelphia, USA: Elsevier, 2020. 2020-651.

11. A 6-year-old girl presented with complaints of bleeding and pallor. On evaluation, Hb—7 g/dL, WBC—45,000/mm^3, and platelets—67,000/mm^3. Flow cytometry confirmed the diagnosis of AML. Samples for cytogenetic and molecular studies were sent. Which of the following is true about cytogenetics/molecular abnormalities in deciding further management?

A. HSCT should be considered in the first remission as a consolidation treatment in children with inv(16)
B. In the presence of t(8;21), the standard of care is induction with intensive chemotherapy followed by consolidation chemotherapy
C. Sorafenib is used in combination with chemotherapy in children with BCR-ABL1 mutation
D. HSCT should be considered in the second remission (postrelapse) in the case of monosomy 7

EXPLANATION

Treatment of AML is mainly based on cytogenetic and molecular abnormalities. t(8;21) and inv(16) are considered good risk cytogenetics and the standard of care is to treat with induction chemotherapy followed by consolidation chemotherapy. HSCT is only considered in case of refractory or relapsed (CR2) disease. Monosomy 7 is considered as poor risk cytogenetics, and HSCT should be considered in the first remission as a consolidation therapy. Sorafenib and midostaurin are used in case of the presence of FLT3-ITD mutation. For children who rarely have BCR-ABL1 positive AML, TKIs (i.e., imatinib and dasatinib) are used in combination with chemotherapy.

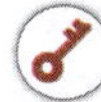

Key: B

BOOST YOUR KNOWLEDGE

Children with AML are classified into good, intermediate, and high-risk groups based on cytogenetic and molecular abnormalities. Postremission therapy is chosen based on a combination of cytogenetic and molecular markers of the leukemia as well as the response to induction chemotherapy (MRD assessment). For selected patients with favorable prognostic features [t(8;21); t(15;17); inv(16)] and improved outcomes with chemotherapy alone, stem cell transplantation is recommended only after a relapse. However, patients with unfavorable prognostic features (e.g., monosomies 7 and 5, 5q–, and 11q23 abnormalities) who have inferior outcomes with chemotherapy might benefit from stem cell transplant in the first remission. Postremission therapy in case of intermediate-risk disease is guided by postinduction MRD.

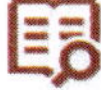

REFERENCES/SOURCES

- Aplenc R, Elgarten CW, Choi J, Meshinchi S. Acute myeloid leukemia and myelodysplastic syndrome. In: Blaney SM, Helman LJ, Adamson PC (Eds). Pizzo and Poplack's Pediatric Oncology, 8th edition. Philadelphia, USA: Lippincott Williams & Wilkins; 2020. pp. 454-95.

- Conneely SE, Stevens AM. Acute myeloid leukemia in children: emerging paradigms in genetics and new approaches to therapy. Curr Oncol Rep. 2021;23(2):16.
- Rubnitz JE, Kaspers GJL. How I treat pediatric acute myeloid leukemia. Blood. 2021;138(12):1009-18.
- Tubergen D, Bleyer A, Ritchey AK, Friehling E. The leukemias. In: Kliegman RM, St Geme III JW (Eds). Nelson Textbook of Pediatrics, 21st edition. Philadelphia, USA: Elsevier, 2020. pp. 2020-651.

12. A 13-year-old boy presented with complaints of pallor and bone pain of 3 months duration. On examination, spleen was 7 cm enlarged. On evaluation, Hb—7.5 g/dL, WBC—650,000/mm^3, neutrophils—55%, lymphocytes—20%, myelocytes—12%, promyelocytes—10%, band cells—3%, and platelets—450,000/mm^3. Bone marrow studies showed 3% blasts, increased myelopoiesis with a high myeloid: erythroid ratio, and a shift to the left with an increase in myeloid precursor cells. Cytogenetic studies showed presence of t(9;22)(q34;q11). Which of the following is true about this condition?

A. Hydroxyurea is a curative treatment for children with this condition
B. In case of a blast crisis, HSCT should be considered in the first remission
C. Splenomegaly and thrombocytosis are considered poor prognostic factors
D. TKIs combined with chemotherapy is a standard of care

EXPLANATION

This boy has a diagnosis of CML chronic phase. TKIs (i.e., imatinib, dasatinib, and nilotinib) are considered standard care for the CML chronic phase, but they are not a curative option. The only curative treatment in children with CML at present is HSCT. Blast crisis and progression to accelerated phase are indications of HSCT in the first remission. Splenomegaly and thrombocytosis are commonly associated with CML; however, they are not associated with prognosis. TKI combined with chemotherapy is considered standard of care in children with Ph+ ALL, and in the context of CML will only be indicated when there is a blast crisis. Hydroxyurea can be started pending the confirmation of diagnosis for cytoreduction. TKI alone is continued once the BCR-ABL1 mutation is confirmed. Hydroxyurea is not a curative treatment.

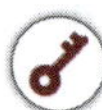

Key: B

BOOST YOUR KNOWLEDGE

Children with CML are considered to have accelerated phase if there are 10–19% blasts in the blood or bone marrow, >20% basophils in peripheral blood, a specific additional chromosomal abnormality in Ph+ cells at diagnosis, persistent increase in WBC or thrombocytosis or thrombocytopenia unresponsive to therapy. The blast phase is diagnosed when there are ≥20% blasts in the blood or bone marrow, extramedullary blast proliferation, or large foci or clusters of blasts on bone marrow biopsy. HSCT is the standard of care in children with blast crisis once remission is achieved.

REFERENCES/SOURCES

- Athale U, Hijiya N, Patterson BC, Bergsagel J, Andolina JR, Bittencourt H, et al. Management of chronic myeloid leukemia (CML) in children and adolescents: Recommendations from the Children's Oncology Group CML Working Group. Pediatr Blood Cancer. 2019;66(9):e27827.
- Hijiya N, Suttorp M. How I treat chronic myeloid leukemia in children and adolescents. Blood. 2019;133(22):2374-84.
- Rau R, Loh M. Myeloproliferative neoplasms of childhood. In: Blaney SM, Helman LJ, Adamson PC (Eds). Pizzo and Poplack's Pediatric Oncology, 8th edition. Philadelphia, USA: Lippincott Williams & Wilkins; 2020. pp. 496-516.
- Smith G, Apperley J, Milojkovic D, Cross NCP, Foroni L, Byrne J, et al. A British Society for Haematology Guideline on the Diagnosis and Management of Chronic Myeloid Leukaemia. Br J Haematol. 2020;191(2):171-93.
- Tubergen D, Bleyer A, Ritchey AK, Friehling E. The leukemias. In: Kliegman RM, St Geme III JW (Eds). Nelson Textbook of Pediatrics, 21st edition. Philadelphia, USA: Elsevier; 2020. pp. 2020-651.

13. A 14-year-old boy presented with pallor, bone pain, and left quadrant fullness of 6 months duration. On examination spleen was 12 cm below the left costal margin. CBCs revealed Hb—7.3 g/dL, WBC—312,000/mm^3, platelets—675,000/mm^3, neutrophils—45%, lymphocytes—30%, basophils—4%, eosinophils—5%, promyelocytes—8%, myelocytes—5%, and band cells—3%. Peripheral smear showed leukocytosis with myeloid cells with all stages of differentiation with basophilia and eosinophilia. What is true about further diagnostic studies for this condition?

A. p190 variant of t(9;22) confirms the diagnosis of CML
B. Molecular studies [reverse transcription (RT)-PCR] are not needed if cytogenetic/fluorescence in situ hybridization (FISH) confirms the presence of t(9;22)(q34;q11)
C. Tyrosine kinase domain mutation analysis should be done when the child presents in an accelerated phase or blast crisis
D. Bone marrow studies are not needed at the time of diagnosis if there are no blasts on the peripheral smear and the presence of t(9;22)(q34;q11) is confirmed

EXPLANATION

This boy has clinical and laboratory features of CML. CML is almost always associated with the p210 variant of t(9;22). P190 variant of t(9;22) is associated with Ph+ ALL. In CML, cytogenetic studies also provide evidence of additional cytogenetic abnormalities apart from t(9;22). Molecular studies (RT-PCR) are necessary at the time of diagnosis to detect BCR-ABL1 mutation variants and also for monitoring and response assessment after starting treatment with TKI. Bone marrow studies should be done at the time of diagnosis to confirm the diagnosis of CML, rule out acute leukemia, and collect samples for cytogenetic studies. Tyrosine kinase domain mutation analysis should be done in children presenting in accelerated phase or blast crisis and in children who fail to achieve molecular remission despite compliant therapy with TKIs.

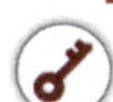

Key: C

BOOST YOUR KNOWLEDGE

The P210 BCR-ABL1 fusion is typical of CML but has also been associated with some forms of Ph1-positive ALL (Ph+ ALL). Over 40% of adults with Ph+ ALL carry the P210 BCR-ABL1 fusion. In 60% of adults and over 80% of children with Ph+ ALL, a different rearrangement occurs, with ABL1 exon 2 spliced to an exon outside the major BCR region [known as the minor BCR region (m-BCR)]. The resultant protein product(P190) has approximately a fivefold higher level of TK activity and higher transforming ability than does P210. A third BCR-ABL1 fusion protein (P230) is the molecular basis for rare chronic neutrophilic leukemia. This translocation involves a third breakpoint cluster region in BCR (μ-BCR). Approximately 5–10% of CML patients in chronic phase (CML-CP) have, in addition to the Ph1 chromosome, other visible karyotypic abnormalities such as a second Ph1 chromosome, lack of the Y chromosome, isochromosome 17, or an extra chromosome 8 or 19; these secondary changes are associated with a worse prognosis.

REFERENCES/SOURCES

- Athale U, Hijiya N, Patterson BC, Bergsagel J, Andolina JR, Bittencourt H, et al. Management of chronic myeloid leukemia in children and adolescents: Recommendations from the Children's Oncology Group CML Working Group. Pediatr Blood Cancer. 2019;66(9): e27827.
- Hijiya N, Suttorp M. How I treat chronic myeloid leukemia in children and adolescents. Blood. 2019;133(22):2374-84.
- Rau R, Loh M. Myeloproliferative neoplasms of childhood. In: Blaney SM, Helman LJ, Adamson PC (Eds). Pizzo and Poplack's Pediatric Oncology, 8th edition. Philadelphia, USA: Lippincott Williams & Wilkins; 2020. pp. 496-516.
- Smith G, Apperley J, Milojkovic D, Cross NCP, Foroni L, Byrne J, et al. A British Society for Haematology Guideline on the Diagnosis and Management of Chronic Myeloid Leukaemia. Br J Haematol. 2020;191(2):171-93.
- Tubergen D, Bleyer A, Ritchey AK, Friehling E. The leukemias. In: Kliegman RM, St Geme III JW (Eds). Nelson Textbook of Pediatrics, 21st edition. Philadelphia, USA: Elsevier, 2020. pp. 2020-651.

14. A 6-month-old boy was brought with complaints of increasing pallor, skin bleeds, and abdominal distension of 4 weeks duration. On evaluation, CBC showed Hb—7 g/dL, WBC—35,000/mm^3, platelets—28,000/mm^3, lymphocytes—30%, neutrophils—45%, and monocytes—25%. Peripheral smear revealed monocytosis without the presence of blasts. Bone marrow studies showed 4% blasts with erythroid and myeloid hyperplasia and increased monocytic precursor cells. Which of the following is not true for this condition?

A. Child should be screened for NF-1 mutation and features of neurofibromatosis
B. Cytogenetic studies should be done to look for mutation of *PTPN11* (protein tyrosine phosphatase non-receptor type 11), *N-RAS* (neuroblastoma RAS viral oncogene homolog), *K-RAS* (Kirsten rat sarcoma virus), and casitas B-cell lymphoma (*CBL*) genes
C. HSCT should be considered in refractory or relapsed cases where chemotherapy is not effective
D. Increased HbF is not a mandatory criterion for the diagnosis

EXPLANATION

Children with neurofibromatosis-1 and Noonan syndrome (PTPN11 mutation) have an increased risk of juvenile myelomonocytic leukemia (JMML). Mutation in *NF1, PTPN11, N-RAS, K-RAS,* and *CBL* genes is a part of the diagnostic criteria for JMML. Increased HbF is one of the criteria for diagnosis of JMML but is not a mandatory criterion. Monosomy 7 is found in approximately 25–33% of patients with features of JMML. HSCT is considered standard care for children with JMML and should be considered as an upfront treatment.

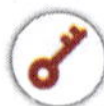

Key: C

BOOST YOUR KNOWLEDGE

Revised diagnostic criteria for JMML:

- *Clinical and hematologic features (all four features mandatory):*
  1. Peripheral blood monocyte count >1 × 10^9/L
  2. Blast percentage in peripheral blood and bone marrow <20%
  3. Splenomegaly
  4. Absence of Philadelphia chromosome (BCR/ABL rearrangement)
- *Oncogenetic studies (one finding is sufficient):*
  1. Somatic mutation in PTPN11* or K-RAS* or N-RAS*
  2. Clinical diagnosis of neurofibromatosis type 1 (NF-1) or germline NF1 mutation
  3. Germline CBL mutation and loss of heterozygosity of CBL[†]
- Only for those patients (10% of the whole number) without any oncogenetic parameter, besides the clinical and hematologic features listed under I, at least two of the following criteria have to be fulfilled:
  1. Monosomy 7 or any other chromosomal abnormality
  2. HbF increased for age
  3. Myeloid precursors on peripheral blood smear
  4. Spontaneous growth or granulocyte-macrophage-colony-stimulating factor (GM-CSF) hypersensitivity in colony assay[£]
  5. Hyperphosphorylation of STAT5 (signal transducer and activator of transcription 5)

*Germline mutations need to be excluded (Noonan syndrome)
[†]Occasional cases with heterozygous splice site mutations
[£]Tests are not routinely available and are rarely done to clinically diagnose JMML

REFERENCES/SOURCES

- Gupta AK, Meena JP, Chopra A, Tanwar P, Seth R. Juvenile myelomonocytic leukemia—A comprehensive review and recent advances in management. Am J Blood Res. 2021;11(1):1-21.
- Locatelli F, Algeri M, Merli P, Strocchio L. Novel approaches to diagnosis and treatment of juvenile myelomonocytic leukemia. Expert Rev Hematol. 2018;11(2):129-43.
- Locatelli F, Niemeyer CM. How I treat juvenile myelomonocytic leukemia? Blood. 2015;125(7):1083-90.
- Mayerhofer C, Niemeyer CM, Flotho C. Current treatment of juvenile myelomonocytic leukemia. J Clin Med. 2021;10(14):3084.
- Rau R, Loh M. Myeloproliferative neoplasms of childhood. In: Blaney SM, Helman LJ, Adamson PC (Eds). Pizzo and Poplack's Pediatric Oncology, 8th edition. Philadelphia, USA: Lippincott Williams & Wilkins; 2020. pp. 496-516.
- Tubergen D, Bleyer A, Ritchey AK, Friehling E. The leukemias. In: Kliegman RM, St Geme III JW (Eds). Nelson Textbook of Pediatrics, 21st edition. Philadelphia, USA: Elsevier, 2020. pp. 2020-651.
- Wintering A, Dvorak CC, Stieglitz E, Loh ML. Juvenile myelomonocytic leukemia in the molecular era: a clinician's guide to diagnosis, risk stratification, and treatment. Blood Adv. 2021;5(22):4783-793.

15. A 5-month-old boy presented with complaints of pallor, abdominal distension, and papulonodular skin rash of 1½ months duration. The liver was 4 cm below the right costal margin and the spleen was 5 cm below the left costal margin. CBCs revealed Hb—6 g/dL, WBC—28,000/mm^3, platelets—43,000/mm^3. Peripheral smear showed monocytosis with 1% immature cells. Bone marrow studies showed 3% blasts with increased monocytic precursor cells. Which of the following is true about this condition?

A. Presence of BCR-ABL1 is a mandatory criteria to diagnose JMML
B. This condition is commonly associated with DS
C. Excellent survival is achieved by HSCT
D. Spontaneous resolution of disease is commonly seen in children with Noonan's syndrome

EXPLANATION

This child has been presented with clinical and laboratory features of JMML. The absence of BCR-ABL1 is a mandatory criterion to diagnose JMML. This condition is not seen in children with DS but is commonly associated with NF-1 and Noonan syndrome. In children with Noonan syndrome and CBL mutation, spontaneous resolution of disease has been observed.

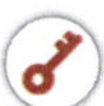

Key: D

BOOST YOUR KNOWLEDGE

JMML is rare, constituting <1% of all cases of childhood leukemia. Patients with this disease do not have the Philadelphia chromosome characteristic of CML. Patients with JMML present with rashes, lymphadenopathy, splenomegaly, and hemorrhagic manifestations. Analysis of the peripheral blood often shows an elevated leukocyte count with increased monocytes, thrombocytopenia, and anemia with the presence of erythroblasts. The bone marrow shows a myelodysplastic pattern, with blasts accounting for <20% of cells. Most patients with JMML have been found to have mutations that lead to activation of the *RAS* oncogene pathway, including *RAS*, *NF1*, and *PTPN11*. Patients with *NF-1* and *Noonan syndrome* have a predilection for this type of leukemia since they have germline mutations involved in *RAS* signaling. JMML in the setting of Noonan syndrome is unique, with most patients having a spontaneous resolution. However, for most patients with JMML, stem cell transplantation offers the best opportunity for cure, but outcomes are still poor.

REFERENCES/SOURCES

- Gupta AK, Meena JP, Chopra A, Tanwar P, Seth R. Juvenile myelomonocytic leukemia—A comprehensive review and recent advances in management. Am J Blood Res. 2021;11(1):1-21.
- Locatelli F, Algeri M, Merli P, Strocchio L. Novel approaches to diagnosis and treatment of juvenile myelomonocytic leukemia. Expert Rev Hematol. 2018;11(2):129-43.

- Locatelli F, Niemeyer CM. How I treat juvenile myelomonocytic leukemia? Blood. 2015;125(7):1083-90.
- Mayerhofer C, Niemeyer CM, Flotho C. Current treatment of juvenile myelomonocytic leukemia. J Clin Med. 2021;10(14):3084.
- Rau R, Loh M. Myeloproliferative neoplasms of childhood. In: Blaney SM, Helman LJ, Adamson PC (Eds). Pizzo and Poplack's Pediatric Oncology, 8th edition. Philadelphia, USA: Lippincott Williams & Wilkins; 2020. pp. 496-516.
- Tubergen D, Bleyer A, Ritchey AK, Friehling E. The leukemias. In: Kliegman RM, St Geme III JW (Eds). Nelson Textbook of Pediatrics, 21st edition. Philadelphia, USA: Elsevier; 2020. pp. 2020-651.
- Wintering A, Dvorak CC, Stieglitz E, Loh ML. Juvenile myelomonocytic leukemia in the molecular era: a clinician's guide to diagnosis, risk stratification, and treatment. Blood Adv. 2021;5(22):4783-93.

16. A 6-year-old boy was diagnosed with a T-ALL and was started on BFM 2009 protocol. Which of the following is not a principle of ALL treatment?

A. Induction chemotherapy lowers the leukemic burden in the bone marrow and eradicates it to achieve remission

B. Consolidation or compartmental chemotherapy contributes to eradicating leukemic cells in CNS and extramedullary sites

C. Maintenance chemotherapy is low dose prolonged duration chemotherapy to eradicate residual leukemic cells and prevent relapse by maintaining remission

D. Delayed induction/reinduction therapy is only given to children with ALL where the disease is not in remission postremission induction treatment

EXPLANATION

Initial therapy, termed *remission induction,* is designed to eradicate the leukemic cells from the bone marrow and to achieve remission and normal blood counts. The second phase of treatment, *consolidation,* focuses on intensive CNS therapy in combination with continued intensive systemic therapy in an effort to prevent later CNS relapses. Intrathecal chemotherapy is given repeatedly by lumbar puncture (LP). The goal of delayed intensification (Delayed induction) is to eradicate residual leukemic cells (postremission). Maintenance chemotherapy is low dose prolonged duration chemotherapy to keep residual leukemic cells in control and prevent relapse by maintaining remission.

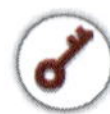

Key: D

BOOST YOUR KNOWLEDGE

During the induction phase, therapy is given for 4 weeks and consists of vincristine weekly, a corticosteroid such as dexamethasone or prednisone, and L-asparaginase (conventional or pegylated). Patients at higher risk also receive daunomycin at weekly intervals. With this approach, 98% of patients achieve remission, as defined by <5% blasts in the marrow and a return of neutrophil and platelet counts to near-normal levels after 4–5 weeks of treatment. Physical examination should be normal postinduction and there should be no evidence of disease at an extramedullary location by light microscopy (i.e., CSF). During delayed intensification, similar multiagent noncross-resistant chemotherapy used during initial induction and consolidation, such as cytarabine, methotrexate, asparaginase, and vincristine, is used again to eradicate residual disease. All children receive the delayed induction or reinduction phase of therapy following the consolidation/interim maintenance phases of therapy. The purpose is quiescent cells are more resistant to chemotherapy than actively dividing cells and the reinduction therapy targets the few leukemic cells that may be quiescent before and by now will enter the cell division phase, becoming sensitive to cytotoxic therapy. Finally, patients enter the *maintenance* phase of therapy, which lasts for 2–3 years, depending on the protocol used. Patients are given daily mercaptopurine and weekly oral methotrexate, in some protocols with intermittent doses of vincristine and corticosteroid. Intrathecal therapy with methotrexate is continued throughout treatment for the CNS sanctuary site. Cranial radiation is currently reserved for patients with CNS involvement at the time of diagnosis.

REFERENCES/SOURCES

- Cooper SL, Brown PA. Treatment of pediatric acute lymphoblastic leukemia. Pediatr Clin North Am. 2015;62(1):61-73.
- Gramatges M, O'Brien M, Rabin K. Acute lymphoblastic leukemia. In: Blaney SM, Helman LJ, Adamson PC (Eds). Pizzo and Poplack's Pediatric Oncology, 8th edition. Philadelphia, USA: Lippincott Williams & Wilkins; 2020. pp. 419-53.
- Tubergen D, Bleyer A, Ritchey AK, Friehling E. The leukemias. In: Kliegman RM, St Geme III JW (Eds). Nelson Textbook of Pediatrics, 21st edition. Philadelphia, USA: Elsevier; 2020. pp. 2020-651.

17. A 10-year-old boy presented with complaints of high-grade fever (102°F), and abdominal distension of 10 days duration. On examination, pallor was present along with multiple petechiae, the liver was palpable 5 cm below the right costal margin and the spleen was 3 cm below the left costal margin. CBCs revealed Hb—6.7 g/dL, WBC—3,100/mm^3, and platelets—25,000/mm^3. Which of the following investigations is least useful for diagnosing the condition in this child?

A. Peripheral smear
B. Rapid malarial antigen test
C. Bone marrow studies
D. Serum ferritin, serum iron and transferrin saturation, vitamin B_{12}, and folate levels

EXPLANATION

This child has presented with fever and abdominal distension which points toward hepatosplenomegaly. The child also has features of pancytopenia. Peripheral smear would help in looking at red blood cell morphology and to rule out the presence of blasts. Bone marrow studies will be useful in ruling out leukemia and looking for erythroid maturation and megaloblastoid pictures in the marrow. Malaria can also present with a similar clinical picture and is known to be associated with anemia, leucopenia, and thrombocytopenia. In iron deficiency anemia hepatosplenomegaly is unusual and platelet counts either remain normal or elevated. megaloblastic anemia can cause pancytopenia and some organomegaly, the high fever, severe cytopenia and significant organomegaly in the index case are unlikely to be attributable to nutritional anemia.

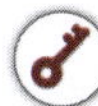

Key: D

BOOST YOUR KNOWLEDGE

Differential diagnoses of pancytopenia associated with fever and hepatosplenomegaly are: (1) infection—malaria, enteric fever, viral infection, such as dengue, chikungunya, cytomegalovirus, Epstein-Barr virus; (2) marrow replacement in leukemia, lymphoma, and myelodysplasia; and (3) sometimes children with vitamin B_{12} or folate deficiency present with acute febrile illness. The presence of hepatosplenomegaly excludes the diagnosis of aplastic anemia.

REFERENCES/SOURCES

- Brix N, Rosthøj S, Glerup M, Hasle H, Herlin T. Identifying acute lymphoblastic leukemia mimicking juvenile idiopathic arthritis in children. PLoS One. 2020;15(8):e0237530.
- Tubergen D, Bleyer A, Ritchey AK, Friehling E. The leukemias. In: Kliegman RM, St Geme III JW (Eds). Nelson Textbook of Pediatrics, 21st edition. Philadelphia, USA: Elsevier, 2020. pp. 2020-651.

18. A 12-year-old boy presented with increasing pallor and skin bleeds. He was diagnosed with B-ALL at the age of 7 years and was treated with BFM 2009 chemotherapy protocol and completed the chemotherapy at the age of 10 years. On evaluation, bone marrow studies revealed 86% blasts and flow cytometry confirmed B-ALL relapse. CSF studies showed the presence of blasts. Which of the following is true about ALL relapse?

A. All children with ALL relapse should be treated with chemotherapy followed by HSCT
B. Isolated CNS relapse (without bone marrow relapse), is treated with intrathecal chemotherapy and cranial/craniospinal radiotherapy, and systemic chemotherapy is usually not required

C. B-ALL relapse is associated with a worse prognosis compared to T-ALL relapse
D. Children with isolated bone marrow relapse have poor prognosis compared to children with combined marrow and CNS relapse

EXPLANATION

Children with ALL relapse are risk stratified at the time of relapse based on prognostic factors and children with low-risk relapse disease can be treated with chemotherapy alone without HSCT. Isolated CNS relapse requires treatment with systemic chemotherapy along with CNS-directed therapy because these patients are at high risk of subsequent marrow relapse if not treated with systemic chemotherapy. B immunophenotype has a better prognosis at the time of relapse compared with T-ALL. Children with isolated marrow relapse have poor prognosis compared to children with combined relapse and isolated extramedullary relapse.

Key: D

BOOST YOUR KNOWLEDGE

Important prognostic factors at the time of ALL relapse are: Time from initial diagnosis, immunophenotype, and medullary or extramedullary relapse. Relapse is classified into very early (<18 months from diagnosis), early (18 months from diagnosis to 6 months post-treatment), and late (6 months post-treatment). Children with very early and early relapse have a worse prognosis compared to late relapse. Children with isolated bone marrow relapse have a worse prognosis compared to combined (medullary and extramedullary) and isolated extramedullary relapse. Patients with a low-risk relapse such as late medullary relapse or isolated extramedullary relapse of B-ALL can be treated with relapse chemotherapy protocols. High-risk relapses are typically offered HSCT after achieving remission.

REFERENCES/SOURCES

- Bhojwani D, Pui CH. Relapsed childhood acute lymphoblastic leukaemia. Lancet Oncol. 2013;14(6):e205-17.
- Gramatges M, O'Brien M, Rabin K. Acute lymphoblastic leukemia. In: Blaney SM, Helman LJ, Adamson PC (Eds). Pizzo and Poplack's Pediatric Oncology, 8th edition. Philadelphia, USA: Lippincott Williams & Wilkins; 2020. pp. 419-53.
- Hunger SP, Raetz EA. How I treat relapsed acute lymphoblastic leukemia in the pediatric population? Blood. 2020;136(16): 1803-12.
- Parker C, Waters R, Leighton C, Hancock J, Sutton R, Moorman AV, et al. Effect of mitoxantrone on outcome of children with first relapse of acute lymphoblastic leukaemia (ALL R3): an open-label randomised trial. Lancet. 2010;376(9757):2009-17.
- Tubergen D, Bleyer A, Ritchey AK, Friehling E. The leukemias. In: Kliegman RM, St Geme III JW (Eds). Nelson Textbook of Pediatrics, 21st edition. Philadelphia, USA: Elsevier; 2020. pp. 2020-651.

19. A 6-month-old infant was presented with complaints of pallor, abdominal distension, and papulonodular skin rash. On evaluation, Hb was 4 g/dL, WBC—310,000/mm^3, and platelets were 24,000/mm^3. Bone marrow studies revealed 82% blasts and flowcytometry confirmed the diagnosis of B-ALL. Which of the following is true about this condition?

A. CNS involvement is uncommon in infant leukemia
B. Similar to older children, infants with ALL have significantly better outcomes compared to AML
C. Blasts are commonly CD10 positive in infants with ALL
D. KMT2A rearrangement in children is associated with hyperleukocytosis, CNS infiltration, and poor prognosis

EXPLANATION

About >80% of infants with leukemia have KMT2A rearrangement (MLL rearrangement) and it is associated with hyperleukocytosis, CNS infiltration, and a high risk of relapse. CNS involvement is more common in infants with ALL compared to older children. In infants, ALL is associated with poor outcomes and there is not much difference in the outcome of infants with ALL and AML. Blasts in infant ALL are commonly CD10 negative.

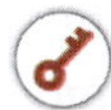

Key: D

BOOST YOUR KNOWLEDGE

Approximately 2% of cases of leukemia during childhood occur before age 1 year. In contrast to the situation in older children, the ratio of ALL in infants to AML is 2:1. Leukemic clones have been noted in cord blood at birth before symptoms appear. Poor prognostic features include diagnosis at a young age [<6 months in Interfant and Japanese Infant Leukemia/Lymphoma Study Group (JILSG) studies; <3 months in COG (Children's Oncology Group) trials], high WBC count (>300 × 10^9/L per Interfant; >50 ×10^9/L/COG), CNS disease (JILSG), and rearrangement of *KMT2A* (all groups). Although most infants are able to achieve morphologic CR with intensive chemotherapy regimens, high relapse rates, and treatment-related mortality led to poor survival. Very intensive chemotherapy programs, including stem cell transplantation, are being explored in infants with *KMT2A* (*MLL*) gene rearrangements, but none has yet been proven satisfactory. Infants with leukemia who lack the 11q23 rearrangements have a prognosis similar to that of older children with ALL.

REFERENCES/SOURCES

- Brown P, Pieters R, Biondi A. How I treat infant leukemia. Blood. 2019;133(3):205-14.
- Brown P. Treatment of infant leukemias: challenge and promise. Hematology Am Soc Hematol Educ Program. 2013;2013:596-600.
- Gramatges M, O'Brien M, Rabin K. Acute lymphoblastic leukemia. In: Blaney SM, Helman LJ, Adamson PC (Eds). Pizzo and Poplack's Pediatric Oncology, 8th edition. Philadelphia, USA: Lippincott Williams & Wilkins; 2020. pp. 419-53.
- Kotecha RS. Updates in infant acute lymphoblastic leukemia and the potential for targeted therapy. Hematology Am Soc Hematol Educ Program. 2022;2022(1):611-7.
- Tubergen D, Bleyer A, Ritchey AK, Friehling E. The leukemias. In: Kliegman RM, St Geme III JW (Eds). Nelson Textbook of Pediatrics, 21st edition. Philadelphia, USA: Elsevier; 2020. pp. 2020-651.

20. A 13-year-old boy presented with complaints of pallor, skin bleeds, and hematuria. On evaluation, Hb was 6 g/dL, WBC—9 × 10^9/L, platelets—19 × 10^9/L, PT—31.2, aPTT—74, INR—2.3, and fibrinogen was 0.7 g/dL. Peripheral smear showed strong MPO-positive blasts. Bone marrow studies revealed 79% MPO-positive blasts with Auer rods. Which of the following is true about this condition?

A. Diagnostic lumbar puncture should be performed to look for CNS involvement
B. This type of leukemia is commonly seen in children <5 years age group
C. Disseminated intravascular coagulation and hemorrhagic complications are not common in these children
D. Differentiation syndrome is commonly seen in children with high initial WBC counts

EXPLANATION

This child was presented with abnormal coagulation and bleeding manifestations. Blasts are MPO positive with the presence of Auer rods which points toward the diagnosis of APML. These children are at increased risk of disseminated intravascular coagulation and hemorrhagic complications. CNS hemorrhage at the time of presentation or during induction therapy is a significant risk factor for relapse. Current therapeutic approaches thus avoid diagnostic lumbar puncture to minimize the risk of bleeding and introduction of leukemic cells into the CNS. Differentiation syndrome is a unique adverse effect of the treatment of APML and is commonly seen in children with high initial WBC counts.

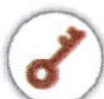

Key: D

BOOST YOUR KNOWLEDGE

The treatment of pediatric APL has several important potential side effects. The first is the APL differentiation syndrome or retinoic acid syndrome, which is characterized by fever, pulmonary infiltrates, pleural pericardial effusions, respiratory distress, fluid retention with weight gain, hypotension, and, sometimes, renal failure. This syndrome is more frequently observed in patients with elevated WBC. Initiation of corticosteroids with the onset of signs and symptoms or prophylactically for patients with WBC of >5,000/μL suggests that a reduction in mortality and morbidity can be achieved, although randomized studies have not been done. Pseudotumor cerebri is another adverse event that appears to occur more frequently in patients <20 years of age. A reduction in the recommended ATRA to 25 mg/m^2 daily (vs. 45 mg/m^2 daily) effectively decreased the incidence of this complication without compromising outcomes.

REFERENCES/SOURCES

- Abla O, Ribeiro RC. How I treat children and adolescents with acute promyelocytic leukaemia. Br J Haematol. 2014;164(1):24-38.
- Aplenc R, Elgarten CW, Choi J, Meshinchi S. Acute myeloid leukemia and myelodysplastic syndrome. In: Blaney SM, Helman LJ, Adamson PC (Eds). Pizzo and Poplack's Pediatric Oncology, 8th edition. Philadelphia, USA: Lippincott Williams & Wilkins; 2020. pp. 454-95.
- Gurnari C, Voso MT, Girardi K, Mastronuzzi A, Strocchio L. Acute promyelocytic leukemia in children: a model of precision medicine and chemotherapy-free therapy. Int J Mol Sci. 2021;22(2):642.
- Sanz MA, Fenaux P, Tallman MS, Estey EH, Löwenberg B, Naoe T, et al. Management of acute promyelocytic leukemia: updated recommendations from an expert panel of the European LeukemiaNet. Blood. 2019;133(15):1630-43.
- Testi AM, Pession A, Diverio D, Grimwade D, Gibson B, de Azevedo AC, et al. Risk-adapted treatment of acute promyelocytic leukemia: results from the International Consortium for Childhood APL. Blood. 2018;132(4):405-12.
- Tubergen D, Bleyer A, Ritchey AK, Friehling E. The leukemias. In: Kliegman RM, St Geme III JW (Eds). Nelson Textbook of Pediatrics, 21st edition. Philadelphia, USA: Elsevier; 2020. pp. 2020-651.

21. A 10-year-old boy was diagnosed with B-ALL relapsed 2 months after completing the first line of treatment for B-ALL. On evaluation at relapse, bone marrow showed 81% blasts, which were positive for CD10, CD19, CD22, and CD34 and negative for CD20. CSF did not show evidence of blasts and testes were normal on examination. He was being evaluated for different treatment options at the relapse. Which of the following is true about novel approaches for the treatment of ALL?

A. Blinatumomab cannot be used here as blasts are CD20-negative
B. Chimeric antigen receptor (CAR) cells are the B cells that are engineered to target leukemia cells with specific antigens on blasts (i.e., CD19 and CD22)
C. Inotuzumab ozogamicin is a targeted agent for leukemia cells expressing CD22 antigen
D. Cytokine release syndrome (CRS) is a nonsignificant toxicity with immunotherapy

EXPLANATION

Blinatumomab is a bispecific T-cell engager antibody (BiTE) with specificity for CD3/CD19 antigens. It binds to CD19-positive blast cells and CD3-positive T-cells and brings T-cells in proximity to blast cells to induce T-cell-induced blast killing. CAR cells are T-cells that are engineered to target leukemia with specificity for single or double antigens on the blast cells. Inotuzumab ozogamicin is an antibody-drug conjugate medicine. The medication consists of a humanized monoclonal antibody against CD22 (inotuzumab), linked to a cytotoxic agent from the class of calicheamicins called ozogamicin. CRS mainly occurs in children with high disease burden at the time of immunotherapy treatment and it can be a life-threatening complication of immunotherapy.

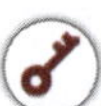

Key: C

BOOST YOUR KNOWLEDGE

Novel approaches including immunotherapy and targeted therapy are being considered in case of relapse/refractory ALL to avoid short- and long-term chemotherapy toxicities and to overcome chemotherapy resistance at the time of relapse. Immunotherapy mainly acts by either bringing T-cells in proximity to blast cells and activating them or by infusing T-cells which are engineered to target specific blast cells. CRS is a form of systemic inflammatory release syndrome, because of the release of inflammatory cytokines by activated T-cells and myeloid cells during treatment with immunotherapy. Risk and severity of CRS increase with increased disease burden, and increased CAR T-cell dose. Patients are regularly monitored for CRS post-CAR T cell and other immunotherapy and considered for anti-interleukin 6 (anti-IL-6) antibodies, anti-interleukin 1 (anti-IL-1) antibodies/inhibitors, or steroids based on the severity of CRS.

REFERENCES/SOURCES

- Brudno JN, Kochenderfer JN. Toxicities of chimeric antigen receptor T-cells: recognition and management. Blood. 2016;127(26):3321-30.
- Freyer CW, Porter DL. Cytokine release syndrome and neurotoxicity following CAR T-cell therapy for hematologic malignancies. J Allergy Clin Immunol. 2020;146(5):940-8.
- Gramatges M, O'Brien M, Rabin K. Acute lymphoblastic leukemia. In: Blaney SM, Helman LJ, Adamson PC (Eds). Pizzo and Poplack's Pediatric Oncology, 8th edition. Philadelphia, USA: Lippincott Williams & Wilkins; 2020. pp. 419-53.
- Inaba H, Pui CH. Immunotherapy in pediatric acute lymphoblastic leukemia. Cancer Metastasis Rev. 2019;38(4):595-610.
- Lv M, Liu Y, Liu W, Xing Y, Zhang S. Immunotherapy for Pediatric Acute Lymphoblastic Leukemia: Recent Advances and Future Perspectives. Front Immunol. 2022;13:921894.
- Murthy H, Iqbal M, Chavez JC, Kharfan-Dabaja MA. Cytokine release syndrome: current perspectives. Immunotargets Ther. 2019;8:43-52.

CHAPTER **18.10**

Lymphomas

Divij Sachdeva

1. A 12-year-old male child was evaluated for complaints of progressive cough, neck swellings, and fever since the last 4 months. He was presumptively started on antitubercular treatment (ATT) by his local pediatrician (no microbial evidence of tuberculosis). His symptoms continued to progress. He also reported to have increased work on breathing and a low oxygen saturation [saturation of peripheral oxygen (SpO_2)—86% on room air] was documented in the emergency room (ER). His complete blood count (CBC) was normal with a normal peripheral smear. A chest X-ray was done which revealed the following. On examination, there were dilated neck veins.

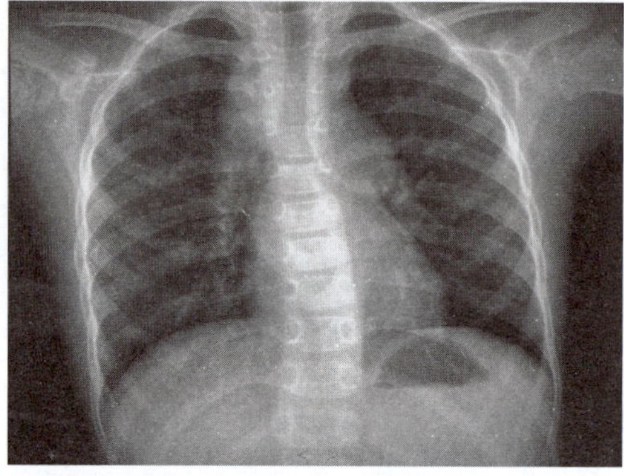

How would you go about the tissue diagnosis of the patient?

A. Sedate and supine biopsy from the mediastinal node
B. Sedate and biopsy in a propped-up position from the neck node
C. Conscious biopsy in the supine position from the mediastinal node
D. Conscious biopsy in a propped-up position from the neck node

EXPLANATION

The aforementioned scenario is that of a child with a mediastinal mass with suspected superior mediastinal syndrome (SMS). It is caused by compression/obstruction to the flow of the superior vena cava along with the compression of the trachea by the mass. A child with an SMS is at further risk of respiratory failure due to sedation and associated decrease in the respiratory muscle tone. They should have a biopsy in the least invasive method from the most accessible site.

Key: D

BOOST YOUR KNOWLEDGE

Children with SMS may require empiric therapy with steroids/chemotherapeutic agents (injection vincristine, injection cyclophosphamide)/radiation therapy even without tissue diagnosis as a life-saving measure.

The differential diagnosis for malignant mediastinal masses in children varies by their site of presentation:

- *Anterior mediastinum:* T-cell acute lymphoblastic leukemia (T-ALL)/T-cell lymphoblastic lymphoma (T-LBL), Hodgkin's lymphoma (HL), primary mediastinal B-cell lymphoma (PMBL), and germ cell tumor
- *Middle mediastinum:* Hodgkin's lymphoma, non-Hodgkin's lymphoma (NHL)
- *Posterior mediastinum:* Neuroblastoma, schwannoma, and malignant peripheral nerve sheath tumor

REFERENCE/SOURCE

- Fisher MJ, Rheingold SR. Oncological emergencies. In: Pizzo PA, Poplack DG (Eds). Principles and Practice of Pediatric Oncology, 7th edition. Philadelphia: Lippincott Williams & Wilkins; 2015. pp. 1125-7.

2. A 15-year-old male walks into your outpatient department (OPD). He has had complaints of progressive weight loss since the last 6 months and swelling on his neck and fever since the last 2 weeks.

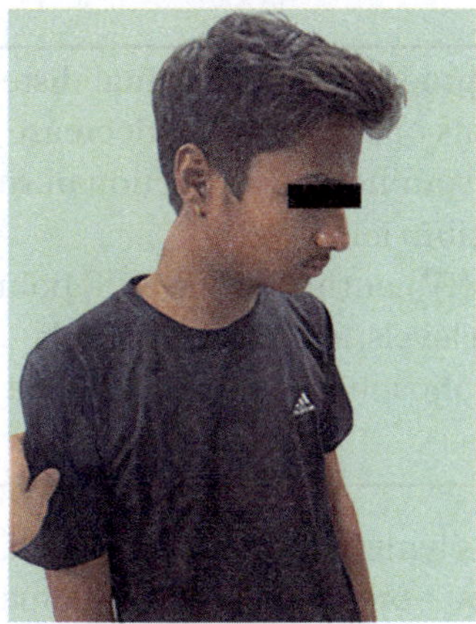

How would you go about the tissue diagnosis of the child?

A. Bone marrow aspiration
B. Start empiric ATT
C. Fine-needle aspiration cytology (FNAC) from the neck swelling
D. Core biopsy/excision biopsy from the neck swelling

EXPLANATION

The above child has a lymph node swelling, the history being chronic and insidious in nature along with the presence of "B-symptoms"

Weight loss of >10% body weight over 6 months
Or,
Drenching night sweats for more than three nights
Or,
Unexplained recurrent fever >38°C

Such a scenario is commonly seen in patients with Hodgkin's lymphoma. Hodgkin's lymphoma has a bimodal age distribution with an early peak around the adolescent and young adult age group and a second peak at around the sixth to eighth decade of life.

Tissue diagnosis for Hodgkin's lymphoma should be in the form of an excision biopsy as the characteristic cells—Reed-Sternberg cells account for only 1–10% of the microscopic mass. The rest of the cells are usually of a mixed inflammatory background. Immunohistochemistry (IHC) confirmation with a cluster of differentiation 30 (CD30), CD15, and CD20 may further delineate the subtype. Fine-needle aspiration usually misses these important findings.

Key: D

BOOST YOUR KNOWLEDGE

Children with non-Hodgkin's lymphoma usually have an acute presentation with rapid onset of symptoms. Hodgkin's lymphoma in contrast has a more indolent presentation with contiguous lymph node involvement, local infiltration, and B-symptoms. Non-Hodgkin's lymphoma can aggressively disseminate to distant sites including the bone marrow and central nervous system (CNS).

REFERENCES/SOURCES

- Alexander S, Ferrando AA. Pediatric lymphoma. In: Orkin SH, Fisher DE, Ginsburg D, Look AT, Lux SE, Nathan DG (Eds). Nathan and Oski's Hematology and Oncology of Infancy and Childhood, 8th edition. Philadelphia, PA: Elsevier Saunders; 2015. pp. 1626-71.
- Sondhi V, Arora B. Hodgkin lymphoma. In: Gupta P, Lodha R, Menon P, Ramji S (Eds). PG Textbook of Pediatrics, 1st edition. New Delhi: Jaypee Brothers Medical Publishers; 2015. pp. 2635-36.

3. An 8-year-old child with complaints of progressive abdominal distension and an abdominal mass since the last 7 days presents to the EM with complaints of a progressive decrease in urine output and 1 episode of generalized tonic-clonic movement. What would be your next step of action in such a scenario?

A. Intubate the child and check magnesium levels
B. Check a creatinine, give intravenous (IV) normal saline (NS) bolus
C. Check serum creatinine, magnesium levels, and chloride levels
D. Check serum creatinine, potassium, phosphorous, uric acid, and calcium levels

EXPLANATION

The above scenario is of a non-Hodgkin's lymphoma, probably Burkitt lymphoma (BL).

Burkitt lymphoma is the most common non-Hodgkin's lymphoma that is seen in pediatrics, it is a malignancy that has a high division rate (as documented with a Ki 67 index higher than 90%). Burkitt lymphoma is known to undergo spontaneous tumor lysis syndrome (TLS) in treatment—naïve patients. TLS is manifested as the biochemical triad of hyperkalemia, hyperuricemia, hyperphosphatemia, and secondary hypocalcemia (reactive to the hyperphosphatemia).

In the above scenario, we would most likely suspect the child to have TLS. TLS if not treated can progress to acute kidney injury. Prompt identification of it with proper hydration, input-output monitoring, and emergent control of dyselectrolytemia is pertinent.

Key: D

BOOST YOUR KNOWLEDGE

Hypocalcemia in TLS is not to be treated unless it is symptomatic. Treatment of asymptomatic hypocalcemia may precipitate the formation of crystalluria (calcium phosphate stones) and further aggravation of TLS.

In addition, patients with TLS need hyperhydration (3,000 $mL/m^2/day$ or 125 $mL/m^2/h$) to flush the metabolites through the kidney. Careful consideration of input and output with regular monitoring of renal function and electrolytes should be done. Dyselectrolytemias are managed through the following pharmacological therapies:

- *Hyperkalemia:* Use of potassium-free fluids, hydration, avoidance of potassium supplements/potassium-rich diet. Therapy with Kayexalate, insulin therapy with dextrose infusion, and salbutamol nebulization are medical measures for hyperkalemia. Refractory hyperkalemia (failing medical therapy) requires dialysis support.
- *Hyperuricemia:* Xanthine oxidase inhibitor (allopurinol) and recombinant urate oxidase (rasburicase) are the common pharmacological therapies that are used to lower increased uric acid levels.
- *Hyperphosphatemia:* Phosphate binders are employed to lower phosphate levels. The common agents used to do so include sevelamer and calcium acetate.

REFERENCES/SOURCES

- Fisher MJ, Rheingold SR. Oncologic emergencies. In: Pizzo PA, Poplack DG (Eds). Principles and Practice of Pediatric Oncology, 7th edition. Baltimore, MD: Wolters Kluwer; 2015. pp. 1143-5.
- Prakash A, Rau A. Oncological emergencies and supportive care. In: Gupta P, Lodha R, Menon P, Ramji S (Eds). PG Textbook of Pediatrics, 1st edition. New Delhi: Jaypee Brothers Medical Publishers; 2015. pp. 2703-5.

4. A 5-year-old male child, presented with complaints of swelling in his axillary region since the last 6 months, he also has complaints of abdominal fullness. He was detected to have a palpable spleen of 6 cm. He, however, did not have any constitutional complaints. On further excision biopsy of the patient, Hodgkin's lymphoma, mixed cellularity was diagnosed. A staging positron emission tomography-computed tomography (PET-CT) was done which revealed fluorodeoxyglucose (FDG)-avid 6 × 6 cm conglomerate axillary nodal mass, 4 × 4 cm sized aortocaval lymph nodes, along with uptake in the spleen. Name the staging method used, and what is the stage of the disease?

A. Ann Arbor staging, stage IIE
B. St Jude's staging, stage III ES
C. Ann Arbor staging, stage IIIS
D. St Jude's staging, stage IIB

EXPLANATION

Ann Arbor staging for Hodgkin's lymphoma

Stage	*Description*
I	Involvement of a single lymphatic site (i.e., nodal region, Waldeyer's ring, thymus, or spleen) (I); or localized involvement of a single extralymphatic organ or site in the absence of any lymph node involvement (IE)
II	Involvement of two or more lymph node regions on the same side of the diaphragm (II); or localized involvement of a single extralymphatic organ or site in association with regional lymph node involvement with or without the involvement of other lymph node regions on the same side of the diaphragm (IIE)
III	Involvement of lymph node regions on both sides of the diaphragm (III), which also may be accompanied by extralymphatic extension in association with adjacent lymph node involvement (IIIE) or by the involvement of the spleen (IIIS) or both (IIIE, S)
IV	Diffuse or disseminated involvement of one or more extralymphatic organs, with or without associated lymph node involvement; or isolated extralymphatic organ involvement in the absence of adjacent regional lymph node involvement, but in conjunction with the disease in distant site(s). Stage IV includes any involvement of the liver or bone marrow, lungs (other than by direct extension from another site), or cerebrospinal fluid
Designations applicable to any stage	
A	No symptoms
B	Fever (temperature >38.0°C), drenching night sweats, unexplained loss of >10% of body weight within the preceding 6 months
E	Involvement of a single extranodal site that is contiguous or proximal to the known nodal site
S	Splenic involvement

As the child has involvement of lymph nodal regions on both sides of the diaphragm, he is already a stage III, and the PET-CT also showed splenic involvement. This cumulatively makes him a stage IIIS.

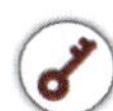

Key: C

BOOST YOUR KNOWLEDGE

The presence of B-symptoms is a prognostic marker, those patients with the presence of B-symptoms tend to do worse off than those who do not. The other prognostic factors that are associated with an inferior outcome include stage IV disease, presence of fever, massive tumor in the mediastinum (>0.33 of the diameter of the chest), and serum albumin <35 g/L.

Positron emission tomography-computed tomography scan is now the standard imaging for staging of Hodgkin's lymphoma and additionally acts as a method to gauge early response assessment post-two cycles of chemotherapy to assess the need of radiation therapy. In centers that have nonavailability of PET-CT, cross-sectional imaging of the thorax, abdomen, and pelvis along with clinical and ultrasonography (USG) examination of the neck region should be done.

REFERENCES/SOURCES

- Cheson BD. Staging and response assessment in lymphomas: the new Lugano classification. Chin Clin Oncol. 2015;4(1):5.
- Metzger M, Krasin MJ, Hudson MM, Onciu M. Hodgkin lymphoma. In: Pizzo PA, Poplack DG (Eds). Principles and Practice of Pediatric Oncology, 7th edition. Baltimore, MD: Wolters Kluwer; 2015. p. 645.

5. A 10-year-old boy, human immunodeficiency virus (HIV) positive on antiretroviral therapy (ART) presents to you with complaints of a lump abdomen. Physical examination reveals a huge periumbilical, diffuse lump around 10 × 12 cm in size, you go forward with a biopsy from the mass abdomen, which was suggestive of the following, what is this characteristic histology known as, and which viral infection is the likely etiology of the condition?

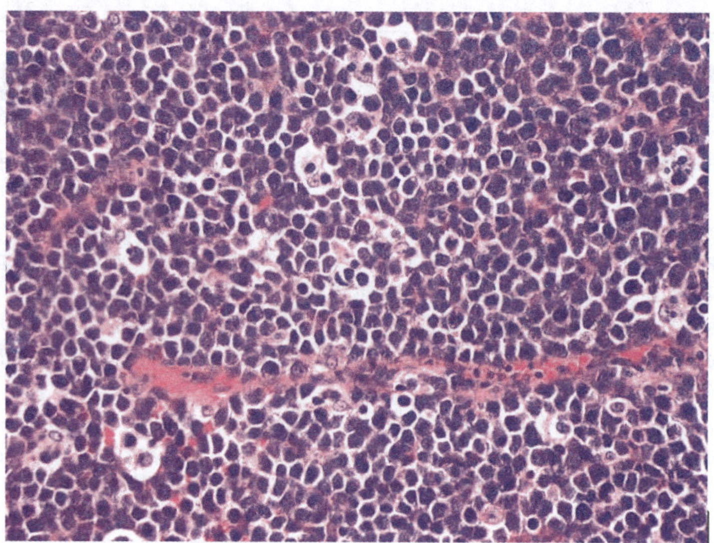

A. Hand mirror cell, *Cytomegalovirus* (CMV) virus
B. Cobblestone appearance, human herpesvirus 6 (HHV-6) virus
C. Starry sky appearance, Epstein–Barr virus (EBV)
D. Tram-track appearance, parvovirus

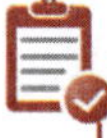

EXPLANATION

Burkitt lymphoma is characterized by cells that are intermediate-sized, homogeneous with round to oval nuclei containing multiple, variable prominent basophilic nucleoli with a modest amount of somewhat basophilic cytoplasm which is vacuolated (due to oil droplets). On tissue sections, because of the rapidly dividing cells with high mitotic activity, this characteristic appearance is known as starry-sky appearance, where the sheets of lymphoma cells constitute the "sky" and the tangible body macrophages appear as "stars."

Epstein–Barr virus infection is a common implicating agent for mature B-cell lymphomas (BCLs), especially in the immunocompromised host (e.g., HIV infection). EBV causes immortalization of B-cell lines. Many nonviral proteins of EBV are implicated, out of which Epstein–Barr nuclear antigen (EBNA) and latent membrane protein (LMP) are essential for B-cell immortalization.

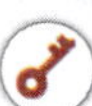

Key: C

BOOST YOUR KNOWLEDGE

Burkitt lymphoma occurs in two forms as far as the presentation is concerned, endemic Burkitt lymphoma and sporadic Burkitt lymphoma.

Children with endemic Burkitt lymphoma are those who are mostly African by race and region, with prominent head and neck involvement. The usual site of involvement here is the Jaw and CNS dissemination is more common. EBV infection can be demonstrated in almost all cases.

Sporadic Burkitt lymphoma is the most common form seen in India. The usual site of involvement being the abdomen. EBV infection is seen in <20% of patients.

Although Burkitt lymphoma can be seen in patients with HIV infection, it is not an acquired immunodeficiency syndrome (AIDS) defining malignancy.

Acquired immunodeficiency syndrome defining malignancies:
- HHV-8-induced Kaposi's sarcoma
- Invasive cervical carcinoma
- Non-Hodgkin's lymphoma (systemic and CNS)

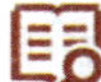

REFERENCES/SOURCES

- Alexander S, Ferrando AA. Pediatric lymphoma. In: Orkin SH, Fisher DE, Ginsburg D, Look AT, Lux SE, Nathan DG (Eds). Nathan and Oski's Hematology and Oncology of Infancy and Childhood, 8th edition. Amsterdam: Elsevier Saunders; 2015. pp. 1658-9.
- Gross TG, Perkins SL. Malignant non-Hodgkin lymphomas in children. In: Pizzo PA, Poplack DG (Eds). Principles and Practice of Pediatric Oncology, 7th edition. Baltimore, MD: Wolters Kluwer; 2015. pp. 665-7.

6. A 14-year-old male came with complaints of a progressively enlarging neck mass, 6 × 7 cm in size. A USG-guided core biopsy was done from the lesion which revealed the following histology, furthermore, IHC was done which revealed negativity for CD15 and CD 30.

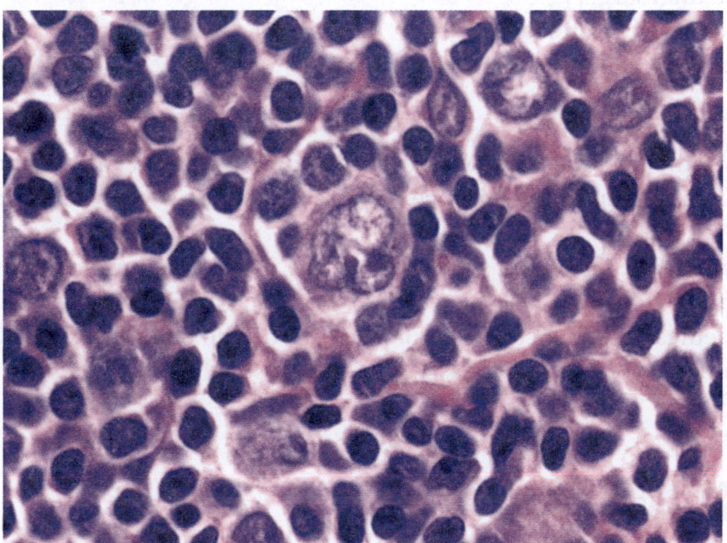

On further testing, IHC revealed positivity for leukocyte common antigen (LCA), CD20. How would you proceed further with therapy?

A. Nodular lymphocyte predominant Hodgkin's lymphoma (NLPHL)
B. Burkitt lymphoma
C. Anaplastic large cell lymphoma (ALCL)
D. *Hodgkin's lymphoma:* Mixed cellularity

EXPLANATION

The child is most likely suffering from NLPHL. This a rare histological subtype of Hodgkin's lymphoma (around 5–10% of cases). NLPHL is characteristically distinct from classical Hodgkin's lymphoma (CHL) with the absence of typical Reed–Sternberg cells and the presence of "Popcorn cells"—cells with multilobed and folded nuclei and single prominent nucleoli. These cells are CD20 positive on IHC in contrast to Reed–Sternberg cells which are CD20 and CD15 positive.

Key: A

BOOST YOUR KNOWLEDGE

Nodular lymphocyte-predominant Hodgkin's lymphoma is known to present at a lower stage than CHL and with a lower risk of systemic spread, mediastinal involvement, and at an earlier age as well (around 10–12 years of age). Management of limited disease is with surgical excision, radiation, or low-dose chemotherapy. Advanced disease is treated with multiagent chemotherapy akin to CHL.

REFERENCE/SOURCE

- Alexander S, Ferrando AA. Pediatric lymphoma. In: Orkin SH, Fisher DE, Ginsburg D, Look AT, Lux SE, Nathan DG (Eds). Nathan and Oski's Hematology and Oncology of Infancy and Childhood, 8th edition. Philadelphia, PA: Elsevier Saunders; 2015.

7. A 15-year-old, male, African by ethnicity, presented you with complaints of cough, dyspnea on exertion, and difficulty in breathing while lying down. He also has neck nodes around 3 × 4 cm in size in the right level III region and a big mediastinal mass on chest X-ray with tracheal compression. After a mediastinal biopsy in a nonsedated state, what would be your next step of action?

A. Start him on IV antibiotics and wait for a biopsy
B. Wait for biopsy and then surgery
C. Empirical administration of steroids
D. Vincristine and emergent radiation to the chest

EXPLANATION

The above child has a mediastinal mass which is causing a SMS. SMS is an oncological emergency and warrants emergent therapy even in the absence of a tissue diagnosis to prevent further worsening of airway compression.

The ideal treatment of SMS in such a scenario is in the form of an empiric institution of corticosteroids, with an expedited approach to establishing a pathological diagnosis. Usually, children will be sick and are unable to take oral medications, hence, IV steroids are used. The choice of steroid is institution-dependent and includes methylprednisolone/dexamtheasone/hydrocortisone.

Key: C

BOOST YOUR KNOWLEDGE

T-cell lymphoblastic lymphoma is the second most common non-Hodgkin's lymphoma seen in the pediatric population; the presentation of a T-cell lymphoblastic lymphoma is usually in the form of an anterior mediastinal mass in around 90% of cases. Patients can present with a significant amount of respiratory distress with worsening tachypnea if not diagnosed in time. Conventionally acute lymphoblastic leukemias and lymphoblastic lymphomas are differentiated based on their level of bone marrow involvement, with ALL having bone marrow involvement >25% of all nucleated cells. Patients with T-cell lymphoblastic lymphoma have more propensity of having dissemination of disease to the CNS than patients with B-cell lymphoblastic lymphoma with signs and symptoms related to cranial nerve palsies and raised intracranial pressure (headaches and early morning vomiting).

REFERENCES/SOURCES

- Prakash A, Rau A. Oncological emergencies and supportive care. In: Gupta P, Lodha R, Menon P, Ramji S (Eds). PG Textbook of Pediatrics, 1st edition. New Delhi: Jaypee Brothers Medical Publishers; 2015. pp. 2703-5.
- Thacker N, Kanwar VS, Nazeer T. Non-Hodgkin lymphoma. In: Gupta P, Lodha R, Menon P, Ramji S (Eds). PG Textbook of Pediatrics, 1st edition. New Delhi: Jaypee Brothers Medical Publishers; 2015. pp. 2643-5.

8. A 10-year-old boy who presented with a swelling in his postauricular region for 3 months, on further examination of the child you found generalized lymphadenopathy in the inguinal region and his axillary region. A CBC was done, which showed a hemoglobin (Hb) of 6 g/dL, white blood cell (WBC)—2,600/mm^3, neutrophil (N)—17%, and platelets—1.4 lac/mm^3. He was further proven to be having Hodgkin's lymphoma. His bone marrow revealed involvement by small round blue cells which were CD15+ and CD30+. What stage would you assign him to?

He further went on to receive two cycles of OEPA (vincristine, etoposide, prednisolone, and adriamycin) chemotherapy, PET-CT post them revealed the disease to be in complete remission (CR), what would be his final plan for therapy?

A. Stage III, OEPA × 2 and radiotherapy (RT) ABVD × 2 cycles + RT
B. Stage III, OEPA ×2, COPDAC 2 and RT
C. Stage IV, OEPA ×2, COPDAC × 4 and no RT
D. Stage IV, OEPA × 2, COPDAC × 2 and RT

EXPLANATION

Treatment for Hodgkin's lymphoma now follows a risk-stratified and response-adapted approach. The above child has stage IV disease as confirmed by the bone marrow biopsy showing involvement. Stage IV disease is considered to be a high-risk disease, this child would benefit from an intensive chemotherapy schedule, typically consisting of six to eight cycles of chemotherapy. In the EuroNet protocol that employs the OEPA/COPDAC regimens, a documented CR after the first two cycles of OEPA translates into the omission of RT.

Key: C

BOOST YOUR KNOWLEDGE

With intensive chemotherapy protocols, cure rates for pediatric Hodgkin's lymphoma have now reached >80%. With the time-tested regimens of ABVD, COPP, ABVE-PC, MOPP, etc., the incidence of anthracycline-induced cardiotoxicity and alkylating agents-induced gonadotoxicity are high. Furthermore, RT can cause secondary malignancies, endocrinopathies, etc.

There is a lot of emphasis now on reducing toxicity due to chemotherapy regimens to prevent long-term morbidity. In the OEPA/COPDAC treatment schema, OPPA, COPP (P: Prednisolone, P: Procarbazine) has been replaced by Etoposide, OEPA, and COPDAC (DAC: Dacarbazine) to reduce the incidence of gonadotoxicity.

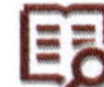

REFERENCES/SOURCES

- Metzger M, Krasin MJ, Hudson MM, Onciu M. Hodgkin lymphoma. In: Pizzo PA, Poplack DG (Eds). Principles and Practice of Pediatric Oncology, 7th edition. Baltimore, MD: Wolters Kluwer; 2015. pp. 650-4.
- Sondhi V, Arora B. Hodgkin lymphoma. In: Gupta P, Lodha R, Menon P, Ramji S (Eds). PG Textbook of Pediatrics, 1st edition. New Delhi: Jaypee Brothers Medical Publishers; 2015. pp. 2638-9.

9. A 10-year-old boy with no B-symptoms and clinical enlargement of only left-sided cervical nodes has been diagnosed with Hodgkin's lymphoma on lymph node biopsy. He has now been referred to you for further management. Which of the following is the best option for staging the child?

A. X-ray survey of the whole body
B. CT chest and CT abdomen along with bone marrow
C. PET-CT alone
D. CT of chest and abdomen, bone marrow, and cerebrospinal fluid (CSF) analysis

EXPLANATION

Staging for a Hodgkin's lymphoma is now been replaced by the advent of PET-CT scanning in most centers, PET-CT has been found to be more sensitive in detecting locations with active disease as compared to CT scan or gallium scanning. There is good concordance between CT images and PET images.

Bone marrow evaluation should be considered as part of staging for Hodgkin's lymphoma especially for individuals with advanced-stage disease (stages III and IV).

Key: C

BOOST YOUR KNOWLEDGE

An early PET-response, rapid early response (RER) is used post two to three cycles of chemotherapy to further customize treatment and avoid radiation therapy on most modern protocols.

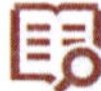

REFERENCES/SOURCES

- Alexander S, Ferrando AA. Pediatric lymphoma. In: Orkin SH, Fisher DE, Ginsburg D, Look AT, Lux SE, Nathan DG (Eds). Nathan and Oski's Hematology and Oncology of Infancy and Childhood, 8th edition. Amsterdam: Elsevier Saunders; 2015. p. 1634.
- Metzger M, Krasin MJ, Hudson MM, Onciu M. Hodgkin lymphoma. In: Pizzo PA, Poplack DG (Eds). Principles and Practice of Pediatric Oncology, 7th edition. Baltimore, MD: Wolters Kluwer; 2015. pp. 644-5.

10. A 10-year-old male child came with complaints of severe pain abdomen. He looks to be in severe pain and is guarding his abdomen on palpation. A USG abdomen is done which shows an intussusception and a mass associated with it in the ileocolic region. The pediatric surgeon operated on the patient and histopathology revealed a Burkitt lymphoma with margins that were negative for the disease. What would be the definitive therapy for such a case?

A. Definitive radiation therapy
B. Radiation therapy with chemotherapy
C. Wait and watch
D. Multiagent chemotherapy

EXPLANATION

In children with Burkitt lymphoma, treatment is in the form of multiagent chemotherapy. In an older child with intussusception, malignant etiology should be highly suspected, and histopathology should be followed for further therapy. Patients with Burkitt lymphoma are staged according to the St Jude's staging:

- *Stage I:* A single tumor (extranodal) or single anatomic area (nodal) with the exclusion of thoracic or abdomen.
- *Stage II:* A single tumor (extranodal) with regional node involvement
  Two or more nodal areas on the same side of the diaphragm.
  Two single (extranodal) tumors with or without regional node involvement on the same side of the diaphragm.
  A primary gastrointestinal tract tumor that is resectable, usually in the ileocecal area, with or without involvement of associated mesenteric nodes.
- *Stage III:* Two single tumors (extranodal) on opposite sides of the diaphragm. Two or more nodal areas above and below the diaphragm. All the primary intrathoracic tumors (mediastinal, pleural, and thymic). All extensive primary intra-abdominal diseases. All paraspinal or epidural tumors, regardless of other tumor site(s).
- *Stage IV:* Any of the above with initial central nervous system and/or bone marrow involvement.

Key: D

BOOST YOUR KNOWLEDGE

Complete surgical excision can downstage disease and reduce the intensity and duration of chemotherapy in Burkitt lymphoma. However, irrespective of stage and surgical resection status, multiagent chemotherapy is mandatory for management.

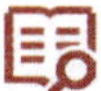

REFERENCES/SOURCES

- Gross TG, Perkins SL. Malignant non-Hodgkin lymphomas in children. In: Pizzo PA, Poplack DG (Eds). Principles and Practice of Pediatric Oncology, 7th edition. Baltimore, MD: Wolters Kluwer; 2015. pp. 673-4.
- Thacker N, Kanwar VS, Nazeer T. Non-Hodgkin lymphoma. In: Gupta P, Lodha R, Menon P, Ramji S (Eds). PG Textbook of Pediatrics, 1st edition. New Delhi: Jaypee Brothers Medical Publishers; 2015. pp. 2643-5.

11. **A 7-year-old child with a CD20+ mature B-cell non-Hodgkin's lymphoma (Burkitt lymphoma) stage IV with bone marrow metastasis has come for post-treatment surveillance after 3 months of completing therapy. His USG of abdomen is normal, chest X-ray does not show any abnormality. His immunoglobulin G (IgG) has come low for his age. How would you manage him further?**

A. Intravenous immunoglobulin (IVIG) infusion
B. Evaluate further for immunodeficiency
C. Repeat IgG post-3 months
D. Granulocyte colony-stimulating factor (G-CSF) injections

EXPLANATION

Most modern-day protocols now employ treatment with the injection of rituximab (a chimeric human-murine monoclonal antibody against CD20). CD20 is positive in mature B-cells. Treatment with rituximab can lead to B-cell aplasia and transient hypogammaglobulinemia ranging up to 1–2 years post-therapy. Children who have completed treatment utilizing rituximab need to be monitored on surveillance for hypogammaglobulinemia. This is usually supported with injection IVIG infusion at 0.4 g/kg/dose.

Key: A

BOOST YOUR KNOWLEDGE

Non-Hodgkin's lymphoma can be associated with primary immunodeficiencies and acquired immunodeficiencies (e.g., HIV/AIDS) as well. Children with earlier age of presentation, syndromic anomalies, and a history of repeated infections need to be evaluated further for immunodeficiency-associated non-Hodgkin's lymphoma.

Defects in genomic stability (e.g., ataxia telangiectasia), humoral immunity [e.g., common variable immunodeficiency (CVID)], apoptosis (e.g., autoimmune lymphoproliferation syndrome), and combined immunodeficiency [e.g., Wiskott–Aldrich syndrome (WAS)] can all be associated with lymphomas. The diagnosis of lymphoma may be the first manifestation of primary immunodeficiency (PID). The most common types of lymphoma observed are mature BCLs, such as diffuse large B-cell lymphoma (DLBCL) and Burkitt lymphoma, followed by Hodgkin's lymphoma.

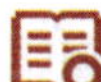

REFERENCE/SOURCE

- Thacker N, Kanwar VS, Nazeer T. Non-Hodgkin lymphoma. In: Gupta P, Lodha R, Menon P, Ramji S (Eds). PG Textbook of Pediatrics, 1st edition. New Delhi: Jaypee Brothers Medical Publishers; 2015. pp. 2640-1.

12. **A 2-year-old girl presents with abdominal distension. Imaging reveals a large abdominal mass, and core needle biopsy of the mass shows monomorphic medium-sized B-lymphoid cells that stain positive for CD20, CD10, and BCL6. What cytogenetic abnormality would you likely see in such a case?**

A. t(8,21)
B. t(11,14)
C. t(10,14)
D. t(8,14)

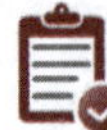

EXPLANATION

Key features of Burkitt lymphoma:

- *Morphology:* Uniform medium-sized B-lymphoid cells with basophilic cytoplasm and numerous mitotic figures. Starry-sky appearance on histology.
- *Immunophenotype:* Cells express B-cell markers CD19, CD20, CD22, and CD79a. Also, express CD10 and BCL6.
- *Genetics:* Characteristic t(8;14) translocation placing MYC under the control of immunoglobulin gene enhancers. This leads to massively increased proliferation. The other cases have positivity for t(2,8) or t(8,22).
- *Clinical:* Very rapid doubling time of 24–48 hours. Can disseminate widely. High risk of tumor lysis with therapy.

In this vignette, a 2-year-old girl presents with an abdominal mass. Biopsy reveals morphology and immunophenotype classic for Burkitt lymphoma.

If untreated, Burkitt lymphoma will progress extremely rapidly given its short doubling time. Spontaneous remission does not occur. The highly proliferative nature puts patients at high risk for TLS with initiation of chemotherapy since rapid cell death releases intracellular contents.

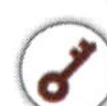

Key: D

BOOST YOUR KNOWLEDGE

Burkitt lymphoma is an aggressive B-cell non-Hodgkin's lymphoma that often presents as an abdominal mass in pediatric patients. It has three clinical variants:

1. *Endemic*—occurs commonly in equatorial Africa, associated with EBV and malaria
2. *Sporadic*—occurs worldwide, usually abdomen in children and adolescents
3. *Immunodeficiency-related*—occurs in HIV or post-transplant immunosuppression

REFERENCES/SOURCES

- Gross TG, Perkins SL. Malignant non-Hodgkin lymphomas in children. In: Pizzo PA, Poplack DG (Eds). Principles and Practice of Pediatric Oncology, 7th edition. Baltimore, MD: Wolters Kluwer; 2015. pp. 665-6.
- Thacker N, Kanwar VS, Nazeer T. Non-Hodgkin lymphoma. In: Gupta P, Lodha R, Menon P, Ramji S (Eds). PG Textbook of Pediatrics, 1st edition. New Delhi: Jaypee Brothers Medical Publishers; 2015. pp. 2642-3.

13. A 16-month-old child with complaints of repeated diarrhea and dysentery comes to your OPD. You note that there are multiple scaling lesions on his body. The parents say that the child is mostly sick and in and out of the hospital. He now has abdominal distension. He has been diagnosed now with a high-grade lymphoma. Which of the following syndromes will you suspect the child to have? What investigations in the CBC analysis can yield a cue to the diagnosis?

A. Ataxia telangiectasia and red cell distribution width (RDW)
B. Common variable immunodeficiency and lymphocyte count
C. Wiskott-Aldrich syndrome and mean platelet volume (MPV)
D. Chédiak-Higashi and RBC count

EXPLANATION

Wiskott-Aldrich syndrome is an X-linked immunodeficiency disorder that is characterized by thrombocytopenia, eczema, and repeated infections.

The platelets in a patient with Wiskott-Aldrich syndrome are small in size. This can be measured as part of a CBC analysis with the help of MPV. An MPV <7 in the above scenario would likely help to investigate further for Wiskott-Aldrich syndrome.

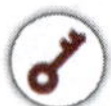

Key: C

BOOST YOUR KNOWLEDGE

Children with multiple immunodeficiency syndromes can present with a non-Hodgkin's lymphoma, most commonly implicated are Wiskott–Aldrich syndrome, Chédiak–Higashi, ataxia telangiectasia, common variable immunodeficiency, and autoimmune lymphoproliferative syndrome.

In Wiskott–Aldrich syndrome, bloody diarrhea is often the initial presenting feature, and eczema can be mild to confluent. The skin lesions can secondarily be affected by staphylococcal infections. Patients usually die of a thrombocytopenic bleed if not picked up early. Recurrent infections in the form of sinopulmonary infections and otitis media are often seen. Autoinflammatory disorders such as autoimmune hemolysis, vasculitis, inflammatory bowel disease, and glomerulonephritis have been seen in patients with Wiskott–Aldrich syndrome. Patients usually have a heightened risk of developing EBV-driven lymphomas.

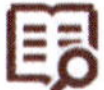

REFERENCES/SOURCES

- Bonilla FA, Notarangelo LD. Primary immunodeficiency diseases. In: Orkin SH, Fisher DE, Ginsburg D, Look AT, Lux SE, Nathan DG (Eds). Nathan and Oski's Hematology and Oncology of Infancy and Childhood, 8th edition. Philadelphia: WB Saunders Co Ltd; 2015. pp. 898-9.
- Thacker N, Kanwar VS, Nazeer T. Non-Hodgkin lymphoma. In: Gupta P, Lodha R, Menon P, Ramji S (Eds). PG Textbook of Pediatrics, 1st edition. New Delhi: Jaypee Brothers Medical Publishers; 2015. pp. 2643-5.

14. A child with stage IIIB Hodgkin's lymphoma has come with new onset nodal swellings 4 months postcompletion of therapy. He was further diagnosed to have a recurrence of the Hodgkins (Stage IV). How would you want to proceed further with his therapy?

A. Surgical excision
B. Involved field radiation therapy (IFRT)
C. Multiagent chemotherapy followed by hematopoietic stem-cell transplantation (HSCT) in remission
D. HSCT

EXPLANATION

In the above scenario, the child has had a recurrence of his malignancy in a very short interval postcompletion of primary therapy.

Relapsed Hodgkin's lymphoma is treated with combination salvage chemotherapy followed by autologous stem cell transplantation.

Key: C

BOOST YOUR KNOWLEDGE

Patients that have recurrence of Hodgkin's lymphoma within 3 months of completion of therapy are known to have a primary refractory Hodgkin's lymphoma in contrast to those that have recurrences three months post-therapy (relapse).

Patients with primary refractory Hodgkin's lymphoma tend to do worse off than those with relapsed disease.

Brentuximab vedotin (anti-CD30 monoclonal antibody) and checkpoint inhibitors such as nivolumab are now being used in salvage therapy in relapsed/refractory Hodgkin's lymphoma.

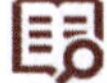

REFERENCES/SOURCES

- Alexander S, Ferrando AA. Pediatric lymphoma. In: Orkin SH, Fisher DE, Ginsburg D, Look AT, Lux SE, Nathan DG (Eds). Nathan and Oski's Hematology and Oncology of Infancy and Childhood, 8th edition. Philadelphia, PA: Elsevier Saunders; 2015. pp. 1652-45.
- Sondhi V, Arora B. Hodgkin lymphoma. In: Gupta P, Lodha R, Menon P, Ramji S (Eds). PG Textbook of Pediatrics, 1st edition. New Delhi: Jaypee Brothers Medical Publishers; 2015. p. 2638.

15. A 12-year-old child has completed therapy for stage IIIA Hodgkin's lymphoma. He had received ABVD × six cycles during his treatment. What all toxicities you would like to screen for in the long term?

A. Cardiotoxicity, pulmonary fibrosis
B. Nephrotoxicity, cardiotoxicity
C. Pulmonary fibrosis, low bone density
D. Pulmonary fibrosis, neurotoxicity

EXPLANATION

Patients with Hodgkin's lymphoma with early-stage disease are treated with ABVD-based chemotherapy.

ABVD stands for A: Adriamycin (Doxorubicin), B (Bleomycin), V (Vinblastine), and D (Dacarbazine). Doxorubicin belongs to the anthracycline dose which is known to cause cardiotoxicity. A patient with cumulative anthracycline exposure exceeding >300 mg/m^2 needs to be monitored postcompletion of therapy. The risk increases even further once it has crossed 375 mg/m^2 of anthracycline cumulative dose. Bleomycin induces pulmonary fibrosis due to the stimulation of oxygen-mediated damage by proinflammatory cytokines.

The child has received six cycles of ABVD chemotherapy, his cumulative anthracycline exposure is 300 mg/m^2 (50 mg/m^2 doxorubicin × six cycles). He has also received bleomycin. Hence, the long-term monitoring for cardiotoxicity and pulmonary toxicity.

Key: A

BOOST YOUR KNOWLEDGE

Patients treated with higher-intensity protocols of topoisomerase inhibitors and alkylating agents are at risk of therapy-related myelodysplasia and myeloid leukemia. Therapy-related myeloid leukemia following topoisomerase inhibitors such as etoposide is associated with KMT2A rearrangements and occurs relatively early, by 2 years postcompletion of therapy. Therapy-related acute myeloid leukemia (AML) after alkylating agents occurs after a latent period of 5 years or more and is associated with chromosome gains/losses. Secondary malignancies after exposure to radiation can occur after a few years to even 10–15 years post-therapy.

REFERENCES/SOURCES

- Metzger M, Krasin MJ, Hudson MM, Onciu M. Hodgkin lymphoma. In: Pizzo PA, Poplack DG (Eds). Principles and Practice of Pediatric Oncology, 7th edition. Baltimore, MD: Wolters Kluwer; 2015. pp. 655-8.
- Sondhi V, Arora B. Hodgkin lymphoma. In: Gupta P, Lodha R, Menon P, Ramji S (Eds). PG Textbook of Pediatrics, 1st edition. New Delhi: Jaypee Brothers Medical Publishers; 2015. p. 2638.

16. A 4-year-old girl came with complaints of fever and right axillary region swelling. On examining her, you noticed a 4 × 4 cm lymphadenopathy in the right axillary region. She underwent a biopsy which showed round blue cells with multiple mitotic figures. Her IHC was positive for CD30 and anaplastic lymphoma receptor tyrosine kinase (ALK). Bone marrow was involved in the malignancy. Cytogenetics done on the biopsy block revealed a t(2,5). What disorder would you suspect in the child? What is the management of the child?

A. DLBCL, multiagent chemotherapy + RT
B. Burkitt lymphoma, multiagent chemotherapy
C. ALCL, multiagent chemotherapy
D. Pediatric follicular lymphoma, multiagent chemotherapy + RT

EXPLANATION

The child has ALCL, and the tumor cells are positive for CD30 and ALK staining on IHC. Furthermore, the cells were harboring the characteristic chromosomal translocation t(2,5) involving the *ALK* gene and nucleophosmin *(NPM)* gene.

Management of ALCL is in the form of multiagent chemotherapy ranging from a duration of 6 months to 1 year. Cure rates with such an approach range up to 60–70% even with metastatic disease.

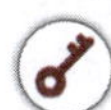 **Key: C**

BOOST YOUR KNOWLEDGE

Anaplastic large-cell lymphoma tends to present in lymph nodes and extranodal sites. The common extranodal sites being the skin, soft tissues, and bone. There are grossly two clinical varieties of ALCL, including: (1) primary cutaneous ALCL (C-ALCL) and (2) systemic ALCL. Fever and weight loss are the common presenting features and around two-thirds of the cases present with disseminated disease. Skin involvement is the most common site of extranodal disease and waxing and waning of the rashes can be seen. Histopathologically, large horseshoe-shaped lymphoma cells are seen in classical ALCL. IHC is positive for CD3, CD45, and CD30 and >90% of pediatric ALCL is ALK-positive.

Anaplastic large cell lymphoma on relapse can be treated with single-agent vinblastine therapy, brentuximab vedotin (CD30 inhibitor), and crizotinib therapy (ALK inhibitor). Salvage rates range from 40 to 60% depending on the stage and the timing of relapse.

REFERENCES/SOURCES

- Alexander S, Ferrando AA. Pediatric lymphoma. In: Orkin SH, Fisher DE, Ginsburg D, Look AT, Lux SE, Nathan DG (Eds). Nathan and Oski's Hematology and Oncology of Infancy and Childhood, 8th edition. Philadelphia, PA: Elsevier Saunders; 2015. pp. 1666-7.
- Thacker N, Kanwar VS, Nazeer T. Non-Hodgkin lymphoma. In: Gupta P, Lodha R, Menon P, Ramji S (Eds). PG Textbook of Pediatrics, 1st edition. New Delhi: Jaypee Brothers Medical Publishers; 2015. pp. 2646-7.

17. A 10-year-old male has been recently diagnosed with stage III DLBCL. Which of the following is true about his disease?

A. Ki Index is likely to be 99% in histopathology
B. Activated B-cell type more common in children
C. Germinal center type is more common in children
D. Radiation therapy is the treatment of choice

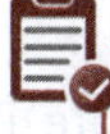

EXPLANATION

Diffuse large B-cell lymphoma are rare non-Hodgkin's lymphomas encountered in the pediatric age group (around 15–20%) cases. They tend to increase in incidence with increasing age. There are multiple morphological variants of DLBCL (immunoblastic, centroblastic, T-cell/histiocyte rich, and anaplastic); however, this does not have clinical implications.

Diffuse large B-cell lymphoma cells are typically positive for CD19, CD20, CD22, paired box protein 5 (PAX5), and CD79A. In contrast to adult DLBCL, pediatric DLBCL has higher mitotic rates and more germinal center immunophenotype with negativity for BCL2 and a higher incidence of positivity for BCL6. Although Ki67 is high, it is not as high as seen in Burkitt lymphoma.

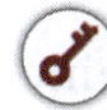 **Key: C**

BOOST YOUR KNOWLEDGE

Treatment for DLBCL on most protocols is with multiagent chemotherapy as for Burkitt lymphoma. DLBCL is a salvageable malignancy with response rates above 80% even in patients with advanced disease.

REFERENCE/SOURCE

- Gross TG, Perkins SL. Malignant non-Hodgkin lymphomas in children. In: Pizzo PA, Poplack DG (Eds). Principles and Practice of Pediatric Oncology, 7th edition. Baltimore, MD: Wolters Kluwer; 2015. pp. 667-8.

18. An 8-year-old boy has presented to you with abdominal distension. He was further diagnosed with Burkitt lymphoma. He received chemotherapy 10 days back. He has now presented you with low urine output. He has a serum uric acid of 11 mg/dL, so you went forward with giving a dose of rasburicase. 3 hours later, he presented with dark urine, difficulty breathing, and fast breathing. A peripheral smear revealed this:

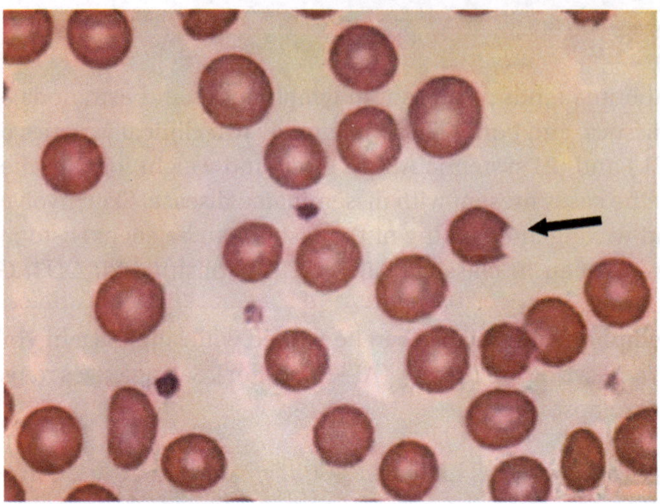

What could be the cause behind this?

A. Intravascular hemolysis, erythrocyte membrane damage due to paraneoplastic phenomenon
B. Intravascular hemolysis, erythrocyte membrane damage due to TLS
C. Intravascular hemolysis, erythrocyte membrane damage due to rasburicase with underlying glucose-6-phosphate dehydrogenase (G6PD) deficiency
D. Intravascular hemolysis, erythrocyte membrane damage due to acute kidney injury

EXPLANATION

Rasburicase is a recombinant urate oxidase, which converts uric acid to allantoin, a less toxic purine metabolite that is excreted by the kidney.

Rasburicase is known to precipitate hemolysis in children with G6PD. Patients should be tested for it before rasburicase therapy is initiated. However, in most acute scenarios, G6PD is sent but rasburicase is usually administered before the results are available.

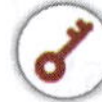

Key: C

BOOST YOUR KNOWLEDGE

There are two enzymes that are pivotal in the management of hyperuricemia, that are: (1) xanthine oxidase and (2) urate oxidase.

Xanthine oxidase catalyzes the conversion of xanthine to uric acid, allopurinol is an inhibitor of xanthine oxidase.

Rasburicase as mentioned above helps in the catalysis of uric acid to allantoin.

Samples testing for uric acid levels postrasburicase therapy should be sent on an ice pack to prevent ongoing drug action on the sample leading to spuriously low uric acid levels.

REFERENCE/SOURCE

- Fisher MJ, Rheingold SR. Oncologic emergencies. In: Pizzo PA, Poplack DG (Eds). Principles and Practice of Pediatric Oncology, 7th edition. Baltimore, MD: Wolters Kluwer; 2015. p. 1145.

19. A 6-year-old girl has presented with complaints of a mass abdomen which has been progressively evolving over the last 2 months. She also complained of severe bony pains. A mass biopsy was done which showed round blue cells with a high nuclear cytoplasmic ratio, one to two nucleoli, Ki67 index was 85%.
The blasts were positive for CD19, CD20, terminal deoxynucleotidyl transferase (TdT), and CD10.
Her bone marrow done revealed atypical cells which amounted to 6% of all cells. What disease is the child suffering from? Mention the stage too.

A. T-cell lymphoblastic lymphoma, stage IV
B. B-cell lymphoblastic lymphoma, stage III
C. T-cell lymphoblastic lymphoma, stage III
D. B-cell lymphoblastic lymphoma, stage IV

EXPLANATION

In the above scenario, the child is having blasts that are positive for B-cell markers (CD19, CD20, TdT, and CD10), TdT is a sensitive marker of differentiating between Burkitt lymphoma and B-cell lymphoblastic lymphoma. TdT adds single nucleotides to double-stranded deoxyribonucleic acid (DNA) breaks during the stages of T-cell rearrangement/immunoglobulin gene rearrangements. This is a process integral for precursor B-cell development.

The child has bone marrow metastasis (presence of >5% involvement), children with >5% involvement of bone marrow are considered to have precursor B-cell acute lymphoblastic leukemia rather than B-cell lymphoblastic lymphoma.

According to St Jude's staging classification, the child has stage IV disease with bone marrow involvement.

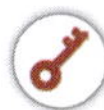

Key: D

BOOST YOUR KNOWLEDGE

Children with B-cell lymphoblastic lymphoma are treated with protocols similar to acute lymphoblastic leukemia overall survival (OS) for them ranges to above 80%.

REFERENCE/SOURCE

- Alexander S, Ferrando AA. Pediatric lymphoma. In: Orkin SH, Fisher DE, Ginsburg D, Look AT, Lux SE, Nathan DG (Eds). Nathan and Oski's Hematology and Oncology of Infancy and Childhood, 8th edition. Philadelphia, PA: Elsevier Saunders; 2015. pp. 1652,1656-7.

20. A 7-year-old male child with a newly diagnosed Burkitt lymphoma also has complaints of severe headaches. You did a CSF analysis at initial evaluation which yielded positivity for L-3 blasts, how would you treat such a child?

A. Cranial irradiation
B. Craniospinal irradiation
C. Multiagent chemotherapy + local intrathecal chemotherapy
D. Multiagent chemotherapy + intrathecal chemotherapy+ cranial irradiation

EXPLANATION

Children with Burkitt lymphoma with CNS involvement are treated with intensive multiagent combination chemotherapy along with triple intrathecal chemotherapy instillation (injection hydrocortisone, injection cytarabine, and injection methotrexate). There is a proven role in increasing methotrexate dose and infusion time in this high-risk cohort. Cranial RT is no longer used in the upfront management of Burkitt lymphoma with CNS involvement.

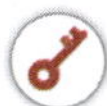

Key: C

BOOST YOUR KNOWLEDGE

Children with CNS-positive disease, especially those that have CSF positivity for blasts are the worst cohort of BL to treat. They tend to do worse off than those with stage IV disease due to bone marrow metastasis. Event-free survival across most studies ranges up to 70% only. Furthermore, when they relapse, the relapse usually is not salvageable.

REFERENCE/SOURCE

- Alexander S, Ferrando AA. Pediatric lymphoma. In: Orkin SH, Fisher DE, Ginsburg D, Look AT, Lux SE, Nathan DG (Eds). Nathan and Oski's Hematology and Oncology of Infancy and Childhood, 8th edition. Philadelphia, PA: Elsevier Saunders; 2015. pp. 1661.

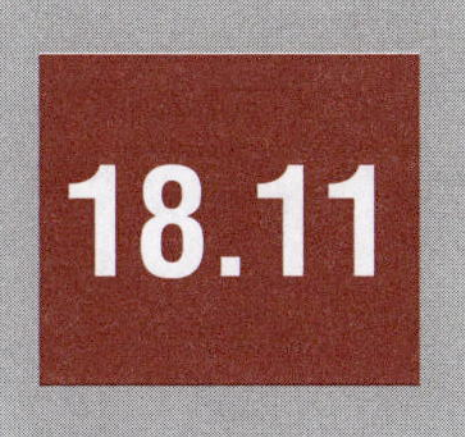

CHAPTER 18.11 Blood Component Therapy

Nidhi Srivastava

1. Red cell concentrate (RCC) transfusion is indicated in which of the following child?

A. A 6-year-old male with Hb 7.4 g/dL and symptomatic chronic anemia
B. A 9-year-old female with Hb 10.5 g/dL and severe cardiopulmonary disease
C. A 4-year-old male with Hb 8 g/dL with diagnosis of aplastic anemia
D. A 3-month-old baby on extracorporeal membrane oxygenation (ECMO) with Hb 12.8 g/dL

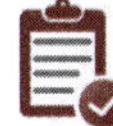

EXPLANATION

In children and adolescents with symptomatic chronic anemia, RCC transfusion is indicated if Hb is <7 g/dL (so option A is wrong). In severe cardiopulmonary disease, Hb should be maintained >12 g/dL. As Hb is only 10.5 g/dL in option B, RCC transfusion is indicated in this child. In marrow failure, Hb should be maintained >7 g/dL. In option C, the child is having Hb of 8 g/dL, so no transfusion needed at this point. Children on ECMO need to maintain Hb >12 g/dL, so option D child is also not an indication for RCC transfusion.

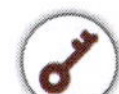

Key: B

BOOST YOUR KNOWLEDGE

The red blood cell (RBC) product of choice to transfuse neonates, infants, children, and adolescents is prestorage leukocyte-reduced RBCs suspended in an anticoagulant/preservative storage solution with hematocrit of approximately 60–70%, and it should be used within 35–45 days of collection.

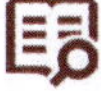

REFERENCE/SOURCE

- Josephson CD, Strauss RG. Red blood cell transfusions and erythropoietin therapy (Table 497.1). In: Kliegman RM, St Geme III JW, Blum NJ, Shah SS, Tasker RC, Wilson KM (Eds). Nelson Textbook of Pediatrics, 21st edition. Elsevier; 2019. pp. 2581-2.

2. A 6-year-old male child came in your OPD with severe pallor. On laboratory investigations, his Hb was found to be 5.5 g/dL; his peripheral smear showed hypochromic microcytic RBCs, and his iron studies were suggestive of iron deficiency anemia (IDA). He was clinically stable. What will be your line of treatment?

A. Oral iron with Hb monitoring
B. Parenteral iron treatment
C. RCC transfusion
D. RCC transfusion followed by oral iron supplement

EXPLANATION

Since the child is clinically stable, transfusion is not indicated in this child. Oral iron at a dose of 3–6 mg/kg/day with monitoring of Hb level is the ideal treatment for clinically stable child. Parenteral iron is only indicated if there is significant intolerance to oral iron or malabsorption syndrome interfering with iron malabsorption.

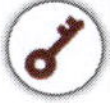

Key: A

BOOST YOUR KNOWLEDGE

Red cell concentrate transfusion is indicated in symptomatic chronic anemia with Hb level <7 g/dL.

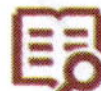

REFERENCE/SOURCE

- Josephson CD, Strauss RG. Red blood cell transfusions and erythropoietin therapy (Table 497.1). In: Kliegman RM, St Geme III JW, Blum NJ, Shah SS, Tasker RC, Wilson KM (Eds). Nelson Textbook of Pediatrics, 21st edition. Elsevier; 2019. p. 2581.

3. Which of the following is not prevented by leukoreduction?

A. Febrile nonhemolytic transfusion reactions
B. Cytomegalovirus (CMV) transmission
C. Alloimmunization
D. Transfusion-associated graft-versus-host disease (TA-GVHD)

EXPLANATION

Leukoreduction reduces the frequency of febrile nonhemolytic transfusion reactions, CMV transmission, and alloimmunization.

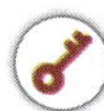

Key: D

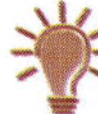

BOOST YOUR KNOWLEDGE

Irradiation of RBC and platelet products is recommended for immunocompromised patients, because it is effective in preventing TA-GVHD by halting donor T-cell replication and engraftment in the host.

REFERENCE/SOURCE

- Blaney SM, Adamson PC, Helman LJ (Eds). Pizzo and Poplack's Pediatric Oncology, 8th edition. Wolters Kluwer; 2020. p. 2795.

4. Recommended threshold for platelet transfusion in children and adolescents:

A. 20×10^9/L with bleeding
B. 20×10^9/L and marrow failure without hemorrhagic risk factors
C. 50×10^9/L and marrow failure with hemorrhagic risk factors
D. 50×10^9/L with major invasive procedure

EXPLANATION

According to guidelines for pediatric platelet transfusion, platelet transfusion is indicated in a bleeding child with platelet count $<50 \times 10^9$/L. In marrow failure, platelet count should be maintained above 10×10^9/L in child without hemorrhagic risk factors and 20×10^9/L in child with hemorrhagic risk factors. Prior to major invasive procedure platelet count should be $>50 \times 10^9$. Therefore only correct option is D.

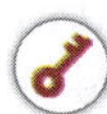

Key: D

BOOST YOUR KNOWLEDGE

In contrast to older children and adult, who respond to situations of increased demands for platelets by first increasing megakaryocyte size and ploidy which is followed in 3–5 days by increased megakaryocyte number, in thrombocytopenic neonates, megakaryocyte numbers increase but no increase in size occurs.

REFERENCE/SOURCE

- Josephson CD, Strauss RG. Platelet transfusions (Table 498.1). In: Kliegman RM, St Geme III JW, Blum NJ, Shah SS, Tasker RC, Wilson KM (Eds). Nelson Textbook of Pediatrics, 21st edition. Elsevier; 2019. p. 2583.

5. Platelet transfusion is indicated in a 2-month-old child with platelet count less than:

A. 100×10^9/L on ECMO
B. 60×10^9/L going for an invasive procedure
C. 70×10^9/L and clinically unstable
D. 25×10^9/L and clinically stable

EXPLANATION

In infants of <4 months on ECMO, platelet count should be maintained >100×10^9/L, so option A is correct. For invasive procedures and clinically unstable infant of <4 months, platelet counts need to be >50×10^9/L, so options B and C child do not need platelet transfusion. In clinically stable infants, platelet count should be maintained above 20×10^9/L.

Key: A

BOOST YOUR KNOWLEDGE

Platelet products generally have 5 days expiration time and should be stored at 20–24°C with constant agitation.

REFERENCE/SOURCE

- Josephson CD, Strauss RG. Platelet transfusions (Table 498.1). In: Kliegman RM, St Geme III JW, Blum NJ, Shah SS, Tasker RC, Wilson KM (Eds). Nelson Textbook of Pediatrics, 21st edition. Elsevier; 2019. pp. 2583-4.

6. In which of the following cases granulocyte transfusion (GTX) is indicated?

A. A 5-year-old male child with fungal sepsis and absolute neutrophil count of 0.4×10^6/L
B. A 2-month-old infant with fulminant bacterial infection and absolute neutrophil count of 1.2×10^6/L
C. A 3-day-old baby girl with bacterial infection and absolute neutrophil count of 3.1×10^6/L
D. A 10-year-old male on maintenance therapy for acute lymphocytic leukemia with febrile neutropenia

EXPLANATION

In a child with bacterial or fungal infection not responding to antimicrobial therapy with neutrophil count below 0.5×10^6/L, GTX is indicated. Therefore, granulocytes transfusion is indicated to option A child with absolute neutrophil count of 0.4×10^6/L. Antimicrobial therapy is the treatment of choice in case of febrile neutropenia.

Guideline for pediatric GTX:

- *Children and adolescence:*
  - Severe neutropenia (blood neutrophil count <0.5×10^9/L) and infection unresponsive and progressive despite antimicrobial therapy
  - Qualitative neutrophil defect, neutropenia not required, and infection unresponsive and progressive despite antimicrobial therapy
- *Infants <4 months old:*
  - Blood neutrophils count <3×10^9/L in first week of life or <1×10^9/L thereafter with fulminant bacterial infection

Key: A

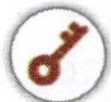

BOOST YOUR KNOWLEDGE

Granulocyte dosing:

- *Neonate and infant (<10 kg):* $1–2 \times 10^9$/kg neutrophils per each GTX
- *Larger infants and small children:* 1×10^{10}/kg neutrophils per each GTX
- *Adolescents:* $5–8 \times 10^{10}$/kg neutrophils per each GTX

REFERENCE/SOURCE

- Josephson CD, Strauss RG. Neutrophil (granulocyte) transfusions (Table 499.1). In: Kliegman RM, St Geme III JW, Blum NJ, Shah SS, Tasker RC, Wilson KM (Eds). Nelson Textbook of Pediatrics, 21st edition. Elsevier; 2019. p. 2585.

7. Fresh frozen plasma transfusion is indicated in all, *except:*

A. For rapid reversal of effect of warfarin in actively bleeding patients
B. Dilutional coagulopathy (massive transfusion) and bleeding
C. Anticoagulant protein (protein AT3, protein C, and protein S) replacement
D. Acquired thrombotic thrombocytopenic purpura (TTP)

EXPLANATION

First three options are absolute indications for plasma transfusion. Congenital TTP can be benefited with fresh frozen plasma as well. But acquired TTP needs plasma exchange.

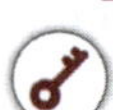

Key: D

BOOST YOUR KNOWLEDGE

Two interchangeable plasma products are available for transfusion, plasma frozen within 8 hours of collection (known as FFP), and plasma frozen within 24 hours of collection (known as F-24). Although levels of factor V and VIII are modestly reduced in F24, they are equally efficacious in all indications.

REFERENCE/SOURCE

- Josephson CD, Strauss RG. Plasma transfusions (Table 500.1). In: Kliegman RM, St Geme III JW, Blum NJ, Shah SS, Tasker RC, Wilson KM (Eds). Nelson Textbook of Pediatrics, 21st edition. Elsevier; 2019. pp. 2585-6.

8. Of the following, which is not an indication of fresh frozen plasma transfusion in newborn?

A. Reconstitution of RBC concentrate to simulate whole blood for use in massive transfusion (exchange transfusion, cardiac bypass, and ECMO)
B. Hemorrhage secondary to vitamin K deficiency
C. Disseminated intravascular coagulation (DIC) with bleeding
D. Prophylactic plasma transfusion to prevent intraventricular hemorrhage (IVH) in premature infants

EXPLANATION

Option A, B, and C are indications of plasma transfusion in neonates. Prophylactic plasma transfusion to prevent IVH in premature infants is not recommended.

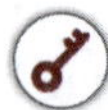

Key: D

BOOST YOUR KNOWLEDGE

Other indications of plasma transfusion in neonates are bleeding in congenital coagulation factor deficiency, when more specific treatment is either unavailable or inappropriate, and purpura fulminans due to congenital protein C/protein S deficiency.

REFERENCE/SOURCE

- Josephson CD, Strauss RG. Plasma transfusions. In: Kliegman RM, St Geme III JW, Blum NJ, Shah SS, Tasker RC, Wilson KM (Eds). Nelson Textbook of Pediatrics, 21st edition. Elsevier; 2019. p. 2586.

9. A 6-year-old boy, known complaint of (k/c/o) B-cell acute lymphoblastic leukemia (ALL), on induction chemotherapy, was transfused with RCC. After 1 hour of starting the transfusion, he developed dyspnea, tachypnea, hypoxemia, and tachycardia. On clinical examination, jugular venous pressure (JVP) and central venous pressure (CVP) were raised. True about this case scenario is:

A. This is acute hemolytic transfusion reaction (AHTR) and treatment is intravenous (IV) hydrocortisone, diuretic, dopamine, and FFP
B. Allergic transfusion reaction and the management is diphenhydramine, epinephrine beta-2 agonist inhalation
C. Elevated brain natriuretic peptide (BNP) is characteristic. Management is to stop transfusion, supportive oxygen, and diuretics
D. Oxygen, pressor support, and steroids may be helpful

EXPLANATION

Acute hemolytic transfusion reaction occurs immediately, within 15 minutes of starting the transfusion. It presents with fever, backache, hypotension, DIC, and renal failure. Allergic transfusion reaction also presents immediately after starting the transfusion. Therefore, the first two options are ruled out. As the child presented after 1 hour of transfusion and clinical features are dyspnea, tachypnea, and hypoxemia, transfusion-associated circulatory overload (TACO) is the most probable diagnosis. Elevated BNP is a characteristic laboratory feature, and treatment is supportive care with oxygen and diuretics. Steroids and pressor support are helpful in transfusion-associated acute lung injury (TRALI).

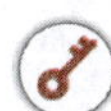

Key: C

BOOST YOUR KNOWLEDGE

Transfusion-associated circulatory overload appears to be much more frequent than TRALI. It occurs when the volume or rate of transfusion overwhelms the patient's cardiovascular system, resulting in pulmonary edema. Clinical and laboratory signs include dyspnea, tachypnea, hypoxemia, orthopnea, new gallop, jugular venous distention, elevated CVP, elevated serum troponin, and elevated BNP. Patients at the highest risk of TACO include pediatric patients, elderly patients, patients with congestive heart failure, and patients with severe anemia. Blood components should be administered slowly in nonbleeding patients, and careful attention should be paid to fluid balance.

Transfusion-associated acute lung injury usually presents within 6 hours of transfusion. Clinical symptoms include dyspnea, tachypnea, fever, and hypotension. Pressor agents may be useful in cases of sustained hypotension. Diuretics are not helpful, because the pathogenesis is microvascular damage rather than fluid overload. The majority of patients recovers within a 48- to 96-hours period.

REFERENCE/SOURCE

- Blaney SM, Adamson PC, Helman LJ (Eds). Pizzo and Poplack's Pediatric Oncology (Table 35.5), 8th edition. Wolters Kluwer; 2020. p. 2810.

10. Fresh frozen plasma:

A. Does not contain all necessary clotting factors required for secondary hemostasis
B. Should be leukoreduced and irradiated before transfusion
C. Should be ABO compatible
D. Typical dose is 5–10 mL/kg

EXPLANATION

Plasma contains all of the necessary clotting factors required for secondary hemostasis, each with a different half-life. Plasma is indicated for factor replacement in patients with coagulopathy and bleeding. Because plasma contains iso-hemagglutinins, it should be ABO compatible with the patient to prevent hemolysis of patient RBCs. The majority of WBCs are killed or nonfunctional because of the freezing process; therefore, leukoreduction and irradiation of plasma products are not recommended. The typical dose ordered is 15–20 mL/kg administered at a rate of 10–20 mL/kg/h (typically over 30–60 minutes). This dosage results in an expected rise in all the coagulation factors by approximately 25%.

Key: C

BOOST YOUR KNOWLEDGE

Plasma is prepared from a whole-blood collection or apheresis collection; the extracted plasma is frozen within 6–24 hours depending on the processing method and stored at –18°C or colder for up to 1 year. Before issuing, plasma requires approximately 30 minutes to thaw.

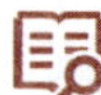

REFERENCE/SOURCE

- Blaney SM, Adamson PC, Helman LJ (Eds). Pizzo and Poplack's Pediatric Oncology, 8th edition. Wolters Kluwer; 2020. p. 2805.

11. True statement about granulocyte concentrate is:

A. Granulocyte colony-stimulating factor (G-CSF) (5 µg/kg) and oral dexamethasone or prednisolone are administered to a healthy donor 12 hours before granulocyte collection
B. Granulocytes are stored at 20–24°C with agitation
C. It expires 48 hours after collection, although, ideally it should be transfused as soon as possible after collection
D. They need not to be ABO compatible

EXPLANATION

Granulocyte colony-stimulating factor (5 µg/kg) and oral dexamethasone (8–12 mg) or prednisone (60 mg) administration to a healthy donor 12 hours before granulocyte collection by apheresis provides an optimal yield of granulocytes. The expected yield with G-CSF and corticosteroid stimulation is 5-7 × 10^{10} granulocytes per product. Granulocytes are most commonly collected via apheresis. Granulocytes are stored at 20–24°C without agitation (not with agitation as mentioned in option B) and expire 24 hours after collection (not 48 hours), although, ideally, they should be transfused as soon as possible after collection, because their viability declines rapidly. Because these preparations contain significant numbers of RBCs, they must be transfused after crossmatching only.

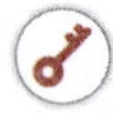

Key: A

BOOST YOUR KNOWLEDGE

Granulocytes are most commonly collected via apheresis. Granulocytes should be collected from CMV-seronegative donors to mitigate the risk of CMV transmission in a CMV-negative patient. Granulocytes should also be irradiated to prevent TA-GVHD. Granulocyte and amphotericin B infusion should be separated as far as possible in time, because severe pulmonary reactions can occur, secondary to granulocyte aggregates. For infants, a dose of 1–2 × 10^9 cells/kg is recommended. For larger children and adults, a dose of 4–8 × 10^{10} granulocytes is recommended. Typically, a granulocyte unit is 200 mL, and the usual dose is the greatest volume that the patient can tolerate given over 1–2 hours, for 5 consecutive days or as clinically indicated.

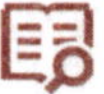

REFERENCE/SOURCE

- Blaney SM, Adamson PC, Helman LJ (Eds). Pizzo and Poplack's Pediatric Oncology, 8th edition. Wolters Kluwer; 2020. pp. 2804-5.

12. Advantages of BCPC (buffy coat platelet concentrates) over PRP-PC (platelet-rich plasma-platelet concentrates) are all of the following, *except:*

A. Minimal red cell contamination
B. Harvesting of platelets on plastic surface hence better in vivo survival
C. Lower leukocyte concentration
D. Improvement and standardization of quality of the product

EXPLANATION

Platelet-rich plasma-platelet concentrates are prepared from whole blood kept at room temperature within 6–8 hours of collection. Blood is centrifuged with a light spin, and PRP is separated into a satellite bag. PRP is centrifuged again and separated into platelet concentrate and FFP. For BCPC, whole blood can be stored at room temperature for up to 24 hours. Hard spin is first done to spin the platelet into the buffy coat on a cushion of red cells and then using a slow spin from the separated buffy coat. Advantages of BCPC over PRP-PC are minimal red blood cell contamination, harvesting of platelet from a biological cell bed (not plastic bed), hence better in vivo survival, lower leukocyte contamination, and improvement and standardization of quality of the product.

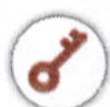

Key: B

BOOST YOUR KNOWLEDGE

One unit platelet concentrate is prepared from single buffy coat while pooled platelet concentrate is prepared from pooling of 4–5 buffy coats.

REFERENCE/SOURCE

- Bhardwaj K (Ed). Transfusion Update (ISBTI), 1st edition. New Delhi: Jaypee Brothers Medical Publishers; 2015. pp. 123-4.

13. One unit of platelet concentrate (PRP-PC) contains:

A. Volume 50–70 mL
B. Platelet $<5.5 \times 10^{10}$
C. pH <6
D. WBC contamination $2 \times 10^7 - 2 \times 10^8$

EXPLANATION

One unit PRPC contain volume 50–70 mL, platelets $>5.5 \times 10^{10}$, RBC contamination in traces, WBC contamination $5.5 \times 10^7 - 5.5 \times 10^8$ and pH >6. Therefore, only option A is correct.

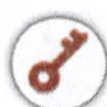

Key: A

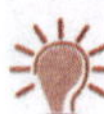

BOOST YOUR KNOWLEDGE

One unit of random donor platelet (RDP)/10 kg BW or 4–6 units in an adult of 70 kg is the ideal dose of RDP.

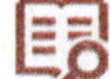

REFERENCE/SOURCE

- Bhardwaj K (Ed). Transfusion Update (ISBTI), 1st edition. New Delhi: Jaypee Brothers Medical Publishers; 2015. pp. 123-4.

14. Which of the following is *not* true about delayed hemolytic transfusion reaction (DHTR)?

A. It occurs more than 24 hours after red cell transfusion (days to about 2 weeks)
B. Presents with unexplained anemia and jaundice
C. *Evidence of extravascular hemolysis:* Spherocytes and reticulocytes on peripheral smear, increase in total and unconjugated bilirubin, increased lactate dehydrogenase (LDH)
D. Usually severe and definitive treatment necessary

EXPLANATION

First three options are right. Option D is wrong as DHTR is usually mild requiring no treatment. Sometimes, after DHTR, patient may require repeat transfusion.

Key: D

BOOST YOUR KNOWLEDGE

Delayed hemolytic transfusion reactions or delayed serologic transfusion reactions (DSTRs) classically present with fever and anemia for days to weeks after an RBC transfusion and are caused by immunoglobulin G (IgG) anti-red cell antibodies directed at minor red cell antigens, such as anti-K. These are typically mild compared with AHTRs, although sometimes patients have jaundice or other signs of hemolysis. Hemoglobinuria, acute renal failure, and DIC are rare.

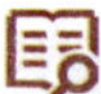

REFERENCE/SOURCE

- Blaney SM, Adamson PC, Helman LJ (Eds). Pizzo and Poplack's Pediatric Oncology, 8th edition. Wolters Kluwer; 2020. p. 2811.

15. The correct statement regarding RDP of the following options is:

A. Dose in children is 4 units/10 kg body weight
B. 4–6 units in adults of 70 kg
C. One unit raises platelet count 2×10^9/L in adult
D. One unit raises platelet count by $30–60 \times 10^9$/L in an adult person

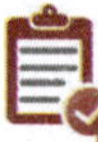

EXPLANATION

One unit of RDP/10 kg BW or 4–6 units in an adult of 70 kg is the ideal dose of RDP, which will raise the platelet count $5–10 \times 10^9$/L.

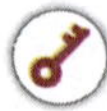

Key: B

BOOST YOUR KNOWLEDGE

One unit of platelet from an apheresis donor [single donor platelet (SDP)] will raise the platelet count of an adult of 70 kg BW by $30–60 \times 10^9$/L.

REFERENCE/SOURCE

- Bhardwaj K (Ed). Transfusion Update (ISBTI), 1st edition. New Delhi: Jaypee Brothers Medical Publishers; 2015. pp. 124-5.

16. Identify the true statement on platelet refractoriness.

A. Condition in which a patient ceases to respond to platelet transfusions with appropriate and sustained increments in the platelet count on two separate occasions as measured by a 1-hour post-platelet transfusion count, regardless of the etiology

B. Can occur secondary to nonimmune and immune causes, the latter being more common
C. Occurs more frequently in children
D. Leukoreduction of platelets before transfusion eliminates the risk of alloimmunization

EXPLANATION

Platelet refractoriness is the condition in which a patient ceases to respond to platelet transfusions with appropriate and sustained increments in the platelet count on two separate occasions as measured by a 1-hour post platelet transfusion count, regardless of the etiology. Platelet refractoriness can occur secondary to nonimmune and immune causes, the former being more common. Platelet refractoriness seems to occur less frequently in children. Leukocyte-contaminating platelet preparations are the primary stimulus for alloimmunization. Leukoreduction of platelets before transfusion has been shown to reduce the frequency of alloimmunization.

Key: A

BOOST YOUR KNOWLEDGE

Nonimmune causes of platelet refractoriness include bleeding, splenomegaly, fever, infection, medications, allogeneic transplantation, and DIC. Immune causes of platelet refractoriness are because of alloimmunization, leading to alloantibody-mediated clearance of transfused platelets. The alloantibody is usually directed to human leukocyte antigen (HLA) class I antigens and, rarely, to human platelet antigens (HPAs) and at times to both. Risk factors for alloimmunization include a patient's underlying disease, immunosuppressive effects of treatment, prior pregnancies, and exposure to leukocytes in previous transfusions. At times, a patient may have concurrent immune and nonimmune causes for platelet refractoriness.

Human leukocyte antigen antibodies can occur as early as 10 days after primary exposure to HLA class I molecules (mainly of the HLA-A and HLA-B locus antigens) present on the platelet surface and 4 days after secondary exposure in patients previously transfused or pregnant.

REFERENCE/SOURCE

- Blaney SM, Adamson PC, Helman LJ (Eds). Pizzo and Poplack's Pediatric Oncology (Table 35.3), 8th edition. Wolters Kluwer; 2020. pp. 2810, 2802.

17. Incorrect about AHTR is:

A. Occurs immediately during the first 15 minutes of transfusion
B. Presents as fever, backache, hypotension, and DIC
C. Can also be caused by infusion of plasma and platelets
D. AHTR occurs predominantly due to Anti A/Anti B IgG antibodies

EXPLANATION

Acute hemolytic transfusion reaction (AHTR) occurs immediately, usually during the first 15 minutes of transfusion. AHTR classically presents with fever with or without chills or rigors. A patient with mild AHTR may also have abdominal, chest, flank, and back pain, while patient with severe AHTR presents with dyspnea, flank pain and hypotension and progresses to shock with or without DIC. AHTRs can also be caused by the infusion of plasma or platelet products containing anti-A or anti-B that reacts with the recipient's RBCs, most commonly a group O platelet into a group A recipient. AHTRs are the result of acute intravascular hemolysis due to preformed complement-fixing anti-red cell antibodies. These reactions are usually owing to immunoglobulin M (IgM) anti-A or anti-B isohemagglutinins but rarely can be caused by complement-fixing IgG or IgM antibodies of other minor RBC antigens, such as anti-Jka.

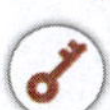

Key: D

BOOST YOUR KNOWLEDGE

The clinical severity is extremely variable. Patient misidentification resulting in infusion of ABO-incompatible RBCs is the most common cause of AHTR. The misidentification occurs at the time of sampling/labeling or when the blood is infused into the wrong patient. Rare cases of acute hemolysis have been reported, however, in patients who received greater amounts of incompatible plasma and/or products containing unusually high titers of anti-A or anti-B. Transfusion services typically have institutional policies to limit the amount of incompatible plasma or platelets transfused, and some screen products for high anti-A, defined by each hospital's transfusion service.

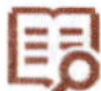

REFERENCE/SOURCE

- Blaney SM, Adamson PC, Helman LJ (Eds). Pizzo and Poplack's Pediatric Oncology (Table 35.3), 8th edition. Wolters Kluwer; 2020. pp. 2810, 2807.

18. Which of the following is incorrect with regards to fibrinogen concentrate (FC) compared to cryoprecipitate?

A. Decreased risk of viral infection
B. Low volume needed
C. Short preparation time
D. Increased risk of immunological/adverse events

EXPLANATION

Fibrinogen concentrates are human-derived, preservative-free, lyophilized fractionated products containing fibrinogen. When compared to cryoprecipitate, benefits include decreased risk of viral infection, low volume, and short preparation time. The viral inactivation process also removes antigens and antibodies, thereby reducing the risk of immunologic and allergic reactions.

Key: D

BOOST YOUR KNOWLEDGE

The viral inactivation process also removes antigens and antibodies, thereby reducing the risk of immunologic and allergic reactions. Serious adverse safety event reports are low, including thromboembolic events.

REFERENCE/SOURCE

- Blaney SM, Adamson PC, Helman LJ (Eds). Pizzo and Poplack's Pediatric Oncology, 8th edition. Wolters Kluwer; 2020. p. 2714.

19. The risk of TA-GVHD is increased in, *if:*

A. Transfusion recipient is immunocompetent
B. Donor and recipient have completely different HLA haplotype
C. Children with malignancies is treated with immunosuppressive drugs or myeloablative therapy
D. Transfusion-dependent thalassemia

EXPLANATION

Transfusion-associated graft-versus-host disease is caused by engraftment of the donor blood T lymphocytes in the transfusion recipient. Usually, the small number of residual T lymphocytes in blood components is eradicated by the competent immune system of the recipient. Therefore, if the recipient is immunocompetent, risk is actually reduced. If the donor is homozygous for an HLA haplotype that a heterozygous immunocompetent recipient also shares (one-way haplotype match), the recipient does not recognize donor cells as foreign and donor cells may be able to engraft in the recipient and cause TA-GVHD. Hence, transfusion from close relatives should be avoided. Children on immunosuppressive drugs or myeloablative therapy are unable to eradicate T lymphocytes in blood components, which get engrafted in recipient bone marrow causing TA-GVHD.

Key: C

BOOST YOUR KNOWLEDGE

Symptoms of TA-GVHD are similar to GVHD in hematopoietic stem cell transplant recipients, with the exception that TA-GVHD almost always results in pancytopenia from marrow aplasia and death within a few weeks in 90% of cases. Patients at increased risk of TA-GVHD include those with hematologic malignancies or other malignancies treated with immunosuppressive drugs or myeloablative chemotherapy, recipients of hematopoietic cell transplants, patients with Hodgkin lymphoma and children with congenital immunodeficiencies, recipients of intrauterine transfusions, and neonatal exchange transfusions. It can be prevented by irradiating cellular blood components (RBCs and platelets) before transfusion, rendering the T lymphocytes unable to proliferate. Irradiation of blood components does not impair their therapeutic efficacy. Irradiation of cellular blood products is performed with either gamma rays from cesium-137 or cobalt-60 sources, or X-rays. T lymphocytes are rendered inactive with a minimum radiation dose of 2,500 cGy. Leukoreduction is not enough. Frozen thawed plasma (FFP, cryoprecipitate) has not been associated with TA-GVHD.

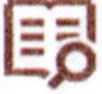

REFERENCE/SOURCE

- Blaney SM, Adamson PC, Helman LJ (Eds). Pizzo and Poplack's Pediatric Oncology, 8th edition. Wolters Kluwer; 2020. p. 2714.

20. All are true regarding preparation prior to transfusion, *except:*

A. Leukoreduction reduces the frequency of febrile nonhemolytic transfusion reactions
B. Crossmatching is not needed prior to the release of platelets, FFP, and cryoprecipitate
C. Irradiation of RBC is recommended for immunocompromised patients to prevent GVHD, but the same is not true for platelets
D. Directed blood donation increases risk of alloimmunization and TRALI

EXPLANATION

There are two mechanisms involved in the manifestation of a FNHTR. The first involves the presence of a white cell antibody in the patient's plasma that interacts with the white cells in the blood product. These antibodies may be directed against granulocyte antigens or HLA. This interaction causes endotoxins to be released, which act on the hypothalamus and stimulate a fever. The second mechanism involves the generation of leukocyte cytokines during product storage. Therefore leukoreduction reduces the frequency of FNHTR.

Irradiation of RBC and platelet products is recommended for immunocompromised patients, because it is effective in preventing TA-GVHD by halting donor T-cell replication and engraftment in the host.

When biological parents serve as directed donors to a child who may later need a hematopoietic stem cell transplantation (HSCT) from a family member, the risk of alloimmunization and TRALI increases.

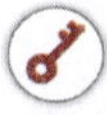

Key: C

BOOST YOUR KNOWLEDGE

Leukoreduction refers to the removal of white blood cells that remain in the RBC or platelet unit after production. Leukoreduction can occur through filtration soon after collection or through the use of a filter at the time of transfusion. Current AABB guidelines state that leukoreduced RBCs must contain $<5 \times 10^6$ leukocytes per unit. Leukoreduction reduces the frequency of febrile nonhemolytic transfusion reactions and CMV transmission.

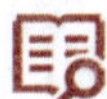

REFERENCE/SOURCE

- Blaney SM, Adamson PC, Helman LJ (Eds). Pizzo and Poplack's Pediatric Oncology, 8th edition. Wolters Kluwer; 2020. pp. 2714, 2715.

21. All are true about packed RBC products, *except:*

A. Prepared from whole blood after centrifugation
B. Additive solutions (ASs) are designed to preserve RBCs and to minimize hemolysis to <1% of RBCs
C. The storage life of RBCs varies based on the type of anticoagulant preservative solution from 21 (AS) to 42 days [citrate phosphate dextrose (CPD)]
D. The hematocrit of AS units ranges from 55% to 65% whereas that of citrate phosphate dextrose-adenine (CPDA) units varies between 70% and 80%

EXPLANATION

Packed RBC products are prepared from whole blood after centrifugation. RBCs can be stored in various anticoagulant-preservative solutions, including acid citrate dextrose (ACD), CPD, CPDA1, or additive solutions (AS-1, AS-3, and AS-5). ASs are designed to preserve RBCs and to minimize hemolysis to <1% of RBCs during prolonged storage. The storage life of RBCs varies based on the type of anticoagulant preservative solution from 21 (CPD) to 42 days (AS). The hematocrit of AS units ranges from 55 to 65%, whereas the hematocrit of CDPA units is between 70 to 80%. In option C, the storage life of RBCs is written wrong.

Key: C

BOOST YOUR KNOWLEDGE

Pretransfusion testing for products includes ABO grouping, Rh typing, and screening for any unexpected antibodies to red blood cell antigen. Before RBC component release, a crossmatch is performed to detect compatibility between recipient plasma and donor RBCs. Crossmatching is not needed prior to release of cryoprecipitate, FFP, and platelets.

REFERENCE/SOURCE

- Blaney SM, Adamson PC, Helman LJ (Eds). Pizzo and Poplack's Pediatric Oncology, 8th edition. Wolters Kluwer; 2020. p. 2714.

SECTION

19 Respiratory Diseases

CHAPTER 19.1

Upper Respiratory Infections including OM, Pharyngotonsillitis, Sinusitis, Croup, LTB, and Stridor

Hema Gupta Mittal

1. An 18-month-old infant presented in emergency department with fever and cough for 5 days and breathing difficulty for 1 day. On examination, the child was toxic and had respiratory distress [respiratory rate (RR) 65 breaths/minute and oxygen saturation (SpO_2) 88%]. The mother also said that child had hoarse cry. There was no drooling of saliva. He started on adrenaline nebulization and one dose of dexamethasone. In view of poor response, a bronchoscopy was done and showed the following. What is the most probable differential diagnosis?

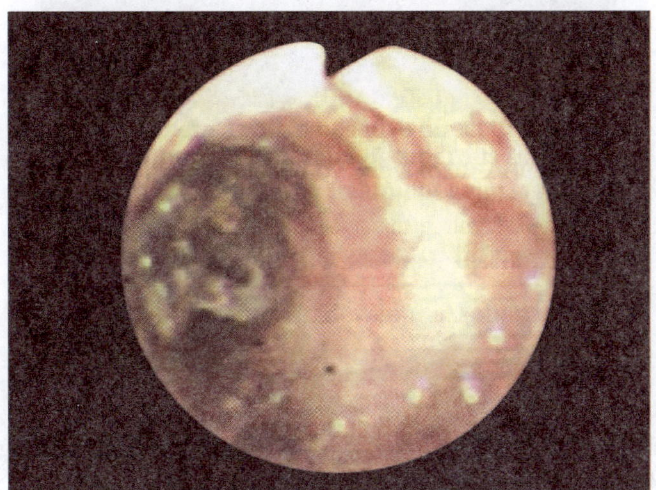

A. Foreign body aspiration
B. Bacterial tracheitis
C. Tuberculosis
D. Epiglottitis

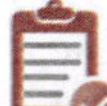

EXPLANATION

This child shows symptoms of upper respiratory tract infection (URI) such as fever and cough. However, there seems to be complication after 5 days of illness. As he developed repeat severe symptoms such as respiratory distress and toxicity with a hoarse voice suggestive of laryngeal involvement. The bronchoscopy image is suggestive of pus spots in trachea (presence of tracheal rings) suggest a diagnosis of tracheitis.

- Absence of drooling and no bronchoscopy abnormalities mentioned rule out epiglottitis.
- Foreign body aspiration is ruled out on absence of sudden onset acute distress with any history of foreign body consumption and choking history. Further bronchoscopy does not reveal any foreign body.
- Tuberculosis is a chronic illness which should be suspected in children with 2 weeks cough, fever, anorexia, and weight loss unlike in this scenario.

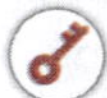

Key: B

BOOST YOUR KNOWLEDGE

Bacterial tracheitis is due to a secondary bacterial infection of the trachea, resulting in the formation of mucopurulent exudates that may acutely obstruct the upper airway, resulting in a life-threatening condition. The only definitive way to diagnose bacterial tracheitis is by direct visualization of the trachea via bronchoscopy.

Children with bacterial tracheitis usually present with a history of a viral respiratory illness (rhinorrhea, cough, fever, and sore throat) that may be present for up to 1 week before presentation. This is followed by acute deterioration characterized by severe upper airway obstruction, high fever, and toxicity. More specific findings include stridor, hoarseness, cough, and tachypnea.

REFERENCE/SOURCE

- Kliegman RM, St Geme JW III, Blum NJ, Shah SS, Tasker RC, Wilson KM. Nelson Textbook of Pediatrics, 21st edition. Amsterdam: Elsevier; 2020. p. 2206.

2. A 5-month-old boy presented with noisy breathing since few days after birth and repeated episodes of fast breathing and wheezing for which he had multiple hospitalizations. There was no response to beta-2 agonist nebulization. Flexible bronchoscopy was done as shown in the given Figure.

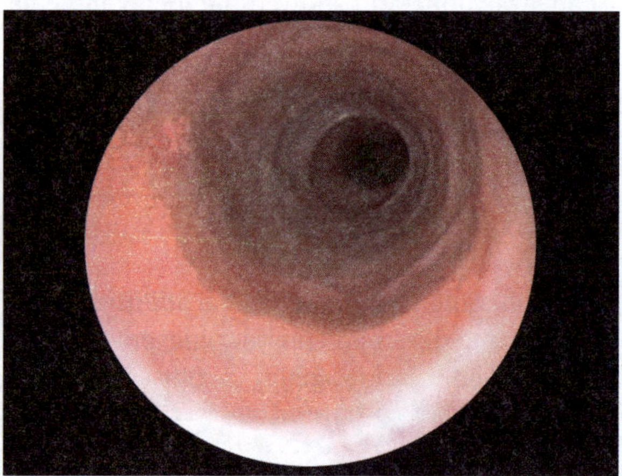

The most probable diagnosis will be:

A. Vascular malformation
B. Complete tracheal rings
C. Subglottic stenosis (SGS)
D. Tracheomalacia

EXPLANATION

This infant has recurrent episodes of wheezing with onset in neonatal period and also severe episodes of wheezing and fast breathing suggesting airway obstruction. Nonresponse to bronchodilators rules out reversible etiologies and suggests structural causes. In this infant, the bronchoscopy image shows complete tracheal rings. A normal trachea (windpipe) has many rings made of cartilage (a strong and flexible tissue) that are C-shaped. The bronchoscopy image clearly rules out SGS as lumen is completely patent. Tracheomalacia is ruled out on absence of any prolapsed of lumen. There is no bulge on tracheal wall in image provided to suggest vascular malformation.

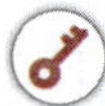

Key: B

BOOST YOUR KNOWLEDGE

Complete tracheal rings are a birth defect in the cartilage rings that keep the trachea, from collapsing. A normal tracheal cartilage is C-shaped with a softer, posterior membrane consisting of muscle. In complete tracheal rings, the trachea is made with several or more O-shaped rings. Symptoms include noisy breathing (stridor), recurring pneumonias, wheezing, retractions, wet-sounding biphasic noise (like a washing machine), cyanosis (blue-spells), apnea (breathing pauses), and chest congestion.

REFERENCE/SOURCE

- Kliegman RM, St Geme JW III, Blum NJ, Shah SS, Tasker RC, Wilson KM. Nelson Textbook of Pediatrics, 21st edition. Amsterdam: Elsevier; 2020. p. 2210.

3. **A 4-year-old child presents with low-grade fever, cough, coryza, and diarrhea for 2 days. On examination, temperature 100°F, RR 35 breaths/minute, and pallor+. *Oral examination:* No exudates on pharynx, painless cervical lymphadenopathy (1.5 cm), and conjunctivitis present. What is the most likely diagnosis?**

A. Viral nasopharyngitis
B. Streptococcal nasopharyngitis
C. Kawasaki diseases
D. Infectious mononucleosis

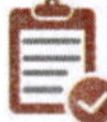

EXPLANATION

In this child, low-grade fever and cold without any tachypnea suggest URI mainly nasopharyngitis. Absence of exudates and presence of diarrhea and conjunctivitis suggests a viral etiology than bacterial. Infectious mononucleosis is associated with pharyngeal exudates and tender lymphadenopathy.

Key: A

BOOST YOUR KNOWLEDGE

Acute nasopharyngitis is a common viral infection, especially in children. It often presents with symptoms such as sore throat, runny or blocked nose, fever, and cough. There are >200 different viruses that can cause this infection, but rhinovirus is the most common cause. The virus can spread through tiny air droplets that are expelled when an infected person sneezes, coughs, blows their nose, or talks. Treatment for acute nasopharyngitis in children is usually symptomatic. Over-the-counter medications such as decongestants, antihistamines, and mucus thinners like guaifenesin are not recommended.

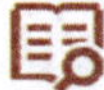

REFERENCE/SOURCE

- Kliegman RM, St Geme JW III, Blum NJ, Shah SS, Tasker RC, Wilson KM. Nelson Textbook of Pediatrics, 21st edition. Amsterdam: Elsevier; 2020. p. 2192.

4. **A 2-year-old boy presented with high-grade fever and slight cough since morning. He was brought to the pediatric emergency in night. Examination revealed a sick looking child, febrile, RR 50 breaths/minute, SpO_2 90% room air, with drooling of saliva and soft stridor. The most probable diagnosis is:**

A. Croup
B. Tracheitis
C. Epiglottitis
D. Retropharyngeal abscess (RPA)

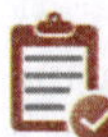

EXPLANATION

This young child with cough and fever and severe rapid progression of symptoms suggest airway involvement. The presence of toxicity, drooling of saliva, and soft stridor are suggestive of epiglottic disease. In croup, there would be absent of drooling and in tracheitis there would be harsh stridor. RPA may have all signs except stridor.

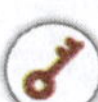

Key: C

BOOST YOUR KNOWLEDGE

Epiglottitis is an infection of the supraglottis that may cause airway compromise due to inflammation and swelling. It is an airway emergency, especially in children and is classically described in children aged 2–6 years of age. In countries that have introduced routine *Haemophilus influenzae* type B (Hib) vaccination, it has become uncommon in children. The most common signs are rapid onset of high fever, sore throat, inability to control secretions, classic tripod positioning, difficult breathing, and irritability, and stridor. These may be associated with difficult and painful swallowing and drooling.

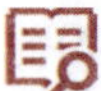

REFERENCE/SOURCE

- Kliegman RM, St Geme JW III, Blum NJ, Shah SS, Tasker RC, Wilson KM. Nelson Textbook of Pediatrics, 21st edition. Amsterdam: Elsevier; 2020. p. 2202.

5. A 3-year-old girl presented with cough, cold, and low-grade fever for 5 days. Since 1 day, the cough has become loud and there is worsening of symptoms at night. On examination, child was active, RR 48 breaths/minute, SpO_2 89%, and chest retractions were present. There was harsh stridor present. The most probable diagnosis is:

A. Pneumonia
B. Croup
C. Epiglottitis
D. RPA

EXPLANATION

In this scenario, the young child with cough, cold, and fever suggesting mild URI possibly viral etiology. On Day 5, there seems to be progression of cough and appearance of stridor suggesting airway obstruction. In an otherwise non-sick child, most probable diagnosis would be croup. Absence of toxicity, drooling, etc., makes epiglottitis and RPA unlikely. Pneumonia does not present with stridor.

Key: B

BOOST YOUR KNOWLEDGE

Croup [laryngotracheobronchitis (LTB)] is a respiratory infection that affects young children. Croup is frequently preceded by 24–72 hours of nonspecific cough, rhinorrhea, coryza and fever, with abrupt onset of barky cough, hoarse voice and, often, inspiratory stridor during the night. Croup is caused by a viral infection of the respiratory tract that causes edema and inflammation of the upper airway, and laryngeal mucosa resulting in narrowing in the subglottic region of the airway. Human parainfluenza virus (types 1 and 3) is the most common pathogen, but other causative viruses include influenza A and B viruses, respiratory syncytial virus (RSV), rhinovirus, coronavirus, human metapneumovirus, and adenovirus.

REFERENCE/SOURCE

- Kliegman RM, St Geme JW III, Blum NJ, Shah SS, Tasker RC, Wilson KM. Nelson Textbook of Pediatrics, 21st edition. Amsterdam: Elsevier; 2020. p. 2202.

6. A 15-month-old unvaccinated child presented with persistent cough for 25 days. The cough was associated with post-tussive vomiting. He has received multiple antibiotics and nebulization's with levosalbutamol from various doctors but of no use. On examination, the child was afebrile, RR 38 breaths/minute and SpO_2 90%. What is the best investigation in this child to diagnose the likely etiology?

A. Blood culture
B. Blood reverse transcription polymerase chain reaction (RT-PCR)
C. *Bordetella pertussis* antibody IgG
D. Chest X-ray

EXPLANATION

In this clinical scenario, this young child who is unvaccinated and has persistent cough which is not responsive to beta-2 agonists is suggestive of pertussoid cough. After 3 weeks of illness the best investigation would be IgG anti-PT as culture would be best up to 2 weeks, and RT-PCR up to 3 weeks. Chest X-ray is not diagnostic and may be normal or have nonspecific infiltrates/atelectasis.

Key: C

BOOST YOUR KNOWLEDGE

Whooping cough (pertussis) is a highly contagious respiratory tract infection. Pertussis, literally meaning "a violent cough", also known as whooping cough or "the cough of 100 days", was first described in the Paris epidemic of 1578. *Bordetella pertussis* and *Bordetella parapertussis* are the causative organisms. In many people, it is marked by a severe hacking cough followed by a high-pitched intake of breath that sounds like "whoop". After an incubation period of 1–3 weeks, pertussis infection typically progresses through three distinct stages, i.e., the catarrhal phase, the paroxysmal phase, and the convalescent phase. Nasopharyngeal culture and polymerase chain reaction (PCR) may yield laboratory confirmation, but the fastidious and slow-growing *Bordetella* organisms require specialized media, and cultures are typically not positive for 3–7 days. By the time the diagnosis is suspected, cultures are typically negative (96%), and overall culture sensitivity is only 20–40%. PCR is more sensitive and specific than culture, but testing is not widely available.

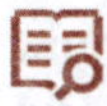

REFERENCE/SOURCE

- Kliegman RM, St Geme JW III, Blum NJ, Shah SS, Tasker RC, Wilson KM. Nelson Textbook of Pediatrics, 21st edition. Amsterdam: Elsevier; 2020. p. 1492.

7. A 4-year-old boy presented with fever and sore throat for 5 days. He also developed difficulty in swallowing food and drooling. On examination, the child was sick, febrile, and had torticollis and cervical lymphadenopathy. On oral examination, uvula was central. The X-ray neck and soft tissue with cervical spine of child was done and shown in given Figure.

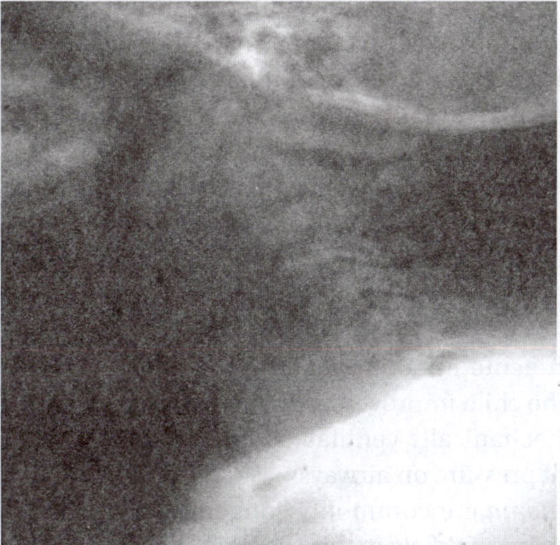

The most likely diagnosis is:

A. Epiglottitis
B. RPA
C. Tracheitis
D. Croup

EXPLANATION

This child had an upper respiratory infection suggested by fever and cough. There seems development of some complications with dysphagia, drooling, and torticollis. Dysphagia and drooling suggest upper airway obstruction. This characteristic X-ray is showing an increase in retropharyngeal space and more than half of C2 vertebra space suggesting a diagnosis of RPA. Children with epiglottitis may present in similar way except the X-ray which will show thumb sign suggesting swollen epiglottis. Similarly, tracheitis and croup may present in similar clinical way except stridor and absence of X-ray findings as mentioned earlier.

Key: B

BOOST YOUR KNOWLEDGE

Retropharyngeal abscess is a relatively uncommon midline deep neck space infection that extends from the base of the skull to the posterior mediastinum, situated between the buccopharyngeal and alar fascia. Usually occurring in children between the ages of 3 and 5 years, it is often preceded by an URI involving the retropharyngeal lymph nodes and leading to suppuration and perforation into the retropharyngeal space. The typical presentation consists of high fever, dysphagia, odynophagia, drooling with decreased oral intake, trismus, and neck stiffness or wry neck. In severe cases, the infection may extend into the mediastinum, and the growing abscess can result in upper airway obstruction and asphyxiation. An inspiratory lateral airway X-ray with neck extension has been reported to be useful as a screening study and shows increased depth of the prevertebral space on the lateral neck X-ray. CT scan remains the gold standard imaging modality for RPA and can provide further insights into the extent of infection and involvement of the carotid sheath and mediastinum. The mainstay of treatment is early transoral or transcervical surgical drainage and empirical antibiotic administration to eliminate infections.

REFERENCE/SOURCE

- Kliegman RM, St Geme JW III, Blum NJ, Shah SS, Tasker RC, Wilson KM. Nelson Textbook of Pediatrics, 21st edition. Amsterdam: Elsevier; 2020. p. 2197.

8. **A 10-month-old infant developed fever, cough followed by severe respiratory distress on day 3 of illness. On examination, he was febrile, RR 57 breaths/minute, cold clammy skin, and had low blood pressure. He was admitted to pediatric intensive care unit (PICU) on D3 of illness. Chest X-ray was suggestive of acute respiratory distress syndrome (ARDS) like picture and infant was put on ventilation and other supportive treatment. After 2 weeks of adequate treatment the chest X-ray of the patient improved, shock resolved, and he became afebrile. However, the infant could not be extubated and was referred for bronchoscopy which clinched the diagnosis. Which of the following is the most likely diagnosis?**

A. Subglottic web
B. Subglottic hemangioma
C. Mucous plug
D. Subglottic stenosis (SGS)

EXPLANATION

The infant was admitted with acute infection leading to sepsis, respiratory failure, and shock and hence required ventilatory support. The child improved with time but persistent difficulty in weaning from ventilator.

- *SGS* is not uncommon in mechanically ventilated children which may occur because of repeated trauma due to intubation or constant pressure on airways.
- *Subglottic web* and *hemangioma* are commonly congenital condition presenting with early onset stridor and respiratory failure and seems unlikely in this scenario.
- Pneumonia, mucus plugs, and collapse are common causes of failure of extubation however in this scenario there was clinical resolution.

Key: D

BOOST YOUR KNOWLEDGE

The subglottis is that portion of the airway located just below the vocal cords. It serves as the entry point of air into the trachea. Narrowing or stenosis of the subglottis can be a "congenital" anomaly that is present at or shortly after birth or an "acquired" condition that most commonly arises in infants who require prolonged airway intubation for ventilation. More than 90% of cases of SGS are secondary to endotracheal intubation. Symptoms of SGS include recurrent croup, shortness of breath, exercise intolerance, and cough. The diagnosis of SGS usually requires "direct laryngoscopy and bronchoscopy" depending on the severity of symptoms and the type of narrowing. Treatment includes observation, balloon dilation, laser excision, and sometimes open surgical airway reconstruction. The most common grading for the diagnosis of SGS is the Myer–Cotton grading scale. Grade 1 stenosis is lumen obstruction <50%. Grade 2 stenosis is lumen obstruction between 51 and 70%. Grade 3 stenosis is lumen obstruction between 71 and 99%.

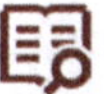

REFERENCE/SOURCE

- Kliegman RM, St Geme JW III, Blum NJ, Shah SS, Tasker RC, Wilson KM. Nelson Textbook of Pediatrics, 21st edition. Amsterdam: Elsevier; 2020. pp. 2208-9.

9. A 5-year-old unvaccinated girl presented with persistent hacking cough and was diagnosed with pertussis. Her 21 days, old male sibling was considered for prophylactic treatment by parents. He was also suspected of pyloric stenosis. Which of the following is the best medication for prophylaxis for pertussis in this neonate?

A. Cotrimoxazole
B. Erythromycin
C. Clarithromycin
D. Azithromycin

EXPLANATION

This is a case scenario where prophylaxis for a neonate with contact with pertussis is to be prescribed. In a neonate for prophylaxis of pertussis with suspected pyloric stenosis, erythromycin is contraindicated. Also cotrimoxazole may not be preferred due to risk of jaundice. Hence, the drug of choice will be azithromycin. Clarithromycin is not indicated for pertussis prophylaxis.

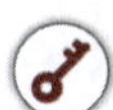

Key: D

BOOST YOUR KNOWLEDGE

Guidelines support targeting postexposure antibiotic use to people at high risk of developing severe pertussis, as well as people who will have close contact with others at high risk of developing severe pertussis. The recommended antimicrobial agents for treatment or chemoprophylaxis of pertussis are azithromycin, erythromycin, and trimethoprim-sulfamethoxazole. Clinicians should choose the antimicrobial after consideration of the potential for adverse events and drug interactions, tolerability, ease of adherence to the regimen prescribed, cost, and age. For infants younger than 1 month of age, use macrolides with caution as an association between orally administered erythromycin and azithromycin with infantile hypertrophic pyloric stenosis (IHPS) has been reported. However, azithromycin remains the drug of choice for treatment or prophylaxis of pertussis in very young infants because the risk of developing severe pertussis and life-threatening complications outweighs the potential risk of IHPS. Clinicians should monitor infants younger than 1 month of age who receive a macrolide for the development of IHPS and for other serious adverse events.

REFERENCE/SOURCE

- Kliegman RM, St Geme JW III, Blum NJ, Shah SS, Tasker RC, Wilson KM. Nelson Textbook of Pediatrics, 21st edition. Amsterdam: Elsevier; 2020. p. 1492.

10. A 10-year-old boy presented with fever, cough, and cold for 4 days. Fever resolved but nasal discharge and slight cough persisted even after 10 days of illness. The child could not concentrate on studies because of constant irritability and headache. On examination, there was nasal congestion and malodorous breath. The most appropriate treatment in this condition will be:

A. Reassurance and symptomatic treatment
B. Amoxicillin
C. Azithromycin
D. Montelukast in view of allergic rhinitis

EXPLANATION

After episode of upper respiratory infection persistent/redevelopment of symptoms such as nasal congestion and headache suggest acute bacterial sinusitis (ABS). *Haemophilus influenzae (nontypeable), Streptococcus pneumoniae*, and *Moraxella catarrhalis* are the major pathogens in uncomplicated ABS in otherwise healthy children. Hence amoxicillin remains the drug of choice. The drug of choice for treating ABS is amoxicillin or amoxiclav if beta-lactamase resistance is expected. This scenario does not indicate any previous history suggestive of allergic rhinosinusitis which may require montelukast.

Key: B

BOOST YOUR KNOWLEDGE

In the pediatric age group, approximately 7.5% of URIs are complicated by ABS. In complicated ABS, polymicrobial infections are common. The diagnosis of acute sinusitis is mainly clinical and based on stringent criteria, including persistent symptoms and signs of a URI beyond 10 days, without appreciable improvement; a URI with high fever and purulent nasal discharge at onset lasting for at least 3 consecutive days; and biphasic or worsening symptoms. The present consensus is that amoxicillin-clavulanate, at a standard dose of 45 mg/kg/day orally, is the drug of choice for most cases of uncomplicated ABS or oral amoxicillin 90 mg/kg/day may be administered.

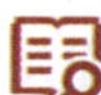

REFERENCE/SOURCE

- Kliegman RM, St Geme JW III, Blum NJ, Shah SS, Tasker RC, Wilson KM. Nelson Textbook of Pediatrics, 21st edition. Amsterdam: Elsevier; 2020. p. 2189.

11. What is true about RSV prophylaxis in children?

A. Nirsevimab is the new drug approved for use
B. Palivizumab prophylaxis prevents both upper and lower respiratory tract infections
C. Palivizumab is IgG4 monoclonal antibody recommended for children under 24 months of age with certain high-risk conditions
D. All of the above

EXPLANATION

Palivizumab is IgG1 antibody not IgG4 to prevent lower respiratory infections in children with high risk to infections. Palivizumab prophylaxis is not recommended for preventing URIs. Hence, answer is nirsevimab is the new drug approved for use.

Key: A

BOOST YOUR KNOWLEDGE

Respiratory syncytial virus is a virus that causes acute respiratory infection in individuals of all age groups. While most infants and young children experience mild, cold-like symptoms, some infants, especially with their first infection, develop lower respiratory tract disease such as pneumonia and bronchiolitis (swelling of the small airway passages in the lungs). Premature infants, and those with chronic lung disease of prematurity or significant congenital heart disease, are at highest risk for severe RSV disease.

Nirsevimab is a long-acting intramuscular recombinant neutralizing human IgG1κ monoclonal antibody to the prefusion conformation of the RSV-F protein that has been modified with a triple amino acid substitution in the Fc region to extend the serum half-life for the prevention of RSV disease. The extended serum half-life allows administration of nirsevimab as a single dose to cover the RSV season. Nirsevimab was approved in the EU and UK in 2022 for the prevention of RSV lower respiratory tract disease in neonates and infants during their first RSV season.

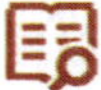

REFERENCE/SOURCE

- Kliegman RM, St Geme JW III, Blum NJ, Shah SS, Tasker RC, Wilson KM. Nelson Textbook of Pediatrics, 21st edition. Amsterdam: Elsevier; 2020. p. 1734.

12. A 2-month-old infant is brought with complaints of noisy breathing for 10 days with worsening on feeding or crying and improves slightly during sleep. On examination, there is inspiratory stridor and some suprasternal retractions. The most likely diagnosis is:

A. Severe SGS
B. Laryngomalacia
C. Lower airway collapse
D. Laryngeal cleft

EXPLANATION

In this scenario, the presence of inspiratory strider suggests airway obstruction. With an early onset of symptoms, the possibility of congenital disease is high. A stridor with improvement during sleep is suggestive of laryngomalacia in an infant. SGS would be associated with respiratory distress which would not improve with change in position. In the laryngeal cleft, a history of choking and aspirations must have been present. Lower airway collapse will not have stridor nut hypoxia and distress as predominant complaints.

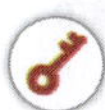

Key: B

BOOST YOUR KNOWLEDGE

Laryngomalacia is a common cause of congenital stridor. In laryngomalacia, the supraglottic structures are weak and they collapse into the airway during the inspiration resulting in stridor. It is a congenital condition although it may not appear until the first several days or weeks of life. Mostly the stridor in laryngomalacia is mild which resolves by itself by 12–24 months. However, the condition must be diagnosed and must be differentiated from other causes of stridor. The stridor in laryngomalacia worsens with agitation and with feeding but typically improves with sleep. Stridor may be the only symptom in mild cases of laryngomalacia. More severe cases also cause difficulty breathing and/or difficulty drinking. The diagnosis of laryngomalacia is best made by flexible fiber-optic laryngoscopy. Laryngomalacia is a "self-limited" condition since infants outgrow it, usually by 12–18 months of age. Approximately 15% of infants with laryngomalacia have severe enough airway or feeding problems requiring surgical treatment "supraglottoplasty".

REFERENCE/SOURCE

- Kliegman RM, St Geme JW III, Blum NJ, Shah SS, Tasker RC, Wilson KM. Nelson Textbook of Pediatrics, 21st edition. Amsterdam: Elsevier; 2020. p. 2207.

13. A 7-year-old boy child developed cough, cold, and fever. After treatment from pediatrician the fever resolved in 5 days but slight cough persisted. His mother complained that even after 4 weeks there is persistent cough with worsening at night leading to poor sleep. There was no past history of recurrent cough or sneezing in child or family. On examination, child had adenoid hypertrophy. The most probable diagnosis is:

A. Upper airway cough syndrome (UACS)
B. Allergic cough
C. Cough variant asthma
D. Somatic cough

EXPLANATION

In this scenario, it suggests that child had a URI which resolved in 5 days except persistence of cough. It is a common condition seen after an episode of URIs characterized by persistent cough worsening at night due to postnasal drip, etc., commonly now labeled as UACS.

Absence of previous history or in family rules out allergic disease/asthma.

Tuberculosis remains unlikely due to absence of fever, weight loss, and anorexia. Also cough in pulmonary tuberculosis usually is a wet cough. Dry cough may be seen in pleural or mediastinal disease.

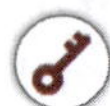

Key: A

BOOST YOUR KNOWLEDGE

In 2006, the American College of Chest Physicians (ACCP) defined UACS, previously referred to as postnasal drip syndrome (PNDS), as one of several critical pathogeneses of chronic cough. In UACS patients, cough can be caused by a variety of upper respiratory disorders, including nasal and sinus diseases. It can also result from anatomic abnormalities and physically- or chemically-induced rhinitis, as well as pharyngeal diseases. The criteria for diagnosing UACS/PNDS are: (1) paroxysmal or persistent cough, often in the daytime and rare after sleep; (2) history and clinical manifestations of nasal and/or throat conditions; (3) auxiliary tests supporting nasal and/or throat conditions; and (4) cough improves after specific therapy. Treatment should be determined based on potential conditions related to UACS/PNDS.

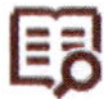

REFERENCE/SOURCE

- Kliegman RM, St Geme JW III, Blum NJ, Shah SS, Tasker RC, Wilson KM. Nelson Textbook of Pediatrics, 21st edition. Amsterdam: Elsevier; 2020. p. 2163.

14. A newborn had birth weight 1.5 kg and had ear anomalies, hypogonadism, and 7th cranial nerve palsy. The child had vigorous attempts to inspire and cyanosis which decreased on crying. What is the best immediate management strategy?

A. Establish oral airway/intubation/tracheostomy
B. Order for an echocardiology and chest X-ray
C. Mitomycin C
D. Oxygenation by nasal continuous positive airway pressure (CPAP)

EXPLANATION

In this case scenario, there is a description in which a neonate is born with low birth weight and has various anomalies in form of ear anomalies, gonadal under development, and respiratory difficulties. Cyanosis which improves on crying suggests rescue by mouth breathing and hence nasal anomalies like choanal atresia possibly bilateral. This child has genetic syndrome with choanal atresia, possibly CHARGE syndrome. In children with bilateral choanal atresia (BCA), priority step is establishing oral airway before definite surgery.

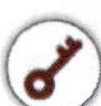

Key: A

BOOST YOUR KNOWLEDGE

Choanal atresia is lack of communication between the nasal cavity and nasopharynx. It is an uncommon condition leading to respiratory distress in a newborn. Unilateral cases are generally more common though asymptomatic and present with unilateral nasal discharge and persistent nasal obstruction after the first episode of URI in a newborn. BCA presents as medical emergency at birth. Newborn with BCA makes vigorous attempts to inspire, often sucks lips, and develops cyanosis. Distressed infant then cries and cyanosis disappears. Emergency airway management includes passage of oropharyngeal airway, orotracheal intubation or tracheostomy. The definitive treatment includes nasal recanalization through transpalatal or transnasal route.

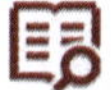

REFERENCE/SOURCE

- Kliegman RM, St Geme JW III, Blum NJ, Shah SS, Tasker RC, Wilson KM. Nelson Textbook of Pediatrics, 21st edition. Amsterdam: Elsevier; 2020.

15. A newborn, diagnosed of Arnold–Chiari malformation, developed respiratory distress, high-pitched inspiratory stridor, and weak cry. Most probable underlying associated condition would be:

A. Bilateral vocal cord palsy
B. Pneumonia
C. Bronchomalacia
D. Laryngomalacia

EXPLANATION

Bilateral vocal cord palsy commonly presents in children with Arnold–Chiari malformation, and meningomyelocele. Bilateral vocal cod palsy presents with respiratory distress, weak cry, and stridor. Vocal cord paralysis with inspiratory stridor during infancy is a complication of the Chiari II malformation associated with meningomyelocele, though rarely found with type I Chiari malformation. This develops with acute downward or upward displacement of the malformed brainstem secondary to increased or decreased intracranial pressure.

Children with bronchomalacia and laryngomalacia may present with stridor and respiratory distress rather than voice abnormalities. Newborns with pneumonia present with fever, fast breathing, and respiratory failure rather voice abnormalities.

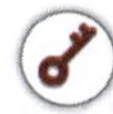

Key: A

BOOST YOUR KNOWLEDGE

The diagnosis of bilateral vocal cord palsy is established by direct laryngoscopy performed without general anesthesia. Most common cause of vocal cord palsy may be iatrogenic trauma during thoracic surgery or underlying neurological condition with documented or suspected intracranial hypertension.

The Chiari malformations are a rare group of congenital abnormalities involving the hindbrain and spinal cord. Herniation of the cerebellar tonsils through the foramen magnum into the cervical spinal canal places the spinal cord under pressure. The type 1 Chiari malformation or adult Chiari malformation has its primary feature herniation of the cerebellar tonsils through the foramen magnum into the cervical spinal canal with obliteration of the cerebellomedullary cistern but no meningomyelocele associated. The type 2 Chiari malformation has a meningomyelocele associated with it and typically presents early in the pediatric population.

REFERENCE/SOURCE

- Kliegman RM, St Geme JW III, Blum NJ, Shah SS, Tasker RC, Wilson KM. Nelson Textbook of Pediatrics, 21st edition. Amsterdam: Elsevier; 2020. p. 2208.

16. **A 16-year-old girl developed cough and cold for 5 days. She remained well for 2 days but then developed fever, throat pain, difficulty in swallowing food, and fast breathing. On examination, she was hypoxic and oral examination showed deviation of uvula and bulge on lateral pharyngeal wall. Despite adequate antibiotics, she developed septic thrombophlebitis of internal jugular vein and lung cavitation. Which of the following is the most likely etiological organism?**

A. *Fusobacterium necrophorum*
B. *Escherichia coli*
C. Adenovirus
D. *Bordetella pertussis*

EXPLANATION

In this scenario, the child had minor upper respiratory infection, redevelopment of symptoms, and clinical picture parapharyngeal abscess (swallowing difficulties, deviation of uvula, and deviation of lateral pharyngeal wall). Development of septic thrombophlebitis of internal jugular vein suggests complication like Lemierre's syndrome. Most common organism for this is *Fusobacterium*.

Group A beta-hemolytic *Streptococcus* is known to cause tonsillopharyngitis and rheumatic fever. Adenovirus may cause infections of respiratory tract both upper and lower but unlikely cause of septic thrombophlebitis of internal jugular vein. *E. coli* is an unusual organism for upper airway infections in otherwise healthy children or causing Lemierre syndrome.

Key: B

BOOST YOUR KNOWLEDGE

Lemierre's syndrome is a rare and potentially severe complication of bacterial infections that usually affects previously healthy adolescents and young adults. It most commonly develops in association with a bacterial throat infection, but it may develop in association with an infection involving the ears, salivary glands (parotitis), sinuses, or teeth; or in association with an Epstein–Barr infection.

In people with Lemierre's syndrome, the initial infection spreads into tissues and deep spaces within the neck, leading to the formation of an infected blot clot (septic thrombophlebitis), sometimes made up of pus, in the internal jugular vein. The infected clot then circulates in the blood, resulting in the infection also spreading to the lungs (most commonly), skeletal system, and/or other parts of the body such as the spleen, liver, kidney, heart, or brain. This can lead to severe complications such as respiratory distress syndrome due to pulmonary embolism damage to other affected organs, and/or septic shock (in about 7% of cases).

Lemierre syndrome may be diagnosed based on signs and symptoms, various blood tests, and imaging studies. The most common causative agent of Lemierre's syndrome is *Fusobacterium necrophorum*, followed by *Fusobacterium nucleatum* and aerobic bacteria such as streptococci, staphylococci, and *Klebsiella pneumoniae*.

REFERENCE/SOURCE

- Kliegman RM, St Geme JW III, Blum NJ, Shah SS, Tasker RC, Wilson KM. Nelson Textbook of Pediatrics, 21st edition. Amsterdam: Elsevier; 2020. p. 2198.

17. **A mother bought his 6-year-old child with a history of pulling of right ear infrequently. On examination, the tympanic membrane was pearly white and mildly retracted; and malleus was visible. Which of the following is the correct diagnosis?**

A. Acute otitis media
B. Normal ear
C. Serous otitis media
D. Chronic otitis media

EXPLANATION

Pulling of ear may also be seen in a normal child. When this is associated with fever and other symptoms such as cough, nasal discharge, earache, and crying it is more suggestive of disease like acute and serous otitis media. In children with chronic otitis media, there is often a history of scant foul-smelling discharge and deafness.

Pearly white tympanic membrane with visible malleus is a normal finding. In diseased condition, the tympanic membrane may be bulging, fluid collections, and perforation with invisible malleus.

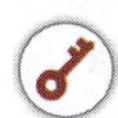

Key: B

BOOST YOUR KNOWLEDGE

Otoscopy is the cornerstone for diagnosing acute and chronic ear conditions. Two types of otoscope heads can be used to evaluate the ears: (1) Surgical or operating and (2) diagnostic or pneumatic. By inspecting the ears, the degree of tympanic membrane mobility in response to negative or positive pressure can be evaluated to assess for fluid in the middle ear, a hallmark of otitis media. Other abnormalities in the tympanic membrane found are erythema, bulging or fullness, or extreme retraction.

In acute otitis media, the tympanic membrane may appear bulging, erythematous with indistinct landmarks, and displacement of the light reflex. Air insufflation (pneumatic otoscopy) shows poor mobility of the tympanic membrane. Spontaneous perforation of the tympanic membrane causes serosanguineous or purulent otorrhea. In chronic suppurative otitis media, the tympanic membrane is perforated and draining, and the auditory canal is macerated and littered with granulation tissue. Symptoms include painless otorrhea with conductive hearing loss. Complications include development of aural polyps, cholesteatoma, and other infections.

REFERENCE/SOURCE

- Kliegman RM, St Geme JW III, Blum NJ, Shah SS, Tasker RC, Wilson KM. Nelson Textbook of Pediatrics, 21st edition. Amsterdam: Elsevier; 2020. p. 3418.

18. Which of the following is the mainstay of treatment in mild croup?

A. Salbutamol nebulization
B. Oral/injectable dexamethasone
C. Subcutaneous epinephrine/nebulization
D. Antibiotics

EXPLANATION

Dexamethasone, given orally as a single dose at 0.6 mg/kg, is highly efficacious in treating croup symptoms and reduces swelling in the airway. Nebulized epinephrine is recommended for moderate-to-severe croup as additional therapy with steroids. As the onset of action of steroids is delayed, epinephrine nebulization with rapid and short-lived onset of action is helpful in moderate and severe cases. Antibiotics agonists have no role. Nebulized salbutamol is also of no use.

Key: B

BOOST YOUR KNOWLEDGE

Croup or viral LTB is one of the frequent causes of stridor. Highest incidence among the preschool children (6 months to 3 years of age) occurs during the autumn and winter months. Less than 5% of children with croup require hospitalization and among those hospitalized only 1–2% require intensive care. It is characterized by sudden onset of barky cough, hoarse voice, inspiratory stridor, and respiratory distress caused by upper airway inflammation secondary to a viral infection. Croup is caused by viral infections of the respiratory tract and most commonly by parainfluenza types 1 and 3 viruses, influenza A and B, adenovirus, RSV, and metapneumovirus.

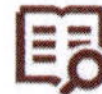

REFERENCE/SOURCE

- Kliegman RM, St Geme JW III, Blum NJ, Shah SS, Tasker RC, Wilson KM. Nelson Textbook of Pediatrics, 21st edition. Amsterdam: Elsevier; 2020. p. 2202.

19. A 13-year-old girl presented with a 2-year history of episodic wheezing, cough, and shortness of breath presented to pediatric emergency. In the past, he had 2 emergency department visits for wheezing. He also had a 1-year history of recurrent otitis media and persistent purulent nasal discharge. He had antineutrophil cytoplasm antibodies (ANCAs) which were proteinase 3-positive. What is the most common abnormality likely to be reported on bronchoscopy?

A. SGS
B. Laryngomalacia
C. Papilloma
D. Hemangiomas

EXPLANATION

This case scenario describes the classical scenario of upper airway involvement with ear and nose involvement in a wheezing child with recurrent symptoms. The most likely diagnosis is granulomatosis with polyangiitis (Wegener's) (GPA). The positivity in serum for antibodies confirms this diagnosis. Hemangioma, papilloma, and laryngomalacia are not classical abnormalities described in GPA.

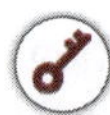

Key: A

BOOST YOUR KNOWLEDGE

Granulomatosis with polyangiitis (Wegener's) is a small vessel necrotizing granulomatous vasculitis. Ear, nose, and throat (ENT), lung, and kidney are the most frequently involved organs. Tracheobronchial stenoses (TBSs) are potentially severe manifestations of GPA. SGS is the most frequent TBS type that could be related to anatomic specificities and pathophysiological mechanisms.

REFERENCE/SOURCE

- Kliegman RM, St Geme JW III, Blum NJ, Shah SS, Tasker RC, Wilson KM. Nelson Textbook of Pediatrics, 21st edition. Amsterdam: Elsevier; 2020. p. 2213.

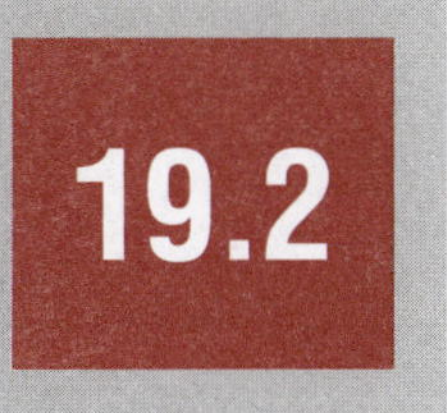

CHAPTER 19.2 Congenital Malformations of the Respiratory Tract and Foreign Bodies

NK Subramanya

1. A 4-year-old child presents with recurrent pneumonia (three episodes in the past 2 years). In the first episode, the child was hospitalized with a history of respiratory distress and X-ray as shown in first figure. The symptoms apparently improved after hospitalization and antibiotics for 1 week. The second episode occurred after 3 months and was again treated in the same hospital with similar plan, and X-ray findings are shown in second figure. The child apparently improved after 1 week. The current hospitalization for fever and respiratory distress with X-ray (third figure) is under evaluation. The growth of the child is apparently normal.

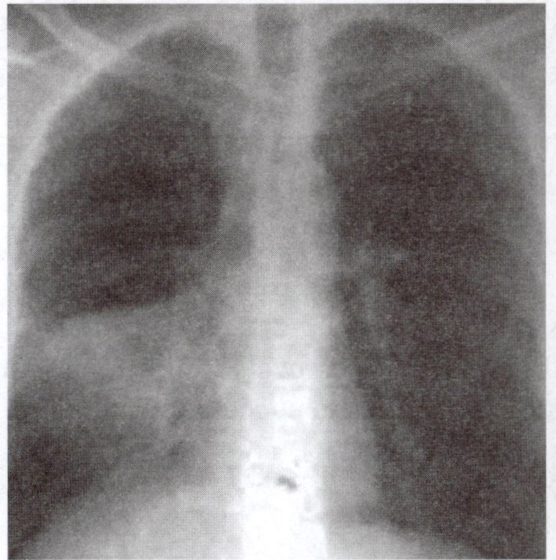

First figure: First admission

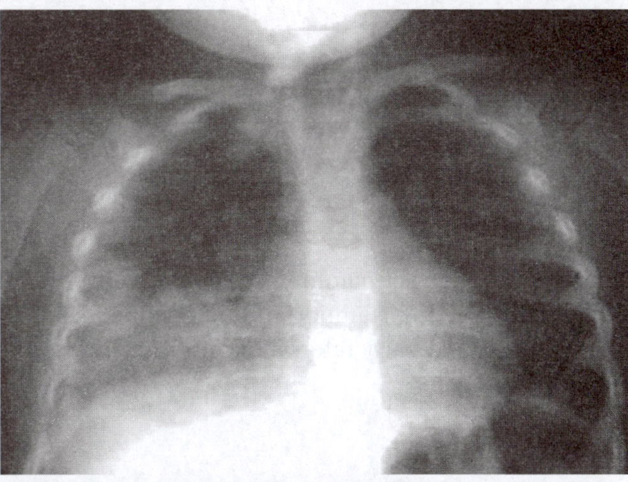

Second figure: Second admission

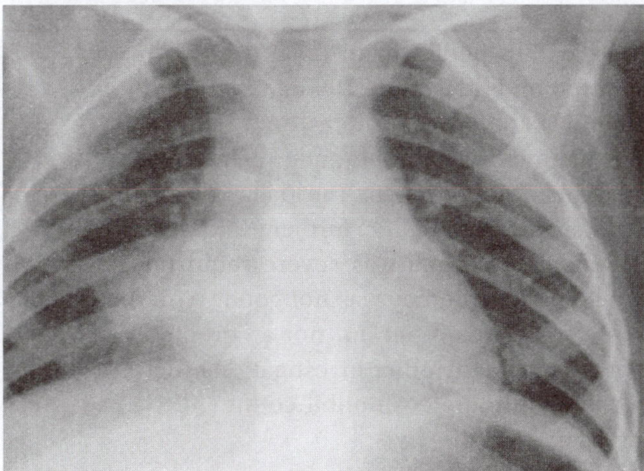

Third figure: Current admission

What is the most probable etiology of recurrent pneumonia?

A. Immunodeficiency
B. Cystic fibrosis
C. Foreign body (FB) in airways
D. Swyer-James syndrome

EXPLANATION

The key features in clinical presentation are: (1) Young age at onset, (2) recurrent pneumonia in the same lobe, and (3) resolution with treatment in each episode.

Let us analyze these characteristics for each of the four options:

Options	*Age of presentation*	*Recurrent pneumonia*	*Typical features*	*Current case*
A. Immunodeficiency	Any age depending on the subtype	Multilobar presentation and multisystem involvement	Recurrent pneumonia, diarrhea, and failure to thrive (FTT)	Unilobar
B. Cystic fibrosis	Newborn to any age	Bilateral airway disease	Recurrent pneumonia, diarrhea, and FTT	Unilobar
C. Foreign body in airways	Toddlers, however, should not be excluded by age	Recurrent pneumonia in same lobe or segment	Acute, subacute, recurrent or persistent symptoms, and signs of lower respiratory disease depending on the type and lodging of the FB	Unilobar
D. Swyer-James syndrome	Pediatric age	Unilateral hyperlucency on X-ray		Unilobar

Foreign body is the only option that satisfies all the parameters needed for the diagnosis.

Key: C

BOOST YOUR KNOWLEDGE

Foreign body aspiration is a common accident among toddlers in our country.

The history of choking is important but may be forgotten by mothers or by evaluating pediatricians. A high index of suspicion and early referral to prevent bronchiectasis are the keys to success. FB should be removed by bronchoscopy.

REFERENCE/SOURCE

- Subramanya NK, Gupta MH. IAP NRC Textbook of Paediatric Pulmonology, 1st edition. Noble Vision; 2023.

2. An 8-year-old child presents with a pediatrician diagnosed with asthma. The pediatrician started on budesonide 100 μg twice daily with metered dose inhaler (MDI) and spacer. The asthma remains uncontrolled despite good technique and adherence to therapy. The recurrent wheezing has been going on for the past 5 years. The pediatrician decided to revisit the diagnosis. On further evaluation, it was found that the first attack of asthma was severe requiring hospitalization. Response to long-term therapy was not good. When the child took relievers, there was some relief but not a complete cure. The chest X-ray is shown here. Many other investigations such as complete blood count (CBC), absolute eosinophil count (AEC), and immunoglobulin E (IgE) were normal.

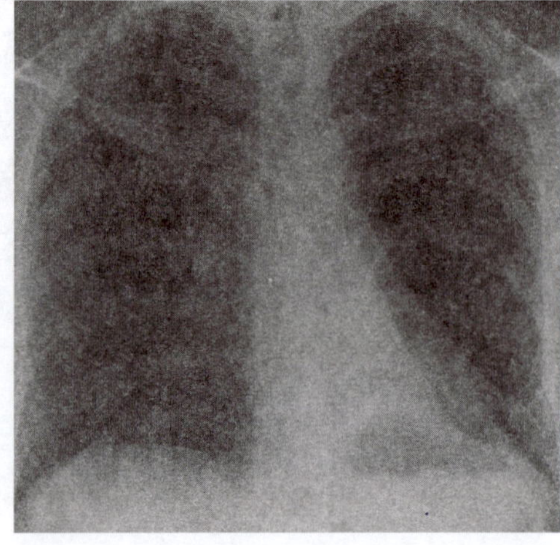

What is the most probable cause of uncontrolled wheezing?

A. Inadequate treatment, needs to step-up the dose of inhalational corticosteroids
B. Poor compliance, needs supervised therapy
C. FB in airways
D. Therapy-resistant asthma

EXPLANATION

The key features in clinical presentation are: (1) age of onset of wheeze, (2) not responding to inhaled corticosteroid (ICS) or bronchodilators, and (3) chest X-ray findings.

Let us analyze these characteristics for each of the four options:

Options	*Typical features*	*Current case*
A. Uncontrolled asthma, needs to step up the dose of inhalational corticosteroids	Check diagnosis, device, drug, dose, technique, and adherence to therapy	Looks that all have been revisited and fine
B. Poor compliance	Only if there are issues listed above	We need to achieve control, which failed, and we should revise the approach
C. Foreign body in airways	Acute, subacute, recurrent, or persistent symptoms and signs of lower respiratory disease depending on the type and lodging of the FB	There is a left lower lobe collapse. The collapsed margin is retrocardiac. Foreign body in left lower lobe bronchus is likely.
D. Therapy-resistant asthma	True therapy-resistant phenotypes are rare and require referral to a pulmonologist	Should be the last resort

Foreign body in left lower lobe bronchus is the only option that satisfies all the parameters for the diagnosis.

Key: C

BOOST YOUR KNOWLEDGE

The diagnosis of uncontrolled asthma should be revisited. Generally, asthma responds well to bronchodilators or steroids if the diagnosis is correct. The evaluation requires a good history and careful examination which may reveal missed information. The onset of wheeze was an acute episode in the toddler age group. Chest X-ray may or may not help in every case but must be done since it can be valuable in this case. Forgotten FB aspiration is more common than we think. A high index of suspicion and early referral are the keys to success. FB should be removed by bronchoscopy.

REFERENCE/SOURCE

- Subramanya NK, Gupta MH. IAP NRC Textbook of Paediatric Pulmonology, 1st edition. Noble Vision; 2023.

3. A 3-year-old child presents with acute respiratory distress following upper respiratory symptoms, including cold and coryza but no fever. The child was started on supportive oxygen in the mask to correct hypoxia. The attending resident calls up the consultant and plans to treat based on the management of croup since there was an audible stridor. However, the child started deteriorating despite dexamethasone and adrenaline nebulization.

Which is the most probable diagnosis *missed* in this situation if the diagnosis of croup is incorrect?

A. Tracheomalacia
B. Subglottic stenosis
C. FB in airways
D. Pertussis

EXPLANATION

The key features in clinical presentation are: (1) acute episode, (2) upper airway obstruction, and (3) clinical deterioration.

Let us analyze these characteristics for each of the four options:

Options	*Typical features*	*Current case*
A. Tracheomalacia	Monophonic wheeze, not stridor. Generally recurrent or persistent symptoms than acute episodes	Not consistent
B. Subglottic stenosis	History of intubation, persistent or chronic symptoms than acute presentation	Acute episode (not chronic or recurrent symptoms)
C. Foreign body in airways	Upper airway FB should be considered a close differential for a croup worsening	Stridor does not respond to therapy and the condition of the child is deteriorating consistently
D. Pertussis	Bouts of cough, whoop, and no stridor	Unlikely

Foreign body is the only option that satisfies all the parameters for the diagnosis.

Key: C

BOOST YOUR KNOWLEDGE

Croup is common; however, it should be revisited for diagnosis if there is a deterioration or severe in presentation. Upper airway obstructions are life-threatening at times. The evaluation requires a good history and careful examination which may reveal missed information. The onset of stridor was an acute episode in the toddler age group. FB aspiration should always be thought of in life-threatening upper airway obstruction. A high index of suspicion and early referral are the keys to success. FB should be removed by bronchoscopy.

REFERENCE/SOURCE

- Subramanya NK, Gupta MH. IAP NRC Textbook of Paediatric Pulmonology, 1st edition. Noble Vision; 2023.

4. A 3-year-old child presents to the emergency room (ER) with a history of choking. The resident suspects FB in the airways. The child has bilateral wheeze not responding to salbutamol inhalation. The resident orders a chest X-ray which is normal. What is the most correct approach to the case?

A. Continue O_2, wait and watch, and repeat X-ray after 6 hours
B. Add steroids and antibiotics
C. Refer for a diagnostic flexible bronchoscopy
D. Call an ENT surgeon for a rigid bronchoscopy

EXPLANATION

In view of the history of choking, FB is most likely. There is no point in waiting. X-ray of chest may be normal in many FBs if they are radiolucent or if they do not cause anatomical changes such as atelectasis or localized emphysema. There is also no role of steroids or antibiotics since there are no pointers to any infection. Therapeutic options for bronchoscopy removal of FB should be sought from an expert in the field. Though there are reports of removal by flexible bronchoscopy, the gold standard is rigid bronchoscopy and removal of FB.

Key: D

BOOST YOUR KNOWLEDGE

Foreign body removal should be done by a rigid bronchoscopy. Some experienced centers or experts report the removal by flexible scopy but should not be the ideal practice. If the FB is found incidentally in a diagnostic flexible bronchoscopic evaluation, an attempt to remove it can be made. If the procedure fails, it should be referred to a surgeon for rigid bronchoscopy.

REFERENCE/SOURCE

- Subramanya NK, Gupta MH. IAP NRC Textbook of Paediatric Pulmonology, 1st edition. Noble Vision; 2023.

5. A 4-year-old child thought to be a suspected case of pulmonary tuberculosis (TB) was referred for a second opinion. The symptoms are persistent wet cough of 3 weeks duration with no findings on chest examination. Routine investigations, or microbiological tests for TB, and chest X-ray were normal.

What is the most correct approach to the case?

A. Do spirometry
B. Repeat all tests again
C. Diagnostic flexible bronchoscopy
D. Start empirical antituberculosis treatment (ATT)

EXPLANATION

The key features in clinical presentation are: (1) TB unlikely situation and (2) wet cough which cannot be ignored.

Let us analyze these characteristics for each of the four options:

Options	*Considerations*	*Current case*
A. Do spirometry	Chronic cough should be considered for spirometry above 6 years of age	• A good option for dry cough, less helpful in wet cough • The age of 4 years makes the option incorrect
B. Repeat all tests again	We should order tests based on history, not repeat tests blindly to get confused	Repeat tests will not help unless the earlier tests are not from a good laboratory or with a good effort
C. Diagnostic flexible bronchoscopy	The flexible bronchoscopy will reveal a diagnosis of FB, protracted bacterial bronchitis, or evidence of endobronchial TB or bronchoalveolar lavage (BAL). Wet cough is also a potential for bronchiectasis if ignored	This case revealed a carinal FB; however, other diagnoses are possible
D. Start empirical ATT	No role in National Tuberculosis Elimination Programme (NTEP) unless it is a "Clinically diagnosed TB" as a last resort after thorough evaluation by an expert or institution	Not advisable

The correct approach is diagnostic flexible bronchoscopy and other options unlikely.

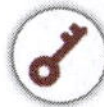

Key: C

BOOST YOUR KNOWLEDGE

A persistent wet cough should be evaluated since ignoring the cause will prove costly as it may end-up having bronchiectasis. Repeated attempts for microbiological diagnosis of TB by sputum evaluation are a good practice even from better specimens like BAL. The confirmation of diagnosis of TB is a prerequisite for starting ATT.

REFERENCE/SOURCE

- Subramanya NK, Gupta MH. IAP NRC Textbook of Paediatric Pulmonology, 1st edition. Noble Vision; 2023.

6. A 3-year-old child was referred to you with "persistent pneumonia" not responding to intravenous (IV) antibiotics after hospitalization for 1 week. The X-ray of the chest is shown below on Days 1 and 8 of the treatment. The child is having minimal symptoms at the end of 1 week. What is the most correct approach to the case?

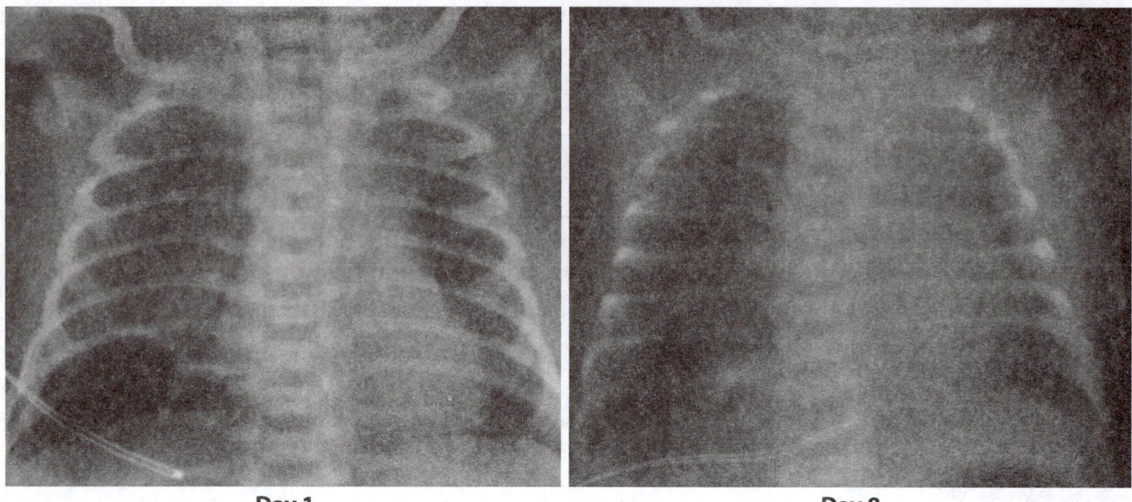

Day 1 Day 8

A. Change antibiotics and work-up for TB
B. Do a bronchoscopy first then a CT scan of the chest
C. Do a CT scan and review
D. Do ultrasonography (USG) of the chest and lateral chest X-ray

EXPLANATION

The key features in clinical presentation are: (1) persistent pneumonia and (2) suggestive chest X-ray.

Let us analyze these characteristics for each of the four options:

A. Any persistent pneumonia can be considered TB in our country. However, we should not change antibiotics without a proper re-evaluation.
B. Airway symptoms (like a persistent cough), and not parenchymal symptoms, should prompt bronchoscopy followed by CT scan.
C. Persistent pneumonia not fitting into a prototype of pneumonia should be considered for alternative diagnosis like congenital cystic adenomatoid malformation. CT is a good option for other considerations.
D. USG of the chest and lateral chest X-ray may not yield more information on Day 8 unless pleuropulmonary diseases or parenchymal diseases are close to the chest wall.

The correct approach is to do a bronchoscopy first then a CT of the chest.

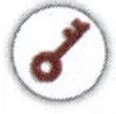

Key: B

BOOST YOUR KNOWLEDGE

Foreign body removal should be done by a rigid bronchoscopy. Some experienced centers or experts report the removal by flexible scope, but this should not be the practice ideally. If the FB is found incidentally in a diagnostic flexible bronchoscopic evaluation, an attempt at removal can be made. If the procedure fails, it should be referred to a surgeon for rigid bronchoscopy.

REFERENCE/SOURCE

- Subramanya NK, Gupta MH. IAP NRC Textbook of Paediatric Pulmonology, 1st edition. Noble Vision; 2023.

7. A 1-year-old child presents with an inspiratory stridor that started from 2 months of age. Noise is heard more during inspiration, while feeding, and with a supine position and flexing of neck. There are no episodes of spells or hypoxia or hospitalizations. Feeding and sleep are without any disturbance. The child is thriving well and immunized. What is the most appropriate diagnosis?

A. Laryngomalacia
B. Choanal atresia
C. Vascular rings
D. Subglottic FB

EXPLANATION

Laryngomalacia refers to a floppy larynx. Mild laryngomalacia is characterized by inspiratory stridor. SpO_2 is 98–100%. There may be occasional regurgitation or cough. There is no hypoxia or feeding disturbance. Choanal atresia presents at birth. Vascular rings are unlikely in a child who is a thriving child. Subglottic FB is also unlikely because of a very young age, and no episodes of recurrent symptoms or the persistence of airway symptoms or hospitalizations.

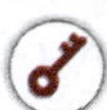

Key: A

BOOST YOUR KNOWLEDGE

Laryngomalacia is the most common cause of stridor and accounts for 60% of all causes of stridor in otherwise healthy infants. Nearly 10–20% of infants with laryngomalacia will have severe symptoms such as feeding problems, recurrent aspiration, cyanosis, apnea, and hypoxemia, resulting in FTT. Mild laryngomalacia, such as in this case, just needs reassurance.

REFERENCE/SOURCE

- Subramanya NK, Gupta MH. IAP NRC Textbook of Paediatric Pulmonology, 1st edition. Noble Vision; 2023.

8. A 4-year-old asymptomatic child has undergone chest X-ray as preoperative evaluation for anesthesia. The chest X-ray is shown here. What is the most likely diagnosis?

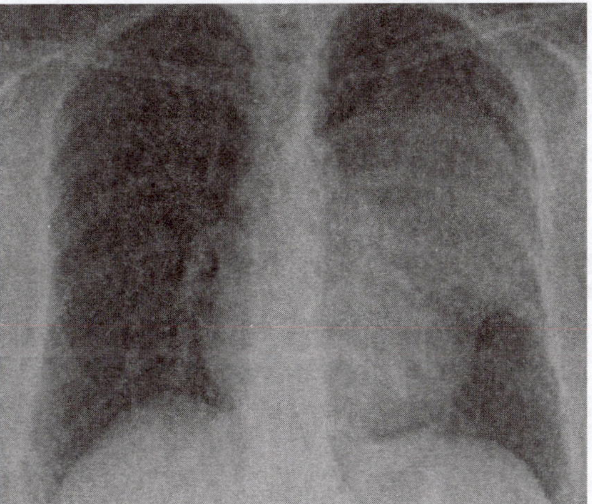

A. Bronchogenic cyst
B. Diaphragmatic hernia
C. Aortic aneurysm
D. Hilar lymphadenopathy

EXPLANATION

The chest X-ray reveals a round shadow on the left side in an asymptomatic child.

- Bronchogenic cysts are usually asymptomatic. It can become symptomatic by infection or obstruction inside the thorax. It is the most likely option for this child because of an asymptomatic, round shadow with well-defined margins.
- Diaphragmatic hernia can be asymptomatic or symptomatic. However, in the X-ray, both hemidiaphragms are clearly seen. The lower part of the shadow is convex, and no intestinal patterns are seen.
- Aortic aneurysm will silhouette the shadow with an aortic configuration. It is X-ray, and the descending aorta can be seen separately, not silhouetting the round shadow.
- Hilar lymphadenopathy is usually symptomatic or may cause airway compressions.

Key: A

BOOST YOUR KNOWLEDGE

A bronchogenic cyst is a closed sac made of respiratory epithelium. It may constitute 14–22% of lung cysts and 10% of mediastinal masses in children. About 20% of bronchogenic cysts can be asymptomatic. Rupture of cyst can cause pneumothorax.

REFERENCE/SOURCE

- Subramanya NK, Gupta MH. IAP NRC Textbook of Paediatric Pulmonology, 1st edition. Noble Vision; 2023.

9. A newborn presented with respiratory distress at birth with cyanosis. Cyanosis improves with intermittent crying. What is the most likely diagnosis?

A. Unilateral choanal atresia
B. Bilateral choanal atresia
C. Bilateral vocal cord palsy
D. Diaphragmatic hernia

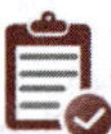

EXPLANATION

Unilateral choanal atresia may be asymptomatic. It can become symptomatic by upper respiratory tract infection. Bilateral choanal atresia is characterized by intermittent cyanosis relieved by crying or mouth opening. Cyanosis relieved by crying makes it to be the most likely diagnosis. Bilateral vocal cord palsy is unlikely as it presents with stridor or phonation abnormalities. In diaphragmatic hernia, neonatal distress worsens with crying than improvement with crying. Bilateral choanal atresia is the most likely diagnosis compared to other options.

Key: B

BOOST YOUR KNOWLEDGE

Choanal atresia can be bony or cartilaginous. The assessment of bony portion requires a CT scan apart from clinical evaluation. Bilateral disease is an emergency while unilateral atresia can be asymptomatic. The management of the oropharyngeal airway followed by surgery is the treatment of choice.

REFERENCE/SOURCE

- Subramanya NK, Gupta MH. IAP NRC Textbook of Paediatric Pulmonology, 1st edition. Noble Vision; 2023.

CHAPTER

19.3 Pneumonia including Air Leaks and Pleural Effusion

Jagdish P Goyal

1. **A 4-year-old human immunodeficiency virus (HIV)-positive child presented in the emergency room (ER) with complaints of cough and fever for 5 days. On examination, the child had tachycardia, tachypnea, and cyanosis. Auscultation revealed bilateral diffuse crackles. What is the most likely etiology of his pneumonia?**

A. *Streptococcus pneumoniae*
B. *Mycoplasma pneumoniae*
C. Respiratory syncytial virus (RSV)
D. *Pneumocystis jirovecii*

EXPLANATION

In HIV-infected patients, *Pneumocystis jirovecii* symptoms are often more abrupt, with fever, tachypnea, dyspnea, and cough, progressing to severe respiratory compromise. This type accounts for most cases, although the severity of clinical expression can vary. The child may sometimes not have crackles on auscultation.

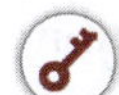

Key: D

BOOST YOUR KNOWLEDGE

Pneumocystis jirovecii is the most common cause of opportunistic pneumonia in HIV-infected children. Chest X-ray reveals bilateral diffuse interstitial or alveolar ground glass infiltrates. Definitive diagnosis requires demonstrating *P. jirovecii* in the lung in the presence of clinical signs and symptoms of the infection. Organisms can be detected in specimens collected by bronchoalveolar lavage (BAL), tracheal aspirate, transbronchial lung biopsy, bronchial brushings, percutaneous transthoracic needle aspiration, and open lung biopsy. Specimen can be stained with Grocott–Gömöri silver stain and toluidine blue stain for the cyst form, polychrome stains such as Giemsa stain or the trophozoites and sporozoites, and the fluorescein-labeled monoclonal antibody stains for both trophozoites and cysts. The recommended treatment for *Pneumocystis jirovecii* pneumonia is trimethoprim-sulfamethoxazole for 3 weeks in HIV-infected patients.

REFERENCE/SOURCE

- Gigliotti F, Wright TW. *Pneumocystis jirovecii*. In: Kliegman RM, St Geme JW III, Blum NJ, Shah SS, Tasker RC, Wilson KM (Eds). Nelson Textbook of Pediatrics, 21st edition. Amsterdam: Elsevier; 2020. pp. 1662-4.

2. **A 7-year-old presented with history of cough, coryza, fever, and headache for 7 days. Examination of the chest reveals crepitations, localized wheeze, and small areas of dullness to percussion over atelectatic areas or fluid collection. The child also had skin rashes, arthralgia, and hemolytic anemia. What is the most likely cause of her pneumonia?**

A. *Staphylococcal pneumoniae*
B. *Mycoplasma pneumoniae*
C. *Streptococcal pneumoniae*
D. *Klebsiella pneumoniae*

EXPLANATION

Usually, *Mycoplasma pneumoniae* starts as influenza-like syndrome with the predominant symptoms being fever, malaise, headache, scratchy sore throat, and cough. The temperature rarely exceeds 38.5°C. The symptoms in mycoplasma infection are much worse than what the physical signs will suggest. Examination of the chest may be unrevealing or reveal crepitations, localized wheeze, and small areas of dullness to percussion over atelectatic areas or fluid collection. Various nonrespiratory features of mycoplásma infection are skin rashes, arthralgia, hemolytic anemia, muscle tenderness, and central nervous system involvement including acute cerebritis, aseptic meningitis, cerebellar ataxia, transverse myelitis, and Guillain–Barré syndrome.

Key: B

BOOST YOUR KNOWLEDGE

Most *M. pneumoniae* infections are asymptomatic, and most of them occur in children and adolescents. Tracheobronchitis and atypical pneumonia are the commonly recognized clinical syndromes associated with *M. pneumoniae*. The best method for diagnosis is a combination of polymerase chain reaction (PCR) from respiratory samples and serology. *M. pneumoniae* is typically sensitive to macrolides (erythromycin, clarithromycin, and azithromycin), tetracyclines, and quinolones.

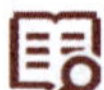

REFERENCE/SOURCE

- Mejias A, Ramilo O. Mycoplasma pneumoniae. In: Kliegman RM, St Geme JW III, Blum NJ, Shah SS, Tasker RC, Wilson KM (Eds). Nelson Textbook of Pediatrics, 21st edition. Amsterdam: Elsevier; 2020. pp. 1609-11.

3. A 3-year-old child presented with history of cough, fever, and respiratory difficulty for 4 days. On examination, you observed bronchial breathing on the right side. Chest X-ray revealed right middle lobe consolidation. Which of the following will be the antibiotic of choice in this case?

A. Aminoglycoside
B. Ciprofloxacin
C. Amoxicillin
D. Azithromycin

EXPLANATION

Pneumococcal pneumonia is the most common cause of pneumonia in children. The typical lobar involvement also suggests the possibility of pneumococcal pneumonia. The drug of choice for pneumococcal pneumonia is amoxicillin.

Key: C

BOOST YOUR KNOWLEDGE

The empiric treatment of suspected bacterial pneumonia in a hospitalized child requires an approach based on local epidemiology, the immunization status of the child, and the clinical manifestations at the time of presentation. In areas without substantial high-level penicillin resistance among *S. pneumoniae*, children who are fully immunized against *Haemophilus influenzae* type b and *S. pneumoniae* and are not severely ill should receive ampicillin or penicillin G.

REFERENCE/SOURCE

- Kelly MS, Sandora TJ. Community-Acquired Pneumonia. In: Kliegman RM, St Geme JW III, Blum NJ, Shah SS, Tasker RC, Wilson KM (Eds). Nelson Textbook of Pediatrics, 21st edition. Amsterdam: Elsevier; 2020. p. 2271.

4. An infant presented with complaints of cough, fever, and difficulty in respiration following viral prodrome. You ordered an X-ray, which revealed hyperinflation, interstitial infiltrates, and peribronchial thickening. What is the most likely etiology of his pneumonia?

A. Respiratory syncytial virus (RSV)
B. *Staphylococcus aureus*
C. *H. influenzae*
D. *Streptococcus pneumoniae*

EXPLANATION

Respiratory syncytial virus is the most common cause of viral pneumonia in an infant. The typical age and characteristic X-ray findings point toward RSV pneumonia. Pneumococcal pneumonia classically presents with a more focal infiltrate with consolidation, is unilateral, and is not associated with wheezing. *Mycoplasma* infections are not expected at this age.

Key: A

BOOST YOUR KNOWLEDGE

Respiratory syncytial virus is the etiologic agent in about 70% of patients with bronchiolitis and results in approximately 70,000 inpatient admissions yearly in the United States. Congestive heart failure likely would be associated with other physical findings such as hepatomegaly or have demonstrable cardiomegaly on the chest radiograph. Respiratory distress syndrome typically has a ground-glass appearance on chest radiography and presents with more severe clinical symptoms.

REFERENCE/SOURCE

- Kelly MS, Sandora TJ. Community-acquired pneumonia. In: Kliegman RM, St Geme JW III, Blum NJ, Shah SS, Tasker RC, Wilson KM (Eds). Nelson Textbook of Pediatrics, 21st edition. Amsterdam: Elsevier; 2020. p. 2271.

5. An immunocompromised infant presented with pneumonia, it was diagnosed as cytomegalovirus (CMV) pneumonia. Which of the following is true regarding CMV pneumonia?

A. CMV-DNA in biopsy tissue can be of great value in establishing CMV
B. Immunoglobulin M (IgM) cannot be used to reliably estimate the duration of infection
C. Intravenous (IV) ganciclovir is used for the treatment of CMV pneumonia
D. All of the above

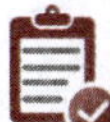

EXPLANATION

The diagnosis of CMV can be established by sequential viral load measurement by PCR in relevant body fluid and measurement of CMV-DNA in biopsy tissue. The presence of immunoglobulin G (IgG) antibody to CMV does not provide evidence of acute infection. In addition, IgM reactivity for CMV can be detected for prolonged periods after acute infection and cannot be used to reliably estimate the duration of infection.

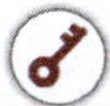

Key: D

BOOST YOUR KNOWLEDGE

Treatment of immunocompromised hosts with invasive CMV disease has been shown to limit both the morbidity and mortality in the patient with disseminated CMV infections with end-organ disease. This has been shown in allograft transplant recipients and patients with HIV/acquired immunodeficiency syndrome (AIDS). Similarly, antiviral prophylaxis can limit the development of clinically important CMV disease in allograft recipients and is the standard of care in most transplant centers. Several agents are currently licensed for CMV infections, including ganciclovir, foscarnet, and cidofovir, and all have appreciable toxicity. Newer agents such as letermovir have been licensed for use in adults and it is expected that indications for this agent will extend into pediatrics.

REFERENCE/SOURCE

- Kelly MS, Sandora TJ. Community-acquired pneumonia. In: Kliegman RM, St Geme JW III, Blum NJ, Shah SS, Tasker RC, Wilson KM (Eds). Nelson Textbook of Pediatrics, 21st edition. Amsterdam: Elsevier; 2020. pp. 2266-74.

6. A 2-year child was admitted with pneumonia, and you have started antibiotics as per your unit protocol. The child had a high grade of fever despite antibiotics. Air entry decreased on the left intrascapular area with stony dull note on percussion. What will you do next?

A. Upgrade the antibiotics
B. CT chest
C. Ultrasonography (USG) chest
D. Intercostal tube drainage

EXPLANATION

If a child is not responding with the usual course of antibiotics, then we need to suspect complications of pneumonia. In the index child, pleural effusion is the most likely possibility. USG chest should be done to determine the quantity of effusion. If there is a small quantity of effusion, then one may continue antibiotics, while moderate to large effusion requires intercostal tube drainage.

Key: C

BOOST YOUR KNOWLEDGE

Ultrasound is a sensitive modality to detect pleural effusion. It detects the size of pleural effusion, loculation, echogenicity, and pleural thickening.

REFERENCE/SOURCE

- Lodha R, Kabra SK. Essential Pediatric Pulmonology, 4th edition. New Delhi: Jaypee Brothers Medical Publishers; 2023. p. 510.

7. A child with spinal muscular atrophy (SMA) has been presented with recurrent pneumonia. What will be the most likely cause of his pneumonia?

A. Recurrent bacterial infection
B. Congestive heart failure
C. Aspiration pneumonia
D. Chest wall deformity

EXPLANATION

As weakness progresses and difficulty handling oral secretions ensues, aspiration pneumonia becomes a problem for patients with spinal muscular dystrophy. Cardiomyopathy is usually present in children with Duchenne muscular dystrophy.

Key: C

BOOST YOUR KNOWLEDGE

Spinal muscular atrophy children usually present with generalized symmetrical weakness. There may be a range of clinical manifestations and courses of respiratory involvement and swallowing and sucking difficulties.

REFERENCE/SOURCE

- Kliegman RM, St Geme JW III, Blum NJ, Shah SS, Tasker RC, Wilson KM. Disorders of neuromuscular transmission and of motor neurons. In: Nelson Textbook of Pediatrics, 21st edition. Amsterdam: Elsevier; 2020. pp. 3310-2.

8. A 2-year-old child presented to a primary care physician. He diagnosed it with pneumonia. What is the most consistent clinical manifestation of pneumonia in these settings?

A. Chest indrawing
B. Tachycardia
C. Tachypnea
D. Presence of crackles

EXPLANATION

Cough, fever, and lethargy are nonspecific clinical manifestations of pneumonia, while tachypnea is the most consistent feature of pneumonia.

Key: C

BOOST YOUR KNOWLEDGE

Tachypnea had the highest sensitivity (74%), with an acceptable specificity (67%), followed by chest indrawing. The association of both these signs improved specificity but not sensitivity. Alveolar rales had a higher specificity than these signs (79%), but a very low sensitivity (46%). Combinations of alveolar rales with tachypnea or chest indrawing or a combination of these three signs improved specificity (80–84%), but still had a very low sensitivity (<46%).

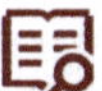

REFERENCES/SOURCES

- Kelly MS, Sandora TJ. Community-acquired pneumonia. In: Kliegman RM, St Geme JW III, Blum NJ, Shah SS, Tasker RC, Wilson KM (Eds). Nelson Textbook of Pediatrics, 21st edition. Amsterdam: Elsevier; 2020. p. 2271.
- Palafox M, Guiscafré H, Reyes H, Munoz O, Martínez H. Diagnostic value of tachypnoea in pneumonia defined radiologically. Arch Dis Child. 2000;82(1):41-5.

9. A 4-year-old child presented with a typical history of pneumonia. Which of the following is true regarding X-rays?

A. It should be done in all children to diagnose pneumonia
B. X-ray is very helpful in differentiating between viral and bacterial pneumonia
C. X-ray helps to determine the choice of antibiotics for pneumonia
D. X-ray should only be done if you suspect any complications

EXPLANATION

Pediatric Infectious Diseases Society-Infectious Diseases Society of America (PIDS-IDSA) guidelines do not recommend chest X-rays for all children with pneumonia. Moreover, X-ray does neither help to differentiate between viral and bacterial pneumonia, nor to choose the antibiotics.

Key: D

BOOST YOUR KNOWLEDGE

The indications for chest X-ray in pneumonia in children are severe pneumonia, a prolonged course of illness, infant age 0–3 months, suspecting complications such as pleural effusion or pneumothorax, children with atypical presentation, children not responding after 48 hours of treatment.

REFERENCE/SOURCE

- Gupta P. Respiratory disorders. In: Gupta P (Eds). UG Textbook of Pediatrics, 1st edition. New Delhi: Jaypee Brothers Medical Publishers; 2023. p. 621.

10. An infant presented with abrupt onset of cough, fever, and respiratory difficulty. On examination, he had tachypnea, hypoxia, and diffuse bilateral crackles. He had a history of skin pustules a few days back. Which of the following antibiotics should be included in the treatment?

A. Ampicillin
B. Erythromycin
C. Ciprofloxacin
D. Vancomycin

EXPLANATION

Because of the abrupt and severe onset of symptoms and the presence of skin pustules points toward *Staphylococcus*. As the child is under 5 years old, it would be wise to start coverage for methicillin-resistant *S. aureus* (MRSA) since the prevalence of MRSA is high in children <5 years.

Key: D

BOOST YOUR KNOWLEDGE

Cloxacillin is the drug of choice for methicillin-sensitive *Staphylococcus pneumonia*. Vancomycin is the drug of choice for MRSA. If clinical features suggest staphylococcal pneumonia, initial antibiotic therapy should include vancomycin.

REFERENCE/SOURCE

- Kelly MS, Sandora TJ. Community-Acquired Pneumonia. In: Kliegman RM, St Geme JW III, Blum NJ, Shah SS, Tasker RC, Wilson KM (Eds). Nelson Textbook of Pediatrics, 21st edition. Amsterdam: Elsevier; 2020. p. 2271.

11. A 12-year-old child living with HIV complained of fever for 20 days, breathlessness for 10 days, and sudden onset left-side chest pain for 1 day. The chest X-ray was suggestive of left-sided pneumothorax. Of the following organisms, which is most likely to be the etiology?

A. CMV
B. *Pneumocystis jirovecii*
C. *Legionella*
D. Herpes simplex

EXPLANATION

The resident should, first, rightly point out the pneumothorax. The key features in this child are underlying secondary immunodeficiency, and in addition, currently, the child is having pneumothorax.

All the organisms in the option can cause infection in HIV children, but the organisms causing secondary pneumothorax should be kept in mind, including measles, *Pneumocystis jirovecii,* tuberculosis (TB), necrotizing pneumonia, or abscess, parasitic, etc.

Pneumocystis jirovecii has classically been considered as causative of pneumothorax, especially when the child is having pneumothorax.

Key: B

BOOST YOUR KNOWLEDGE

Cytomegalovirus, *Legionella*, herpes, and *Pneumocystis* pneumonia (PCP), all of these can cause interstitial pneumonia, especially in Immunodeficiency.

REFERENCE/SOURCE

- Prentice B, Jaffé A. Air and fluid in the pleural space. In: Wilmott RW, Bush A, Deterding RR, Ratjen F, Sly P, Zar H, Li A (Eds). Kendig's Disorders of Respiratory Tract in Children, 9th edition. Amsterdam: Elsevier; 2019.

12. A 17-year-old boy of cystic fibrosis on follow-up presented to the ER with right side pneumothorax. The child is otherwise asymptomatic. Which of the following management is appropriate?

A. Since it is asymptomatic, to observe with antibiotics
B. Since there is a pneumothorax, to give 100 % oxygen
C. Considering underlying lung disease, to put intercostal drainage (ICD) even asymptomatic
D. To do needle aspiration as it may evolve into tension pneumothorax

EXPLANATION

The case is cystic fibrosis. Hence, it is a secondary pneumothorax. Any secondary pneumothorax child simple observation can cause further deterioration. Giving 100% O_2 is an initial management in any secondary pneumothorax; however, it is not the definite one. 100% oxygen hastens the resolution of pneumothorax by decreasing nitrogen concentration in pleural space. Needle aspiration is an emergent procedure done when tension pneumothorax develops. Here, the index child does not have any hemodynamic instability.

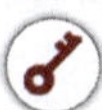

Key: C

BOOST YOUR KNOWLEDGE

If the pneumothorax is recurrent, secondary, or under tension, or there is more than a small collapse, chest tube drainage is necessary.

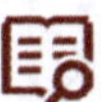

REFERENCE/SOURCE

- Prentice B, Jaffé A. Air and fluid in the pleural space. In: Wilmott RW, Bush A, Deterding RR, Ratjen F, Sly P, Zar H, Li A (Eds). Kendig's Disorders of Respiratory Tract in Children, 9th edition. Amsterdam: Elsevier; 2019.

13. While calculating the size of a pneumothorax, which of the following is correct regarding a large pneumothorax? (The size mentioned here is between the lung and parietal pleural margin)

A. Distance to the cupola or apical dome of the lung is >2 cm
B. Presence of a visible rim of >2 cm at the level of hilum
C. Distance to the lateral edge is >2 cm
D. Tension pneumothorax

EXPLANATION

According to the American College of Chest Physicians, larger pneumothorax is mentioned as:

- If the distance to the cupola or apical dome of the lung is >3 cm
- Distance to the lateral edge is >3 cm

According to the British Thoracic Society (BTS), the presence of a visible rim of >2 cm at the level of the hilum is considered a large pneumothorax.

Any hemodynamic stable patient may or may not have a large pneumothorax. Large does not mean tension pneumothorax. Large means the volume here.

Key: B

BOOST YOUR KNOWLEDGE

Other methods to measure the volume of pneumothorax are the light method, Rhea method, and Collin method.

Light method: Volume (%) = 100 – [Average diameter of lung^3/(Average diameter hemithorax)^3 × 100]

Rhea method: Average of interpleural distance (cm) at three points on chest X-ray

1. Apex
2. Midpoint of upper half of lung
3. Midpoint of lower half of lung

Note: Use nomogram to convert into volume

Collin's method: Size (%) = 4.2 + 4.7 (sum of interpleural distance at apex, midpoint of upper half of lung, and midpoint of lower half of lung)

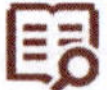

REFERENCES/SOURCES

- Baumann MH, Strange C, Heffner JE, Light R, Kirby TJ, Klein J, et al. Management of spontaneous pneumothorax: An American College of Chest Physicians Delphi consensus statement. Chest. 2001;119(2):590-602.
- MacDuff A, Arnold A, Harvey J; BTS Pleural Disease Guideline Group. Management of spontaneous pneumothorax: British Thoracic Society Pleural Disease Guideline 2010. Thorax. 2010;65(Suppl 2):ii18-31.

14. A healthy 7-year-old boy presents to the ER with sudden onset difficulty in breathing, chest pain, palpitation, and facial swelling. No previous significant history. What is the likely diagnosis?

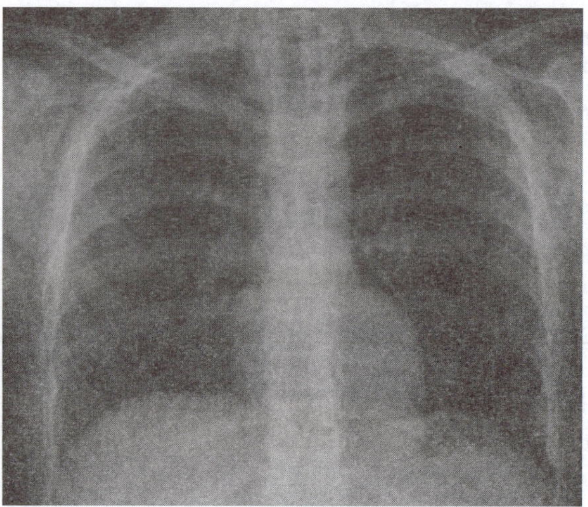

A. Pneumothorax
B. Subcutaneous emphysema
C. Pneumopericardium
D. Pneumomediastinum

EXPLANATION

Pneumothorax will have air inside the pleural cavity with or without collapse of the lung margin from the periphery toward the hilum.

Subcutaneous emphysema is a distractor here since there is facial swelling. It is present, but it is because of underlying pneumomediastinum, which can be traced through vascular sheaths and present with additional subcutaneous emphysema.

The pneumopericardium is a rim of air between the parietal and visceral pericardium. Here air can be traced everywhere.

Key: D

BOOST YOUR KNOWLEDGE

Causes of pneumomediastinum include Valsalva maneuver, vomiting, Boerhaave syndrome (esophageal perforation), weightlifting and choking events, lower respiratory tract infections, and asthma exacerbations. Other causes of secondary pneumomediastinum are anorexia nervosa, normal menses, and diabetes mellitus with ketoacidosis. Traumatic causes dental extractions, adenotonsillectomy, high flow nasal cannula therapy, esophageal perforation, and inhalation of helium gas, and noniatrogenic-inhaled foreign body, penetrating chest trauma, and illicit drug use.

REFERENCE/SOURCE

- Winnie GB, Vemana AP, Haider SK. Pneumomediastinum. In: Kliegman RM, St Geme JW III, Blum NJ, Shah SS, Tasker RC, Wilson KM (Eds). Nelson Textbook of Pediatrics, 21st edition. Amsterdam: Elsevier; 2020.

15. A 10-year-old child with a history of chronic fever, weight loss, and loss of appetite presented to the ER with the following X-ray. Ultrasound showed pleural fluid of 400 mL. The child is having minimal distress and maintains saturation with an oxygen mask. Which of the mentioned management is appropriate regarding the next line of management?

A. Urgent chest tube insertion
B. To do a diagnostic tap
C. Ultrasound-guided pigtail catheter insertion
D. To plan for bronchoscopy

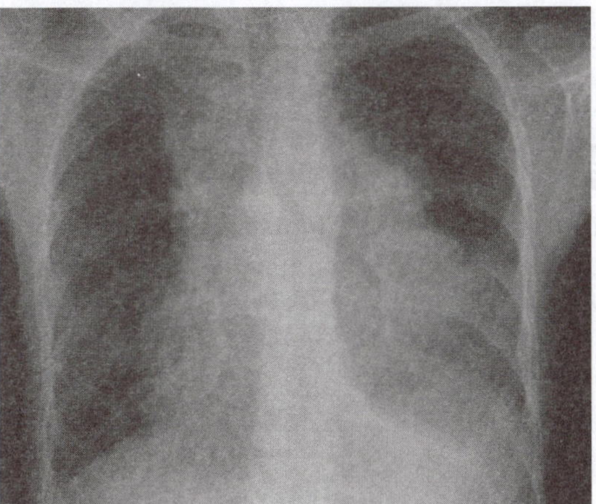

EXPLANATION

- X-ray showed huge mediastinal lymphadenopathy. USG shows the presence of fluid (could be effusion or empyema). Considering history and X-ray the foremost differentials include TB and malignancy.
- The next step will be a diagnostic tap to look for how the pleural fluid looks like and order its cytological and biochemical examination. Also look for malignant cells. ICD insertion/pigtail has no role if there is no significant distress, considering the fistula in TB and continuous leak in malignancy.
- Bronchoscopy may have a role in the form of BAL for TB once malignancy is ruled out and after CT is taken. As such, there is no urgent indication of bronchoscopy.
- An ICD is indicated only if empyema is confirmed. In that case also, look for an underlying condition.

Key: B

BOOST YOUR KNOWLEDGE

In TB effusion, the fluid is secondary to hypersensitivity. Hence, acid-fast bacillus (AFB) or cartridge-based nucleic acid amplification test (CBNAAT) positivity in pleural fluid is unlikely.

REFERENCE/SOURCE

- Balfour-Lynn IM, Abrahamson E, Cohen G, Hartley J, King S, Parikh D, et al. BTS guidelines for the management of pleural infection in children. Thorax. 2005;60:i1-21.

16. A 3-year-old child present with a history of prodrome followed by fever, breathlessness, and decreased feeding. The child was started on amikacin, metronidazole, azithromycin, and oseltamivir by a practitioner. After 5 days of treatment, the child did not improve. Pleural fluid analysis showed frank pus. Which of the following is appropriate for etiology and management?

A. Anti-*Pneumococcus* cover is mandatory in all cases
B. To cover for *Pneumococcus, Streptococcus*, influenza and to continue azithromycin and oseltamivir
C. Viral infection should be considered in etiology
D. Atypical organism coverage (azithromycin) should be included

EXPLANATION

Viral prodrome indicates infection started as a viral respiratory pathogen. But pleural tapping showed frank pus. Viral infections, *Legionella, Mycoplasma*, and other atypical organisms rarely cause empyema. They can cause pleural effusion. Hence, there is no role of azithromycin and oseltamivir here. Hence, option B is also eliminated. The most common causes of empyema are *S. aureus* and *S. pneumoniae*. Since *Staphylococcus* is not one of the options above, the next best option is "A" to give anti-*Pneumococcus* cover.

Key: A

BOOST YOUR KNOWLEDGE

All cases should be treated with IV antibiotics and must include cover for *Streptococcus pneumoniae*. And the most common cause of pleural effusion is *Pneumococcus*, followed by beta-hemolytic streptococci and *Staphylococcus aureus*. Common causes of empyema were listed in the explanation.

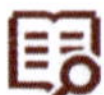

REFERENCE/SOURCE

- Balfour-Lynn IM, Abrahamson E, Cohen G, Hartley J, King S, Parikh D, et al. BTS guidelines for the management of pleural infection in children. Thorax. 2005;60:i1-21.

17. Which of the following is correct regarding chylothorax?

A. Fluid triglyceride level is >110 mg/dL and pleural fluid : serum cholesterol ratio is <1.0
B. Fluid cholesterol level is >200 mg/dL, the pleural fluid : serum triglyceride ratio is <2.0
C. Fluid triglyceride level is >200 mg/dL and pleural fluid : serum cholesterol ratio is >1.0
D. Fluid cholesterol level is >110 mg/dL and pleural fluid : serum triglyceride ratio is >2.0

EXPLANATION

Chylothorax characteristics:

- Fluid triglyceride level is >110 mg/dL
- Pleural fluid : serum triglyceride ratio is >1.0
- Pleural fluid : serum cholesterol ratio is <1.0
- Lipoprotein analysis reveals chylomicrons
- Fluid immunoglobulin levels are elevated
- The cells are primarily (>80%) T-lymphocytes and often exceed 1,000 cells per mm^3
- Positive Sudan III test

Key: A

BOOST YOUR KNOWLEDGE

Pseudochylothorax is the presence of pleural fluid cholesterol >200 mg/dL. It can be seen in any long-standing chronic pleural effusion, such as chronic heart failure, chronic kidney diseases, or connective tissue disorders.

REFERENCE/SOURCE

- Winnie GB, Haider SK, Vemana AP, Lossef SV. Chylothorax. In: Kliegman RM, St Geme JW III, Blum NJ, Shah SS, Tasker RC, Wilson KM (Eds). Nelson Textbook of Pediatrics, 21st edition. Amsterdam: Elsevier; 2020.

18. A 2-month-old child presented with respiratory distress for 10 days. Examination showed syndromic facies with nonpitting pedal edema. There was no history of fever. X-ray showed right-side effusion. Ultrasound confirmed the same. IV antibiotics were started, and ICD was inserted considering distress. There was no improvement in condition. Which of the following is the correct line of management?

A. Give fibrinolytic (urokinase) as distress is not improving
B. Give IV immunoglobulin
C. Plan for video-assisted thoracoscopy (VATS) as the condition is not improving
D. Plan for contrast-enhanced computed tomography (CECT) to check for alternative diagnosis

EXPLANATION

- Since there was no fever, nonpitting edema, and poor response to antibiotics, the diagnosis of empyema or parapneumonic effusion was unlikely. The syndromic child with gradual onset distress with edema favors chylothorax with lymphatic malformations.
- Hence, urokinase has no role unless frank pus was documented in pleural fluid analysis and USG shows septation. VATS has a role if done early in empyema or if there is no response to fibrinolytics.
- CECT has no role in diagnosing chylothorax; rather, MR lymphatics or lymphoscintigraphy has a role in diagnosis.
- Regarding management, as chylothorax causes secondary immunodeficiency by chronic loss of Immunoglobulins and T-cells, intravenous immunoglobulin has a role.

Key: B

BOOST YOUR KNOWLEDGE

Syndromes associated with chylothorax include Noonan syndrome, Turner syndrome, and Down syndrome.

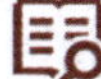

REFERENCE/SOURCE

- Winnie GB, Haider SK, Vemana AP, Lossef SV. Chylothorax. In: Kliegman RM, St Geme JW III, Blum NJ, Shah SS, Tasker RC, Wilson KM (Eds). Nelson Textbook of Pediatrics, 21st edition. Amsterdam: Elsevier; 2020.

19. A case of neonatal chylothorax was diagnosed yesterday and referred to you for a dietary plan and next management. Which of the following is correct?

A. Start feeds at 100 mL/kg and increase feeds with medium-chain triglycerides (MCT)
B. Keep nil per orally (NPO) and start total parenteral nutrition (TPN) with long-chain fatty acid supplementation
C. MCT has a role, and spontaneous recovery can be expected
D. NPO, start TPN, start octreotide, and restrict protein diet

EXPLANATION

- Any child diagnosed with chylothorax has to be kept NPO as fat in the diet leads to further leakage and worsening.
- MCT is absorbed directly in the intestine and hence it can be supplemented and so a protein-rich diet. The child has to be started on TPN to prevent malnutrition from ongoing loss.
- 50% of neonatal chylothorax is expected to have spontaneous recovery.
- Also, octreotide and somatostatin help in splanchnic vasoconstriction, causing a decrease in intestinal blood flow and gastrointestinal secretions, thus ultimately diminishing lymph production.

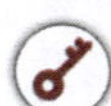

Key: C

BOOST YOUR KNOWLEDGE

Medical treatment is considered failed if there is no improvement after the earlier mentioned measures after 4 weeks. Surgical options include thoracic duct ligation and embolization. Therapy of refractory chylothorax includes pleurodesis and pleuroperitoneal shunt.

REFERENCE/SOURCE

- Winnie GB, Haider SK, Vemana AP, Lossef SV. Chylothorax. In: Kliegman RM, St Geme JW III, Blum NJ, Shah SS, Tasker RC, Wilson KM (Eds). Nelson Textbook of Pediatrics, 21st edition. Amsterdam: Elsevier; 2020.

20. According to the BTS guidelines of pleural infection, which of the following is correct regarding pleural fibrinolytic?

A. Shortens hospital stay and is recommended for thick fluid with locations or empyema
B. Urokinase is more effective than streptokinase in children
C. In necrotizing pneumonia, fibrinolytics help in decreased mortality
D. Fibrinolytic have a better role in organized empyema than surgery

EXPLANATION

- No fibrinolytics have proven to be better than each other. In children, only urokinase has been studied; hence, it is commonly used.
- Fibrinolytics are contraindicated in necrotizing pneumonia and bronchopleural fistula. In organized empyema, surgical options are better than fibrinolytic.

Key: A

BOOST YOUR KNOWLEDGE

Urokinase dosage: It should be given twice daily for 3 days (six doses in total) 40,000 units in 40 mL 0.9% saline for children aged 1 year or above. 10,000 units in 10 mL 0.9% saline for children aged under 1 year.

REFERENCE/SOURCE

- Balfour-Lynn IM, Abrahamson E, Cohen G, Hartley J, King S, Parikh D, et al. BTS guidelines for the management of pleural infection in children. Thorax. 2005;60:i1-21.

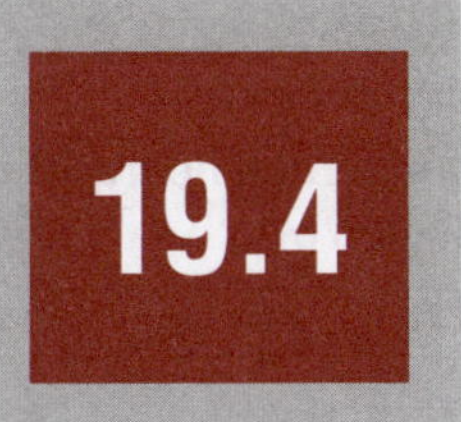

CHAPTER 19.4

Wheezy Illnesses including Bronchiolitis, Multitrigger Wheeze, and Asthma

Prawin Kumar

1. A 6-month-old infant presented in emergency with complaints of fever, cold, cough for 3 days, and fast breathing for 1 day. The mother also noticed noisy breathing. On examination, he had respiratory rate (RR) = 66/minute, SpO_2 = 84% in room air, and bilateral expiratory polyphonic wheeze was heard. Which of the following is true regarding the pathophysiology of hypoxia in the given condition?

A. Consolidation in multiple lung fields
B. Pulmonary microthrombi formation
C. Ventilation-perfusion mismatch
D. Diffuse bronchospasm

EXPLANATION

The index child is suffering from bronchiolitis as he had upper respiratory tract infection followed by lower respiratory tract infection. On examination, there was diffuse expiratory polyphonic wheeze; it is due to the narrowing of small airways, one of the characteristic features of bronchiolitis. The RR and hypoxemia depend on the severity of the disease. Consolidation is usually a feature of pneumonia. The narrowing of small airways in bronchiolitis is due to airway edema and necrosis rather than bronchospasm. Pulmonary microthrombi is a feature of sepsis with disseminated intravascular coagulation disorder. Hypoxemia in bronchiolitis is a consequence of ventilation-perfusion mismatch.

Key: C

BOOST YOUR KNOWLEDGE

In bronchiolitis, the primary pathophysiology mechanism is widespread small airway (bronchiole) obstruction due to airway edema, mucus secretion, and cellular debris. We know that the airway resistance is inversely proportional to the fourth power of radius ($\propto 1/r^4$); therefore, even a small decrease in airway diameter leads to a significant increase in resistance. The resistance increases during both inspiration and expiration; however, the airway is partially collapsed during expiration so wheezing first appears during expiration (with increased severity also occurring in inspiration). Airway obstruction also leads to air trapping and hyperinflation. If obstruction becomes complete, the air distal to obstruction gets absorbed and causes atelectasis. It results in ventilation-perfusion mismatch leading to hypoxemia and respiratory acidosis. The extent of hypoxemia will depend on the severity of the disease.

REFERENCES/SOURCES

- Kabra SK. Disorder of the respiratory tract (Chapter 15). In: Paul VK, Bagga A (Eds). Ghai Essential Pediatrics, 9th edition. New Delhi: CBS Publishers and Distributors (P) Ltd; 2013. p. 381.
- Kliegman RM, St Geme III JW. Nelson Textbook of Pediatrics, 21st edition. Elsevier; 2019. Chapter 418: Wheezing, bronchiolitis, and bronchitis. pp. 2217-20.

2. Which of the following is a true statement about risk factors of severe bronchiolitis in children?

A. Age >6 months
B. Hemodynamically stable congenital heart disease
C. Single child
D. Living at higher altitude (>2,500 m)

EXPLANATION

The most common etiology of bronchiolitis is respiratory syncytial virus (RSV). It is more severe in infants 6–12 weeks of age, so option A is incorrect. Hemodynamically unstable congenital heart disease (CHD) is a risk factor—not stable CHD, so option B is also incorrect. Having an older sibling is a risk factor, so option C is also wrong. Infants living at higher altitudes (>2,500 m) are at risk for severe disease, so option D is correct.

Key: D

BOOST YOUR KNOWLEDGE

The risk factors for severe bronchiolitis are both host and environment related. They are described in given box:

Host related	*Environmental*
• Prematurity (gestational age ≤36 weeks) • Low birth weight • Age <6–12 weeks • Chronic pulmonary disease • Airway malacias • Hemodynamically significant congenital heart disease • Immunodeficiency • Neurologic disease	• Passive smoking • Crowded household • Higher altitude (>2,500 m) • Daycare attendance • Older siblings

REFERENCES/SOURCES

- Kliegman RM, St Geme III JW. Nelson Textbook of Pediatrics, 21st edition. Elsevier; 2019. Chapter 418: Wheezing, bronchiolitis, and bronchitis. pp. 2217-20.
- Tungal S, Lodha R. Acute bronchiolitis. In: Lodha R, Kabra SK (Eds). Essential Pediatric Pulmonology, 4th edition. New Delhi: Jaypee Brothers Medical Publishers; 2023. pp. 117-27.
- UpToDate. (2024). Bronchiolitis in infants and children: treatment, outcome, and prevention. [online] Available from https://www.uptodate.com/contents/bronchiolitis-in-infants-and-children-treatment-outcome-and-prevention [Last accessed June, 2024].

3. An 8-week-old infant delivered at 33 weeks, immunized to date developed fever, cough, and cold for 2 days. He had a 3-year-old sister who also had similar complaints. On day 3 of illness, he developed apnea at home, his mother gave him mouth-to-mouth breathing and brought him to the emergency. On examination, he had RR = 68/minute, SpO_2 = 92% at room air, and bilateral diffuse wheezing. Which of the following is the most possible clinical diagnosis?

A. Community-acquired pneumonia (CAP)
B. Bronchiolitis
C. Pertussis
D. Foreign body (FB) aspiration

EXPLANATION

In this case, the infants developed upper respiratory symptoms followed by features of the lower respiratory tract infection (LRTI) which is characteristic of bronchiolitis (option B). There is also a history of upper respiratory infection (URI) symptoms in older siblings, which also favors the diagnosis of viral infection. CAP usually has a sudden onset and on examination more of a localized finding. Since, the child is immunized and has B/L polyphonic wheeze, pertussis is less likely here. There is no history of choking and with bilateral diffuse findings, the FB is less likely. However, in 30% one will not find the history of FB aspiration.

Key: B

BOOST YOUR KNOWLEDGE

Bronchiolitis usually first presents with URI symptoms (cough, rhinorrhea, sneezing, nasal block, fever, etc.) followed by LRTI (tachypnea with or without retraction, on examination polyphonic wheeze, and hypoxemia). There may be fever, decreased oral intake, nausea, vomiting, loose stool, dehydration, or symptoms of urinary tract infection. On auscultation, one may get crepitation wheezing, or both but it will be diffuse in nature. Apnea may be the clinical presentation in young infants with a prevalence of 5–20%. Apnea may be the only symptom preceding LRTI. Premature and young infants are prone to recurrent apnea.

REFERENCES/SOURCES

- Kliegman RM, St Geme III JW. Nelson Textbook of Pediatrics, 21st edition. Elsevier; 2019. Chapter 418: Wheezing, bronchiolitis, and bronchitis. pp. 2217-20.
- Tungal S, Lodha R. Acute bronchiolitis. In: Lodha R, Kabra SK (Eds). Essential Pediatric Pulmonology, 4th edition. New Delhi: Jaypee Brothers Medical Publishers; 2023. pp. 117-27.
- UpToDate. (2024). Bronchiolitis in infants and children: Treatment, outcome, and prevention. [online] Available from https://www.uptodate.com/contents/bronchiolitis-in-infants-and-children-treatment-outcome-and-prevention [Last accessed June, 2024].

4. **A 2-month-old girl presented with cough, fast breathing, and chest retraction for 5 days. The duty residents suspected bronchiolitis in her. Which of the following statements is correct for establishing a diagnosis of bronchiolitis?**

A. Hemogram with differential counts may help in making a diagnosis
B. Polymerase chain reaction (PCR) in nasopharyngeal aspirate should be done to document the etiology
C. Chest X-ray may lead to increased use of antibiotics
D. Procalcitonin differentiates viral from bacterial infection

EXPLANATION

The diagnosis of bronchiolitis is mainly clinical. Laboratory investigations do not help in making a diagnosis. Hemogram may show leukocytosis which does not differentiate viral from bacterial infection. PCR may help in documenting viral etiology, but it is not necessary for routine care. Procalcitonin and CRP do not differentiate viral from bacterial infection and hence not recommended. A chest X-ray is not helpful in making a diagnosis and may lead to increased inappropriate use of antibiotics.

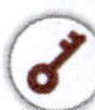

Key: C

BOOST YOUR KNOWLEDGE

Bronchiolitis is a clinical diagnosis. Laboratory investigation and chest X-ray is not helpful in making a diagnosis and are not recommended in routine care; however, they may be required to exclude other differential and to evaluate complication. Procalcitonin and CRP are not specific for bacterial infection and may be raised in viral infection. They are not helpful in making the diagnosis. Chest X-ray finding is variable and non-specific, which includes hyperinflation and peribronchial thickening. There may be patchy atelectasis. It would be difficult to differentiate viral from bacterial infection by chest X-ray. Chest X-rays may lead to increased inappropriate use of antibiotics. The X-ray indications are moderate-to-severe respiratory distress, atypical findings, having cardiac murmur, or to exclude alternative diagnosis.

REFERENCES/SOURCES

- Kliegman RM, St Geme III JW. Nelson Textbook of Pediatrics, 21st edition. Elsevier; 2019. Chapter 418: Wheezing, bronchiolitis, and bronchitis. pp. 2217-20.
- Tungal S, Lodha R. Acute bronchiolitis. In: Lodha R, Kabra SK (Eds). Essential Pediatric Pulmonology, 4th edition. New Delhi: Jaypee Brothers Medical Publishers; 2023. pp. 117-27.
- UpToDate. (2024). Bronchiolitis in infants and children: Treatment, outcome, and prevention. [online] Available from https://www.uptodate.com/contents/bronchiolitis-in-infants-and-children-treatment-outcome-and-prevention [Last accessed June, 2024].

5. A 10-week-old child presented in emergency with fast breathing, irritability, and refusal to feed for 36 hours. There was a history of cold and fever for 4 days. On examination, RR = 74/minute, SpO_2 = 90% on room air, chest retraction, and diffuse polyphonic wheeze were heard. What is your next step in management?

A. Start oral antibiotic and ask to review after 48 hours
B. Start O_2 with nasal cannula, nasal suction, and maintenance IV fluid
C. Start nebulization with salbutamol
D. Start O_2 and nebulization with inhaled budesonide

EXPLANATION

The given condition is bronchiolitis, which is mostly caused by viruses. Here age <12 weeks, hypoxemia (SpO_2 <92%) and RR >70/minute are risk factors for severe bronchiolitis and hence, this child required hospital admission. In option A, there is OPD-based treatment which is incorrect. Supportive therapy is the mainstay of treatment for bronchiolitis, so option B is correct. Nebulization with bronchodilator and steroid are not useful and so not recommended, so both options C and D are incorrect.

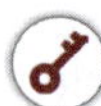

Key: B

BOOST YOUR KNOWLEDGE

- First look for risk factors for severe disease, if any risk factors are present child needs hospitalization otherwise can be managed on OPD-basis.
- Supportive therapy such as O_2 supplementation, maintenance of hydration (IV fluid), and gentle nasal suctioning are the mainstay of therapy.
- Most guidelines do not support the use of a nebulized bronchodilator (salbutamol or epinephrine) for routine use in bronchodilators.
- There are some benefits of nebulized hypertonic saline in admitted children, but routine use is not recommended.
- High-flow nasal cannula (HFNC) or continuous positive airway pressure (CPAP) may be helpful in children not improving with supportive therapy.
- Close clinical monitoring is the key.

REFERENCES/SOURCES

- Florin TA. Viral bronchiolitis. Lancet. 2017;389:211-24.
- Kliegman RM, St Geme III JW. Nelson Textbook of Pediatrics, 21st edition. Elsevier; 2019. Chapter 418: Wheezing, bronchiolitis, and bronchitis. pp. 2217-20.
- Tungal S, Lodha R. Acute bronchiolitis. In: Lodha R, Kabra SK (Eds). Essential Pediatric Pulmonology, 4th edition. New Delhi: Jaypee Brothers Medical Publishers; 2023. pp. 117-27.

6. A 3-year-old child presented with recurrent wheezing episodes since 1 year of age and required multiple hospitalizations. These symptoms worsen during the winter seasons. The episode responded with inhaled bronchodilators. On examination, he is growing well, RR = 34/minute, SpO_2 = 95% on room air, and bilateral polyphonic wheeze was heard. There is a history of atopic dermatitis since infancy. There was no family history of atopy; however, his grandfather smoked at home. Of them, which is the most significant risk factor for the development of asthma at 6 years of age?

A. Multiple hospitalizations
B. Worsening during winter
C. Atopic dermatitis
D. Passive smoke exposure

EXPLANATION

The child is a case of preschool wheezing. Multiple hospitalizations (option A) are an indicator of disease severity and deciding current therapy but not for predicting future asthma. Seasonal variation is a characteristic feature of asthma and not for predicting future asthma. Atopic dermatitis and parental history of asthma are major risk factors for predicting future asthma, so option C is correct. Passive exposure to smoke (option D) is a precipitating factor for the recurrent episode but not for predicting future asthma.

Key: C

BOOST YOUR KNOWLEDGE

There are several predictive models aimed at predicting future asthma in children based on different risk factors. However, none of these predictive models was validated in different populations from the study population. The modified Asthma Predictive Index (mAPI) is the most widely used.

Modified Asthma Predicting Index

Children with ≥4 episodes of wheezing episode per year and having one major or two minor factors have an increased risk of having asthma at 6, 8, 11, and 13 years of age.

Primary	
≥4 wheezing episodes in a year	
Secondary	
Major	***Minor***
• Physician diagnosed atopic dermatitis • A physician diagnosed parental asthma • Aeroallergen sensitization to at least one antigen	• Food allergy (milk, peanut, or eggs) • Wheezing unrelated to the cold • Eosinophil ≥4%

REFERENCES/SOURCES

- Kumar VU, Jat KR. Preschool wheeze. In: Lodha R, Kabra SK (Eds). Essential Pediatric Pulmonology, 4th edition. New Delhi: Jaypee Brothers Medical Publishers; 2023. pp. 300-09.
- National Asthma Education and Prevention Program. Expert Panel Report 3 (EPR-3): Guidelines for the Diagnosis and Management of Asthma-Summary Report 2007. J Allergy Clin Immunol. 2007;120(5 Suppl):S94-138.

7. A 12-year-old boy presented with a cough for the last 3 years. The cough was dry in nature and increased at night and in winter months. It was associated with chest pain, breathing difficulty, and noisy breathing. He was hospitalized 1 year back for the same episode. There was a family history of asthma and a history of exposure to smoke at home. Which of the following is a characteristic feature for the diagnosis of asthma?

A. Symptoms vary in time and intensity
B. Chest pain
C. History of hospitalization
D. Exposure to smoke

EXPLANATION

The characteristic feature of asthma is having more than one symptom, and they vary in time and intensity, so option A is correct. Chest pain is not a characteristic feature of asthma. History of hospitalization may help in deciding the severity and starting asthma therapy but not helpful in making a diagnosis as it could be due to various reasons. Exposure to smoke is a risk factor for respiratory disease and may lead to worsening of asthma symptoms but not helpful in making the diagnosis.

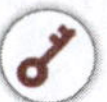

Key: A

BOOST YOUR KNOWLEDGE

The characteristic symptoms of asthma are dry cough, shortness of breath, wheezing, and/or chest tightness.

The following features *increase the probability* of asthma:

- Presence of more than one symptom
- Symptoms vary in time and intensity
- Symptoms often worse at night or in early morning
- Symptoms are often triggered by viral infection (cold), exercise, change in weather, exposure to smoke, or strong smell.

The following features *decrease the probability* of asthma:

- Isolated cough in the absence of other respiratory symptoms
- Productive cough
- Chest pain
- Shortness of breath associated with dizziness or light-headedness
- Exercise-induced dyspnea or noisy breathing

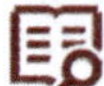

REFERENCES/SOURCES

- Ginasthma.org. (2023). Global Initiative for Asthma (GINA). [online] Available from https://ginasthma.org/2023-gina-main-report/ [Last accessed June, 2024].
- Goyal JP, Thakur C. Clinical presentation and diagnosis of asthma. In: Lodha R, Kabra SK (Eds). Essential Pediatric Pulmonology, 4th edition. New Delhi: Jaypee Brothers Medical Publishers; 2023. pp. 253-60.
- Kliegman RM, St Geme III JW. Nelson Textbook of Pediatrics, 21st edition. Elsevier; 2019. Chapter 169: Childhood asthma. pp. 1186-209.
- Kumar P. Bronchial asthma. In: Gupta P (Ed). The Textbook of Pediatrics, 1st edition. New Delhi: Jaypee Brothers Medical Publishers; 2023. pp. 214-24.

8. A 9-year-old girl presented to pediatrics OPD with symptoms suggestive of asthma. She was asked to perform spirometry pre- and post-bronchodilator. Which of the following spirometry findings suggests the diagnosis of asthma in her?

A. >10% increase in FEV1/FVC
B. >12% increase in FEV1
C. >12% increase in PEFR
D. >20% Increase in FE25-75

EXPLANATION

Post-bronchodilator >12% increase in forced expiratory volume 1 (FEV1) supports the diagnosis of asthma (B). Change in FEV1/FVC (forced vital capacity) is not taken for the diagnosis of asthma (A). For peak expiratory flow rate (PEFR), >15% post-bronchodilator increase is helpful in making the diagnosis (C). Post-bronchodilator change in FEF25-75 is highly variable and so not very helpful in making a diagnosis (D).

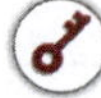

Key: B

BOOST YOUR KNOWLEDGE

Asthma is diagnosed by characteristics symptoms and documentation of expiratory flow limitation and variability. Spirometry is an important tool for the diagnosis of asthma in children. The variability in expiratory flow limitation can be done with a bronchodilator or bronchoprovocation test. The bronchodilator reversibility test is most performed in clinical practice. The following spirometer indices are helpful in making an asthma diagnosis:

To document expiratory airflow limitation	
FEV1/FVC <80% of the predicted value	
To document variable expiratory airflow limitation	
Positive bronchodilator responsiveness test	• >12% increase in FEV1 from baseline • >15% increase in PEFR from baseline
Positive bronchoprovocation test	>20% decrease in FEV1 from baseline with a standard dose of methacholine
Positive exercise challenge test	>12% decrease in FEV1 from baseline
Daily variability in PEFR over 2 weeks	>13% average daily variability in PEFR

REFERENCES/SOURCES

- Ginasthma.org. (2023). Global Initiative for Asthma (GINA). [online] Available from https://ginasthma.org/2023-gina-main-report/ [Last accessed June, 2024].
- Goyal JP, Thakur C. Clinical presentation and diagnosis of asthma. In: Lodha R, Kabra SK (Eds). Essential Pediatric Pulmonology, 4th edition. New Delhi: Jaypee Brothers Medical Publishers; 2023. pp. 253-60.
- Kliegman RM, St Geme III JW. Nelson Textbook of Pediatrics, 21st edition. Elsevier; 2019. Chapter 169: Childhood asthma. pp. 1186-209.

9. An 11-year-old girl presented with a dry cough for 1 year. There was no diurnal and seasonal variation in symptoms. The physician performed spirometry and got the following graph. Which of the following is the correct interpretation of the spirometry findings?

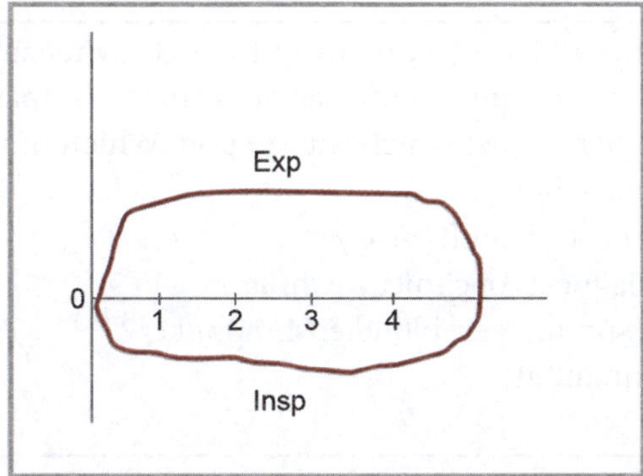

A. Severe peripheral airway obstruction (asthma)
B. Extrathoracic airway obstruction
C. Intrathoracic airway obstruction
D. Both extra- and intrathoracic obstruction

EXPLANATION

The given image represents the fixed airflow limitation of both the extrathoracic and intrathoracic airway. Asthma is characterized by expiratory flow limitation, which is recognized by scooping the descending arm of the expiratory phase, it is not here, and so option A is incorrect. Extrathoracic airway obstruction shows a flattening of inspiratory limbs whereas intrathoracic obstruction shows flattening of expiratory limbs. Here, both expiratory and inspiratory limbs are flattened, so option D is the correct answer.

Key: D

BOOST YOUR KNOWLEDGE

Spirometry gives rise to two graphs: flow volume loop and volume-time graph. The visual inspection of these graphs is very informative.

- First, look for the *acceptability* of the test. It can be done by close observation of graphs.
    - There should be a sharp rise, smooth descending and free from artifacts (cough, premature termination, glottis closure, etc.) in the expiratory limb.
    - In the volume-time graph, a plateau should be achieved (>3 seconds in children).
    - *The start should be from zero:* Back extrapolated volume (BEV) and should be less than <5% of FVC or <100 mL, whichever is greater.
- Then look for *repeatability*—difference between the two largest FEV1 or FVC should be <150 mL or <10% of the highest value.
- In asthma, there will be scooping of the expiratory limbs, the greater the scooping the more severe the disease.
- In restrictive lung disease—there will be an overall small flow-volume loop.
- In extrathoracic obstruction—flattening of inspiratory limbs
- In intrathoracic obstruction—flattening of expiratory limbs
- In both intrathoracic and extrathoracic obstruction—flattening of both inspiratory and expiratory limbs

REFERENCES/SOURCES

- Graham BL, Steenbruggen I, Miller MR, Barjaktarevic IZ, Cooper BG, Hall GL, et al. Standardization of Spirometry 2019 Update. An Official American Thoracic Society and European Respiratory Society Technical Statement. Am J Respir Crit Care Med. 2019;200(8): e70-e88.
- Stanojevic S, Kaminsky DA, Miller MR, Thompson B, Aliverti A, Barjaktarevic I, et al. ERS/ATS technical standard on interpretive strategies for routine lung function tests. Eur Respir J. 2022;60(1):2101499.

10. An 8-year-old girl presented with a history of recurrent cough, wheezing, and breathing difficulties for the last 2 years. Asthma was suspected and spirometry was performed but that was within normal limits. Fractional exhaled nitric oxide (FeNO) was performed which was 39 ppb. Which of the following is correct about the role of FeNO in the diagnosis of asthma in her?

A. It has no role in the diagnosis of childhood asthma
B. FeNO >20 ppb supports the diagnosis of clinical asthma
C. FeNO does not correlate with sputum and blood eosinophilia
D. It reflects type-1 airway inflammation

EXPLANATION

Nitric oxide is a noninvasive test to measure type-2 airway inflammation (option D incorrect). A value >20 ppb supports the clinical diagnosis of asthma in children (B). It modestly correlates with sputum and blood eosinophilia (C). It helps in the diagnosis of clinical asthma (A). In this case, PPB was 39 ppb, so it supports the clinical diagnosis of asthma and option B is correct.

Key: B

BOOST YOUR KNOWLEDGE

Nitric oxide is a noninvasive test. It measures type-2 airway inflammation. It is considered an emerging biomarker of asthma. It does not require much effort so it can be performed even in children <5 years of age. It helps in the diagnosis of asthma, assessment of asthma control, and response to inhaled corticosteroids (ICS). However, FeNO value may increase in many other allergic conditions such as allergic rhinitis, atopic dermatitis etc. It could be normal during exacerbation or early phase of inflammation. Therefore, it should be interpreted cautiously.

- FeNO value >20 ppb supports the clinical diagnosis of childhood asthma.
- FeNO value also predicts response to ICS:
    - <20 ppb—low—unlikely to respond to ICS
    - 20–35 ppb—intermediate—may respond to ICS
    - >35 ppb—high—likely to respond to ICS

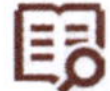

REFERENCES/SOURCES

- Ginasthma.org. (2023). Global Initiative for Asthma (GINA). [online] Available from https://ginasthma.org/2023-gina-main-report/ [Last accessed June, 2024].
- Kliegman RM, St Geme III JW. Nelson Textbook of Pediatrics, 21st edition. Elsevier; 2019. Chapter 169: Childhood asthma. pp. 1186-209.
- Maitra A. Assessment of airway inflammation. In: Lodha R, Kabra SK (Eds). Essential Pediatric Pulmonology, 4th edition. New Delhi: Jaypee Brothers Medical Publishers; 2023. pp. 261-9.
- National Heart, Lung, and Blood Institute. (2020). 2020 Focused Updates to the Asthma Management Guidelines: A Report from the National Asthma Education and Prevention Program Coordinating Committee Expert Panel Working Group. [online] Available from https://www.nhlbi.nih.gov/resources/2020-focused-updates-asthma-management-guidelines [Last accessed June, 2024].

11. A 14-year-old girl presented with recurrent episodes of cough, wheezing, shortness of breath, and chest tightness. She has almost daily symptoms and wakes up at night with symptoms at least once a week. Spirometry showed FEV1 72% of predicted and 13% increase in FEV1 after bronchodilator reversibility test. You have decided to start asthma therapy. Which step of therapy would you start in this child?

A. Step-II
B. Step-III
C. Step-IV
D. Step-V

EXPLANATION

Here the child has characteristics asthma symptoms as well as expiratory flow limitation with a positive bronchodilator reversibility test. Therefore, she is a candidate to start asthma therapy. She has daily symptoms during the daytime and night-time symptoms once a week. She has decreased FEV1 but no low lung function (<60%). Hence, Step-III is appropriate therapy for this child (option B).

Key: B

BOOST YOUR KNOWLEDGE

Global Initiative for Asthma (GINA) has given guidelines to start therapy in adults, adolescents, and children. The step of therapy depends upon the frequencies of symptoms both during day and night-time and spirometry findings. It is given in the box below. Previous hospitalization, intensive care unit (ICU) admission, and previous therapy taken should also be considered before choosing the step of therapy.

Guide to start initial asthma therapy:

Symptoms frequency			
Daytime	***Night-time***	***FEV1***	***Step of treatment***
Symptoms once a month or less	No	60–80%	I
Symptoms once a week but not daily	Once a month	60–80%	II
Daily symptoms	Once a week	60–80%	III
Daily symptoms	Once a week	<60%	IV

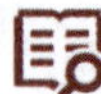

REFERENCES/SOURCES

- Ghimre JJ, Kabra SK. Long-term treatment of asthma. In: Lodha R, Kabra SK (Eds). Essential Pediatric Pulmonology, 4th edition. New Delhi: Jaypee Brothers Medical Publishers; 2023. pp. 280-94.
- Ginasthma.org. (2023). Global Initiative for Asthma (GINA). [online] Available from https://ginasthma.org/2023-gina-main-report/ [Last accessed June, 2024].
- Kliegman RM, St Geme III JW. Nelson Textbook of Pediatrics, 21st edition. Elsevier; 2019. Chapter 169: Childhood asthma. pp. 1186-209.
- National Heart, Lung, and Blood Institute. (2020). 2020 Focused Updates to the Asthma Management Guidelines: A Report from the National Asthma Education and Prevention Program Coordinating Committee Expert Panel Working Group. [online] Available from https://www.nhlbi.nih.gov/resources/2020-focused-updates-asthma-management-guidelines [Last accessed June, 2024].

12. An 11-year-old boy was diagnosed with asthma and started on step III treatment as per the latest GINA guideline. In the last 4 weeks, he had asthma symptoms 3–4 times per week, which require the use of reliever therapy. However, he did not have night-time symptoms or any active limitations. What is the next step of management?

A. Symptoms are well controlled, the same treatment should be continued
B. He has exacerbation and requires short-term oral corticosteroid therapy
C. Symptoms are partly controlled, need optimization of therapy
D. Symptoms are uncontrolled and need a step-up of therapy

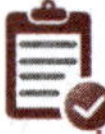

EXPLANATION

Asthma control is assessed with the frequency of day- and night-time symptoms, the need for reliever therapy, and the limitation of activity due to asthma. In this vignette, the child had symptoms frequency more than twice a week and required reliever therapy for the same. Therefore, he had partly controlled asthma. He just needs optimization of therapy and follow-up.

Key: C

BOOST YOUR KNOWLEDGE

The level of asthma control is based on symptom frequency, activity limitation, and need for reliever therapy. It can be performed clinically or numeric asthma control score. GINA assessment of asthma control is a simpler one and suited for routine use in clinical practice. Many validated questionnaires available give objective evidence of asthma control.

Global Initiative for Asthma Assessment of Asthma Control

Symptoms frequency	*Well-controlled*	*Partly controlled*	*Uncontrolled*
Symptoms more than twice a week	None of these	Yes to 1–2 of these	Yes to 3–4 of these
Night-time symptoms more than once a month			
Use of reliever more than twice a week			
Activity limitation due to asthma symptoms			

Numeric asthma assessment score
- *Asthma control test (ACT):* In children >12 years
- *Childhood asthma control test (C-ACT):* In children 4–11 years
- *Asthma control questionnaire (ACQ):* In children >4 years

REFERENCES/SOURCES

- Ghimre JJ, Kabra SK. Long-term treatment of asthma. In: Lodha R, Kabra SK (Eds). Essential Pediatric Pulmonology, 4th edition. New Delhi: Jaypee Brothers Medical Publishers; 2023. pp. 280-94.
- Ginasthma.org. (2023). Global Initiative for Asthma (GINA). [online] Available from https://ginasthma.org/2023-gina-main-report/ [Last accessed June, 2024].

- Kliegman RM, St Geme III JW. Nelson Textbook of Pediatrics, 21st edition. Elsevier; 2019. Chapter 169: Childhood asthma. pp. 1186-209.
- National Heart, Lung, and Blood Institute. (2020). 2020 Focused Updates to the Asthma Management Guidelines: A Report from the National Asthma Education and Prevention Program Coordinating Committee Expert Panel Working Group. [online] Available from https://www.nhlbi.nih.gov/resources/2020-focused-updates-asthma-management-guidelines [Last accessed June, 2024].

13. A 13-year-old boy presented with recurrent episodes of cough, breathing difficulty, and wheezing. He has episodes once a month and improves with oral medication and/or nebulization in 3–4 days. He has no night symptoms, but it aggravated with exertion and cold foods. Spirometry showed FEV1/FVC was 78% and a 14% increase in FEV1 on the bronchodilator reversibility test. Which of the following is the preferred management of his condition?

A. As needed salbutamol (SABA)
B. Low-dose budesonide + formoterol combination as needed
C. Low-dose daily budesonide
D. Low-dose daily budesonide + salbutamol combination

EXPLANATION

In this case, the boy has mild intermittent symptoms (step I). As per the latest guideline, Salbutamol alone therapy is not recommended at any stage of the disease (Option A—incorrect). As needed budesonide + formoterol is now the preferred recommended therapy for both step I and II (B). Daily ICS with or without long-acting beta agonist (LABA) is not recommended therapy for step I (C and D).

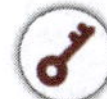

Key: B

BOOST YOUR KNOWLEDGE

The latest GINA guideline no longer recommends SABA-alone therapy in adults, adolescents, and children 6–11 years. It increases the risk of:

- Severe exacerbation
- Asthma-related death

The latest recommendation for step I therapy is:

- Low-dose budesonide + formoterol combination as needed for symptom relief (preferred)
- Use low-dose budesonide whenever salbutamol is taken (alternative).

Evidence has shown that ICS-containing therapy reduces the risk of severe exacerbation, gives a simpler regimen, and avoids confusion.

In different studies, a needed ICS + LABA combination in comparison to daily ICS showed a similar or greater reduction in symptom exacerbation and no difference in the level of asthma control or lung function.

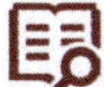

REFERENCES/SOURCES

- Ghimre JJ, Kabra SK. Long-term treatment of asthma. In: Lodha R, Kabra SK (Eds). Essential Pediatric Pulmonology, 4th edition. New Delhi: Jaypee Brothers Medical Publishers; 2023. pp. 253-60.
- Ginasthma.org. (2023). Global Initiative for Asthma (GINA). [online] Available from https://ginasthma.org/2023-gina-main-report/ [Last accessed June, 2024].
- Kliegman RM, St Geme III JW. Nelson Textbook of Pediatrics, 21st edition. Elsevier; 2019. Chapter 169: Childhood asthma. pp. 1186-209.
- National Heart, Lung, and Blood Institute. (2020). 2020 Focused Updates to the Asthma Management Guidelines: A Report from the National Asthma Education and Prevention Program Coordinating Committee Expert Panel Working Group. [online] Available from https://www.nhlbi.nih.gov/resources/2020-focused-updates-asthma-management-guidelines [Last accessed June, 2024].

14. A 15-year-old girl presented with asthma symptoms almost daily and night-time once a week. Her baseline FEV1 was 74% and there was a positive bronchodilator reversibility test. Which is the preferred treatment for her?

A. Daily low-dose ICS + formoterol as maintenance and salbutamol as reliever therapy
B. Daily medium-dose ICS + formoterol for both maintenance and reliever therapy
C. Daily medium-dose ICS as maintenance and salbutamol as reliever therapy
D. Daily low-dose ICS + formoterol for both maintenance and reliever therapy

EXPLANATION

In the given case, child has both asthma symptoms and expiratory flow limitation with a positive reversibility test. He requires step-3 therapy. The preferred therapy in step-3 is daily low-dose ICS + formoterol for both maintenance and reliever therapy (MART), so option D is correct. Option A can also be used in step-3 therapy but that is not the preferred treatment. Options B and C are preferred as alternative therapy for step-4.

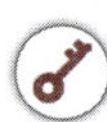

Key: D

BOOST YOUR KNOWLEDGE

Maintenance and reliever therapy is the use of an ICS + formoterol combination for maintenance, and also for the relief of asthma symptoms in step-3 onwards in children >12 years and in adults. MART is also known as SMART (single maintenance and reliever therapy). Either budesonide-formoterol (≥12 years) or beclomethasone-formoterol (≥18 years) can be used as MART. However, other LABA has not been studied and not recommended as MART. The maximum recommended dose of budesonide-formoterol (100/6) in a single day is eight puffs.

Stepwise treatment of asthma in children >12 years

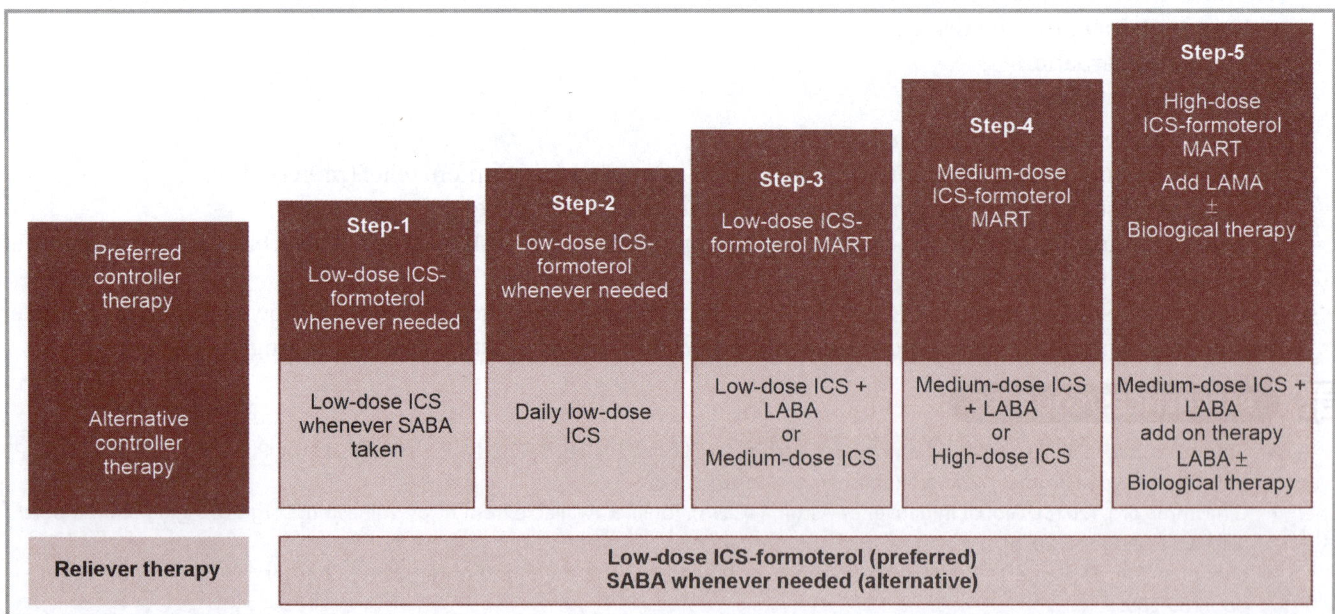

(ICS: inhaled corticosteroid; LABA: long-acting beta agonist; LAMA: long-acting muscarinic antagonist; MART: maintenance and reliever therapy; SABA: short-acting beta agonist)

Source: Adapted from Ginasthma.org. (2022). 2022 GINA Report, Global Strategy for Asthma Management and Prevention. [online] Available from https://ginasthma.org/gina-reports/ [Last accessed June, 2024].

REFERENCES/SOURCE

- Ghimre JJ, Kabra SK. Long-term treatment of asthma. In: Lodha R, Kabra SK (Eds). Essential Pediatric Pulmonology, 4th edition. New Delhi: Jaypee Brothers Medical Publishers; 2023. pp. 253-60.
- Ginasthma.org. (2023). Global Initiative for Asthma (GINA). [online] Available from https://ginasthma.org/2023-gina-main-report/ [Last accessed June, 2024].
- Kumar P. Bronchial asthma. In: Gupta P (Ed). UG Textbook of Pediatrics, 1st edition. New Delhi: Jaypee Brothers Medical Publishers; 2023. pp. 214-24.
- National Heart, Lung, and Blood Institute. (2020). 2020 Focused Updates to the Asthma Management Guidelines: A Report from the National Asthma Education and Prevention Program Coordinating Committee Expert Panel Working Group. [online] Available from https://www.nhlbi.nih.gov/resources/2020-focused-updates-asthma-management-guidelines [Last accessed June, 2024].

15. **A 10-year-old boy diagnosed with asthma was started on budesonide (100 µg) and formoterol (6 µg) combination two puffs twice a day along with salbutamol as reliever therapy. After 8 weeks of therapy, he had daytime symptoms 3 times/week requiring reliever therapy. There were also night-time symptoms once a week. He often missed school and avoid going to play. What is the next best step of management?**

A. Check compliance with therapy and technique
B. Add short-term systemic steroid
C. Increase budesonide to 200 µg two puffs twice a day
D. Add long-acting muscarinic antagonist (tiotropium)

EXPLANATION

In the given vignette, the child has uncontrolled symptoms as per the GINA assessment of asthma control. The first step is to confirm the diagnosis of asthma. The second step is to optimize adherence to therapy and check the inhalation technique. Therefore, option A is correct. The child is not in exacerbation right now, so no need for adding systemic steroid (B). Just increasing the dose of inhaled steroids without optimizing adherence and technique will less likely to work, and at risk of adverse effects (C). Tiotropium is not recommended in children <12 years of age (D). Moreover, we need to optimize adherence and technique before considering stepping up therapy.

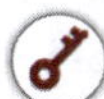

Key: A

BOOST YOUR KNOWLEDGE

Uncontrolled asthma is defined as the presence of one or both of the following:

- Poor symptom control, and/or
- Frequent exacerbation (>2/year) requiring oral corticosteroid or serious exacerbation (>1/year) requiring hospitalization

The steps to approach uncontrolled asthma are as follows:

- First, confirm the diagnosis—is it really asthma?
- Look for factors contributing to symptoms:
  - Inhalation technique
  - Adherence to therapy
  - Comorbidities
  - Modifiable risk factors and triggers
- Review and optimize the therapy:
  - Optimize therapy
  - Step-up
- Review response after 3–6 months—if poor response moves to next step, or else optimize the therapy and keep on follow-up.

- Investigate further and give patients support.
- Assess the severe asthma phenotype (high Th2 vs. low Th2 inflammation)
  - *High Th2 inflammation:* Consider biological therapy if affordable and recommended for the age.
  - *Low Th2 inflammation:* Add other therapy.
- Consider other therapy if non-T2 inflammation
- Response to therapy
- Continue collaborative optimization of therapy

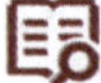

REFERENCES/SOURCES

- Agrawal S, Kabra SK. Difficult asthma. In: Lodha R, Kabra SK (Eds). Essential Pediatric Pulmonology, 4th edition. New Delhi: Jaypee Brothers Medical Publishers; 2023. pp. 295-300.
- Ginasthma.org. (2023). Global Initiative for Asthma (GINA). Difficult to treat or severe asthma. [online] Available from https://ginasthma.org/2023-gina-main-report/ [Last accessed June, 2024].
- Kliegman RM, St Geme III JW. Nelson Textbook of Pediatrics, 21st edition. Elsevier; 2019. Chapter 169: Childhood asthma. pp. 1186-209.
- National Heart, Lung, and Blood Institute. (2020). 2020 Focused Updates to the Asthma Management Guidelines: A Report from the National Asthma Education and Prevention Program Coordinating Committee Expert Panel Working Group. [online] Available from https://www.nhlbi.nih.gov/resources/2020-focused-updates-asthma-management-guidelines [Last accessed June, 2024].

16. A 9-year-old girl is diagnosed with asthma since infancy. She was on a high dose of inhaled corticosteroid therapy. Her symptoms remain uncontrolled despite the optimization of therapy, and she has two exacerbations in the last 6 months and needed oral steroids therapy. On further investigations, her total immunoglobulin E (IgE) level was 1,500 IU/L, FeNO 25 ppb, and peripheral eosinophilic counts were 200/mcL. The treating physician wanted to start omalizumab. Which of the following is a good predictor of response to omalizumab?

A. Disease for prolonged duration
B. High total IgE level
C. Eosinophil 200/mcL
D. FeNO–25 ppb

EXPLANATION

The given vignette has uncontrolled asthma even after optimization of therapy and a high dose of ICS. A high total IgE level is not a predictor of a good response to omalizumab (B). Eosinophil >260/mcL has good prediction (C). FeNO >20 ppb has a good prediction of response to therapy (D). Prolonged duration (A) is not a predictive factor for response to omalizumab.

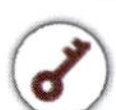

Key: D

BOOST YOUR KNOWLEDGE

Omalizumab is a monoclonal antibody that binds the Fc portion of free IgE to its receptors on mast cells. It reduces the free IgE and down regulates its receptors.

The *eligibility criteria* to start omalizumab in children ≥6 years having uncontrolled asthma and with one or more of the following:

- Total IgE level and weight should be in dosage range.
- Sensitization to inhalant allergens
- More than a specified number of exacerbations

The factors predicting good response to omalizumab are:

- Baseline total IgE does not predict response.
- Blood eosinophilia >260/mcL
- FeNO >20 ppb
- Childhood onset
- Clinical history suggests allergy to inhalant allergens.

REFERENCES/SOURCES

- Agrawal S, Kabra SK. Difficult asthma. In: Lodha R, Kabra SK (Eds). Essential Pediatric Pulmonology, 4th edition. New Delhi: Jaypee Brothers Medical Publishers; 2023. pp. 295-306.
- Ginasthma.org. (2023). Global Initiative for Asthma (GINA). Difficult to treat or severe asthma. [online] Available from https://ginasthma.org/2023-gina-main-report/ [Last accessed June, 2024].
- Kliegman RM, St Geme III JW. Nelson Textbook of Pediatrics, 21st edition. Elsevier; 2019. Chapter 169: Childhood asthma. pp. 1186-209.
- National Heart, Lung, and Blood Institute. (2020). 2020 Focused Updates to the Asthma Management Guidelines: A Report from the National Asthma Education and Prevention Program Coordinating Committee Expert Panel Working Group. [online] Available from https://www.nhlbi.nih.gov/resources/2020-focused-updates-asthma-management-guidelines [Last accessed June, 2024].

17. A 14-year-old boy, known case of asthma, is on low-dose maintenance and reliever therapy (MART). What advice will you give him in case of worsening of symptoms at home?

A. Increase the dose of maintenance ICS-budesonide combination for symptom relief
B. Add short-acting beta2-agonist (SABA) along with MART
C. Add leukotriene receptor antagonist along with MART
D. Start short course of oral corticosteroid

EXPLANATION

In adults and adolescents on MART, increase the frequency of same ICS-LABA combination with worsening of symptoms. It causes rapid symptomatic relief (A). There is no need to add SABA to existing MART; however, it can be used in children who is not on MART rather on only maintenance ICS-LABA combination (B). There is no role of adding montelukast during worsening of symptoms (C). Short course of oral corticosteroid is given when MART as reliever therapy failed to response (D).

Key: A

BOOST YOUR KNOWLEDGE

Asthma action plan aims to educate parents or patients to recognize the worsening of symptoms and institute the appropriate therapy. It is a very important step in the long-term management of asthma. All patients should be provided with written asthma management plans either in printed form or digitally. It helps to recognize and respond appropriately in case of worsening symptoms. It has been shown that asthma action plans reduce serious exacerbation and hence mortality.

Asthma action plan:

- *General plan:*
  - Know how to self-monitored asthma symptoms/or lung function (PEFR)
  - Written asthma action plan
  - Regular follow-up
- *With worsening of symptoms:*
  - *Increase reliever therapy:*
    - If on MART therapy, increases the frequency of same ICS-LABA combination (maximum eight puffs in children)
    - If on ICS-LABA + SABA, start SABA as needed
  - *If no improvement/worsening:*
    - Visit nearby healthcare center
    - Short course of oral corticosteroid

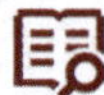

REFERENCES/SOURCES

- Ginasthma.org. (2023). Global Initiative for Asthma (GINA). [online] Available from https://ginasthma.org/2023-gina-main-report/ [Last accessed June, 2024].
- Kliegman RM, St Geme III JW. Nelson Textbook of Pediatrics, 21st edition. Elsevier; 2019. Chapter 169: Childhood asthma. pp. 1186-209.
- Kumar P. Bronchial asthma. In: Gupta P (Ed). UG Textbook of Pediatrics, 1st edition. New Delhi: Jaypee Brothers Medical Publishers; 2023. pp. 214-24.
- National Heart, Lung, and Blood Institute. (2020). 2020 Focused Updates to the Asthma Management Guidelines: A Report from the National Asthma Education and Prevention Program Coordinating Committee Expert Panel Working Group. [online] Available from https://www.nhlbi.nih.gov/resources/2020-focused-updates-asthma-management-guidelines [Last accessed June, 2024].

18. A 16-year-old boy, diagnosed case of asthma on step-4 therapy, presented in emergency with worsening of symptoms. On examination, he talks in phrases, RR = 38/minute, HR = 132/minute, SpO_2 = 92% on room air, B/L air entry was good but polyphonic wheeze was heard throughout the expiration. He was started on O_2 with a mask and continuous salbutamol nebulization for 1 hour but there was no improvement. What is the next step of management?

A. IV magnesium sulfate infusion
B. IV aminophylline
C. IM epinephrine
D. Systemic corticosteroids

EXPLANATION

In this case, the child has exacerbation of asthma. First, take care of airway, breathing, and circulation (ABC). Next step is to start inhaled salbutamol (pMDI or nebulized) with or without ipratropium bromide. If patient does not improve, start oral or IV steroid (D). Magnesium sulfate is usually administered after use of systemic steroids (A). IV aminophylline is only given for severe asthma (B). Epinephrine is given if the child has concurrent anaphylaxis (C).

Key: D

BOOST YOUR KNOWLEDGE

Asthma exacerbation is characterized by progressive increase in asthma symptoms and/or decrease in lung function. In children, the most common triggers are viral respiratory tract infections. The diagnosis of asthma exacerbation is mainly clinical. Pulmonary function test (PFT) if performed may assist in diagnosis. The management of exacerbation depends upon the severity of episodes, which is assessed clinically. There are many numerical scores available which give objective evidence of severity. Modified pulmonary index score (MPIS) is most used in clinical practice.

Modified pulmonary index score:

Parameters	***0***	***1***	***2***	***3***
SpO_2	>95%	>93–95%	>90–92%	<90%
Accessory muscle use	None	Mild	Moderate	Severe
Inspiratory-to-expiratory flow ratio	2:1	1:1	1:2	1:3
Wheezing	None	End expiration only	• Both in inspiratory and expiratory • Good air entry	• Both in inspiratory and expiratory • Poor air entry
HR (/minute): <3 years ≥3 years	 <120 <100	 120–140 100–120	 141–160 121–140	 >160 >140

Contd...

Contd...

Parameters	*0*	*1*	*2*	*3*
RR (/minute): <6 years ≥6 years	 ≤30 ≤20	 31–45 21–35	 46–60 36–50	 >60 >50
Mild: <7, moderate: 7–11, severe: ≥12				

REFERENCES/SOURCES

- Ginasthma.org. (2023). Global Initiative for Asthma (GINA). Difficult to treat or severe asthma. [online] Available from https://ginasthma.org/2023-gina-main-report/ [Last accessed June, 2024].
- Kumar K, Shankar J. Acute exacerbation of asthma. In: Lodha R, Kabra SK (Eds). Essential Pediatric Pulmonology, 4th edition. New Delhi: Jaypee Brothers Medical Publishers; 2023. pp. 270-280.
- National Heart, Lung, and Blood Institute. (2020). 2020 Focused Updates to the Asthma Management Guidelines: A Report from the National Asthma Education and Prevention Program Coordinating Committee Expert Panel Working Group. [online] Available from https://www.nhlbi.nih.gov/resources/2020-focused-updates-asthma-management-guidelines [Last accessed June, 2024].

19. A 4-year-old child presented in OPD with cough, cold, wheezing, and breathing difficulty. He had a similar episode 6 months back which lasted for 7 days and improved with nebulization. There was no personal or family history of atopy. His symptoms also worsen with play, cold food, and laughing/crying. Which of these increases the probability of asthma diagnosis in him?

A. Absence of family history of atopy
B. Symptoms in between episodes
C. Duration of episode 7 days
D. Two episodes/year

EXPLANATION

In this case, the baby has two episodes of wheezing in 6 months. In preschool wheeze, it is difficult to perform spirometry, thus the probability of asthma is decided by clinical history and examination. Each episode lasting for ≥10 days increases the probability of asthma (C). Family history of atopy (asthma, allergic rhinitis, or dermatitis) increases the probability (A). It is very important to ask about how is the symptoms in between episodes. If symptoms trigger other than viral infection such as play (exertion), crying/laughing, exposure to dust/smoke, etc., increases the probability of asthma (B). The number of episodes also has influence on the probability of asthma; ≥3 episodes/year increases the probability (D).

Key: B

BOOST YOUR KNOWLEDGE

Wheezing in preschool children is a prevalent condition and almost 50% of the children develop at least one episode by their 6th birthday. As we know the diagnosis of asthma depends upon characteristics symptoms pattern and expiratory flow limitation, however, this age group is not cooperative and so difficult to perform spirometry. These symptoms are very common in this age group even without asthma. Moreover, these children are growing, their symptoms widely vary with age. GINA has provided a probability based on clinical history, which guide the clinician in decision-making.

Probability of asthma in preschool wheezing:

Low probability (few have asthma)	*Intermediate (some have asthma)*	*High probability (most have asthma)*
• Symptoms (cough, wheezing, difficulty in breathing, and shortness of breath) last for <10 during viral respiratory infection	• Symptoms (cough, wheezing, difficulty in breathing, and shortness of breath) last for >10 during viral respiratory infection	• Symptoms (cough, wheezing, difficulty in breathing, and shortness of breath) last for >10 during viral respiratory infection

Contd...

Contd...

Low probability (few have asthma)	*Intermediate (some have asthma)*	*High probability (most have asthma)*
• 2–3 episodes/year • No symptom between episodes	• >3 episodes/year or severe episode or worsening at night • Episode last for >10 days • Between episode child may have the symptoms	• >3 episodes/year or severe episode or worsening at night • Between episodes child has symptoms, trigger by exertion (play), exposure to dust/ smoke, laughing, etc. • Allergic sensitization, family history of atopy

REFERENCES/SOURCES

- Ginasthma.org. (2023). Global Initiative for Asthma (GINA). Difficult to treat or severe asthma. [online] Available from https://ginasthma.org/2023-gina-main-report/ [Last accessed June, 2024].
- Kliegman RM, St Geme III JW. Nelson Textbook of Pediatrics, 21st edition. Elsevier; 2019. Chapter 169: Childhood asthma. pp. 1186-209.
- National Heart, Lung, and Blood Institute. (2020). 2020 Focused Updates to the Asthma Management Guidelines: A Report from the National Asthma Education and Prevention Program Coordinating Committee Expert Panel Working Group. [online] Available from https://www.nhlbi.nih.gov/resources/2020-focused-updates-asthma-management-guidelines [Last accessed June, 2024].

20. A 3-year-old child had recurrent episodes of cough, wheezing, and breathing difficulty for 1 year. The symptoms occur almost every month and each episode lasts for ≥10 days. Apart from viral infection, his symptoms also worsen by cold food and during play. His mother has a history of allergic rhinitis. Which is the preferred treatment for this patient?

A. Daily low-dose ICS
B. Daily low-dose ICS + formoterol
C. As needed inhaled salbutamol
D. Oral leukotriene receptor blocker

EXPLANATION

This child has a high probability of having asthma and need controller therapy. Daily low-dose ICS (budesonide here) is the preferred treatment for him (A). ICS-LABA combination is not recommended in children ≤4 years of age (B). Since, child has symptoms almost every month and symptom last for >10 days, only inhaled salbutamol is not helpful (C). Oral leukotriene receptor antagonist (LTRA) may be effective in a subset of children, but it is an alternative treatment not the preferred one (D).

Key: A

BOOST YOUR KNOWLEDGE

In preschool wheeze, we should have probability-based approach. If the child has low probability of asthma, giving inhaled salbutamol during the viral respiratory infection will be sufficient. In high probability, the preferred treatment is daily low-dose ICS. Daily LTRA is an alternative to daily low-dose ICS. Whatever the treatment started it is very important to follow-up these children regularly. After 8–12 weeks if there is symptomatic improvement the treatment can be stopped and kept on follow-up. If symptoms do not improve or partly improve, treat him like an asthma after excluding other possible differential diagnosis.

REFERENCES/SOURCES

- Ginasthma.org. (2023). Global Initiative for Asthma (GINA). Difficult to treat or severe asthma. [online] Available from https://ginasthma.org/2023-gina-main-report/ [Last accessed June, 2024].
- Kumar P. Bronchial asthma. In: Gupta P (Ed). UG Textbook of Pediatrics, 1st edition. New Delhi: Jaypee Brothers Medical Publishers; 2023. pp. 214-24.
- National Heart, Lung, and Blood Institute. (2020). 2020 Focused Updates to the Asthma Management Guidelines: A Report from the National Asthma Education and Prevention Program Coordinating Committee Expert Panel Working Group. [online] Available from https://www.nhlbi.nih.gov/resources/2020-focused-updates-asthma-management-guidelines [Last accessed June, 2024].

CHAPTER 19.5

Aerosol Therapy

Kamal Kumar Singhal

1. Which one of the following is true regarding the usage of spacer along with a metered dose inhaler (MDI)?

A. Spacer should be used only in young children and not adolescents
B. Spacer reduces systemic and local side effects of drugs
C. Only commercially available spacers should be used and not homemade spacers
D. The use of a spacer alongside a mask is imperative for children under the age of 5 years

EXPLANATION

- Many patients find it challenging to use pressurized metered dose inhalers (pMDIs) effectively without spacers or holding chambers. Hence, it is recommended that individuals prescribed an inhaled corticosteroid (ICS) in a pMDI should utilize spacers.
- Spacer devices reduce the total body dose of inhaled drugs, thereby reducing both systemic and local side effects of the drugs.
- Any spacer is better than no spacer. Homemade spacers have been found to be as effective as commercial spacers.
- The selection of the inhaler device ought to consider the child's age and proficiency. Transitioning children from a face mask to a mouthpiece should occur once they exhibit good technique.

Key: B

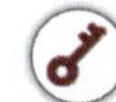

BOOST YOUR KNOWLEDGE

The effectiveness of the drug for inhalation can be influenced by the size of the spacer, which depends on the prescribed medication and the type of pMDI used. Although young children can use spacers of different sizes, theoretically, a smaller volume spacer (<350 mL) is considered advantageous for very young children.

REFERENCES/SOURCES

- Global Initiative for Asthma. (2022). 2022 GINA Main Report. [online] Available from https://ginasthma.org/gina-reports/ [Last accessed July, 2024].
- Kliegman R, Stanton B, St Geme JW, Schor NF, Behrman RE (Eds). Nelson Textbook of Pediatrics, 20th edition. Philadelphia, PA: Elsevier Inc.; 2016.
- Wilmott RW. Kendig and Chernick's Disorders of the Respiratory Tract in Children, 9th edition. Philadelphia, PA: Elsevier; 2019.

2. The most effective breathing pattern for pMDI inhalation along with a spacer is:

A. Deep tidal breathing
B. Tidal breathing
C. Slow deep inhalation and hold
D. Deep and rapid breathing

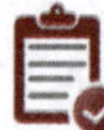

EXPLANATION

The recommended optimal inhalation technique when using a pMDI without a spacer is a slow maximal inhalation with actuation of the pMDI as the slow inhalation is commenced.

Key: C

BOOST YOUR KNOWLEDGE

For infants and young children who cannot perform the recommended maneuver, inhalation through a spacer using tidal breathing (though less efficient) may be considered. The optimal inhalation technique for each puff of MDI-delivered medication is a slow (5 seconds) inhalation, then a 5–10 seconds breath hold. No waiting time is required between puffs of medication. Preschool-age children cannot perform this inhalation technique. Hence, for children in this age bracket, MDI medications are delivered with a spacer and mask, employing a unique method: Each puff is administered during regular breathing for around 30 seconds or 5–10 breaths, maintaining a tight seal is crucial, avoiding speaking, coughing, or crying (may cause the medication to be expelled from the spacer). Nevertheless, this approach may not yield as much medication per puff as the optimal MDI technique utilized by older children and adults.

REFERENCES/SOURCES

- Global Initiative for Asthma. (2022). 2022 GINA Main Report. [online] Available from https://ginasthma.org/gina-reports/ [Last accessed July, 2024].
- Kliegman R, Stanton B, St Geme JW, Schor NF, Behrman RE (Eds). Nelson Textbook of Pediatrics, 20th edition. Philadelphia, PA: Elsevier Inc.; 2016.
- Wilmott RW. Kendig and Chernick's Disorders of the Respiratory Tract in Children, 9th edition. Philadelphia, PA: Elsevier; 2019.

3. Which of the following is true?

A. When MDI is used appropriately, most of the drug reaches the lower airway
B. When using nebulizers, a large proportion of the drug reaches the lower airways
C. Autohalers (breath actuated) with spacers are more effective than the combination of MDI with spacers
D. Dry powder inhalers (DPIs) are to be used with deep and forceful inhalation

EXPLANATION

- All the common aerosol delivery devices (MDI, DPI, and nebulizer) show lung deposition of approximately 10–15% of the total nominal dose. Even when used appropriately, only a small proportion reaches the lower airway.
- The delivery method with the highest cost-effectiveness and efficiency is via pMDI when used with a spacer.
- With nebulizers compared to pMDIs, a much smaller proportion of drugs will reach the lower airway, thus are inefficient compared to MDIs.
- Autohalers cannot be used with a spacer.

Key: D

BOOST YOUR KNOWLEDGE

- Nebulizers, the only practical alternative delivery systems for children, are reserved for the minority who are unable to effectively use a spacer device. If a nebulizer is used to administer ICS, it should be equipped with a mouthpiece to prevent the medication from reaching the eyes.

- For the majority of children, the combination of pMDI and spacer is preferred due to its greater efficiency compared to a nebulizer for delivering bronchodilators.
- The utilization of nebulizers can disperse aerosols and potentially contribute to the transmission of respiratory viral infections.
- The issue of coordination can be addressed through the utilization of breath-actuated pMDIs, such as the autohaler. Nonetheless, they necessitate a minimum inspiratory flow for activation, posing challenges for younger children, and leading to increased oropharyngeal deposition, as these devices cannot be paired with spacers.

REFERENCES/SOURCES

- Global Initiative for Asthma. (2022). 2022 GINA Main Report. [online] Available from https://ginasthma.org/gina-reports/ [Last accessed July, 2024].
- Kliegman R, Stanton B, St Geme JW, Schor NF, Behrman RE (Eds). Nelson Textbook of Pediatrics, 20th edition. Philadelphia, PA: Elsevier Inc.; 2016.
- Wilmott RW. Kendig and Chernick's Disorders of the Respiratory Tract in Children, 9th edition. Philadelphia, Pennsylvania: Elsevier; 2019.

4. Which of the following is correct about spacer usage?

A. It should be scrubbed with a dry cloth to remove the deposited drug on the inner walls
B. It should be dipped in dilute liquid soap and allowed to air dry without rinsing
C. Spacer should not be washed with detergent
D. Deposition of a thin layer of detergent on the inner surface of spacer increases the static charge on the spacer walls and reduces the proportion of drug available

EXPLANATION

- Due to static charge, certain spacers may need to be washed with detergent (without rinsing) and left to air dry prior to use.
- Some plastic spacers may accumulate static charge, which can attract drug particles and diminish lung delivery. A thin layer of detergent may reduce the static charge on the spacer wall.
- Whenever a patient or healthcare provider gets a new plastic spacer for emergency purposes, it is advisable to wash it regularly with detergent (e.g., on a monthly basis) to minimize static charge.

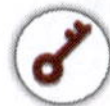

Key: B

BOOST YOUR KNOWLEDGE

Reducing static charge involves washing the spacer with detergent (without rinsing) and letting it air dry; however, it may gradually reaccumulate. Spacers crafted from antistatic materials or metals are less prone to this issue.

REFERENCES/SOURCES

- Global Initiative for Asthma. (2022). 2022 GINA Main Report. [online] Available from https://ginasthma.org/gina-reports/ [Last accessed July, 2024].
- Kliegman R, Stanton B, St Geme JW, Schor NF, Behrman RE (Eds). Nelson Textbook of Pediatrics, 20th edition. Philadelphia, PA: Elsevier Inc.; 2016.
- Wilmott RW. Kendig and Chernick's Disorders of the Respiratory Tract in Children, 9th edition. Philadelphia, PA: Elsevier; 2019.

5. Which of the following is true regarding the use of face mask with a spacer with MDI?

A. Must be used in all children <3 years of age, even if the child is able to make good seal around the mouthpiece of the spacer and breathes through it rather than the nose
B. A tight seal over the face should not be used in children

C. The use of face mask along with a spacer, compared to the spacer alone, reduces the proportion of drug reaching the lower airway
D. The movement of the valve, while the child is breathing through the valved spacer, is not important

EXPLANATION

- The selection of the inhaler device should depend on the child's age and proficiency in using the device. Transitioning children from a face mask to a mouthpiece should occur promptly once they exhibit good technique.
- When utilizing a face mask, it should be snugly fitted around the child's mouth and nose to prevent drug loss. The nose is significantly more effective than the mouth in filtering out particles.
- Ensure that the valve moves as the child breathes through the spacer.

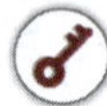

Key: C

BOOST YOUR KNOWLEDGE

- In selecting an inhaler device, consider the child's age and ability. The recommended choice is a pMDI with a spacer, using a face mask for children under 3 years old and a mouthpiece for most children aged 3–5. Transitioning from a face mask to a mouthpiece should occur once the child can demonstrate a good technique.
- Using a face mask that permits nasal inhalation or a nasal mask during administration has demonstrated significantly reduced lung deposition. This is because the nose is far more effective than the mouth in filtering out particles >1 μm in diameter.

REFERENCES/SOURCES

- Global Initiative for Asthma. (2022). 2022 GINA Main Report. [online] Available from https://ginasthma.org/gina-reports/ [Last accessed July, 2024].
- Kliegman R, Stanton B, St Geme JW, Schor NF, Behrman RE (Eds). Nelson Textbook of Pediatrics, 20th edition. Philadelphia, PA: Elsevier Inc.; 2016.
- Wilmott RW. Kendig and Chernick's Disorders of the Respiratory Tract in Children, 9th edition. Philadelphia, PA: Elsevier; 2019.

6. Which of the following is a correct statement regarding pMDI usage in children?

A. Always prime the pMDI before use
B. Multiple actuations into the spacer before inhalation may increase the amount of drug inhaled
C. Connect the pMDI to the spacer and exhale inside the spacer
D. Actuate the pMDI and take deep and slow breathing, followed by breath-hold for 5–10 seconds

EXPLANATION

- Prime your inhaler if this is the first time you are using it, if you have not used it for several days, or if you have dropped it. Priming a MDI usually involves shaking it and spraying it into the air (away from your face) up to four times.
- Multiple actuations into the spacer before inhalation may markedly reduce the amount of drug inhaled.
- With traditional spacers, the child must breathe in through the spacer and breathe out away from the spacer.

Key: D

BOOST YOUR KNOWLEDGE

- The delay between actuating the pMDI into the spacer and inhalation could decrease the available drug amount. To optimize drug delivery, inhalation should commence promptly after actuation.
- If a healthcare provider or caregiver is administering the medication to the child, they should only actuate the pMDI when the child is prepared, and the spacer is positioned in the child's mouth.

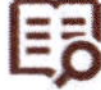

REFERENCES/SOURCES

- Global Initiative for Asthma. (2022). 2022 GINA Main Report. [online] Available from https://ginasthma.org/gina-reports/ [Last accessed July, 2024].
- Kliegman R, Stanton B, St Geme JW, Schor NF, Behrman RE (Eds). Nelson Textbook of Pediatrics, 20th edition. Philadelphia, PA: Elsevier Inc.; 2016.
- Wilmott RW. Kendig and Chernick's Disorders of the Respiratory Tract in Children, 9th edition. Philadelphia, PA: Elsevier; 2019.

7. Which of the following is correct regarding the inhaled route of drug delivery?

A. It permits the use of drugs which are not readily absorbed by the oral route
B. DPIs are suitable for preschool children
C. It has no systemic side effects
D. It has slower onset of action

EXPLANATION

- The inhaled entry route ensures a more rapid onset of action within the target organ.
- Aerosol delivery has the advantage of reducing systemic side effects.
- At present, DPIs rely on forceful inhalation to aerosolize the drug, making them unsuitable for preschool children.

Key: A

BOOST YOUR KNOWLEDGE

Utilizing an inhaled entry route offers relatively unimpeded access to the actively exchanging capillary beds in the lungs. This results in a faster onset of drug action within the target organ compared to alternative administration methods such as oral (solid or liquid doses swallowed) and subcutaneous or intramuscular injections. Consequently, a lower dose is required for an equivalent effect, and aerosol delivery offers the advantage of minimizing systemic side effects.

REFERENCES/SOURCES

- Global Initiative for Asthma. (2022). 2022 GINA Main Report. [online] Available from https://ginasthma.org/gina-reports/ [Last accessed July, 2024].
- Kliegman R, Stanton B, St Geme JW, Schor NF, Behrman RE (Eds). Nelson Textbook of Pediatrics, 20th edition. Philadelphia, PA: Elsevier Inc.; 2016.
- Wilmott RW. Kendig and Chernick's Disorders of the Respiratory Tract in Children, 9th edition. Philadelphia, PA: Elsevier; 2019.

8. Which of the following is correct regarding drug administration by inhalation compared with oral or parenteral administration?

A. Portable metered dose devices do not require specific inhalation techniques for optimal delivery
B. If demonstrated well initially, repeated training is not needed for optimal use
C. Drug delivery is impaired in diseased regions of the lungs
D. Health professionals need to assess the best drug-device "fit" for patients, depending on the age and disease condition

EXPLANATION

- Patients who exhibit errors in inhalation technique experience reduced clinical benefits compared to those with proficient technique, particularly noticeable in individuals with poor coordination.
- Fewer patients demonstrate errors in inhaler technique with a DPI when compared to a standard pMDI.
- Various inhaler devices are currently accessible for delivering inhaled drugs. The field of inhaled drug delivery is dynamic, with numerous inhalers already available and new ones continually being introduced. The abundance of available inhaler devices, each requiring distinct inhalation techniques for optimal drug delivery, may lead to confusion among both patients and healthcare providers, a phenomenon termed "device dementia." It is essential to reinforce the technique during subsequent visits after initial instruction.

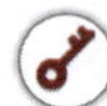

Key: C

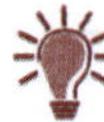

BOOST YOUR KNOWLEDGE

Devices utilized for aerosol drug delivery exhibit diverse designs, which can be customized for application or dosage. However, instructions for usage and optimal inhalation techniques vary significantly depending on the type of device, potentially leading to confusion and misuse if patients are prescribed multiple devices for various medications. Consequently, achieving optimal benefits necessitates receiving instructions for device usage through personalized professional guidance. Consistency in dosing can be challenging due to numerous factors, including tissue and systemic absorption, airway obstruction, patient training, and the ability to perform the required inhalation technique. Furthermore, a patient's cognitive capacity to operate the device and anatomical considerations specific to their age or medical condition may impact drug delivery efficacy.

A thorough comprehension of the principles governing aerosol particle deposition within the lungs empowers healthcare professionals to evaluate the most suitable drug-device combination for patients across different age groups and medical conditions.

REFERENCES/SOURCES

- Global Initiative for Asthma. (2022). 2022 GINA Main Report. [online] Available from https://ginasthma.org/gina-reports/ [Last accessed July, 2024].
- Kliegman R, Stanton B, St Geme JW, Schor NF, Behrman RE (Eds). Nelson Textbook of Pediatrics, 20th edition. Philadelphia, PA: Elsevier Inc.; 2016.
- Wilmott RW. Kendig and Chernick's Disorders of the Respiratory Tract in Children, 9th edition. Philadelphia, PA: Elsevier; 2019.

9. Which of the following is correct regarding the use of DPIs?

A. There is a need for coordinated actuation and breath inhalation
B. They lack portability
C. They do not require a mid to high peak inspiratory flow (PIF) rate
D. They are breath-driven

EXPLANATION

- The predominant commercially utilized DPIs operate on a breath-driven mechanism, eliminating the need for coordination between actuation and inhalation, unlike pMDIs.
- DPIs offer numerous benefits, notably their portability.
- Typically, DPIs necessitate a mid-to-high peak inspiratory flow to effectively disperse and suspend the drug particles within the airflow.

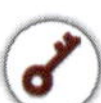

Key: D

BOOST YOUR KNOWLEDGE

Flow rates below the minimum required for dispersing the drug and excipient will result in inadequate pulmonary deposition. Children, particularly those who are ill, frequently lack the ability to generate adequate flow to effectively disperse the powder. Moreover, the total volume of inspiration may not be adequate to draw the powder deep into the lungs to the desired therapeutic site of action. Therefore, DPIs are not advisable for children under 5 years of age.

REFERENCES/SOURCES

- Global Initiative for Asthma. (2022). 2022 GINA Main Report. [online] Available from https://ginasthma.org/gina-reports/ [Last accessed July, 2024].
- Kliegman R, Stanton B, St Geme JW, Schor NF, Behrman RE (Eds). Nelson Textbook of Pediatrics, 20th edition. Philadelphia, PA: Elsevier Inc.; 2016.
- Wilmott RW. Kendig and Chernick's Disorders of the Respiratory Tract in Children, 9th edition. Philadelphia, PA: Elsevier; 2019.

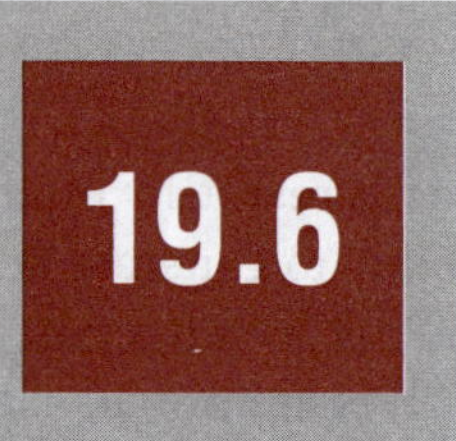

CHAPTER 19.6 Suppurative Lung Disease

Lokesh Guglani

1. A 3-year-old boy presents with history of chronic wet cough since early infancy. He was born full term and had a history of neonatal respiratory distress requiring oxygen support in the neonatal intensive care unit (NICU) for 2 days and was discharged home at 1 week of age. He had respiratory syncytial virus (RSV) bronchiolitis at 2 months of age, and his parents report that his cough has never resolved since then. In addition, he has also daily nasal drainage since early infancy that is present year-round. He has had appropriate weight gain and has no gastrointestinal complaints. There is no history of coughing or choking while drinking liquids. He has been reported to have frequent otitis media episodes requiring frequent antibiotics, especially during the winter months. Examination reveals a healthy toddler with normal vital signs, weight at 50th percentile, and bilateral basilar crackles on auscultation.

Which of the following would be the most useful next test in diagnostic evaluation of this patient?

A. Modified barium swallow study
B. Nasal ciliary brush biopsy
C. Echocardiogram
D. Throat swab

EXPLANATION

The patient described in this clinical vignette has all the classical features of primary ciliary dyskinesia (PCD) and satisfies at least two out of the four clinical criteria that have been reported to be highly predictive of a diagnosis of PCD. These four clinical criteria are:

1. History of neonatal respiratory distress
2. Onset of chronic, year-round wet cough before 6 months of age
3. Onset of chronic, year-round nasal drainage before 6 months of age
4. Laterality defects

The presence of any two out of the above four criteria has a sensitivity of 80% and a specificity of 72% for the diagnosis of PCD.

A swallow study would be helpful for the diagnosis of dysphagia and aspiration, but this patient has no suggestive history of coughing or choking with liquids. An echocardiogram would not be helpful in this patient with recurrent respiratory complaints in the absence of any heart murmurs or suggestive symptoms. A throat swab could help assess for bacterial colonization of the airways but will not provide any assistance with diagnostic testing in this patient.

Key: B

BOOST YOUR KNOWLEDGE

Primary ciliary dyskinesia is an inherited disorder characterized by motile ciliary dysfunction, resulting in an array of clinical manifestations, including chronic rhinosinusitis, middle ear effusions, laterality defects, infertility, and chronic bronchitis, leading to bronchiectasis. Historically, the diagnosis of PCD relied on the combination of clinical features and ultrastructural analysis of respiratory cilia, which can be done by collecting nasal epithelial cells using a nasal ciliary brushing procedure that can be done in clinic. Other additional tests that can be done include nasal nitric oxide measurement and molecular genetic testing for known PCD-associated genes.

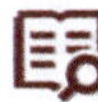

REFERENCES/SOURCES

- Goutaki M, Shoemark A. Diagnosis of primary ciliary dyskinesia. Clin Chest Med. 2022;43(1):127-40.
- Horani A, Ferkol TW. Understanding primary ciliary dyskinesia and other ciliopathies. J Pediatr. 2021;230:15-22.e1.
- Leigh MW, Ferkol TW, Davis SD, Lee HS, Rosenfeld M, Dell SD, et al. Clinical features and associated likelihood of primary ciliary dyskinesia in children and adolescents. Ann Am Thorac Soc. 2016;13(8):1305-13.

2. A 12-year-old boy with PCD (homozygous for *CCDC39* gene variants) has been hospitalized for an acute pulmonary exacerbation and is being treated with intravenous antibiotics and airway clearance therapies. His forced expiratory volume in 1 second (FEV1) at admission was 58% of predicted with no bronchodilator response, and it has now improved to 81%. This is his third admission for acute pulmonary exacerbation this year, and his fifth one in the last 2 years. He has not had any evidence of chronic colonization with *Pseudomonas aeruginosa* or infection with atypical mycobacteria on his prior respiratory cultures. His chest computed tomography (CT) scan shows significant mucus plugging and airway wall thickening in the right and left lower lobe bronchi with some areas of cylindrical bronchiectasis.

Which of the following therapies should be added to prevent ongoing recurrence of acute pulmonary exacerbations?

A. Inhaled steroids
B. Recombinant human DNase (Pulmozyme)
C. Antireflux medications
D. Azithromycin

EXPLANATION

Patients with PCD can have periodic infectious exacerbations that require hospitalization and treatment with intravenous antibiotics. Patients with PCD with specific gene variants that cause inner dynein arm and central apparatus defects in their ciliary ultrastructure (such as those with *CCDC39* or *CCDC40* gene variants) tend to have greater rates of decline of lung function and are at risk for recurrent pulmonary exacerbations.

The use of inhaled steroids in patients with PCD has not been associated with any significant improvement in the lung function or the reduction in the number of pulmonary exacerbations. Recombinant human DNase (Pulmozye) has not been shown to be effective in adults with noncystic fibrosis bronchiectasis, and there is limited evidence for its utility in pediatric patients with PCD. Antireflux medication can be helpful in patients who have gastroesophageal reflux disease as a comorbidity, but it may not help to reduce the frequency of pulmonary exacerbations in patients with PCD.

Azithromycin has been used as three times a week therapy (every Monday, Wednesday, and Friday) for its anti-inflammatory properties in patients with PCD. Prior to initiation of long-term azithromycin therapy, it is important to exclude infections with atypical mycobacteria and to assess for risk of prolongation of QT interval (if there is suggestive family history, or if patients are on other medications that also prolong QT interval) with a baseline electrocardiogram (EKG) prior to starting therapy. The optimal duration of this therapy is not known, and most patients continue this treatment long term with re-evaluations every 6 months to decide on the continuation of this therapy.

Key: D

BOOST YOUR KNOWLEDGE

The patient in this vignette has had multiple acute pulmonary exacerbations requiring hospitalization for intravenous antibiotics. Most patients with PCD tend to have a daily wet cough that improves with airway clearance treatments. This patient has been screened for chronic colonization with *P. aeruginosa* and atypical mycobacterial infections through periodic screening respiratory cultures and does not have any other daily medications that prolong the QT interval. Treatment with thrice weekly azithromycin therapy can help to reduce the frequency of her pulmonary exacerbations in this patient.

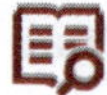

REFERENCES/SOURCES

- Horani A, Ferkol TW. Understanding primary ciliary dyskinesia and other ciliopathies. J Pediatr. 2021;230:15-22.e1.
- Kobbernagel HE, Buchvald FF, Haarman EG, Casaulta C, Collins SA, Hogg C, et al. Efficacy and safety of azithromycin maintenance therapy in primary ciliary dyskinesia (BESTCILIA): a multicentre, double-blind, randomised, placebo-controlled phase 3 trial. Lancet Respir Med. 2020;8(5):493-505.
- Shapiro AJ, Zariwala MA, Ferkol T, Davis SD, Sagel SD, Dell SD, et al; Genetic Disorders of Mucociliary Clearance Consortium. Diagnosis, monitoring, and treatment of primary ciliary dyskinesia: PCD foundation consensus recommendations based on state of the art review. Pediatr Pulmonol. 2016;51(2):115-32.

3. An 8-year-old boy presents with a history of recurrent pneumonia and chronic wet cough that is present year-round. He also has a history of poor weight gain and nasal polyps. His parents bring a chest CT scan that was done recently.

Which of the following radiologic findings on his chest CT would be the most sensitive indicators for the development of bronchiectasis?

A. Bilateral upper lobe infiltrates
B. Tree-in-bud opacities
C. Airway-to-artery ratio >1
D. Mucus plugging

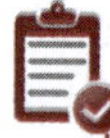

EXPLANATION

Chest imaging, specifically CT scanning, is required to make the diagnosis of bronchiectasis. In a patient with persistent wet cough and a history of frequent acute exacerbations, there should be at least one of the following findings on high-resolution CT with a slice thickness of 1 mm or less: (1) A ratio of the inner or outer airway diameter to the artery diameter of 1.0 or more, (2) a lack of tapering of the airways as they are tracked to the periphery, and (3) the presence of radiographically visible airways in the outer periphery.

The presence of bilateral upper lobe infiltrates is not specific for bronchiectasis. The presence of a tree in bud opacities can be an associated finding due to infections or inflammation that affect the small airways but is not considered a diagnostic feature of bronchiectasis. Similarly, mucus plugging of the airways can be present in many chronic respiratory conditions and is not specific for bronchiectasis.

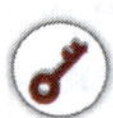

Key: C

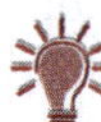

BOOST YOUR KNOWLEDGE

Bronchiectasis is a clinical syndrome that is characterized by chronic wet cough and sputum production in the presence of abnormal thickening and dilation of the bronchial wall that is visible on lung imaging. Bronchiectasis is a heterogeneous condition and may be encountered as a stand-alone pulmonary disease or occurs due to a number of congenital and hereditary diseases, including cystic fibrosis, PCD, Mounier–Kuhn syndrome, and alpha-1 antitrypsin deficiency. It may also develop in patients with autoimmune disorders and immune deficiency syndromes, including common variable immunodeficiency and human immunodeficiency virus infection.

Several scoring systems have been developed for the assessment of the severity and extent of bronchiectasis. These include the Brody score, disease-specific scores such as the CF-CT (cystic fibrosis–specific computed tomography) score (for children >6 years of age), or PRAGMA-CF score (for children <6 years of age), or the Bhalla score. However, scoring may be affected by the heterogeneity in CT scan settings and the different lung volumes at which these images are acquired.

REFERENCES/SOURCES

- Barbosa M, Chalmers JD. Bronchiectasis. Presse Med. 2023;52(3):104174.
- Cohen R, Shteinberg M. Diagnosis and evaluation of bronchiectasis. Clin Chest Med. 2022;43(1):7-22.
- O'Donnell AE. Bronchiectasis: a clinical review. N Engl J Med. 2022;387(6):533-45.

4. A 4-year-old girl has been reported to have a chronic wet cough and recurrent otitis media since she started elementary school at 3 years of age. Prior to that, she had a few colds, but it did not cause any persistent cough or wheezing. During the first month of starting school at the age of 3 years, she developed frequent colds. On evaluation, you find a normal growth pattern, no history of eczema or environmental allergies, no history of chronic nasal congestion, no reported coughing or choking with liquids, and there is no concern for any gastrointestinal complaints or malabsorption. There is no significant nocturnal cough or wheezing reported. There is no prior history of exposure to anyone with tuberculosis. On examination, there are no signs of respiratory distress or noisy breathing and no lymphadenopathy. On auscultation, there are coarse rhonchi bilaterally, but no wheezing or prolonged expiratory phase. Parents report that her cough has not resolved over the past 4 weeks despite ongoing intermittent use of salbutamol on an as-needed basis.

Which of the following is the next step in the management of this patient?

A. Amoxicillin-clavulanic acid for 14 days
B. Fluticasone nasal spray
C. Famotidine therapy for 6 weeks
D. Wait and watch

EXPLANATION

The patient described in this vignette has protracted bacterial bronchitis (PBB). It is defined as a wet cough of at least 4-week duration with no identified specific cause of cough that resolved following 2–4 weeks of appropriate antibiotics. PBB can be treated with a prolonged course of empiric antibiotics. Further evaluation is necessary if a child with suspected PBB does not adequately respond to antibiotics as chronic suppurative lung disease or bronchiectasis must be considered. The general approach is to choose an antibiotic that would adequately treat pathogens such as *Haemophilus influenzae*, *Streptococcus pneumoniae*, and *Moraxella catarrhalis*.

The use of fluticasone nasal spray would not help much in this patient with PBB as postnasal drip may not be the cause of this child's persistent cough, and there is no reported history of chronic nasal congestion. This patient does not have any reported symptoms of gastroesophageal reflux, and hence famotidine therapy may not help much. A wait-and-watch approach may be considered for postviral cough for up to 2 weeks, but due to the persistent wet character of the cough that has now gone on for 4 weeks, treatment with an antibiotic is warranted in this patient.

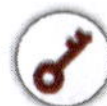

Key: A

BOOST YOUR KNOWLEDGE

Considering PBB in the differential diagnosis of chronic wet cough in children allows an early and adequate antibiotic treatment to eradicate the infection. Bronchoalveolar lavage (BAL) and respiratory cultures generally are not required, as well as chest X-ray and clinical diagnosis are enough to start an empiric 2-week therapy with amoxicillin-clavulanate acid. This therapy is mostly effective against the bacterial species involved, such as *H. influenzae* [nontypeable *Haemophilus influenzae* (NTHi)], *S. pneumoniae*, and *M. catarrhalis*. Moreover, an adequate therapy prevents the onset of a prolonged inflammatory process potentially associated with structural damage of the lower airways, which may be involved in bronchiectasis. Several studies provide evidence to support a link between PBB and bronchiectasis in children, and this emphasizes the necessity to consider this possibility of progression and to carry out some more detailed investigations in the case of a clinical suspicion.

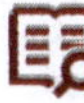

REFERENCES/SOURCES

- How to manage protracted bacterial bronchitis. Arch Dis Child. 2021;106(11):1074.
- O'Grady KF, Mahon J, Arnold D, Grimwood K, Hall KK, Goyal V, et al. Predictors of the development of protracted bacterial bronchitis following presentation to healthcare for an acute respiratory illness with cough: analysis of three cohort studies. J Clin Med. 2021;10(24):5735.

- Ruffles TJC, Goyal V, Marchant JM, Masters IB, Yerkovich S, Buntain H, et al. Duration of amoxicillin-clavulanate for protracted bacterial bronchitis in children (DACS): a multi-centre, double blind, randomised controlled trial. Lancet Respir Med. 2021;9(10):1121-9.
- Ruffles TJC, Marchant JM, Masters IB, Yerkovich ST, Wurzel DF, Gibson PG, et al. Outcomes of protracted bacterial bronchitis in children: a 5-year prospective cohort study. Respirology. 2021;26(3):241-8.

5. A 2-year-old child is brought to the emergency room with persistent bouts of coughing that started 6 hours ago when he was playing unattended. His mother heard him developing a sudden onset cough and noted that he had opened one of the jars with chickpeas and was red in the face from the coughing. Since then, he has been noted to have persistent retractions and nasal flaring and has been coughing without relief. There is no audible stridor on examination, but there is diminished air entry on right side of the chest on auscultation.

What would be the least invasive test to confirm the diagnosis of foreign-body aspiration in this patient?

A. Anteroposterior and lateral neck radiographs
B. Right and left lateral decubitus chest radiographs
C. Chest CT
D. Nasal endoscopy

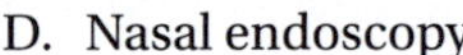

EXPLANATION

The patient in his clinical scenario has presented with foreign body (FB) aspiration into the lower airways. This patient will require an airway endoscopy for identification and removal of the FB.

For evaluation, radiologic imaging with right and left lateral decubitus films helps to identify areas of air trapping on chest radiographs. A neck soft tissue X-ray will not be helpful in identifying the FB. A chest CT can provide more detailed imaging but cannot be easily done in a 2-year-old agitated patient without using sedation. Nasal endoscopy will further irritate the child and cause worsening of respiratory distress without allowing visualization of the FB.

Key: B

BOOST YOUR KNOWLEDGE

Most aspirated FBs in children are in the bronchi. Laryngeal and tracheal FBs are less common. In a large case series of foreign body aspirations (FBAs) in children, the sites of the FB were as follows:

- Larynx—3%
- Trachea/carina—13%
- Right lung—60% (52% in the main bronchus, 6% in the lower lobe bronchus, and <1% in the middle lobe bronchus)
- Left lung—23% (18% in the main bronchus and 5% in the lower bronchus)
- Bilateral—2%

Although most aspirated FBs are located in the bronchi, large, bulky FBs (e.g., food), or those with sharp, irregular edges may become lodged in the larynx. This is particularly common in infants younger than 1 year. Tracheal narrowing or weak respiratory effort may predispose to tracheal FB. Compared with bronchial FBs, laryngotracheal FBs are associated with increased morbidity and mortality.

REFERENCES/SOURCES

- Eren S, Balci AE, Dikici B, Doblan M, Eren MN. Foreign body aspiration in children: experience of 1160 cases. Ann Trop Paediatr. 2003;23(1):31-7.
- Keil O, Schwerk N. Foreign body aspiration in children: being safe and flexible. Curr Opin Anaesthesiol. 2023;36(3):334-9.
- White JJ, Cambron JD, Gottlieb M, Long B. Evaluation and management of airway foreign bodies in the emergency department setting. J Emerg Med. 2023;64(2):145-55.

CHAPTER 19.7

Primary Ciliary Dyskinesia and Interstitial Lung Disease

Jijo Joseph John, Reny Joseph

1. A 7-year-old boy presents with a chronic wet cough, which started in early infancy, for which he has received regular controller asthma therapy, without significant improvement. He also has a history of recurrent rhinitis. He was born at term and had respiratory distress soon after birth for which he required mechanical ventilation for 3 days. His chest X-ray is given here. What is the most likely diagnosis?

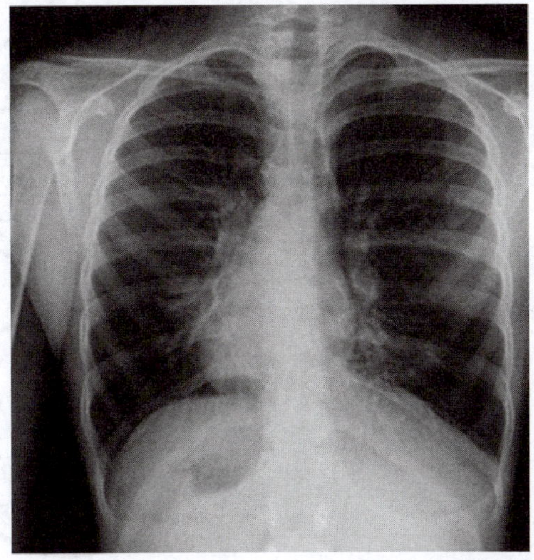

A. Cystic fibrosis
B. Asthma/allergic rhinitis
C. Primary ciliary dyskinesia (PCD)
D. Inhaled foreign body

EXPLANATION

Key features in this case are a chronic cough beginning in early infancy, neonatal respiratory distress, and chronic rhinosinusitis. The chest X-ray is suggestive of dextrocardia with hyperinflation. A computed tomography (CT) scan would be suggestive of bronchiectasis in this child.

	PCD	*Cystic fibrosis*	*Asthma*	*Inhaled foreign body*
Age at onset	Early infancy	Early infancy	Variable	Variable
Neonatal symptoms	+	±	–	–
Chronic respiratory symptoms	+	+	+	±
Chronic rhinosinusitis	+	+	–	–
Dextrocardia	+	–	–	–

Key: C

BOOST YOUR KNOWLEDGE

Situs inversus is seen in 50% of patients with PCD due to impaired ciliary movement (nodal cilia) during embryonic development.

Kartagener syndrome is a subset of PCD with a triad of situs inversus, bronchiectasis, and sinusitis. Young's syndrome (YS) is a triad of bronchiectasis, chronic rhinosinusitis, and infertility due to vas deferens obstruction, in which case cystic fibrosis (CF) and PCD are excluded.

The respiratory symptoms in CF can start at any age depending on the mutation; however, it is characterized by progressive loss of lung function along with recurrent respiratory infections.

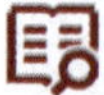

REFERENCE/SOURCE

- Ferkol TW. Primary ciliary dyskinesia (immotile cilia syndrome, Kartagener syndrome). In: Kliegman RM, St Geme III JW, Blum NJ, Shah SS, Tasker RC, Wilson KM (Eds). Nelson Textbook of Pediatrics, 21st edition. Elsevier; 2019. p. 2298.

2. A 6-year-old child presents with chronic rhinosinusitis, a chronic wet cough, and failure to thrive. In view of a significant neonatal history of respiratory distress, the pediatrician makes a provisional diagnosis of PCD. Which of the following represents a normal motile cilium in the respiratory epithelium?

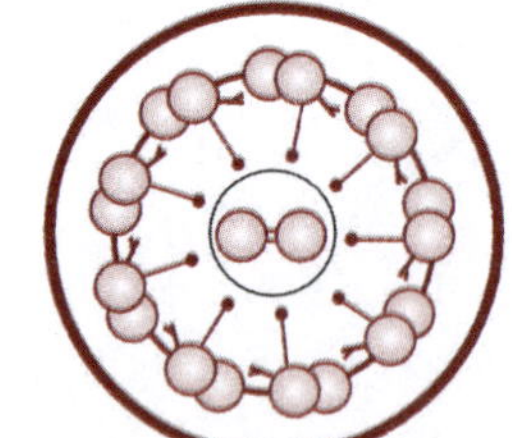

A.

B.

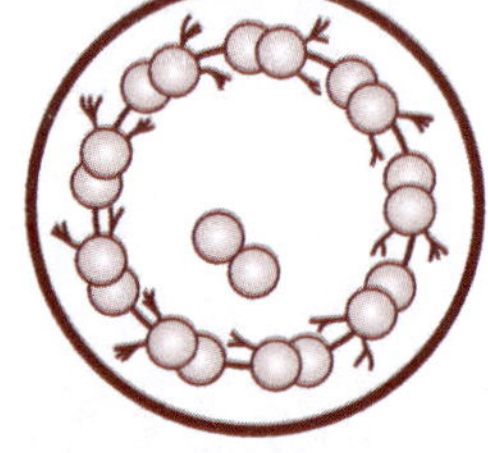

C.

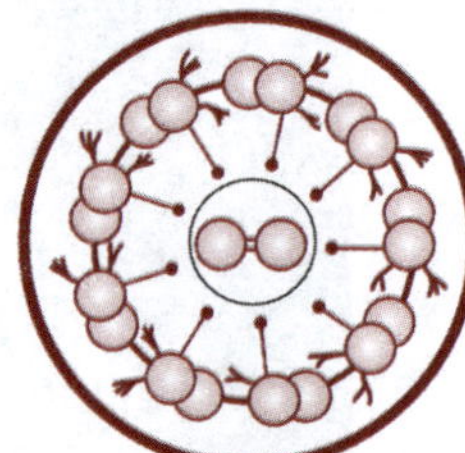

D.

EXPLANATION

The normal motile cilia in the respiratory epithelium have a (9 + 2) structure as seen under the electron microscope. There is a cylinder of microtubule doublets arranged around a pair of central microtubules. Each microtubule has an inner and outer dynein arm. Outer dynein arms are responsible for beat frequency, while inner dynein arms influence the bent shape of the cilium. The outer microtubules are connected by nexin links. These microtubules are connected to the central microtubule by radial spokes.

In this stem, option A has an outer dynein arm defect, which is the most common structural defect seen in PCD (43%). Option B lacks both outer and inner dynein arms. Option C lacks radial spokes. Option D is the normal motile cilia.

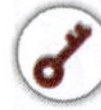

Key: D

BOOST YOUR KNOWLEDGE

Primary cilia and nodal cilia are the other types of cilia—both of which have a 9 + 0 configuration. Primary cilia are mainly sensory and nodal cilia are essential to determine laterality during embryogenesis.

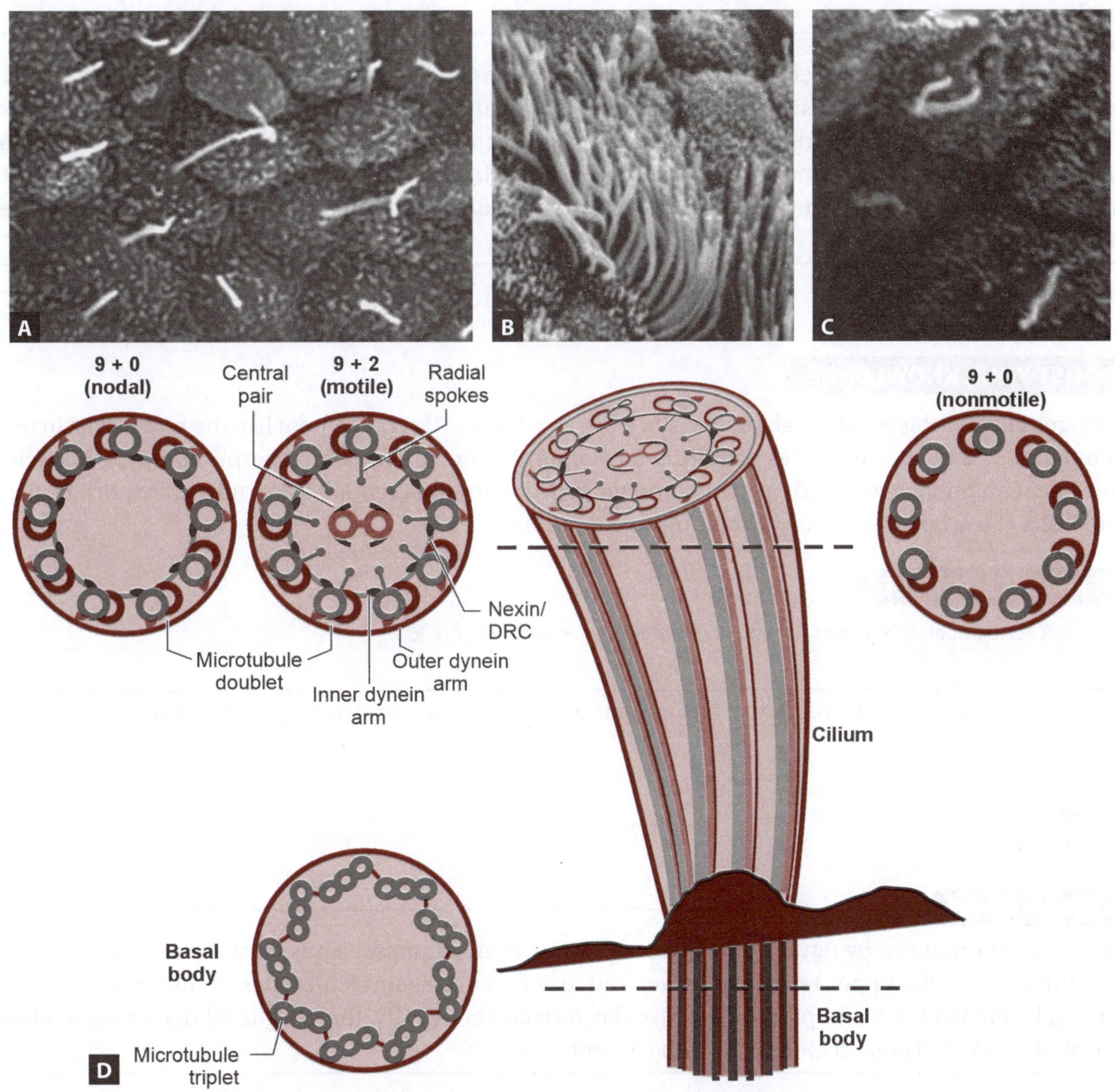

Source: Praveen K, Davis EE, Katsanis N. Unique among ciliopathies: primary ciliary dyskinesia, a motile cilia disorder. F1000Prime Rep. 2015;7:36.

REFERENCE/SOURCE

- Ferkol TW. Primary ciliary dyskinesia (immotile cilia syndrome, Kartagener syndrome). In: Kliegman RM, St Geme III JW, Blum NJ, Shah SS, Tasker RC, Wilson KM (Eds). Nelson Textbook of Pediatrics, 21st edition. Elsevier; 2019. p. 2298.

3. A 30-year-old male is being evaluated for infertility. On examination, he is noted to be thin, with digital clubbing and a prominent Harrison sulcus. He also informs that he has recurrent sinusitis and needs special vaccinations due to lack of a spleen. Which of the following is the likely cause of his infertility?

A. Testicular degeneration
B. Decreased sperm motility
C. Low testosterone levels
D. Congenital absence of vas deferens

EXPLANATION

This patient in question had recurrent respiratory infections/hypoxia (digital clubbing and Harrison sulcus), associated with recurrent sinusitis and asplenia. While CF and PCD can produce these symptoms, asplenia is not a feature of CF. Male infertility in PCD is caused by decreased sperm motility while in CF, male infertility is caused by congenital absence of vas deferens. Testicular degeneration is a cause of male infertility in Klinefelter syndrome where there is progressive testicular degeneration, leading to replacement of the testis with fibrous tissue.

Key: B

BOOST YOUR KNOWLEDGE

Sperm motility is achieved through motile cilia which have a (9 + 2) arrangement like the motile cilia in respiratory epithelium. 50% of affected males with PCD have infertility due to impaired sperm motility, while females are subfertile with an increased risk of ectopic pregnancy due to impaired fallopian tube transport. Defects in the motile cilia cause both respiratory symptoms and infertility in PCD.

REFERENCE/SOURCE

- Gupta P. PG textbook of Pediatrics, 1st edition, Volume 2, Chapter 39.27, p.1886.

4. Which of the following is the most appropriate cut-off level of nasal nitric oxide (nNO) to exclude PCD?

A. >150 ppb
B. >150 ppm
C. >180 ppb
D. >200 ppm

EXPLANATION

Nitric oxide is produced by nitric oxide synthase mainly from paranasal sinus epithelium. It is present in high concentrations in the upper respiratory tract and as a defense against microbes. It also plays a role in cilia motility, bronchial tone, and pulmonary vascular resistance. In PCD, the nNO level decreases to about 10% of normal. nNO >150 ppb excludes PCD with certainty.

Key: A

BOOST YOUR KNOWLEDGE

Nitric oxide (NO), a small gaseous molecule, is produced in various body cells, affecting processes such as muscle relaxation, blood vessel regulation, neurotransmission, and immune defense. In the respiratory system, NO is created from L-arginine by three types of NO synthase (NOS): Neuronal NOS, inducible NOS, and endothelial NOS. Exhaled NO levels are mainly controlled by inducible nitric oxide synthase (iNOS), which is induced by inflammation, primarily in the nose and sinuses. Nasal NO plays a vital role in the sinuses enhancing the body's local defense mechanism, promoting ciliary motility, and acting as an aerocrine mediator to regulate reduction in pulmonary vascular resistance and enhanced oxygen absorption. Low nasal NO levels can serve as a noninvasive diagnostic marker of PCD.

REFERENCE/SOURCE

- Gupta P. PG textbook of Pediatrics, 1st edition, Volume 2, Chapter 39.27, p.1887.

5. A 6-year-old child is referred to an ENT specialist for evaluation of recurrent otitis media and hearing loss. There is a history of chronic sinusitis and recurrent wet cough. Which of the following treatments should be avoided?

A. Treat the otitis media with antibiotics
B. Audiometry and hearing aid assessment
C. Ear toileting
D. Grommet insertion

EXPLANATION

Children with PCD can present with recurrent middle ear infections. The mainstay of treatment includes antibiotics for acute otitis media, regular audiometry monitoring for effusions, and evaluation of hearing with hearing aid placement. Grommet insertion in children with PCD can present with persistent otorrhea in 33% of cases and should be avoided.

Key: D

BOOST YOUR KNOWLEDGE

A grommet is a small tube placed in the tympanic membrane in children with recurrent or persistent otitis media. A type B curve on the tympanogram suggests the diagnosis of otitis media with effusion (OME). (*Types of tympanogram readings*: Type A—normal, type B—fluid accumulation, type C—Eustachian tube dysfunction, type As—hypomobile TM, type Ad—hypermobile TM)

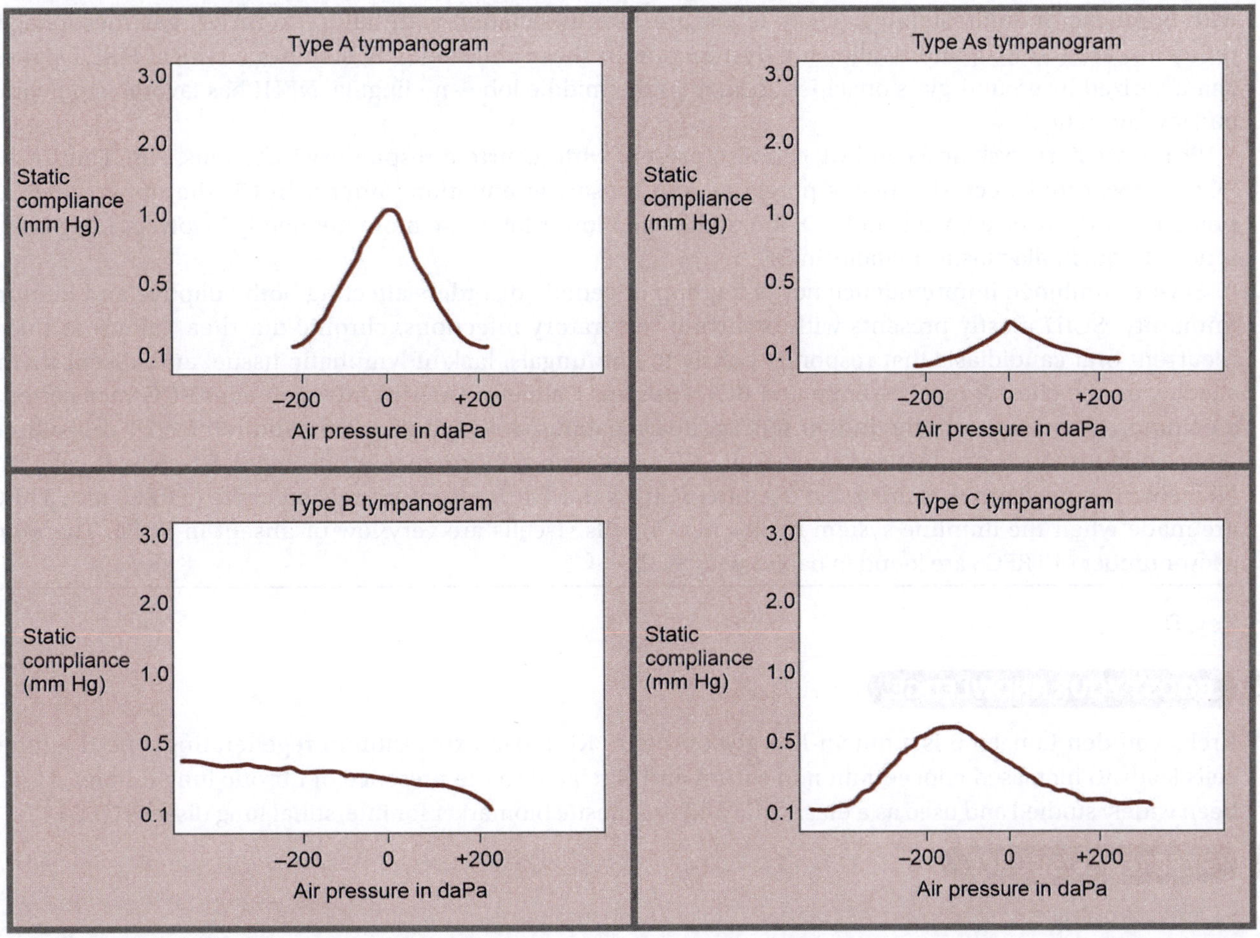

Type A tympanogram
Static compliance (mm Hg): 3.0, 2.0, 1.0, 0.5, 0.1
Air pressure in daPa: −200, 0, +200

Type As tympanogram
Static compliance (mm Hg): 3.0, 2.0, 1.0, 0.5, 0.1
Air pressure in daPa: −200, 0, +200

Type B tympanogram
Static compliance (mm Hg): 3.0, 2.0, 1.0, 0.5, 0.1
Air pressure in daPa: −200, 0, +200

Type C tympanogram
Static compliance (mm Hg): 3.0, 2.0, 1.0, 0.5, 0.1
Air pressure in daPa: −200, 0, +200

The incidence of recurrent otitis media and otorrhea reduces as the child grows older. Children can develop conductive hearing loss due to recurrent ear infections; however, sensorineural hearing loss is uncommon.

Central complex defects in the cilia are related to worse otological and pulmonary manifestations in PCD.

REFERENCE/SOURCE

- Gupta P. PG Textbook of Pediatrics, 1st edition, Volume 2, Chapter 39.27, p.1888.

6. A 6-month-old boy presents with respiratory distress, failure to thrive, and frequent chest infections since birth. On examination, the child appears tachypneic with bilateral inspiratory crackles. High-resolution computed tomography (HRCT) of chest shows bilateral diffuse lung involvement with ground-glass opacities. Laboratory investigations show a high level of serum KL-6 (Krebs von den Lungen 6), and lung biopsy shows increased staining with bombesin immunostaining. What is the most likely diagnosis?

A. CF
B. PCD
C. Severe combined immunodeficiency (SCID)
D. Neuroendocrine cell hyperplasia of infancy

EXPLANATION

Neuroendocrine hyperplasia of infancy (NEHI) is a childhood interstitial lung disease (chILD), presenting in infancy with chronic tachypnea, retractions, and hypoxemia in the first months to years of life. Lung biopsy demonstrated near normal histology with an increased number of neuroendocrine cells staining with bombesin immunostaining. There is a significant association with failure to thrive, gastroesophageal reflux disease (GERD), and swallowing dysfunction in these children. NEHI shows a typical HRCT pattern characterized by ground-glass opacities, located in the middle lobe and lingula. NEHI has favorable outcomes and low mortality.

Primary ciliary dyskinesia and CF can also present with recurrent respiratory infections. HRCT in CF and PCD shows bronchiectasis, mucus plugging, and mosaic attenuation pattern. In CF, the upper lobes are predominantly involved, while in PCD, the middle and lower lobes are more frequently involved. Lung biopsy is not a frequent diagnostic modality in CF.

Severe combined immunodeficiency is a group of genetic disorders affecting both adaptive and humoral immunity. SCID mostly presents with recurrent respiratory infections, chronic diarrhea, failure to thrive, recurrent oral candidiasis that responds poorly to antifungals, lack of lymphatic tissue, and absent thymic shadow on the chest X-ray. Disseminated BCG (Bacillus Calmette-Guerin) infection after BCG vaccination is a common presentation in the Indian setting. Investigations show lymphopenia and reduced T-cell subsets. Flow cytometry tests can be used to classify SCID based on the presence or absence of T-cells, B-cells, and NK-cells. The newborn screening test used for SCID is the T-cell receptor excision circle (TREC) test. TRECs are made when the immune system makes new T-cells. T-cells are very low or absent in SCID. Therefore, a low number of TRECS are found in babies with SCID.

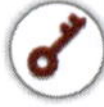

Key: D

BOOST YOUR KNOWLEDGE

Krebs von den Lungen 6 is a mucin-like glycoprotein. KL-6 overexpression in regenerating type II epithelial cells leads to increased concentration in serum and is related to the presence of fibrotic lung lesions. KL-6 has been widely studied and used as a diagnostic and prognostic biomarker for interstitial lung disease (ILD).

REFERENCE/SOURCE

- Textbook of Pediatric Pulmonology (AAP), Chapter 26 (Intersitial lung disease), p.540, ISBN: 978-1-58110-492-9.

7. A 1-month-old girl in the neonatal intensive care unit (NICU) is noted to have persistent respiratory distress and ventilator requirement. The baby was born at term by normal vaginal delivery and developed respiratory distress soon after birth. On Day 3 of her life, in view of low-volume lungs and respiratory distress, she received surfactant therapy, but her oxygen requirement persisted. On examination, she is noted to have bilateral crackles and increased work of breathing. ECHO is normal. What is the most likely diagnosis?

A. Respiratory distress syndrome (RDS) of the newborn
B. Surfactant protein A deficiency
C. Surfactant protein B deficiency
D. CF

EXPLANATION

Genetic disorders affecting normal surfactant metabolism include surfactant protein B deficiency, surfactant protein C deficiency, and *ABCA3* mutation. Of these Sp-B deficiency presents in the newborn period with severe respiratory distress mimicking hyaline membrane disease which presents in the preterm child. Sp-C deficiency can present in an older child, and *ABCA3* mutation can have a varied phenotype. Sp-B deficiency is a fatal disease with the only cure being lung transplantation.

Respiratory distress syndrome of newborns has a similar clinical presentation but is most commonly seen in preterm babies due to lack of production of surfactant. Inactivation of surfactant can be seen in certain conditions such as infants of diabetic mothers, and these term babies can present with features similar to RDS.

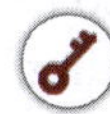

Key: C

BOOST YOUR KNOWLEDGE

A CT chest in Sp-B deficiency shows diffuse ground-glass opacities with septal thickening. Histopathology reveals alveolar proteinosis with interstitial widening, and electron microscopy shows disorganized lamellar bodies. Diagnosis can be made by genetic testing.

In fetal life, surfactant is produced by alveolar type 2 cells, starting from around 20 weeks of gestation. The surfactant consists of four surfactant-specific proteins (SP): SP-A, SP-B, SP-C, and SP-D. Sp-A and Sp-D are involved in regulating inflammatory processes in the lung. Sp-B is required for the formation of normal lamellar bodies in the alveolar cells.

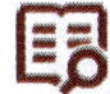

REFERENCE/SOURCE

- Textbook of Pediatric Pulmonology (AAP), Chapter 26 (Intersitial lung disease), p.539, ISBN: 978-1-58110-492-9.

8. A 16-year-old boy presents with chronic cough and two episodes of hemoptysis, which started after an episode of upper respiratory tract infection. On examination, his pulse is 88 beats/min, and his BP is 142/88 mm Hg. He has bibasilar crackles. His investigations show the following results:

Hemoglobin	10 g%
Total WBC counts	18,000/mm^3
Platelet count	2.6 lakh/mm^3
Bleeding time	4 minutes
Serum creatinine	1 mg/dL
Urine routine	Protein 1+, RBCs++

Which of the following investigations will lead to a diagnosis in this child?

A. Chest X-ray and CT chest
B. Thromboelastogram
C. Renal biopsy
D. Urine protein–creatinine ratio

EXPLANATION

This 16-year-old boy is presenting with features suggestive of pulmonary and renal involvement and a diagnosis of Goodpasture syndrome [anti-glomerular basement membrane (anti-GBM) disease] should be considered. The serologic detection of anti-GBM antibodies is positive in >90% of patients. Renal biopsy yields better results than lung biopsy in these children. Light microscopy will show crescentic glomerulonephritis. Over time, the crescents turn fibrotic, and frank glomerulosclerosis with interstitial fibrosis and tubular atrophy may be appreciated. Immunofluorescence will show the linear deposition of immunoglobulin G (IgG) and complement (C3) along the basement membrane.

Radiological features of Goodpasture syndrome include nonspecific reticular opacities in the chest X-ray and ground-glass and airspace opacities that progress to reticular "crazy paving" pattern.

Key: C

BOOST YOUR KNOWLEDGE

Goodpasture syndrome is a type II hypersensitivity reaction with antibodies directed against type IV collagen in the basement membrane. Close differentials are granulomatosis with polyangiitis, microscopic polyangiitis, and Henoch-Schönlein purpura (HSP). Goodpasture syndrome appears to result from environmental insults in a genetically predisposed person, and triggers can include smoking, infections, and drugs like alemtuzumab and cocaine.

Thromboelastography (TEG) is a noninvasive test, which quantitatively measures the ability of whole blood to form a clot. TEG shows the interaction of platelets with the coagulation cascade (aggregation, clot strengthening, fibrin crosslinking, and fibrinolysis). Its use has been demonstrated in cardiac surgery and liver transplantation, to guide the need for transfusion.

Normal TEG Graph

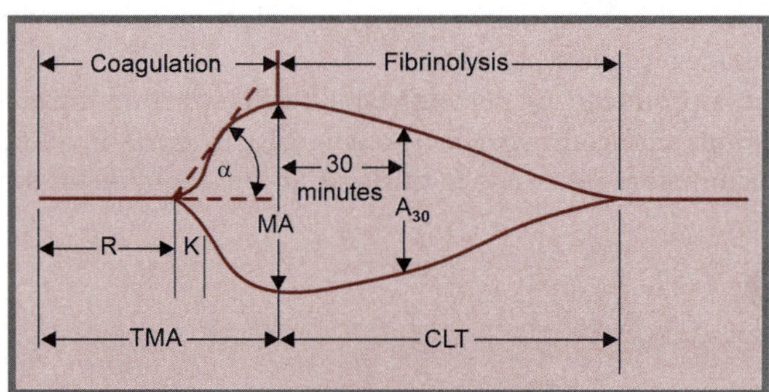

R—reaction time	Time of latency from the start of the test to initial fibrin formation	Dependent on clotting factors
K—kinetics	Time taken to achieve a particular clot strength	Dependent on fibrinogen
Alpha—angle (slope of the line between R and K)	Measures the speed at which fibrin build-up and crosslinking take place, hence assesses the rate of clot formation	Dependent on fibrinogen
MA—maximum amplitude (mm)	Represents the ultimate strength of the fibrin clot, i.e., overall stability of the clot	Dependent on platelets (80%) and fibrin (20%) interacting via GPIIb/IIIa
CLT—clot lysis time		

REFERENCE/SOURCE

- Kelly KJ, Vece TJ. Interstitial lung disease. In: Kliegman RM, St Geme III JW, Blum NJ, Shah SS, Tasker RC, Wilson KM (Eds). Nelson Textbook of Pediatrics, 21st edition. Chapter 427.5 (Interstitial Lung Disease), p.2262.

9. A 7-year-old boy presents with a chronic dry cough and exertional dyspnea. On examination, he is noted to have finger clubbing and bilateral inspiratory crackles. He also complained of knee and elbow pain and swelling for the past 1 year. The HRCT of the chest shows ground-glass opacities with honey-combing pattern. Pulmonary function tests show a restrictive pattern. What is the most likely diagnosis?

A. Juvenile interstitial pulmonary fibrosis
B. Uncontrolled asthma
C. Recurrent community-acquired pneumonia
D. Systemic-onset juvenile inflammatory arthritis

EXPLANATION

This 7-year-old child presents with features of ILD associated with arthritis. Juvenile interstitial pulmonary fibrosis is a rare cause of childhood ILD, which can present in association with connective tissue disorders. Various other causes of pulmonary fibrosis in children are pulmonary hemorrhage, alveolar proteinosis, and idiopathic pulmonary fibrosis. None of the other options in the stem would fulfill both respiratory and rheumatological symptoms in the child.

Key: A

BOOST YOUR KNOWLEDGE

Juvenile idiopathic arthritis (JIA)-associated lung damage can present in a variety of ways including pleurisy, diffuse lung disease (lipoid pneumonia, pulmonary interstitial lesions, pulmonary hemosiderosis, and pulmonary arterial hypertension), and secondary infections. ILD can be severe and fatal.

10. A 1-year-old girl presented with worsening of respiratory distress following an upper respiratory infection. She had wheeze, retractions, and hypoxemia on examination. An upper respiratory polymerase chain reaction (PCR) panel was positive for adenovirus. However, her symptoms persisted beyond 3 weeks, and she continued to be oxygen dependent. Chest X-ray appeared normal, but her HRCT of chest demonstrated a mosaic pattern of hyperlucency, air-trapping, and bronchiectasis. Which of the following will be most likely to give a clue to her diagnosis?

A. Induced sputum for culture
B. Quanti-FERON TB gold
C. Barium swallow to rule out a reflux
D. Transbronchial lung biopsy

EXPLANATION

The clinicoradiological picture suggests a diagnosis of bronchiolitis obliterans (BO), and transbronchial lung biopsy will be the most appropriate diagnosis investigation for this girl. Sputum induction with hypertonic nebulized saline is an option to obtain respiratory cultures in chronic conditions such as CF and tuberculosis.

Quanti-FERON TB test is an interferon-gamma release assay (IGRA), which measures in vitro cell-mediated immune response to *Mycobacterium tuberculosis*, in whole blood incubated with *M. tuberculosis* antigens (*ESAT-6, CFP-10, and TB 7.7*).

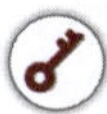

Key: D

BOOST YOUR KNOWLEDGE

Bronchiolitis obliterans is a histopathologic diagnosis characterized by chronic obstructive lung disease of the bronchioles and smaller airways, resulting from an insult to the lower respiratory tract, leading to inflammation and fibrosis of the small airways. In the nontransplant patient, BO most commonly occurs in the pediatric population after respiratory infections, particularly adenovirus, but also *M. pneumonia*, measles, *Legionella pneumophila*, influenza, and pertussis; other causes include inflammatory diseases (JIA and systemic lupus erythematosus). BO is the most common cause of morbidity and transplant rejection following lung transplantation.

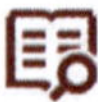

REFERENCE/SOURCE

- Boas SR. Bronchiolitis obliterans. In: Kliegman RM, St Geme III JW, Blum NJ, Shah SS, Tasker RC, Wilson KM (Eds). Nelson Textbook of Pediatrics, 21st edition. Chapter 442.1 (Bronchiolitis Obliterans), p.2226.

SECTION 20

Cardiology

Section Editor: *Sakshi Sachdeva*

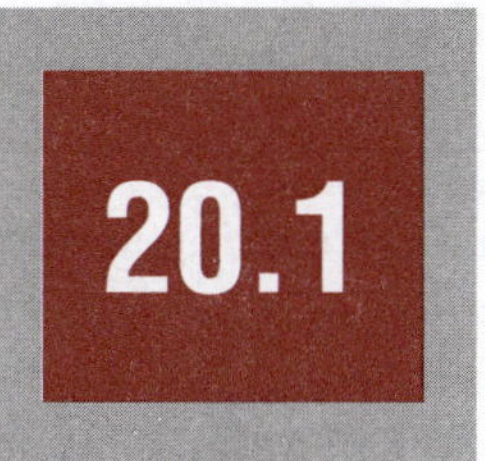

CHAPTER 20.1

Acute Rheumatic Fever, Infective Endocarditis, Rheumatic Heart Diseases, Pericardial Diseases

Sakshi Sachdeva

1. What is the dose of aspirin for treating acute rheumatic fever (ARF)?

A. 3–5 mg/kg/day
B. 20–30 mg/kg/day
C. 40–60 mg/kg/day
D. 80–100 mg/kg/day

EXPLANATION

High-dose anti-inflammatory therapy is given to patients of ARF.

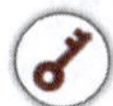

Key: D

BOOST YOUR KNOWLEDGE

Treatment of acute carditis in ARF includes following measures:

- *General measures*:
  - *Restrict activity:* Bed/chair rest for ~4–6 weeks
  - Initiate secondary prophylaxis with intramuscular (IM) benzathine penicillin 2–3 weekly
  - *Anti-inflammatory therapy:*
    - Mild-to-moderate carditis
    - *Aspirin:* 80–100 mg/kg/day in QID dose
  - *Severe carditis:*
    - Initial steroids (prednisone 2 mg/kg/day) for approximately 2 weeks, then taper
    - Aspirin is initiated 1 week before stopping steroids to prevent rebound
    - Follow acute phase reactants [erythrocyte sedimentation rate (ESR), C-reactive protein (CRP)]
- *Other treatments depend on the severity of involvement and symptoms*:
  - *Moderate-to-severe carditis:* Anti-heart failure measures such as salt and fluid restriction, diuretics, inotropes, and afterload reducing agents
  - *Intractable heart failure:* Surgery if refractory heart failure; surgery is best avoided in ARF due to risk of residual valvar lesions.

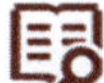

REFERENCE/SOURCE

- Penny DJ, Cetta F, Allen HD, Shaddy RE, Feltes TF (Eds). Moss and Adam's Heart Disease in Infants, Children, and Adolescents: Including the Fetus and Young Adult, 9th edition, Volume 2. Argentina: Wolters Kluwer; 2016. p. 1390.

2. Which of the following valves is most commonly involved in RF?

A. Tricuspid valve
B. Pulmonary valve
C. Mitral valve
D. Aortic valve

EXPLANATION

Mitral regurgitation (MR) is the most common cardiac abnormality in patients with RF occurring in approximately 95% of cases with acute rheumatic carditis. Mechanism of MR is a combination of dilation of mitral annulus and elongation of chordae resulting in abnormal and inadequate coaptation of leaflet tips. Leaflet tip prolapse happens and in extreme cases the mitral valve chordate can rupture leading to flail mitral valve leaflet and severe acute MR, which can be catastrophic.

Key: C

BOOST YOUR KNOWLEDGE

Majority of patients with acute MR do not have any symptoms. However, with acute severe MR, there is sudden volume loading on the left ventricle, which increases the left ventricular (LV) filling pressures, left atrial (LA) mean pressure, and pulmonary venous pressure culminating in pulmonary edema. Presenting features in such patients include dyspnea, orthopnea, paroxysmal nocturnal dyspnea (PND), cough, and hemoptysis in most severe cases. Right heart failure can occur due to secondary pulmonary hypertension.

REFERENCE/SOURCE

- Penny DJ, Cetta F, Allen HD, Shaddy RE, Feltes TF (Eds). Moss and Adam's Heart Disease in Infants, Children, and Adolescents: Including the Fetus and Young Adult, 9th edition, Volume 2. Argentina: Wolters Kluwer; 2016. p. 1382.

3. Which of the following is *correct* regarding the pathophysiology of rheumatic chorea?

A. Antibodies to surface M protein cross-reacting with basal ganglia dopaminergic neurons
B. Antibodies to surface G protein cross-reacting with basal ganglia serotonergic neurons
C. Antibodies to surface M protein cross-reacting with basal ganglia serotonergic neurons
D. Antibodies to surface G protein cross-reacting with basal ganglia dopaminergic neurons

EXPLANATION

Sydenham chorea occurs in approximately 10–30% of cases of RF. It occurs due to cross-reaction of antibodies against streptococcal M protein cross-reacting with basal ganglia dopaminergic neurons.

Key: A

BOOST YOUR KNOWLEDGE

Sydenham chorea is equally common in prepubertal males and female. But postpuberty females are more commonly affected in comparison to males. It is characterized by involuntary purposeless movements and emotional lability. The findings that can be elicited on physical examination include spooning of hands, pronator sign, milkmaid's grip, and jack-in-the-box tongue. Usually the findings are bilateral, but hemichorea is also known to occur. The symptoms tend to resolve by 6 weeks.

REFERENCE/SOURCE

- Penny DJ, Cetta F, Allen HD, Shaddy RE, Feltes TF (Eds). Moss and Adam's Heart Disease in Infants, Children, and Adolescents: Including the Fetus and Young Adult, 9th edition, Volume 2. Argentina: Wolters Kluwer; 2016. p. 1381.

4. Which of the following set of clinical signs/symptoms is *not* associated with streptococcal pharyngitis?

A. Throat pain, high-grade fever, odynophagia
B. Nausea, vomiting, pain abdomen
C. Tender lymphadenopathy, toxic look
D. Diarrhea, conjunctivitis, rhinorrhea

EXPLANATION

Symptoms in streptococcal pharyngitis are less common as compared to signs. In viral sore throat, the symptoms of diarrhea, rhinorrhea, and conjunctivitis are common. In Group A *Streptococcus* (GAS) pharyngitis, there is high fever, throat pain, and red strawberry tongue. There are enlarged cervical nodes and red enlarged tonsils, which may be covered with membrane. Diarrhea, cough, coryza, ulcerations, croup/laryngitis/hoarseness, and conjunctivitis are not associated with GAS pharyngitis and increase the likelihood of viral etiology.

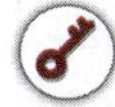

Key: D

BOOST YOUR KNOWLEDGE

Streptococcal pharyngitis is very common in children between the age groups of 5 and 15 years. Approximately 15–30% of pharyngitis in school children are due to GAS.

REFERENCE/SOURCE

- Tanz RR. Acute pharyngitis. In: Kliegman RM, Stanton BF, St Geme J, Schor NF (Eds). Nelson Textbook of Pediatrics, 20th edition, Volume 2. Philadelphia: Elsevier; 2016. p. 2018.

5. Which of the following is the *correct* criterion for labeling "Pathological" MR in ARF?

A. Seen in at least three views on echocardiography
B. Jet length ≥1 cm in at least two views
C. Peak velocity >3 m/s
D. Pansystolic jet in both the envelopes

EXPLANATION

Subclinical carditis refers exclusively to the circumstance where classic auscultatory findings of valvar dysfunction either are not present or are not recognized by the diagnosing clinician, but echocardiography/Doppler studies reveal mitral or aortic valvulitis. The World Heart Federation (WHF) has laid the standard criteria to differentiate subclinical carditis due to ARF from other conditions. The box provides the WHF criteria for subclinical carditis.

Pathological mitral regurgitation (all four criteria met):

1. Seen in at least two views
2. Jet length ≥2 cm in at least one view
3. Peak velocity >3 m/s
4. Pansystolic jet in at least one envelope

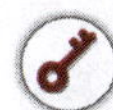

Key: C

BOOST YOUR KNOWLEDGE

Pathological aortic regurgitation (all four criteria met):

1. Seen in at least two views
2. Jet length ≥1 cm in at least one view
3. Peak velocity >3 m/s
4. Pandiastolic jet in at least one envelope

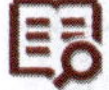

REFERENCE/SOURCE

- Reményi B, Wilson N, Steer A, Ferreira B, Kado J, Kumar K, et al. World Heart Federation criteria for echocardiographic diagnosis of rheumatic heart disease: an evidence-based guideline. Nat Rev Cardiol. 2012;9(5):297-309.

6. Which of the following is *not* a major criterion for ARF?

A. Polyarthritis
B. Polyarthralgia
C. Monoarthritis
D. Monoarthralgia

EXPLANATION

Monoarthralgia is a minor criterion, remaining other options constitute major criteria in diagnosis of ARF as per the new Jones criteria.

Key: D

BOOST YOUR KNOWLEDGE

Revised Jones criteria 2015 for diagnosis of ARF:

- *Low-risk population:* Defined as ARF incidence ≤2 per 100,000 school-aged children or all-age rheumatic heart disease (RHD) prevalence of ≤1 per 1,000 population per year.
- *Moderate-high risk population:* Defined as ARF incidence >2 per 100,000 school-aged children or all-age RHD prevalence of >1 per 1,000 population per year.

A. For all patient populations with evidence of preceding GAS infection	
Diagnosis: Initial ARF	2 major manifestations or 1 major plus 2 minor manifestations
Diagnosis: Recurrent ARF	2 major or 1 major and 2 minor or 3 minor
B. Major criteria	
Low-risk populations:	*Moderate- and high-risk populations:*
Carditis: Clinical and/or subclinical	*Carditis:* Clinical and/or subclinical
Arthritis: Polyarthritis only	*Arthritis:* • Monoarthritis or polyarthritis • Polyarthralgia
Chorea	Chorea
Erythema marginatum	Erythema marginatum
Subcutaneous nodules	Subcutaneous nodules
C. Minor criteria	
Low-risk populations:	*Moderate- and high-risk populations:*
Polyarthralgia	Monoarthralgia
Fever (≥38.5°C)	Fever (≥38°C)
ESR ≥60 mm in the first hour and/or CRP ≥3.0 mg/dL	ESR ≥30 mm/h and/or CRP ≥3.0 mg/dL
Prolonged PR interval, after accounting for age variability (unless carditis is a major criterion)	Prolonged PR interval, after accounting for age variability (unless carditis is a major criterion)

(ARF: acute rheumatic fever; CRP: C-reactive protein; ESR: erythrocyte sedimentation rate)

REFERENCE/SOURCE

- Gewitz MH, Baltimore RS, Tani LY, Sable CA, Shulman ST, Carapetis J, et al; American Heart Association Committee on Rheumatic Fever, Endocarditis, and Kawasaki Disease of the Council on Cardiovascular Disease in the Young. Revision of the Jones Criteria for the diagnosis of acute rheumatic fever in the era of Doppler echocardiography: a scientific statement from the American Heart Association. Circulation. 2015;131(20):1806-18.

7. Which of the following electrocardiogram (ECG) abnormalities can occur in ARF?

A. PR prolongation
B. Heart block
C. ST-T changes
D. All of the above

EXPLANATION

Patients with suspected RF should have an ECG because conduction abnormalities are not uncommon. Although first-degree atrioventricular (AV) block is a minor Jones criterion, it should be noted that a prolonged PR interval occurs in up to one-third of patients who have GAS infections, regardless of whether they develop RF.

Key: D

BOOST YOUR KNOWLEDGE

Complete heart block (CHB) due to ARF is a reversible cause of CHB. ST-T changes due to pericarditis are also reversible. Tall R waves due to LV dilation and deep negative P-terminal forces in V1 due to LA dilation are also common findings.

REFERENCE/SOURCE

- Penny DJ, Cetta F, Allen HD, Shaddy RE, Feltes TF (Eds). Moss and Adam's Heart Disease in Infants, Children, and Adolescents: Including the Fetus and Young Adult, 9th edition, Volume 2. Argentina: Wolters Kluwer; 2016. p. 1385.

8. What is a MacCallum patch?

A. Scar in LA roof where MR jet hits
B. Scar in LV apex where AR jet hits
C. Fibrosis in anterior mitral leaflet (AML)
D. Fibrosis in aortic valve cusp

EXPLANATION

MacCallum patch is located in the roof of the left atrium in patients with MR.

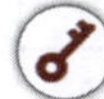

Key: A

BOOST YOUR KNOWLEDGE

Mural endocardial lesions can be seen as MacCallum plaques in RHD. These are map-like areas of thick, rough endocardium caused by jet effect of MR hitting the roof of the left atrium. This is a characteristic but uncommon finding.

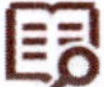

REFERENCE/SOURCE

- Schoen FJ, Mitchell RN. The heart. In: Kumar V, Abbas AK, Aster JC (Eds). Robbins and Cotran Pathologic Basis of Disease, 9th edition. Philadelphia: Elsevier; 2014. p. 558.

9. Which of the following is *not* correct about rheumatic nodules?

A. Nodules are freely mobile
B. Occur at extensor surfaces
C. Grouped lesions occur
D. They are painful

EXPLANATION

The nodules are 0.5–2.0 cm in diameter, round, firm, freely movable, painless, and nontender, with no evidence of inflammation. They occur in crops over extensor surfaces of joints or bony prominences of the elbows, wrists, knees, ankles, scalp, and spinous processes of the back. They persist for a few days to as long as 1–2 weeks and are not evanescent. However, as they are small and are not associated with symptoms, they may be easily overlooked.

Key: D

BOOST YOUR KNOWLEDGE

Subcutaneous nodules are relatively uncommon in ARF, reported in 0–10% of cases. They are not pathognomonic of ARF and may occur with systemic lupus erythematosus (SLE) or rheumatoid arthritis. Similar to erythema marginatum, subcutaneous nodules in ARF are almost always associated with carditis, and rarely occur as the sole major Jones manifestation.

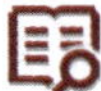

REFERENCE/SOURCE

- Penny DJ, Cetta F, Allen HD, Shaddy RE, Feltes TF (Eds). Moss and Adam's Heart Disease in Infants, Children, and Adolescents: Including the Fetus and Young Adult, 9th edition, Volume 2. Argentina: Wolters Kluwer; 2016. p. 1384.

10. Which of the following is *true* for juvenile mitral stenosis (MS)?

A. Occurs in <5 years age group
B. Mitral stenosis is never severe
C. Atrial fibrillation is commonly associated
D. Valve calcifications are characteristically absent

EXPLANATION

Juvenile MS is a term coined by Sujoy B Roy et al. in 1963. It involved very severe MS in the age group <20 years. Patients had severe pulmonary hypertension, and congestive heart failure occurred due to severe MS and pulmonary arterial hypertension (PAH) in the absence of ARF. Atrial fibrillation is less common in this entity, and mitral valve does not have calcification.

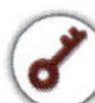

Key: D

BOOST YOUR KNOWLEDGE

Features in lung biopsy specimens include pronounced medial hypertrophy and intimal thickening of small muscular pulmonary arteries, arterioles, and venules; alveolar capillary sclerosis; and hypertrophic smooth muscle bands in the distal respiratory passages.

REFERENCE/SOURCE

- Roy SB, Bhatia ML, Lazaro EJ, Ramalingaswami V. Juvenile mitral stenosis in India. Lancet. 1963;2(7319):1193-5.

11. Which of the following is a characteristic feature of cardiac tamponade?

A. Heart block
B. Hypertension
C. Kussmaul sign
D. Friedreich sign

EXPLANATION

Cardiac tamponade is characterized by Beck triad: (1) Muffled heart sounds, (2) hypotension, and (3) elevated central venous pressure (CVP) with raised jugular venous pressure (JVP). Patients have tachycardia, tachypnea, and a narrow pulse pressure with pulsus paradoxus.

During inspiration in normal patients, intrathoracic pressure decreases with an increase in venous return to the right atrium. In patients with cardiac tamponade, however, expansion of the right atrium is limited by pericardial pressure. Thus, there may be a paradoxical increase in central venous pressure as evident by Kussmaul sign; a rise in JVP during inspiration.

Friedrick sign is a sharp and deep y descent of the jugular venous waveform. It can be a clue to the diagnosis of constrictive pericarditis.

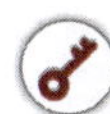

Key: C

BOOST YOUR KNOWLEDGE

During the initial stages of tamponade, cardiac output is preserved by increased ejection fraction and heart rate. As these physiologic mechanisms are unable to maintain cardiac output, the patient will become unstable as systemic vascular resistance increases to maintain systemic blood pressure. This will cause the pulse pressure to narrow, with compromised systemic perfusion. Ultimately, decreased coronary perfusion pressure will result in decreased myocardial function, cardiac output, and blood pressure.

REFERENCE/SOURCE

- Penny DJ, Cetta F, Allen HD, Shaddy RE, Feltes TF (Eds). Moss and Adam's Heart Disease in Infants, Children, and Adolescents: Including the Fetus and Young Adult, 9th edition, Volume 2. Argentina: Wolters Kluwer; 2016. p. 1428.

12. Which of the following is a characteristic feature of constrictive pericarditis?

A. Minimal ventricular interdependence
B. Septal bounce
C. Limited early diastolic filling
D. Decreased septal mitral annulus velocity compared to lateral mitral annulus velocity

EXPLANATION

In constrictive pericarditis, there is a limitation of diastolic expansion of ventricles. Early diastolic filling is normal, but mid and delayed filling is classically hampered. Pulmonary wedge pressure and CVP is raised due to raised LV and right ventricular (RV) end-diastolic pressure (EDP). Systemic and pulmonary congestion features are present. Echocardiography shows paradoxical septal motion with a septal "bounce." The "bounce" refers to the septum shifting leftward with increased RV filling during inspiration, and then shifting back toward the right with expiration due to improved LV filling. Doppler echocardiography shows marked respiratory variation of both left- and right-sided inflows. With inspiration, there is an exaggerated decrease in the mitral inflow velocity (mitral E velocity) and an exaggerated increase in the tricuspid inflow velocity (tricuspid E velocity). Conversely, in expiration, there is an exaggerated increase in mitral inflow velocity and an exaggerated decrease in tricuspid inflow velocity. This is called increased ventricular interdependence.

In normal hearts, the lateral mitral annulus e′ velocity is greater than the septal mitral annulus e′ velocity. In constriction, the septal mitral annulus e′ velocity can be greater than or equal to the lateral mitral annulus e′ velocity, a paradoxical finding called mitral annulus reversus.

Key: B

BOOST YOUR KNOWLEDGE

Tissue Doppler imaging can be helpful in the differentiation of constriction and restriction. In normal children beyond infancy, the early diastolic septal mitral annulus velocity (e′) should be between 9 and 16 cm/s. In constriction, the septal e′ velocity may be increased. In restriction, the septal e′ velocity often is <8 cm/s (similar to other cardiomyopathies).

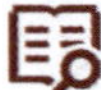

REFERENCE/SOURCE

- Penny DJ, Cetta F, Allen HD, Shaddy RE, Feltes TF (Eds). Moss and Adam's Heart Disease in Infants, Children, and Adolescents: Including the Fetus and Young Adult, 9th edition, Volume 2. Argentina: Wolters Kluwer; 2016. p. 1436.

13. Which of the following JVP findings is present in constrictive pericarditis?

A. Prominent x descent
B. Prominent y descent
C. Prominent x and y descent
D. None of the above

EXPLANATION

Jugular venous pressure waveform has four clinically observable components: a wave, x descent, v wave, and y descent. In pericardial constriction, both x and y descents are prominent. Normally, x descent is more prominent than y descent.

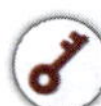

Key: C

BOOST YOUR KNOWLEDGE

In constrictive pericarditis, the thickened pericardium causes elevated atrial pressure and limits ventricular filling to the early diastolic period. The resultant brisk and enhanced early diastolic filling produces a sharp and deep y descent, known as Friedreich sign. The prominent y descent occurs in combination with a prominent x descent, creating two steep troughs known as the "W" sign. This finding may be helpful in distinguishing constrictive pericarditis from restrictive cardiomyopathy, in which the x descent is typically diminished.

REFERENCE/SOURCE

- Sharma I, Nugent JG, Sullivan PD, Mansoor AM. Jugular venous pulse in constrictive pericarditis. BMJ Case Rep. 2020;13(4): e233078.

14. Which of the following conditions can be associated with chylopericardium?

A. Pericardial lymphangioma
B. Postcardiac surgery
C. Cystic hygroma
D. All of the above

EXPLANATION

During surgery for congenital heart disease (CHD), the thoracic duct may get damaged or there can be raised CVP. These can lead to chylous pericardial effusion. Other reasons could be post-traumatic, or mediastinal masses, which hamper drainage of lymph such as cystic hygroma and postradiation therapy. Chylopericardium can occur as a consequence to all of the options mentioned here.

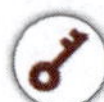

Key: D

BOOST YOUR KNOWLEDGE

The pericardial fluid is milk-colored, with elevated triglyceride and protein levels. Management of chylo-pericardium includes low fat, medium chain triglyceride (MCT) rich diet. Some patients may need to be kept NPO (nil per os), on parenteral nutrition. Octreotide infusion, pericardial window, and pericardiopleural or pericardioperitoneal shunts are the last options.

REFERENCE/SOURCE

- Penny DJ, Cetta F, Allen HD, Shaddy RE, Feltes TF (Eds). Moss and Adam's Heart Disease in Infants, Children, and Adolescents: Including the Fetus and Young Adult, 9th edition, Volume 2. Argentina: Wolters Kluwer; 2016. p. 1433.

15. Which of the following ECG changes is *not* seen in pericarditis?

A. ST segment elevation
B. PR segment depression
C. T-wave inversion
D. Low voltage complexes

EXPLANATION

There are four stages of ECG changes in pericarditis:

1. ST segment elevation in the lateral/inferior leads (I, II, aVF, aVL, and V4–V6). Reciprocal ST segment depression in leads aVR and V1. PR interval depression.
2. ST segment normalizes, and T-wave amplitude diminishes.
3. ST segment remains normal, T waves become inverted in the lateral/inferior leads (aVF, aVL, and V4–V6)
4. Relative normalization of the ECG, some T-wave changes may persist.

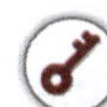

Key: D

BOOST YOUR KNOWLEDGE

Low voltage complexes are a feature of cardiac tamponade.

REFERENCE/SOURCE

- Penny DJ, Cetta F, Allen HD, Shaddy RE, Feltes TF (Eds). Moss and Adam's Heart Disease in Infants, Children, and Adolescents: Including the Fetus and Young Adult, 9th edition, Volume 2. Argentina: Wolters Kluwer; 2016. p. 1429.

16. Infective endocarditis (IE) prophylaxis may *not* be prescribed in which of the following conditions?

A. Prosthetic cardiac valves
B. Unrepaired cyanotic CHDs
C. Unrepaired acyanotic CHDs
D. Previous history of infective endocarditis

EXPLANATION

Because of the high rates of morbidity and mortality associated with IE, any measure that can prevent the disease is desirable. It is thought that daily activities like eating and tooth brushing produce significant bacteremia and good dental hygiene is the most important factor in preventing IE. Abolition of risk factors like repair of CHDs is important. A prosthetic cardiac valve or other prosthetic material, and/or a history of previous IE are significant risk factors for IE.

Key: C

 BOOST YOUR KNOWLEDGE

Prophylaxis is limited to dental procedures that involve manipulation of gingival tissue or the periapical region of teeth or perforation of the oral mucosa. Prophylaxis is not appropriate for shedding of deciduous teeth and bleeding from trauma to the lips or oral mucosa. Prophylaxis for most procedures involving the upper or lower respiratory tract, upper or lower gastrointestinal (GI) tract, or genitourinary (GU) tract is recommended routinely.

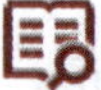 REFERENCE/SOURCE

- Penny DJ, Cetta F, Allen HD, Shaddy RE, Feltes TF (Eds). Moss and Adam's Heart Disease in Infants, Children, and Adolescents: Including the Fetus and Young Adult, 9th edition, Volume 2. Argentina: Wolters Kluwer; 2016. p. 1452.

17. Which of the following conditions predisposes to *fungal* endocarditis?

A. Postcardiac surgery
B. Neonates
C. Narcotic addicts
D. All of the above

 EXPLANATION

Risk factors for fungal endocarditis include narcotic addicts, postcardiac surgery status, immunocompromised individuals, and neonates.

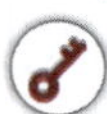 **Key:** D

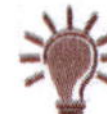 BOOST YOUR KNOWLEDGE

Fungal endocarditis is relatively unusual in children although it is one of the most feared forms of endocarditis. Complications, especially embolization, are frequent. *Candida* species are the most common organisms recovered; *Aspergillus* species, *Torulopsis glabrata*, and some other fungi (*Histoplasma, Coccidioides,* and *Cryptococcus*) also have been reported. The mortality rate from fungal endocarditis is high, even with intensive medical and surgical therapy.

 REFERENCE/SOURCE

- Penny DJ, Cetta F, Allen HD, Shaddy RE, Feltes TF (Eds). Moss and Adam's Heart Disease in Infants, Children, and Adolescents: Including the Fetus and Young Adult, 9th edition, Volume 2. Argentina: Wolters Kluwer; 2016. p. 1442.

18. Which of the following is *not* an immunological phenomenon in patients with infective endocarditis?

A. Glomerulonephritis
B. Osler nodes
C. Roth spots
D. Janeway lesions

 EXPLANATION

Janeway lesions are microabscesses that occur due to embolic phenomenon and are not immunological phenomenon. The immunologic consequence of endocarditis is the development of circulating immune complexes in the sera of patients. This is due to extended exposure to foreign antigen, and these immune complexes disappear after successful antimicrobial therapy. All other three lesions occur due to immune complexes.

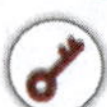 **Key:** D

BOOST YOUR KNOWLEDGE

Modified Dukes criteria for IE diagnosis

Definite IE:

- *Pathologic criteria:*
    - Microorganisms demonstrated by culture or histologic examination of a vegetation, a vegetation that has embolized, or an intracardiac abscess specimen; or
    - Pathologic lesions; vegetation or intracardiac abscess confirmed by histologic examination showing active endocarditis
- *Clinical criteria (see definitions):*
    - Two major criteria; or
    - One major criterion and three minor criteria; or
    - Five minor criteria

Possible IE:

- One major criterion and one minor criterion; or
- Three minor criteria

Rejected IE:

- Firm alternative diagnosis explaining evidence of IE; or
- Resolution of IE syndrome with antibiotic therapy for ≤4 days; or
- No pathologic evidence of IE at surgery or autopsy, with antibiotic therapy for ≤4 days; or
- Does not meet criteria for possible IE as above

REFERENCE/SOURCE

- Penny DJ, Cetta F, Allen HD, Shaddy RE, Feltes TF (Eds). Moss and Adam's Heart Disease in Infants, Children, and Adolescents: Including the Fetus and Young Adult, 9th edition, Volume 2. Argentina: Wolters Kluwer; 2016. p. 1447.

19. Which of the following is *not* an alternative to intramuscular 3 weekly depot penicillin prophylaxis for RHD?

A. Oral penicillin
B. Oral sulfadiazine
C. Oral erythromycin
D. Oral ciprofloxacin

EXPLANATION

Although less effective at least in part due to compliance, oral penicillin may be considered as an alternative, especially in parts of the world where RF is less common and in low-risk cases. It is worth noting that most individuals labeled as being allergic to penicillin are not, with such labeling leading to use of an antibiotic with greater cost and/or side effect profile along with the possibility of treatment failure. For patients with a history of nonanaphylactic allergic reactions to penicillin, formal drug allergy testing should strongly be considered (where possible). Sulfadiazine is recommended for patients allergic to penicillin. In penicillin and sulfa-allergic patients macrolide antibiotics may be used.

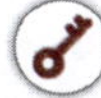

Key: D

BOOST YOUR KNOWLEDGE

Intramuscular benzathine penicillin (1.2 million units) is the most effective secondary prophylaxis regimen. There is pharmacokinetic evidence that penicillin levels fall between 21 and 28 days after administration in a significant number of patients. Thus, in areas where RF is endemic, every 3-week administration of intramuscular penicillin may be preferable (Indian Academy of Pediatrics recommends every 2 weeks for some patients).

REFERENCE/SOURCE

- Penny DJ, Cetta F, Allen HD, Shaddy RE, Feltes TF (Eds). Moss and Adam's Heart Disease in Infants, Children, and Adolescents: Including the Fetus and Young Adult, 9th edition, Volume 2. Argentina: Wolters Kluwer; 2016. p. 1395.

20. Long-term penicillin prophylaxis is advised till what age in a 12-year-old boy who underwent mitral valve repair due to severe rheumatic mitral regurgitation?

A. Till 15 years of age
B. Till 18 years of age
C. Till 21 years of age
D. Till 40 years of age

EXPLANATION

Prophylaxis duration in established RHD is till 40 years of age or lifelong.

Key: D

BOOST YOUR KNOWLEDGE

In the absence of specific and effective treatment for RF, preventing RF recurrences (termed secondary prophylaxis) is the most effective means of decreasing the likelihood and severity of long-term chronic RHD. Recurrence of ARF could be to the tune of 40–60% in patients with carditis in previous episodes. Recurrence risk gradually decreases as the age advances. Recurrence pattern is also mimetic. Recurrence causes more severe valvar dysfunction. Thus, all patients who have had RF should receive secondary prophylaxis to prevent recurrences.

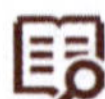

REFERENCE/SOURCE

- Penny DJ, Cetta F, Allen HD, Shaddy RE, Feltes TF (Eds). Moss and Adam's Heart Disease in Infants, Children, and Adolescents: Including the Fetus and Young Adult, 9th edition, Volume 2. Argentina: Wolters Kluwer; 2016. p. 1394.

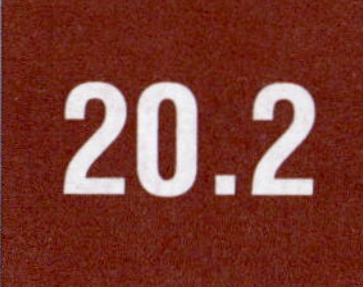

CHAPTER 20.2 Acyanotic Congenital Heart Defects

Lamak Kadiyani

1. A neonatologist hears a murmur in a 1-week-old baby. Electrocardiogram (ECG) shows left axis deviation. Which of the following is the most likely diagnostic cause of the left axis deviation?

A. Complete atrioventricular (AV) canal defect
B. Total anomalous pulmonary venous connection
C. Concentric left ventricular hypertrophy (LVH)
D. Secundum atrial septal defect

EXPLANATION

The normal QRS axis in frontal plane in neonatal period between 3 days and 7 days ranges from +76° to +191°. All options except A cause right axis deviation. In children, left axis deviation is not a criterion for LVH.

Key: A

BOOST YOUR KNOWLEDGE

Common causes of left axis deviation in infants include the AV canal defects (complete or partial) and tricuspid atresia, with or without transposition of the great vessels. Many patients with AV canal defects may have a more superior axis (–60° to –100°). Right axis deviation may be indicative of right ventricular hypertrophy in certain patients.

REFERENCE/SOURCE

- Allen HD, Shaddy RE, Penny DJ, Feltes TF, Cetta F. Moss and Adams' Heart Disease in Infants, Children, and Adolescents: Including the Fetus and Young Adult, 9th edition. Wolters Kluwer; 2016. pp. 551, 553, 767.

2. A 3-year-old boy is noted to have a murmur on school screening. His peripheral pulses are normal. The first and second heart sounds are normal. There is a grade 2/6 low-to-mid frequency "vibratory" murmur along the left sternal border.

When would one expect this murmur to increase in intensity?

A. When going from sitting to supine position
B. When going from sitting to standing position
C. With deep inhalation
D. During the third phase of the Valsalva maneuver

EXPLANATION

Considering, it is a low-grade systolic murmur, without any antecedent history suggestive of heart disease and heart sounds are normal, it is less likely to be a pathogenic murmur.

Key: A

BOOST YOUR KNOWLEDGE

The most common innocent systolic murmur of childhood is Still's murmur. It has many descriptions, including innocent, vibratory, functional, normal, and physiologic murmur. It is a systolic ejection murmur heard loudest somewhere between the left lower sternal border and the apex. Described as having a vibratory, musical, or twanging string quality, its usual intensity is grade I to III/VI. It is a low-frequency murmur in the range of 150 Hz. The murmur is heard best with the patient supine. This murmur also varies significantly with respiration, becoming softer and less vibratory during inspiration.

REFERENCE/SOURCE

- Allen HD, Shaddy RE, Penny DJ, Feltes TF, Cetta F. Moss and Adams' Heart Disease in Infants, Children, and Adolescents: Including the Fetus and Young Adult, 9th edition. Wolters Kluwer; 2016. p. 767.

3. A 2-year-old patient is referred to you with post-axial polydactyly, dwarfism, and fingernail dysplasia. Which of the following is the most likely to be detected if an echocardiogram is performed?

A. Interrupted aortic arch
B. Transposition of great arteries
C. Atrial septal defect
D. Coarctation of aorta

EXPLANATION

The question describes syndromic association of congenital heart defect (CHD). Option A is associated with DiGeorge syndrome (22q11 microdeletion). Option D is associated with Turner syndrome. Option B is almost never associated with genetic syndrome.

Key: C

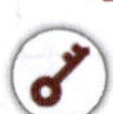

BOOST YOUR KNOWLEDGE

Holt–Oram syndrome is an autosomal dominant disorder caused by mutations of the *TBX5* gene. Patients most often present with abnormalities of the carpal bones of the wrist, which can include a malformed or missing thumb. Approximately 75% of patients have cardiac manifestations, with the most common form being atrial septal defects.

REFERENCE/SOURCE

- Allen HD, Shaddy RE, Penny DJ, Feltes TF, Cetta F. Moss and Adams' Heart Disease in Infants, Children, and Adolescents: Including the Fetus and Young Adult, 9th edition. Wolters Kluwer; 2016. p. 93

4. An 8-month-old child with a large membranous ventricular septal defect (VSD) develops complete heart block shortly after surgical repair. A suture "bite" placed too deep in which of the following sites is most likely responsible for the heart block?

A. Posterior-inferior rim of the VSD
B. Anterior-superior rim of the VSD
C. Superior right atrial free wall
D. Inferior right atrial free wall

EXPLANATION

A significant concern during the repair of membranous VSDs, particularly when performed on young infants, is damaging the AV node when suturing the patch in place. The AV node courses along the posterior–inferior rim of membranous VSDs. Damage to the node could result in high-grade AV block immediately or shortly after surgical repair.

Key: A

BOOST YOUR KNOWLEDGE

The conduction bundle runs along the antero-superior border of the inlet VSD. Surgical injury in this area can result in complete heart block (CHB) during inlet VSD closure. Superior right atrial free wall in the region of superior vena cava-right atrium (SVC-RA) junction houses the sinoatrial node. Injury to this area during superior cavopulmonary shunt or atrial switch (Senning's) surgery may lead to sinus node dysfunction and bradycardia.

REFERENCE/SOURCE

- Allen HD, Shaddy RE, Penny DJ, Feltes TF, Cetta F. Moss and Adams' Heart Disease in Infants, Children, and Adolescents: Including the Fetus and Young Adult, 9th edition. Wolters Kluwer; 2016. p. 1338.

5. A 5-year-old girl is found to have a murmur during evaluation for an upper respiratory tract infection (RTI). Echocardiogram reveals a secundum atrial septal defect (ASD) with continuous left to right shunt. Which of the following factors would be the strongest indication for surgical repair rather than percutaneous closure of the ASD?

A. Patient's age
B. Deficient retro-aortic rim
C. Moderate tricuspid valve regurgitation
D. Estimated pulmonary artery systolic pressure = 40 mm Hg

EXPLANATION

Device closure of atrial septal defects has been performed from children weighing <10 kg to elderly. Deficient retro-aortic rim is not a contraindication to device closure. Pulmonary artery systolic pressure would likely indicate mild pulmonary artery hypertension.

Key: C

BOOST YOUR KNOWLEDGE

Most centrally located secundum ASDs can be closed safely and effectively in the cardiac catheterization laboratory. Indications for surgical repair of a secundum ASD include deficiency of the posterior-inferior septal rim and the presence of coexisting abnormalities that would benefit from surgical repair. Specific recommendations for surgical repair include moderate or severe tricuspid valve regurgitation, which would benefit from annuloplasty or repair of the valve.

REFERENCE/SOURCE

- Allen HD, Shaddy RE, Penny DJ, Feltes TF, Cetta F. Moss and Adams' Heart Disease in Infants, Children, and Adolescents: Including the Fetus and Young Adult, 9th edition. Wolters Kluwer; 2016. p. 1299.

6. The pulse wave Doppler obtained in the descending thoracic aorta of a patient shows early diastolic reversal. Which of the following is *not* a probable diagnosis?

A. PDA (patent ductus arteriosus)
B. Truncus arteriosus
C. Aortic regurgitation
D. Coarctation of aorta

EXPLANATION

Coarctation of aorta results in narrowing in the isthmus leading to obstruction in flow across the same causing systolic gradient. In severe cases, narrowing causes obstruction flow across the segment even in diastole causing diastolic gradient ("spill").

Key: D

BOOST YOUR KNOWLEDGE

Reversal in descending thoracic aorta (DTA) is a feature of diastolic run off. Truncus arteriosus, and PDA have a systemic to pulmonary communication leading to diastolic run off. In AR, the run-off happens into the left ventricle during diastole.

7. Which of the following statements is *false* about the ECG in congenital heart disease?

A. First-degree atrioventricular (AV) block can be a feature in AV septal defects, congenitally corrected transposition of the great arteries, or Ebstein anomaly
B. Atrial fibrillation is more common than atrial flutter in young patients with congenital heart disease
C. The presence of right ventricular hypertrophy suggests pulmonary hypertension or right ventricular outflow tract obstruction
D. Deep Q waves in the left chest leads can be caused by left ventricular volume overload in a young person with aortic or mitral regurgitation

EXPLANATION

The ECG is helpful in the assessment of congenital heart disease. In particular, evaluation for right-axis deviation and right ventricular hypertrophy, and rhythm and conduction disturbances, is important. For example, right ventricular hypertrophy may be a sign of pulmonary hypertension or right ventricular outflow tract obstruction or other disorders causing right-sided pressure or volume overload, including septal defects.

Atrial arrhythmias commonly accompany congenital heart disease. Atrial flutter is much more frequent in young patients than atrial fibrillation. It often arises in patients with a history of surgical repair and can be challenging to treat. Pharmacologic agents are generally ineffective, and catheter ablation is usually necessary; recurrence is common. Conduction disturbances such as first-degree AV block, are often evident in patients with AV septal defects, congenitally corrected transposition of the great arteries, and Ebstein anomaly.

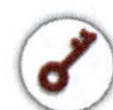

Key: B

BOOST YOUR KNOWLEDGE

The electrocardiographic findings of myocardial infarction in an infant suggest the presence of an anomalous origin of a coronary artery. Left ventricular volume overload due to aortic or mitral regurgitation can result in deep Q waves in the left precordial leads.

REFERENCES/SOURCES

- Khairy P, Van Hare GF, Balaji S, Berul CI, Cecchin F, Cohen MI, et al. PACES/HRS expert consensus statement on the recognition and management of arrhythmias in adult congenital heart disease: developed in partnership between the Pediatric and Congenital Electrophysiology Society (PACES) and the Heart Rhythm Society (HRS). Heart Rhythm. 2014;11(10):102-65.
- Mondésert B, Abadir S, Khairy P. Arrhythmias in adult congenital heart disease: The year in review. Curr Opin Cardiol. 2014;28:8354.

8. Which of the following statements about atrial septal abnormalities is *not* correct?

A. The sinus venosus-type ASD is almost always accompanied by anomalous pulmonary venous connections
B. The most common presenting symptoms of ASDs in adults are exercise intolerance and palpitations
C. Children with ASDs typically experience easy fatigability and exertional dyspnea
D. Atrial arrhythmias are uncommon in children with ASDs

EXPLANATION

- The sinus venosus defect is often accompanied by anomalous pulmonary venous return. The ostium secundum type of ASD, which appears in the mid-interatrial septum, should be distinguished from patent foramen ovale, which occurs in up to 25% of adults.

- Patients with ASDs are usually asymptomatic in early life, and only rare children with this disorder experience exertional dyspnea and easy fatigability. Atrial arrhythmias are uncommon. Children with ASDs do tend to be underdeveloped physically and prone to respiratory tract infections.
- The diagnosis of ASD in the young is most often prompted by detection of a heart murmur on routine physical examination.
- In adults, the most common manifesting symptoms are exercise intolerance and palpitations.

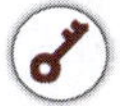

Key: C

BOOST YOUR KNOWLEDGE

The common anatomic types of ASD include the sinus venosus or "high" ASD, the ostium secundum ASD, and the ostium primum ASD. Ostium primum ASDs are a type of atrioventricular septal defect, discussed in a subsequent question.

REFERENCE/SOURCE

- Geva T, Martins JD, Wald RM. Atrial septal defects. Lancet. 2014;383:145.

9. Which of the following statements regarding ventricular septal defects (VSDs) is *not* correct?

A. Small VSDs pose a high risk of endocarditis

B. A restrictive VSD does not cause significant hemodynamic derangement and may close spontaneously during childhood

C. Infants with large, non-restrictive VSDs have less symptom and more signs than those with restrictive defects

D. The ECG after VSD repair usually demonstrates right bundle branch block

EXPLANATION

The size of a VSD relates to the consequent pathophysiology and potential complications. A restrictive VSD is small (Qp/Qs <1.4) and thus produces a significant pressure gradient between the left and right ventricles. It typically does not cause hemodynamic impairment and may eventually spontaneously close, but the turbulence of the high-pressure jet across the defect presents a high risk of endocarditis.

Because of the high gradient, infants with a restrictive VSD demonstrate a loud murmur but are asymptomatic. Conversely, infants with large nonrestrictive defects have softer murmurs but have significant feeding issues, failure to thrive (FTT), and recurrent lower respiratory tract infection (LRTIs). A large, nonrestrictive VSD (Qp/Qs >2.2) is accompanied by a substantial left-to-right shunt, with subsequent development of an elevated pulmonary artery systolic pressure. Such patients may eventually develop left ventricular volume overload, heart failure, and Eisenmenger syndrome (related to the progressive rise in pulmonary artery pressure). Closure of the defect, either surgically or by transcatheter device placement, is the treatment of choice for those with a significant VSD in the absence of contraindications (e.g., irreversible pulmonary hypertension). After repair, the ECG is usually notable for right bundle branch block.

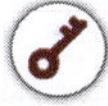

Key: C

BOOST YOUR KNOWLEDGE

Ventricular septal defects (VSDs) may be classified by their locations and margins. Muscular VSDs are bordered entirely by myocardium and may be found in the trabecular septum, inlet septum, or outlet septum. Membranous VSDs are bordered in part by fibrous continuity between an atrioventricular valve and an arterial valve. Doubly committed subarterial VSDs, which are more common in Asian and South American patients, are situated in the outlet. Septum and bordered by fibrous continuity of the aortic and pulmonary valves.

REFERENCE/SOURCE

- Penny DJ, Vick GW. Ventricular septal defect. Lancet. 2011;377:1103

10. Which of the following statements regarding ASDs is *true*?

A. Percutaneous device closure of ASDs improves functional status in symptomatic patients and exercise capacity in both asymptomatic and symptomatic patients

B. Children who have undergone repair of an isolated secundum defect should receive lifelong endocarditis prophylaxis

C. Murmurs are not typically present in patients with uncomplicated ASDs

D. Left-axis deviation of the QRS complex on the ECG suggests the presence of a sinus venosus ASD

EXPLANATION

Atrial septal defect repair is advised for patients with a Qp/Qs ≥1.5, particularly if the anatomy is suitable for percutaneous transcatheter device closure. Repair improves New York Heart Association functional class in symptomatic patients.

For adults who are asymptomatic or mildly symptomatic, device closure improves exercise capacity. In patients who undergo successful repair of an isolated secundum defect (by surgery or by transcatheter device), lifelong endocarditis prophylaxis is not required. Prophylaxis is appropriate for the first 6 months after device closure, while the device endothelializes.

Key: A

BOOST YOUR KNOWLEDGE

- Although atrial septal defects are frequently asymptomatic, children may experience exertional dyspnea or frequent chest infections. Physical examination usually demonstrates wide fixed splitting of the second heart sound.
- Other common findings include a systolic murmur of increased flow across the pulmonic valve or a mid-diastolic rumble due to increased flow through the tricuspid valve.
- The ECG may be helpful in determining the type of ASD. Secundum ASD patients often exhibit right-axis deviation on the ECG, whereas those with primum ASD characteristically
- Exhibit left-axis deviation. Patients with sinus venosus ASD exhibit left-axis deviation of the P wave.

REFERENCES/SOURCES

- Akagi T. Current concept of transcatheter closure of atrial septal defect in adults. J Cardiol. 2015;65:17.
- Humenberger M, Rosenhek R, Gabriel H, Rader F, Heger M, Klaar U, et al. Benefit of atrial septal defect closure in adults: impact of age. Eur Heart J. 2011;32(5):553-60.
- Vasquez A, Lasala J. Atrial septal defect closure. Cardiol Clin. 2013;31:385-400.

11. A 2-year-old, is quite friendly, has stellate irises, a long philtrum, depressed nasal bridge, prominent lower lip, and enamel hypoplasia. There is a 3/6 systolic ejection murmur and no click. Which of the following deletions is most likely in this patient?

A. 18q

B. 22p

C. 8p23

D. 7q11.23

EXPLANATION

The features described are suggestive of Williams syndrome (option D). Approximately 90% of patients with the clinical diagnosis of Williams syndrome have a deletion at chromosome 7q11.23, which is not generally apparent on a routine karyotype but can be detected by fluorescence in situ hybridization (FISH).

18q deletion is associated with ASD, VSD, and pulmonary stenosis and is associated with cleft palate and genitourinary (GU) anomalies. Tetrasomy 22p is known as "cat eye syndrome" and is associated with anorectal anomalies, coloboma, GU anomalies, and preauricular pits/tags. Deletion of 8p23 is associated with septal defects, GU anomalies, abnormally formed ears, and minor hand anomalies. Chromosome 22q11 deletion is known as DiGeorge syndrome or velocardiofacial syndrome and is characterized by hypocalcemia, immunodeficiency, and severe CHD, most commonly interrupted aortic arch (IAA) type B, truncus arteriosus, or tetralogy of Fallot (TOF).

Key: D

BOOST YOUR KNOWLEDGE

Williams syndrome is characterized in part by CHDs, hypercalcemia in infancy, skeletal and renal anomalies, cognitive deficits, social personality, and so-called "elfin facies."

Approximately 55–80% of patients with Williams syndrome have CHDs, which typically include supravalvar aortic stenosis and/or supravalvar pulmonary stenosis. Therefore, a click may not be present despite a murmur and significant gradient across the involved outflow tract.

REFERENCE/SOURCE

- Allen HD, Shaddy RE, Penny DJ, Feltes TF, Cetta F. Moss and Adams' Heart Disease in Infants, Children, and Adolescents: Including the Fetus and Young Adult, 9th edition. Wolters Kluwer; 2016. p. 85.

12. **You receive a call from the neonatal intensive care unit (NICU) regarding a child with feeding difficulty. His serum calcium is 5.4 mg/dL and total leukocyte count (TLC) 14,000 (N-89%, L-6%). In addition, he has a cleft palate. FISH testing is positive for 22q11 deletion. Among the following, what is his echocardiogram most likely to demonstrate?**

A. Pulmonary atresia + VSD
B. Interruption of aortic arch between the left common carotid and left subclavian artery
C. Interruption of aortic arch just beyond the left subclavian artery
D. Interruption of aortic arch between the innominate artery and the left carotid artery

EXPLANATION

The blood work-up is suggestive of hypocalcemia and lymphopenia. FISH analysis confirms suspicion of DiGeorge syndrome. The most common CHDs associated with a 22q11 deletion include TOF, IAA type B, truncus arteriosus, perimembranous VSD, and aortic arch anomalies.

Key: B

BOOST YOUR KNOWLEDGE

A wide range of CHDs has been reported in patients with a 22q11 deletion, including pulmonary valve stenosis, atrial septal defect, heterotaxy syndrome, and hypoplastic left heart syndrome.

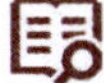

REFERENCE/SOURCE

- Allen HD, Shaddy RE, Penny DJ, Feltes TF, Cetta F. Moss and Adams' Heart Disease in Infants, Children, and Adolescents: Including the Fetus and Young Adult, 9th edition. Wolters Kluwer; 2016. p. 145.

13. Which of the following is true regarding left ventricular outflow tract (LVOT) obstruction in patients with atrioventricular septal defects (AVSDs)?

A. Obstruction may be due to displacement of the left AV valve annulus, resulting in shortening and narrowing of the LVOT
B. Nearly 30% of patients with AVSDs will require reoperation for LVOT obstruction
C. Progressive LVOT obstruction is more common in patients with two AV valve orifices
D. Preoperative LVOT obstruction is often progressive, while postoperative obstruction is frequently static

EXPLANATION

In the normal heart, the aortic valve is wedged between the mitral and the tricuspid annuli. In AVSD, the aortic valve is displaced or "sprung" anteriorly. This anterior displacement creates an elongated, so-called gooseneck deformity of the LVOT.

Left ventricular outflow tract obstruction may occur in all forms of AVSD. It is more frequent when two atrioventricular valve orifices are present than when there is a common orifice. 10% of patients with AVSD may require reoperation to relieve LVOT obstruction (while the most common indication for reoperation is left AV valve regurgitation or stenosis). Progressive LVOT obstruction is more common in partial than in complete AVSD. Obstruction may develop de novo after initial repair of the AVSD and closure of the mitral valve cleft. The gooseneck deformity of left ventricular outflow tract is characteristic of atrioventricular septal defect.

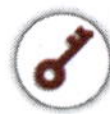

Key: C

BOOST YOUR KNOWLEDGE

Mechanisms of LVOT obstruction include attachments of superior bridging leaflet to ventricular septum, extension of the anterolateral papillary muscle into the LVOT, discrete fibrous subaortic stenosis, and tissue from an aneurysm of the membranous septum bowing into the LVOT.

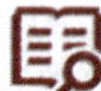

REFERENCE/SOURCE

- Allen HD, Shaddy RE, Penny DJ, Feltes TF, Cetta F. Moss and Adams' Heart Disease in Infants, Children, and Adolescents: Including the Fetus and Young Adult, 9th edition. Wolters Kluwer; 2016. p. 1328.

14. An 18-month-old boy undergoes operative repair of a moderate-sized ASD and moderate-sized mid-muscular VSD. His preoperative chest X-ray revealed borderline cardiomegaly and an ECG at the same time was normal. He remains intubated on postoperative day 2, at which time you note a new finding of a fixed split S2 with no murmur. Which of the following is the most likely reason for your findings?

A. Residual ASD
B. Postoperative decrease in pulmonary artery pressure
C. Right bundle branch block
D. Mechanical ventilation

EXPLANATION

Residual ASD would likely not be the cause of a newly split S2, a residual VSD would be accompanied by a murmur. Ventilation changes would not result in a newly split S2.

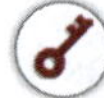

Key: C

BOOST YOUR KNOWLEDGE

Right bundle branch block is common and may be due to ventriculotomy or direct injury to the right bundle itself. Delayed depolarization leads to delayed ejection and subsequently delayed second heart sound. However, right bundle branch block occurs after a transatrial repair as well.

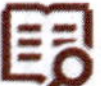

REFERENCE/SOURCE

- Abrams J. Synopsis of Cardiac Physical Diagnosis. 2nd edition. Butterworth-Heinemann Ltd.; 2001. p. 72.

15. An adolescent girl was lost to follow up after a childhood diagnosis of hole in the heart. The patient presents for evaluation of a murmur that was noted during her required physical for her new job. She is asymptomatic. There is a grade III/IV high-pitched decrescendo diastolic murmur at the left sternal border. What is the most likely explanation for the murmur?

A. Prolapse of left aortic cusp has closed the VSD, and the aortic valve is insufficient
B. Prolapse of the right aortic cusp has closed the VSD, and the aortic valve is insufficient
C. Prolapse of the septal leaflet of the tricuspid valve has closed the VSD, and the tricuspid valve is insufficient
D. RV and LV pressures have equalized, and new PR has developed

EXPLANATION

An early diastolic murmur in the setting of an intracardiac shunt lesion in infancy is suggestive of aortic regurgitation secondary to ventricular septal defect. The murmur of an incompetent tricuspid valve or mitral valve would be systolic. The patient is asymptomatic and acyanotic; hence, Eisenmenger physiology is not present. Therefore, RV and LV pressures have not equalized.

Key: B

BOOST YOUR KNOWLEDGE

Prolapse of one of the aortic valve cusps may occur with outlet or perimembranous VSDs. Patients with outlet defects usually have deficiency of muscular or fibrous support below the aortic valve with herniation of the right coronary leaflet through the VSD. The aortic commissures themselves are usually normal. In contrast, patients with perimembranous VSDs and aortic insufficiency have herniation of the right or much less commonly the noncoronary cusp, have frequent abnormalities of aortic commissures (usually the right/noncoronary), and may have associated infundibular pulmonary stenosis. Echocardiography and angiography can show that the prolapsed aortic leaflet partially closes a moderate-to-large VSD and limits the left-to-right shunt. The associated aortic valve insufficiency is progressive.

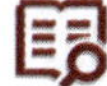

REFERENCE/SOURCE

- Allen HD, Shaddy RE, Penny DJ, Feltes TF, Cetta F. Moss and Adams' Heart Disease in Infants, Children, and Adolescents: Including the Fetus and Young Adult, 9th edition. Wolters Kluwer; 2016. p. 799.

16. What is the theoretical benefit of ibuprofen over indomethacin for closure of PDA in premature infants?

A. Decreased risk of intraventricular hemorrhage
B. Decreased risk of pulmonary hypertension
C. Decreased risk of gastrointestinal (GI) bleeding
D. Less effect on cerebral blood flow

EXPLANATION

Ibuprofen may have fewer negative effects on cerebral vasculature and cerebral blood flow than indomethacin, although the risk of intraventricular hemorrhage is equivocal. Of note, using ibuprofen for prophylaxis is associated with increased risk of pulmonary hypertension.

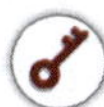

Key: D

BOOST YOUR KNOWLEDGE

Ibuprofen has been evaluated as a possible alternative to indomethacin in preterm infants. Studies have shown a similar rate of ductal closure after ibuprofen treatment with fewer negative effects on renal function. Of late, paracetamol has been shown non-inferior to other nonsteroidal anti-inflammatory drugs (NSAIDs).

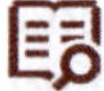

REFERENCE/SOURCE

- Allen HD, Shaddy RE, Penny DJ, Feltes TF, Cetta F. Moss and Adams' Heart Disease in Infants, Children, and Adolescents: Including the Fetus and Young Adult, 9th edition. Wolters Kluwer; 2016. p. 813.

17. An infant presents in acute cardiovascular collapse on day 3 of life. Physical examination reveals absence of all limb pulses with strong carotid pulses bilaterally.
Echocardiogram is most likely to reveal which of the following?

A. Critical aortic stenosis
B. Interruption of the aortic arch, type A, with anomalous subclavian artery
C. Interruption of the aortic arch type B
D. Interruption type B with anomalous subclavian artery

EXPLANATION

Presentation at Day 3 of life correlates with the closure of ductus arteriosus. Absence of all limb pulses suggests a type B interruption with an anomalous subclavian artery. In this situation, both carotid arteries are proximal to the interruption, while both subclavians are distal to the interruption. Strong carotid pulses help to differentiate interrupted arch from critical aortic stenosis in which all pulses are diminished.

Key: D

BOOST YOUR KNOWLEDGE

Interrupted aortic arch (IAA) is defined as a complete separation of ascending and descending aorta. Celoria and Patton classified IAA into three types—type A if the interruption was distal to the left subclavian artery, type B if between carotid and subclavian arteries, and type C if between carotid arteries. These patients typically present with acute cardiovascular collapse or heart failure after spontaneous closure of the ductus arteriosus in the first days of life.

REFERENCE/SOURCE

- Allen HD, Shaddy RE, Penny DJ, Feltes TF, Cetta F. Moss and Adams' Heart Disease in Infants, Children, and Adolescents: Including the Fetus and Young Adult, 9th edition. Wolters Kluwer; 2016. p. 859.

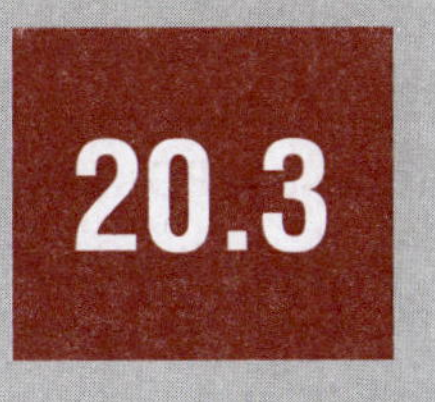

CHAPTER 20.3 Congenital Cyanotic Heart Defect

Nidhi Rawal

1. A 5-day-old cyanotic neonate with no murmur, chest X-ray (CXR) revealed decreased pulmonary vascular markings and electrocardiogram (ECG) showed left-axis deviation. The most likely diagnosis is:

A. Tetralogy of Fallot (TOF)
B. Truncus arteriosus
C. Transposition of great arteries (TGA)
D. Tricuspid atresia

EXPLANATION

- All congenital heart diseases with pulmonary stenosis (PS) have decreased pulmonary vascularity on CXR. In the options, TOF and tricuspid atresia with PS have decreased pulmonary vascularity.
- CXR of truncus arteriosus and TGA shows increased pulmonary vascularity.
- Characteristic left-axis deviation is seen in tricuspid atresia and endocardial cushion defect (ECD).

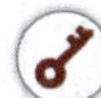

Key: D

BOOST YOUR KNOWLEDGE

- The normal QRS axis variation is seen with age.
- *The significance of abnormal QRS axis:*
  - Left-axis deviation (with the QRS axis lesser than the normal range) is seen in left ventricular hypertrophy (LVH), left bundle branch block (LBBB), and left anterior hemiblock (or superior QRS axis, *characteristic of ECD and tricuspid atresia).*
  - Right-axis deviation (RAD; with the QRS axis greater than the normal range) is seen in right ventricular hypertrophy (RVH) and right bundle branch block (RBBB).

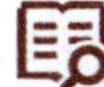

REFERENCE/SOURCE

- Park MK. Park's Pediatric Cardiology Handbook, 5th edition. United Kingdom: Elsevier Health Sciences; 2014. p. 36.

2. A newborn on day 2 of life presented with marked cyanosis, respiratory distress, and increased vascularity on a CXR. Echo could not be done due to technical reasons. What should be the first line of treatment?

A. Indomethacin
B. Digoxin
C. Prostaglandin E1 (PGE1)
D. Epinephrine

EXPLANATION

Any neonate with respiratory distress and severe cyanosis is duct-dependent lesion, unless proven otherwise. Even before echo is available, PG infusion should be started. If baby's color starts improving and urine output increases, it is diagnostic that the child has duct-dependent pulmonary circulation. Echocardiography is confirmatory.

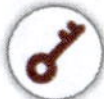

Key: C

BOOST YOUR KNOWLEDGE

Prostaglandin E1 is used to open and dilate the ductus arteriosus in patent ductus arteriosus (PDA)-dependent newborns to maintain either pulmonary or systemic blood flow or to improve mixing [e.g., D-transposition of the great arteries (D-TGA)]. The indications for PGE1 therapy include critical aortic stenosis, interrupted aortic arch, coarctation of the aorta, hypoplastic left heart syndrome (HLHS), pulmonary atresia, critical PS, and TGA.

Whenever a duct-dependent cardiac defect is in the differential diagnosis, administration of PGE1 should be strongly considered very early in the management of infants, especially for infants with possible congenital heart disease born at a peripheral center without cardiac services. Although there are side effects of PGE1 administration, the potential benefits outweigh its risks in these conditions.

REFERENCES/SOURCES

- Fulton DR, Fyler DC. D-transposition of the great arteries. In: Keane JF, Fyler DC, Lock JE (Eds). Nada's Pediatric Cardiology, 2nd edition. Philadelphia: Elsevier; 2006. p. 653.
- Penny DJ, Cetta F, Allen HD, Shaddy RE, Feltes TF (Eds). Moss and Adam's Heart Disease in Infants, Children, and Adolescents: Including the Fetus and Young Adult, 9th edition, Volume 2. Argentina: Wolters Kluwer; 2016. p. 3427.

3. Treatment of cyanotic spells include all of the following, *except*:

A. Digoxin

B. Morphine

C. Propranolol

D. Sodium bicarbonate

EXPLANATION

Cyanotic spells are characteristic of TOF-like physiology. They are due to spasm of infundibulum. So, all maneuvers and medication are targeted at the relaxation of right ventricular (RV) infundibulum and promote more blood flow into the pulmonary artery (PA) and prevent right-to-left shunt through ventricular septal defect (VSD). This can be achieved by calming the child, preventing any precipitating event, and correcting acidosis, if spell cycle has set in. Positioning such as knee chest position in infants and squatting in toddlers helps. Medication that is helpful is morphine. It calms the baby, relaxes the vasculature, and decreases the oxygen requirement. Propranolol relaxes the infundibular spasm, decreases the heart rate, and vasodilates pulmonary vasculature. Treat acidosis by sodium bicarbonate to prevent the perpetuation of spell cycle. Other important inclusions are normal saline bolus and oxygen.

Digoxin is used to treat heart failure and not spell.

Key: A

BOOST YOUR KNOWLEDGE

- The mainstay of the management is to break the vicious circle of hypoxic spell. One or more of the following may be employed:
    - Hold the infant in a knee-chest position
    - Morphine sulfate in the dose of 0.1–0.2 mg/kg SC or IM suppresses the respiratory center and also hyperpnea
    - Acidosis is treated with sodium bicarbonate, 1 mEq/kg IV, reducing the respiratory center-stimulating effect of acidosis
    - Oxygen therapy
- If less responsive with the above measures, the following may be attempted:
    - Ketamine 1–3 mg/kg (average of 2 mg/kg) slow IV push [helps by increasing the systemic vascular resistance (SVR) and sedating the infant]
    - Propranolol 0.01–0.25 mg/kg (average 0.05 mg/kg) slow IV push works well by reducing the heart rate and may even reverse the spell.

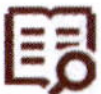

REFERENCE/SOURCE

- Park MK. Park's The Pediatric Cardiology Handbook, 5th edition. United Kingdom: Elsevier Health Sciences; 2014. p. 145.

4. A 1-year-old child brought to emergency room (ER) with marked cyanosis and rapid breathing. CXR showed reduced pulmonary vascularity. Venous blood gas (VBG) analysis was done, which revealed decreased pH, decreased pO_2, and increased pCO_2. What is the most likely diagnosis?

A. TGA
B. TOF
C. Truncus arteriosus
D. Total anomalous pulmonary venous connection (TAPVC)

EXPLANATION

This is a characteristic picture of cyanotic spell. Most common cyanotic heart disease is TOF. Fallot physiology has marked cyanosis and spells. CXR showed reduced vascularity and VBG showed marked acidosis with decreased pO_2. TGA, truncus, and TAPVC have cyanosis with increased lung vascularity with cardiomegaly.

Key: B

BOOST YOUR KNOWLEDGE

In cyanotic spells, the increased right-to-left shunt leads to a fall in systemic arterial pO_2 and pH and a rise in pCO_2. Resulted blood gas composition stimulates a sleep-sensitive respiratory center and carotid body, provoking hyperpnea. This in turn further increases the cardiac output and the cycle perpetuates.

REFERENCES/SOURCES

- Park MK. Park's The Pediatric Cardiology Handbook, 5th edition. United Kingdom: Elsevier Health Sciences; 2014. p. 145.
- Perloff JK, Marelli A (Eds). Perloff's Clinical Recognition of Congenital Heart Disease, 6th edition. Philadelphia: Elsevier Health Sciences; 2012. p. 325.

5. An infant at the age of 2 months was admitted with history of recurrent pneumonia and saturations of 88%. A CXR showed increased vascularity. Echo revealed single ventricle with increased blood flow in pulmonary circulation. What is the first line of treatment after the infection control?

A. PGE1 infusion
B. PA band
C. Bidirectional Glenn shunt
D. BT shunt

EXPLANATION

All the congenital heart diseases with increased flow in pulmonary circulation need reduction of PA blood to protect the lungs and prevent recurrent pneumonia. All the correctable shunt lesions, such as atrial septal defect (ASD), VSD, and PDA, should have shunt closure. Lesions that are not correctable, such as single ventricle, should undergo early PA band surgery to protect lungs and prepare them for next stage surgery.

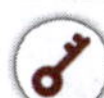

Key: B

BOOST YOUR KNOWLEDGE

Patients with single ventricle eventually require palliative single staged repair (i.e., Glenn and Fontan operation). The purpose of the PA band surgery is to make them suitable candidates for the bidirectional Glenn procedure.

- *First stage surgery:*
  - *No PS + unobstructed biventricular flow [with large pulmonary blood flow and congestive heart failure (CHF)]:* PA banding is done.

- *No PS + obstructed systemic blood flow:* Damus-Kaye-Stansel operation [transection of the main PA (MPA), anastomosis of the proximal PA to the aorta] and bidirectional Glenn operation or a BT shunt.

- *Second-stage palliative procedures*: The bidirectional Glenn operation is carried out between the age of 3 and 6 months.
- *The Fontan-type* operation is performed when the child is aged 4 years.

REFERENCE/SOURCE

- Park MK. Park's The Pediatric Cardiology Handbook, 5th edition. United Kingdom: Elsevier Health Sciences; 2014. pp. 179-80.

6. A cyanotic infant was referred to the emergency with history of pneumonia. Examination revealed saturation of 80%, with loud "to and fro" murmur on auscultation. CXR revealed prominent hilar pulmonary arteries. The likely diagnosis is:

A. TOF with aortic regurgitation (AR)
B. TOF, severe PS
C. TOF, absent pulmonary valve
D. TOF with large PDA

EXPLANATION

Child with TOF as a diagnosis has small PAs. Murmur heard is of PS, which is ejection systolic murmur. TOF along with PDA, AR do not have loud diastolic murmur. Only TOF with absent pulmonary valve have loud to and fro murmur with large hilar PAs.

Key: C

BOOST YOUR KNOWLEDGE

Clinical manifestations of TOF with absent pulmonary valve:

- At a neonatal age, mild cyanosis may be present. As pulmonary vascular resistance (PVR) falls, cyanosis disappears and signs of CHF may develop.
- On auscultation, a to-and-fro murmur ("sawing-wood sound") audible at the upper and middle left sternal border [resulting from PS and pulmonary regurgitation (PR)] is characteristic of the condition. The S2 is loud and single, and the right ventricle is hyperactive on palpation.
- RAD and RVH seen on ECG.
- Chest radiographs divulge markedly dilated MPA and hilar PAs. The heart size may be normal or mildly enlarged, and pulmonary vascular markings either normal or slightly increased. The lung fields may show atelectatic or hyperinflated zone.
- Infants with severe pulmonary complications mostly die during infancy if not treated surgically.

The surgical mortality is as high as 40% in infants with pulmonary complications. Therefore, it is recommended that surgery should be performed in early infancy.

REFERENCE/SOURCE

- Park MK. Park's The Pediatric Cardiology Handbook, 5th edition. United Kingdom: Elsevier Health Sciences; 2014. pp. 152-3.

7. An infant of diabetic mother, delivered by cesarean section, was noticed to have cyanosis with minimal tachypnea on Day 1. Cyanosis started worsening from 90 to 65% in one day. Saturations improved after starting PG infusion. What is the immediate intervention required?

A. Right ventricular outflow tract (RVOT) stenting
B. PDA ligation
C. PDA stenting
D. Balloon atrial septostomy

EXPLANATION

As per the description, the child seems to have TGA. Presentation starts after PDA starts closing. If there are no adequately sized ASD/VSD, PDA is the main source of oxygenated flow to the aorta. Once PDA starts closing, the child starts developing cyanosis and worsening of symptoms. At that stage, PG infusion is lifesaving and next procedure required is balloon atrial septostomy for proper atrial level mixing.

Very soon arterial switch operation will have to be planned.

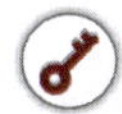

Key: D

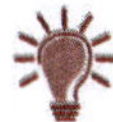

BOOST YOUR KNOWLEDGE

Balloon atrial septostomy (Rashkind procedure) is a procedure wherein a special balloon-tipped catheter is used to create an opening or enlarge ASD in the atrial septum to improve atrial level shunting in patients with serious congenital heart diseases such as TGA, pulmonary atresia, tricuspid atresia, and total anomalous pulmonary venous return (TAPVR). In infants older than 6–8 weeks of age, blade atrial septostomy is done as the atrial septum is very thick and does not allow an effective balloon septostomy.

REFERENCES/SOURCES

- Fulton DR, Fyler DC. D-transposition of the great arteries. In: Keane JF, Fyler DC, Lock JE (Eds). Nada's Pediatric Cardiology, 2nd edition. Philadelphia: Elsevier; 2006. p. 653.
- Park MK. Park's The Pediatric Cardiology Handbook, 5th edition. United Kingdom: Elsevier Health Sciences; 2014. p. 135.
- Schneider DS. Cyanotic congenital heart disease. In: Schuh AM, Marcdante K, Kliegman RM (Eds). Nelson Essentials of Pediatrics, 9th edition. Netherlands: Elsevier Health Sciences; 2022. pp. 570-1.

8. A cyanotic child was diagnosed with D-TGA, VSD, and PS at the age of 1 month. What is the suggested surgery for him?

A. BT shunt
B. Rastelli operation
C. Glenn shunt
D. Fontan operation

EXPLANATION

Children with diagnosis of D-TGA, VSD with PS come under Fallot physiology. They are cyanotic and prone to cyanotic spells. They need early BT shunt to improve the pulmonary blood flow and relieve cyanosis. At a later stage, around 1 year of age, they undergo complete repair, that is, Rastelli operation. Rastelli operation is VSD closure with routing of aorta to LV and right ventricle to PA via conduit.

Glenn shunt and Fontan operation are done for single ventricle physiology at around 6 months and 4 years of age, respectively.

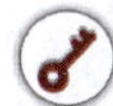

Key: A

BOOST YOUR KNOWLEDGE

The definitive surgery in TGA are atrial switch (Senning operation)—the right- and left-sided structures are switched at the atrial level; Rastelli operation—switching at the ventricular level; or arterial switch operation—switch done at the great artery level.

- *Rastelli operation*, wherein PA flow is directed to RV and aorta to LV. It is carried out in patients with VSD and severe PS. VSD is closed, committing aorta to LV. A valved conduit or a homograft is placed between the RV and the PA. Two alternative procedures available are REV procedure and Nikaidoh procedure.
- *The Damus-Kaye-Stansel operation* may be performed in infants with a large VSD and significant subaortic stenosis around the age of 1–2 years.

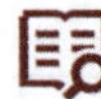

REFERENCE/SOURCE

- Park MK. Park's The Pediatric Cardiology Handbook, 5th edition. United Kingdom: Elsevier Health Sciences; 2014. pp. 135-40.

9. A term baby was brought to ER with cyanosis and respiratory distress. CXR revealed white out lungs. What is the likely diagnosis?

A. Infracardiac TAPVC
B. HLHS
C. Hypoplastic right heart syndrome
D. Large VSD, severe PS

EXPLANATION

White out lungs could be due to respiratory or cardiac causes. Respiratory causes could be respiratory distress syndrome (RDS) or congenital B/L pneumonia. Cardiac cause is obstructive TAPVC. RDS is more commonly seen in preterm babies. In term babies, more common is TAPVC.

- Most common obstructive TAPVC in newborn period is infracardiac TAPVC. Infracardiac TAPVC is always obstructive, so needs urgent surgical correction.
- HLHS kids present with shock.
- Children with hypoplastic right heart and VSD PS present with cyanosis and oligemic lung fields.

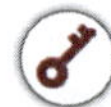

Key: A

BOOST YOUR KNOWLEDGE

Clinical presentation with obstructive TAPVR:

- Neonate presents with significant cyanosis and respiratory distress.
- A loud and single S2 and gallop rhythm present. No heart murmur is usually heard. Pulmonary crepts may be audible.
- The ECG findings are RAD and RVH.
- Chest radiograph shows usually a normal-sized heart with findings of pulmonary venous congestion or edema in lung fields.
- Echo is diagnostic and shows anomalous PV return below the diaphragm and relatively hypoplastic LA and LV.
- Cardiac catheterization, magnetic resonance imaging (MRI), or cardiac CT are confirmatory to complete the diagnosis.
- Patients with the infracardiac type are an emergency and they do not survive more than a few weeks without surgery.

Children with nonobstructive TAPVR: Chest radiographs show cardiomegaly, mainly involving right atrium (RA) and RV with increased pulmonary vascular markings. Supracardiac type TAPVC shows a "snowman" sign and is seen in older infants (usually after 4 months of age).

REFERENCES/SOURCES

- Park MK. Park's The Pediatric Cardiology Handbook, 5th edition. United Kingdom: Elsevier Health Sciences; 2014. pp. 154-5.
- Perloff JK, Marelli A (Eds). Perloff's Clinical Recognition of Congenital Heart Disease, 6th edition. Philadelphia: Elsevier Health Sciences; 2012. p. 247.

10. A child came walking to emergency with severe cyanosis and no respiratory distress. Echo revealed structurally normal heart. Contrast echo also did not reveal any shunt. The most probable diagnosis is:

A. Trauma
B. Methemoglobinemia
C. Multiple pulmonary arteriovenous fistula
D. Interstitial lung disease

EXPLANATION

- Central cyanosis with structurally normal heart is most seen in methemoglobinemia and next in line is pulmonary arteriovenous (AV) fistulas. Children with multiple pulmonary AV fistulas will have cyanosis with tachypnea.
- There can be a history of certain drug intake, such as antimalarial—chloroquine; antibiotics such as dapsone and nitrofurantoin; or certain painkillers which can cause methemoglobinemia. Diagnosis is established by laboratory investigation and arterial blood gas (ABG) analysis, which can reveal methemoglobin level.
- Diagnosis of pulmonary AV fistula is established by contrast echo and computed tomography (CT) chest with contrast.

Key: B

BOOST YOUR KNOWLEDGE

Methemoglobinemia is a combination of low oxygen saturation and normal oxygen tension. It is a very uncommon condition where blood has a chocolate-brown color and does not become red when exposed to air.

Pulmonary AV fistulas may be:

- Multiple, tiny, and diffusely scattered throughout in both the lungs, as in Osler-Weber-Rendu syndrome or after Glenn shunt surgery or
- Localized malformations confined to a single lobe. They are mostly congenital and increase with time.
- The pulmonary arteriovenous malformations (PAVMs) formed following surgical Glenn shunt result from exclusion of a hepatic factor directly reaching the pulmonary circulation. The diffuse variety is also seen in patients with liver disease. They are reversible in both cases by connecting hepatic venous return to the lungs following Glenn shunt and liver transplantation in cases of liver disease.

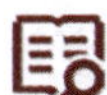

REFERENCE/SOURCE

- Keane JF, Fyler DC, Lock JE (Eds). Nada's Pediatric Cardiology, 2nd edition. Philadelphia: Elsevier; 2006. pp. 141-2, 801.

11. A child was diagnosed as a case of truncus arteriosus type 1. He became inoperable at the age of 1 year. What is a likely reason?

A. Severe pulmonary vascular obstructive disease (PVOD)
B. Recurrent pneumonia
C. Truncal valve regurgitation
D. Severe failure to thrive

EXPLANATION

Child with truncus arteriosus have PAs arising from the large trunk, which is giving rise to the aorta, PA, and coronary artery. All the arteries are at systemic pressures. PA when exposed to such a high pressure for long time develops early PVOD. Therefore, truncus repair should be done early within 6 weeks to 6 months of age.

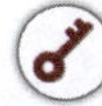

Key: A

BOOST YOUR KNOWLEDGE

Due to prolonged exposure of the pulmonary vasculature to systemic arterial pressure, hypertensive pulmonary vascular disease (plexogenic pulmonary arteriopathy) may develop. The arteriolar lesions develop more rapidly and to a severe extent in truncus arteriosus than in isolated ventricular septal defect or PDA.

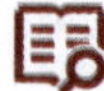

REFERENCE/SOURCE

- Penny DJ, Cetta F, Allen HD, Shaddy RE, Feltes TF (Eds). Moss and Adam's Heart Disease in Infants, Children, and Adolescents: Including the Fetus and Young Adult, 9th edition, Volume 2. Argentina: Wolters Kluwer; 2016. pp. 1054-8.

12. A child was brought to pediatric outpatient department (OPD) with history of one episode of syncope. There was no prior history of heart disease. ECG showed complete heart block. What is the likely heart disease associated with it?

A. AV canal defect
B. Congenitally corrected TGA (C-TGA)
C. D-TGA
D. Large VSD

EXPLANATION

Corrected TGA is the most common heart disease associated with complete heart block in children. Even in fetal life, if heart block is detected, screening for C-TGA should be done. The position of the atrioventricular node and course of the atrioventricular conduction bundle is very unusual due to which disorders of cardiac conduction are commonly seen.

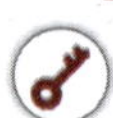

Key: B

BOOST YOUR KNOWLEDGE

Causes of congenital heart block:

- Neonatal lupus erythematosus accounts for 60–90% of the cases. Heart block is caused by maternal antibodies for autoimmune connective tissue diseases crossing the placenta to the fetus.
- Among all, 25–33% cases are associated with CHDs, most commonly with C-TGA, single ventricle, or left isomerism syndrome.
- It is also seen in cases of neonatal myocarditis and various genetic disorders such as familial ASD and Kearns–Sayre syndrome.

REFERENCES/SOURCES

- Park MK. Park's The Pediatric Cardiology Handbook, 5th edition. United Kingdom: Elsevier Health Sciences; 2014. pp. 140-2, 297.
- Perloff JK, Marelli A (Eds). Perloff's Clinical Recognition of Congenital Heart Disease, 6th edition. Philadelphia: Elsevier Health Sciences; 2012. pp. 63-6.

13. A newborn was detected to have pulmonary atresia with intact ventricular septum with coronary sinusoids. Which of the following is the correct sequence of management?

A. PGE1→ BT shunt→ Glenn shunt→ Fontan operation
B. PGE1→PDA stenting→RV to PA conduit repair
C. RVOT ballooning and stenting
D. Pulmonary valvotomy

EXPLANATION

Pulmonary atresia with intact ventricular septum has small RV under high pressure. If coronary sinusoids have developed, this RV is not opened, rather pulmonary circulation is established by PGE1 infusion followed by BT shunt. Glenn shunt and Fontan follow later.

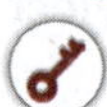

Key: A

BOOST YOUR KNOWLEDGE

In patients with hypoplastic RV (monopartite RV) with or without coronary sinusoids, surgery performed is a staged Fontan operation. A BT shunt/PDA stenting is performed initially, followed by Bidirectional Glenn shunt at 3–6 months of age and Fontan operation at 4 years of age. For patients with RV sinusoids, the sinusoids may be left alone, or the tricuspid valve is closed (Starnes operation).

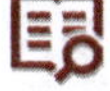

REFERENCE/SOURCE

- Park MK. Park's The Pediatric Cardiology Handbook, 5th edition. United Kingdom: Elsevier Health Sciences; 2014. pp. 164-6.

14. A child underwent Glenn shunt operation at the age of 8 months. Post-Glenn surgery, the child was noticed to have irritability and swelling over the face after waking up. What is the most likely reason behind it?

A. Obstruction in the superior vena cava (SVC) PA anastomosis
B. High PA pressures
C. Clot in SVC
D. All of the above

EXPLANATION

Glenn shunt, also known as cavopulmonary connection, is a communication created between SVC and right PA. If there is an increase in PA pressures or there is any obstruction in SVC, it leads to an increase in SVC pressures proximal to obstruction, resulting in venous congestion in the head and neck area and upper limbs, commonly seen as facial congestion. Due to the increase in venous congestion in the head, the child becomes very irritable.

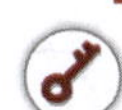

Key: D

BOOST YOUR KNOWLEDGE

The superior cavopulmonary shunt, that is, bidirectional Glenn shunt, reduces the load of single ventricle and, at the same time, provides a more reliable source of pulmonary blood flow than the pre-existent BT shunt/PDA stenting/RV to PA shunt. In the younger ages, routinely a bidirectional Glenn shunt is performed above the age of 3 months.

There are known incremental risk factors for a bidirectional Glenn shunt: (1) Reduced systemic ventricular function, (2) uncorrected significant AV valve regurgitation, (3) pulmonary vein stenosis (PVS), (4) uncorrected subaortic obstruction, and (5) anomalies of PA arborization.

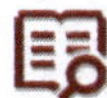

REFERENCE/SOURCE

- Sharma R. The bidirectional Glenn shunt for univentricular hearts. Indian J Thorac Cardiovasc Surg. 2018;34(4):453-6.

15. Master C, 4-year-old boy, underwent Glenn shunt at the age of 9 months for tricuspid atresia, ASD, VSD, and mild PS. He underwent cardiac catheterization study to plan for Fontan operation. Cath data revealed PA pressures of 36/18/24 and pulmonary vascular resistance index (PVRI) 2.8 Wood units. Fontan was deferred. What was the most likely reason?

A. He is late for the surgery
B. He is early for the surgery
C. PA pressures and PVRI high
D. He was planned for tricuspid valve implantation

EXPLANATION

Fontan operation is done in cases of single ventricle palliation. It is done after Glenn operation after the age of 4 years. The Fontan tube is placed between inferior vena cava (IVC) and PA. There are stringent criteria for Fontan operation. If they are not fulfilled, operation may fail and child lands up in deep trouble.

First and foremost, the criteria are normal PA pressures (it should be <18–20 mm Hg, ideal is 15 mm Hg and PVRI should be <2 Wood units). If PA pressures are high, IVC blood will not flow into PA, and there will be pooling in the lower limbs and ascites.

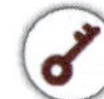

Key: C

BOOST YOUR KNOWLEDGE

The risk factors for the Fontan operation are:

- A high PVR (>2 U/m^2) or high mean PA pressure (>18 mm Hg)
- Distorted or stenotic PAs postprevious shunt operations
- Reduced LV systolic and diastolic functions (LV end-diastolic pressure >12 mm Hg or an ejection fraction <50%)

REFERENCE/SOURCE

- Park MK. Park's The Pediatric Cardiology Handbook, 5th edition. United Kingdom: Elsevier Health Sciences; 2014. pp. 160-4.

16. A 6-month-old baby presented to the emergency with shock, respiratory distress, and cyanosis. Echo diagnosis was supracardiac TAPVC with unrestricted flow in the vertical vein and restrictive ASD. ABG revealed acidosis, decreased PO_2, and increased lactate. What is the most likely reason for her deterioration?

A. Unrestricted flow in the vertical vein
B. Restrictive ASD
C. Increasing lactate
D. Age <1 year

EXPLANATION

- TAPVC is total anomalous drainage of pulmonary veins to the right side. It could be supracardiac (via vertical vein to innominate to SVC), cardiac (RA/coronary sinus), or infracardiac (below the diaphragm, to IVC, or hepatic veins). All the blood is reaching the RA. Source of blood to LA and LV is through ASD. In cases of no obstruction to pulmonary venous drainage, the child usually presents with heart failure and signs of pulmonary congestion.
- If ASD becomes small, the child goes into shock, urine output decreases, develops acidosis, and lactate increases. Other causes of deterioration are any obstruction in the vertical vein, coronary sinus opening, or individual pulmonary vein obstruction.
- In this case scenario, the culprit is restrictive ASD.

Key: B

BOOST YOUR KNOWLEDGE

Clinical presentation in a child with diagnosis of TAPVC, without obstruction:

- Failure to thrive, mild cyanosis/duskiness, and signs of CHF (tachypnea, tachycardia, and hepatomegaly) are common.
- RV impulse is palpable and quadruple or quintuple rhythm is characteristic. The S2 is wide split and fixed, and the P2 may be loud and palpable. A grade 2 to 3/6 systolic ejection murmur is present at the upper left sternal border.

Clinical presentation in a child with obstruction:

- Neonate presents with severe cyanosis and respiratory distress.
- A loud and single S2 along with gallop rhythm present. Heart murmur is usually absent. Pulmonary crepts may be audible.

REFERENCE/SOURCE

- Park MK. Park's The Pediatric Cardiology Handbook, 5th edition. United Kingdom: Elsevier Health Sciences; 2014. pp. 164-6.

17. A child presented to emergency with a cyanotic spell. Which of the following is the correct approach to management?

A. Increasing SVR and increasing pulmonary resistance
B. Decreasing SVR and decreasing pulmonary resistance
C. Increasing SVR and decreasing pulmonary resistance
D. Increasing heart rate to increase the stroke volume

EXPLANATION

Hypercyanotic spells are a result of RVOT (infundibular spasm) decreasing blood flow into pulmonary circulation and increasing cyanosis. Increased right-to-left shunts occur through the VSD leading to increased desaturating blood reaching the aorta. So, the aim of therapy is to increase the SVR and decrease PVR, so that more and more blood enters PA and increase in SVR also reduces right-to-left shunt and promotes left-to-right shunt.

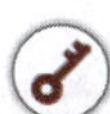

Key: C

BOOST YOUR KNOWLEDGE

A typical spell starts with a progressively increase in the rate and depth of breathing and ends up in paroxysmal hyperpnea, worsening of cyanosis, limpness, syncope, and occasionally leads to convulsions, cerebrovascular accidents, and death. Five mechanisms are involved in the pathogenesis of spell in TOF: (1) increase in heart rate; (2) an increase in cardiac output and venous return; (3) an increase in right-to-left shunt; (4) stimulation of respiratory control centers; and (5) infundibular spasm (contraction of RVOT).

Pathophysiology of hypoxic spell: In TOF, the RV and LV can be viewed as a single pumping chamber, as pressures in both the ventricles are equalized by a large VSD. Lowering the SVR or increasing resistance at the RVOT will accelerate the right-to-left shunting. This in turn stimulates the respiratory center to produce hyperpnea. Hyperpnea results in an increase in systemic venous return, which in turn increases the right-to-left shunt through the VSD, as there is an obstruction at the RVOT. A vicious circle becomes established.

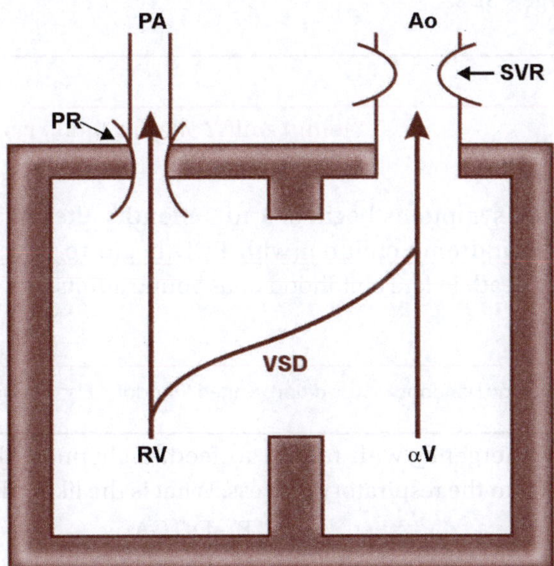

Schematic diagram to show how change in the SVR affects the direction and the volume of the ventricular shunt.

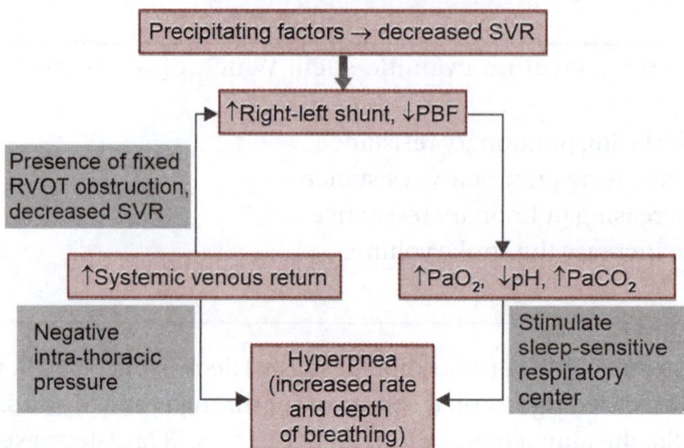

REFERENCES/SOURCES

- Park MK. Park's The Pediatric Cardiology Handbook, 5th edition. United Kingdom: Elsevier Health Sciences; 2014. pp. 145-6.
- Perloff JK, Marelli A (Eds). Perloff's Clinical Recognition of Congenital Heart Disease, 6th edition. Philadelphia: Elsevier Health Sciences; 2012. pp. 325-6.

18. Eisenmenger syndrome develops early in which one of the following condition?

A. TGA, PS
B. Tricuspid atresia, VSD, PS
C. Complete AV canal defect
D. TOF

EXPLANATION

- Eisenmenger syndrome develops secondary to huge left-to-right shunts over a long period leading to irreversible obstructive changes in pulmonary vascular bed, leading to raised PA pressures and PVR.
- Heart lesions prone for early development of Eisenmenger syndrome are truncus, AV canal defect, large AP window, large PDA, and large VSDs.
- Presence of PS is protective.

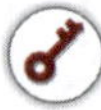

Key: C

BOOST YOUR KNOWLEDGE

In AV canal defect, heart failure symptoms begin at 1 to 2 months after birth, and recurrent pneumonia is a common presentation. Down syndrome children with ECD begin to develop PVOD in the 1st year of life. Development of PVOD leads to death in late childhood or as young adults.

REFERENCE/SOURCE

- Park MK. Park's The Pediatric Cardiology Handbook, 5th edition. United Kingdom: Elsevier Health Sciences; 2014. pp. 112-3.

19. A newborn presented to the emergency with refusal to feed, tachypnea, deep cyanosis, and was lethargic. The cyanosis is out of proportion to the respiratory distress. What is the likely diagnosis?

A. Congenital pneumonia
B. D-TGA
C. Truncus arteriosus
D. Large VSD, PDA

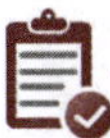

EXPLANATION

- Newborns presenting to emergency with cyanosis most commonly have duct-dependent lesion, most commonly it is D-TGA.
- Truncus, AV canal defect, large VSD, and PDA present with heart failure.
- Congenital pneumonia presents respiratory distress.

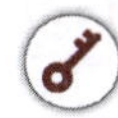

Key: B

BOOST YOUR KNOWLEDGE

- 5% of all CHDs are constituted by TGA, with preponderance in boys (3:1).
- ASD, VSD, and PDA are necessary for mixing of the two circulations for survival, VSD is seen in almost 40% of cases. No associated defect is present in about 50% of patients other than patent foramen ovale (PFO), small ASD, or small PDA.
- Presents as cyanosis and signs of CHF in the newborn period. Neonates with poor mixing present as severe arterial hypoxemia unresponsive to oxygen inhalation and acidosis. Occasionally, hypoglycemia and hypocalcemia are present.
- The clinical recognition of TGA is based on the following features: (1) male gender; (2) large weight of the baby; (3) cyanosis soon after birth; (4) radiologic evidence of increased pulmonary blood flow in the presence of cyanosis and an egg-shaped cardiac silhouette with a narrow vascular pedicle; (5) absent thymic shadow; and (6) echocardiographic identification of aortic alignment with the morphologic right ventricle, pulmonary trunk alignment with the morphologic left ventricle, right atrial alignment with the right ventricle, and left atrial alignment with the left ventricle.

REFERENCES/SOURCES

- Park MK. Park's The Pediatric Cardiology Handbook, 5th edition. United Kingdom: Elsevier Health Sciences; 2014. pp. 133-4.
- Perloff JK, Marelli A (Eds). Perloff's Clinical Recognition of Congenital Heart Disease, 6th edition. Philadelphia: Elsevier Health Sciences; 2012. pp. 488-9.

20. A 6-month-old baby was brought to emergency in respiratory distress and cyanosis. CXR revealed cardiomegaly with increased lung vascularity. Clinical examination revealed single S2, ejection clicks, and ejection systolic murmur. ABG done revealed pH 7.3, pO_2 52 mm Hg, pCO_2 42 mm Hg, and saturation 80%. What is the most likely possibility?

A. TOF
B. TGA
C. Truncus arteriosus
D. Tricuspid atresia

EXPLANATION

- Common causes of heart failure in a 6-month-old child are large shunt lesion.
- Cyanosis with heart failure is seen in truncus arteriosus, D-TGA with large VSD, or single ventricle physiology with unrestrictive pulmonary blood flow.
- Truncus has single second heart sound with ejection click and ejection systolic murmur with large heart size and increased pulmonary vascularity on CXR.
- ABG picture is also suggestive of truncus.
- TOF will not have cardiomegaly. Child with tricuspid atresia or D-TGA will have lesser saturations and pO_2 will also be less. Ejection click will also be not there.

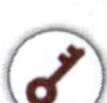

Key: C

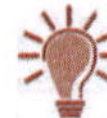

BOOST YOUR KNOWLEDGE

Single arterial trunk (with a truncal valve) arising from both the ventricles and gives rise to the pulmonary, systemic, and coronary circulations. A large VSD is mandatory. A right aortic arch is seen in 30% of patients.

Collette and Edwards classification classifies this anomaly into four types: *type I* (most common, 60%); *type II* (20%); *type III* (10%); and *type IV* (10%). Type IV is not a true truncus arteriosus; it is now considered as a severe form of TOF with pulmonary atresia with aortopulmonary collaterals supplying the lungs. About 30% of patients have DiGeorge syndrome with hypocalcemia, it is associated with interrupted aortic arch.

REFERENCE/SOURCE

- Park MK. Park's The Pediatric Cardiology Handbook, 5th edition. United Kingdom: Elsevier Health Sciences; 2014. pp. 175-6.

21. Cyanosis with increased pulmonary vascularity is *not* seen in which of the following conditions?

A. TOF
B. TAPVR
C. Truncus arteriosus
D. TGA

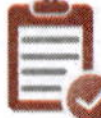

EXPLANATION

TOF presents with cyanosis with decreased lung vascularity. TAPVR, TGA, and truncus have cyanosis but with increased lung vascularity.

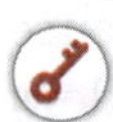

Key: A

BOOST YOUR KNOWLEDGE

- *Increased pulmonary vascularity in chest radiograph:*
  - Increased pulmonary vascular markings in a child with no cyanosis suggest a left-to-right shunt lesion such as ASD, VSD, PDA, ECD, partial anomalous pulmonary venous drainage, or any combination of these.
  - In an infant with cyanosis with increased pulmonary vascular markings, differential diagnoses are TGA, TAPVR, HLHS, persistent truncus arteriosus, or single ventricle.
- Decreased pulmonary vascular markings in a cyanotic baby suggest critical stenosis or pulmonary atresia, tricuspid atresia, or TOF.
- Pulmonary venous congestion is a feature of left-sided lesion such as HLHS, MS, TAPVR, and cor triatriatum.
- Normal pulmonary vasculature is seen in patients with mild-to-moderate PS and in patients with small left-to-right shunt lesions.

REFERENCE/SOURCE

- Park MK. Park's The Pediatric Cardiology Handbook, 5th edition. United Kingdom: Elsevier Health Sciences; 2014. pp. 59-60.

22. Increased pulmonary vascularity along with cyanosis and cardiomegaly is seen in:

A. TGA
B. TOF
C. Large VSD, PAH
D. Eisenmenger syndrome

EXPLANATION

- Cyanosis, cardiomegaly, and increased pulmonary vascularity are features of D-TGA, truncus arteriosus, TAPVR, and complete AV canal defect.
- Large VSD with PAH develops cyanosis very late and by that time heart size starts becoming smaller and pulmonary vasculature reduces. Same is true with Eisenmenger syndrome.
- TOF also presents with decreased pulmonary vascularity and no cardiomegaly.

Key: A

BOOST YOUR KNOWLEDGE

Covered in Question 21.

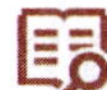

REFERENCE/SOURCE

- Park MK. Park's The Pediatric Cardiology Handbook, 5th edition. United Kingdom: Elsevier Health Sciences; 2014. pp. 59-60.

23. A 1-year-old child with the diagnosis of pink TOF presented to the ER with excessive irritability, hyperpnea, cyanosis, and unresponsiveness. What is the likely cause?

A. Convulsions
B. Cyanotic spell
C. Brain abscess
D. Aspiration

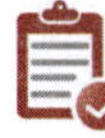

EXPLANATION

Pink TOF kids are very much prone for cyanotic spells. Sometimes their first presentation is a cyanotic spell. Child with brain abscess with cyanosis usually presents with fever, deep cyanosis, convulsions, and unconsciousness. Cyanotic spell if left untreated can lead to convulsions.

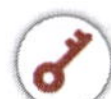

Key: B

BOOST YOUR KNOWLEDGE

Children with the pink TOF gradually become cyanotic form by 1 to 3 years of age. Hypoxic spells may develop in infants. Brain abscess, cerebrovascular accident, and subacute bacterial endocardiitis (SBE) are rare complications.

Hypoxic spell (also called cyanotic spell or "tet" spell) is characterized by: (1) a paroxysm of hyperpnea (rapid and deep respiration), (2) irritability and inconsolable crying, (3) worsening cyanosis, and (4) heart murmur becomes less intensive. A severe spell may progress to limpness, convulsion, cerebrovascular accident, or even death. It occurs in young infants, with peak incidence between 2 and 6 months of age. Hypoxic spell requires early recognition and prompt appropriate treatment.

REFERENCE/SOURCE

- Park MK. Park's The Pediatric Cardiology Handbook, 5th edition. United Kingdom: Elsevier Health Sciences; 2014. pp. 145-7.

24. DiGeorge syndrome in association with hypocalcemia is seen in 30% of patients with one of the following conditions. Name it.

A. TGA
B. Coarctation of aorta
C. Truncus arteriosus
D. Tricuspid atresia

EXPLANATION

DiGeorge syndrome with hypocalcemia is seen in about 30% of patients. 13% have interrupted aortic arch (type B interruption between the left carotid and left subclavian arteries).

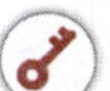

Key: C

BOOST YOUR KNOWLEDGE

Serious CHDs are seen in great majority of patients (85%) with the syndrome:

- *Heart anomalies:* With decreasing frequency—TOF (25%), interrupted aortic arch (15%), VSD (15%), persistent truncus arteriosus (9%), and less commonly isolated aortic arch anomalies (5%).

- Abnormal facial deformities seen are hypertelorism, micrognathia, fish-mouth appearance with short philtrum, antimongoloid slant, telecanthus with short palpebral fissures, and low-set ears often with defective pinna.
- Thymic anomaly (hypoplasia or aplasia) with mild-to-moderate reduction in T-cell number
- Cleft palate (70–80%) with speech and disorders of feeding
- Hypocalcemia present in around 60% of syndromic children due to hypoparathyroidism.
- *General appearance:* Frequently have short stature, mental retardation, and hypotonia. Occasionally, can present with psychiatric disorders (e.g., schizophrenia and bipolar disorder)

On suspicion or confirmation of DiGeorge syndrome, following precautions should be followed:

- Get serum Ca and Mg levels.
- For transfusion, always use irradiated blood products.
- As it is a thymus-based immune deficiency, it is important to start treatment and prophylaxis against pneumococcal and streptococcal infection.
- Avoid immunization with live vaccine.

REFERENCE/SOURCE

- Park MK. Park's The Pediatric Cardiology Handbook, 5th edition. United Kingdom: Elsevier Health Sciences; 2014. pp. 175-6.

25. Following congenital cardiac defects is associated with infant of diabetic mother:

A. TOF
B. TGA
C. Truncus
D. TAPVC

EXPLANATION

Infants of diabetic mothers have higher incidence of ASD, VSD, TGA/LVH/asymmetrical septal hypertrophy, and PAH along with hypocalcemia and hypoglycemia.

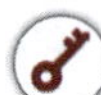

Key: B

BOOST YOUR KNOWLEDGE

Common malformations in infants of diabetic mothers are congenital heart defects (such as ASD, VSD, TGA, tricuspid atresia, and COA), severe neural tube anomalies (anencephaly and myelomeningocele), and sacral dysgenesis or agenesis.

In addition to the congenital anomalies, they have a high prevalence of hypertrophic cardiomyopathy (reversible) and persistent pulmonary hypertension of newborn (PPHN).

REFERENCE/SOURCE

- Park MK. Park's The Pediatric Cardiology Handbook, 5th edition. United Kingdom: Elsevier Health Sciences; 2014. p. 259.

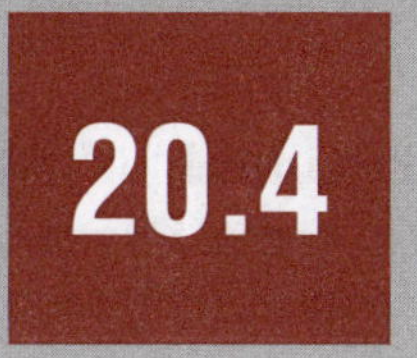

CHAPTER 20.4

Obstructive Lesions, Admixture Lesions, and Pulmonary Arterial Hypertension

Sakshi Sachdeva

1. Which of the following is the correct definition of pulmonary hypertension?

A. mPAP >10 mm Hg
B. mPAP >15 mm Hg
C. mPAP >20 mm Hg
D. mPAP >25 mm Hg

EXPLANATION

The definition of pulmonary hypertension has been lowered from the previous cut-off of mean pulmonary artery (PA) pressure 25 mm Hg to the present cut-off of 20 mm Hg.

Key: C

BOOST YOUR KNOWLEDGE

Studies on normal subjects have revealed that resting mean PA pressure is approximately 14.0 ± 3.3 mm Hg. Two standard deviations above this mean value derive the upper limit of normal as mean pulmonary artery pressure (PAP) >20 mm Hg. This raised mean PAP could be due to increased cardiac output, hence to define pulmonary vascular disease, pulmonary vascular resistance (PVR) ≥3 WU (Wood units) is included to define pre-capillary pulmonary arterial hypertension (PAH) in presence of mPAP >20 mm Hg, irrespective of etiology.

REFERENCE/SOURCE

- Galiè N, McLaughlin VV, Rubin LJ, Simonneau G. An overview of the 6th World Symposium on Pulmonary Hypertension. Eur Respir J. 2019;53(1):1802148.

2. What is the mechanism of action of riociguat?

A. Soluble guanylate cyclase stimulator
B. Phosphodiesterase 5 inhibitor
C. Endothelin receptor antagonist
D. Prostaglandin analogue

EXPLANATION

The options include all the pathways by which the anti-PAH medications act. Riociguat is a novel soluble guanylate cyclase stimulator. The stimulation of soluble guanylate cyclase increases the level of cyclic guanosine monophosphate (cGMP). Riociguat also sensitizes soluble guanylate cyclase (sGC) to endogenous nitric oxide by stabilizing nitric oxide–sGC binding and directly stimulating sGC via a different binding site, independently of nitric oxide resulting in increased production of cyclic GMP (cGMP).

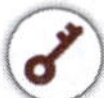

Key: A

BOOST YOUR KNOWLEDGE

The nitric oxide pathway is an important pharmacologic target for anti-PAH medications. Riociguat is the first drug which has been found efficacious in two separate pulmonary hypertension subsets, i.e., PAH and chronic thromboembolic pulmonary hypertension (CTEPH). It causes vasodilation and anti-proliferation in the pulmonary vascular intima and media.

REFERENCE/SOURCE

- Allen HD, Shaddy RE, Penny DJ, Feltes TF, Cetta F. Moss and Adams' Heart Disease in Infants, Children, and Adolescents: Including the Fetus and Young Adult, 9th edition, Volume 2. Wolters Kluwer; 2016. p. 1542.

3. Which of the following drugs is given parenterally for PAH?

A. Macitentan
B. Tadalafil
C. Selexipag
D. Treprostinil

EXPLANATION

All the options given here are anti-PAH drugs. Prostanoids are parenteral medications. Treprostinil is a prostanoid.

Key: D

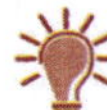

BOOST YOUR KNOWLEDGE

There are three target pathways by which anti-PAH drugs act:

1. *Nitric oxide (NO) pathway:* Phosphodiesterase 5 (PDE-5), which breaks down cGMP, protein activity is increased in PH. Specific PDE-5 inhibitors, such as sildenafil, promote an increase in cGMP levels and thus promote pulmonary vasodilation and remodeling. Sildenafil and tadalafil are oral PDE-5 inhibitors. Riociguat, a direct oral soluble guanylate cyclase (sGC) stimulator, increases cGMP directly in a non-NO (nitric oxide) dependent manner but also increases the sensitivity of sGC to NO.
2. *Endothelin pathway:* The endothelins are a family of isopeptides consisting of ET-1, ET-2, and ET-3. ET-1 is a potent vasoactive peptide produced primarily in the vascular endothelial cell, but also may be produced by smooth muscle cells. Two receptor subtypes, endothelin A (ETA) and endothelin B (ETB), mediate the activity of ET-1. ETA and ETB receptors on vascular smooth muscle mediate vasoconstriction, whereas ETB receptors on endothelial cells cause release of NO and prostacyclin (PGI2), and act as clearance receptors for circulating ET-1. ET-1 expression is increased in the pulmonary arteries of patients with PH. Bosentan, ambrisentan, and macitentan act by this mechanism and all are oral drugs.
3. *Prostacyclin pathway:* Prostacyclin is an arachidonic acid metabolite that stimulates adenylyl cyclase in vascular smooth muscle cells and causes an increase in intracellular cyclic adenosine monophosphate (AMP) leading to vasodilation of the systemic and pulmonary circulatory systems. Adults with IPAH and children with congenital heart disease (CHD) demonstrate an imbalance in the biosynthesis of thromboxane A2 and PGI2. Likewise, adults and children with severe PH show diminished PGI2 synthase expression in the lung vasculature. All prostacyclins are administered parenterally except selexipag which is an oral prostanoid.

REFERENCE/SOURCE

- Allen HD, Shaddy RE, Penny DJ, Feltes TF, Cetta F. Moss and Adams' Heart Disease in Infants, Children, and Adolescents: Including the Fetus and Young Adult, 9th edition, Volume 2. Wolters Kluwer; 2016. p. 1542.

4. Which of the following is a therapeutic modality for pulmonary hypertension?

A. Central shunt
B. Potts shunt
C. Waterston shunt
D. Blalock–Taussig–Thomas (BTT) shunt

EXPLANATION

All the options given here are aorta-pulmonary shunts. Historically, these surgeries were carried out in patients with tetralogy of Fallot (TOF). But these days only BTT shunt is done. In all the surgeries for TOF, the blood in the shunt flows from aorta to PA. Potts shunt has become a modality of treatment for PAH where the blood flows from PA to aorta to decompress the PA.

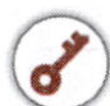

Key: B

BOOST YOUR KNOWLEDGE

Creation of a Potts shunt (anastomosis between the left pulmonary artery and the descending aorta) may allow a decrease in right ventricular afterload with subsequent improvement in right ventricular function. The Potts shunt allows a "systolic" pop-off whereas atrial septostomy offers a "diastolic" pop-off. A potential advantage of the Potts shunt is maintenance of upper body saturation with lower extremity desaturation.

REFERENCE/SOURCE

- Allen HD, Shaddy RE, Penny DJ, Feltes TF, Cetta F. Moss and Adams' Heart Disease in Infants, Children, and Adolescents: Including the Fetus and Young Adult, 9th edition, Volume 2. Wolters Kluwer; 2016. p. 1549.

5. Which of the following is the most appropriate indication for atrial septostomy in PAH?

A. Markedly elevated PVR
B. RV dysfunction
C. RA pressure >20 mm Hg
D. Suprasystemic PA pressure

EXPLANATION

Atrial septostomy is one of the procedures carried out for PAH. There are few contraindications for atrial septostomy. Patients with severe PAH, right heart failure, and markedly elevated PVR may not tolerate atrial septostomy because of a massive intracardiac right-to-left shunting and secondary severe hypoxemia. Hereditary PAH is one of the indications for atrial septostomy when pharmacologic interventions do not provide symptom relief.

Key: D

BOOST YOUR KNOWLEDGE

Atrial septostomy may benefit patients with severe PAH with recurrent syncope and intractable right heart failure. Right-to-left shunting through an interatrial defect allows to maintain the cardiac output at the expense of increased hypoxemia and alleviates signs of right heart failure by decompression of the right heart. Improvement of symptoms and increased survival have been reported.

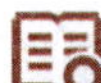

REFERENCE/SOURCE

- Allen HD, Shaddy RE, Penny DJ, Feltes TF, Cetta F. Moss and Adams' Heart Disease in Infants, Children, and Adolescents: Including the Fetus and Young Adult, 9th edition, Volume 2. Wolters Kluwer; 2016. p. 1549.

6. Which of the following drugs can be used if acute vasoreactivity testing (AVT) result is positive in PAH?

A. Calcium channel blockers
B. Angiotensin receptor blockers
C. Beta blockers
D. Angiotensin-converting enzyme (ACE) inhibitors

EXPLANATION

Out of all the four options, only calcium channel blockers are one of the treatment options for PAH if AVT is positive. An acute trial of calcium channel blocker therapy should be performed only in those patients who are acutely responsive to either NO or PGI2. Likewise, patients who do not have an acute vasodilatory response to short-acting agents and who are then placed on calcium channel blocker therapy are unlikely to benefit from this form of therapy.

Key: A

BOOST YOUR KNOWLEDGE

A total of 80% of children with severe PH are nonresponsive to acute vasodilator testing, and therefore require therapy other than calcium channel antagonists. Amlodipine, nifedipine, and diltiazem are the preferred agents. The use of calcium channel antagonists to evaluate vasoreactivity is dangerous, as these drugs can cause a decrease in cardiac output or a marked drop in systemic blood pressure. Such deleterious effects may be prolonged due to the relatively long half-life of calcium channel blockers. Consequently, elevated right atrial pressure and low cardiac output are contraindications to acute or chronic calcium channel blockade. The number of patients treated with calcium channel blockers is steadily decreasing.

REFERENCE/SOURCE

- Allen HD, Shaddy RE, Penny DJ, Feltes TF, Cetta F. Moss and Adams' Heart Disease in Infants, Children, and Adolescents: Including the Fetus and Young Adult, 9th edition, Volume 2. Wolters Kluwer; 2016. p. 1543.

7. GRIPHON trial established the use of which of the following drug for PAH?

A. Macitentan
B. Beraprost
C. Selexipag
D. Tadalafil

EXPLANATION

Stimulation of the IP receptor alone may decrease systemic side effects caused by the EP receptor. GRIPHON [prostacyclin (PGI_2) **R**eceptor agonist **I**n **P**ulmonary arterial **H**ypertensi**ON**] was a randomized, multicenter, double-blind, placebo-controlled trial evaluating the long-term efficacy and safety of oral selexipag in patients with pulmonary arterial hypertension. Selexipag decreased the risk of a morbidity/mortality event versus placebo by 40% (p <0.0001).

Key: C

BOOST YOUR KNOWLEDGE

Selexipag is an orally available and selective prostacyclin receptor (IP receptor) agonist.

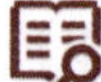

REFERENCE/SOURCE

- Allen HD, Shaddy RE, Penny DJ, Feltes TF, Cetta F. Moss and Adams' Heart Disease in Infants, Children, and Adolescents: Including the Fetus and Young Adult, 9th edition, Volume 2. Wolters Kluwer; 2016. p. 1546.

8. What is the mechanism of action of ambrisentan?

A. Endothelin A receptor antagonist
B. Endothelin B receptor antagonist
C. Endothelin C receptor antagonist
D. Endothelin D receptor antagonist

EXPLANATION

Selective ETA receptor blockade is possible using ambrisentan, an ET-receptor antagonist with high oral bioavailability and a long duration of action, and high specificity for the ETA receptor. Selective ETA receptor blockade may benefit patients with PAH by blocking the vasoconstrictor effects of ETA receptors while maintaining the vasodilator/clearance functions of ETB receptors.

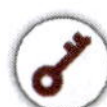

Key: A

BOOST YOUR KNOWLEDGE

Bosentan and macitentan are dual ET-receptor antagonists.

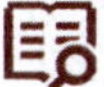

REFERENCE/SOURCE

- Allen HD, Shaddy RE, Penny DJ, Feltes TF, Cetta F. Moss and Adams' Heart Disease in Infants, Children, and Adolescents: Including the Fetus and Young Adult, 9th edition, Volume 2. Wolters Kluwer; 2016. p. 1547.

9. Which of the following is the operability criterion for large post-tricuspid shunt with severe PAH?

A. PVRI <6 Wood unit m^2, PVR:SVR <0.3
B. PVRI <3 Wood unit m^2, PVR:SVR <0.2
C. PVRI <6 Wood unit m^2, PVR:SVR <0.2
D. PVRI <3 Wood unit m^2, PVR:SVR <0.3

EXPLANATION

For preoperative evaluation and management of pediatric patients with congenital cardiac shunts, the following approach is followed. Clinical features of pulmonary overcirculation, failure to thrive, oxygen saturation >95%, and shunt direction only left to right are taken as criteria for operability. In the absence of such scenario, cardiac catheterization is carried out and PVRI and PVR : SVR ratio is calculated. If PVRI <6 Wood unit m^2, and PVR : SVR <0.3 is there patient is considered operable. If PVRI >6 Wood unit m^2, and PVR:SVR >0.3, then acute vasoreactivity testing is done. Proposed criteria for a pulmonary vasodilator response to be considered as positive: ≥20% decrease in PVRI and PVR : SVR ratio from baseline, with respective final (lowest) values of <6 Wood units × m^2 and <0.3.

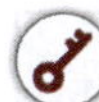

Key: A

BOOST YOUR KNOWLEDGE

The algorithm is not applicable to complex conditions such as the absence of a subpulmonary ventricle (candidates to cavopulmonary anastomoses).

REFERENCE/SOURCE

- Allen HD, Shaddy RE, Penny DJ, Feltes TF, Cetta F. Moss and Adams' Heart Disease in Infants, Children, and Adolescents: Including the Fetus and Young Adult, 9th edition, Volume 2. Wolters Kluwer; 2016. p. 1535.

10. In a patient with pulmonary stenosis, electrocardiogram (ECG) shows pure R wave in V_1 with 14 mV amplitude. What shall be RVSP (right ventricular systolic pressure)?

A. 50 mm Hg
B. 60 mm Hg
C. 70 mm Hg
D. 80 mm Hg

EXPLANATION

It is possible to estimate the right ventricular pressure in patients between 2 and 20 years of age if a pure R wave is present in lead V4R or V_1. The height of the R wave in millimeters, multiplied by 5, approximates the right ventricular systolic pressure in millimeters of mercury.

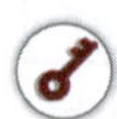

Key: C

BOOST YOUR KNOWLEDGE

The ECG can be somewhat useful in assessing the severity of obstruction in patients with pulmonary valve stenosis. As many as 40–50% of patients with mild stenosis have a normal ECG. Slight rightward deviation of the QRS frontal axis is often the only abnormality. The R wave amplitude in the right precordial leads rarely exceeds 10–15 mm. A right ventricular conduction delay is commonly present.

In moderate pulmonary stenosis, the ECG is almost always abnormal, with only 10% of patients having a normal tracing. Right axis deviation is usually present. The R:S ratio in V_1 is usually >4:1, and the R wave is typically <20 mm. The T waves in the right precordial leads are upright in approximately 50% of patients.

In severe pulmonary stenosis, the ECG is rarely normal. The mean frontal QRS axis is usually >110°, and not uncommonly, extreme right axis deviation is seen. A pure R, RS, or QR is the usual pattern in the right precordial leads, and the R wave is usually >20 mm. The R:S ratio in V_6 may be <1.0. The T waves may be upright or inverted in the right precordial leads, and the P waves are abnormally tall and peaked in lead 2 and in the right precordial leads, indicating right atrial enlargement.

REFERENCE/SOURCE

- Allen HD, Shaddy RE, Penny DJ, Feltes TF, Cetta F. Moss and Adams' Heart Disease in Infants, Children, and Adolescents: Including the Fetus and Young Adult, 9th edition, Volume 2. Wolters Kluwer; 2016. p. 986.

11. What is "hemodynamic vise" in total anomalous pulmonary venous connection (TAPVC)?

A. Obstruction of vertical vein between aorta and pulmonary artery
B. Obstruction of vertical vein between pulmonary artery and left bronchus
C. Obstruction of vertical vein between aorta and vertebral column
D. Obstruction of vertical vein between SVC and pulmonary artery

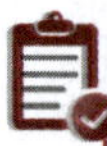

EXPLANATION

Obstruction of the vertical vein in supracardiac TAPVC is caused by a "hemodynamic vise" formed posteriorly by the left bronchus and anteriorly by the pulmonary trunk. Vertical veins get compressed between the two structures and cause obstruction to pulmonary venous flow.

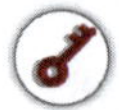

Key: B

BOOST YOUR KNOWLEDGE

There are different types of TAPVC, and the "hemodynamic vise" is associated with supracardiac TAPVC.

In supracardiac TAPVC, the abnormal connection between the pulmonary veins and the right atrium occurs above the diaphragm. This type of TAPVC can be further classified based on the location of the vertical vein that drains blood from the anomalous connection.

- In most cases, there is a left-sided vertical vein which goes up along the left side of the spine (paravertebral gutter) and joins the left brachiocephalic vein. This connection with the brachiocephalic vein, which then drains into the superior vena cava (SVC), produces a characteristic "snowman" appearance on a chest X-ray.

- In this scenario, a left-sided "hemodynamic vise" can occur. This happens when the vertical vein is squeezed between the left pulmonary artery (LPA) and the left main bronchus. This compression can obstruct blood flow through the vertical vein.
- Less commonly, there can be a right-sided ascending vertical vein, which is a rare variation. In this case, a right-sided "hemodynamic vise" can develop when the vertical vein passes between the right pulmonary artery (RPA) and the carina (the point where the trachea splits into the left and right main bronchi).

The presence of a hemodynamic vise can worsen the complications associated with TAPVC, such as decreased blood flow to the lungs and congestive heart failure. Treatment for TAPVC typically involves surgery to create a normal connection between the pulmonary veins and the left atrium.

REFERENCE/SOURCE

- Perloff JK, Marelli A. Perloff's Clinical Recognition of Congenital Heart Disease, 6th edition. Elsevier; 2012. p. 245.

12. The vertical vein in infracardiac TAPVC descends through which opening in the diaphragm?

A. Vena caval hiatus
B. Esophageal hiatus
C. Aortic hiatus
D. Vertebral hiatus

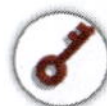

EXPLANATION

The pulmonary veins from both lungs join to form a confluence immediately behind the LA. A common vessel originates from this confluence, descends immediately anterior to the esophagus, and penetrates the diaphragm through the esophageal hiatus.

Key: B

BOOST YOUR KNOWLEDGE

Most commonly, the anomalous descending vessel then joins the portal vein at the confluence of the splenic and superior mesenteric veins. Less often, the anomalous vessel connects to the ductus venosus, to one of the hepatic veins, or to the IVC. When the anomalous connection is to the umbilicovitelline system, pulmonary venous obstruction is usually present.

REFERENCE/SOURCE

- Allen HD, Shaddy RE, Penny DJ, Feltes TF, Cetta F. Moss and Adams' Heart Disease in Infants, Children, and Adolescents: Including the Fetus and Young Adult, 9th edition, Volume 2. Wolters Kluwer; 2016. p. 896.

13. Which of the following lesions *does not* have wide pulse pressure?

A. TOF with aortic regurgitation
B. Truncus arteriosus
C. Tricuspid atresia with large aorta-pulmonary collaterals
D. Transposition of great arteries

EXPLANATION

Aortic regurgitation, truncus arteriosus, large patent ductus arteriosus (PDA), or large aorta-pulmonary collaterals cause diastolic run-off into the ventricle in case of AR, and into the pulmonary vascular bed in case of PDA and aorta-pulmonary collaterals (APCs).

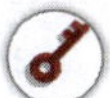

Key: D

BOOST YOUR KNOWLEDGE

In truncus arteriosus, the pulse pressure is wide because low pulmonary vascular resistance permits a diastolic runoff from the truncus into the pulmonary bed. The rate of rise of the arterial pulse is brisk because of rapid ejection of a large left ventricular stroke volume. A brisk arterial pulse is especially noteworthy in the context of left ventricular failure and pulsus alternans. Truncal valve regurgitation independently causes a bounding arterial pulse analogous to the water-hammer pulse of aortic regurgitation.

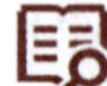

REFERENCE/SOURCE

- Perloff JK, Marelli A. Perloff's Clinical Recognition of Congenital Heart Disease, 6th edition. Elsevier; 2012. p. 496.

14. A 2-year-old child with TAPVC underwent cardiac catheterization. SpO_2 was 67% and 87% in arterial blood gas (ABG) obtained from right atrium and right femoral artery, respectively. What shall be the Qp:Qs?

A. 1.5
B. 2
C. 2.5
D. 3

EXPLANATION

Qp/Qs = (AO saturation – systemic venous saturation)/(PV saturation – PA saturation)
= (87 – 67)/(100 – 87) = 20/13 = 1.53:1.

Key: A

BOOST YOUR KNOWLEDGE

It is safe to assume that for a normal cardiac index, the arteriovenous oxygen difference will be around 25% in the basal state. In admixture lesions, the aortic saturation and the pulmonary saturation will be identical. If the aortic saturation is 85%, PA saturation can be assumed as 85% and pulmonary venous saturation as 100%. If we assume normal cardiac index, then the arteriovenous oxygen difference will be approximately 25%, that is, the systemic venous saturation will be around 60%. QP/QS = (AO saturation – systemic venous saturation)/(PV saturation – PA saturation) = (85 – 60)/(100 – 85) = 25/15 = 1.67:1.

REFERENCE/SOURCE

- Tharakan JA. Admixture lesions in congenital cyanotic heart disease. Ann Pediatr Card. 2011;4:53-9.

15. Which of the following syndromes is commonly associated with common atrium?

A. Ellis–Van Creveld syndrome
B. Down syndrome
C. Kabuki syndrome
D. Andersen–Tawil syndrome

EXPLANATION

Ellis–Van Creveld syndrome, chondroectodermal dysplasia, is an important phenotype because 50% of patients with this syndrome have congenital heart disease and half of them have a common atrium.

Key: A

BOOST YOUR KNOWLEDGE

Ellis–Van Creveld syndrome is autosomal recessive and is characterized by dwarfism with polydactyly of the hands that is invariable, but polydactyly of the feet occurs in only 10% of cases. Polycarpaly (a ninth or tenth carpal bone), clinodactyly (bent fingers), syndactyly (interdigital webbing), and hypoplasia of the nails are common features. Premature eruption of malformed maxillary incisors, gingival hypertrophy, and multiple frenula is distinctive.

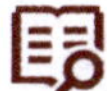

REFERENCE/SOURCE

- Perloff JK, Marelli A. Perloff's Clinical Recognition of Congenital Heart Disease, 6th edition. Elsevier; 2012. p. 241.

16. Which of the following lesions is *not* an admixture lesion?

A. Common atrium
B. TAPVC
C. Common arterial trunk
D. TGA

EXPLANATION

Congenital cyanotic heart disease (CCHD) with admixture physiology is a cardiac defect which facilitates complete mixing of the deoxygenated systemic venous (SV) blood returning from the tissues and the fully oxygenated pulmonary venous blood from the lungs in a common receiving chamber. TGA belongs to transposition physiology. All other options mentioned are admixture lesions.

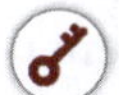

Key: D

BOOST YOUR KNOWLEDGE

The common CCHD with admixture physiology includes TAPVC, atresia of one of the atrioventricular valves (tricuspid atresia, mitral atresia), single ventricle physiology (double inlet ventricle), semilunar valve atresia (pulmonary atresia including hypoplastic right heart syndrome, aortic atresia including hypoplastic left heart syndrome), double outlet RV or double outlet LV, complete deficiency of atrial septum as in common atrium, and complete deficiency of conotruncal and truncoaortic septum as in truncus arteriosus.

REFERENCE/SOURCE

- Tharakan JA. Admixture lesions in congenital cyanotic heart disease. Ann Pediatr Card. 2011;4:53-9.

17. Blood pressure difference between right arm and left arm in case of supravalvar aortic stenosis is known as:

A. Coanda effect
B. Nyquist limit
C. Reverberation artefact
D. Suzman sign

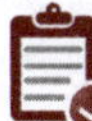

EXPLANATION

Coanda effect and Suzman sign are clinical signs. Rest both options are echocardiographic phenomenon. Suzman sign is seen in cases of coarctation of aorta.

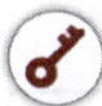

Key: A

BOOST YOUR KNOWLEDGE

In cases of supravalvar aortic stenosis, there may be a discrepancy in blood pressure between arms, with the right arm often demonstrating a systolic pressure 15–20 mm Hg higher than the left. This finding is thought to be related to streaming of blood due to the Coanda effect, a phenomenon in fluid dynamics in which a jet stream adheres to a boundary wall. Patients with supravalvar stenosis may also present with systolic hypertension and a widened pulse pressure due to reduced elasticity of the aorta.

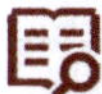

REFERENCE/SOURCE

- Allen HD, Shaddy RE, Penny DJ, Feltes TF, Cetta F. Moss and Adams' Heart Disease in Infants, Children, and Adolescents: Including the Fetus and Young Adult, 9th edition, Volume 2. Wolters Kluwer; 2016. p. 1093.

18. Coronary artery ostial stenosis is commonly associated with which of the following?

A. Subvalvar aortic stenosis
B. Valvar aortic stenosis
C. Supravalvar aortic stenosis
D. Coarctation of aorta

EXPLANATION

All the options are examples of obstruction to left ventricle outflow. In supravalvar AS, coronary ostial stenosis is associated. While stenosis or obstruction is the most concerning coronary manifestation of supravalvar aortic stenosis, coronary artery dilation is also well described and is likely more common. Generally, the dilation is not severe, but case reports of large coronary artery aneurysms in the setting of supravalvar stenosis have been documented along with an increased potential risk for thrombosis.

Key: C

BOOST YOUR KNOWLEDGE

Supravalvar aortic stenosis is a form of ELN (elastin) arteriopathy. The coronary arteries are an important potential site of disease in patients with ELN arteriopathy. As ELN-containing arteries, the coronaries do develop thickened walls with the potential for diffuse luminal narrowing, but there are several other mechanisms that also contribute to impaired coronary artery perfusion in patients with supravalvar aortic stenosis. The most common coronary anomaly in this population is ostial stenosis, which is present in up to 45% of patients with supravalvar aortic stenosis referred for surgery. More commonly affecting the left coronary artery than the right, ostial stenosis can be caused by adhesion of an aortic valve cusp to the supravalvar ridge immediately above the coronary orifice. In extreme cases, the ostium can be completely excluded from the aortic lumen by the valve tissue. Alternatively, ostial stenosis or even atresia can be due to pathologic thickening of the aortic or proximal coronary artery wall that impinges on the orifice.

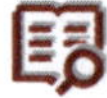

REFERENCE/SOURCE

- Allen HD, Shaddy RE, Penny DJ, Feltes TF, Cetta F. Moss and Adams' Heart Disease in Infants, Children, and Adolescents: Including the Fetus and Young Adult, 9th edition, Volume 2. Wolters Kluwer; 2016. p. 1089.

19. Most of the congenital heart diseases have an embryologic or anatomical basis. Coarctation of aorta primarily occurs due to which of the following reasons?

A. Ductal sling theory
B. Dilated vein compressing the aorta
C. Hemodynamic theory in presence of pulmonary valve stenosis
D. Bronchus compressing the aorta

EXPLANATION

Coarctation typically occurs at the site of insertion of the ductus arteriosus. The ductus tissue theory proposes that coarctation develops as the result of migration of ductal smooth muscle cells into the periductal aorta, with subsequent constriction and narrowing of the aortic lumen.

Key: A

BOOST YOUR KNOWLEDGE

The hemodynamic theory proposes that coarctation develops because of hemodynamic disturbances that reduce the volume of blood flow through the fetal aortic arch such as ventricular septal defect, aortic stenosis, and hypoplasia of the transverse aortic arch. An interesting variation of the hemodynamic theory explains coarctation in girls with Turner syndrome.

It is suggested that fetal lymphatic obstruction, which may cause the webbed neck in Turner syndrome, also leads to distended thoracic ducts that compress the fetal aorta and promote the development of coarctation.

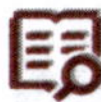

REFERENCE/SOURCE

- Allen HD, Shaddy RE, Penny DJ, Feltes TF, Cetta F. Moss and Adams' Heart Disease in Infants, Children, and Adolescents: Including the Fetus and Young Adult, 9th edition, Volume 2. Wolters Kluwer; 2016. p. 1108.

20. Coarctation of aorta classically has difference in blood pressure between arm and leg. In which of the following situations this finding is present?

A. CoA with large collaterals
B. CoA with ARSA
C. CoA with large PDA
D. CoA with hypertension

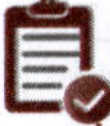

EXPLANATION

In coarctation with PDA, collaterals, or ARSA (aberrant left subclavian artery), the BP difference may not be found.

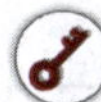

Key: D

BOOST YOUR KNOWLEDGE

Systolic blood pressure is elevated proximal to the coarctation, and a systolic pressure gradient is present between the arm and leg. In several clinical circumstances, detection of difference in arterial pulse and pressure is difficult.

These situations include:

- Mild coarctation
- Coarctation with heart failure
- Coarctation with large PDA or collaterals
- *Variations in brachiocephalic artery anatomy:*
  - Anomalous right subclavian artery arises distal to the coarctation—the arterial pulse and blood pressure are identical in the right arm and leg, and discrepancies are detected only in the left arm.
  - Left subclavian artery arises adjacent to the coarctation, and its orifice may be stenotic—a bounding arterial pulse and elevated systolic pressure will be detected only in the right arm.
  - Anomalous right subclavian artery and a stenotic left subclavian artery, arterial differences in the four extremities will not be detected, although carotid artery pulsations can be bounding.

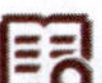

REFERENCE/SOURCE

- Allen HD, Shaddy RE, Penny DJ, Feltes TF, Cetta F. Moss and Adams' Heart Disease in Infants, Children, and Adolescents: Including the Fetus and Young Adult, 9th edition, Volume 2. Wolters Kluwer; 2016. p. 1111.

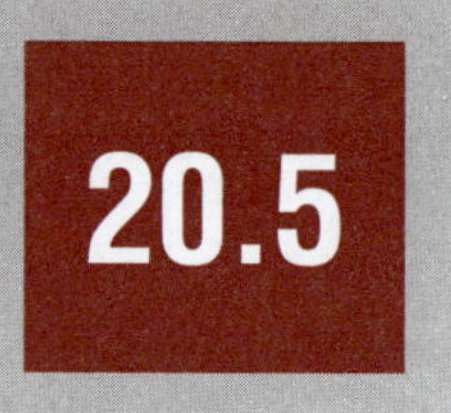

CHAPTER 20.5

Congestive Heart Failure, Myocardial Diseases, and Cardiomyopathies

Sataroopa Mishra

1. Which of the following is the most common cause of restrictive cardiomyopathy (RCM) in children?

A. Endomyocardial fibroelastosis
B. Idiopathic
C. Amyloidosis
D. Loffler endocarditis

EXPLANATION

Restrictive cardiomyopathy may result from myocardial diseases including noninfiltrative or infiltrative processes, storage diseases, endomyocardial diseases, myocarditis, etc. In the pediatric population, however, the most common cause is idiopathic. Amyloidosis is an infiltrative disorder that causes RCM in adults and is rarely reported in children. Endomyocardial fibrosis is the most common cause of RCM in tropical countries and is often associated with hypereosinophilia. Loffler's syndrome, also known as hypereosinophilic syndrome, is seen in temperate regions and presents with persistent eosinophilia, which involves other organs such as lungs and bone marrow, which may be primary or secondary.

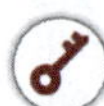

Key: B

BOOST YOUR KNOWLEDGE

Other causes of RCM are storage diseases such as lysosomal disorders such as Hurler's syndrome, Gaucher's disease, Fabry's disease, glycogen storage diseases, and hemochromatosis. Mediastinal radiation, anthracyclines, serotonin, busulfan, ergotamine, and methysergide have been reported to cause RCM.

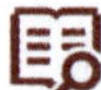

REFERENCE/SOURCE

- Restrictive cardiomyopathy. In: Shaddy RE, Penny DJ, Feltes TF, Cetta F, Mittal S, Kailin J (Eds). Moss and Adams' Heart Disease in Infants, Children, and Adolescents, 10th edition. Philadelphia: Wolters Kluwer Health; 2021. pp. 1304-14.

2. Which is the most important pathophysiology underlying RCM?

A. Systolic dysfunction of ventricles
B. Pulmonary hypertension
C. Increased pulmonary wedge pressure
D. Diastolic dysfunction of ventricles

EXPLANATION

Diastolic function is primarily affected by ventricular compliance/stiffness and relaxation. In RCM, increased stiffness of ventricles and delayed relaxation causes increased ventricular pressure during diastole and impairs ventricular filling in diastole. In the normal heart, the phase of rapid or early filling occurs as the left ventricular pressure falls below that in the left atrium, just after the mitral valve opens and accounts for most of the ventricular filling. In RCM the elevated ventricular pressure, in turn, leads to increased left atrial pressure, pulmonary wedge pressure, and pulmonary hypertension. Therefore, the primary problem is diastolic dysfunction of ventricles (option D), while options B and C are the results of option D. Systolic dysfunction is seen in dilated cardiomyopathy.

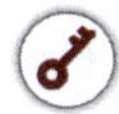

Key: D

BOOST YOUR KNOWLEDGE

Pulmonary hypertension is frequently present at the time of initial cardiac catheterization in addition to elevated left and/or right ventricular end-diastolic pressures. Elevated pulmonary vascular resistance may preclude cardiac transplantation and is a marker of poor prognosis.

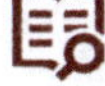

REFERENCE/SOURCE

- Restrictive cardiomyopathy. In: Shaddy RE, Penny DJ, Feltes TF, Cetta F, Mittal S, Kailin J (Eds). Moss and Adams' Heart Disease in Infants, Children, and Adolescents, 10th edition. Philadelphia: Wolters Kluwer Health; 2021. pp. 1304-14.

3. A 6-month-old infant presented with a history of feeding difficulty for the last 4 months. The baby takes pauses in between feeding while taking a long time to feed associated with excessive sweating. He weighs 4 kg (birth weight 2.8 kg). The mother has noticed persistent chest indrawing. Which functional class does the baby fall into?

A. Ross class III heart failure (HF)
B. New York Heart Association (NYHA) class III heart failure
C. Ross class II heart failure
D. American College of Cardiology Foundation (ACCF)/American Heart Association (AHA) stage B heart failure

EXPLANATION

Several classification schemes are used to define the clinical severity of chronic heart failure in children. The NYHA functional classification widely used for adults and older children can be used only in children >7 years of age. The Ross classification was developed to make NYHA criteria more relevant to young children. The ACCF and AHA have proposed staging criteria for heart failure that incorporate functional and risk factor criteria. The baby will fall into the stage C of congestive heart failure (CHF) as per this classification (structural heart disease with prior or current symptoms of heart failure). Of Ross class II and III, this baby is best classified into class III since the baby has significant growth failure along with marked symptoms of heart failure.

Key: A

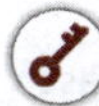

BOOST YOUR KNOWLEDGE

Ross classification for heart failure in children:

- *Class I:* Asymptomatic
- *Class II:* Mild tachypnea or diaphoresis with feeding in infants; dyspnea on exertion in older children
- *Class III:* Marked tachypnea or diaphoresis with feeding in infants; prolonged feeding times with growth failure resulting from heart failure; marked dyspnea on exertion in older children
- *Class IV:* Symptoms such as tachypnea, retractions, grunting, and diaphoresis at rest

REFERENCE/SOURCE

- Chronic Heart Failure in Children. In: Shaddy RE, Penny DJ, Feltes TF, Cetta F, Mittal S, Kailin J (Eds). Moss and Adams' Heart Disease in Infants, Children, and Adolescents, 10th edition. Philadelphia: Wolters Kluwer Health; 2021. pp. 1652-73.

4. A term, newborn with a birth weight of 2.8 kg has respiratory distress at birth. There is history of birth asphyxia with meconium-stained liquor. At 6 hours of life, her respiratory rate (RR) is 90 breaths/min, heart rate (HR) is 280 beats/min, change to capillary refill time (CRT) >5 seconds, saturation of peripheral oxygen ($SpPO_2$) is 95% (preductal and postductal), and femoral pulses are well felt. There is tender hepatomegaly. Her blood sugar is 68 mg% and ionized calcium is normal. Cord blood thyroid stimulating hormone (TSH) is normal. What is the next appropriate step in management?

A. Stabilize the baby and ask for an electrocardiography (ECG)
B. The chest X-ray (CXR) shows evidence of meconium aspiration syndrome, hence continue the mechanical ventilation and other supportive care
C. Stabilize the baby and ask for an echocardiogram as you strongly suspect a structural congenital heart disease (CHD)
D. Birth asphyxia is likely to cause such a presentation, hence you continue supportive care and ask for a sepsis screen

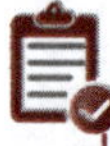

EXPLANATION

This baby has features of CHF seen at 6 hours of life. The causes include duct-dependent systemic circulation CHD, obstructed total anomalous pulmonary venous connection (TAPVC), total anomalous pulmonary circulation, and Ebstein anomaly. However, SpO_2 95% makes TAPVC unlikely. The femoral pulses are normal ruling out severe aortic stenosis, coarctation of the aorta, interrupted aortic arch, and hypoplastic left heart syndrome. Hence, option C is less useful. Option B is ruled out since heart failure symptoms cannot be explained by meconium aspiration only. Birth asphyxia can cause heart failure in newborns and sepsis can further worsen it by increasing the demand on the failing heart. But HR of 280 beats/min (>220 beats/min) in a newborn is a strong indicator of an underlying arrhythmia and not sinus tachycardia. Hence, option A is the preferred modality. Tachyarrhythmia leading to ventricular dysfunction is a potentially reversible condition when treated on time and should be suspected in a patient with CHF. Other causes of CHF in newborns such as hypoglycemia, hypocalcemia, and hypothyroidism have been ruled out in the case.

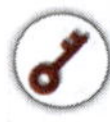

Key: A

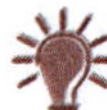

BOOST YOUR KNOWLEDGE

Other causes of heart failure in neonates include myocarditis, congenital heart block, atrioventricular (AV) valve insufficiency, and anomalous left coronary artery from the pulmonary artery.

REFERENCE/SOURCE

- Chronic Heart Failure in Children. In: Shaddy RE, Penny DJ, Feltes TF, Cetta F, Mittal S, Kailin J (Eds). Moss and Adams' Heart Disease in Infants, Children, and Adolescents, 10th edition. Philadelphia: Wolters Kluwer Health; 2021. pp. 1652-73.

5. A 6-month-old baby presented with fast breathing, feeding difficulty, and failure to thrive for the last 4 months. The mother has noticed episodes of excessive crying, sweating, and the baby turning pale on feeding which resolves in 5–10 minutes. Chest X-ray showed cardiomegaly. Below is the ECG of the baby. What is the diagnosis?

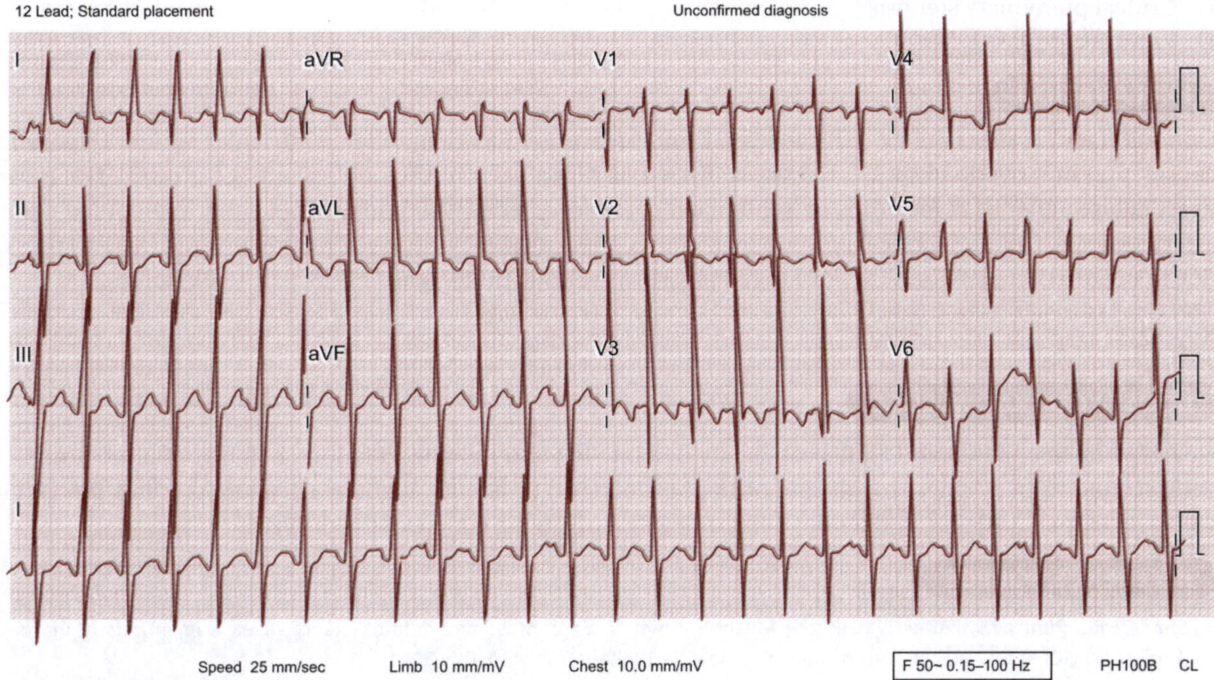

A. Tetralogy of Fallot (TOF)
B. Aortic stenosis
C. Anomalous origin of the left coronary artery from the pulmonary artery (ALCAPA)
D. Myocarditis

EXPLANATION

Option A, TOF does not usually have heart failure, and the description given is not characteristic of a cyanotic spell. ECG of TOF has right ventricular hypertrophy (RVH). ECG of aortic stenosis has left ventricular hypertrophy (LVH) with strain pattern in left lateral leads but deep Q waves in I and aVL are not explained. Option C myocarditis has features, such as ST-T changes, tachycardia, bradycardia, and heart block. But the ECG here has very deep Q waves like a dagger which are >2.5 mm deep and wide with T wave inversion in I and aVL suggestive of infarction on the left ventricle (LV) lateral region. The baby has characteristic episodic crying, suggestive of intermittent myocardial ischemia which is equivalent to angina in adults. Hence, option C is the answer.

Key: C

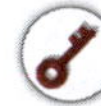

BOOST YOUR KNOWLEDGE

Anomalous origin of the left coronary artery from the pulmonary artery should be considered in infants presenting with CHF since timely surgery results in a complete cure. The primary surgery for ALCAPA is direct coronary reimplantation. Other surgeries include the Takeuchi procedure and coronary artery bypass graft.

REFERENCE/SOURCE

- Shaddy RE, Penny DJ, Feltes TF, Cetta F, Mittal S, Kailin J (Eds). Restrictive Cardiomyopathy. Moss and Adams' Heart Disease in Infants, Children, and Adolescents (Chapters 32, 41, 44, 55, 72), 10th edition. Philadelphia: Wolters Kluwer Health; 2021.

6. Which of the following predominantly causes right heart failure in a 12-year-old child?

A. Mitral regurgitation (MR) due to acute rheumatic fever
B. CHF due to hypertensive emergency
C. Critical pulmonary stenosis
D. Kawasaki disease

EXPLANATION

Options A and B affect the LV. MR causes LV volume overload leading to left ventricular failure. Hypertension causes pressure overload on LV. Kawasaki disease is rarely seen in the adolescent age group. Also, it causes heart failure either by myocarditis or ischemia of coronary arteries which may affect either right or left coronary artery systems. Option C critical pulmonary stenosis presents with supra-systemic right ventricle (RV) pressures due to obstruction to RV outflow. Prolonged pressure overload on RV leads eventually to RV failure.

Key: C

BOOST YOUR KNOWLEDGE

Heart failure in children and adults can be divided into left and right heart failure. Left heart failure presents with early symptoms of dyspnea, cough, and orthopnea followed by edema. Right heart failure presents predominantly with ascites, pedal edema, and tender hepatomegaly early in the course of the disease.

REFERENCE/SOURCE

- Shaddy RE, Penny DJ, Feltes TF, Cetta F, Mittal S, Kailin J (Eds). Moss and Adams' Heart Disease in Infants, Children, and Adolescents (Chapters 38, 72), 10th edition. Philadelphia: Wolters Kluwer Health; 2021.

7. Which of the following cardiac biomarkers is most commonly used in pediatric heart failure?

A. Troponin
B. N-terminal pro b-type natriuretic peptide (NT-proBNP)
C. High-sensitivity C-reactive protein (Hs-CRP)
D. Galectin-3

EXPLANATION

All the aforementioned options are cardiac biomarkers. Troponin is a marker of ischemia useful for myocarditis. Brain natriuretic peptide (BNP) is the most useful cardiac biomarker useful for the diagnosis and treatment of chronic heart failure. NT-proBNP is a clinically inactive form of BNP. Both are released from the ventricular myocardium in response to increased myocardial stretch. Hs-CRP is a marker of low-level inflammation associated with coronary artery disease in adults. ST2 and galectin are biomarkers not commonly used in clinical practice.

Key: B

BOOST YOUR KNOWLEDGE

The level of BNP and NT-proBNP vary with age with very high in neonates up to day 2 of life then decreased with age. Some of the clinical utilities of BNP and NT-proBNP include differentiating lung disease from heart disease, anthracycline-treated children, follow-up of patients with heart failure, prognostication, and guiding therapy in heart failure.

REFERENCE/SOURCE

- Chronic Heart Failure in Children. In: Shaddy RE, Penny DJ, Feltes TF, Cetta F, Mittal S, Kailin J (Eds). Moss and Adams' Heart Disease in Infants, Children, and Adolescents, 10th edition. Philadelphia: Wolters Kluwer Health; 2021. pp. 1652-73.

8. What is the most appropriate role of diuretics in the management of chronic heart failure in children?

A. Use them in acute exacerbations of chronic heart failure for control of symptoms of extravascular volume overload
B. Diuretics have shown survival benefits and hence should be given to all patients for maintenance therapy
C. Should be routinely given in patients with hypertrophic cardiomyopathy (HCM) with heart failure
D. Use diuretics for favorable remodeling of cardiac tissue

EXPLANATION

Conventional diuretics other than aldosterone antagonists, such as loop diuretics, thiazide diuretics reduce systemic, and pulmonary venous congestion. Hence, they are useful to control symptoms and signs of extravascular volume overload, such as orthopnea, dyspnea, peripheral edema, hepatomegaly, and ascites. They may also be used as a part of chronic medical regimens in patients who are dependent on their administration for the maintenance of the euvolemic state. Several adult studies have shown that diuretics do not improve survival. Option D is not true. Diuretics activate the renin-angiotensin-aldosterone system (RAAS) and lead to adverse remodeling of the ventricular myocardium. In HCM, diuretics should be avoided as decreased ventricular volume increases the LV outflow tract obstruction.

Key: A

BOOST YOUR KNOWLEDGE

Adverse effects of loop diuretics include excessive contraction of extracellular volume, hyponatremia, hypokalemia, and ototoxicity. Torsemide is a more potent loop diuretic than furosemide, hence requires a lower dose, and it also prevents adverse remodeling.

REFERENCE/SOURCE

- Shaddy RE, Penny DJ, Feltes TF, Cetta F, Mittal S, Kailin J (Eds). Moss and Adams' Heart Disease in Infants, Children, and Adolescents (Chapters 52, 72, 81), 10th edition. Philadelphia: Wolters Kluwer Health; 2021.

9. Which of the following drugs have been shown to have survival benefits in patients with chronic CHF?

A. Diuretics, digoxin, ACE inhibitors
B. ACE inhibitors, digoxin, and aldosterone receptor antagonists
C. Calcium channel blockers, beta-blockers, and angiotensin-converting enzyme (ACE) inhibitors
D. ACE inhibitors, beta-blockers, and aldosterone receptor antagonists

EXPLANATION

Digoxin has been shown to reduce the rate of heart failure hospitalization, but it does not improve survival hence it is recommended only in patients refractory to guideline-directed medical therapy (GMDT). Calcium channel blockers are used as antihypertensives or antiarrhythmic drugs. These three classes (option D) are a part of GMDT and should be given to all patients with chronic heart failure. They have been proven to have survival benefits in several trials in adults. ACE inhibitors and angiotensin receptor blockers (ARBs) reduce afterload, preload, and wall stress on the myocardium by systemic vasodilatation. It prevents adverse remodeling of the ventricular myocardium. Beta-blockers primarily prevent and reverse adrenergically-mediated myocardial dysfunction and remodeling. Aldosterone receptor antagonists prevent aldosterone-mediated fluid retention and myocardial fibrosis, ventricular dilation, and dysfunction.

Key: D

BOOST YOUR KNOWLEDGE

Angiotensin receptor blocker and neprilysin inhibitor (valsartan-sacubitril) is a novel therapy for heart failure approved in children. Valsartan blocks angiotensin receptors and inhibition of neprilysin prevents degradation of BNP which counteracts adverse neurohormonal effects in chronic heart failure. PANORAMA-HF (Prospective Trial to Assess the Angiotensin Receptor Blocker Neprilysin Inhibitor LCZ696 Versus Angiotensin-Converting Enzyme Inhibitor for the Medical Treatment of Pediatric HF) is a randomized controlled trial (RCT) for valsartan-sacubitril in children. Ivabradine is an f-receptor blocker on sinus nodes and is another novel therapy used for dilated cardiomyopathy in children.

REFERENCE/SOURCE

- Shaddy RE, Penny DJ, Feltes TF, Cetta F, Mittal S, Kailin J. Moss and Adams' Heart Disease in Infants, Children, and Adolescents (Chapters 72, 81), 10th edition. Philadelphia: Wolters Kluwer Health; 2021.

10. Which of the following is a known adverse effect of ACE inhibitors and is seen more often in infants and children?

A. Bradycardia
B. Tachycardia
C. Ototoxicity
D. First dose hypotension

EXPLANATION

Angiotensin-converting enzyme inhibitor causes systemic vasodilation without affecting the HR. Hence, options A and B are ruled out. Ototoxicity is a known adverse effect of loop diuretics. Significant hypotension may occur in volume-depleted patients or in patients with high basal renin activity. When starting ACE inhibitors in infants and young children, a low first dose is given, and blood pressure (BP) is monitored. If the drug is well tolerated, then the dose is increased gradually.

Key: D

BOOST YOUR KNOWLEDGE

Other adverse effects of ACEI are neutropenia, proteinuria, especially in children with renal impairment, hyperkalemia, teratogenicity, dry nonproductive cough, rash, taste impairment, and minor gastrointestinal (GI) disturbances.

REFERENCE/SOURCE

- Shaddy RE, Penny DJ, Feltes TF, Cetta F, Mittal S, Kailin J (Eds). Moss and Adams' Heart Disease in Infants, Children, and Adolescents (Chapters 72, 81), 10th edition. Philadelphia: Wolters Kluwer Health; 2021.

11. What is the recommended therapeutic serum digoxin level?

A. 1–2 ng/mL
B. 3–4 ng/mL
C. 4–5 ng/mL
D. 5–6 ng/mL

EXPLANATION

Digoxin has a large volume of distribution therefore it requires a loading dose. Loading dose is associated with higher toxic effects, especially in newborns. Since digoxin is rarely required in an emergency, it is better to avoid the loading dose and start with the maintenance dose. $T^{1/2}$ is 20 and 40 hours in infants and older children, respectively. Because of the lack of higher serum levels and greater therapeutic effect, trough serum digoxin level should be 1–2 ng/mL.

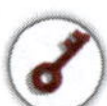

Key: A

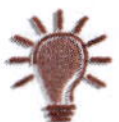

BOOST YOUR KNOWLEDGE

Digoxin has a narrow therapeutic index. Toxicity signs include anorexia, vomiting visual and central nervous system (CNS) disturbances (seen commonly in adults), apathy or intolerance to feeding, second and third-degree AV block (infants), and tachyarrhythmias. Prolonged PR interval is an expected effect (not toxicity). Treatment of toxicity includes temporary cardiac pacing if required, antiarrhythmic drugs, normalization of potassium levels, and specific Fab antibodies.

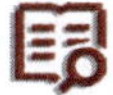

REFERENCE/SOURCE

- Shaddy RE, Penny DJ, Feltes TF, Cetta F, Mittal S, Kailin J. Moss and Adams' Heart Disease in Infants, Children, and Adolescents (Chapters 72, 81), 10th edition. Philadelphia: Wolters Kluwer Health; 2021.

12. Identify the device (A) used for heart failure.

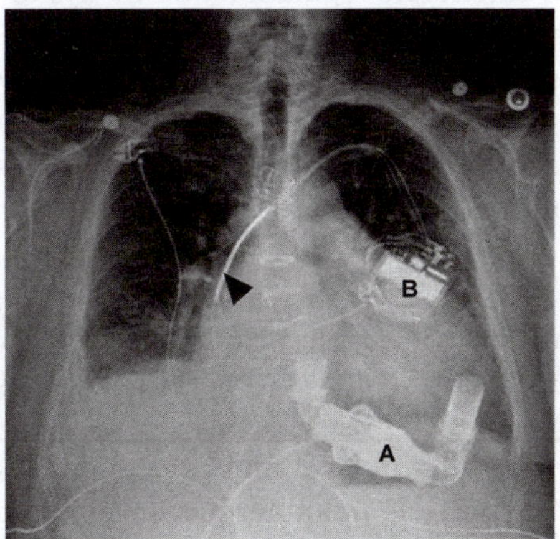

A. Endocardial permanent pacemaker
B. Epicardial permanent pacemaker
C. Ventricular assist device (VAD)
D. CRT

EXPLANATION

This is a chest X-ray of a child with CHF, showing cardiomegaly and pulmonary venous congestion. Device A is a left ventricular assist device (LVAD) HeartMate II with inflow and outflow limbs. Device B is an intracardiac defibrillator (ICD) can that has an electrode (black arrow) placed in the heart. An epicardial and endocardial pacemaker will not have thick electrodes as seen here. CRT will have electrodes on both ventricles (biventricular pacing). Of these, VADs and CRT are device therapy for heart failure.

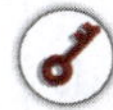

Key: C

BOOST YOUR KNOWLEDGE

The main indications for mechanical circulatory support [extracorporeal membrane oxygenation (ECMO)/VAD] include bridge to transplant and bridge to recovery. ECMO is short term and VAD are long-term mechanical circulatory support (MCS). Berlin Heart EXCOR was approved by the FDA in 2012 for use in children. The devices used for larger children and adults are HeartMate II and HeartWare HVAD.

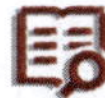

REFERENCE/SOURCE

- Shaddy RE, Penny DJ, Feltes TF, Cetta F, Mittal S, Kailin J (Eds). Moss and Adams' Heart Disease in Infants, Children, and Adolescents (Chapters 25, 72), 10th edition. Philadelphia: Wolters Kluwer Health; 2021.

13. Which of the following is the predominant neurohormonal pathway underlying heart failure?

A. Endothelin pathway
B. Prostacyclin pathway
C. RAAS
D. Nitric oxide pathway

EXPLANATION

Options A, B, and D are pathways involved in pulmonary hypertension. Option C, the RAAS pathway plays an important role in heart failure syndrome and is also a target of therapeutic options, such as ACE inhibition.

Key: C

BOOST YOUR KNOWLEDGE

Pathophysiology of heart failure: In the neurohormonal model of heart failure, there is an index injury event to the myocardium leading to loss of adrenergic regulation and LV dysfunction. This leads to activation of renin angiotensin aldosterone pathway (RAAS), the adrenergic nervous system, and other inflammatory cytokines. Various biochemical abnormalities include vascular dysfunction, renal dysfunction, and oxidative stress. Initially compensatory, many of these are maladaptive in nature and lead to more myocardial stress, LV dilatation, and heart failure. Blocking these maladaptive RAAS and adrenergic nervous systems using ACE inhibitors and beta-blockers respectively, has led to improved survival.

REFERENCE/SOURCE

- Shaddy RE, Penny DJ, Feltes TF, Cetta F, Mittal S, Kailin J (Eds). Moss and Adams' Heart Disease in Infants, Children, and Adolescents (Chapters 65, 72, 81), 10th edition. Philadelphia: Wolters Kluwer Health; 2021.

14. A 1-year-old child presented with a history of fever and cold 15 days back followed by cough, fast breathing, and poor feeding for the last 2 days. He is irritable, has severe respiratory distress, RR 80 breaths/min, HR 170 beats/min, cold peripheries, CRT >5 seconds, BP is 88/54 mm Hg (in both upper and lower limb), and feeble pulses. He appears pale and edematous. There are bilateral crackles heard over the chest and tender hepatomegaly. What is the most appropriate initial line of management?

A. IV diuretics, vasodilators (dobutamine), consider mechanical ventilation
B. IV diuretics, norepinephrine, consider mechanical ventilation
C. Liberal IV fluid boluses, broad-spectrum antibiotics, and consider mechanical ventilation
D. Liberal IV fluids boluses, epinephrine infusion, and intravenous (IV) immunoglobulin

EXPLANATION

This patient has acute heart failure with BP maintained. As per the classification below, the patient has congestion (respiratory distress and crackles) and critical perfusion (cold peripheries), hence, option A—IV diuretics and vasodilators are the preferred regimen which allows for reduction in preload and afterload. If he does not respond to this regimen or his BP reduces, then option B is the treatment of choice. Liberal fluids cannot be given as it is cardiogenic shock.

Perfusion	***Congestion***	
Adequate perfusion	*A* *Warm and dry* Rx: Goal of HF therapy	*B* *Warm and wet* Rx: Diuretics with the continuation of STD therapy
Critical hypoperfusion	*L* *Cold and dry* Rx: Limited options, consider inodilators and/or vasopressors	*C* *Cold and wet* • If BP normal—inodilators and diuresis • If BP is low—vasopressors

 **Key: A**

 **BOOST YOUR KNOWLEDGE**

Epinephrine's (adrenaline) main indication is cardiovascular collapse that is refractory to dopamine and/or dobutamine. The major side effect is life-threatening ventricular arrhythmias. Epinephrine increases myocardial oxygen requirements. High doses may produce myocardial ischemia and tissue ischemia. Norepinephrine infusion increases systolic and diastolic pressure systemic vascular resistance and contractility. HR is largely unaffected. Hence, the rate of arrhythmias is less than epinephrine.

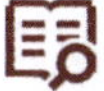 **REFERENCE/SOURCE**

- Shaddy RE, Penny DJ, Feltes TF, Cetta F, Mittal S, Kailin J (Eds). Moss and Adams' Heart Disease in Infants, Children, and Adolescents (Chapters 53, 55, 72), 10th edition. Philadelphia: Wolters Kluwer Health; 2021.

15. What is the cause of left ventricular outflow tract obstruction in hypertrophic cardiomyopathy?

A. Systolic anterior motion of mitral leaflets
B. Subaortic membrane
C. Subaortic hypertrophied muscle bundle
D. Accessory mitral tissue

 **EXPLANATION**

Subaortic obstruction is dynamic in nature in HCM produced by the mitral valve, causing contact between the mitral valve and hypertrophied ventricular septum. A characteristic of this disease is an abrupt anterior motion in which the elongated mitral valve leaflets move toward the septum in early systole. This anterior motion occurs by virtue of the high-velocity jet streaming through the narrowed outflow tract and pulling the mitral valve leaflets toward the septum (venturi effect). Longer duration of contact indicates severe obstruction. The options B, C, and D are causes of fixed obstruction.

 **Key: A**

 **BOOST YOUR KNOWLEDGE**

The subaortic gradient in HCM being dynamic shows spontaneous variability that is reduced or abolished by interventions that decrease myocardial contractility (beta-blockers) or increase ventricular volume or arterial pressure (e.g., squatting, isomeric handgrip, or phenylephrine). Alternatively, outflow gradient or murmur can be augmented by factors that decrease ventricular volume or arterial pressure (Valsalva maneuver and nitroglycerine) or increase contractility (standing, amyl nitrite, exercise, isoproterenol, and premature ventricular contraction). This forms the basis of dynamic auscultation in HCM.

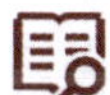 **REFERENCE/SOURCE**

- Hypertrophic cardiomyopathy. In: Shaddy RE, Penny DJ, Feltes TF, Cetta F, Mittal S, Kailin J (Eds). Moss and Adams' Heart Disease in Infants, Children, and Adolescents, 10th edition. Philadelphia: Wolters Kluwer Health; 2021. pp. 1221-54.

16. Which is of the following is the most common nontraumatic cause of sudden death in young?

A. Myocarditis
B. Coronary artery anomalies
C. HCM
D. Ventricular tachycardia

EXPLANATION

All the choices are causes of sudden death in adolescents and young adults. Sudden death in HCM most commonly occurs during adolescence and young adulthood (12–35 years) and rarely before 10 years of age. Most sudden death events occur while sedentary or during normal/modest physical exertion or during or just following vigorous physical activity. Clinical risk markers for high-risk of sudden death in HCM include prior cardiac arrest or sustained ventricular tachycardia, family history of ≥1 premature HCM-related death, unexplained syncope, massive LVH [intraventricular septum (IVS) thickness ≥30 mm for all ages and sizes]. These patients are candidates for ICD therapy.

Key: C

BOOST YOUR KNOWLEDGE

Young patients with HCM are disqualified from intense competitive sports to reduce their risk of sudden death (36th Bethesda Conference).

REFERENCE/SOURCE

- Shaddy RE, Penny DJ, Feltes TF, Cetta F, Mittal S, Kailin J (Eds). Moss and Adams' Heart Disease in Infants, Children, and Adolescents (Chapters 20, 52), 10th edition. Philadelphia: Wolters Kluwer Health; 2021.

17. What is the diagnosis for a 7-month-old infant with CHF, whose ECG is shown below?

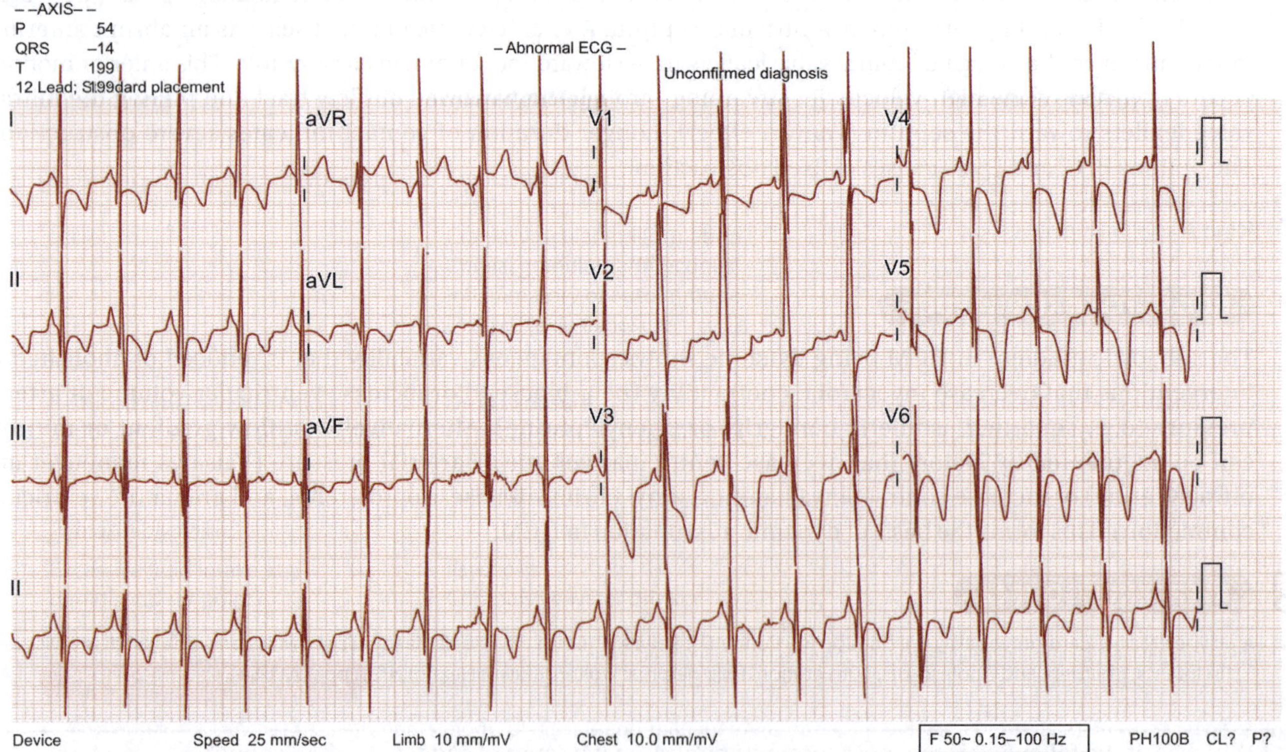

A. Aortic stenosis
B. Pompe's disease
C. TOF
D. Acute rheumatic fever with MR and tricuspid regurgitation (TR)

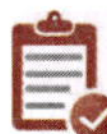

EXPLANATION

The above ECG shows increased voltages suggestive of LVH and RVH, ST-T changes including marked T wave inversions in both anterior and lateral leads. Additionally, the PR interval is short indicating a diagnosis of biventricular HCM associated with storage disease such as Pompe's disease, option B. Infants, often ECG show RVH which may or may not be related to right ventricular outflow tract obstruction. Aortic stenosis shows LVH dominantly and PR is normal. TOF has dominant RVH. Acute rheumatic fever is unlikely at the age of 7 months and the ECG will show a pattern of volume overload and not pressure overload as seen in this ECG.

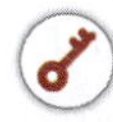

Key: B

BOOST YOUR KNOWLEDGE

Early onset HCM in infants has an unfavorable course. A large proportion of infants with HCM have non-sarcomeric HCM (true HCM is caused by a mutation in genes encoding sarcomeric proteins). This includes Noonan's syndrome, glycogen storage disease, transient and nonfamilial cardiomyopathy in infants of insulin-dependent diabetic mothers, primary mitochondrial myopathies, abnormalities of fatty acid oxidation (acyl-CoA dehydrogenase deficiency) and carnitine deficiency and infiltrative cardiomyopathies, such as Hunter and Hurler disease. Hence, a metabolic screening panel is required in infants with cardiomyopathy.

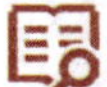

REFERENCE/SOURCE

- Shaddy RE, Penny DJ, Feltes TF, Cetta F, Mittal S, Kailin J (Eds). Moss and Adams' Heart Disease in Infants, Children, and Adolescents (Chapters 41, 44, 52, 59), 10th edition. Philadelphia: Wolters Kluwer Health; 2021.

18. Which is the most common form of cardiomyopathy associated with the following disease shown in the picture?

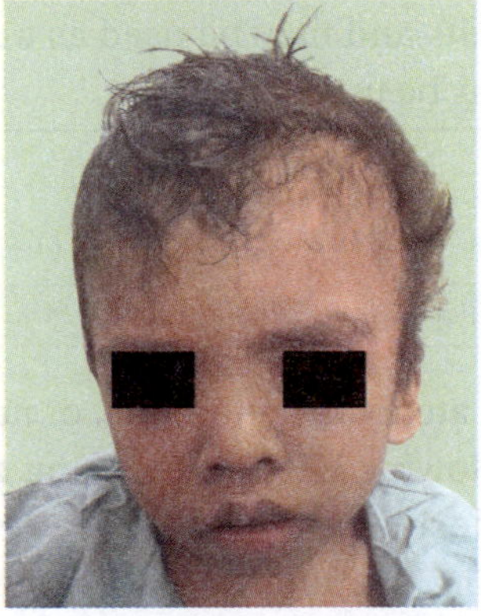

A. HCM

B. Dilated cardiomyopathy

C. RCM

D. LV noncompaction cardiomyopathy

EXPLANATION

The child here has features of Noonan's syndrome, viz., large and tall forehead with narrow temples, hypertelorism, downward slant of the palpebral fissure, epicanthal folds, short broad nose with depressed root and full nasal tip, deeply grooved philtrum, full lips with high wide peaks to the vermillion border of the upper lip, small chin, short neck. 80% of Noonan's syndrome patients have a cardiovascular abnormality, of which 60% are CHD [pulmonary valve stenosis, atrial septal defect (ASD), ventricular septal defect (VSD), TOF, and coarctation of the aorta (CoA)], 20% are HCM [especially those with rapidly accelerated fibrosarcoma-1 (RAF1), uncommonly with protein tyrosine phosphatase non-receptor type 11 (PTPN11) mutation].

Key: A

BOOST YOUR KNOWLEDGE

Genetic diseases that have significant LVH mimics HCM include protein kinase AMP-activated non-catalytic subunit gamma 2 (PRKAG2) mutation, Fabry's disease (α-galactosidase deficiency), and lysosome-associated membrane protein (LAMP2) mutation (Danon's disease). Diagnosis of Fabry's disease is important since enzyme replacement therapy is available for it.

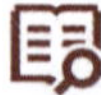

REFERENCE/SOURCE

- Shaddy RE, Penny DJ, Feltes TF, Cetta F, Mittal S, Kailin J (Eds). Moss and Adams' Heart Disease in Infants, Children, and Adolescents (Chapters 3, 52), 10th edition. Philadelphia: Wolters Kluwer Health; 2021.

19. An 8-year-old boy presented with dyspnea on exertion for the last 1 year. There was no history of syncope or sudden death in the family. The echocardiogram showed HCM with no LV outflow tract obstruction. Holter study did not reveal arrhythmia. What is the first line of management in this patient?

A. Propranolol
B. ICD
C. Surgical myectomy
D. Verapamil

EXPLANATION

Option C; surgical myectomy is a treatment modality used for drug-refractory HCM with LV obstruction 50 mm Hg in basal state or with physiologic exercise. This patient has no left ventricular outflow tract obstruction (LVOT). Prevention of sudden death in HCM is done by the use of an ICD. However, since ICD has complications, especially in a young child, it is recommended only with HCM with high-risk features. Drug therapy is the mainstay of treatment of HCM. Beta-blockers are first-line therapy. Verapamil is a calcium channel blocker used more often in adults and may be used as a second-line drug. If refractory to both beta-blocker and verapamil, disopyramide may be used.

Key: A

BOOST YOUR KNOWLEDGE

Long-acting preparations of propranolol, atenolol, metoprolol, or nadolol are now the most commonly used beta-blockers. They improve symptoms by slowing HR and reducing the force of LV contraction, thus augmenting ventricular filling and relaxation, and decreasing myocardial consumption, as well as inhibiting sympathetic stimulation of the heart, thereby reducing the outflow gradient under conditions of exercise, and augmenting sympathetic stimulation.

REFERENCE/SOURCE

- Hypertrophic Cardiomyopathy. In: Shaddy RE, Penny DJ, Feltes TF, Cetta F, Mittal S, Kailin J (Eds). Moss and Adams' Heart Disease in Infants, Children, and Adolescents, 10th edition. Philadelphia: Wolters Kluwer Health; 2021. pp. 1221-54.

20. What is the recommended screening strategy for cardiomyopathy in patients with Duchenne muscular dystrophy (DMD)?

A. Yearly ECHO after diagnosis
B. 2 yearly ECHO from 6 years onward, then yearly after 10 years of age
C. Yearly ECHO from 6 years onward, then 2 yearly after 10 years of age
D. 2 yearly ECHO after 10 years of age

EXPLANATION

Cardiac involvement is universal in DMD with an estimated incidence of cardiomyopathy 25% by age 6 years and 59% by age 10 years. The median age of diagnosis of cardiomyopathy is 14–15 years. Hence, the recommended screening by guidelines is option B with more frequent screening after 10 years of age.

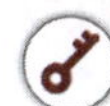

Key: B

BOOST YOUR KNOWLEDGE

Other muscular dystrophies with clinical cardiac disease include Becker's muscular dystrophy, Emery–Dreifuss muscular dystrophy (joint contractures, cardiomyopathy, complete heart block), and limb-girdle muscular dystrophy. All of the above are X-linked diseases. Myotonic muscular dystrophy and Friedreich ataxia are also associated with cardiomyopathy.

REFERENCE/SOURCE

- The Heart in Muscular Dystrophies. In: Shaddy RE, Penny DJ, Feltes TF, Cetta F, Mittal S, Kailin J (Eds). Moss and Adams' Heart Disease in Infants, Children, and Adolescents, 10th edition. Philadelphia: Wolters Kluwer Health; 2021. pp. 1315-27.

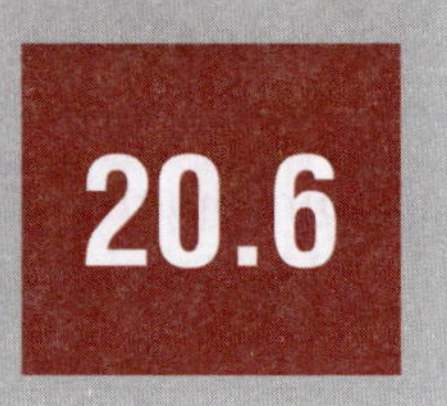

CHAPTER 20.6 Cardiac Dysrhythmias

Uma Devi Karuru

1. The triangle of Koch is *not* bounded by:

A. Septal tricuspid annulus
B. Ostium of the coronary sinus
C. Tendon of Todaro
D. Inferior vena cava orifice

EXPLANATION

The triangle of Koch delineates the atrioventricular (AV) node location. It is bounded anteriorly by the annulus of the septal tricuspid leaflet, posteriorly by the tendon of Todaro, and inferiorly by the coronary sinus orifice along with the vestibule immediately anterior to it.

Key: D

BOOST YOUR KNOWLEDGE

The triangle of Koch was first described by Walter Koch. AV node lies subendocardially in contrast to the sinus node, which is located subepicardially. The tendon of Todaro is a subendocardial fibrous cord traversing from thebesian–eustachian valvular commissure to the membranous septum. Thebesian valve is a coronary sinus valve, and the eustachian valve is an inferior vena caval valve.

REFERENCE/SOURCE

- Shaddy RE, Penny DJ, Feltes TF, Cetta F, Mital S. Moss and Adams' Heart Disease in Infants, Children and Adolescents (Chapter 18), 10th edition. Wolters Kluwer; 2021.

2. Wolff-Parkinson-White (WPW) syndrome is *not* associated with which of the following heart diseases?

A. Ebstein anomaly
B. Congenitally corrected transposition of great arteries
C. Hypertrophic cardiomyopathy
D. D-transposition of great arteries

EXPLANATION

Wolff-Parkinson-White syndrome is associated with structural cardiac diseases including Ebstein anomaly of the tricuspid valve, congenitally corrected transposition of great arteries, hypertrophic cardiomyopathy, and noncardiac diseases including glycogen storage disease and tuberous sclerosis.

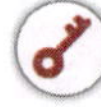

Key: D

BOOST YOUR KNOWLEDGE

Wolff-Parkinson-White syndrome has an association with congenital heart diseases in 9–32% of the patients. So, echocardiography is indicated in the confirmed cases of the WPW. More than one accessory pathway is seen in approximately 9% of the patients. In patients with underlying congenital heart disease, the incidence of multiple accessory pathways is as high as 20%.

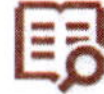

REFERENCE/SOURCE

- Shaddy RE, Penny DJ, Feltes TF, Cetta F, Mital S. Moss and Adams' Heart Disease in Infants, Children and Adolescents (Chapter 22), 10th edition. Wolters Kluwer; 2021.

3. The following condition is *not* associated with surgery of which of the following defects?

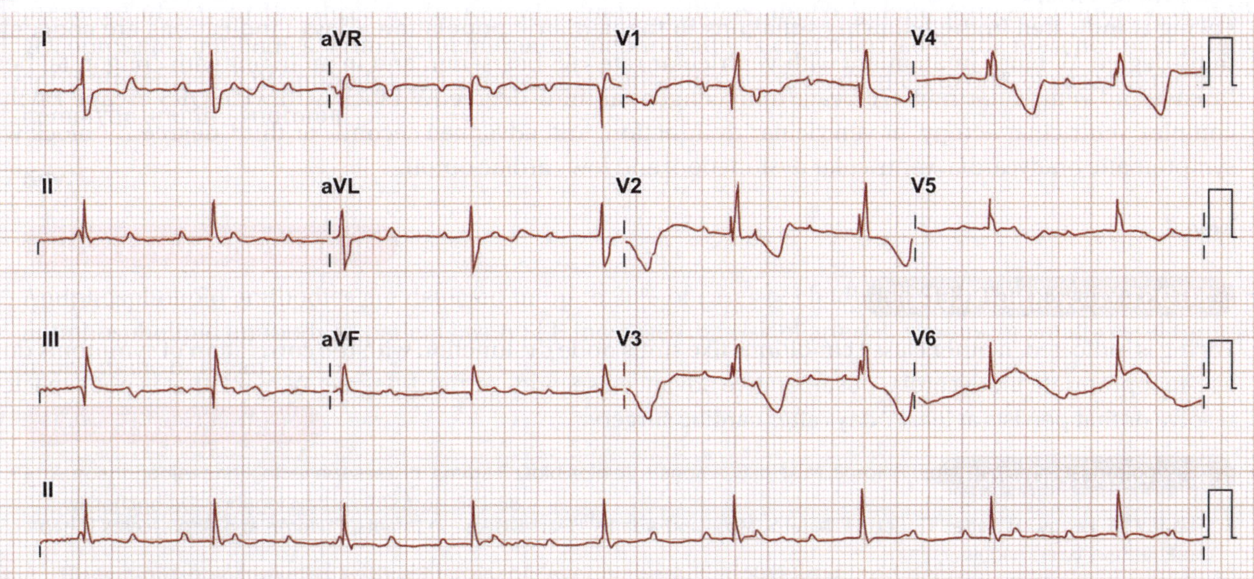

A. Ventricular septal defects (VSD)
B. Ostium secundum atrial septal defects (OS-ASD)
C. Atrioventricular septal defects (AVSD)
D. Aortic valve replacement (AVR)

EXPLANATION

The electrocardiogram (ECG) is showing AV dissociation with atrial rate more than the ventricular rate. This rules out AV dissociation caused by junctional and ventricular rhythm. There are constant P-P and R-R intervals, but varying P-R intervals. This confirms complete AV block or third-degree AV block. There is a complete failure of sinus atrial impulses to conduct to the ventricles. Any surgery which involves damage to the AV node causes this condition like perimembranous VSD, AVSD repairs, and ccTGA with VSD. In aortic and mitral valve replacements, impingement of the prosthetic valve on normal AV conduction system causes AV block.

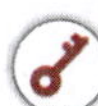

Key: B

BOOST YOUR KNOWLEDGE

Nowadays, AV block is a relatively rare complication following surgery affecting less than 3% of cases. Risk factors include younger age, low-weight babies, longer aortic cross-clamp time, or cardiopulmonary bypass. These blocks are temporary and do not need long-term treatment. Temporary pacing can be used in perioperative period until normal conduction is established. Permanent pacing is rarely required.

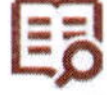

REFERENCE/SOURCE

- Shaddy RE, Penny DJ, Feltes TF, Cetta F, Mital S. Moss and Adams' Heart Disease in Infants, Children and Adolescents (Chapter 22), 10th edition. Wolters Kluwer; 2021.

4. Pacemaker implantation is indicated in which of the following conditions?

A. Congenital third-degree AV block in an infant with ventricular rate >55 bpm
B. Congenital third-degree AV block in an infant with congenital heart disease and ventricular rate >70 bpm
C. Congenital third-degree AV block with wide QRS escape rhythm, complex ventricular ectopy, or ventricular dysfunction
D. Asymptomatic type I second-degree AV block

EXPLANATION

Pacing is indicated in the following situations in the pediatric population. Class I indications are congenital third-degree AV block in an infant with ventricular rate <55 beats/min and in an infant with congenital heart disease and ventricular rate <70 beats/min; congenital third-degree AV block with wide QRS escape rhythm, complex ventricular ectopy, or ventricular dysfunction; and advanced second- or third-degree AV block with symptomatic bradycardia, ventricular dysfunction, and low cardiac output.

Key: C

BOOST YOUR KNOWLEDGE

Pacing is indicated in other class I conditions like sinus node dysfunction with the correlation of symptoms during age-inappropriate bradycardia, postoperative advanced second- or third-degree AV block that is not expected to resolve or that persists at least 7 days after cardiac surgery.

REFERENCE/SOURCE

- Shaddy RE, Penny DJ, Feltes TF, Cetta F, Mital S. Moss and Adams' Heart Disease in Infants, Children and Adolescents (Chapter 22), 10th edition. Wolters Kluwer; 2021.

5. Which of the following conditions *does not* cause this ECG change?

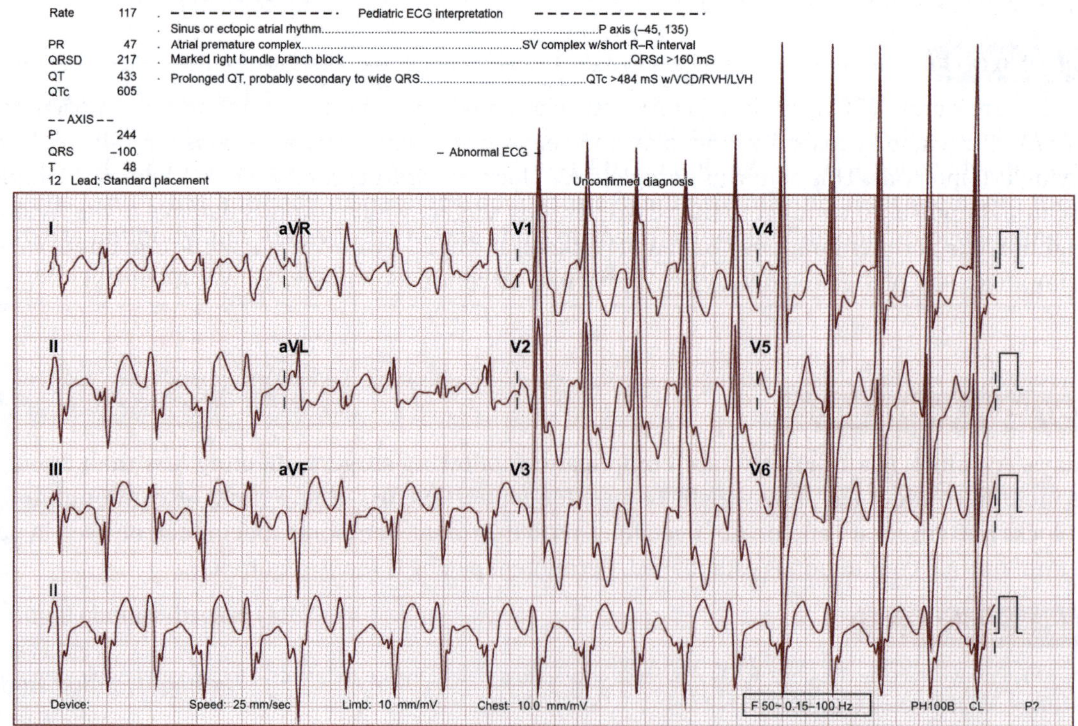

A. Catecholaminergic polymorphic ventricular tachycardia (CPVT)
B. Long QT syndrome (LQTS)
C. Andersen–Tawil syndrome
D. Digitalis toxicity

EXPLANATION

The electrocardiogram is showing wide complex tachycardia. The frontal plane axis alternatively changes by 180° with each successive beat, which is a characteristic of bidirectional ventricular tachycardia (VT). This is seen in severe digoxin toxicity, familial CPVT, and Andersen–Tawil syndrome.

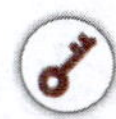

Key: B

BOOST YOUR KNOWLEDGE

Catecholaminergic polymorphic ventricular tachycardia causes progressively worsening ventricular arrhythmias during exercise. Typical bidirectional VT develops after 1 minute of exercise with a sinus heart rate of approximately 120 beats/min, and arrhythmias rapidly recede during recovery. LQTS is characterized by prolonged QTc interval and is due to the mutations of potassium and sodium channels. Andersen–Tawil syndrome is characterized by the triad of periodic paralysis, variable developmental abnormalities, and frequent ventricular ectopy/arrhythmias (mostly ventricular bigeminy, polymorphic VT, and rarely bidirectional VT). Digoxin toxicity causes multifocal tachycardia, regularization of atrial fibrillation (AF), and bidirectional VT.

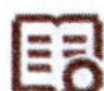

REFERENCE/SOURCE

- Giudicessi JR, Tester DJ, Ackerman MJ. Genetics of cardiac arrhythmias. In: Libby P, Bonow RO, Mann DL, Tomaselli GF, Bhatt DL, Solomon Scott D, et al. (Eds). Braunwald's Heart Disease: A Textbook of Cardiovascular Medicine, 12th edition. Elsevier; 2022. pp.1191-207.

6. A 5-year-old boy was brought to pediatric OPD with the following ECG. Identify the abnormality.

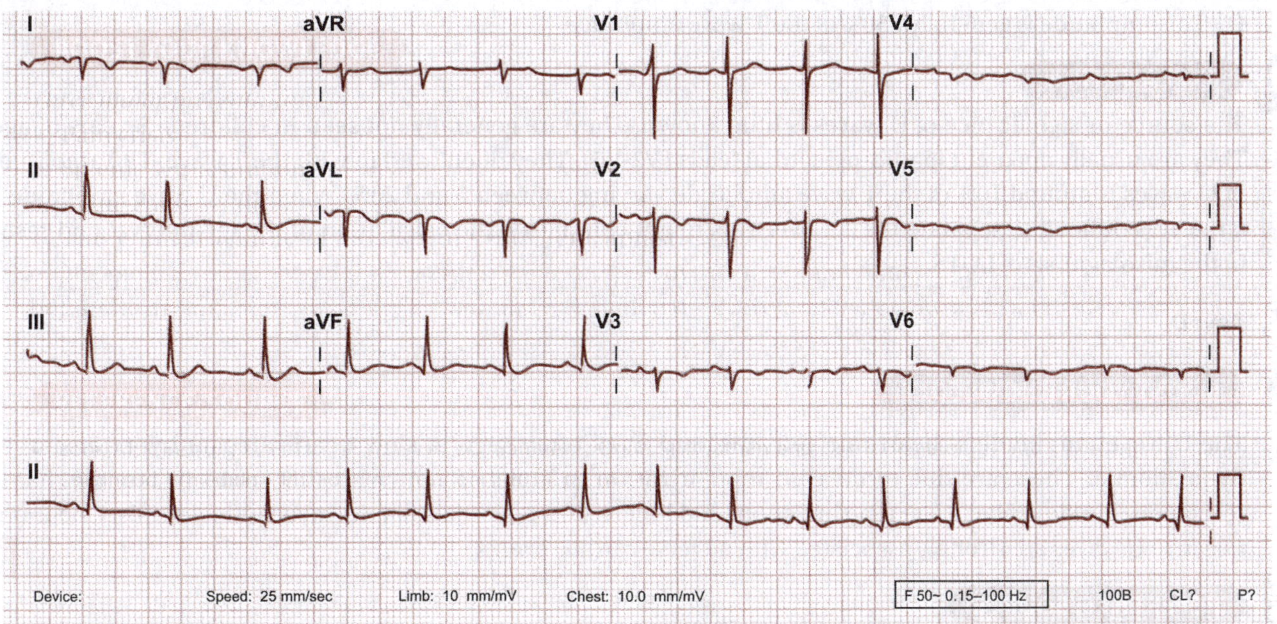

A. Right-left arm lead reversal
B. Left atrial ectopic origin
C. Situs inversus dextrocardia
D. Isolated dextrocardia

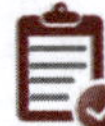

EXPLANATION

The ECG features are: In lead I and aVL, p and T waves are inverted, and major QRS deflections are negative. aVR and aVL are mirror images. Inverted P wave in lead I and aVL and upright P wave in aVR suggest atrial depolarization from left sinus node. In chest leads, there is poor R wave progression and absence of septal Q waves in left lateral leads, which suggests dextrocardia. All these features are suggestive of situs inversus dextrocardia. ECG can be corrected when limb leads are reversed, and chest leads are recorded from right precordial leads.

Key: C

BOOST YOUR KNOWLEDGE

- In right-left arm lead reversal, there is an inversion of lead I and reversal of lead II, III, aVR, and aVL. The arm lead reversal and dextrocardia are differentiated by precordial R wave progression. Normal R wave progression is seen in arm lead reversal, whereas it is lost in dextrocardia.
- The left atrial ectopic rhythm is manifested by a negative P wave in lead I, isoelectric or a negative P wave in precordial leads.
- In situs solitus with dextrocardia, septal depolarization proceeds from left to right as in a normally positioned heart. Q waves are present in standard left precordial leads. In addition, depolarization of the frontal plane is counterclockwise so Q waves appear in lead I and aVL.

REFERENCE/SOURCE

- Cardiac malpositions. In: Perloff JK, Marelli AJ. Perloff's Clinical Recognition of Congenital Heart Disease, 6th edition. Elsevier; 2012. pp. 15-40.

7. Which of the following is *incorrect* about the U wave?

A. Not seen in children <8 years of age
B. Seen in the mid-precordial leads V2-V5
C. Misdiagnosed as LQTS in the presence of prominent U waves
D. The amplitude is generally >50% of the T wave amplitude

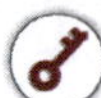

EXPLANATION

The source or significance of U waves is little known. They are generally not seen in children <8 years of age. They are usually apparent in mid-precordial leads (V2-V5). They often overlap with the T wave. The amplitude of U waves is around 10% of the T wave amplitude varying between 5 and 28%. When the U wave amplitude is large, it is difficult to separate the T wave. This might complicate the calculation of the QT interval and result in the misdiagnosis of LQTS.

Key: D

BOOST YOUR KNOWLEDGE

The U wave amplitude is heart rate sensitive and most often seen at slow heart rates, in hypertension and hypokalemia. These are due to delayed repolarization in areas of ventricles that undergo late mechanical relaxation, Purkinje fiber's late repolarization, and long action potentials of mid-myocardial M cells. Uncommon negative U waves are strongly associated with adverse cardiac events.

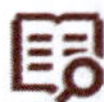

REFERENCE/SOURCE

- Shaddy RE, Penny DJ, Feltes TF, Cetta F, Mital S. Moss and Adams' Heart Disease in Infants, Children and Adolescents (Chapter 19), 10th edition. Wolters Kluwer; 2021.

8. Which of the following is *not* a feature of digitalis toxicity?

A. AF with fast ventricular rate
B. Paroxysmal atrial tachycardia with varying AV block
C. Regularization of rate in patients of AF
D. Biventricular tachycardia

EXPLANATION

Digoxin causes a multitude of arrhythmias by causing increased automaticity and decreased AV conduction. The arrhythmias seen in digoxin toxicity are: Ventricular bigeminy, paroxysmal atrial tachycardia with block, regularized AF, and bidirectional VT. The ST depression of digoxin toxicity is characteristically scooped and often referred to as reverse tick or Salvador Dali's moustache ST depression.

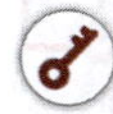

Key: A

BOOST YOUR KNOWLEDGE

Digoxin reversibly inhibits sodium-potassium ATPase and has a very narrow therapeutic window. Digoxin can be used intravenous (IV) to control ventricular rate in AF and atrial flutter. Various factors such as worsening of renal function, hypokalemia, chronic lung disease, hypothyroidism, amyloidosis, and advanced age-precipitate digoxin-induced arrhythmias.

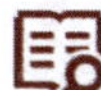

REFERENCE/SOURCE

- Djohan AH, Sia CH, Singh D, Lin W, Kong WK, Poh KK. A myriad of electrocardiographic findings associated with digoxin use. Singapore Med J. 2020;61(1):9-14.

9. Congenital forms of LQTS are most commonly due to abnormality of which ion channel?

A. Sodium
B. Potassium
C. Calcium
D. Ryanodine receptor

EXPLANATION

Nearly 75% of patients with LQTS host either gain or loss of function of pathogenic variants. In LQT1, there is loss of KCNQ1-encoded potassium (Kv 7.1) channel (seen in 35% of patients). There is loss of KCNH-2–encoded potassium (Kv 11.1) channel (30% of patients) and gain-of-function mutation in SCN5A-encoded sodium channel in 10% of patients.

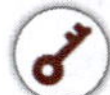

Key: B

BOOST YOUR KNOWLEDGE

Congenital LQTS comprises a distinct group of cardiac channelopathies characterized by delayed repolarization of myocardium. Clinically, these patients have the symptoms of syncope, seizures, and sudden cardiac death in the setting of a structurally normal heart. Most of the LQTS disorders are of autosomal dominant pattern, and rarely some of them are recessive. LQTS results from the loss of some of the channels or gain of some of the mutated channel functions. For example, the gain of function of mutations of SCN5A sodium-encoding channel is responsible for the development of Brugada syndrome, cardiac conduction disease, and sick sinus syndrome. Similarly, the gain of function of mutated calcium channels can result in Timothy syndrome. Gain of mutation of ryanodine receptor abnormalities results in catecholaminergic polymorphic VT.

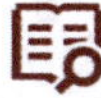

REFERENCE/SOURCE

- Giudicessi JR, Tester DJ, Ackerman MJ. Genetics of cardiac arrhythmias. In: Libby P, Bonow RO, Mann DL, Tomaselli GF, Bhatt DL, Solomon Scott D, et al. (Eds). Braunwald's Heart Disease: A Textbook of Cardiovascular Medicine, 12th edition. Elsevier; 2022. pp.1191-207.

10. An adolescent male presented to OPD with complaints of palpitations. ECG was done which is given here. Identify the abnormality.

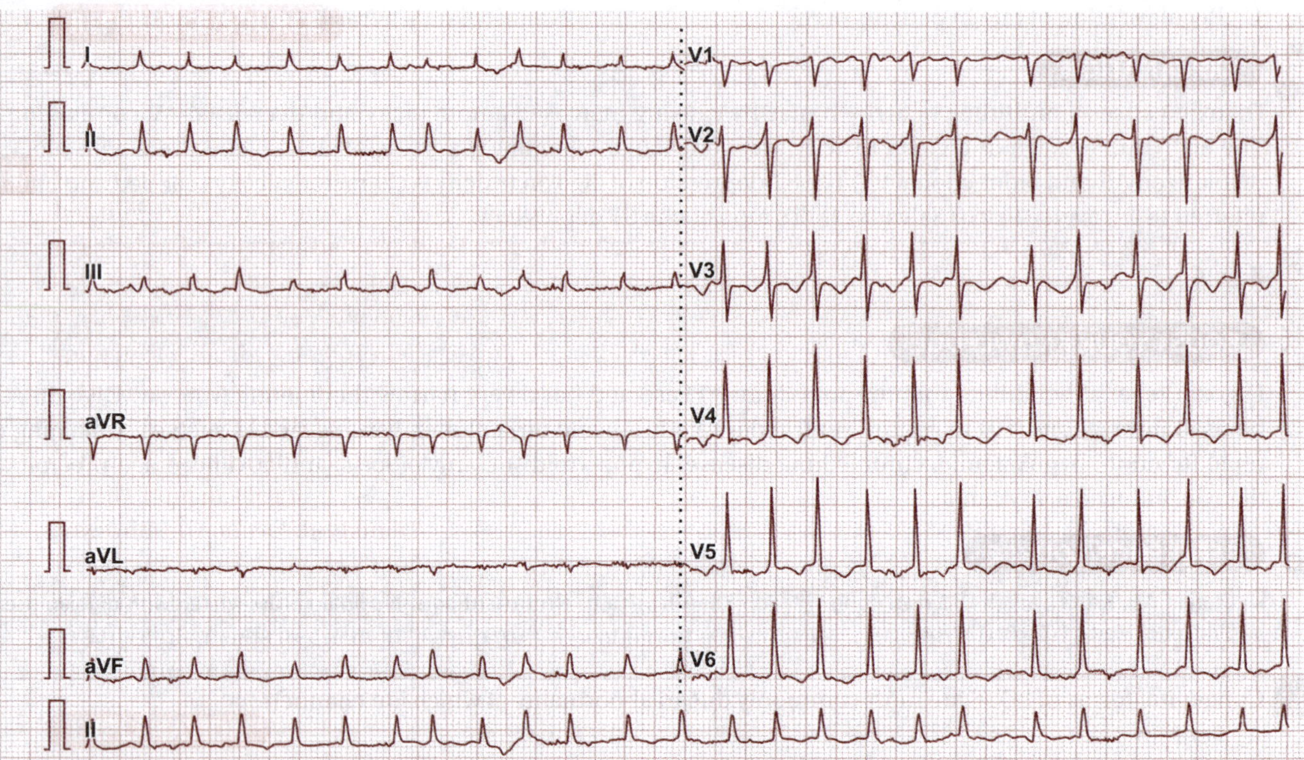

A. Ectopic atrial tachycardia
B. AF
C. Atrial flutter
D. Multifocal atrial tachycardia

EXPLANATION

The electrocardiogram is showing narrow complex tachycardia with an irregularly irregular rhythm. The atrial rate is more than the ventricular rate. So, *differentials are:* Atrial flutter with variable block, multifocal atrial tachycardia, and AF. There are no visible P waves and fibrillatory waves seen (F waves). These features differentiate AF from the other two tachycardias. Focal atrial tachycardia is characterized by regular atrial tachycardia with P wave morphology different from that in sinus tachycardia. Multifocal atrial tachycardia requires at least three distinct P waves morphologies in the rhythm strip. Atrial flutter has a typical sawtooth pattern.

Key: B

BOOST YOUR KNOWLEDGE

Atrial fibrillation is a very uncommon arrhythmia in children. It occurs in the context of WPW syndrome or following extensive atrial surgeries like total cavopulmonary correction or atrial switch surgery. If AF occurs in a structurally normal heart, further evaluation is mandatory and should be looked at for re-entrant supraventricular tachycardia (SVT), channelopathies, or drug abuse. It may be an initial presentation in cases of hyperthyroidism, myocarditis, and digoxin toxicity.

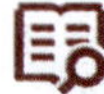

REFERENCE/SOURCE

- Shaddy RE, Penny DJ, Feltes TF, Cetta F, Mital S (Eds). Moss and Adams' Heart Disease in Infants, Children and Adolescents (Chapter 22), 10th edition. Wolters Kluwer; 2021.

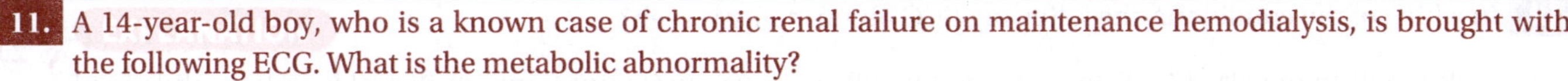

11. A 14-year-old boy, who is a known case of chronic renal failure on maintenance hemodialysis, is brought with the following ECG. What is the metabolic abnormality?

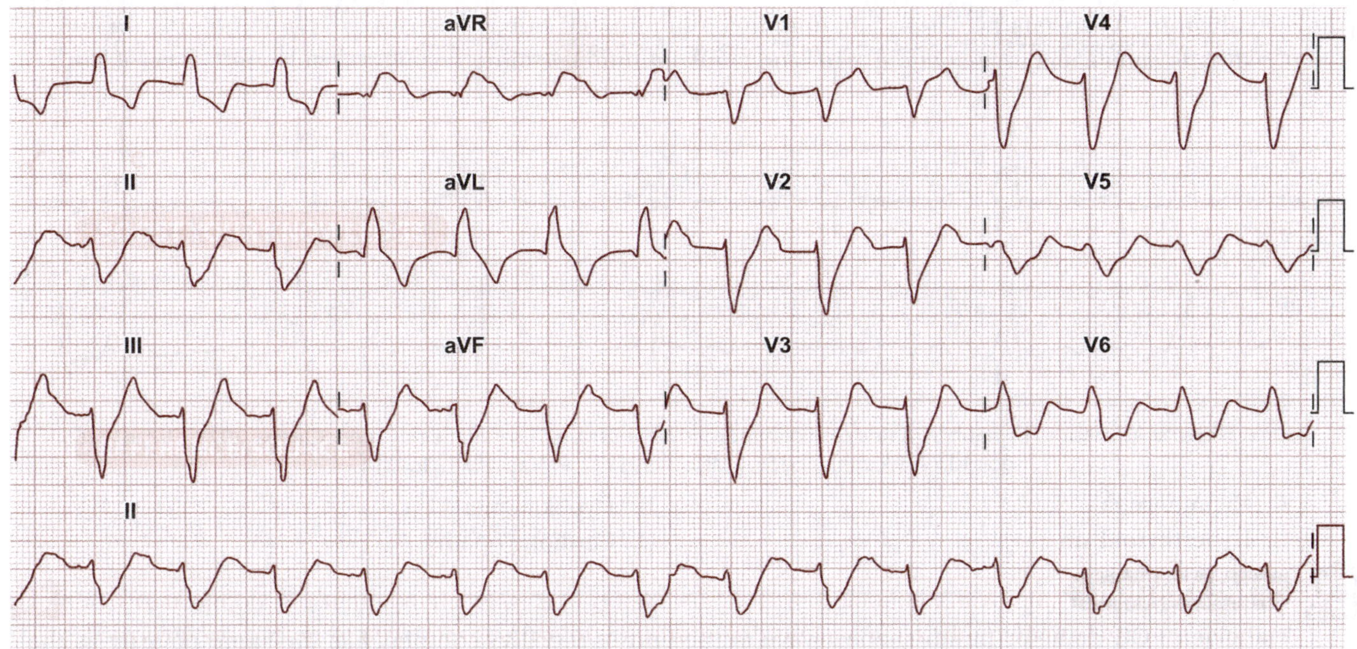

Source: Buttner R, Burns E. (2022). Hyperkalaemia. [online] Available from https://litfl.com/hyperkalaemia-ecg-library/ [Last accessed July, 2024].

A. Hypercalcemia
B. Hypokalemia
C. Hyperkalemia
D. Hypocalcemia

EXPLANATION

The electrocardiogram is showing tall, peaked T waves, QRS widening, and PR prolongation. All these findings suggest hyperkalemia. Hypercalcemia shortens the QT interval, and hypocalcemia lengthens the QT interval. Hypokalemia is associated with decreased T-wave amplitude.

Key: C

BOOST YOUR KNOWLEDGE

Hyperkalemia produces tall, peaked T waves. This is a nonspecific and insensitive finding because normal children may have peaked T waves, and hyperkalemic children may not have peaked T waves. As potassium levels rise, T waves become more peaked, and there is intraventricular conduction delay. This results in widened QRS and PR prolongation resembling sine wave or wide VT. At potassium levels of 9 mEq/L, atrial standstill, AV block, and ventricular fibrillation occur.

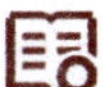

REFERENCE/SOURCE

- Shaddy RE, Penny DJ, Feltes TF, Cetta F, Mital S (Eds). Moss and Adams' Heart Disease in Infants, Children and Adolescents (Chapter 19), 10th edition. Wolters Kluwer; 2021.

12. In which of the conditions, the following ECG abnormality is seen?

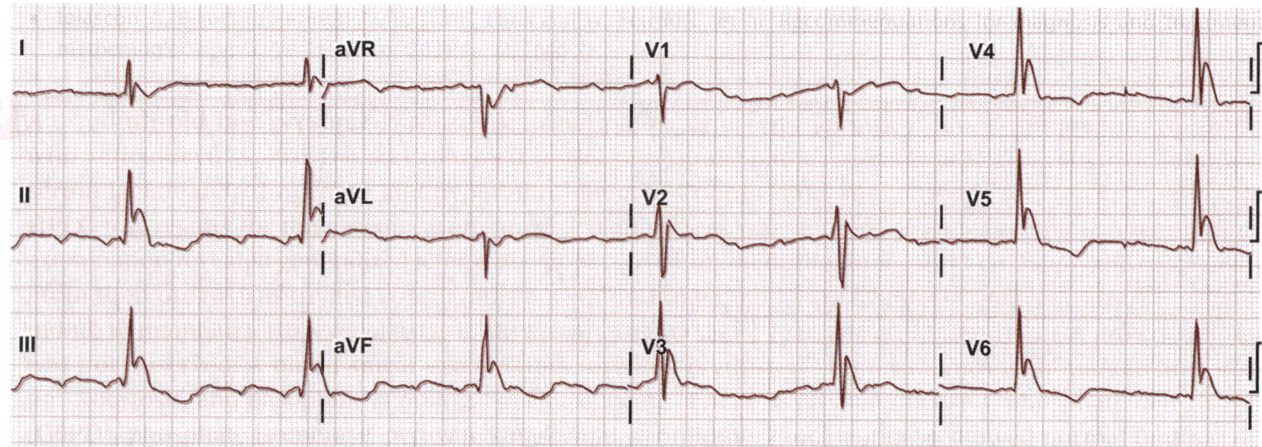

Source: Forlemu AN, Sarma H, Khatib M. A rare case of hypothermia-induced ST segment elevation. Cureus. 2021;13(7):e16365. doi: 10.7759/cureus.16365. PMID: 34395142; PMCID: PMC8360314.

A. Hypothermia
B. Hypokalemia
C. Hyperthyroidism
D. Cardiomyopathy

EXPLANATION

The given ECG dome or hump-shaped wave at the end of the QRS complex has the same polarity as the preceding QRS complex. This is typical of J wave or Osborn wave, which is seen in hypothermia.

Key: A

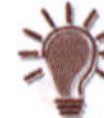

BOOST YOUR KNOWLEDGE

Osborn waves/J waves appear in hypothermic patients at the end of the QRS complex and the beginning of the ST-T wave resulting in QRS notching and ST elevation, which is due to transmural potential gradient. Other J wave syndromes include Brugada pattern and early repolarization pattern. Epsilon wave is another repolarizing wave which occurs in right cardiomyopathy.

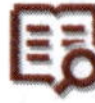

REFERENCE/SOURCE

- Mirvis DM, Goldberger AL. Electrocardiography. In: Libby P, Bonow RO, Mann DL, Tomaselli GF, Bhatt DL, Solomon Scott D, et al. (Eds). Braunwald's Heart Disease: A Textbook of Cardiovascular Medicine, 12th edition. Elsevier; 2022. pp. 141-74.

13. Identify the ECG abnormality.

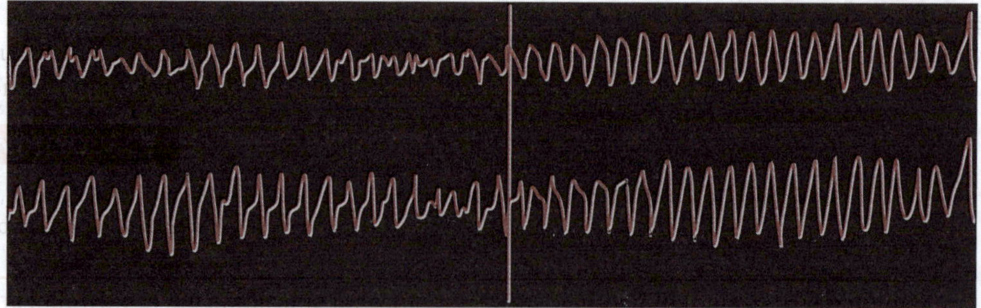

A. Ventricular fibrillation
B. Sine wave pattern
C. AF
D. Torsades de pointes

EXPLANATION

The electrocardiogram shows polymorphic VT with characteristic twisting of the QRS complex around the isoelectric baseline. It is always initiated by a specific electrical ventricular complex. It continues with progressive, regular, and successive inversions of the trace and ends spontaneously after a ventricular pause. This uncommon form of polymorphic VT is called Torsades de pointes (TDP). Ventricular fibrillation appears as continuous oscillations resembling a fine tremor, and amplitude varies progressively to form bulges. A sine wave pattern is seen in hyperkalemia.

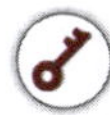

Key: D

BOOST YOUR KNOWLEDGE

Torsades de pointes episodes are paradoxical and terminate spontaneously. Longer episodes may progress to ventricular fibrillation and cause rapid hemodynamic compromise and sudden cardiac death. This tachycardia is unique as it may respond to treatment with isoproterenol or magnesium. It commonly occurs in Brugada syndrome or LQTS. Sometimes, it may be associated with myocardial ischemia, myocarditis, hypokalemia, hypomagnesemia, hypothyroidism, hyperparathyroidism, and pheochromocytoma.

REFERENCE/SOURCE

- Shaddy RE, Penny DJ, Feltes TF, Cetta F, Mital S (Eds). Moss and Adams' Heart Disease in Infants, Children and Adolescents (Chapter 22), 10th edition. Wolters Kluwer; 2021.

14. Which of the following features is *not* favoring the ECG abnormality shown here?

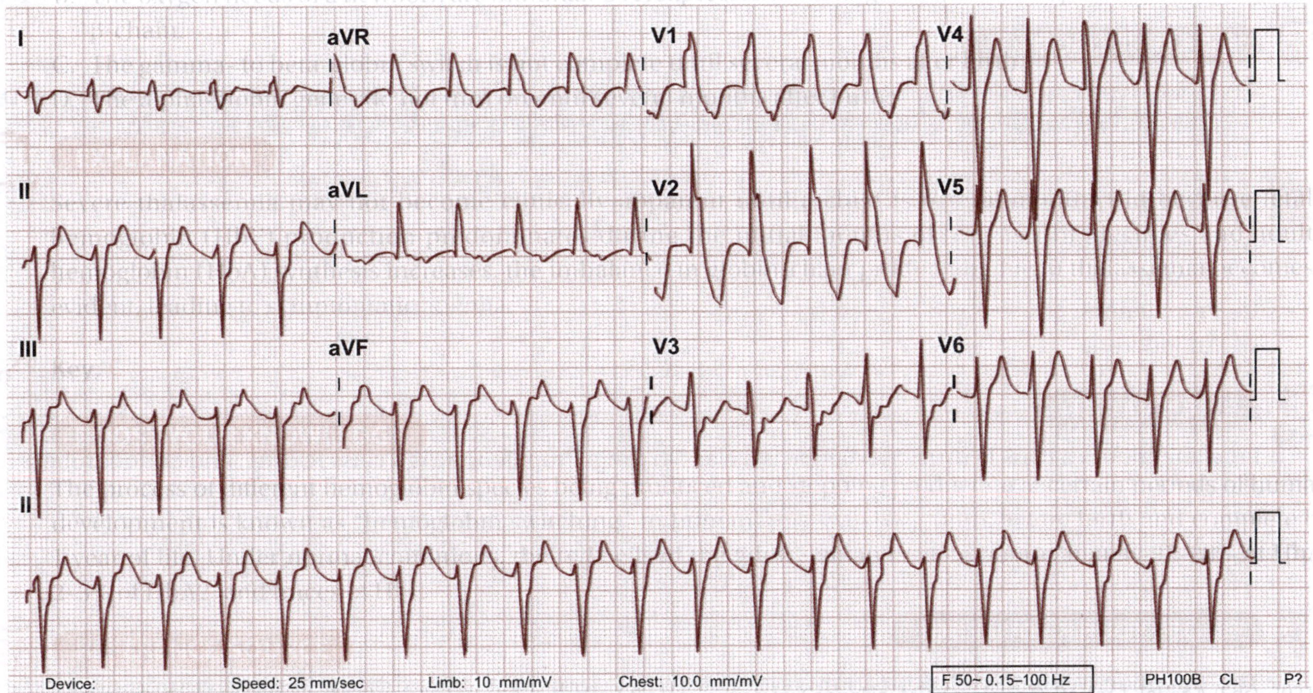

A. Irregularly irregular rhythm

B. QRS >140 m/sec

C. Northwest axis

D. AV dissociation

EXPLANATION

The ECG shows regular, wide complex tachycardia. Other findings seen are the superior axis, AV dissociation, and right bundle branch block (RBBB) pattern. These features are suggestive of monomorphic VT. Irregularly irregular rhythm favors SVT with aberrancy.

Key: A

BOOST YOUR KNOWLEDGE

The following Brugada algorithm is used to differentiate VT from SVT.

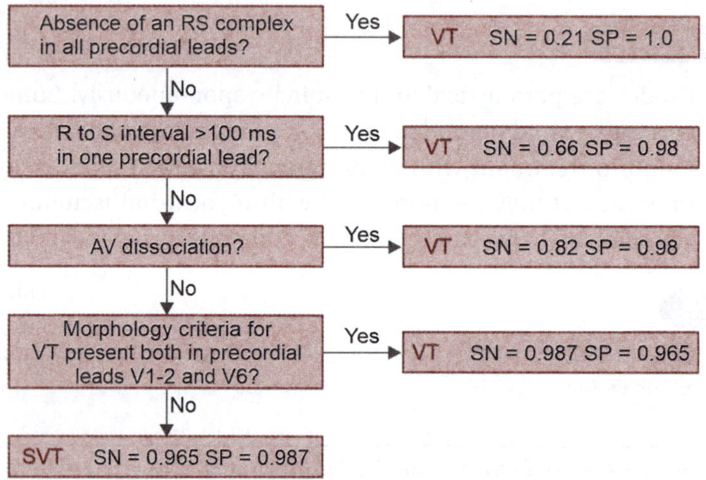

REFERENCE/SOURCE

- Stevenson WG, Zeppenfeld K. Ventricular arrhythmias. In: Libby P, Bonow RO, Mann DL, Tomaselli GF, Bhatt DL, Solomon Scott D, et al. (Eds). Braunwald's Heart Disease: A Textbook of Cardiovascular Medicine, 12th edition. Elsevier; 2022. pp. 1288-311.

15. Which of the following is a class Ic antiarrhythmic drug?

A. Procainamide
B. Mexiletine
C. Propafenone
D. Amiodarone

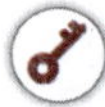

EXPLANATION

Procainamide is a class Ia drug. Mexiletine is a class Ib drug. Propafenone is a class Ic drug, and amiodarone is a class III drug.

Key: C

BOOST YOUR KNOWLEDGE

The Vaughan William's classification system was developed for categorizing antiarrhythmic drugs. This classification is based on the mechanism of action. They affect the cardiac cell membrane and the cardiac action potential. These changes will subsequently change the conduction velocity, refractoriness, and automaticity.

Class	*Actions*	*Drugs*
I	*Sodium channel blockade*	
IA	Prolong repolarization	Quinidine, procainamide, and disopyramide
IB	Shorten repolarization	Lidocaine, mexiletine, tocainide, and phenytoin
IC	Little effect on repolarization	Flecainide, encainide, and propafenone
II	*Beta-adrenergic blockade*	*Propanolol and esmolol*
III	*Prolong repolarization potassium channel blockade*	*Sotalol and amiodarone*
IV	*Calcium channel blockade*	*Verapamil and diltiazem*

REFERENCE/SOURCE

- Shaddy RE, Penny DJ, Feltes TF, Cetta F, Mital S (Eds). Moss and Adams' Heart Disease in Infants, Children and Adolescents (Chapter 22), 10th edition. Wolters Kluwer; 2021.

16. Which of the following is a long RP tachycardia?

A. Sinus tachycardia
B. Atrial flutter
C. Fascicular VT
D. Atrioventricular nodal reentrant tachycardia (AVNRT) with block

EXPLANATION

Sinus tachycardia, atrial flutter, AVNRT with block, and fascicular VT are regular narrow complex tachycardias. These are classified based on atrial rate (A) and ventricular rate (V). A > V tachycardias are atrial flutter, AVNRT with block, and focal AT. V > A tachycardias are junctional ectopic tachycardia (JET), fascicular VT, concealed nodofascicular AP, and AVNRT with block to A. A = V are the most common tachycardias.

Key: A

BOOST YOUR KNOWLEDGE

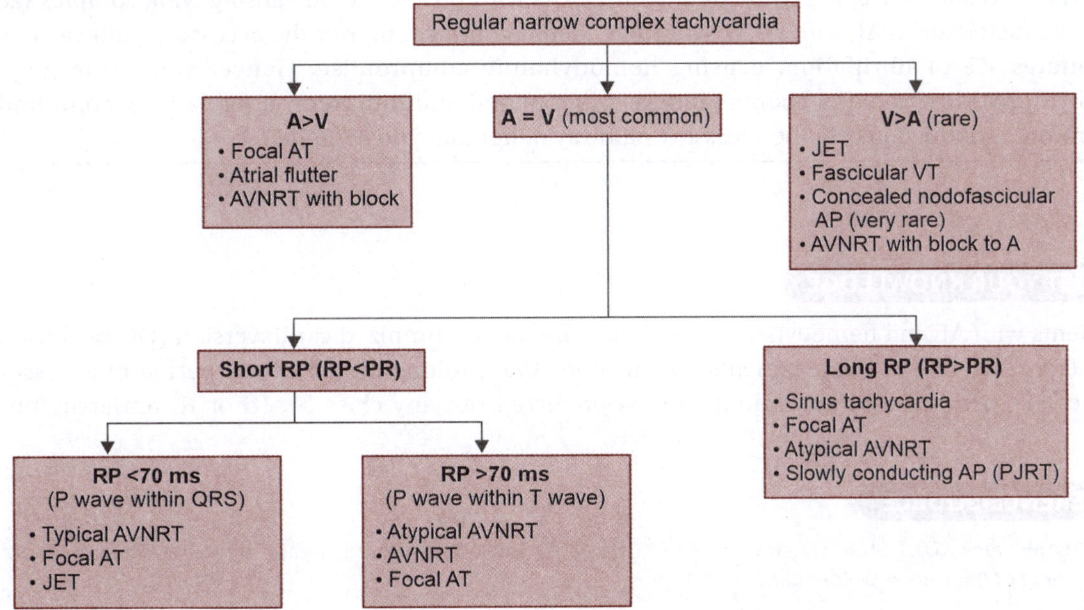

REFERENCE/SOURCE

- Kalman JM, Sanders P. Supraventricular tachycardias. In: Libby P, Bonow RO, Mann DL, Tomaselli GF, Bhatt DL, Solomon Scott D, et al. (Eds). Braunwald's Heart Disease: A Textbook of Cardiovascular Medicine, 12th edition. Elsevier; 2022. pp. 1245-71.

17. Which of the following drugs should not be given in the condition characterized by this ECG?

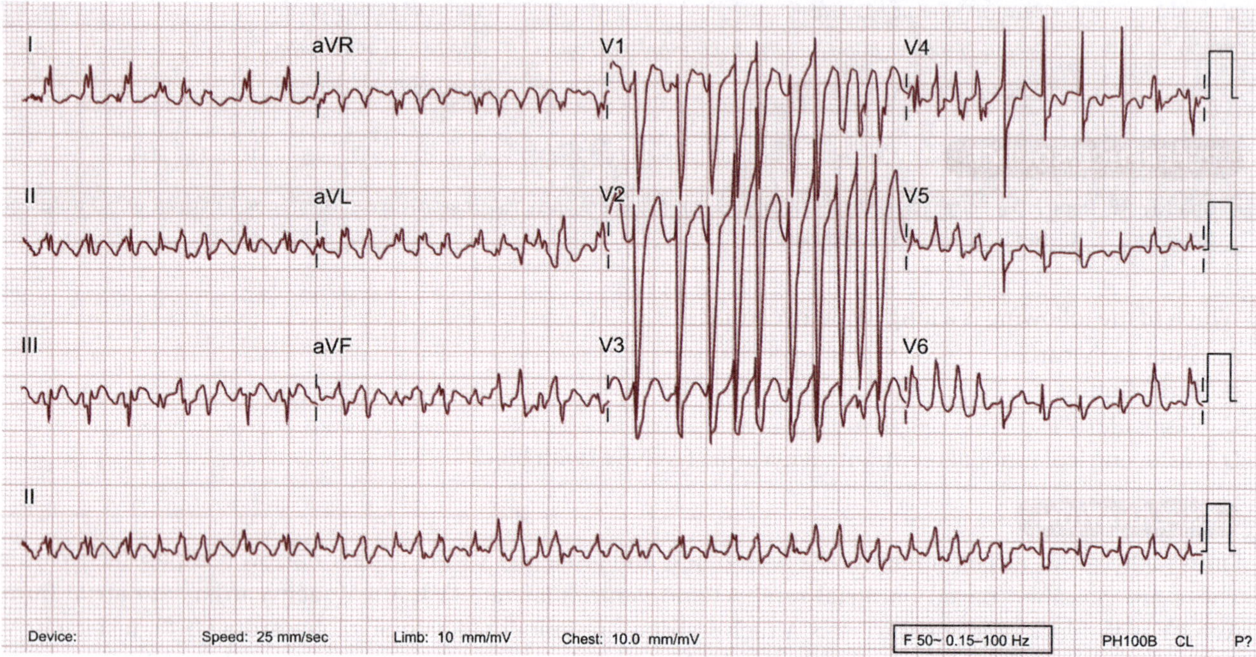

A. Beta blockers
B. Procainamide
C. Digoxin
D. Amiodarone

EXPLANATION

The given ECG shows irregularly irregular tachycardia with pre-excitation causing wide complex tachycardia. This is characteristic of AF with WPW syndrome. Rapid conduction, over the accessory pathway to ventricles, precipitates VT or fibrillation, causing hemodynamic compromise. Hence, adenosine, digoxin, and nondihydropyridine calcium channel blockers (verapamil and diltiazem) are relatively contraindicated as they promote conduction over the accessory pathway rather than the AV node.

Key: C

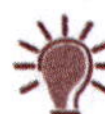

BOOST YOUR KNOWLEDGE

In patients with AF and hemodynamic instability, urgent synchronized cardioversion (DC cardioversion) is the treatment of choice. In stable patients, medications that prolong the refractory period of accessory pathway are used. IV procainamide or amiodarone is preferred but any class IA, IC or III antiarrhythmics can be used.

REFERENCE/SOURCE

- Shaddy RE, Penny DJ, Feltes TF, Cetta F, Mital S (Eds). Moss and Adams' Heart Disease in Infants, Children and Adolescents (Chapter 22), 10th edition. Wolters Kluwer; 2021.

18. What is the generic code of pacing for pacemaker which paces, senses both atria and ventricles, and has triggered and inhibitory responses with rate modulation?

A. DDD
B. DDDR
C. AAIR
D. VVIR

EXPLANATION

NASPE/BPEG generic code for bradycardia pacing depends on the chambers paced, chambers sensed, response to sensing, and rate modulation.

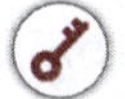

Key: B

BOOST YOUR KNOWLEDGE

NASPE/BPEG Generic Code for Bradycardia Pacing:

	Position			
	I	*II*	*III*	*IV*
Category	***Chamber(s) paced***	***Chamber(s) sensed***	***Response to sensing***	***Rate modulation***
	O = None	O = None	O = None	O = None
	A = Atrium	A = Atrium	T = Triggered	R = Rate modulation
	V = Ventricle	V = Ventricle	I = Inhibited	
	D = Dual (A + V)	D = Dual (A + V)	D = Dual (T + I)	
Manufacturers' designation only	S = Single (A or V)	S = Single (A or V)		

REFERENCE/SOURCE

- Chung MK, Daubert JP. Pacemakers and implantable cardioverter-defibrillators. In: Libby P, Bonow RO, Mann DL, Tomaselli GF, Bhatt DL, Solomon Scott D, et al. (Eds). Braunwald's Heart Disease: A Textbook of Cardiovascular Medicine, 12th edition. Elsevier; 2022. pp. 1321-48.

19. Which of the following beta blockers is avoided in lactating mother?

A. Metoprolol
B. Labetalol
C. Propranolol
D. Atenolol

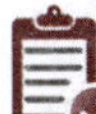

EXPLANATION

Drugs that are considered safe during pregnancy are: Metoprolol, propranolol, labetalol, bisoprolol, nadolol, and carvedilol.

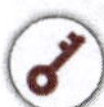

Key: D

BOOST YOUR KNOWLEDGE

Drugs that are considered contraindicated during pregnancy are: Atenolol, amiodarone, and ivabradine.

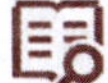

REFERENCE/SOURCE

- Siu SC, Silversides CK. Pregnancy and heart disease. In: Libby P, Bonow RO, Mann DL, Tomaselli GF, Bhatt DL, Solomon Scott D, et al (Eds). Braunwald's Heart Disease: A Textbook of Cardiovascular Medicine, 12th edition. Elsevier; 2022. pp. 1723-42.

CHAPTER

20.7 Cardiac Dysrhythmias

Mily Ray

1. What is the normal resting heart rate (beats/min) of a child aged 1 year?

A. 60–120
B. 90–150
C. 120–160
D. 75–135

EXPLANATION

Heart rate (beats/min)		
Age	***Awake***	***Asleep***
Neonate (<28 days)	100–205	90–160
Infant (1–12 months)	100–190	
Toddler (1–2 years)	98–140	80–120
Preschool (3–5 years)	80–120	65–100
School-age (6–11 years)	75–118	58–90
Adolescent (12–15 years)	60–100	50–90

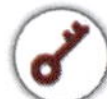

Key: B

BOOST YOUR KNOWLEDGE

Pediatric Vital Signs Reference Chart				
Heart rate (beats/min)			***Respiratory rate (breaths/min)***	
Age	***Awake***	***Asleep***	***Age***	***Normal***
Neonate (<28 days)	100–205	90–160	Infant (<1 year)	30–53
Infant (1–12 months)	100–190			
Toddler (1–2 years)	98–140	80–120	Toddler (1–2 years)	22–37
Preschool (3–5 years)	80–120	65–100	Preschool (3–5 years)	20–28
School-age (6–11 years)	75–118	58–90	School-age (6–11 years)	18–25
Adolescent (12–15 years)	60–100	50–90	Adolescent (12–15 years)	12–20

Source: PALS Guidelines, 2015

Contd...

Contd...

Blood Pressure (mm Hg)				
Age		***Systolic***	***Diastolic***	***Systolic hypotension***
Birth (12 hours)	<1 kg	39–59	16–36	<40–50
	3 kg	60–76	31–45	<50
Neonate (96 hours)		67–84	35–53	<60
Infant (1–12 months)		72–104	37–56	<70
Toddler (1–2 years)		86–106	42–63	<70 + (age in years × 2)
Preschool (3–5 years)		89–112	46–72	
School-age (6–9 years)		97–115	57–76	
Preadolescent (10–11 years)		102–120	61–80	<90
Adolescent (12–15 years)		110–131	64–83	

Source: PALS Guidelines, 2015
For diagnosis of hypertension, refer to the 2017 AAP guidelines Tables 4 and 5
http://pediatrics.aappublications org/content/early2017708/21/peds.2017–1904.

Temperature (°C)	
Method	***Normal***
Rectal	36.6–38.0
Tympanic	35.8–38.0
Oral	35.5–37.5
Axillary	36.5–37.5

Ranges do not vary with age.
Screening: Axillary, temporal, and tympanic (↓ accuracy)
Definitive: Rectal and oral (↑ reflection of core temperature)
Source: CPS Position Statement on Temperature Measurement in Pediatrics (2015)

Oxygen saturation (SpO_2)

SpO_2 is lower in the immediate newborn period. Beyond this period, a SpO_2 of *<90–92%* may suggest a *respiratory condition* or *cyanotic heart disease.*

REFERENCE/SOURCE

- Dr Chris Novak and Dr Peter Gill for www.pedscases.com (Edited March 2020 by Richard He).

2. What is the characteristic of abnormal rhythms originating in the atrium?

A. P waves have abnormal configuration, caused by an inverted P or different number of P waves per QRS complex
B. QRS complexes are usually of normal shape and narrow
C. ST segment is elevated
D. Presence of tall T waves

EXPLANATION

If the P wave has a different shape and size from the typical sinus rhythm, it is termed ectopic, meaning coming from somewhere other than the sinus node. Examples of ectopic atrial rhythms are multifocal atrial tachycardia and junctional rhythms in which P waves are not of sinus morphology.

Key: A

BOOST YOUR KNOWLEDGE

Determining Rhythm

Sinus rhythm refers to the origination of the electrical activity coming from the sinus node. This results in an upright P wave in lead II on the electrocardiogram (ECG).

If there is a P wave before every QRS complex, and it has a sinus morphology, then it is called normal sinus rhythm, or NSR. A sinus morphology is an upright P wave in lead II and a biphasic (up and down) P wave in lead V1 as in the first ECG strip. The second ECG strip below shows an ectopic atrial rhythm. Note that the P wave is down in lead II and only up (not biphasic) in lead V1.

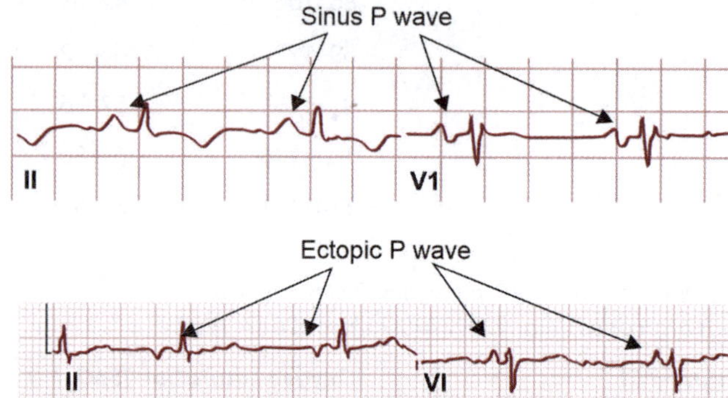

REFERENCE/SOURCE

- ECG Tutorial: Basic principles of ECG analysis—UpToDate.

3. What is the characteristic of abnormal rhythms originating in the ventricle?

A. P waves have an abnormal configuration, caused by an inverted P or a different number of P waves per QRS complex.
B. QRS are broad and wide complex and bizarre.
C. ST segment is elevated.
D. Presence of tall T waves

EXPLANATION

When a rhythm originates from within the ventricles, it is termed a ventricular rhythm.

Since ectopic electrical activity does not pass through the normal conduction system, it can only slowly depolarize the myocardium, leading to a broad QRS (>120 ms). This helps us differentiate it from a supraventricular rhythm, which is essentially a narrow complex.

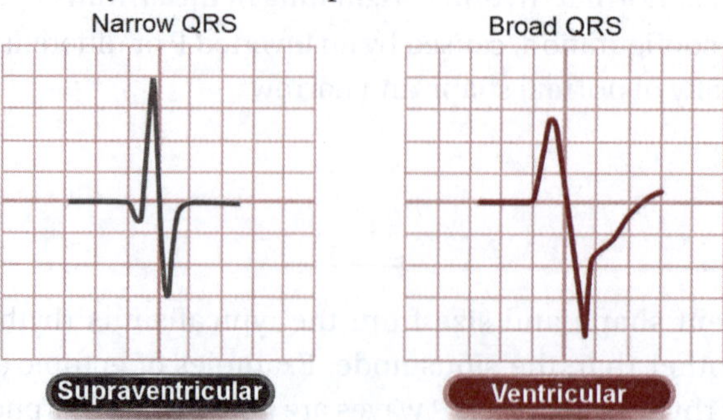

Key: B

BOOST YOUR KNOWLEDGE

Why the Ventricular Rhythm?

Ventricular rhythm may arise as an escape rhythm due to the failure of propagation of electrical activity from the atria to the ventricles.

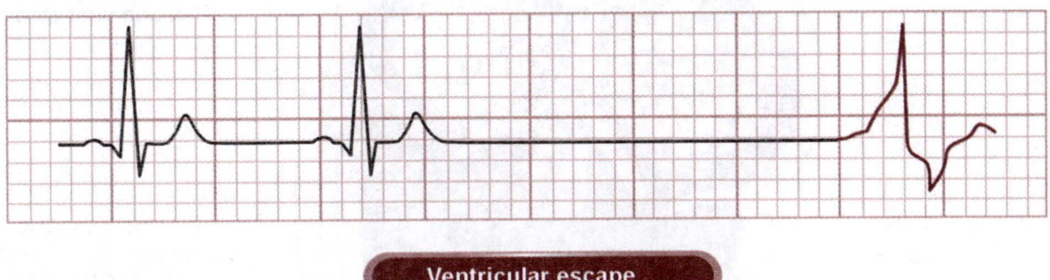

Ventricular escape

REFERENCE/SOURCE

- Rate & rhythm. [online] Available from https://app.pulsenotes.com/clinical/ecgs/notes/2-rate-rhythm [Last accessed July, 2024].

4. Which of the following ions is required for rhythm origination and propagation in the heart?

A. Na^+ B. Ca^+
C. K^+ D. All of the above

EXPLANATION

For cardiac cells to propagate action potentials, they need an electrochemical potential gradient across cellular membranes. Ions, mainly sodium (Na^+), potassium (K^+), and calcium (Ca^{2+}), are present in different concentrations inside the cells and surrounding environments.

Key: D

BOOST YOUR KNOWLEDGE

The sinoatrial (SA) node contains the most excitable cells in the heart so the pacemaker. They have an unstable resting membrane potential that spontaneously depolarizes. This is caused by the Na^+ current and a decrease in the conductance K^+ channel. On reaching a threshold of about –55 mV, an action potential starts which also requires the Ca ion. The slope of the pacemaker potential and the resting membrane potential determine the time necessary to reach the threshold: The sooner the threshold is reached, the sooner an action potential is fired and the faster the heart rate.

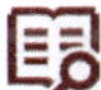

REFERENCE/SOURCE

- The cardiac action potential. In: Feher J (Ed). Quantitative Human Physiology. Elsevier; 2012.

5. What are the steps in the cardiac conduction pathway?

A. Sinoatrial node → Bundle of His → Atrioventricular node → Purkinje fibers
B. Sinoatrial node → Atrioventricular node → Bundle of His → Purkinje fibers
C. Sinoatrial node → Purkinje fibers → Atrioventricular node → Bundle of His
D. Atrioventricular node → Sinoatrial node → Purkinje fibers → Bundle of His

EXPLANATION

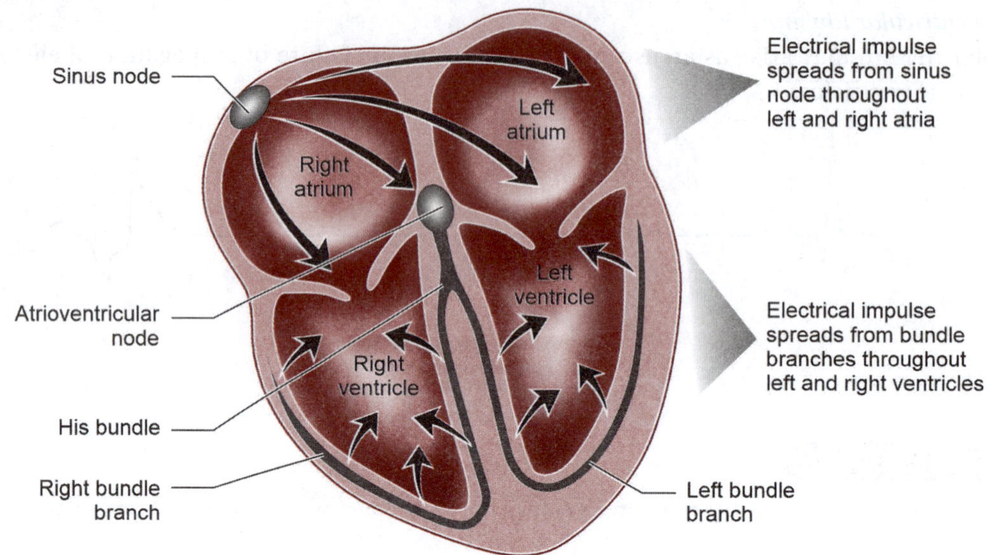

The proper order is (A) SA node → AV node → Bundle of His → Purkinje fibers. The SA node is the heart rate-determining structure, because it is the fastest self-depolarizing set of cells in the heart.

Key: B

BOOST YOUR KNOWLEDGE

The electrical signals, or impulses, of the heart are generated by a clump of specialized tissue called the sinus node. Each time the sinus node generates a new electrical impulse, it spreads across the two atria, stimulating them to contract and pumping blood into the right and left ventricles, in a coordinated way.

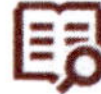

REFERENCE/SOURCE

- Park DS, Fishman GI. Development and function of the cardiac conduction system in health and disease. J Cardiovasc Dev Dis. 2017;4(2):7.

6. Which of the following is known as the gatekeeper of the heart?

A. SA node
B. AV node
C. Bundle of His
D. Purkinje fibers

EXPLANATION

The AV node, which is located at the AV junction of the heart, acts as a gatekeeper and briefly delays the impulses coming from the SA node, which allows the atria to contract completely and empty all of the blood into the ventricles.

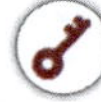

Key: B

BOOST YOUR KNOWLEDGE

The atrioventricular node (AVN) is made up of several compartments that transmit electrical stimulus from the atria to the ventricles via the fast or slow pathways. These varied electrophysiological characteristics of the fast and slow pathways stem from their unique structural and molecular composition (tissue and cellular geometry, ion channels, and gap junctions.

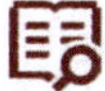

REFERENCE/SOURCE

- George SA, Faye NR, Murillo-Berlioz A, Lee KB, Trachiotis GD, Efimov IR. Trachiotis GD, Efimov IR. At the atrioventricular crossroads: dual pathway electrophysiology in the atrioventricular node and its underlying heterogeneities. Arrhythm Electrophysiol Rev. 2017;6(4):179-85.

7. What is the recurrence rate for pregnancies following the birth of a child with a complete heart block (CHB)?

A. 1%
B. 5%
C. 0%
D. 15%

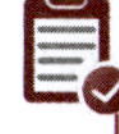

EXPLANATION

Outcome	*Percentage of pregnancies*
Healthy	73%
CHB	16%
Fetal demise	2%
Neonatal death	2%

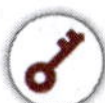

Key: D

BOOST YOUR KNOWLEDGE

Neonatal lupus is due to passively acquired autoimmunity of transplacental passage of maternal immunoglobulin G (IgG) autoantibodies to SSA/Ro and/or SSB/La intracellular ribonuclear proteins. The mother may have systemic lupus erythematosus (SLE) or Sjögren's syndrome or maybe asymptomatic herself. Maternal antibodies that begin crossing the placenta as early as 11 weeks of gestation are associated with the development of cardiac abnormalities, rash, and/or various liver and blood cell abnormalities in the newborn. Skin, liver, and blood cells are regenerative and, as such, the effect of passively acquired antibodies on these systems disappears with the clearance of the antibodies in the 6th to 8th month of postnatal life. But this does not happen in the heart, so the permanent reversal of third-degree CHB is not there.

REFERENCE/SOURCE

- Capone C, Buyon JP, Friedman DM, Frishman WH. Cardiac manifestations of neonatal lupus: a review of autoantibody-associated congenital heart block and its impact in an adult population. Cardiol Rev. 2012;20(2):72-6.

8. A term baby had a normal vaginal delivery, cried well soon after birth, and the Apgar score was 8 at both 1 and 5 minutes after birth. The amniotic fluid was clear. The birth body weight was 2,615 g. He was admitted to the neonatal intensive care unit for bradycardia (heart rate: 75 beats/min), but the pulse volume was normal, and no hypotension was detected (blood pressure: 70/29 mm Hg). The peripheral saturation was 97% in room air. Echocardiography showed a normal heart structure with a normal left ventricular (LV) systolic function.

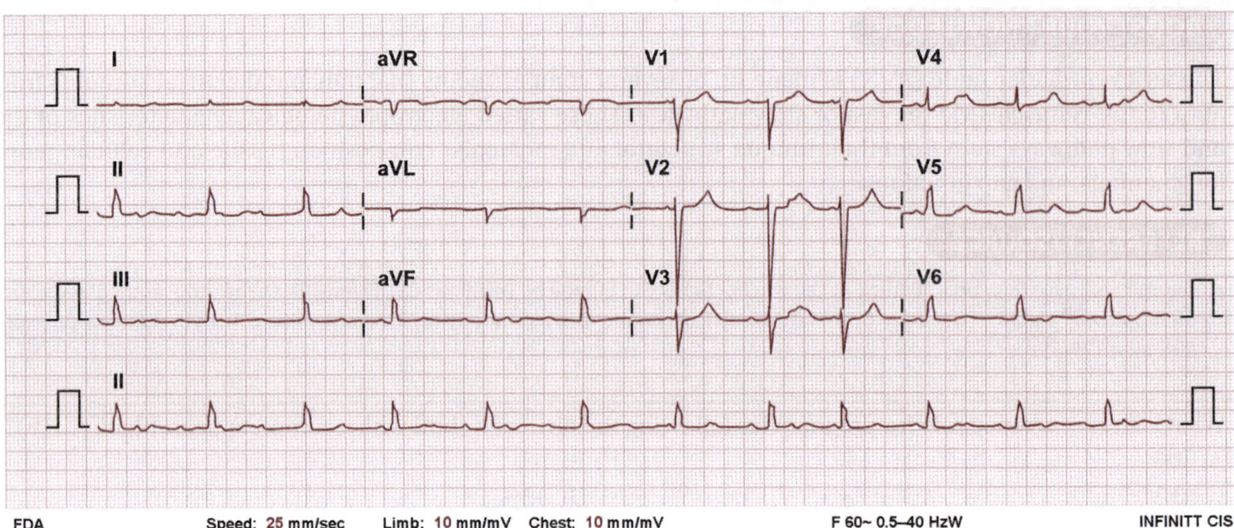

What should be done now?

A. Permanent pacemaker implantation
B. Medications like salbutamol and terbutaline
C. Steroids
D. Wait and watch with a close follow-up

EXPLANATION

The above ECG is that of complete heart block with a ventricular rate of 75 beats/min. With the term baby without any congenital heart defects, the cut-off value of HR is 55 beats/min for any kind of intervention. Meanwhile, continue to follow-up closely with serial ECGs and signs of congestive heart failure (CHF).

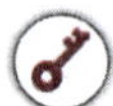

Key: D

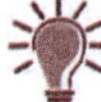

BOOST YOUR KNOWLEDGE

Isolated Congenital Complete Atrioventricular Block:

COR	Recommendations isolated congenital complete atrioventricular block
I	Permanent pacemaker implantation is indicated for patients with congenital complete atrioventricular block (CCAVB) with symptomatic bradycardia
I	Permanent pacemaker implantation is indicated for patients with CCAVB with a wide QRS escape rhythm, complex ventricular ectopy, or ventricular dysfunction
I	Permanent pacemaker implantation is indicated for CCAVB in asymptomatic neonates or infants when the mean ventricular rate is <50 beats/min. Ventricular rate alone should not be used as implant criteria, as symptoms due to low cardiac output may occur at faster heart rates
IIa	Permanent pacemaker implantation is reasonable for asymptomatic CCAVB beyond the first year of life when the mean ventricular rate is <50 beats/min or there are prolonged pauses in ventricular rate

REFERENCES/SOURCES

- Martin TA. Congenital heart block: current thoughts on management, morphologic spectrum, and role of intervention. Cardiol Young. 2014;24(Suppl S2):41-6.
- Silka MJ, Shah MJ, Silva JN, Balaji S, Beach CM, Benjamin MN, et al. 2021 PACES expert consensus statement on the indications and management of cardiovascular implantable electronic devices in pediatric patients: Executive summary. Ann Pediatr Cardiol. 2022;15(3):323-46.

9. A 15-year-old boy complains of palpitations. Most episodes developed when exercising. During the episodes, he experienced dizziness, rapid heartbeats, heavy sweating, and intense fear. Otherwise, he reported hardly any physical complaints. During one of these episodes, the 12-lead ECG revealed the following. What is the diagnosis?

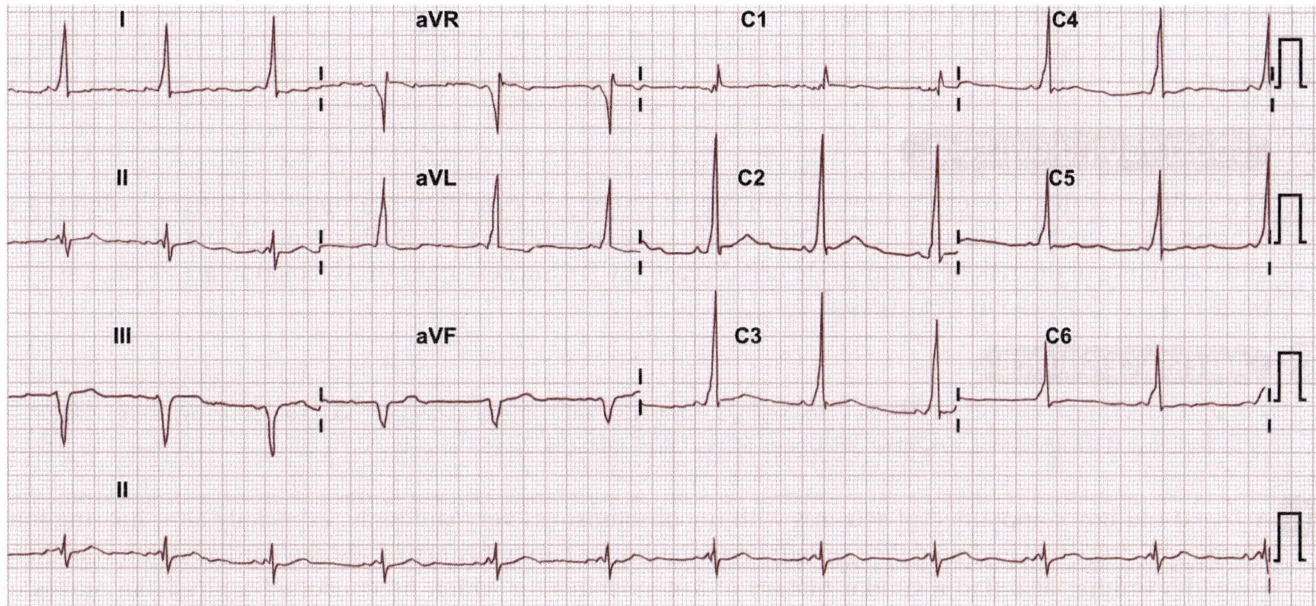

A. Long QT syndrome
B. Wolff-Parkinson-White (WPW) syndrome
C. Heart block
D. Ventricular tachycardia

EXPLANATION

Wolff-Parkinson-White syndrome or preexcitation may not always be evident on ECG, potentially obscuring the presence of an aberrant pathway (AP). This young patient is experiencing hemodynamically significant episodes. The prevalence of preexcitation on ECG is reported to range from 0.1% to 0.3%. Sometimes the patient remains asymptomatic. So, it is always better to do a Holter monitoring.

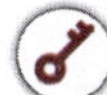

Key: B

BOOST YOUR KNOWLEDGE

Preexcitation of the ventricle may also, on rare occasions, lead to the development of dilated cardiomyopathy secondary to dyssynchronous ventricular contraction.

Between 15% and 25% of asymptomatic patients will go on to develop reentrant supraventricular tachycardias (SVTs). The patients that are asymptomatic may be termed "WPW pattern." The presence of an AP is also associated with the development of atrial fibrillation (AF) in later life.

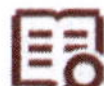

REFERENCE/SOURCE

- Chubb H, Ceresnak SR. A proposed approach to the asymptomatic pediatric patient with Wolff-Parkinson-White pattern. HeartRhythm Case Rep. 2020;6(1):2-7.

10. What should be the next course of action for the patient mentioned in Question 9?

A. Start beta blockers
B. Insert implantable cardioverter-defibrillator (ICD)
C. Perform electrophysiological study
D. Wait and watch

EXPLANATION

Firstly, the presence of AP has to be confirmed by electrophysiology (EP) studies. Only then a diagnosis of WPW can be made. Medical therapy for WPW syndrome, targeting the AV node, AP, or both, includes antiarrhythmics like B-blockers, flecainide, and amiodarone. Radiofrequency ablation is the treatment of choice. Absolute contraindication is digoxin and verapamil.

Key: C

BOOST YOUR KNOWLEDGE

The children with accessory pathways with robust antegrade conduction properties, generally defined as shortest preexcited R-R interval in AF (SPERRI-AF) <250 ms, ablation is usually necessary based upon current understanding of the risk of future sickle cell disease (SCD). Success rates of AP ablation are as high as 95%, while recurrence is seen in <5% of cases.

REFERENCE/SOURCE

- Garg J, Shah N, Krishnamoorthy P, Mehta K, Bozorgnia B, Boyle NG, et al. Catheter ablation of accessory pathway: 14-year trends in utilization and complications in adults in the United States. Int J Cardiol. 2017;248:196-200.

11. A 7-year-old boy complained of seizures with unconsciousness very suddenly, especially after hearing loud noises, i.e., dog's barking, no deficit, mental retardation, or family history of sudden cardiac death was there. His elder brother also had a similar history of 3–4 episodes for which he consulted a physician and is on anticonvulsants. This boy was also started on anticonvulsants, but repeated episodes are still present. What is the boy suffering from? His ECG is shown here.

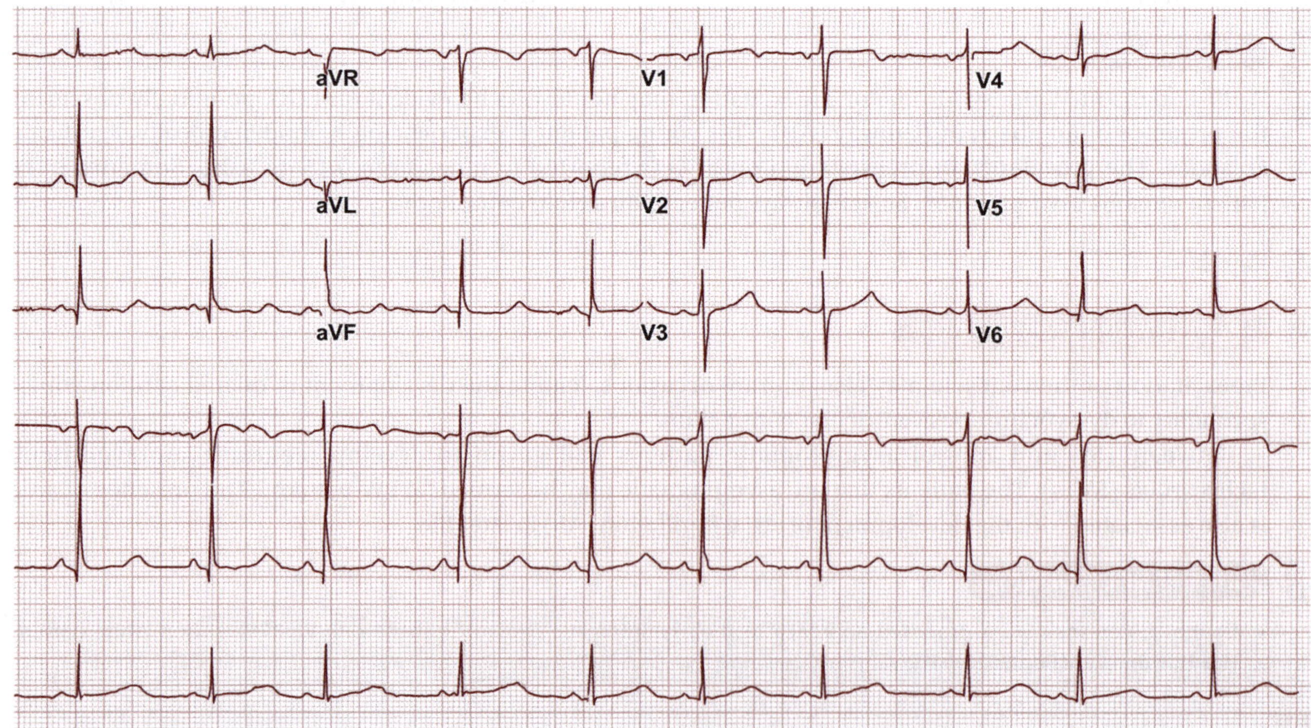

A. Vasovagal attack
B. Epilepsy
C. Long QT syndrome
D. Globus hystericus

EXPLANATION

For males and females below 15 years of age:
- *Normal QT interval:* 0.35–0.44 seconds
- *Borderline QT interval:* 0.44–0.46 seconds
- *Prolonged QT interval:* More than 0.46 seconds

Clinically, it may present with unexplained syncope, seizures, or sudden cardiac arrest preceded by emotion or exercise.

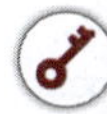

Key: C

BOOST YOUR KNOWLEDGE

Criteria for Long QT syndrome:

Schwartz incorporated clinical and ECG findings in probability-based diagnostic criteria for long QT syndrome. The maximum score is 9, and a score of >3 indicates a high probability of long QT syndrome. The criteria are as follows:

ECG findings (without medications or disorders known to affect ECG features) include the following:
- QT corrected for heart rate (QTc), calculated using Bazett's formula, of >480 ms—3 points
- QTc of 460–470 ms—2 points
- QTc of 450 ms in male patients—1 point
- Torsades de pointes—2 points
- T wave alternans—1 point
- Notched T wave in 3 leads—1 point
- Low heart rate for age—0.5 point

Clinical history includes the following:
- Syncope with stress—2 points
- Syncope without stress—1 point
- Congenital deafness—0.5 point

Family history includes:
- Family member with definite long QT syndrome—1 point
- Unexplained sudden cardiac death (age <30 years) in an immediate family member—0.5 point

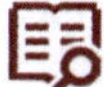

REFERENCE/SOURCE

- Raghavan SS. (2020). Pediatric Long QT Syndrome. [online] Available from https://emedicine.medscape.com/article/891571-overview?form=fpf [Last accessed July, 2024].

12. Which of the following is the most dreaded complication/outcome of long QT syndrome?

A. Seizures
B. Neurological deficit
C. Sudden cardiac death
D. Congestive cardiac failure

EXPLANATION

Some patients (9%) presented with sudden cardiac arrest and no preceding symptoms. So may be prophylactic treatment in asymptomatic children is indicated.

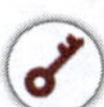

Key: C

BOOST YOUR KNOWLEDGE

The prognosis for patients with long QT syndrome who have been treated with beta blockers and other therapeutic measures is not bad. Fortunately, episodes of torsades de pointes are usually self-terminating in patients with long QT syndrome; only about 4–5% of cardiac events are fatal.

Patients at high risk, e.g., with recurrent cardiac events despite beta-blocker therapy have a markedly increased risk of sudden death. Treat these patients with an ICD.

REFERENCE/SOURCE

- Garson Jr A, Dick 2nd M, Fournier A, Gillette PC, Hamilton R, Kugler JD, et al. The long QT syndrome in children. An international study of 287 patients. Circulation. 1993;87(6):1866–72.

13. Magnesium sulfate belongs to which class of antiarrhythmics and is used in which arrhythmia?

A. Class II; SVT
B. Class I; ventricular tachycardia (VT)
C. Class III; AF
D. Class V; torsades de pointes (TdP)

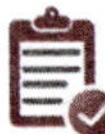

EXPLANATION

Intravenous magnesium sulfate, a relatively new mode of therapy for torsades de pointes, was proven to be extremely effective and is now regarded as the treatment of choice for this arrhythmia.

Key: D

BOOST YOUR KNOWLEDGE

The five main classes in the Vaughan Williams classification of antiarrhythmic agents are:

1. Class I agents interfere with the sodium (Na^+) channel.
2. Class II agents are antisympathetic nervous system agents. Most agents in this class are beta blockers.
3. Class III agents affect potassium (K^+) efflux.
4. Class IV agents affect calcium channels and the AV node.
5. Class V agents work by other or unknown mechanisms.

   Classes I and III are used in rhythm control as medical cardioversion agents, while classes II and IV are used as rate-control agents.

REFERENCE/SOURCE

- Lei M, Wu L, Terrar DA. Modernized classification of cardiac antiarrhythmic drugs. Circulation. 2018;138:1879-96.

14. Adenosine, used intravenously for terminating SVTs, belongs to which class of antiarrhythmics?

A. Class II
B. Class III
C. Class IV
D. Class V

EXPLANATION

The European Society of Cardiology guidelines advocate using vagal maneuvers and adenosine as first-line therapies in diagnosing and treating SVT.

Key: D

BOOST YOUR KNOWLEDGE

Supraventricular tachycardias, which can be successfully terminated with adenosine, include any reentrant arrhythmias that require the AV node for the re-entry, e.g., AV re-entrant tachycardia (AVRT) and AV nodal reentrant tachycardia (AVNRT).

Fast rhythms of the heart that are confined to the atria (e.g., AF and atrial flutter) or ventricles and do not involve the AV node as part of the reentrant circuit, are not typically converted by adenosine. However, the ventricular response rate is temporarily slowed with adenosine in such cases, and it is normal for the heart to enter ventricular asystole for a few seconds. Since the effects of adenosine on AV node-dependent SVTs, adenosine is considered a class 5 antiarrhythmic agent.

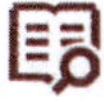

REFERENCE/SOURCE

- Antiarrhythmic agent. [online] Available from https://en.wikipedia.org/wiki/Antiarrhythmic_agent#cite_note-pmid7882485-13 [Last accessed July, 2024].

15. A 12-year-old boy was presented to the emergency department with palpitations and almost a syncopal attack. He had some breathing difficulty. His heart rate was 186 beats/min, had hypotension, and was hemodynamically compromised. The monitor showed arrhythmia, so a 12-lead ECG was done quickly. Identify the rhythm in the ECG.

– Abnormal ECG –

>>> Very high heart rate <<<

12 Lead: Standard placement

Unconfirmed diagnosis

I aVR V1 V4 II aVL V2 V5 III aVF V3 V6 II

Device: 506295 Speed: 25 mm/sec Limb: 10 mm/mV Chest: 10 mm/mV F 50~ 0.15–100 Hz PH100B CL P?

A. Monomorphic ventricular tachycardia
B. Ventricular fibrillation (VF)
C. Torsades de pointes
D. SVT with aberrancy

EXPLANATION

ECG features of monomorphic VT:

- Regular, broad complex tachycardia
- Uniform QRS complexes within each lead that is each QRS is identical

Key: A

BOOST YOUR KNOWLEDGE

Ventricular tachycardia is a broad complex tachycardia originating from the ventricles. There are several different forms of VT—the most common is monomorphic VT.

Clinical significance:

- VT can decrease cardiac output resulting in hypotension and cardiac failure because of very high heart rates and loss of coordinated atrial contraction, resulting or pre-existing poor ventricular function which is the main contributory factor for cardiovascular compromise.
- Decreased cardiac output may result in decreased myocardial perfusion with degeneration into VF.
- Prompt recognition and initiation of treatment (e.g., electrical cardioversion) are required in all cases of VT.

REFERENCE/SOURCE

- Robert B, Burns E. (2023). Ventricular Tachycardia – Monomorphic VT. [online] Available from https://litfl.com/ventricular-tachycardia-monomorphic-ecg-library/ [Last accessed July, 2024].

16. What is the immediate treatment of choice for ventricular tachycardia with hemodynamic compromise?

A. Defibrillation
B. Synchronized direct current cardioversion
C. IV adenosine
D. Magnesium sulfate infusion

EXPLANATION

PALS Tachycardia Initial Management Algorithm

For synchronized cardioversion, begin with an electrical dose of 0.5–1 J/kg of the child's body weight. If ineffective, increase to 2 J/kg. For defibrillation (cardiac arrest with a shockable rhythm), the first shock should be given at 2 J/kg, and the second shock should be given at 4 J/kg. Subsequent shocks may be higher, up to the adult maximum of 10 J/kg body weight.

Key: B

BOOST YOUR KNOWLEDGE

Ventricular tachycardia classification is based on:

- *Clinical presentation:*
  - Hemodynamically stable
  - Hemodynamically unstable, e.g., hypotension, chest pain, cardiac failure, and decreased conscious level

This is the most important classification clinically and influences immediate management.

- *Duration:*
  - Sustained = Duration >30 seconds, or requiring intervention due to hemodynamic compromise
  - Nonsustained = Three or more consecutive ventricular complexes, terminating spontaneously in <30 seconds
- *Morphology:*
  - Monomorphic
  - Polymorphic VT
  - Torsades de pointes (polymorphic with QT prolongation)
  - Right ventricular outflow tract tachycardia
  - Fascicular tachycardia
  - Bidirectional VT
  - Ventricular flutter
  - Ventricular fibrillation (VF)

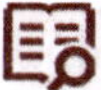

REFERENCES/SOURCES

- https://acls-Algorithms.com>PALS made simple.
- Pellegrini CN, Scheinman MM. Clinical management of ventricular tachycardia. Curr Probl Cardiol. 2010;35(9):453-504.

17. A 7-year-old child has H/o deafness and repeated syncope. He reported to triage as unresponsive. Identify the rhythm in his ECG given here.

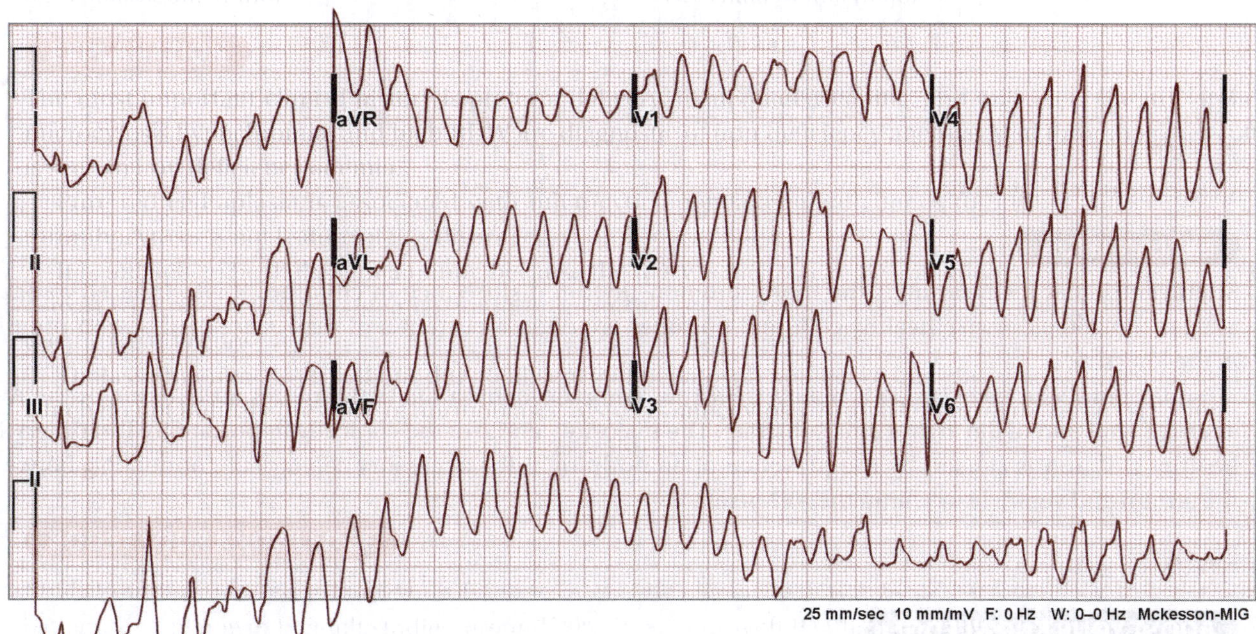

A. Monomorphic ventricular tachycardia
B. Polymorphic ventricular tachycardia (TdP)
C. VF
D. SVT with aberrancy

EXPLANATION

Torsades de pointes is a type of polymorphic ventricular arrhythmia that is characterized by its hallmark "twisting of peaks" waxing and waning QRS amplitude. TdP may terminate spontaneously or degenerate into VF, with the potential to result in sudden cardiac death.

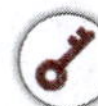

Key: B

BOOST YOUR KNOWLEDGE

Torsades de pointes is a special form of VT in that it shows a cyclic pattern in which the wave heights of the QRS wave in the ECG vary in a progressive and repeating manner to produce an undulating pattern. It may occur in case of prolonged QT interval on the ECG, a slow heart rate, and/or disturbances in blood electrolyte balance. This can be an iatrogenic arrhythmia due to drugs or may be genetic in origin.

REFERENCE/SOURCE

- Torsade de pointes, ventricular fibrillation, and differential diagnosis of wide QRS tachycardias. In: Surawicz B, Knilans T (Eds). Chou's Electrocardiography in Clinical Practice, 6th edition. Elsevier; 2008.

18. A 2-month-old infant had complaints of decreased feeds, incessant crying, and some breathing difficulty. Saturation was 94% with tachycardia (>220/min) with no beat-to-beat variation even on crying. There was no H/o cough or fever in the past few days. Identify the rhythm in the strip.

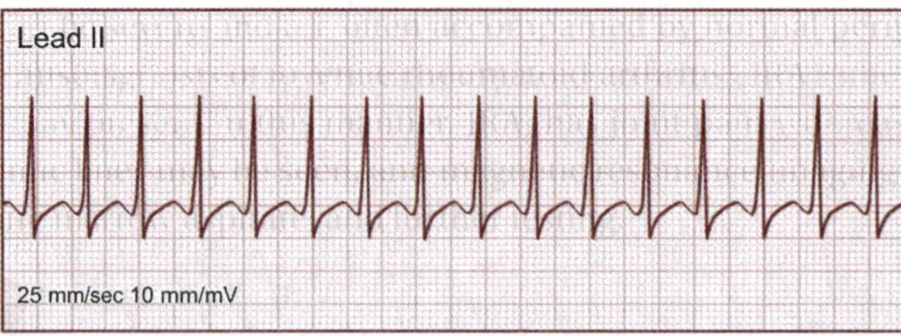

A. SVT
B. AF
C. Ventricular tachycardia
D. VF

EXPLANATION

Supraventricular tachycardia is the most common rhythm disturbance in children. It is estimated to occur almost 1 in 250 otherwise healthy children. Episodes are often recurrent and may cause cardiac compromise in the long run.

Supraventricular tachycardia is mainly a narrow, complex tachycardia that requires atrial tissue or the AVN as an integral part of the arrhythmia substrate. The majority (>90%) of the clinically important SVT in otherwise healthy children is caused by the presence of an additional (or accessory) electrical connection between the atrium and ventricle or within the AVN itself.

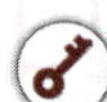

Key: A

BOOST YOUR KNOWLEDGE

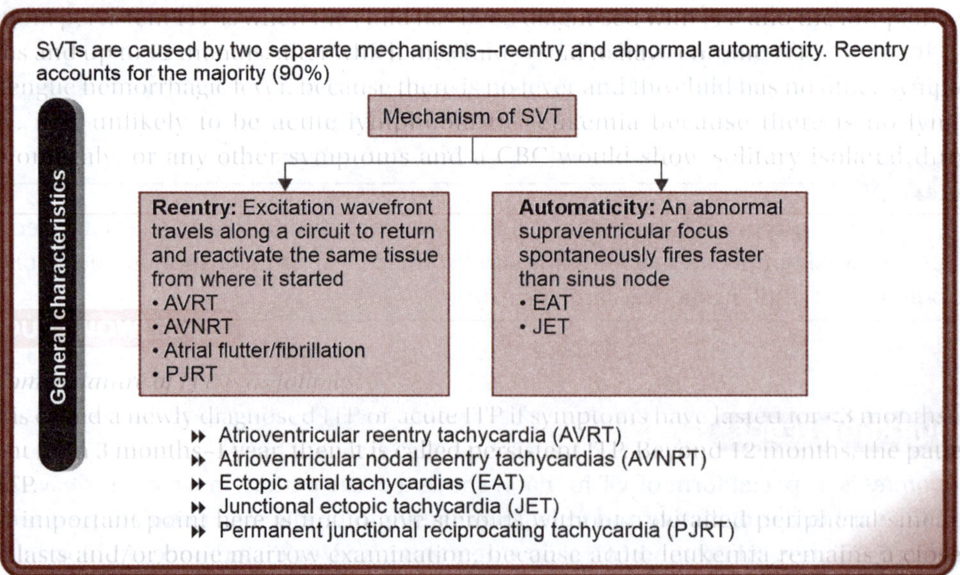

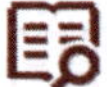

REFERENCES/SOURCES

- Bibas L, Levi M, Essebag V. Diagnosis and management of supraventricular tachycardias. CMAJ. 2016;188(17-18):E466-73.
- Supraventricular tachycardia. In: Chattopadhyay A (Ed). Indian Academy of Pediatrics: Standard Treatment Guidelines; 2022.

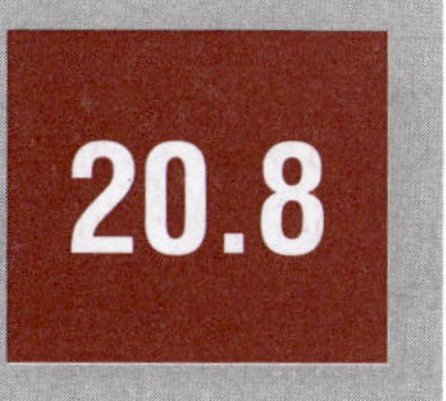

CHAPTER 20.8

Systemic Disorders with Heart Diseases, Genetics in Heart Disease, Surgical Consideration

Mrigank Choubey

1. A 10-year-old boy presented with joint pains involving knees, ankles, and hands of 4 weeks duration, with continuous fever. On examination, he is found to have fever, arthritis, and cardiac friction rub. Which of the following electrocardiogram (ECG) findings is most likely in this child?

A. Prolonged PR interval
B. Diffuse ST-T changes
C. Complete heart block
D. Prolonged QT interval

EXPLANATION

Commonly, joint pain and heart involvement raises suspicion of acute rheumatic fever. However, the presence of small joint involvement is strongly against acute rheumatic fever. The scenario describes a child with polyarticular juvenile idiopathic arthritis (JIA), as indicated by the small joint involvement, with pericarditis.

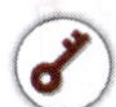

Key: B

BOOST YOUR KNOWLEDGE

The presence of a cardiac friction rub indicates pericarditis, which is the most common cardiac involvement in JIA, with clinical evidence in 7–36% of patients. ECG findings of pericarditis include PR depression, diffuse ST segment elevation and T wave inversion, and electrical alternans in cases of large effusions.

Prolonged PR interval is a feature of acute rheumatic fever. Complete heart block is only rarely seen.

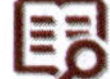

REFERENCES/SOURCES

- ILAR Criteria for JIA. In: Kliegman RM, St Geme III JW (Eds). Nelson Textbook of Pediatrics, 21st edition. Amsterdam: Elsevier; 2019. p. 1160.
- Inflammatory and Immune-Mediated Noninfectious Cardiovascular Diseases. In: Shaddy RE, Penny DJ, Feltes TF, Cetta F, Mittal S, Kailin J (Eds). Moss and Adams' Heart Disease in Infants, Children, and Adolescents Including the Fetus and Young Adult, 10th edition. Philadelphia: Wolters Kluwer Health; 2021. pp. 1373-92.

2. A 6-month-old girl with Down syndrome is admitted with complaints of failure to thrive, suck rest suck cycles, and a history of two hospital admissions at 3 and 4 months of age. During an examination, she is found to have cardiomegaly, S3 gallop, and grade 3/6 pansystolic murmur at the left lower sternal edge. ECG shows extreme left-axis deviation. What is the most likely origin of the murmur?

A. Primum atrial septal defect (ASD)
B. Inlet ventricular septal defect (VSD)
C. Subaortic VSD
D. Regurgitation across the atrioventricular (AV) valve

EXPLANATION

The most common congenital heart disease associated with Down syndrome is complete AV Canal defect, characterized by the presence of large inlet VSD, large primum ASD, and Common AV valve. Since the VSD is usually large, it does not produce a murmur. The most likely origin of the murmur is AV valve regurgitation.

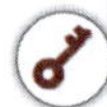

Key: D

BOOST YOUR KNOWLEDGE

Pansystolic murmurs originate due to abnormal blood flow between chambers which have pressure differences right from the isovolumic contraction. Common causes of pansystolic murmurs are: Small VSDs, mitral regurgitation, and tricuspid regurgitation. The other options represent components of AV canal defect but are not the reason for the presence of the murmur. Shunt across Ostium primum ASD does not produce a murmur. Inlet VSDs are large, causing equalization of pressure between LV and right ventricle (RV), and are therefore also silent. Subaortic VSDs are not a component of endocardial cushion defect.

REFERENCE/SOURCE

- Left-to-Right Shunt Lesions. In: Myung KP (Ed). Park's Pediatric Cardiology for Practitioners, 6th edition. Maryland Heights, MO: Mosby; 2014. p. 176.

3. A 2-month-old infant is brought in status epilepticus, responsive to calcium administration. On examination, they found to have elongated facies, almond-shaped eyes, and absent thymus. His saturation of peripheral oxygen (SpO_2) is 85% in all four limbs, has clinical evidence of cardiomegaly, single, loud S2, and election click. What is the most likely underlying heart disease?

A. Truncus arteriosus
B. Tetralogy of Fallot
C. Pulmonary atresia
D. Interrupted aortic arch

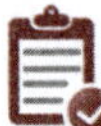

EXPLANATION

The scenario describes velocardiofacial syndrome, with characteristic facies, hypocalcemia, and absent thymus. The most common cyanotic cardiac anomaly with velocardiofacial syndrome is truncus arteriosus. The clinical findings mentioned arise due to a single outflow tract, with pulmonary hypertension and cardiac failure.

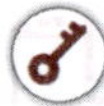

Key: A

BOOST YOUR KNOWLEDGE

Truncus arteriosus is a type of conotruncal defect, in which failure of development of spiral septum in developing fetal heart leads to the development of common outflow for the aortic as well as pulmonary flow. Clinical presentation is characterized by cyanosis soon after birth due to a complete admixture of left and right-sided blood. Cyanosis is mild because of increased pulmonary blood flow. Increased pulmonary blood flow causes left ventricular (LV) diastolic volume overload, causing cardiomegaly. S2 is single due to the presence of a single truncal valve. The truncal valve is commonly abnormal, and the ejection of combined outflow of the left and RV through one valve produces an ejection click.

Newborns with dysmorphism and conotruncal heart defects should be evaluated for the velocardiofacial syndrome.

REFERENCE/SOURCE

- Physical Examination. In: Myung KP (Ed). Park's Pediatric Cardiology for Practitioners, 6th edition. Maryland Heights, MO: Mosby; 2014. p. 9-40.

4. A 6-year-old boy is brought with complaints of episodic rapid regular palpitations, which are sudden in onset and offset, associated with dizziness. There is no history of syncope. A clinical cardiac examination is within normal limits. Which of the following ECG abnormalities is most likely to clinch the diagnosis?

A. Prolonged PR interval
B. Narrow PR interval
C. Complete heart block
D. Long QT

EXPLANATION

The case scenario describes Wolff-Parkinson-White (WPW) syndrome with paroxysmal supraventricular tachycardia. On a resting nontachyarrhythmia ECG, short PR intervals and delta waves are commonly seen. Individuals with first-degree heart block (prolonged PR interval) are usually asymptomatic, and complete heart block presents with syncope (with long pauses), or cardiac failure (slow ventricular escape rate without pauses). Long QT syndrome presents with ventricular tachycardia, with syncope/sudden cardiac death.

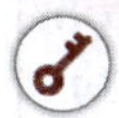

Key: B

BOOST YOUR KNOWLEDGE

During cardiac development, the development of a cardiac fibrous skeleton causes electrical isolation between the atria and the ventricles. Therefore, normally, an impulse generated into the atria cannot directly depolarize the ventricles, except through the AV node, inducing a delay—the PR interval. In WPW syndrome, the persistence of abnormal electrical connections (pathways) between the atria and ventricles leads to direct conduction of the impulse—short PR interval, and relatively slower depolarization of the ventricles (the impulse conducts through the ventricular muscle rather than going through the faster conduction tissue), causing a slow rise of the R wave—delta wave.

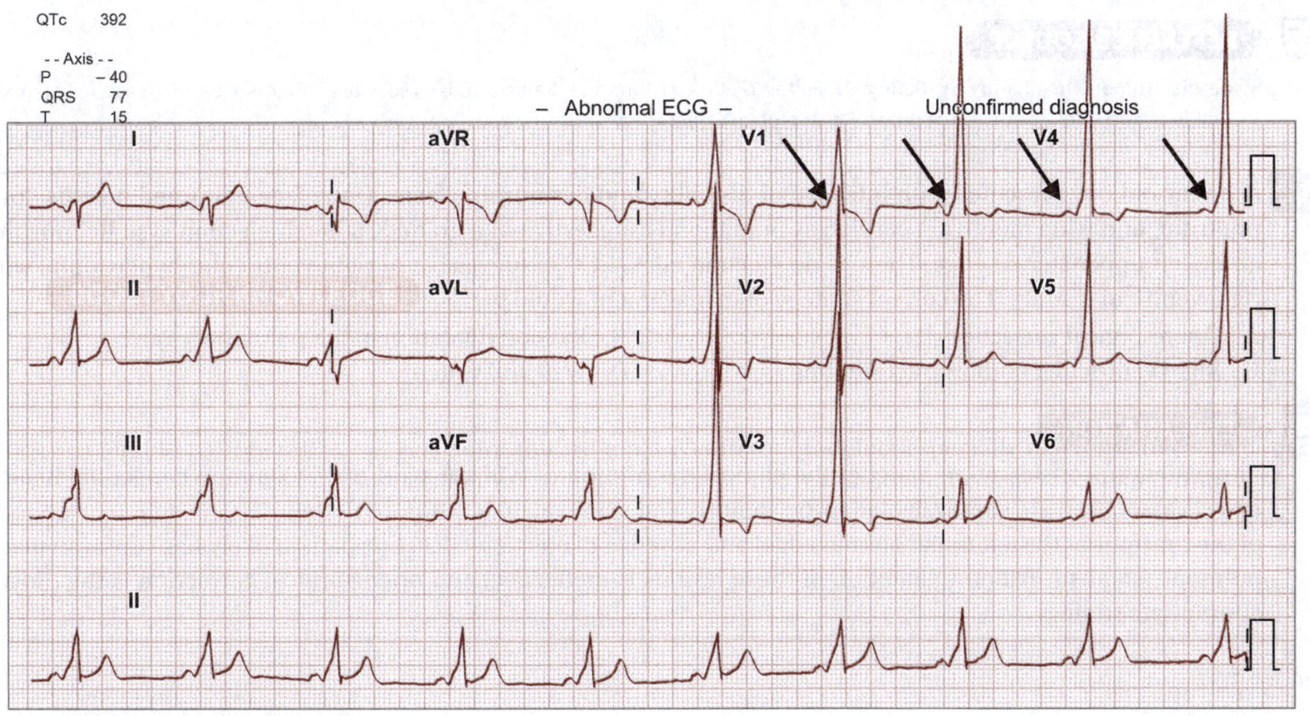

REFERENCE/SOURCE

- Kliegman RM, St Geme III JW (Eds). Nelson Textbook of Pediatrics, 21st edition. Amsterdam: Elsevier; 2019. p. 2254.

5. A newborn has been brought to you for a "second opinion," as she was detected to have "multiple cardiac tumors" on echocardiography, located in the atria as well as ventricles. The child is asymptomatic, and cardiac examination is unremarkable. General examination reveals a lesion characteristic of connective tissue nevus in the axilla. What advice would you have for your parents?

A. The cardiac tumors need intensive follow-up and management due to the high risk of embolization
B. Child needs 3 monthly echocardiography as there is a significant risk of enlargement with obstruction to outflow tracts
C. Surgical excision of the largest tumor, serving as confirmatory tissue diagnosis as well as management
D. 3 monthly follow-up for cardiac tumors with parental reassurance

EXPLANATION

Cardiac rhabdomyomas are the most common cardiac tumors, accounting for about 70% of all cardiac tumors. Diagnosis is suggested by intramyocardial origin, multiple tumors occurring in atria and ventricles, and on examination, other features of Tuberous sclerosis complex. These tumors have a strong tendency to regress on their own with time. As our patient is asymptomatic, and cardiac examination is not suggestive of any obstructive features, the correct strategy is to wait and watch.

Key: D

BOOST YOUR KNOWLEDGE

The management of cardiac rhabdomyoma depends upon the hemodynamic effect of the tumors, including mammalian target of rapamycin (mTOR) inhibitors and surgical resection when the tumors are obstructive or causing refractory arrhythmias.

REFERENCE/SOURCE

- Cardiac tumors. In: Shaddy RE, Penny DJ, Feltes TF, Cetta F, Mittal S, Kailin J (Eds). Moss and Adams' Heart Disease in Infants, Children, and Adolescents, 10th edition. Philadelphia: Wolters Kluwer Health; 2021. pp. 1635-51.

6. A 2-year-old boy presented with intellectual disability and dysmorphic facies (long face, upturned nostrils, long philtrum, and wide mouth). A cardiac examination is suggestive of a grade 3/6 harsh ejection systolic murmur at the left upper sternal edge. There is no ejection click. ECG is suggestive of right ventricular hypertrophy with right ventricular strain. The correct strategy of management would be:

A. Open surgical correction
B. Balloon dilatation of the pulmonary valve
C. Right ventricular outflow tract stenting
D. Wait and watch

EXPLANATION

The patient in consideration matches the clinical description of William syndrome. Common congenital heart defects associated are supravalvular aortic stenosis and supravalvular pulmonary stenosis. Due to the presence of the murmur at the left upper sternal edge, and absence of ejection click, our patient likely has supravalvular pulmonic stenosis. Balloon dilatation of these lesions is ineffective, and open surgical correction is the most appropriate strategy.

Key: A

BOOST YOUR KNOWLEDGE

Valvular aortic or pulmonic stenosis is usually due to commissural fusion of the valve leaflets during valvular development. The valves are therefore bicuspid and offer obstruction to blood flow during systole. Clinically, there is an ejection systolic murmur, with an ejection click (a feature of valvular stenosis). These valves are amenable to balloon dilatation. Balloon dilatation causes mechanical separation of fused commissures, opening the valve. Supravalvular aortic or pulmonary stenosis is fibrous in nature and does not respond to balloon dilatation.

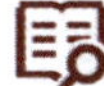

REFERENCE/SOURCE

- Tricuspid Valve Disorders: Atresia, Dysplasia, and Ebstein Anomaly. In: Shaddy RE, Penny DJ, Feltes TF, Cetta F, Mittal S, Kailin J (Eds). Moss and Adams' Heart Disease in Infants, Children, and Adolescents, 10th edition. Philadelphia: Wolters Kluwer Health; 2021. pp. 914-39.

7. All of the following surgeries are done for dextro-transposition of the great arteries (d-TGA) repair, *except*:

A. Senning procedure
B. Nikaidoh procedure
C. Damus–Kaye–Stansel operation
D. Double switch procedure

EXPLANATION

Dextro-transposition of great arteries requires correction in the neonatal age group. The surgery of choice is arterial switch operation, which is done in the neonatal age group if the left ventricle (LV) is adequately prepared. Without treatment, if the patient survives, the LV regresses with age, and an atrial switch (Senning procedure) is performed. Nikaidoh and Damus–Kaye–Stensel procedures are done for patients with d-TGA/VSD/pulmonary stenosis (PS). A double switch procedure is done for congenitally corrected TGA and not d-TGA.

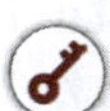

Key: D

BOOST YOUR KNOWLEDGE

In d-TGA, the aorta arises from RV and pulmonary artery (PA) arises from LV. The rest of the anatomic connections are normal. Blood flow in d-TGA is from LA to LV to PA. Systemic veins drain deoxygenated blood to the right atrium (RA), then the RV, and then again to the aorta. LV pumps blood at pulmonary pressures, which are significantly lower than systemic blood pressure. Therefore, the LV regresses. Regression is rather fast, and for patients presenting beyond the first few weeks of life, "LV preparedness" is assessed on echocardiography, by checking the LV posterior wall thickness and LV mass index.

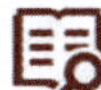

REFERENCE/SOURCE

- Cyanotic Congenital Heart Defects. In: Myung KP (Ed). Park's Pediatric Cardiology for Practitioners, 5th edition. Maryland Heights, MO: Mosby; 2014. p. 206-89.

8. A 2-day-old cyanotic infant with a grade 3/6 ejection systolic murmur is noted to have decreased pulmonary vascular markings on the chest X-ray and left axis deviation on the ECG. The most likely diagnosis is:

A. Tetralogy of Fallot
B. Transposition of great vessels
C. Truncus arteriosus
D. Tricuspid atresia

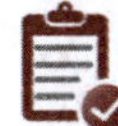

EXPLANATION

In cyanotic neonates with left axis deviation on ECG, tricuspid atresia is the most likely diagnosis.

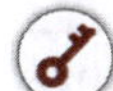

Key: D

BOOST YOUR KNOWLEDGE

Most congenital cyanotic heart diseases have right axis deviation on ECG. Characteristic ECG abnormalities in some congenital heart diseases are as under:

- *Extreme left axis:* Also called "Northwest Axis": Endocardial cushion defect
- *Crochetage sign:* ASD

- *Early transition in precordial leads:* Tetralogy of Fallot
- *Absence of septal q waves:* Situs inversus/ventricular inversion
- *Gerbode defect:* Right atrial enlargement (RAE) with LV volume overload

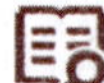

REFERENCE/SOURCE

- Cyanotic Congenital Heart Defects. In: Myung KP (Ed). Park's Pediatric Cardiology for Practitioners, 5th edition. Maryland Heights, MO: Mosby; 2014. p. 206-89.

9. A 12-year-old previously normal boy presents with a history of syncope. On examination, there is an ejection systolic murmur in the left parasternal region without associated valvar click. Echocardiography is suggestive of severe LV hypertrophy with an LV outflow gradient of 90 mm Hg. Which of the following is the most correct statement?

A. The most common inheritance pattern is X-linked dominant
B. Cardiac MRI is the most appropriate modality of diagnosis
C. Echo will reveal the systolic anterior motion of the mitral leaflet
D. Aortic valvular stenosis is commonly associated

EXPLANATION

In patients with hypertrophic cardiomyopathy, anterior movement of AML, approaching the interventricular septum causes left ventricular outflow tract (LVOT) obstruction and gradient on echocardiography. There is evidence suggesting mitral valve anterior leaflet abnormalities in hypertrophic cardiomyopathy. AML is known to have an overall higher surface area than normal. This increase is predominantly due to the increase in the length of the leaflets. This longer leaflet gets pulled into the LVOT due to the venturi effect and increases the LVOT gradient. This is called the systolic anterior motion of the mitral valve anterior leaflet.

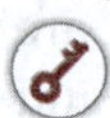

Key: C

BOOST YOUR KNOWLEDGE

- Other morphologic abnormalities seen in hypertrophic cardiomyopathy (HCM) include the following:
  - *Diverse patterns of left ventricular hypertrophy (LVH):*
    - There is no single or classic morphologic form, and virtually all possible patterns of LVH have been observed. Even close relatives with similar genetic patterns may have different patterns of LVH.
    - LVH is characteristically asymmetric (nonuniform).
- Secondary thickening of the area of the mitral valve that comes in contact with the LV septum
- Hypertrophy of anterolateral papillary muscle
- Coronary artery bridging

REFERENCE/SOURCE

- Hypertrophic cardiomyopathy. In: Shaddy RE, Penny DJ, Feltes TF, Cetta F, Mittal S, Kailin J (Eds). Moss and Adams' Heart Disease in Infants, Children, and Adolescents, 10th edition. Philadelphia: Wolters Kluwer Health; 2021. pp. 1221-54.

10. A 2-month-old "floppy infant" has been sent to you for cardiovascular evaluation. His clinical examination is within normal limits. ECG shows biventricular hypertrophy. Echo findings are commensurate. Which of the following statements is *true* about the patient?

A. This condition typically presents within the first year of life
B. Intracavitary gradient in the LV ventricle is commonly seen on echocardiography
C. Muscle biopsy reveals excess vacuolar glycogen
D. Sudden cardiac death is commonly seen

EXPLANATION

Pompe's disease is characterized by biventricular myocardial infiltration giving the appearance of muscle hypertrophy, with reduced ventricular function [as opposed to increased contractility in hypertrophic obstructive cardiomyopathy (HOCM)]. There is an accumulation of glycogen in the lysosomes. Intracavitary gradient and sudden cardiac death are not common in Pompe's disease.

Key: C

BOOST YOUR KNOWLEDGE

Pompe's disease is an inherited disorder of carbohydrate metabolism, caused due to the deficiency of the enzyme lysosomal acid α-1,4-glucosidase, or simply acid maltase. This leads to the accumulation of glycogen in lysosomes. It is an autosomal recessive disorder. The characteristic features of this condition are as under:

- *Infantile Pompe's disease:* Early onset condition, infants present with hypotonia in the first few weeks to months of life.
- *Juvenile or adult-onset disease:* Progressive skeletal muscle dysfunction starting any time after the first year of age.

Cardiomegaly may be the first clue to Pompe's disease in the infantile form. ECG findings include a high-voltage QRS complex and a shortened PR interval.

Management of this condition is with enzyme replacement therapy with recombinant human alpha-glucosidase enzyme.

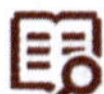

REFERENCE/SOURCE

- Kliegman RM, St Geme III JW (Eds). Nelson Textbook of Pediatrics, 21st edition. Amsterdam: Elsevier; 2019. p. 723.

11. Collett and Edwards classification is used for:

A. Hypoplastic left heart syndrome
B. Endocardial cushion defect
C. Truncus arteriosus
D. Partial anomalous pulmonary venous connection

EXPLANATION

Collett and Edwards are used for the classification of subtypes of truncus arteriosus. The anatomy is classified based on the site of origin of pulmonary arteries and their confluence.

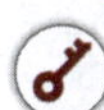

Key: C

BOOST YOUR KNOWLEDGE

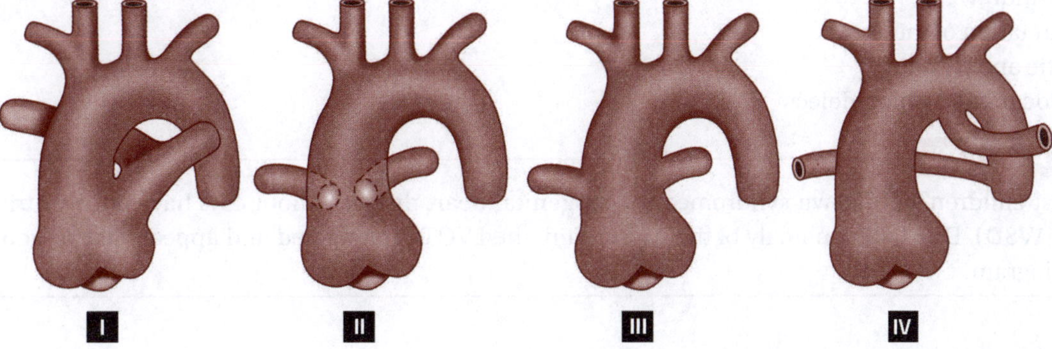

- *Type I:* A short pulmonary trunk originating from the truncus arteriosus gives rise to both pulmonary arteries.
- *Type II:* Both pulmonary arteries are separate from the truncus arteriosus, ostia are located close to each other.
- *Type III:* Both pulmonary arteries separate from the truncus arteriosus, and ostia are located at some distance from each other.
- *Type IV:* Now considered to represent a form of pulmonary atresia with ventricular septal defect.

REFERENCE/SOURCE

- Cyanotic Congenital Heart Defects. In: Myung KP (Ed). Park's Pediatric Cardiology for Practitioners, 6th edition. Maryland Heights, MO: Mosby; 2014. p. 206-89.

12. Which of the following conditions has the highest recurrence risk in the next sibling?

A. Pulmonary stenosis
B. Coarctation of the aorta
C. Transposition of great arteries
D. Endocardial fibroelastosis

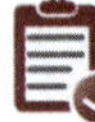

EXPLANATION

The risk of recurrence of common congenital heart diseases if a *sibling* has a cardiovascular anomaly is as under:

Condition in the sibling	***Recurrence risk (%)***
Ventricular septal defect	3.0
Patent ductus arteriosus (PDA)	3.0
ASD	2.5
Pulmonary stenosis	2.0
TGA	1.5
Endocardial fibroelastosis	4.0

Key: D

BOOST YOUR KNOWLEDGE

Endocardial fibroelastosis (EFE) is characterized by diffuse thickening of the LV endocardium secondary to a proliferation of fibrous and elastic tissue. Two forms have been described: (1) a dilated form (DCM phenotype), in which the LV is enlarged, and (2) a contracted form (RCM phenotype), in which the LV cavity is small.

REFERENCE/SOURCE

- Miscellaneous. In: Myung KP (Ed). Park's Pediatric Cardiology for Practitioners, 6th edition. Maryland Heights, MO: Mosby; 2014. p. 581.

13. Gooseneck deformity on an angiogram is seen in which of the following conditions:

A. AP window
B. Coarctation of the aorta
C. Aortic aneurysm
D. Endocardial cushion defect

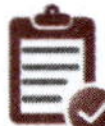

EXPLANATION

Amongst children with Down syndrome and congenital heart disease, about 45% have atrioventricular septal defect (AVSD). Due to an anomaly of the AV septum, the LVOT is elongated and appears like a "gooseneck" on the angiogram.

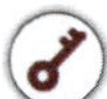

Key: D

BOOST YOUR KNOWLEDGE

Atrioventricular septal defects are a group of anomalies that share a defect of the AV septum and abnormalities of the AV valves. The terms "AV canal defects" or "endocardial cushion defects" are also used synonymously.

These lesions are divided into partial and complete forms. In partial AVSD, a primum ASD is present and there are two distinct but focally contiguous, right and left AV valve orifices within the same plane. The left AV valve invariably appears cleft where the anterior and posterior bridging leaflets coaptation. The complete AVSD also includes a primum ASD, but it is contiguous with a large inlet ventricular septal defect (VSD), and the common AV valve has a single orifice.

REFERENCE/SOURCE

- Left-to-Right Shunt Lesions. In: Myung KP (Ed). Park's Pediatric Cardiology for Practitioners, 5th edition. Maryland Heights, MO: Mosby; 2014. p. 230.

14. Which of the following formulas is used to calculate QTc in an ECG?

A. Gault's formula
B. Bazett's formula
C. Franklin theorem
D. Jone's law of voltages

EXPLANATION

QT interval varies with the heart rate. Standard formulae have been derived to compensate for the variation in heart rate (HR). Bazett's formula is a commonly used formula.

QTc = QT/ÖRR

Where the RR interval of the preceding beat has been taken.

Key: C

BOOST YOUR KNOWLEDGE

Other formulae used for QTc calculation are:

- *Fridericia formula:*
  $QTc = QT/RR^{1/3}$
- *Framingham formula:*
  $QTcFra = QT + 0.154\,(1 - RR)$
- *Rautaharju formula:*
  $QTc = QT - 0.185\,(RR - 1) + k$

Bazett's formula being the simplest, is most used.

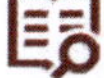

REFERENCE/SOURCE

- Electrocardiography. In: Myung KP (Ed). Park's Pediatric Cardiology for Practitioners, 5th edition. Maryland Heights, MO: Mosby; 2014. p. 82.

15. Which of the following is *false* about Taussig–Bing's anomaly?

A. Pulmonary-mitral continuity is a characteristic manifestation
B. Severe cyanosis is a rule in this condition
C. DORV + Subpulmonic VSD are typical lesions
D. Senning operation is the procedure of choice for treatment

EXPLANATION

The Taussig–Bing anomaly is a variant of double outlet right ventricle (DORV). The DORV, in 20% of cases is "Transposition type". This category includes DORV with subpulmonic VSD or the Taussig–Bing anomaly.

These patients are present with severe cyanosis in the newborn period. The degree of hypoxemia depends on the degree of streaming. These neonates are amongst the bluest patients with DORV. Management is with definitive surgical repair, with closure of the VSD and arterial switch.

Key: D

BOOST YOUR KNOWLEDGE

In this type, the aorta is pushed anteriorly and superiorly, resulting in the rightward positioning of the aorta relative to the pulmonary artery (PA). There is usually no pulmonary-mitral continuity. The pathophysiology is determined by the streaming of blood such that most of the highly oxygenated blood from the LV passes through the VSD into the pulmonary artery, whereas most of the deoxygenated blood from the RV flows directly into the aorta. Thus, there is transposition physiology with a pulmonary arterial oxygen saturation that is higher than the aortic oxygen saturation.

Senning operation, or the "atrial switch" is the procedure of choice for late presenters with d-TGA, and not Taussig–Bing anomaly.

REFERENCE/SOURCE

- Cyanotic Congenital Heart Defects. In: Myung KP (Ed). Park's Pediatric Cardiology for Practitioners, 5th edition. Maryland Heights, MO: Mosby; 2014. p. 364.

16. Which of the following represents a modified Blalock–Taussig (BT) shunt?

A. End-to-side anastomosis between the right subclavian and right pulmonary artery
B. Side-to-side anastomosis between descending thoracic aorta and main pulmonary artery
C. Right pulmonary artery to the RV anastomosis
D. Graft anastomosis between the right pulmonary artery and subclavian artery

EXPLANATION

Anastomosis between the right pulmonary artery and right subclavian using a GORE-TEX graft is called a modified BT shunt. Option A (end-to-side anastomosis between right subclavian and right pulmonary artery) represents a classical BT shunt.

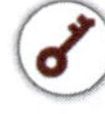

Key: D

BOOST YOUR KNOWLEDGE

Shunt surgeries are done in congenital cyanotic heart diseases with decreased pulmonary blood flow, in order to augment the amount of blood flowing into the pulmonary arteries. Historically, this has been achieved using multiple techniques.

Other types of shunt surgeries:

- *Waterston shunt:* Anastomosis between the ascending aorta and pulmonary artery
- *Potts shunt:* Anastomosis between the descending aorta and pulmonary artery
- *Mee shunt:* For VSD/pulmonary atresia, with small-sized pulmonary arteries: Small branch pulmonary arteries are connected directly to the aorta, aiming at the growth of pulmonary arteries.

REFERENCE/SOURCE

- Cyanotic Congenital Heart Defects. In: Myung KP (Ed). Park's Pediatric Cardiology for Practitioners, 5th edition. Maryland Heights, MO: Mosby; 2014. p. 206-89.

17. A 6-year-old, asymptomatic boy is brought to you, with a history of genetic and symptomatic hypertrophic cardiomyopathy in his father. Which of the following represents the correct management strategy?

A. Immediate baseline echocardiography and genetic testing are indicated
B. The child should not participate in contact sports due to high risk of sudden cardiac death
C. Parental reassurance presently, and screening (genetic/clinical) 10 years onward
D. Screening is not indicated as only one parent is affected

EXPLANATION

Hypertrophic cardiomyopathy is a heritable disorder. The most common age group for symptoms is late adolescence or adulthood. Screening in childhood is recommended only for symptomatic patients. There is a small risk of clinically significant events in the pediatric age group.

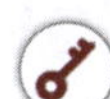

Key: C

BOOST YOUR KNOWLEDGE

European Society of Cardiology (ESC) (2014) Guidelines for Genetic and Clinical Screening Children with a Family History of HCM

Recommendations	***Class* and Level†***
Cascade genetic screening, after pretest counseling, is recommended in first-degree adult relatives of patients with a definite disease-causing mutation	IB
Clinical evaluation, employing ECG and echocardiography, and long-term follow-up, is recommended in first-degree relatives who have the same definite disease-causing mutation as the proband††	IC
First-degree relatives who do not have the same definite disease-causing mutation as the proband†† should be discharged from further follow-up but advised to seek reassessment if they develop symptoms or when new clinically relevant data emerge in the family	IIaB
When no definite genetic mutation is identified in the proband†† or genetic testing is not performed, clinical evaluation with ECG and echocardiography should be considered in first-degree adult relatives and repeated every 2–5 years (or 6–12 monthly if nondiagnostic abnormalities are present)	IIaC

*Class of recommendation
†Level of evidence
††Proband =usually the first family member to be diagnosed with the condition
(ECG: electrocardiogram)

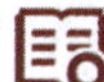

REFERENCE/SOURCE

- Elliott PM, Anastasakis A, Borger MA, Borggrefe M, Cecchi F, Charron P, et al. 2014 ESC Guidelines on diagnosis and management of hypertrophic cardiomyopathy: The Task Force for the Diagnosis and Management of Hypertrophic Cardiomyopathy of the European Society of Cardiology (ESC). Eur Heart J. 2014;35(39):2733-79.

18. Which of the following is *true* about permanent pacemaker implantation (PPI) in children?

A. Common mode of implantation is surgical
B. Leadless pacemakers provide better longevity due to the absence of lead-related complications
C. In neonates/infants, an HR <80 beats/min in cases with complete heart block is an indication of PPI
D. Right pectoral placement is preferred over left-sided placement

EXPLANATION

Permanent pacemaker implantation in infants is epicardial, commonly implanted surgically. Leadless pacemakers require large diameter sheaths, so cannot be implanted in neonates. In neonates/infants with complete heart block, HR <50 is an indication of PPI.

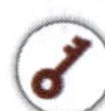

Key: A

BOOST YOUR KNOWLEDGE

Neonates born to mothers with systemic lupus erythematosus (SLE) are the most common scenario with complete heart block. The overall clinical picture depends on the ventricular "escape" rate, that is the rate that determines the "pulse rate" of the baby. If the escape rate is low, the baby may develop symptoms of heart failure or even syncope. Immediate management consists of drugs to increase HR: Salbutamol nebulization, injection isoprenaline infusion, to increase the HR, as a bridge to surgical pacemaker implantation. Recently, guidelines have been published for PPI therapy in children.

Class of recommendation (COR)	*Recommendations* *Isolated congenital complete atrioventricular block (CCAVB)*
I	PPI is indicated for patients with CCAVB with symptomatic bradycardia
I	PPI is indicated for patients with CCAVB with a wide QRS escape rhythm, complex ventricular ectopy, or ventricular dysfunction
I	PPI is indicated for CCAVB in asymptomatic neonates or infants when the mean ventricular rate is <50 beats/min. Ventricular rate alone should not be used as implant criteria, as symptoms due to low cardiac output may occur at faster heart rates
IIa	PPI is reasonable for asymptomatic CCAVB beyond the first year of life when the mean ventricular rate is <50 beats/min or there are prolonged pauses in ventricular rate
IIa	PPI is reasonable for CCAVB with LV dilation (z-score ≥3) associated with significant mitral insufficiency or systolic dysfunction
IIb	PPI may be considered for CCAVB in asymptomatic adolescents with an acceptable ventricular rate, a narrow QRS complex, and normal ventricular function, based on individualized consideration of the risk/benefit ratio

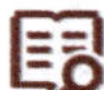

REFERENCE/SOURCE

- Silka MJ, Shah MJ, Silva JNA, Balaji S, Beach CM, Benjamin MN, et al. 2021 PACES Expert Consensus Statement on the Indications and Management of Cardiovascular Implantable Electronic Devices in Pediatric Patients: Executive Summary. Hear Rhythm. 2021;18(11):1925-50.

19. Which of the following is the most common coronary artery abnormality seen in patients with Transposition of Great arteries?

A. Left anterior descending coronary artery from right coronary artery (RCA)
B. Left circumflex coronary artery from RCA
C. Single coronary artery
D. Intramural course of coronary arteries

EXPLANATION

The most common coronary distribution in cases with TGA is the left anterior descending coronary artery and left circumflex coronary artery from the left posterior facing sinus and the RCA from the right posterior facing sinus. The most common anomaly is the left circumflex coronary artery from RCA.

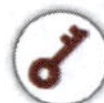

Key: B

BOOST YOUR KNOWLEDGE

Coronary artery patterns in TGA are variable. Defining the coronary origin patterns and course is important for surgical planning. There are many systems of classification of coronary arterial abnormalities in TGA. Yacoub and Radley-Smith classification is the most commonly used system.

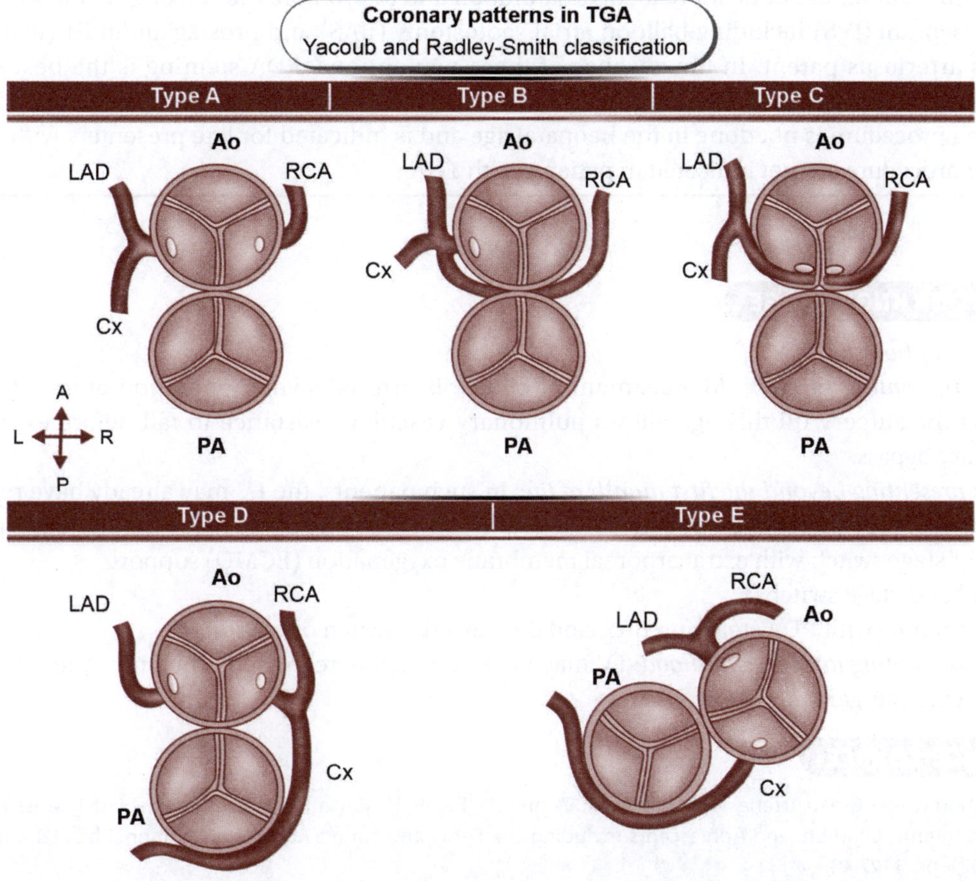

- *Type A:* The most common coronary distribution, with the left circumflex coronary artery and left anterior descending coronary artery from the left posterior facing sinus and the RCA from the right posterior facing sinus.
- *Type B:* Single coronary ostium from a posterior-facing sinus.
- *Type C:* Separate close origins of the left and right coronary arteries from the posterior facing sinuses (often with intramural courses).
- *Type D:* Circumflex coronary artery from the RCA.
- *Type E:* Circumflex coronary artery from right posterior sinus and left anterior descending and RCA from the left posterior facing sinus.

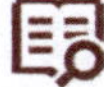

REFERENCE/SOURCE

- Congenitally Corrected Transposition of the Great Arteries. In: Shaddy RE, Penny DJ, Feltes TF, Cetta F, Mittal S, Kailin J (Eds). Moss and Adams' Heart Disease in Infants, Children, and Adolescents Including the Fetus and Young Adult, 10th edition. Philadelphia: Wolters Kluwer Health; 2021. pp. 1145-58.

20. Which of the following strategies is used for the management of severely cyanotic neonates with TGA?

A. Senning procedure
B. PDA stenting
C. BT shunt
D. Fontan procedure

EXPLANATION

Emergency procedures are done for relief of desaturation and to promote the "mixing" of blood in d-TGA/intact ventricular septum (IVS) including balloon atrial septostomy (BAS) and prostaglandin E1 (PGE1) for keeping the ductus arteriosus patent. In the absence of these two options, PDA stenting is the best-suited answer, as this strategy is deployed in increasing the volume overload to regressing LV and also improving saturation. The Senning procedure is not done in the neonatal age and is indicated for late presenters with TGA. BT shunt and Fontan procedure are not indicated in patients with TGA.

Key: B

BOOST YOUR KNOWLEDGE

Management options for TGA:

- *Patients presenting at birth:* Management of choice is arterial switch operation at about 3 weeks of age. Delaying the surgery till this age allows pulmonary vascular resistance to fall before exposure to cardiopulmonary bypass.
- *Patients presenting beyond the first month of life:* In such patients, the LV may already have regressed. Careful assessment of the same is done by echocardiography, and then one of the following strategies is adopted:
    - Single-stage switch with extracorporeal membrane oxygenation (ECMO) support
    - Rapid two-stage switch
    - LV retraining with PDA stent and BAS, and then arterial switch operation
- *Patients presenting later in childhood:* LV may have completely regressed. The only option for these children is atrial switch surgery.

REFERENCE/SOURCE

- Transposition of the Great Arteries. In: Shaddy RE, Penny DJ, Feltes TF, Cetta F, Mittal S, Kailin J (Eds). Moss and Adams' Heart Disease in Infants, Children, and Adolescents Including the Fetus and Young Adult, 10th edition. Philadelphia: Wolters Kluwer Health; 2021. pp. 1122-44.

SECTION

21

Nephrology

Section Editor: *Priyanka Khandelwal*

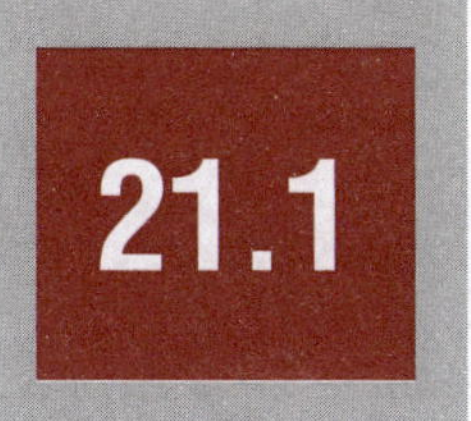

CHAPTER 21.1

Anatomy, Physiology of Kidneys, Investigations for Disorders of Kidney and Urinary Tract

Abhijeet Saha

1. A 6-year-old boy with nephrotic syndrome develops fever, abdominal pain, and vomiting. Physical examination reveals, heart rate 110 beats/minute, respirations 26/minute, temperature 39.8°C, BP 84/52 mm Hg, pallor, and edema. On auscultation chest is clear, without murmur, gallop, or rub. The abdomen has generalized tenderness and guarding. Laboratory values include hemoglobin 10.8 g/dL, WBC 18,000/mm^3, platelet 190,000/mm^3, serum Na^+ 135 mEq/L, K^+ 3.4 mEq/L, Cl^- 101 mEq/L, HCO_3^- 16 mEq/L, and albumin 0.8 g/dL. Arterial blood gases are pH 7.44, pCO_2 24 mm Hg, and pO_2 88 mm Hg. Which of the following best describes the acid-base disturbance in this patient?

A. Normal
B. Normal anion gap metabolic acidosis without compensation
C. High anion gap metabolic acidosis with non-anion gap acidosis and respiratory alkalosis
D. High anion gap metabolic acidosis and metabolic alkalosis and respiratory alkalosis

EXPLANATION

The anion gap is only 18 [135 – (101 + 16)]. The patient has severe hypoalbuminemia, hence causing the true anion gap to be underestimated. The albumin-corrected AG = AG + 2.5 (4.4 – albumin in g/dL) = 12 + 2.5 (4.4 – 0.8) = 27. The albumin-corrected AG indicates that the patient has a high anion gap metabolic acidosis. Delta ratio = (anion gap – 10) ÷ (24 – HCO_3^-) for this child would be (27 – 12) ÷ (24 – 16) = 1.87 suggestive of additional metabolic alkalosis most likely due to vomiting. The pCO_2 is low (24) than expected (ΔpCO_2 = 1.2 × ΔHCO_3^- = 1.2(24– 16) = 9.6, thus the expected pCO_2 should be 40 – 10.8 = 30.4 mm Hg, thus the additional respiratory alkalosis is also present as compensation.

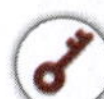

Key: D

BOOST YOUR KNOWLEDGE

Acid-base disorders should be thought of as a process. The history, physical examination, review of medications, suspicion for toxic substances, and an inquiring mind will determine the presence and likely causes of most disturbances in acid-base balance, particularly when there is only one aberration in pH physiology (i.e., the simple acid-base disorders). However, a single patient may have several disparate and opposite metabolic disturbances at the same time. There may be several mechanisms producing metabolic acidosis at the same time, as well as different processes producing metabolic alkalosis. There is certainly no special limit to the number of metabolic disturbances one particular patient may have. Many different acids, pathologic abnormalities, and metabolic processes can contribute to the metabolic component of acid-base alterations.

Decreases in albumin is common in children and can affect the anion gap. In patients with chronic illness, glomerulonephritis, malnutrition and so on, it is useful to correct the anion gap according to the Figge equation. Normal albumin is assumed as 4.4 g/dL.

Corrected AG = AG + 2.5 × (4.4 – observed serum albumin).

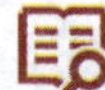

REFERENCES/SOURCES

- Fall PJ. A stepwise approach to acid-base disorders, Postgrad Med. 2000;107(3):249-63.
- Shaw KN, Bachur RG (Eds). Fleisher and Ludwig's Textbook of Pediatric Emergency Medicine, 7th edition. Philadelphia; Wolters Kluwer; 2016. p. 977.

2. A 2-year-old girl complained of weakness. Parents denied any history of loose stools, vomiting or the use of any medications. Physical examination revealed a thin, anxious child with a BP of 84/68 mm Hg. Her serum sodium was 139 mEq/L, potassium 2.2 mEq/L, chloride 80 mEq/L, and bicarbonate 47 mEq/L. Her urine sodium was 58 mEq/L, urine potassium was 128 mEq/L, and her urine chloride was 190 mEq/L. Which of the following is the most likely cause of her hypokalemia with metabolic alkalosis?

A. Bartter syndrome
B. Primary hyperaldosteronism
C. Cushing syndrome
D. Liddle syndrome

EXPLANATION

The findings of hypokalemia, metabolic alkalosis, a high rate of urinary potassium excretion, and a normal BP suggests the diagnosis of Bartter syndrome. Other forms of mineralocorticoid excess, primary hyperaldosteronism, adrenal enzyme defects, Cushing's syndrome, or licorice ingestion) are excluded by the normal BP. The high urine chloride is most consistent with either diuretic abuse or Bartter syndrome. Hence, a history of medication intake is very important.

Key: A

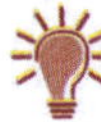

BOOST YOUR KNOWLEDGE

Bartter syndrome is a rare familial defect of chloride reabsorption in the ascending limb of loop of Henle—associated with salt and potassium wasting and secondary (hyperreninemic) hyperaldosteronism. The hypokalemia induced by both a defect in potassium reabsorption in the thick ascending limb, and an increased secretion of potassium in the cortical collecting tubule due to high rates of distal sodium delivery, is particularly resistant to treatment, even with high doses of potassium chloride. The hypokalemia is probably responsible for the decreased response to angiotensin 2 and high levels of urinary prostaglandins, which are characteristics of this disease. Treatment of Bartter syndrome includes adequate hydration and potassium chloride supplementation (1–3 mEq/kg/day), and benefit with therapy with indomethacin (2–3 mg/kg/day) or ibuprofen (30 mg/kg/day) that reduces prostaglandin levels and polyuria. Some patients with Bartter syndrome also exhibit urinary magnesium wasting requiring magnesium supplementation.

REFERENCE/SOURCE

- Schaefer F, Greenbaum LA (Eds). Pediatric Kidney Disease, 3rd edition. Springer International Publishing AG; 2023. pp. 996-9.

3. A 3-year-old previously healthy boy is admitted with a 10-day history of fever, abdominal distension, and pain. In the ER his BP was 128/60 mm Hg, pulse 116 beats/minute, respirations 24/minute. There is bilateral cervical lymphadenopathy, liver 3 cm and spleen 4.0 cm below costal margin, both kidneys are palpable. Laboratory data showed hemoglobin 8.7 g/dL, white blood count 20,600 cells/uL, platelet count 80,000/mm^3, urea 86 mg/dL, creatinine 2.9 mg/dL, sodium 136 mEq/L, potassium 2.9 mEq/L, chloride 97 mEq/L, HCO_3^- 20 mEq/L, calcium 6.9 mg/dL, phosphate 7.8 mg/dL, uric acid 18.6 mg/dL, and albumin 3.7 g/dL. Urinalysis revealed pH 5.0, but no blood or protein. Peripheral smear is awaited. What is most likely cause of the kidney disease?

A. Tumor lysis syndrome due to acute leukemia
B. Urinary tract obstruction and pyonephrosis with underlying posterior urethral valve (PUV)
C. Atypical hemolytic uremic syndrome due to anti-factor H antibodies
D. Acute glomerulonephritis due to falciparum malaria

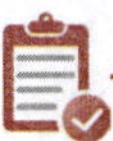

EXPLANATION

Urinary stream is thin or poor in PUV with additional features of growth failure; organomegaly is not explained in PUV with urinary tract infection. Atypical HUS will not have lymphadenopathy and hepatosplenomegaly. Cola-colored urine, anasarca along with urinary findings of proteinuria and hematuria are cardinal features of acute glomerulonephritis. Tumor lysis syndrome (TLS) typically presents with hypocalcemia, hypophosphatemia, metabolic acidosis, and acute kidney injury with marked hyperuricemia. It is rare in solid tumors, and usually occurs in patients with leukemia/lymphoma. Nephromegaly due to infiltration of malignant cell can be a feature of acute leukemia. The diagnosis is certainly consistent with his physical examination.

Key: A

BOOST YOUR KNOWLEDGE

Tumor lysis syndrome is characterized by a group of acute electrolyte and metabolic disturbances caused by massive and abrupt release of intracellular contents such as nucleic acids, uric acid, phosphorus, and potassium into the circulation due to breakdown of tumor cells. It is most seen in the first few days after the start of cytotoxic therapy especially in hematological malignancies such as acute lymphoblastic leukemia and high-grade lymphomas (particularly, Burkitt lymphoma). As a result of breakdown of tumor cells, potentially fatal metabolic derangements such as hyperkalemia, hyperphosphatemia, hypocalcemia, and hyperuricemia may develop. First manifestations of TLS could be subtle and are commonly seen in oncologic patients without TLS, such as nausea, vomiting, diarrhea, muscle cramps, and paresthesia. Edema, arrhythmias, and seizures are often late presentation. A grading system for severity of TLS is also proposed by Cairo–Bishop.

REFERENCES/SOURCES

- Kliegman RM, Stanton BF, Schor NF, St Geme III JW (Eds). Nelson Textbook of Pediatrics, 21st South East Asia edition. Elsevier Health Sciences; 2015. p. 2432.
- Shaw KN, Bachur RG (Eds). Fleisher and Ludwig's Textbook of Pediatric Emergency Medicine, 7th edition. Philadelphia; Wolters Kluwer; 2016. p. 905.

4. An 8-year-old girl presents with growth failure (weight 12 kg, height 110 cm) and easy fatigability. Blood pressure is 116/84 mm Hg. Investigations show serum creatinine 1.0 mg/dL, hemoglobin 7 g/dL, calcium 8.3 mg/dL, phosphorus 5.7 mg/dL, sodium 137 mEq/L, potassium 3.5 mEq/L with urine protein, and creatinine ratio of 1.7 mg/mg. Kidney ultrasound showed bilateral hypo-dysplastic kidneys with increased echogenicity and poor corticomedullary differentiation. What is the most appropriate medication for the management of hypertension in this patient?

A. Amlodipine
B. Enalapril
C. Furosemide
D. Prazosin

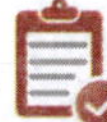

EXPLANATION

The findings are suggestive of chronic kidney disease stage 3 in this patient due to hypo-dysplastic kidneys. Antihypertensive agents that inhibit the renin-angiotensin system provide superior renoprotection in these patients owing to their additional antiproteinuric, anti-inflammatory, and antifibrotic properties. Hence, enalapril, an angiotensin-converting enzyme inhibitor, is the drug of choice for the management of patients with estimated glomerular filtration rate (eGFR) >30 mL/1.73/m^2/day. eGFR of this child is $0.413 \times 110/1.0 = 45.5$ mL/min/1.73m^2

Key: B

BOOST YOUR KNOWLEDGE

Systemic hypertension and glomerular hyperfiltration lead to progressive nephron damage. Both hypertension and increased proteinuria are predictors of the progression of kidney disease among children with chronic kidney disease. This provides a rationale for the selection of pharmacologic therapy to control blood pressure and proteinuria. Intensified antihypertensive therapy with ACE inhibitors delays the progression of kidney disease by controlling both blood pressure and proteinuria in these children. These effects are mediated through decrease in glomerular vascular tone that decreases intraglomerular pressure, proteinuria, and local release of cytokines and chemokines, while attenuating activation of inflammatory pathways. The ESCAPE trial showed that children with CKD with 24-hour mean ambulatory BP < 50th percentile were 35% less likely to attain the composite study endpoint (50% estimated GFR decline or estimated GFR < 10 mL/min/1.73 m^2 or the start of kidney replacement therapy) during 5-year follow-up than children in patients with significant proteinuria, the benefit of intensified BP control was greater than in patients without proteinuria. Intensified BP control has been shown to be effective in preventing cardiac remodeling in children with CKD enrolled in the HOT-KID trial.

REFERENCE/SOURCE

- Schaefer F, Greenbaum LA (Eds). Pediatric Kidney Disease, 3rd edition. Springer International Publishing AG; 2023. pp. 1348-54.

5. A previously healthy 12-year-old girl presents with history of gross hematuria and decreased urine output for 5 days. She also has cough and hemoptysis for 7 days. On examination, her blood pressure is 130/90 mm Hg. She has mild periorbital and pedal edema. Investigations showed urea 120 mg/dL, serum creatinine 6.0 mg/dL, sodium 133 mEq/L, potassium 5.5 mEq/L, and hemoglobin 7.5 g/dL. Her urine routine showed plenty of RBCs and urine protein to creatinine ratio of 4.5 mg/mg. Her X-ray of paranasal sinuses suggests pansinusitis. Which of the following serological tests will be most useful in making a diagnosis in this child?

A. Complement levels
B. Antinuclear antibodies (ANA) titer
C. Antineutrophil cytoplasmic antibodies (ANCA) titer
D. Antistreptolysin (ASO) titer

EXPLANATION

This patient presents with rapidly progressive glomerulonephritis with significant proteinuria and deranged kidney functions. Timely initiation of immunosuppression is very important in the management of this patient. Inflammation of upper respiratory tract with glomerulonephritis and positive cANCA is typical for granulomatosis with polyangiitis (Wegener granulomatosis). Therefore, serological testing with ANCA titers will help in diagnosing this child.

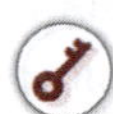

Key: C

BOOST YOUR KNOWLEDGE

Granulomatosis with polyangiitis (Wegener granulomatosis) is characterized by granulomatous inflammation of the respiratory tract with necrotizing vasculitis affecting small to medium-sized vessels and a necrotizing glomerulonephritis. Upper airway involvement is common and often causes sinusitis, otitis media, epistaxis, septal perforation, and subglottic stenosis. It is frequently associated with elevated titers of ANCA directed at PR3 that leads to cytoplasmic staining of neutrophils (c-ANCA). Kidney biopsy shows segmental necrotizing glomerulonephritis with absence of immune deposits. IV and oral steroids, cyclophosphamide, and plasmapheresis are used for the treatment of this condition.

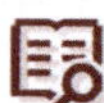

REFERENCE/SOURCE

- Schaefer F, Greenbaum LA (Eds). Pediatric Kidney Disease, 3rd edition. Springer International Publishing AG; 2023. pp. 58-60.

6. A postnatal ultrasound was performed on a baby boy with history of right sided antenatal hydronephrosis on Day 7 of life. It shows normal-sized kidneys on both the sides, right renal pelvis anteroposterior diameter of 8 mm with mild ureteric dilatation and no hydronephrosis on left side. Urinary bladder is of normal shape with normal lining. What is the most appropriate next step in the management of this infant?

A. Start antibiotic prophylaxis and repeat ultrasound at 4 weeks
B. Urgent micturating cystourethrogram (MCU)
C. Dimercaptosuccinic acid (DMSA) scan followed by diethylenetriamine pentaacetic acid (DTPA) scan
D. Referral to pediatric surgeon

EXPLANATION

This patient has mild antenatal hydronephrosis with ureteric dilatation. He will require a repeat kidney ultrasound at the age of 4–6 weeks. As per ISPN (Indian Society of Pediatric Nephrology) guidelines, all infants with postnatally confirmed moderate or severe hydronephrosis [kidney anteroposterior diameter (APD) >10 mm, Society for Fetal Urology (SFU) 3–4] or dilated ureter should receive antibiotic prophylaxis while awaiting evaluation.

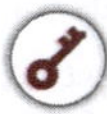

Key: A

BOOST YOUR KNOWLEDGE

Widespread antenatal screening has resulted in increased detection of anomalies of the kidney and urinary tract. Antenatal hydronephrosis is transient and resolves in almost one-half cases by the third trimester. All patients with antenatal hydronephrosis should undergo postnatal ultrasonography within the first week of life. In neonates with suspected posterior urethral valves, oligohydramnios or severe bilateral hydronephrosis, ultrasound should be performed within 24–48 hours of birth, followed by MCU if needed. In all other cases, the ultrasound should be preferably done within 3–7 days of life. Repeat ultrasound should be done at 4–6 weeks of life even with ultrasound is normal at birth. All those infants who have isolated mild unilateral or bilateral hydronephrosis should be followed by sequential ultrasound alone, for resolution or progression of findings. MCU should be performed in patients with unilateral or bilateral hydronephrosis with kidney APD >10 mm, SFU grade 3–4 or ureteric dilatation at 4–6 weeks of age. Diuretic renogram should be done in patients with significant hydronephrosis who do not show vesicoureteral reflux on MCU.

REFERENCE/SOURCE

- Sinha A, Bagga A, Krishna A, Bajpai M, Srinivas M, Uppal R, et al. Revised guidelines on management of antenatal hydronephrosis. Indian Pediatr. 2013;50(2):215-31.

7. A 5-month-old infant presented with a history of generalized body swelling and decreased urine output since the age of 2 months. He has history of multiple admissions for intravenous medications to decrease edema. His examination revealed generalized anasarca and ambiguous genitalia. He had onset of symptoms at the age of 2 months. His investigations showed massive proteinuria (urine protein to urine creatinine ratio of 5 mg/mg) and hypoalbuminemia (serum albumin 1.5 g/dL). Which of the following genes is most likely affected in this patient?

A. *NPSH1*
B. *NPSH2*
C. *WTI*
D. *LAMB2*

EXPLANATION

This patient has congenital nephrotic syndrome (edema, low albumin, and nephrotic range proteinuria with onset before 3 months of life). Since he also has associated ambiguous genitalia, this appears to be a case of Denys-Drash syndrome. The gene responsible for this syndrome is Wilms' tumor suppressor gene (*WT1*).

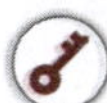

Key: C

BOOST YOUR KNOWLEDGE

Denys–Drash syndrome is characterized by nephrotic syndrome, ambiguous genitalia (male pseudo-hermaphroditism) and Wilms' tumor. It often develops during first year of life and may have a rapid progression to end-stage kidney disease. The syndrome is predominantly caused by missense genetic variants in exon 8 or 9 of *WT1*. Kidney biopsy shows diffuse mesangial sclerosis. Wilms' tumor risk is >90%; screening is recommended by ultrasound every 3 months till 7 years of age. The treatment is unsatisfactory. Most experts recommend bilateral nephrectomy once the patient reaches end-stage kidney disease to avoid emergence of Wilms' tumor.

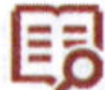

REFERENCE/SOURCE

- Schaefer F, Greenbaum LA (Eds). Pediatric Kidney Disease, 3rd edition. Springer International Publishing AG; 2023. p. 1117.

8. A 4-year-old girl presents with complains of failure to gain weight and height since infancy. There is a history of polyuria, polydipsia, and photophobia. One sibling with similar history has died at the age of 6 years. Liver was just palpable, and spleen was not palpable. Her investigations showed normal anion gap metabolic acidosis with increased fractional urinary excretion of bicarbonate and phosphate. Her CBC shows Hb 11.0 g/dL, TLC 4,500/mm^3, platelet count 1.56 lakh/mm^3. What is the most likely underlying inherited disorder responsible for her condition?

A. Cystinosis
B. Wilson disease
C. Marfan syndrome
D. Pierson syndrome

EXPLANATION

This patient shows features suggestive of renal tubular disorder (failure to thrive, polyuria, and polydipsia). Her investigations revealed normal anion gap metabolic acidosis with bicarbonaturia and phosphaturia, indicating towards type 2 renal tubular acidosis (proximal RTA). Since she has a family history of similar disorder in her sibling and photophobia, it points toward the diagnosis of inherited disorder called cystinosis. Photophobia can be a striking feature in some cases of cystinosis, noted by 2–3 years of age and progress to blepharospasm, superficial punctate keratopathy, and recurrent corneal erosions. Marfan syndrome has tall stature. Pierson syndrome is characterized by narrowing of pupils, lens, and corneal abnormalities.

Key: A

BOOST YOUR KNOWLEDGE

Cystinosis is an autosomal recessive inherited condition characterized by deposition of cystine crystals in the cornea, conjunctiva, bone marrow, leukocytes, lymph nodes, and other organs. Three clinical forms are recognized—infantile, juvenile, or late onset nephropathic cystinosis. Patients with infantile form present at 4–6 months with features of renal tubular disorder with biochemical evidence of proximal tubular dysfunction. In absence of therapy, kidney injury progresses to end stage kidney disease by the age of 10–12 years. Specific therapy with cysteamine enables cystine depletion and should be initiated early and continued lifelong. Kidney transplantation is successful but does not correct the systemic disorder and cystine continues to accumulate in non-kidney tissues and result in multisystem dysfunction.

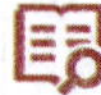

REFERENCE/SOURCE

- Schaefer F, Greenbaum LA (Eds). Pediatric Kidney Disease, 3rd edition. Springer International Publishing AG; 2023. pp. 820-36.

9. **A 7-years-old boy presented with history of decreased urine output, generalized swelling, and loose motions for 3 days. Blood pressure was 132/88 mm Hg. His hemoglobin was 8.8 g/dL, platelet 99,000/mm^3, blood urea 200 mg/dL, serum creatinine 2.2 mg/dL, and schistocyte index was 2.5%. Anti-factor H antibody level was 2500 AU/mL (normal <150 AU/mL). He was treated with steroids and plasmapheresis. However, patient did not achieve hematological remission following 7 daily sessions of plasmapheresis, each of 60 mL/kg volume. Which of the following should be the next step in the management for this patient?**

A. Stop plasma exchange and switch to IV methylprednisolone pulse
B. Give intravenous cyclophosphamide and repeat anti-FH titer
C. Continue plasmapheresis and perform genetic analysis; consider anti-C5 blockade
D. Give injection Rituximab and repeat anti-FH titer

EXPLANATION

The patient is suffering with atypical hemolytic uremic. Anti-factor H antibody titers should be rechecked, and dose/frequency of plasmapheresis should be increased if titers are high. Cyclophosphamide or rituximab should be added only after hematological remission has been achieved. Genetic analysis should be performed next to look for additional defects, although only ~10% Indian children with anti-FH aHUS have concomitant genetic variants. In case a genetic variant is detected or the patient is refractory to plasma exchange, complement blockade with eculizumab may be considered.

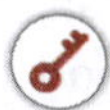

Key: C

BOOST YOUR KNOWLEDGE

Hemolytic uremic syndrome is a triad of microangiopathic hemolytic anemia, acute kidney injury, and thrombocytopenia. It can result from infections [*Shigella, Escherichia coli (E. coli), Pneumococcus,* dengue, malaria, and *Leptospira*] or may be secondary to vasculitis (SLE), solid organ transplant, drugs such as calcineurin inhibitors, oral contraceptives, defective cobalamin metabolism. Atypical HUS results from defects in complement pathway inhibitors or antibody to factor H (FH). Results on anti-FH antibody levels are not available at admission, but usually after a few days. In the interim, the standard of care for patients with aHUS has chiefly been with intensive plasma exchanges in the first week of illness, followed by tapering over the next 2–3 weeks. Immunosuppressive medications are administered once anti-FH antibody levels are shown to be elevated and administered for periods ranging between 6 months and 2 years. There is limited availability of eculizumab in less resourced regions, and this strategy is therefore not used. Therapy with eculizumab should be considered in patients who are refractory to plasma exchange (PEX), show life-threatening features, or have concomitant defect(s) in complement regulation. Given that patients with anti-FH antibodies do not show genetic abnormalities in genes of the complement pathway in almost 90% cases, detailed next-generation studies are not *routinely* carried out in such patients. Almost one-quarter of patients with anti-FH associated HUS show persistent urinary abnormalities, sustained systemic hypertension, and progressive kidney disease (CKD3 or more). This represents an appreciable quantum of disease morbidity that might have implications during long-term follow-up.

REFERENCES/SOURCES

- Bagga A, Khandelwal P, Mishra K, Thergaonkar R, Vasudevan A, Sharma J, et al. Hemolytic uremic syndrome in a developing country: Consensus guidelines. Pediatr Nephrol. 2019;34:1465-82.
- Schaefer F, Greenbaum LA (Eds). Pediatric Kidney Disease, 3rd edition. Springer International Publishing AG; 2023. pp. 1892-5.

10. A 5-year-old girl presented with complaints of reduced growth and appetite. She had a history of recurrent episodes of fever without focus. On examination, she had pallor with blood pressure 110/70 mm Hg. Investigations revealed hemoglobin 7.0 g/dL, blood urea 222 mg/dL, serum creatinine 1.8 mg/dL, urine R/M - 2+ protein without any RBC and WBC. Serum 25(OH)D was 30 ng/mL, serum PTH 82 pg/mL, serum iron 20 μg/dL, serum transferrin saturation 10%, and serum ferritin 12 ng/mL. Ultrasonography (USG) kidneys, ureters, and bladder (KUB) showed bilateral small-sized kidneys with complete loss of corticomedullary junction. Which of the following is correct regarding management of anemia in this patient?

A. Oral iron therapy should be initiated as first line therapy
B. Injection erythropoietin should be the first line therapy
C. Both oral iron and injection erythropoietin should be given simultaneously
D. Packed red cell transfusion should be given immediately

EXPLANATION

Erythropoietin stimulates bone marrow to produce red blood cells. In a patient with chronic kidney disease, iron stores need to be replete before red cell production is enhanced so that there is enough iron available to be carried by red blood cells. Once patient is iron replete but still has anemia, erythropoietin may be added if no other cause for anemia is found. Blood transfusion is avoided unless there is significant blood loss or impending surgical procedure due to risk of development of antibodies which may hamper the future process of kidney transplant. This patient has chronic kidney disease as depicted by presence of short stature, anemia, hyperparathyroidism, and hypoplastic kidneys. Also, she is iron deficient without evidence of significant blood loss or need for surgical procedure, hence oral iron therapy is the most appropriate treatment.

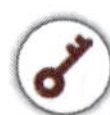

Key: A

BOOST YOUR KNOWLEDGE

Anemia in children with CKD is defined as hemoglobin <11.0 g/dL in children 0.5–5 years, hemoglobin <11.5 g/dL in children 5–12 years and hemoglobin <12.0 g/dL in children 12–15 years. It can result from poor appetite leading nutritional deficiency of iron/vitamin B_{12}/folate, lack of erythropoietin production, uremic or hyperparathyroidism induced suppression of bone marrow, recurrent infections, increase in hepcidin resulting in decreased intestinal absorption of iron. Oral (3–5 mg/kg/day)/IV iron (1–2 mg/kg) therapy and vitamin B_{12}/folate supplementation form the first line of management. Iron replete patients should be checked for evidence of hemolysis [peripheral smear, lactate dehydrogenase (LDH), and direct Coombs test (DCT)] and parvovirus infection. If no other treatable cause for anemia is found, therapy with erythropoietin stimulating agent (ESA) is initiated. ESA are of two types—short acting (100–300 IU/kg/week) or long acting (darbepoetin - 0.45 μg/kg/week).

REFERENCE/SOURCE

- Schaefer F, Greenbaum LA (Eds). Pediatric Kidney Disease, 3rd edition. Springer International Publishing AG; 2023. pp. 1607-22.

11. A 10-year-old boy came with chief complaints of cola colored urine, reduced urine output, and generalized swelling for 5 days. He had suffered an episode of sore throat about a month ago. He was hypertensive with blood pressure 128/80 mm Hg. Urine showed 220 RBC (40% dysmorphic) with RBC cast and 2+ protein. Urine protein creatinine ratio was 1.2, hemoglobin 11.0 g/dL, urea 110 mg/dL, creatinine 1.5 g/dL, sodium 132 mEq/L, and potassium 5.2 mEq/L. Which is the most appropriate first-line antihypertensive of choice?

A. Furosemide
B. Amlodipine
C. Labetalol
D. Enalapril

EXPLANATION

This is a patient of acute glomerulonephritis, most likely secondary to streptococcal infection due to prior history of sore throat. These patients develop hypertension due to activation of renin angiotensin aldosterone system leading to salt retention and fluid overload which responds best to loop diuretics such as furosemide which inhibit Na-K-2Cl channel in ascending limb of loop of Henle causing natriuresis and diuresis. Hence, the most appropriate answer is furosemide.

Key: A

BOOST YOUR KNOWLEDGE

Acute glomerulonephritis affects school-going children of age 5–12 years, occurring most commonly due to streptococcal infection. It presents with oliguria, hematuria, and hypertension. Sometimes, it can present with atypical features of congestive heart failure due to volume overload and encephalopathy due to hypertensive crisis. It is diagnosed with presence of blood and protein in urine with positive antistreptolysin O (ASO) or anti-DNase B titer and low C3. Kidney biopsy shows mesangial proliferation, mesangial hypercellularity, and infiltration with leukocytes along with IgG and C3 deposits in glomerular capillaries and mesangium. Treatment is supportive with management of hypertension and antibiotics to prevent the spread of infection. It can result in acute kidney injury (AKI) requiring kidney replacement therapy. Children with non-resolving AKI, presence of systemic features such as fever, rash, joint pains at presentation, persistent nephrotic range proteinuria, gross hematuria beyond 2 weeks, hypertension >4 weeks or hypocomplementemia >12 months require kidney biopsy to look for alternative cause of glomerulonephritis.

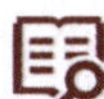

REFERENCE/SOURCE

- Schaefer F, Greenbaum LA (Eds). Pediatric Kidney Disease, 3rd edition. Springer International Publishing AG; 2023. pp. 555-66.

12. A 5-year-old boy presented with complaint of pain abdomen for 5 days. There was no history of fever, loose motion, vomiting, and jaundice. Ultrasound revealed small dysplastic right kidney with few cysts and normal functioning slightly hypertrophied left kidney. Blood pressure was 90/64 mm Hg and urine routine examination was normal. Which is the next best investigation for this child for further management?

A. Computed tomography of abdomen
B. Dimercaptosuccinic acid (DMSA) scan
C. Diethylenetriamine pentaacetic acid (DTPA) scan
D. Micturating cystourethrogram (MCU)

EXPLANATION

This is a case of right multicystic dysplastic kidney with normal left kidney. It is of utmost importance to look for presence of scars in the normally functioning left kidney which will determine if the subsequent worsening of kidney function in this patient. Scars can be best demonstrated using DMSA scan, hence B is the most suitable answer.

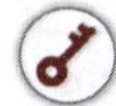

Key: B

BOOST YOUR KNOWLEDGE

Multicystic dysplastic kidney is a congenital defect in the development of kidney wherein large non communicating cysts of varying sizes replace the normal parenchyma in one of the kidneys during the antenatal period. The affected kidney remains non-functional and gradually shrinks to a very small size. However, contralateral vesicoureteral reflux is present in up to 20% of patients. It is important to look for presence of scars in the opposite kidney.

Normal functioning of the single kidney is essential for patient survival. These patients should be monitored for development of proteinuria and hypertension and advised not to engage in contact sports to prevent injury to the single functioning kidney. Routine MCU is not recommended children in all multicystic dysplastic kidney (MCDK).

REFERENCE/SOURCE

- Schaefer F, Greenbaum LA (Eds). Pediatric Kidney Disease, 3rd edition. Springer International Publishing AG; 2023. p. 1489.

13. **A 3-year-old girl presented with complaints of multiple episodes of generalized tonic clonic movements for 1 week. There was history of frequent falls and incoordination while walking, and poor hearing. Blood pressure was 88/52 mm Hg. Investigations revealed blood urea—22 mg/dL, serum creatinine—0.2 mg/dL, sodium—130 mEq/L, potassium—3.4 mEq/L, calcium—6.5 mg/dL, and magnesium—1.2 mg/dL. Further evaluation showed abnormal records on electroencephalogram. Which of the following channel genetic variants is responsible for this disease?**

A. TRPM6
B. Claudin 19
C. KCNJ 10
D. CaSR

EXPLANATION

This patient has ataxia, hearing defect, hypocalcemia, and hypomagnesemia with evidence of epilepsy. These five defects are classically seen in EAST (Epilepsy, Ataxia, Sensorineural deafness and Tubulopathy) syndrome which results from genetic variant in KCNJ 10 potassium channel which is found in renal tubules, cochlea, and glial cells. TRPM6 and Claudin 19 channels are localized to renal tubules only and involved in magnesium and calcium transport. CaSR is a calcium-sensing channel found in renal tubules only unlike KCNJ 10. Its mutation results in urinary loss of sodium, potassium, and calcium but does not result in seizures or hearing loss. The most suitable answer is C.

Key: C

BOOST YOUR KNOWLEDGE

EAST syndrome, also known as SeSAME (Seizures, Sensorineural deafness, Ataxia, Mental retardation and Electrolyte imbalance) syndrome, is an autosomal recessive disorder caused by variants in the gene encoding the KCNJ10 potassium channel resulting in severe early onset of seizures, sensorineural deafness, intellectual disability, and electrolyte imbalance. Abnormality in this channel prevents potassium uptake in glial cells, cochlea, and distal renal tubules and results in the clinical syndrome. Diagnosis is suspected based on clinical syndrome and confirmed with genetic analysis. Treatment involves correction of electrolyte imbalance, antiepileptics to control seizures and hearing aids or cochlear implantation to manage sensorineural hearing loss.

REFERENCE/SOURCE

- Schaefer F, Greenbaum LA (Eds). Pediatric Kidney Disease, 3rd edition. Springer International Publishing AG; 2023. pp. 1000-01.

14. **A 7-year-old girl was diagnosed to have hypodysplastic kidneys and progressed to end-stage kidney disease requiring hemodialysis. Her parents are poor and hence getting dialysis once or twice a week instead of three times a week. She presents with vomiting and proximal muscle weakness in the emergency room. The serum potassium is 7.5 mEq/L, and an electrocardiogram (EKG) shows peaked T-waves. Her blood pH is 7.31. Which of the following agents would lower her serum potassium concentration most quickly?**

A. Calcium gluconate intravenously
B. Glucose and insulin intravenously
C. Sodium bicarbonate intravenously
D. Kayexalate orally

EXPLANATION

Treatment of hyperkalemia includes antagonizing the cell membrane effects of hyperkalemia, shifting potassium to the intracellular space, and removing it from the body. The effect of intravenous calcium is quickest among all the treatments, however, it does not lower the potassium concentration. Insulin drives movement of potassium into the cells. The time of onset is 15–30 minutes. Sodium bicarbonate is most effective in patients having metabolic acidosis, the pH of this child is near normal, hence not likely to cause significant lowering of potassium. Answer to this question is B.

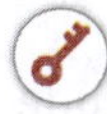

Key: B

BOOST YOUR KNOWLEDGE

Management of acute hyperkalemia includes an electrocardiogram to assess for cardiac toxicity, and intravenous calcium should be administered if electrocardiographic changes are present. The second step involves shifting potassium from the extracellular space to the intracellular space using insulin and beta agonist therapy. This therapy increases potassium uptake through the Na^+/K^+-ATPase into muscle. Interestingly, even in patients with insulin resistance in terms of glucose uptake in response to insulin, potassium uptake is not impaired. Because most potassium excretion is through the kidney, in a patient who is not oliguric or anuric, loop diuretics can be effective in eliminating potassium by increasing the distal delivery of sodium and distal flow rates.

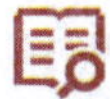

REFERENCE/SOURCE

- Shaw KN, Bachur RG (Eds). Fleisher and Ludwig's Textbook of Pediatric Emergency Medicine, 7th edition. Philadelphia; Wolters Kluwer; 2016. pp. 972-3.

15. A 6-year-old boy presented with anasarca and altered sensorium. On examination, he his GCS was 13/15 and BP was 150/100 mm Hg suggestive of stage 2 hypertension. His biochemistry report was suggestive of nephrotic syndrome. His C3 was 45 mg/dL and ANA was negative. His blood pressure was controlled initially by intravenous labetalol, followed by oral drugs. His sensorium improved and magnetic resonance imaging (MRI) was suggestive of posterior reversible encephalopathy syndrome (PRES). He subsequently required multiple drugs to control his blood pressure along with immunosuppressive medications for nephrotic syndrome. His picture is shown below.

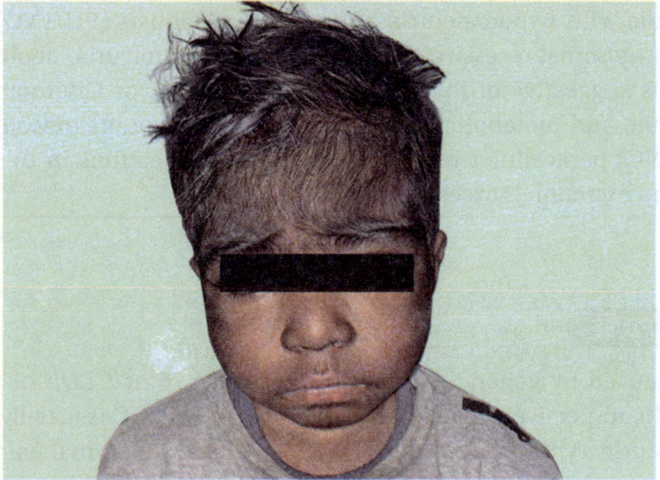

Which of the following drugs this child has most likely received?

A. Methylprednisolone
B. Tacrolimus
C. Minoxidil
D. Amlodipine

EXPLANATION

Methylprednisolone and amlodipine do not cause extensive hypertrichosis. Among calcineurin inhibitors, cyclosporin causes hypertrichosis. Cosmetic side effects of tacrolimus are much less as compared to cyclosporin. Minoxidil causes marked facial hair growth as shown in this picture.

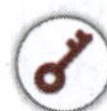

Key: C

BOOST YOUR KNOWLEDGE

Vasodilators are used as add on drugs for the management of refractory hypertension. This class of drugs include hydralazine and minoxidil, which act directly on vascular smooth muscle to reduce vascular wall tension and peripheral vascular resistance. Their side effect profile limits their use in the management of long-term hypertension. Common automated external defibrillators (AEDs) include headache, tachycardia, flushing, fluid retention, and palpitations. Hydralazine is associated with a lupus-like syndrome, and minoxidil causes hypertrichosis, which often affects compliance.

REFERENCE/SOURCE

- Schaefer F, Greenbaum LA (Eds). Pediatric Kidney Disease, 3rd edition. Springer International Publishing AG; 2023. pp. 858-72.

16. A 6-year-old boy presented with increased urine output. His blood pressure was 80/50 mm Hg in left arm supine. On evaluation, his urine output was 5.5 mL/kg/hour. His ultrasonography of the kidneys revealed nephrocalcinosis and urine analysis showed hypercalciuria, and he was suspected to have hereditary syndrome associated with defect in paracellular calcium transport in the thick ascending limb of Henle's loop. What could be the most likely metabolic abnormality in this child?

A. Hypokalemic metabolic alkalosis
B. Salt-wasting
C. Hypocalciuria
D. Hypomagnesemia

EXPLANATION

Familial hypomagnesemia with hypercalciuria and nephrocalcinosis (FHHNC) is associated with genetic variants in paracellin-1 (autosomal recessive). The combination of polyuria, nephrocalcinosis, hyperuricemia, and hypomagnesemia, is suggestive of this diagnosis. The Bartter or Gitelman's syndromes present with salt-wasting, hypokalemia, and metabolic alkalosis. In familial hypomagnesemia with hypercalciuria and nephrocalcinosis (FHHNC) paracellular reabsorption of divalent cations in the loop of Henle is defective. Therefore, urinary calcium excretion is excessive in FHHNC.

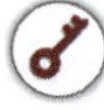

Key: D

BOOST YOUR KNOWLEDGE

The kidney disease is caused by genetic variants in the *CLDN16* or *CLDN19* genes encoding the proteins claudin-16 and claudin-19, respectively. The initial symptoms of FHHNC is usually failure to thrive, polyuria and polydipsia, and recurrent urinary tract infections (UTI). Many have abdominal pain, vomiting, feeding problems, enuresis, nephrolithiasis, or rickets. Hypomagnesemia, hypercalciuria, and nephrocalcinosis are prominent findings in FHHNC patients at the time of diagnosis. The most common imaging finding is the presence of medullary bilateral nephrocalcinosis due to calcium deposits in almost every patient at diagnosis, regardless of the degree of kidney function. An approach to a patient with hypomagnesemia is shown here:

Approach to a patient with hypomagnesemia:

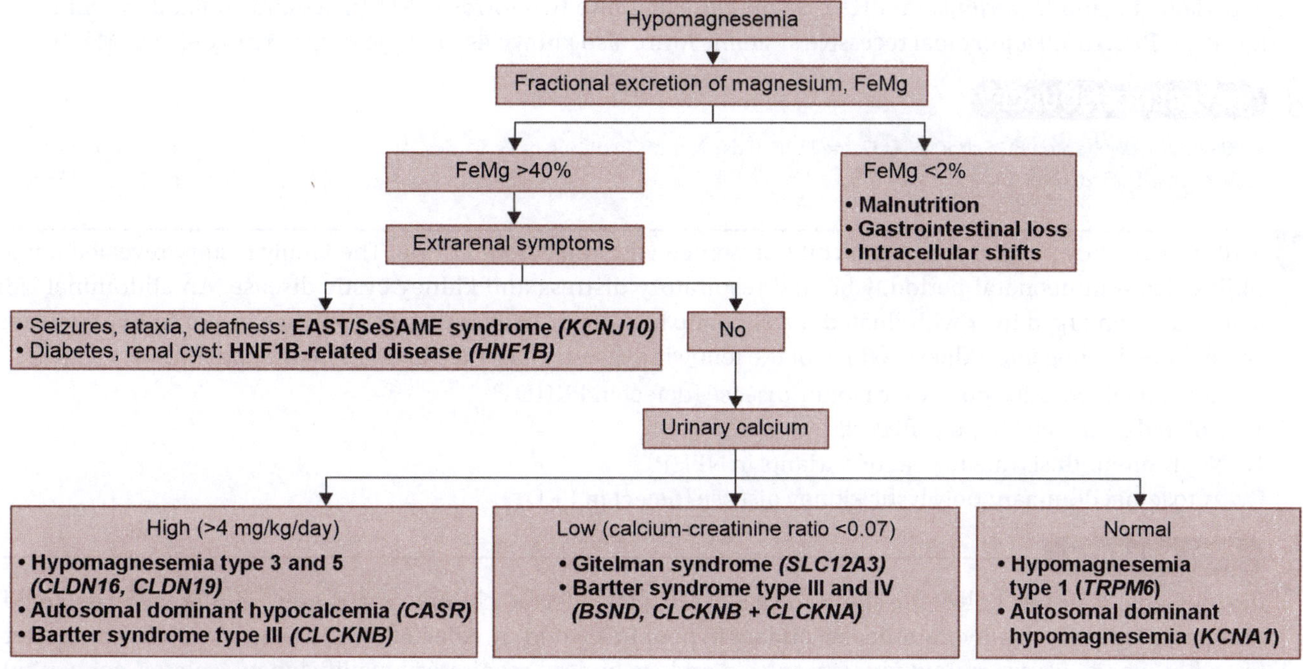

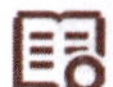

REFERENCE/SOURCE

- Schaefer F, Greenbaum LA (Eds). Pediatric Kidney Disease, 3rd edition. Springer International Publishing AG; 2023. pp. 1026-8.

17. A 6-day-old child presented with vomiting and respiratory distress. In the emergency room the capillary refill time (CRT) was >3 seconds. On evaluation, his sodium was 123 mEq/L, potassium 7.8 mEq/L, pH 7.1, pCO_2 = 22 and HCO_3 = 18 mEq/L. What could be the most likely diagnosis?

A. Liddle syndrome
B. Autosomal recessive pseudohypoaldosteronism type I
C. Pseudohypoaldosteronism type II (Gordon syndrome)
D. Glucocorticoid-remediable aldosteronism (primary hyperaldosteronism)

EXPLANATION

In a neonate, the combination of hyperkalemia, volume depletion, and metabolic acidosis with respiratory distress is suggestive of pseudohypoaldosteronism (autosomal recessive form of pseudohypoaldosteronism type I). There is lack of function of the epithelial sodium channel (ENaC) expressed in respiratory epithelium. In pseudohypoaldosteronism type II, hypertension is an important feature and also known as Gordon syndrome. In glucocorticoid-remediable aldosteronism, the clinical features reflect aldosterone excess and presents with hypertension, hypokalemia, and metabolic alkalosis. Liddle syndrome is associated with hypertension, hypokalemia, and metabolic alkalosis.

Key: B

BOOST YOUR KNOWLEDGE

Pseudohypoaldosteronism (PHA) is a rare heterogeneous disorder characterized by renal electrolyte transport dysfunctions due to mineralocorticoid resistance. Two different forms of PHA have been described—type 1 PHA (PHA1) characterized by hyponatremia, hyperkalemia, and metabolic acidosis with paradoxically increased serum aldosterone concentration and type 2 PHA (PHA2) also known as Gordon syndrome characterized by hyperkalemia and hypertension. PHA1 is sub-classified into two forms—PHA1a, an autosomal dominant renal form and PHA1b, an autosomal recessive systemic form, also known as multiple target organ defects (MTOD).

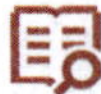

REFERENCE/SOURCE

- Kliegman RM, Stanton BF, Schor NF, St Geme III JW (Eds). Nelson Textbook of Pediatrics, 21st South East Asia edition. Elsevier Health Sciences; 2015. pp. 358-59.

18. A 10-year-old boy previously normal child presented with red colored urine. The family history revealed a male sibling death in neonatal period, who had respiratory distress and kidney cystic disease. An abdominal USG revealed an enlarged liver with dilated intrahepatic bile ducts, splenomegaly, evidence of portal hypertension, and enlarged echogenic kidneys. Which of the following disorders is most likely in this patient?

A. Autosomal recessive polycystic kidney disease (defect in PKHD1)
B. Isolated congenital hepatic fibrosis
C. Nephronophthisis due to genetic variants in NPHP1
D. Autosomal dominant polycystic kidney disease (defect in PKD1)

EXPLANATION

In autosomal recessive polycystic kidney disease (ARPKD), affected children can present in utero with enlarged echogenic kidneys, oligohydramnios secondary to poor urine output. Affected neonates may expire shortly after birth because of severe pulmonary hypoplasia and secondary respiratory insufficiency. Isolated congenital hepatic fibrosis classically involves the biliary tract. Defects in NPHP1 and PKD1 represent kidney cystic diseases *not* typically associated with symptomatic congenital hepatic fibrosis.

Key: A

BOOST YOUR KNOWLEDGE

Autosomal recessive polycystic kidney disease is caused by genetic variants in *PKHD1*, a large ~500-kb gene with a complex splicing pattern located on chromosome 6p21.1-p12. The product of PKHD1, fibrocystin/polyductin (FPC), is a single membrane spanning protein with multiple isoforms expressed predominantly in the kidneys (collecting ducts and thick ascending loops of Henle), liver (in bile duct epithelia), and pancreas. In renal tubular and biliary epithelial cells, FPC localizes to apical membranes, which are the primary cilia/basal body. Management of early ARPKD remains a challenge in pediatric nephrology.

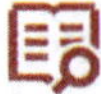

REFERENCE/SOURCE

- Schaefer F, Greenbaum LA (Eds). Pediatric Kidney Disease, 3rd edition. Springer International Publishing AG; 2023. pp. 303-4.

19. An 11-year-old girl is evaluated for enlarged and cystic kidney disease. Her serum creatinine level is 0.6 mg/dL. Identify the below investigation shown in **Figures 1 and 2**. Which of the following statements is correct about these investigations?

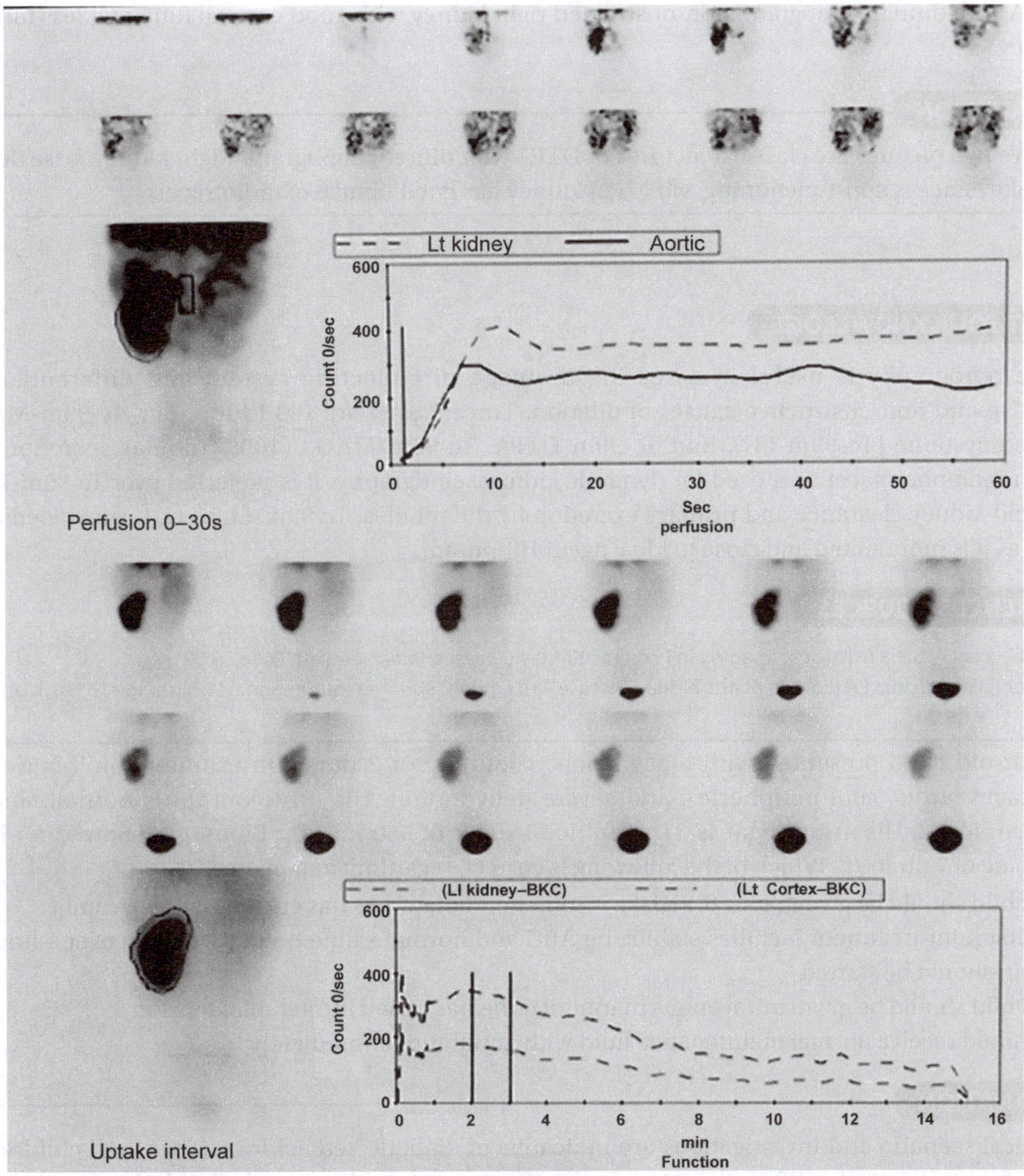

Fig. 1

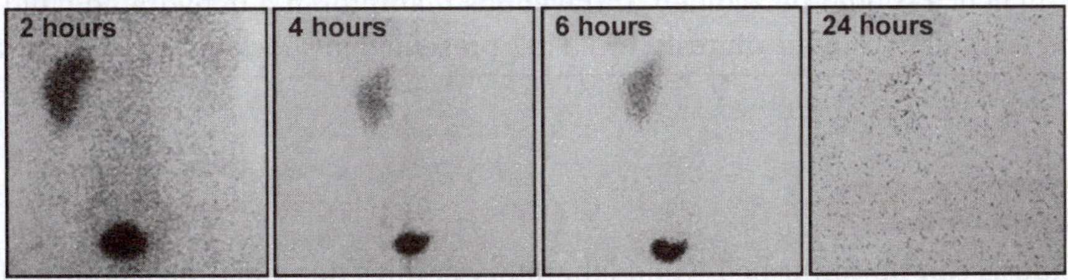

Fig. 2

A. DTPA with diuretic renogram, non-obstructed left kidney with good cortical function, non-functioning right kidney
B. DMSA with cortical scars, bilateral obstructed system, non-functioning right kidney
C. DRCG with reflux nephropathy, right kidney has more reflux than left
D. DPTA with diuretic renogram, non-obstructed right kidney with good cortical function, less functioning right kidney

EXPLANATION

The above two pictures are classical pictures of DTPA with diuretic renogram. Right kidney fossa does not show any uptake hence is non-functioning, while left kidney has good uptake of radiotracer.

Key: A

BOOST YOUR KNOWLEDGE

Diuretic renography is useful in assessing drainage of collecting system and differentiation between obstructive and non-obstructive causes of dilation. Tracers used are 123 I-hippuran, Tc-99m-MAG3, Tc-99m-ethylenedicysteine (Tc-99m-EC), and Tc-99m-DTPA. Tc-99m-MAG3 (100% tubular secretion) is the most common radiopharmaceutical used for dynamic kidney scintigraphy. It is preferred over Tc-99m-DTPA because of its rapid kidney clearance and primary excretion by the tubules. Tc-99m-LLEC (L,L, ethylenedicysteine) may also use as it is more suited and close to ideal agent Hippuran.

REFERENCES/SOURCES

- Dhull RS, Joshi A, Saha A. Nuclear Imaging in Pediatric Kidney Diseases. Indian Pediatr. 2018;55:591-7.
- Schaefer F, Greenbaum LA (Eds). Pediatric Kidney Disease, 3rd edition. Springer International Publishing AG; 2023. pp. 78-82.

20. A 10-year-old child presented with loose stools, vomiting for 2 days. On examination, his weight is 30 kg, he has tachycardia, cool peripheries, and severe dehydration. His urine output is normal, and he appears slightly confused. His urine sugar is 3+ with blood sugar of 550 mg/dL. Blood gas showed a pH of 7.01 and bicarbonate of 7 mmol/L. Which of the following is correct, regarding management?

A. The child should be given bolus 0.1 IU/kg insulin immediately as has critical hyperglycemia
B. His first hour treatment includes stabilizing ABC and normal saline bolus 10 mL/kg over 1 hour after which insulin should be started
C. The child should be given intravenous mannitol as he has raised intracranial tension
D. He should receive normal maintenance fluid with antibiotics immediately

EXPLANATION

The clinical scenario and investigations are indicative of diabetic ketoacidosis (DKA). All children with DKA need stabilization in the ER with assessment of airway, breathing and circulation, and simultaneous management of shock. Insulin bolus within the first hour of management is associated with raised indirect Coombs test (ICT) hence should be avoided. Intravenous mannitol in a dehydrated child will lead to further deterioration and will add to osmotic diuresis. Child has presented in shock hence need intravenous bolus.

Key: B

BOOST YOUR KNOWLEDGE

Diabetic ketoacidosis can be confirmed when laboratory studies demonstrate a serum glucose concentration above 200 mg/dL, a venous pH <7.30 (or serum bicarbonate concentration <15 mmol/L), and ketonuria.

The severity of DKA is classified according to the severity of acidosis, with mild DKA corresponding to a venous pH <7.30 (or serum bicarbonate concentration <15 mmol/L); moderate DKA to a pH <7.2 (or serum bicarbonate <10 mmol/L); and severe DKA to a pH <7.1 (or serum bicarbonate <5 mmol/L). An initial bolus of isotonic intravenous fluids (10–20 mL/kg of 0.9% saline or other isotonic fluid) is often needed to restore adequate perfusion. Treatment with bicarbonate is rarely indicated as children are generally able to tolerate even severe acidosis without hemodynamic instability. Bicarbonate administration does not result in more rapid recovery from DKA, may lead to hypokalemia, and is associated with a four-fold increase in the risk of cerebral edema. Therefore, bicarbonate should not routinely be used in children with DKA. In rare clinical circumstances such as symptomatic hyperkalemia or hemodynamic instability due to extreme acidosis, bicarbonate therapy may be necessary.

REFERENCE/SOURCE

- Kliegman RM, Stanton BF, Schor NF, St Geme III JW (Eds). Nelson Textbook of Pediatrics, 21st South East Asia edition. Elsevier Health Sciences; 2015. pp. 2772-6.

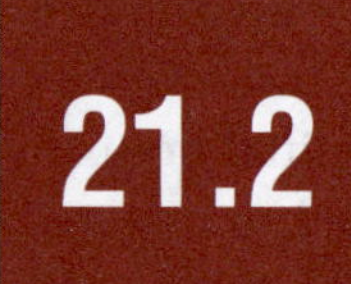

Cystic Diseases of the Kidney

Shilpa Sharma

1. Which is the most common cause of cystic lesion of the kidney in a 3-month-old child?

A. Mesonephric blastoma
B. Wilms tumor
C. Hydronephrosis
D. Simple cyst of kidney

EXPLANATION

Mesonephric blastoma is rare but represents the most common renal neoplasm in neonates. It is most often diagnosed in the first 3–6 months of life with 90% being discovered by the age of 1 year.

Key: A

BOOST YOUR KNOWLEDGE

Differential diagnosis of Wilms tumor can be tricky. While Wilms is the most common childhood kidney tumor, it is typically found in children <5 years old (median age of diagnosis ~3.5 years).

The second most common kidney tumor is clear cell renal sarcoma. The prognosis is not as good as Wilms as it has higher mortality and relapse rates. It often metastasizes to bone. Histological appearance can sometimes be similar to Wilms which can lead to a misdiagnosis.

Rhabdoid renal tumors are rare, highly malignant and are most often seen before age of 2 years and almost never in children >5 years. It is often widely metastatic at the time of initial presentation and has a very poor prognosis with an 80% mortality rate within 1 year of diagnosis.

Congenital mesoblastic nephroma is typically found in the first year of life, most often by ultrasound. Hypertension and elevated renin levels usually accompany it.

Renal cell carcinoma is rare in the pediatric age group. Renal medullary carcinoma is an aggressive carcinoma that is found almost exclusively in individuals with sickle cell disease, usually trait.

REFERENCE/SOURCE

- Gupta P, Menon PSN, Ramji S, Lodha R. PG Textbook of Pediatrics, 3rd edition. New Delhi: Jaypee Brothers Medical Publishers; 2022.

2. Which of the following typically presents between age of 30 and 40 years?

A. Autosomal dominant polycystic kidney disease
B. Autosomal recessive polycystic kidney disease
C. Chromosome-related polycystic kidney disease
D. None of above

EXPLANATION

Polycystic kidney disease (PKD) is an inherited disorder in which clusters of cysts develop primarily within the kidney. It can be transmitted as autosomal dominant (AD) or autosomal recessive (AR).

Autosomal dominant polycystic kidney disease (ADPKD): Signs and symptoms of ADPKD often develop between the ages of 30 and 40. Only one parent needs to have the disease for it to pass to the children. If one parent has ADPKD, each child has a 50% chance of getting the disease. This form is more common.

Key: A

BOOST YOUR KNOWLEDGE

Autosomal recessive polycystic kidney disease (ARPKD): The signs and symptoms often appear shortly after birth. Sometimes, symptoms do not appear until later in childhood or during adolescence. Both parents must have abnormal genes to pass on this form of the disease. If both parents carry a gene for this disorder, each child has a 25% chance of getting the disease.

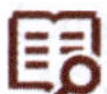

REFERENCE/SOURCE

- Gupta P, Menon PSN, Ramji S, Lodha R. PG Textbook of Pediatrics, 3rd edition. New Delhi: Jaypee Brothers Medical Publishers; 2022.

3. Multicystic dysplastic kidney disease is associated with which of the following abnormality in the ureter?

A. Ureter is dilated
B. Ureter is abnormality inserted in bladder
C. Ureter is atretic
D. Ureter is stenotic

EXPLANATION

Multicystic dysplastic kidney (MCDK) is a condition in which fluid-filled sacs, called cysts, replace normal kidney tissue and prevent the affected kidney from working. MCDK is commonly associated with an atretic or absent ureter.

Key: C

BOOST YOUR KNOWLEDGE

Multicystic dysplastic kidney is the most common cause of kidney cysts in children. An antenatal ultrasound can reveal multiple small cysts in the affected kidney as early as the 15th week of gestation. The condition occurs more commonly in males than females (2.4:1) and the left kidney is more affected than the right kidney. Multicystic dysplastic kidney is mostly an isolated condition; however, the contralateral urinary tract could be affected by other abnormalities such as vesicoureteral reflux (VUR), ureteropelvic junction obstruction (UPJO), and ureterovesical junction obstruction (UVJO).

In a rare occurrence, MCDK may associated with persistent ureteric bud structures. Unilateral MCDK is usually asymptomatic due to the compensatory hypertrophy of the contralateral kidney.

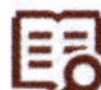

REFERENCE/SOURCE

- Gupta P, Menon PSN, Ramji S, Lodha R. PG Textbook of Pediatrics, 3rd edition. New Delhi: Jaypee Brothers Medical Publishers; 2022.

4. A 1-week-old boy presented with poor stream of urine. The kidneys are dilated on ultrasonography. What is the most likely diagnosis?

A. Anterior urethral valve
B. Bladder neck hypertrophy
C. Neurogenic bladder
D. Posterior urethral valves

EXPLANATION

Posterior urethral valves (PUV) are the commonest cause of bladder outlet obstruction that leads to backflow changes in the kidney with an incidence of approximately 1:5,000 live male births and almost 50% progressing to end-stage kidney disease within 10 years.

Key: D

BOOST YOUR KNOWLEDGE

Ultrasound findings consistent with posterior urethral valves include bilateral hydroureteronephrosis, dilated prostatic urethra (keyhole sign), and a distended bladder with thickened wall >3 mm, with poor emptying over 30 minutes. Focal renal parenchymal cysts demonstrate renal dysplasia. Other findings include oligohydramnios, fetal ascites, or urinoma. An enlarged fetal bladder on ultrasound may indicate obstruction and reflux but may also be a normal variant, and repeated scans are critical to the accurate antenatal diagnosis of posterior urethral valves.

Neonates with undiagnosed posterior urethral valves can present in a variety of ways. These could be an apparent urinary tract pathology such as delayed voiding, weak stream, urosepsis, or a palpable bladder. However, the presentation may also be more indolent with lethargy, poor feeding, or failure to thrive. In severe cases, they may present with respiratory distress due to pulmonary hypoplasia. Infants and older boys may present with similar complaints to neonates, with either specific urinary symptoms such as urinary retention and urinary tract infection or with secondary symptoms related to sepsis or azotemia. Posterior urethral valves may also be identified during the work-up of kidney failure, proteinuria, or hydronephrosis.

Postnatal management is cystoscopic valve ablation as early as possible. There is no international agreement on the degree of kidney function required for antenatal intervention, but evidence of preserved kidney function is required—fetal urinary biochemistry of Na <100 mEq/L, Cl <90 mEq/L, osmolality <210 mOsm/L, and β_2 microglobulin <6 g/L.

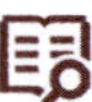

REFERENCE/SOURCE

- Gupta P, Menon PSN, Ramji S, Lodha R. PG Textbook of Pediatrics, 3rd edition. New Delhi: Jaypee Brothers Medical Publishers; 2022.

5. Which of the following is *not* a presentation of hydatid cyst of the kidney?

A. Absence of symptoms
B. Poor stream of urine
C. Shock
D. Flank pain

EXPLANATION

Hydatid cyst of kidneys might remain asymptomatic for many years, and presentations may be nonspecific and vary widely. Symptoms may include palpable mass, hematuria, flank pain, and dysuria; anaphylactic shock may occur.

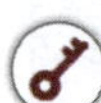

Key: B

BOOST YOUR KNOWLEDGE

Hydatid cyst of the kidneys are rare (4%). The cyst may rupture and grape-like structures may be seen in urine, also known as hydatiduria or presence of daughter vesicle in urine. This is pathognomonic for hydatid cyst of the kidney but occurs in 10–20% of all cases. Eosinophilia occurs in about 50% of cases; and serology in primary kidney hydatidosis is usually negative. Radiological imaging is diagnostic. Surgical kidney sparing cyst removal is performed through cystectomy and pericystectomy; however, nephrectomy is needed when the hydatid cyst invades a major renal part or in cases of hydatiduria. Perioperative albendazole is useful for the prevention of further spread of the infection.

REFERENCE/SOURCE

- Gupta P, Menon PSN, Ramji S, Lodha R. PG Textbook of Pediatrics, 3rd edition. New Delhi: Jaypee Brothers Medical Publishers; 2022.

6. Which of the following is correct for multiloculated cyst of kidney?

A. Absence of normal kidney tissue
B. It is typically bilateral
C. Is a neoplastic lesion
D. Characterized by multiple communicating cysts

EXPLANATION

Multilocular renal cyst is a distinct renal tumor whose gross external appearance and absence of normal renal tissue within the septa of loculi distinguish it clearly from other renal cystic lesions.

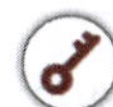

Key: A

BOOST YOUR KNOWLEDGE

Interlocular septa may contain either: (1) fibrous tissue alone or (2) embryonic tissue separating adjacent loculi. Multiloculated kidney cyst is characterized by a typically unilateral, solitary, multiloculated cystic mass consisting of small, noncommunicating cysts with flat, cuboidal, or hobnail epithelial lining, separated by fibrous septa.

REFERENCE/SOURCE

- Gupta P, Menon PSN, Ramji S, Lodha R. PG Textbook of Pediatrics, 3rd edition. New Delhi: Jaypee Brothers Medical Publishers; 2022.

7. Which of the following is correct about a cystic Wilms tumor?

A. Is a common renal tumor
B. May have a solid component
C. Presents below 2 years of age
D. Has female predisposition

EXPLANATION

Cystic Wilms tumor is distinguished from other cystic lesions of kidney by identification of solid nodular components within.

Key: B

BOOST YOUR KNOWLEDGE

Cystic renal tumors of childhood are relatively rare and are believed to be part of spectrum with cystic nephroma (CN) at the benign end, cystic partially differentiated nephroblastoma (CPDN) the intermediate region, and cystic Wilms tumor (CWT) at the malignant end. The only discriminating clinical factor is age at presentation as most patients with CN and CPDN present before 1 year of age, whereas patients of Wilms tumor are often older. Pathologically, CN consist of cysts and septa with cysts lined by flattened, cuboidal, or hobnail epithelium and septa that may be composed of fibrous tissue containing mature tubules but no immature elements. Immature mesenchymal/epithelial tissue or blastemal cells are found in the septa of the lesions classified as CPDN. CWT contains more solid structures between the cysts which bulge into the cystic spaces and also contain blastemal/mesenchymal/epithelial elements.

REFERENCE/SOURCE

- Gupta P, Menon PSN, Ramji S, Lodha R. PG Textbook of Pediatrics, 3rd edition. New Delhi: Jaypee Brothers Medical Publishers; 2022.

8. Dietl's crisis is a feature of which of the following?

A. Pelvi-ureteric junction obstruction (PUJO)
B. Renal calculus
C. Wilms tumor
D. Polycystic kidney disease

EXPLANATION

Dietl's crisis is a feature of pelvi-ureteric junction obstruction.

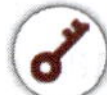

Key: A

BOOST YOUR KNOWLEDGE

The obstruction in PUJO causes collection of urine in the pelvis. This is followed by pain that is relieved as soon as the patient passes urine, this phenomenon is known as Dietl's crisis.

REFERENCE/SOURCE

- Gupta P, Menon PSN, Ramji S, Lodha R. PG Textbook of Pediatrics, 3rd edition. New Delhi: Jaypee Brothers Medical Publishers; 2022.

9. Which of the following is the investigation of choice to see the flow of urine from a hydronephrotic kidney?

A. DTPA
B. DMSA
C. USG
D. IVP

EXPLANATION

Diethylenetriaminepentaacetic acid (DTPA) renal scan assesses the function of the kidney and its flow.

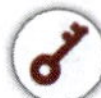

Key: A

BOOST YOUR KNOWLEDGE

Dimercaptosuccinic acid (DMSA) renal scan is better to see the renal scars. Intravenous pyelogram (IVP) is more invasive and not the investigation of choice anymore.

REFERENCE/SOURCE

- Gupta P, Menon PSN, Ramji S, Lodha R. PG Textbook of Pediatrics, 3rd edition. New Delhi: Jaypee Brothers Medical Publishers; 2022.

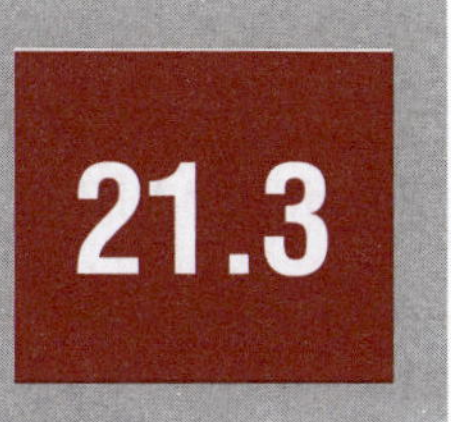

Urinary Tract Infection and Vesicoureteral Reflux

Kirtisudha Mishra

1. In children between 2 months and 2 years of age, presenting with urinary tract infection (UTI), an underlying vesicoureteral reflux (VUR) is expected to be detected in:

A. 7% B. 10%
C. 15% D. 30%

EXPLANATION

The Urinary Tract Subcommittee of the American Academy of Pediatrics Committee on quality improvement compiled 77 studies and found a wide variation in the prevalence of VUR among children with UTI. However, on further analysis, it was observed that the prevalence of VUR was a function of study size. The variation in the reported prevalence of VUR decreased among studies of larger size. As the sample size increased, the prevalence reported converged at 30–40%.

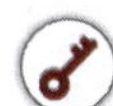

Key: D

BOOST YOUR KNOWLEDGE

Vesicoureteral reflux is the most common congenital anomaly of the urinary tract in children. Most of the primary VUR is diagnosed after a UTI, others being diagnosed during postnatal evaluation of antenatally diagnosed hydronephrosis or other congenital anomalies of the kidney and urinary tract (CAKUT). Children with VUR detected after UTI are predominantly females, while those with VUR diagnosed during follow-up of antenatally diagnosed hydronephrosis are mostly males. Secondary VUR occurs due to anatomical obstruction such as posterior urethral valves, urethral or meatal stenosis, and a functional bladder abnormality, such as neurogenic bladder and nonneurogenic neurogenic bladder.

Not all children with a first febrile UTI need a voiding cystourethrogram (VCUG), but it should be considered in those with abnormal ultrasound findings, recurrent UTIs, and/or an atypical causative pathogen.

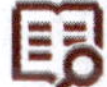

REFERENCES/SOURCES

- Downs SM. Technical report: urinary tract infections in febrile infants and young children. The Urinary Tract Subcommittee of the American Academy of Pediatrics Committee on Quality Improvement. 1999;103(4):e54.
- Mattoo TK, Gupta IR. Vesicoureteral Reflux in Children. In: Emma F, Goldstein SL, Bagga A, Bates CM, Shroff R (Eds). Pediatric Nephrology, 8th edition. Switzerland: Springer Nature; 2022. pp. 1344-51.

2. What is the approximate risk of recurrence of UTI, in children with underlying VUR not on prophylaxis?

A. 10% B. 15%
C. 25% D. 50%

EXPLANATION

Children with VUR have been found to have higher rates of recurrent UTI than children with no VUR. But the overall risk of UTI in children even without VUR is also considerably high.

Key: C

BOOST YOUR KNOWLEDGE

In a large follow-up study of 176 children, post-UTI, Keren, et al. found that at 2 years, the children with grade I to IV VUR had a higher risk of recurrent UTI (25%) compared to those without (17%). None of the children received antimicrobial prophylaxis for the duration of the study.

It is to be noted that though the difference in rates of recurrence was significant, the study created awareness that the risk of recurrent UTIs is not negligible in children without VUR. This is one of the reasons for not being too aggressive in detecting underlying VUR in every child who develops a UTI.

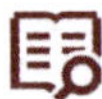

REFERENCES/SOURCES

- Keren R, Shaikh N, Pohl H, Gravens-Mueller L, Ivanova A, Zaoutis L, et al. Risk factors for recurrent urinary tract infection and renal scarring. Pediatrics. 2015;136(1):e13-21.
- Montini G, Spencer JD, Hevitt LK. Urinary tract infections in children. In: Emma F, Goldstein SL, Bagga A, Bates CM, Shroff R (Eds). Pediatric Nephrology, 8th edition. Switzerland: Springer Nature; 2022. pp. 1324-34.

3. Which of the following is *not* an indication for performing micturating cystourethrogram in children following a UTI [as per the Indian Society of Pediatric Nephrology (ISPN) 2024 guidelines]?

A. Any UTI in children <2 years
B. Abnormal ultrasound scan
C. History of recurrent UTI
D. Non-*Escherichia coli* UTI in children <2 years

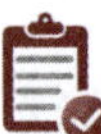

EXPLANATION

The recent ISPN 2023 guidelines suggest performing micturating cystourethrography (MCU) in children with one of the following: (1) UTI caused by non-*E. coli* uropathogens in children <2 years, (2) abnormal ultrasound scan, or (3) history of recurrent UTI.

Key: A

BOOST YOUR KNOWLEDGE

Micturating cystourethrography is the gold standard for the diagnosis and grading of VUR, although it involves discomfort to the child and exposure to radiation. Other imaging modalities to detect primary VUR include contrast-enhanced ultrasonography (CE-USG), direct radionuclide cystography (DRCG), indirect radionuclide cystography (IRCG), and magnetic resonance urography (MRU). VUR is present in approximately one-third of children with UTI. This implies that if imaging for VUR is performed in all children with UTI, two-thirds will undergo the inconvenience and hazards of imaging with negative results. Hence, the MCU study should be reserved for children with high suspicion of VUR. Low-quality evidence suggests that the yield of MCU will increase without much loss of sensitivity if it is restricted to children with UTI caused by non-*E. coli* organisms, abnormal USG findings, and recurrent UTI. MCU can be performed at any time after completion of therapy with antibiotics. The procedure should be performed using a protocol involving fluoroscopy and minimal radiation exposure, keeping the principles of ALARA (as low as reasonably achievable).

REFERENCE/SOURCE

- Hari P, Meena J, Kumar M, Sinha A, Thergaonkar RW, Iyengar A, et al. Evidence-based clinical practice guideline for management of urinary tract infection and primary vesicoureteric reflux. Pediatr Nephrol. 2024;39(5):1639-68.

4. Which of the following clinical scenarios is associated with an increased likelihood of detecting an underlying VUR?

A. Infants with UTI caused by *E. coli*
B. Infants with UTI caused by organisms other than *E. coli*
C. Boys with UTI above 5 years of age
D. Females with UTI in the adolescent age group

EXPLANATION

It has been reported in literature, by various studies, that neonates and infants with non-*E. coli* UTIs are more likely to have an underlying VUR. This is the reason that voiding cystourethrography is indicated in infants with atypical UTI, which includes non-*E. coli* UTI.

Males with VUR are usually detected at an early age during follow-up of antenatally diagnosed hydronephrosis. The etiology of UTI in adolescent females is more likely to be bladder-bowel dysfunction (BBD).

Key: B

BOOST YOUR KNOWLEDGE

The study by Cleper et al., 2004, including 64 neonates (55 males, 9 females) with UTI, found that the incidence of UTI was 6 times more common in males than females, while the incidence of VUR was equal between the sexes. Underlying VUR was detected at a fourfold higher rate in neonates with *Klebsiella*-induced UTI, compared to those with *E. coli*—UTI.

Not only in neonates but also in infants, the likelihood of an underlying VUR is higher in those with UTI due to non-*E. Coli* UTI.

Some of the large studies include:

- Pauchard JY et al., in 2017: In the study of 122 infants <3 months of age, with first febrile UTI, a striking difference was observed in the prevalence of underlying high-grade UTI between *E. coli* UTI (3%) and non-*E. coli* UTI (26%).
- Chong et al., in 2023 a study of 190 infants <3 months of age, with first febrile UTI, showed that non-*E. coli* UTI was independently associated with imaging abnormalities.
- Larger studies involving 607 children in the RIVUR trial by Carpenter et al., in 2013, further confirmed that non-*E. coli* UTI is associated with higher grades of VUR.

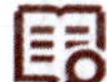

REFERENCES/SOURCES

- Chong SL, Leow EH, Yap CJY, Chao SM, Ganesan I, Ng YH. Risk factors for imaging abnormalities after the first febrile urinary tract infection in infants ≤3 months old: a retrospective cohort study. BMJ Paediatr Open. 2023;7(1):e001687.
- Cleper R, Krause I, Eisenstein B, Davidovits M. Prevalence of vesicoureteral reflux in neonatal urinary tract infection. Clin Pediatr (Phila). 2004;43(7):619-25.
- Mathews RI, Hansson S. Vesicoureteral reflux. In: Geary DF, Schaefer F (Eds). Pediatric Kidney Disease, 2nd edition. Heidelberg: Springer Nature; 2016. p. 1109.
- Pauchard JY, Chehade H, Kies CZ, Avoidance of voiding cystourethrography in infants younger than 3 months with *Escherichia coli* urinary tract infection and normal renal ultrasound. Arch Dis Child. 2017;102(9):804-8.

5. **Which of the following is NOT true regarding the dipstick nitrite test for diagnosing UTI?**

A. Nitrite test is usually false-negative in young infants who pass urine frequently
B. Nitrite test is negative in asymptomatic bacteriuria (ABU)
C. Nitrite test is negative in infections with *Enterococcus*
D. Nitrite test has excellent specificity in children >2 years

EXPLANATION

A positive nitrite test in the urine dipstick indicates bacterial conversion of endogenous nitrates to nitrites. This may be a sign of UTI. Most gram-negative uropathogens produce nitrite from nitrate, thus giving a positive nitrite test. However, it may take up to 4 hours to generate sufficient nitrite. Thus, in young infants and children who cannot hold urine for long in the bladder, even though pathogenic bacteria are present in urine, they may not get sufficient time to convert nitrate to nitrite, thereby giving a false negative reading in dipstick.

- A nitrite test does not detect organisms that are not capable of reducing nitrate to nitrite, such as enterococci and staphylococci.
- Nitrite test can be positive with asymptomatic bacteriuria.
- The meta-analysis by Williams et al., 2010, including studies comparing the accuracy of dipsticks for detecting UTI, found that nitrite-only positive dipsticks had a pooled specificity of 98% [95% confidence interval (CI) 96–99]; sensitivity varies depending on the age groups with up to ~80% sensitivity reported in children >2 years.

Key: B

BOOST YOUR KNOWLEDGE

Antibiotic treatment commenced within 2 days of onset of symptoms of UTI is important to prevent scarring. Therefore, rapid urine tests, such as urine dipsticks are used widely for presumptive diagnosis and a decision to start antibiotics for UTI. Urine dipsticks are quick, easy to perform, and cost-effective; while leukocyte esterase positivity is an indicator of pyuria, the presence of nitrite in urine indicates the conversion of endogenous nitrate to nitrite by bacteria. These tests are, however, not meant to replace urine culture because they neither identify the organism nor give information about antibiotic sensitivities.

REFERENCES/SOURCES

- Montini G, Spencer JD, Hevitt LK. Urinary tract infections in children. In: Emma F, Goldstein SL, Bagga A, Bates CM, Shroff R (Eds). Pediatric Nephrology, 8th edition. Switzerland: Springer Nature; 2022. p. 1330.
- Williams GJ, Macaskill P, Chan SF, Turner RM, Hodson E, Craig JC. Absolute and relative accuracy of rapid urine tests for urinary tract infection in children: a meta-analysis. Lancet Infect Dis. 2010;10(4):240-50.

6. **A 4-year-old boy diagnosed with first febrile UTI at 1.5 years of age, was found to have VUR grade IV on VCUG and was put on antibiotic prophylaxis with nitrofurantoin. Subsequently, he had two more episodes of febrile UTI over the next year and had associated bowel bladder dysfunction. Which of the following is the most appropriate strategy for such a patient?**

A. To change the antibiotic used for continuous prophylaxis
B. To repeat VCUG and dimercaptosuccinic acid (DMSA) to see the status of reflux and scarring
C. To perform surgery for ureter reimplantation
D. To perform endoscopic correction for VUR

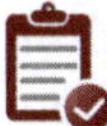

EXPLANATION

The child has a high-grade reflux, for which he was rightly started on antibiotic prophylaxis, which is the preferred first-line therapy for high-grade VUR. Despite prophylaxis, he had breakthrough UTIs. So, in this case, the best strategy is to go for surgical correction of VUR. Ureter reimplantation has been found to be more effective than endoscopic correction, as per Cochrane Systematic Review, 2019.

Key: C

BOOST YOUR KNOWLEDGE

Surgical correction of VUR is usually reserved for patients with high-grade VUR, and recurrent UTI despite antibiotic prophylaxis, noncompliance, or intolerance to prophylactic antibiotics. Open ureteral reimplantation remains the gold standard of surgical correction for VUR. Endoscopic treatment consisting of subureteral or intraureteral injection of a bulking agent such as dextranomer and hyaluronic acid, is also widely used. When surgery is indicated, open ureteric reimplantation is preferred to endoscopic correction as it has a higher success rate of resolution of VUR and a lower complication rate. It is the preferred modality for those with bowel bladder dysfunction and following failure of endoscopic correction. However, longer hospital stays, the need for postoperative analgesia, and the risk of postoperative complications need to be explained to the parents. For those with grade 3 VUR and in case of parental preference, endoscopic correction may be offered.

REFERENCES/SOURCES

- Mattoo TK, Gupta IR. Vesicoureteral reflux in children. In: Emma F, Goldstein SL, Bagga A, Bates CM, Shroff R (Eds). Pediatric Nephrology, 8th edition. Switzerland: Springer Nature; 2022. p. 1359.
- Salih EM, Eldamanhory H, Selmy GI, Galal HA. Comparison of subureteral endoscopic injection of dextranomer/hyaluronic acid and Lich-Gregoir ureteral reimplantation in the treatment of pediatric primary vesicoureteral reflux: a prospective randomized study. J Laparoendosc Adv Surg Tech A. 2021;31(6):719-23.

7. Which of the following patients would benefit most with circumcision for the prevention of UTI?

A. 3-year-old boy with first episode of UTI
B. 1-year-old boy with grade 2 VUR
C. 2-year-old-boy with recurrent UTI
D. Circumcision is never indicated for UTI prevention due to the high complication rate

EXPLANATION

Estimates show that circumcision reduces the risk of UTI by 82% in children. In normal, healthy, uncircumcised boys, the risk of UTI is almost 1–2%, and complications following circumcision are low (0.3–0.5%) in trained hands but can be as high as 1.5–2%. Since the risk of UTI is significantly higher (10–30%) in at-risk children (high-grade VUR and children with previous history of UTI), the benefit from circumcision outweighs the harm associated with it.

Key: C

BOOST YOUR KNOWLEDGE

The role of prophylactic circumcision in all healthy boys for the prevention of UTI is not yet clear due to contradictory results from studies. While one systematic review concluded that routine circumcision to prevent UTI was not indicated in normal boys, as the number needed to treat to prevent one UTI was 111, a second review concluded that circumcision was indicated in all boys, as it reduced the lifetime risk of UTI, with only about four procedures required to prevent one UTI.

In normal healthy uncircumcised boys, the risk of UTI is only about 2%, though, in at-risk children (high-grade VUR, recurrent UTI), the risk of UTI is significantly higher, so the latter are expected to benefit from circumcision. Thus, prophylactic circumcision is suggested only in children with significant risk factors for UTI like high-grade reflux or recurrent UTI by the Indian Society of Pediatric Nephrology 2024 guidelines.

REFERENCES/SOURCES

- Montini G, Hewitt LK. Diagnosis and management of urinary tract infection. In: Geary DF, Schaefer F (Eds). Pediatric Kidney Disease, 2nd edition. Heidelberg: Springer Nature. 2016. p. 1100.
- Morris BJ, Wiswell TE. Circumcision and lifetime risk of urinary tract infection: a systematic review and meta-analysis. J Urol. 2013;189(6):2118-24.
- Singh-Grewal D, Macdessi J, Craig J. Circumcision for the prevention of urinary tract infection in boys: a systematic review of randomised trials and observational studies. Arch Dis Child. 2005;90(8):853-8.
- Wahyudi I, Raharja PAR, Situmorang GR, Rodjani A. Circumcision reduces urinary tract infection in children with antenatal hydronephrosis: systematic review and meta-analysis. J Pediatr Urol. 2023;19(1):66-74.

8. A 5-year-old girl was diagnosed with cystitis. She was prescribed oral amoxicillin for 5 days, following which she recovered and remained well thereafter. After 3 months, the parents got her urine sample tested in a local laboratory and found growth of *E. coli* $>10^5$ colony forming unit (CFU)/mL. What is the most appropriate management strategy for the child now?

A. Restart antibiotics as per sensitivity pattern in culture report
B. Ignore the culture report, considering it to be asymptomatic bacteriuria
C. Restart antibiotics as per the sensitivity pattern in the culture report and put the child on continuous antibiotic prophylaxis, after completion of treatment
D. Restart antibiotics as per sensitivity pattern in culture report and perform ultrasound of the kidneys and urinary tract

EXPLANATION

The child was treated appropriately for cystitis and recovered clinically. She was well without any symptoms, so the urine culture report showing the growth of bacteria is suggestive of asymptomatic bacteriuria, which is not to be treated because avirulent commensal organisms colonizing bladders in children do not cause symptomatic UTI or decline in kidney function. UTI is to be suspected in a child, and urine is to be tested only if the child shows some symptoms suggestive of the infection.

Key: B

BOOST YOUR KNOWLEDGE

The prevalence of asymptomatic bacteriuria (ABU) is <1% in full-term infants, 3% in school-aged children, and about 1% in older children. Follow-up studies of children with ABU have shown that there was no significant difference in the development of symptomatic infection or permanent renal damage among those treated with antibiotics versus placebo. Rather, the treatment of ABU has been shown to be counterproductive with a risk of symptomatic UTI with a different bacterial strain.

However, treatment of ABU may be considered in children who have received renal transplants or who are undergoing invasive procedures involving the urogenital tract.

REFERENCES/SOURCES

- Dahiya A, Goldman RD. Management of asymptomatic bacteriuria in children. Can Fam Physician. 2018;64(11):821-4.
- Montini G, Spencer JD, Hevitt LK. Urinary tract infections in children. In: Emma F, Goldstein SL, Bagga A, Bates CM, Shroff R (Eds). Pediatric Nephrology, 8th edition. Switzerland: Springer Nature; 2022. p. 1336.

9. Which of the following statements regarding congenital reflux nephropathy is, *true*?

A. Predominantly seen in males
B. Associated renal dysplasia is uncommon
C. Mostly includes low-grade reflux
D. History of UTI is always present before diagnosis

EXPLANATION

Kidney damage/scarring associated with VUR is called reflux nephropathy (RN). Pyelonephritis-induced renal injury in the presence of VUR is called acquired RN. On the other hand, congenital RN is a result of abnormal renal development and is not secondary to injury from pyelonephritis.

Congenital RN is more common in boys, usually seen at younger ages, whereas acquired RN occurs after febrile UTI and is more common in girls, seen in all pediatric age groups. Renal dysplasia is commonly seen in congenital RN.

Key: A

BOOST YOUR KNOWLEDGE

Children have been diagnosed with VUR and renal scars even in the absence of UTI, thereby suggesting that the scarring is due to congenital hypodysplasia, rather than acquired after pyelonephritis. The VUR and the renal hypodysplasia are a result of a congenital developmental anomaly, with abnormal ureteric budding being the key factor in the pathogenesis of both. Such congenital hypodysplasia/scarring associated with VUR leads to end-stage renal failure. On the other hand, acquired renal scars following UTI are generally small and innocuous. The majority of hypodysplasia associated with VUR are seen as large areas of parenchymal damage.

REFERENCES/SOURCES

- Mattoo TK, Gupta IR. Vesicoureteral reflux in children. In: Emma F, Goldstein SL, Bagga A, Bates CM, Shroff R (Eds). Pediatric Nephrology, 8th edition. Switzerland: Springer Nature; 2022. p. 1348.
- Meena J, Hari P. Vesicoureteral reflux and recurrent urinary tract infections. Asian J Pediatr Nephrol. 2019;2:61-70.

10. Which of the following landmark trials, *does not* pertain to antibiotic prophylaxis in UTI?

A. PRIVENT (Prevention of Recurrent Urinary Tract Infection in Children with Vesicoureteric Reflux and Normal Renal Tracts)
B. PREDICT (Personalised Responses to Dietary Composition Trial)
C. DUTY (Diagnosis of Urinary Tract infection in Young children)
D. RIVUR (Randomized Intervention for Children with Vesicoureteral Reflux)

EXPLANATION

- *DUTY study clinical rule:* Economic Evaluation study, published in 2017, aimed to estimate the cost-effectiveness of a two-step clinical rule using symptoms, signs, and dipstick testing to guide the diagnosis and antibiotic treatment of UTI in acutely unwell young children presenting to primary care. It was not regarding antibiotic prophylaxis for the prevention of UTI.
- *PRIVENT* was a placebo-controlled trial from four Australian centers which examined whether low-dose, continuous oral antibiotic therapy prevents UTIs in children under the age of 18 years who had had one or more microbiologically proven UTIs.

- *RIVUR* was a multisite, randomized, placebo-controlled trial involving children with VUR that was diagnosed after a first or second febrile or symptomatic UTI, to evaluate the efficacy of trimethoprim/sulfamethoxazole (TMP/SMZ) prophylaxis in preventing recurrences.
- *PREDICT trial* was an open-label randomized controlled trial to evaluate the efficacy of continuous antibiotic prophylaxis in infants with grade III, IV, or V VUR and no previous UTIs in preventing the first UTI over 24-months follow-up.

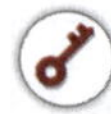

Key: C

BOOST YOUR KNOWLEDGE

Many prospective studies have evaluated the effect of long-term low-dose prophylactic antibiotics administered following an uncomplicated first febrile UTI. The two largest placebo-controlled studies, the PRIVENT (576 children, 64% female, and 61% absent or grade I–II VUR) and RIVUR (607 children, 92% female, and 92% grade I–III VUR) trials, showed a significant reduction in breakthrough UTIs in the antibiotic prophylaxis arm. PREDICT is a recently published open-label trial in infants that showed a small but significant benefit in preventing a first UTI despite an increased occurrence of non–*E. coli* organisms and antibiotic resistance.

REFERENCES/SOURCES

- Montini G, Spencer JD, Hevitt LK. Urinary tract infections in children. In: Emma F, Goldstein SL, Bagga A, Bates CM, Shroff R (Eds). Pediatric Nephrology, 8th edition. Switzerland: Springer Nature; 2022. p. 1335.
- Morello W, Baskin E, Jankauskiene A, Yalcinkaya F, Zurowska A, Puccio G, et al. Antibiotic prophylaxis in infants with grade III, IV, or V vesicoureteral reflux. N Engl J Med. 2023;389(11):987-97.

11. A 10-year-old girl studying in 5th standard with a busy study and activity schedule, presented with constipation, pain in the abdomen, and increased frequency of micturition for a few days. She was diagnosed with cystitis due to *E. coli*. The physician performed an ultrasonography which showed no abnormality in her kidneys and urinary tract. After 6 months, the girl again had a similar presentation, was diagnosed with a second episode of UTI, and treated in the same manner as earlier. From the management's point of view, what was missed in the first episode?

A. Further imaging by DMSA scan to look for permanent scarring post-UTI
B. Starting continuous prophylaxis
C. Asking a child to make a 2-day voiding diary
D. Repeating urine cultures at regular intervals

EXPLANATION

In older children and adolescents, voiding problems including hyperactive and dysfunctional bladder emptying may cause recurrent cystitis. Thus, in these children, a proper history of voiding patterns including frequency, urgency, holding maneuvers, and bowel habits needs to be taken. A 24-hour voiding diary provides information regarding these aspects and some clues regarding a dysfunctional voiding aspect of BBD, which has a strong association with UTI.

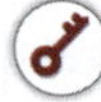

Key: C

BOOST YOUR KNOWLEDGE

Constipation and improper voiding technique are the main features of BBD, without any neuronal or congenital anatomical abnormalities. BBD results in increased voiding pressures, incomplete voiding, and defecation. Constipation compresses adjacent bladder neck-detrusor overactivity and voiding dysfunction.

Incomplete voiding and stasis of urine results in UTI. While the dysfunctional voiding scoring system is a useful tool to detect BBD, functional constipation is diagnosed based on the Rome IV criteria. BBD has been found in 30–50% of patients with primary VUR, which is significantly higher than that in healthy children.

REFERENCES/SOURCES

- Montini G, Spencer JD, Hevitt LK. Urinary tract infections in children. In: Emma F, Goldstein SL, Bagga A, Bates CM, Shroff R (Eds). Pediatric nephrology, 8th edition. Switzerland: Springer Nature; 2022. p. 1325.
- Shaikh N, Hoberman A, Keren R, Gotman N, Docimo SG, Mathews R, et al. Recurrent urinary tract infections in children with bladder and bowel dysfunction. Pediatrics. 2016;137(1):e20152982.

12. Which of the following statements is true regarding the RIVUR trial, which is one of the largest trials evaluating the role of TMP/SMZ prophylaxis in children with VUR?

A. It was found that TMP/SMZ prophylaxis reduced the risk of UTI recurrence by 50%
B. It was found that TMP/SMZ prophylaxis reduced the rate of renal scarring by 50%
C. It was found that TMP/SMZ prophylaxis had no effect on the recurrence of UTI
D. It was found that TMP/SMZ prophylaxis reduced the rate of UTI recurrence by 10%

EXPLANATION

The RIVUR trial was a 2-year, multisite, randomized, placebo-controlled trial involving 607 children with VUR, diagnosed after a first or second febrile UTI. Recurrent UTI developed in 39/302 children receiving prophylaxis compared to 72/305 children receiving placebo (relative risk, 0.55; 95% CI 0.38–0.78). Thus, they concluded that prophylaxis reduced the risk of recurrences by 50% (hazard ratio, 0.50; 95% CI, 0.34–0.74). However, there was no significant difference in the occurrence of renal scarring between the prophylaxis and placebo groups (11.9 and 10.2%, respectively).

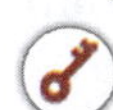

Key: A

BOOST YOUR KNOWLEDGE

While the RIVUR trial showed a 50% decrease in the risk of UTI recurrence in children with reflux receiving continuous antibiotic prophylaxis, on reanalyzing the RIVUR data after stratifying the children into risk groups, it was found that high-risk children benefit more. The high-risk group included: (1) uncircumcised males with VUR Grade I-III with or BBD or (2) females with VUR Grade I-III and BBD, or (3) females and males with VUR Grade IV with or without BBD. The low-risk group included circumcised males and females with VUR Grade I-III and no BBD.

The Cochrane Systematic Review (2019) evaluating studies dealing with interventions for VUR found that there was little or no difference in the risk of recurrent symptomatic UTI between those receiving low-dose antibiotic prophylaxis compared to those on no treatment/placebo. Further, it was found that at 1–3 years, antibiotic prophylaxis made little or no difference to the risk of new or progressive renal damage detected on the DMSA scan.

Based on these latest evidences, a selective approach is now advised for administering antibiotic prophylaxis in children with VUR.

REFERENCES/SOURCES

- Mattoo TK, Gupta IR. Vesicoureteral reflux in children. In: Emma F, Goldstein SL, Bagga A, Bates CM, Shroff R (Eds). Pediatric Nephrology, 8th edition. Switzerland: Springer Nature; 2022. pp. 1357-58.
- Wang ZT, Wehbi E, Alam Y, Khoury A. A reanalysis of the RIVUR trial using a risk classification system. J Urol. 2018;199(6): 1608-14.
- Williams G, Hodson EM, Craig JC. Interventions for primary vesicoureteric reflux. Cochrane Database Syst Rev. 2019;2(2):CD001532.

13. Which of the following is *not* an indication for administering continuous antibiotic prophylaxis?

A. Presence of posterior urethral valves
B. Recurrent UTI in a child with normal urinary tract
C. Grade IV VUR in a child without BBD
D. Grade II VUR in a child with BBD

EXPLANATION

Antibiotic prophylaxis is not advised in patients with urinary tract obstructions like posterior urethral valves. However, high-grade reflux and BBD are independent risk factors for recurrent UTI and thus warrant antibiotic prophylaxis. A child with recurrent UTI, even with a normal urinary tract, should be considered for antibiotic prophylaxis.

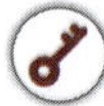

Key: A

BOOST YOUR KNOWLEDGE

Antibiotic prophylaxis is not advised in patients with urinary tract obstruction (e.g., posterior urethral valves), urolithiasis, and neurogenic bladder, and in patients on clean intermittent catheterization.

In a randomized controlled trial including children <6 years of age, followed up for 2 years after the first or second UTI, 51% of those with both BBD and VUR experienced recurrent UTIs, compared with 20% of those with VUR alone, and 35% with BBD alone. Also, it has been demonstrated that children with BBD and any degree of VUR had the highest risk of recurrent UTI (Keren et al., 2015) A study by Wang et al., found that children with VUR in the high-risk group benefit more from antibiotic prophylaxis than those in the low-risk group. The high-risk group included: (1) uncircumcised males with VUR Grade I–III with or without BBD, or (2) females with VUR Grade I–III and BBD, or (3) females and males with VUR Grade IV with or without BBD. The low-risk group included circumcised males and females with VUR Grade I–III and no BBD.

REFERENCES/SOURCES

- Hari P, Meena J, Kumar M, Sinha A, Thergaonkar RW, Iyengar A, et al. Evidence-based clinical practice guideline for management of urinary tract infection and primary vesicoureteric reflux. Pediatr Nephrol. 2024;39(5):1639-68.
- Wang ZT, Wehbi E, Alam Y, Khoury A. A reanalysis of the RIVUR trial using a risk classification system. J Urol. 2018;199(6): 1608-14.

14. Which of the following statements is *true* regarding the prevention of renal scarring with antibiotic prophylaxis?

A. Among the major trials published in the literature in children, all except the Swedish reflux study failed to show a reduction in renal scarring with antibiotic prophylaxis
B. Among the major trials published in the literature in children, all except the RIVUR trial failed to show a reduction in renal scarring with antibiotic prophylaxis
C. All studies have shown a significant reduction of renal scarring with antibiotic prophylaxis
D. The Cochrane Systematic Review, 2019 found significant benefits with antibiotic prophylaxis on long-term scarring and development of end-stage renal disease

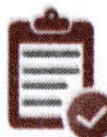

EXPLANATION

The Swedish Reflux Trial IV, by Brandstrom et al., published in 2010, had results differing from most other trials in terms of the effect of antibiotic prophylaxis on renal scarring. A total of 203 children from 1 to 2 years of age with grade III–IV reflux, were randomized to receive antibiotic prophylaxis, endoscopic treatment, or surveillance. New renal damage was seen in 13 girls and 2 boys. None of the children receiving antibiotic prophylaxis developed scars.

On the other hand, the RIVUR trial along with all major well-known trials of the world failed to show a reduction in the development of new scars with antibiotic prophylaxis, which was also demonstrated in the Cochrane Systematic Review, 2019.

Key: A

BOOST YOUR KNOWLEDGE

Based on the pooled evidence in the literature (Cochrane Systematic Review, 2019) shows an overall lack of benefit from antibiotic prophylaxis in children with VUR, in terms of the most critical outcome—renal scarring, which is a surrogate marker of progression to end-stage renal disease, recent guidelines across the world have recommended a selective approach for doing voiding cystourethrography after UTIs.

REFERENCES/SOURCES

- Brandström P, Nevéus T, Sixt R, Stokland E, Jodal U, Hansson S. The Swedish reflux trial in children: IV. Renal damage. J Urol. 2010;184(1):292-7.
- Mattoo TK, Gupta IR. Vesicoureteral reflux in children. In: Emma F, Goldstein SL, Bagga A, Bates CM, Shroff R (Eds). Pediatric Nephrology, 8th edition. Switzerland: Springer Nature; 2022. pp. 1357-58.
- Williams G, Hodson EM, Craig JC. Interventions for primary vesicoureteric reflux. Cochrane Database Syst Rev. 2019;2(2):CD001532.

15. What should be the first-line management of a child diagnosed with UTI, having associated symptoms of enuresis, constipation, and intermittent dribbling during daytime?

A. Desmopressin and lactulose
B. Tamsulosin and lactulose
C. Urotherapy and bowel habit training
D. Urotherapy along with oxybutynin

EXPLANATION

Features of constipation, enuresis, and voiding symptoms in the daytime such as increased frequency, urgency, and incontinence are indicative of BBD, which has a strong association with UTI. Appropriate management of BBD is warranted as the latter is a risk factor for recurrent UTI.

Initial management of BBD is urotherapy—which includes a voiding diary, optimum fluid intake, reduced intake of caffeine and chocolates, timed, frequent (2–4 hourly), and complete or double voiding, pelvic floor exercises, and biofeedback. Constipation is to be treated by dietary measures, laxatives, and proper posture supporting both feet on a stool/flat surface. This first-line therapy should be continued for at least 6 months. If unsuccessful, drugs such as oxybutynin and tamsulosin, or even clean-intermittent catheterization may be required.

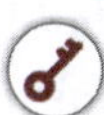

Key: C

BOOST YOUR KNOWLEDGE

Constipation and improper voiding technique are the main features of BBD, in toilet-trained children without any neurological or congenital anatomical abnormalities. This condition results from the poorly learned voiding technique in which the child attempts to suppress impending or active bladder contractions by inappropriately contracting the pelvic floor muscles and tightening the external sphincter, thereby causing an increase in bladder pressure and incomplete bladder emptying. Bladder dysfunction is often associated with constipation. BBD can be assessed using a questionnaire called the dysfunctional voiding scoring system.

REFERENCE/SOURCE

- Mattoo TK, Gupta IR. Vesicoureteral reflux in children. In: Emma F, Goldstein SL, Bagga A, Bates CM, Shroff R (Eds). Pediatric Nephrology, 8th edition. Switzerland: Springer Nature; 2022. p. 1359.

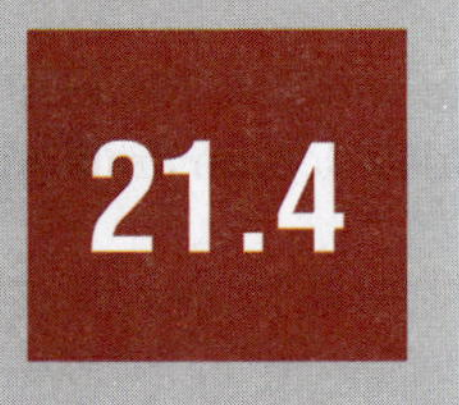

CHAPTER 21.4 Hematuria and Glomerulonephritis

Kanika Kapoor

1. A 13-year-old boy is referred for evaluation of persistent microscopic hematuria with urine routine microscopy showing 30–50 red blood cells (RBCs)/HPF in three instances over a period of 4 months. Urine protein was 2+ on the dipstick. There is a past history of gross hematuria following cough and cold episodes. The elder brother had deafness and a similar history and died at the age of 17 years due to kidney failure. Laboratories reveal blood, urea, and nitrogen (BUN) 40 mg/dL, serum creatinine 1.2 mg/dL, and normal complement. Skin biopsy histopathology would reveal which of the following findings?

A. Absence of epidermal basement membrane staining for the α_5 chain of type IV collagen
B. Leukocytoclastic vasculitis with immunoglobulin A (IgA), C3, and fibrin deposition
C. Rectangular, birefringent, yellowish-brown, polarizable crystalline crystals within the dermis, subcutaneous, and medium-sized vessels along with areas of focal epidermal and superficial dermal necrosis
D. Granular deposits of immunoglobulin M (IgM) and C3 in dermal-epidermal junction

EXPLANATION

The child is presenting in the second decade of life with persistent microscopic hematuria, subnephrotic range proteinuria, deranged kidney functions, gross hematuria following upper respiratory tract infections with a family history of the death of a male sibling who suffered chronic kidney disease and had probably sensorineural deafness. The provisional diagnosis is X-linked Alport syndrome.

Skin histopathological examination (HPE) showing leukocytoclastic vasculitis with IgA, C3, and fibrin deposition is a feature of Henoch–Schönlein purpura.

Skin HPE showing rectangular, birefringent, yellowish-brown, polarizable crystalline crystals within the dermis, subcutaneous, and medium-size vessels along with areas of focal epidermal and superficial dermal necrosis is found in primary hyperoxaluria. Direct immunofluorescence (DIF) demonstrates a granular deposition of immunoglobulins and complement at the dermal-epidermal junction in acute cutaneous lupus (lupus band).

Key: A

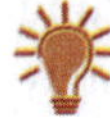

BOOST YOUR KNOWLEDGE

Alport syndrome occurs in three genetic forms: X-linked (80% of all patients), autosomal recessive (15%), and dominant illness (5%). The X-linked form is more severe and results from mutations in the *COL4A5* gene localized to the X chromosome (Xq22). The α5α5α6 trimer is a normal component of the epidermal basement membrane. Most patients with X-linked disease can be diagnosed by lack of immunostaining for α5 (IV) on skin biopsy. The onset usually is below 10 years of age with persistent microscopic hematuria or recurrent episodes of gross hematuria that may follow upper respiratory tract infections. Extrarenal manifestations include high-frequency sensorineural hearing loss, anterior lenticonus, and hypoparathyroidism.

Characteristic histopathological findings are thickening, splitting, and basket weave patterns of the glomerular basement membrane (GBM) demonstrated on electron microscopy.

REFERENCE/SOURCE

- Srivastava RN, Bagga A. Pediatric Nephrology, 6th edition. New Delhi: Jaypee Brothers Medical Publishers; 2016.

2. **A 12-year-old girl presented with fever, recurrent episodes of gross hematuria, and swelling of the body for the last 1 month. On examination (O/E), blood pressure (BP) is 150/95 mm Hg, and oral ulcers, alopecia, and anasarca are present. A urinalysis reveals 50–100 erythrocytes per high-power fields (50% dysmorphic), several erythrocyte casts, and 4+ proteinuria. The random urine protein/creatinine ratio is 2.0. Serum creatinine is 1.9 mg/dL. Which of the following lesions is most likely on kidney biopsy?**

A. Glomeruli are enlarged and show accentuated lobular pattern with endocapillary and mesangial proliferation, capillary walls are thickened, double contour on silver methenamine stain. Immunofluorescence (IF) shows C3 deposits along the peripheral capillary walls

B. Focal segmental proliferative lesions with cellular crescents. IF shows IgA1 deposits in mesangium

C. Glomeruli show hypercellularity, cellular crescents in a few glomeruli, and endothelial proliferation with wire loops. The basement membrane shows focal thickening on the silver methenamine stain. IF shows granular deposits of immunoglobulin G (IgG), C3, immunoglobulin M (IgM), and immunofluorescence microscopy

D. Crescents, focal segmental fibrinoid necrosis, and thrombosis of glomerular tuft with no deposits on IF

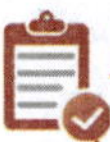

EXPLANATION

An adolescent girl presenting with edema, gross hematuria, hypertension, systemic features of fever, oral ulcers, laboratory tests showing deranged renal function tests, active urinary sediment, and nephrotic range proteinuria, the most probable diagnosis is systemic lupus erythematosus (SLE). A kidney biopsy done in a case of lupus nephritis (LN) would most commonly reveal diffuse mesangial, endocapillary, or mesangiocapillary proliferation and/or extensive subendothelial deposits. The hypercellularity is due to an increase in mesangial matrix and cellularity and infiltration of polymorphs. The capillary walls are thickened due to subendothelial deposits giving the appearance of wire loops. IF reveals a "full house" pattern, i.e., staining for IgM, IgA, C3, and C4 with dominant IgG and often C1q which is characteristic of LN even if serology is negative.

- Option A is typical histology of membranoproliferative glomerulonephritis (GN) with splitting and double contouring of the basement membrane.
- Option B is histopathology of IgA nephropathy with selective IgA deposition
- Option D is suggestive of pauci-immune vasculitis with necrotizing GN and few or no immune deposits on IF.

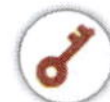

Key: C

BOOST YOUR KNOWLEDGE

Systemic lupus erythematosus is a chronic multisystem autoimmune disorder characterized by widespread inflammation of connective tissues affecting skin, joints, kidneys, heart, lungs, and nervous system. The peak incidence in children is at puberty and the condition is uncommon under the age of 10 years. Clinical features include fever, arthritis, characteristic malar rash, oral ulcers, alopecia, hepatosplenomegaly, and lymphadenopathy. Arthritis is polyarticular, nondeforming, and involves both large and small joints. Cardiac and neuropsychiatric involvement is less common but more serious. Kidney involvement is present in 60–80%, is often severe with deranged kidney functions in more than half the patients at onset and determines the prognosis and therapy of the disease. The World Health Organization (WHO) classification of LN is shown below; kidney biopsy typically reveals class 3 or 4 LN in 60–70% of patients at onset.

WHO classification of lupus nephritis

WHO class	International Society of Nephrology/Renal Pathology Society (ISN/RPS) nomenclature	Clinical features
I	Minimal mesangial LN	No renal findings
II	Mesangial proliferative LN	Mild clinical renal disease; minimally active urinary sediment; mild to moderate proteinuria (never nephrotic) but may have active serology
III	Focal proliferative LN <50% glomeruli involved A—Active A/C—Active and chronic C—Chronic	More active sediment changes; often active serology; increased proteinuria (>25% nephrotic); hypertension may be present; some evolve into class IV pattern; active lesions require treatment; chronic do not
IV	Diffuse proliferative LN (>50% glomeruli involved); all may be with segmental or global involvement (S or G) A—Active A/C—Active and chronic C—Chronic	Most severe renal involvement with active sediment, hypertension, heavy proteinuria (frequent nephrotic syndrome), often reduced glomerular filtration rate, serology very active. Active lesions require treatment
V	Membranous LN GN	Significant proteinuria (often nephrotic) with less active lupus serology
VI	Advanced sclerosing LN	>90% glomerulosclerosis; no treatment prevents renal failure

REFERENCE/SOURCE

- Srivastava RN, Bagga A (Eds). Pediatric Nephrology (Chapters 7, 8), 6th edition. New Delhi: Jaypee Brothers Medical Publishers; 2016.

3. A 5-year-old boy has developed palpable purpura of the lower extremities, abdominal pain, arthralgia of the knee joint, and melena over the last 7 days. The child had one episode of seizure 12 hours back before the child was brought to emergency. On examination, BP is 130/90 mm Hg, and pedal edema is present. Blood investigations revealed a platelet count of 3.45 lac/mm^3 and serum creatinine of 0.6 mg/dL. Urinalysis reveals 3+ protein, 30–40 RBCs/HPF. Kidney biopsy reveals focal proliferative GN with predominant mesangial IgA deposits. What is the most appropriate next step in management?

A. Rest and nonsteroidal anti-inflammatory drugs (NSAIDs) for joint pains
B. Angiotensin-converting enzyme (ACE) inhibitors or angiotensin receptor blockers (ARBs) for proteinuria
C. Oral corticosteroids at 1–2 mg/kg/day for a week followed by tapering
D. Pulse methylprednisolone and intravenous (IV) cyclophosphamide

EXPLANATION

A 5-year-old boy presenting with classical tetrad of nonthrombocytopenic purpura, gastrointestinal (GI) involvement as abdominal pain and bleeding, and joint and kidney involvement is suggestive of IgA vasculitis (Henoch-Schönlein purpura). Rarely cerebral involvement may be seen with seizures. Treatment is usually symptomatic with rest and analgesia for joint pains. Indications for using corticosteroids include severe GI manifestations, orchitis, and severe kidney involvement. In this case, oral steroids are the most appropriate management as there is severe GI involvement in the form of bleed. IV pulse methylprednisolone and IV cyclophosphamide are indicated for rapidly progressive GN (rapidly worsening kidney functions, crescents on biopsy) or pulmonary hemorrhage.

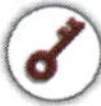

Key: C

BOOST YOUR KNOWLEDGE

Immunoglobulin A vasculitis previously known as Henoch–Schönlein purpura is an acute small-vessel vasculitis, characterized clinically by a nonthrombocytopenic purpuric rash predominantly affecting the lower limbs, arthralgia, and nondeforming arthritis affecting large joints such as ankles and knees, GI involvement as abdominal pain and in severe cases as GI hemorrhage, and nephritis. 90% of cases are found in those <10 years of age, with the median age at presentation being 6 years.

Kidney involvement is usually in the form of isolated microscopic hematuria with or without mild proteinuria. Nephrotic range proteinuria can also occur occasionally. Rarely the course can be rapidly progressive GN. Rarely pulmonary hemorrhage and neurological manifestations in the form of seizures, stroke, and change in mental status may be present. In two-thirds of the children, the disease runs its entire course within 4 weeks of onset.

A patient is considered to have IgA vasculitis in the presence of purpura (commonly palpable) or petechiae with lower limb predominance *and* one of the four following criteria:

1. Abdominal pain.
2. Histopathology showing leukocytoclastic vasculitis with predominant IgA deposits or proliferative GN with predominant IgA deposits.
3. Arthritis or arthralgia.
4. Kidney involvement (proteinuria or hematuria or presence of RBC casts).

Punch biopsy at the edge of a fresh cutaneous lesion can assist in the diagnosis of difficult cases by showing leukocytoclastic vasculitis with deposition of IgA and C3. Kidney biopsy is performed if renal function is deranged, or heavy proteinuria is present. Focal, segmental proliferative GN is typical, occasionally diffuse changes and crescent formation are seen. IF studies show prominent mesangial deposition of chiefly IgA1.

REFERENCES/SOURCES

- Hahn D, Hodson EM, Craig JC. Interventions for preventing and treating kidney disease in IgA vasculitis. Cochrane Database Syst Rev. 2023;2(2):CD005128.
- Srivastava RN, Bagga A (Eds). Pediatric Nephrology (Chapter 8), 6th edition. New Delhi: Jaypee Brothers Medical Publishers; 2016.

4. The risk factors for kidney involvement in IgA vasculitis include all of the following, *except:*

A. Low factor XIII activity
B. Severe abdominal symptoms
C. Persistent rash
D. Arthritis of large joints

EXPLANATION

In children with IgA vasculitis nephritis is associated with older age at presentation, persistent rash, severe abdominal symptoms, and low factor XIII activity. Arthritis affects large joints and is usually oligoarticular and self-limited. It is one of the clinical features of IgA vasculitis but is not a risk factor for kidney involvement.

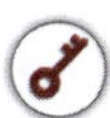

Key: D

BOOST YOUR KNOWLEDGE

Renal involvement of variable severity occurs in about one-third of patients within the first 4–6 weeks and almost always within 6 months. In studies, it has been found that age of >4 years at the onset, severe abdominal pain with GI bleeding, persistent purpura over a month, coagulation factor XIII activity <80%, and treatment with factor XIII concentrate were associated with developing kidney involvement. Coagulation factor XIII is a transglutaminase that cross-links fibrin monomers thereby forming the stable insoluble fibrin clot. The mechanism of the decreased level of factor XIII activity in IgA vasculitis has not yet been clarified, but a hypothesis has been proposed that factor XIII may be broken down by proteases of infiltrating leukocytes or be excessively consumed during fibrin formation around affected vessels.

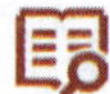

REFERENCES/SOURCES

- Sano H, Izumida M, Shimizu H, Ogawa Y. Risk factors of renal involvement and significant proteinuria in Henoch-Schönlein purpura. Eur J Pediatr. 2002;161(4):196-201.
- Srivastava RN, Bagga A (Eds). Pediatric Nephrology (Chapter 8), 6th edition. New Delhi: Jaypee Brothers Medical Publishers; 2016.

5. A 10-year-old boy presents with cola-colored urine for 2 weeks and swelling of the body for 2 weeks. There is no prior history of sore throat or boils. Examination shows anasarca and BP of 140/90 mm Hg. Labs reveal urine protein 3+, full-field RBCs, urine spot protein creatinine ratio of 3.6 mg/mg. Blood urea of 84 mg/dL and serum creatinine of 0.7 mg/dL. Blood levels of C3, C4, antistreptolysin O (ASO) antibody titers, ANA, anti-GBM antibody, cytoplasmic antineutrophil cytoplasmic antibodies (c-ANCA), and antineutrophil cytoplasmic antibodies (p-ANCA) are normal. What would be the most appropriate next step in management?

A. Start oral corticosteroids @2 mg/kg/day
B. Give IV methylprednisolone for 3 days followed by oral steroids
C. Perform a kidney biopsy
D. Initiate plasmapheresis

EXPLANATION

The child presented with nephritic syndrome with nephrotic range proteinuria with normal kidney function. In the presence of normal complement levels and negative ASO, ANA. Anti-GBM, c-ANCA, and p-ANCA, the most appropriate step would be to do a kidney biopsy to know the etiology. The above evaluation suggests the possibility of IgA nephropathy, pauci-immune vasculitis (ANCA negative), or rarely C3 glomerulopathy (with normal C3).

Key: C

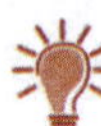

BOOST YOUR KNOWLEDGE

Indications of kidney biopsy in acute GN include:
- *Systemic features:* Fever, rash, joint pain, heart disease
- Absence of serologic evidence of streptococcal infection; normal levels of C3
- Mixed features of GN and nephrotic syndrome
- Severe anemia
- Very high levels of blood creatinine or anuria (suspected rapidly progressive GN)
- *Delayed resolution:*
    - Oliguria, hypertension, and/or azotemia persisting past 7–10 days
    - Gross hematuria persisting past 3–4 weeks
    - Nephrotic range proteinuria beyond 2 weeks
    - Low C3 levels beyond 12 weeks
    - Persistent proteinuria beyond 6 months
    - Persistent microscopic hematuria beyond 12–18 months

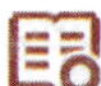

REFERENCE/SOURCE

- Srivastava RN, Bagga A (Eds). Pediatric Nephrology (Chapter 7), 6th edition. New Delhi: Jaypee Brothers Medical Publishers; 2016.

6. What is the most common histopathology seen in patients with nephropathy associated with the hepatitis C virus?

A. Membranous nephropathy
B. Membranoproliferative GN
C. Mesangioproliferative GN
D. Focal segmental glomerulosclerosis

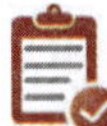

EXPLANATION

Hepatitis C virus infection is more commonly associated with membranoproliferative GN; some also show cryoglobulinemia.

Key: B

BOOST YOUR KNOWLEDGE

Viral infections are associated temporally with the onset of many glomerular diseases, particularly in children. In other cases of GN, when an infection is clinically silent, viral syndromes can still be implicated as a trigger. Kidney involvement in hepatitis B infection generally manifests as nephrotic syndrome but patients may also present with acute GN. The usual glomerular lesion associated with hepatitis B is membranous nephropathy; membranoproliferative GN, mesangial proliferative GN, and vasculitis may occasionally occur.

Immunosuppressive therapy is not indicated in the treatment of hepatitis B or C-associated GN since it impairs the host's ability to clear the virus from circulation and may stimulate viral replication. The role of antiviral drugs is not clear in children. Chronic disease in adults has been treated with regular or pegylated interferon for 6–12 months. The role of lamivudine or ribavirin in the treatment of these conditions is not clear.

REFERENCE/SOURCE

- Srivastava RN, Bagga A (Eds). Pediatric Nephrology (Chapter 7), 6th edition. New Delhi: Jaypee Brothers Medical Publishers; 2016.

7. Nutcracker syndrome (NCS) is *most* likely to occur due to the entrapment of the left renal vein between the abdominal aorta and:

A. Inferior vena cava
B. Superior mesenteric artery
C. Left renal artery
D. Splenic artery

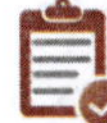

EXPLANATION

Unilateral bleeding of varicose veins of the left ureter, resulting from compression of the left kidney vein between the aorta and superior mesenteric artery (mesoaortic compression), is referred to as the *nutcracker syndrome*. A kidney ultrasound with Doppler sonography would be necessary to diagnose nutcracker syndrome.

Key: B

BOOST YOUR KNOWLEDGE

Patients with nutcracker syndrome typically present with persistent microscopic hematuria (and, occasionally, recurrent gross hematuria) that may be accompanied by proteinuria, left lower abdominal pain, left flank pain, or orthostatic hypotension. The diagnosis requires a high degree of suspicion and is confirmed by Doppler ultrasonography, computed tomography (CT) scanning, phlebography of the left kidney vein, or magnetic resonance imaging (MRI). Conservative approach (e.g., "watch-and-wait" strategy) represents a valid first-line treatment for children diagnosed with NCS.

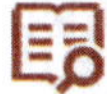

REFERENCE/SOURCE

- Vascular diseases associated with hematuria. In: Kliegman RM, St Geme III JW (Eds). Nelson Textbook of Pediatrics, 21 edition. Amsterdam: Elsevier; 2019.

8. As per the classification jointly proposed by the European Alliance of Associations for Rheumatology (EULAR)/ Paediatric Rheumatology European Society (PRES) in 2005, all of the following are causes of nongranulomatous small vessel vasculitis, *except.*

A. Henoch–Schönlein purpura
B. Microscopic polyangiitis
C. Wegener's granulomatosis
D. Cutaneous leukocytoclastic vasculitis

EXPLANATION

All of the above are causes of nongranulomatous small vessel vasculitis except Wegener's granulomatosis which causes granulomatous small vessel vasculitis.

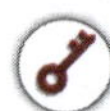

Key: C

BOOST YOUR KNOWLEDGE

Classification of childhood vasculitis:

- *Predominantly large vessel vasculitis:* Takayasu arteritis
- *Predominantly medium-sized vessel vasculitis:* Childhood polyarteritis nodosa (PAN), cutaneous polyarteritis, and Kawasaki disease
- *Predominantly small vessel vasculitis:*
  - *Granulomatous:* Wegener's granulomatosis and Churg–Strauss syndrome
  - *Nongranulomatous:* Henoch–Schönlein purpura, microscopic polyangiitis, hypocomplementemic urticarial vasculitis, and isolated cutaneous leukocytoclastic vasculitis
- *Other vasculitides:* Behçet disease, isolated vasculitis of the central nervous system, secondary to infection (e.g., hepatitis B-associated PAN), malignancy and drugs, including hypersensitivity vasculitis, and Cogan's syndrome

REFERENCE/SOURCE

- Srivastava RN, Bagga A (Eds). Pediatric Nephrology (Chapter 8), 6th edition. New Delhi: Jaypee Brothers Medical Publishers; 2016.

9. All of the following kidney diseases are correctly matched with their eponyms, *except:*

A. *IgA vasculitis:* Henoch–Schönlein purpura
B. *Wegener's granulomatosis:* Granulomatosis with polyangiitis
C. *Churg–Strauss syndrome:* Microscopic PAN
D. *Goodpasture syndrome:* Anti-GBM disease

EXPLANATION AND BOOSTER

Same as in Question 8.

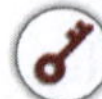

Key: C

10. Which of the following is the classical histopathological lesion of human immunodeficiency virus (HIV)-associated nephropathy?

A. Membranoproliferative GN
B. Membranous nephropathy
C. Necrotizing GN
D. Focal segmental glomerulosclerosis

EXPLANATION

The classic histopathologic lesion of HIV-associated nephropathy (HIVAN) is *focal segmental glomerulosclerosis (FSGS)*. Hepatitis C virus infection is more commonly associated with membranoproliferative GN. The usual glomerular lesion associated with hepatitis B is membranous nephropathy.

Key: D

BOOST YOUR KNOWLEDGE

Human immunodeficiency virus is associated with several kidney syndromes including HIV nephropathy, HIV-associated immune complex GN, thrombotic microangiopathy, and vasculitis-associated nephropathy. Medications used in management can cause nephrolithiasis (indinavir). HIVAN is characterized by nephrotic range proteinuria, azotemia, and normal to large kidneys on ultrasonography and FSGS. Subjects with collapsing glomerulopathy, a variant of FSGS with shrunken glomerular tufts and prominent visceral epithelial cells, show rapid progression to kidney failure.

REFERENCE/SOURCE

- Srivastava RN, Bagga A (Eds). Pediatric Nephrology (Chapter 8), 6th edition. New Delhi: Jaypee Brothers Medical Publishers; 2016.

11. A 10-year-old child presented with repeated episodes of gross hematuria. Which of the following is the *least likely* etiology?

A. IgA nephropathy
B. Hemolytic uremic syndrome (HUS)
C. Alport syndrome
D. Idiopathic hypercalciuria

EXPLANATION

Recurrent gross hematuria after upper respiratory infection (URI) is the typical presentation in IgA nephropathy.

Alport syndrome there may be repeated episodes of gross hematuria following URI or persistent microscopic hematuria with or without proteinuria. Idiopathic hypercalciuria is often detected in children with recurrent gross or microscopic hematuria.

Key: B

BOOST YOUR KNOWLEDGE

Idiopathic hypercalciuria, characterized by a normal concentration of serum calcium but excess urinary calcium, is the most common cause of kidney calculi. Idiopathic hypercalciuria may be a familial, autosomal dominant condition. The cause of this abnormality is not clear. An increased intestinal absorption of calcium is responsible in most cases. Idiopathic hypercalciuria is often detected in children with recurrent gross hematuria or microscopic hematuria. It may also be associated with the "frequency dysuria" syndrome. The management includes ensuring high fluid intake, moderate salt and protein restriction, citrate supplementation, and in some cases thiazide diuretics.

REFERENCES/SOURCES

- Isolated glomerular diseases associated with recurrent gross hematuria. In: Kliegman RM, St Geme III JW (Eds). Nelson Textbook of Pediatrics, 21st edition. Amsterdam: Elsevier; 2019.
- Srivastava RN, Bagga A (Eds). Pediatric Nephrology (Chapter 23), 6th edition. New Delhi: Jaypee Brothers Medical Publishers; 2016.

12. A 14-year-old boy was presented with anasarca, gross hematuria, and oliguria and was found to have normal BP. He had one episode of hemoptysis. Labs reveal urea of 124 mg/dL, serum creatinine of 3.5 mg/dL, urine R/M 2+ protein, and full-feed RBCs on microscopy. C3, C4, c-ANCA, p-ANCA, and ASO titers are normal. What is the most likely histopathological lesion on IF in kidney biopsy?

A. Fine granular deposition of IgG along capillary loops
B. Diffuse mesangial IgA deposits
C. Linear IgG deposits along the GBM
D. Codominant C3 and IgG along capillary loops

EXPLANATION

Fine granular deposition of IgG along capillary loops is found in acute poststreptococcal GN. Diffuse mesangial IgA deposits are found in IgA nephropathy. Linear IgG and C3 deposits are found in Goodpasteur syndrome.

Key: C

BOOST YOUR KNOWLEDGE

Goodpasture disease is an autoimmune disease characterized by pulmonary hemorrhage, rapidly progressive GN, and elevated anti-GBM antibody titers. The disease results from an attack on these organs by antibodies directed against certain epitopes of type IV collagen, located within the alveolar basement membrane in the lung and GBM in the kidney. Patients usually present with hemoptysis from pulmonary hemorrhage that can be life-threatening. Concomitant kidney manifestations include acute GN with hematuria, nephritic urinary sediment with cellular casts, proteinuria, and hypertension, which usually follow a rapidly progressive course. Kidney biopsy shows crescentic GN in most patients. IF microscopy demonstrates the pathognomonic continuous linear deposition of immunoglobulin G along the GBM.

Diagnosis is made by a combination of the clinical presentation of pulmonary hemorrhage with acute GN, the presence of serum antibodies directed against GBM (antitype IV collagen in GBM), and characteristic kidney biopsy findings. The prompt institution of plasmapheresis, high-dose IV methylprednisolone, and cyclophosphamide often induce remission and improve survival times.

REFERENCE/SOURCE

- Multisystem disease associated with hematuria. In: Kliegman RM, St Geme III JW (Eds). Nelson Textbook of Pediatrics, 21st edition. Amsterdam: Elsevier; 2019.

13. An 8-year-old previously healthy girl presents with rapid deterioration of kidney function, oliguria, and bilateral pulmonary infiltrates. There are no neurologic symptoms or fever. Serum creatinine is 5.4 mg/dL, and the urine shows 2+ proteinuria and moderate blood. Hematocrit is 28%, the platelet count is 46,000/mm^3, and numerous schistocytes are seen in the peripheral blood smear. Complement levels are normal. Kidney size is normal by ultrasound. Which of the following laboratory tests would be most useful to identify the cause of her disease?

A. Antiphospholipid antibodies
B. Direct and indirect Coombs test
C. C-reactive protein test
D. Anti-GBM antibody assay

EXPLANATION

The constellation of findings in this patient (acute kidney failure, microangiopathic hemolytic anemia, and thrombocytopenia) is suggestive of thrombotic microangiopathy (TMA). Of the choices given catastrophic anti-phospholipid syndrome would present with TMA, often with normal levels of complement.

Key: A

BOOST YOUR KNOWLEDGE

Catastrophic antiphospholipid syndrome is a rare and potentially fatal disorder characterized by rapid onset of multiorgan thrombosis and/or thrombotic microangiopathies.

Antiphospholipid antibody syndrome (APS) is a well-described syndrome in adults characterized by recurrent fetal loss and/or thrombosis. Antiphospholipid antibodies are associated with both venous and arterial thrombosis. A diagnosis of APS requires the presence of both clinical and laboratory abnormalities. Testing for APS includes evaluation for the lupus anticoagulant as well as anticardiolipin and anti-β_2-glycoprotein antibodies. The laboratory abnormalities must be persistent for 12 weeks. Because of the high risk of recurrence, patients with APS often require long-term anticoagulation. APS can be primary or secondary as is noted in patients with SLE.

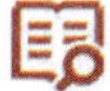

REFERENCE/SOURCE

- Thrombotic disorders in children. In: Kliegman RM, St Geme III JW (Eds). Nelson Textbook of Pediatrics, 21st edition. Amsterdam: Elsevier; 2019.

14. All of the following are additive criterion for classifying as SLE in the recent guidelines by the European League Against Rheumatism and the American College of Rheumatology, *except:*

A. Acute pericarditis
B. Class III/IV LN
C. Nonscarring alopecia
D. Autoimmune hepatitis

EXPLANATION

Autoimmune hepatitis is not a clinical criterion in the 2019 European League Against Rheumatism/American College of Rheumatology classification criteria for SLE.

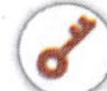

Key: D

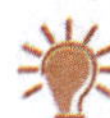

BOOST YOUR KNOWLEDGE

- As per EULAR criteria if the score is 10 points or more SLE is classified as an entry criterion, i.e., ANA titers of >1:80 on human epithelial type 2 (HEp-2) cells or an equivalent positive test.
- Within each domain only the highest weighed criteria are counted towards the total score.

Entry criterion

Antinuclear antibodies at a titer of ≥1:80 on HEp-2 cells or an equivalent positive test (ever)

If absent, do not classify as SLE
If present, apply additive criteria

Additive criteria

- Do not count a criterion if there is a more likely explanation than SLE. The occurrence of a criterion on at least one occasion is sufficient.
- SLE classification requires at least one clinical criterion and ≥10 points.
- Criteria need not occur simultaneously.
- Within each domain, only the highest weighted criterion is counted toward the total score.[§]

Clinical domains and criteria	***Weight***	***Immunology domains and criteria***	***Weight***
Constitutional: Fever	 2	*Antiphospholipid antibodies:* Anti-cardiolipin antibodies OR Anti-β_2 glycoprotein 1 (β_2GP1) antibodies OR Lupus anticoagulant	 2

Contd...

Contd...

Clinical domains and criteria	*Weight*	*Immunology domains and criteria*	*Weight*
Hematologic:		*Complement proteins:*	
• Leukopenia	3	Low C3 OR low C4	3
• Thrombocytopenia	4	Low C3 AND low C4	4
• Autoimmune hemolysis	4		
Neuropsychiatric:		*SLE-specific antibodies:*	
• Delirium	2	Anti-double-stranded deoxyribonucleic acid	
• Psychosis	3	(dsDNA) antibody* OR	
• Seizure	5	Anti-Smith antibody	6
Mucocutaneous:			
• Nonscarring alopecia	2		
• Oral ulcers	2		
• Subacute cutaneous OR discoid lupus	4		
• Acute cutaneous lupus	6		
Serosal:			
• Pleural or pericardial effusion	5		
• Acute pericarditis	6		
Musculoskeletal:			
• Joint involvement	6		
Renal:			
• Proteinuria >0.5 g/24 hour	4		
• Renal biopsy class II or V lupus nephritis	8		
• Renal biopsy class III or IV lupus nephritis	10		
Total score			
↓			
Classify as systemic lupus erythematosus with a score of 10 or more if the entry criterion is fulfilled			

§Additional criteria items within the same domain will not be counted
*In an assay with ≥90% specificity against relevant disease controls

REFERENCE/SOURCE

- Aringer M, Costobander K, Daikh D, Brinks R, Mosca M, Ramsey-Goldman R, et al. 2019 European League Against Rheumatism/ American College of Rheumatology Classification Criteria for Systemic Lupus Erythematosus. Arthritis Rheumatol. 2019;71(9):1400-12.

15. A 5-year-old child is being evaluated for asymptomatic persistent microscopic hematuria. Her hearing is normal. There is no prior history over counter medications. Her elder sibling was also evaluated for the same and no etiology was found. However, a kidney biopsy was not done. She had normal BP. Urinalysis shows trace protein and 10–15 RBCs/HPF. Investigations done were all reported normal. Which one of the following is the most likely pathogenesis of her hematuria?

A. Immune complexes deposit on the subepithelial side of the GBM
B. An inherited disorder involving the α_3 and α_4 chains of type IV collagen
C. The formation of immune complexes containing under-galactosylated IgA1 and antibody to the peptide residues on IgA1 heavy chain
D. An inherited disorder involving the α_5 and α_6 chains of type IV collagen

EXPLANATION

This patient has persistent isolated microscopic hematuria with normal BP and kidney function and a family history of hematuria. This is most compatible with a diagnosis of thin basement membrane nephropathy.

This disorder is now recognized as being due to a genetic abnormality affecting the α_3 and α_4 chains of type IV collagen. IgA nephropathy is less likely, because of the absence of bouts of macroscopic hematuria and the absence of proteinuria.

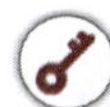

Key: B

BOOST YOUR KNOWLEDGE

Thin basement membrane nephropathy is an autosomal dominant condition. Heterozygous mutations in the genes *COL4A3* or *COL4A4* are seen in 40% of cases. Immunostaining for type IV collagen α_3 and α_4 chains on histology is normal. Clinical presentation is an incidental finding of microscopic hematuria without proteinuria. Some patients have episodic gross hematuria in association with acute infections. There is no evidence of proteinuria, hypertension, and progression to kidney failure, nor hearing or ocular defects. On ultrastructure, diffuse attenuation of the GBM (<200–250 nm) is characteristic. The prognosis is favorable, but patients should be monitored annually for proteinuria or hypertension.

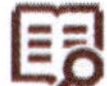

REFERENCE/SOURCE

- Srivastava RN, Bagga A (Eds). Pediatric Nephrology (Chapter 23), 6th edition. New Delhi: Jaypee Brothers Medical Publishers; 2016.

16. A 10-year-old boy was recently diagnosed with IgA nephropathy. Kidney biopsy reveals mesangial hypercellularity, no crescents, and <5% tubulointerstitial damage. IF showed mesangial deposition of IgA. On examination, weight is 40 kg, height is 134 cm, BP is 138/90 mm Hg. Serum creatinine is 0.7 mg/dL. Serum albumin is 4 g/dL. 24-hour urinary protein excretion is 0.8 g/day. Which of the following options is recommended as per Kidney Disease: Improving Global Outcomes (KDIGO) guidelines for initial management?

A. Fish oil, 4 g daily
B. Prednisone 40 mg daily, slowly tapering to10 mg/day over 6 months
C. Enalapril
D. Amlodipine

EXPLANATION

The patient has a *mild* form of IgA nephropathy with abnormal proteinuria (<1.0 g/day), presumably normal kidney function, and mild hypertension. The recommended initial approach to therapy would be to try angiotensin inhibition for 6 months. The use of ACE inhibitors has been recommended for the reduction of proteinuria and improved long-term outcomes in these patients. As per KDIGO guidelines, patients with persistent proteinuria ≥1 g/day, despite 3–6 months of optimized supportive care (including ACE-I or ARBs and BP control), and glomerular filtration rate (GFR) >50 mL/min/1.73 m^2, receive a 6-month course of corticosteroid therapy. While fish oil is not contraindicated, its benefits are unclear.

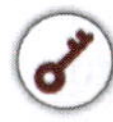

Key: C

BOOST YOUR KNOWLEDGE

IgA nephropathy is the most common form of primary GN worldwide although there are marked differences in its prevalence in different regions. The underlying abnormality appears to be a defect in the glycosylation of IgA1, which leads to the formation of the immune complex. The condition is diagnosed by demonstration of deposits of IgA in the mesangium, usually on IF examination or by immunohistochemistry. Deposits of IgG and C3 might be present, but IgA is predominant (2+ or more). Recurrent gross hematuria is the typical presentation that immediately follows a throat infection. Rarely, heavy proteinuria and impairment of kidney function may be present. Patients with microscopic hematuria and mild proteinuria may not need specific drugs. Those with heavy proteinuria or reduced kidney function should be treated with corticosteroids along with azathioprine or mycophenolate mofetil.

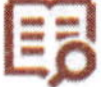

REFERENCE/SOURCE

- Chapter 10. KDIGO Clinical Practice Guideline for Glomerulonephritis. Kidney Int Suppl. 2012;2.

17. A 2-year-old boy presents with oliguria, hematuria, and one episode of seizure. He had bloody stools one week back which have resolved. On examination, severe pallor, BP is 118/84 mm Hg laboratory reveals Hb of 5 g/dL, platelet of 1 lac/mm^3, and total leukocyte count of 7,500/mm^3. Blood urea is 190 mg/dL, serum creatinine is 4 mg/dL. The peripheral smear is shown below:

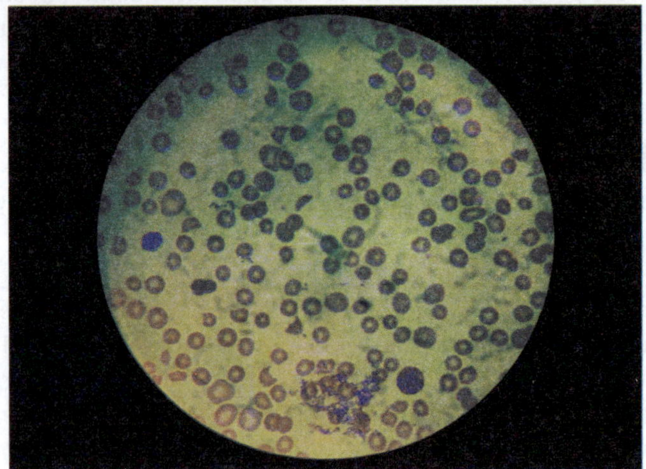

What is the likely diagnosis?

A. Henoch–Schönlein purpura
B. HUS
D. IgA nephropathy
D. Poststreptococcal GN

EXPLANATION

Peripheral smear showing schistocytes in a child with thrombocytopenia, anemia, and deranged kidney functions is suggestive of shiga toxin-associated HUS.

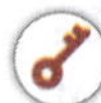

Key: B

BOOST YOUR KNOWLEDGE

Features of HUS include microangiopathic hemolytic anemia, thrombocytopenia, and acute kidney failure. HUS is classified into two broad groups: Shiga toxin-associated HUS (STEC-HUS) which is more common and occurs in young children caused by virulent strains of *Shigella dysenteriae* that produce shiga toxin 1, and verocytotoxin-producing *Escherichia coli*. *Atypical* HUS is heterogeneous and can be due to mutations causing abnormality in complement regulation, presence of inhibitory autoantibodies, familial or drug-induced.

REFERENCE/SOURCE

- Srivastava RN, Bagga A (Eds). Pediatric Nephrology (Chapter 13), 6th edition. New Delhi: Jaypee Brothers Medical Publishers; 2016.

18. A 14-year-old girl presents with gross hematuria and oliguria. In a span of 3 days, a child had progressive deranged kidney functions needing dialysis. She suffered from pharyngitis 1 week before getting admitted. Immunologic tests showed the presence of c-ANCA with antiproteinase 3 specificity and kidney biopsy revealed crescentic focal necrotizing GN with negative IF. What should be the next step in treatment?

A. Five to seven sessions of daily plasmapheresis
B. IV methylprednisolone pulse
C. Two doses of IV rituximab
D. Oral cyclophosphamide for 3 months

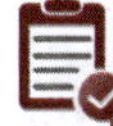

EXPLANATION

It is a case of granulomatosis with polyangiitis (GPA) as it fulfills 3 out of 6 criteria required to diagnose GPA or Wegener's granulomatosis:

1. Histopathology showing granulomatous inflammation within the arterial wall
2. Upper airway involvement (nasal discharge, serum perforation, and sinus inflammation)
3. Laryngeal, tracheal, or bronchial involvement (subglottic, tracheal, and bronchial stenosis)
4. ANCA positivity by IF or enzyme-linked immunosorbent assay (ELISA) for proteinase 3 (PR3) ANCA or myeloperoxidase (MPO)-ANCA
5. Pulmonary involvement (evident on chest X-ray or CT)
6. Kidney involvement

   Proteinuria, hematuria, RBC casts, necrotizing pauci-immune GN

   Combined treatment with corticosteroids and cyclophosphamide induces improvement in over 90% of patients and complete remission in 75%.

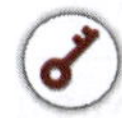

Key: B

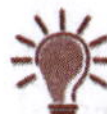

BOOST YOUR KNOWLEDGE

Induction therapy comprises of IV methylprednisolone for four to six doses followed by oral prednisolone (beginning at 2 mg/kg/day for 4 weeks, with gradual tapering for 12–18 months). This is combined with cyclophosphamide administered IV (500–750 mg/m^2 per dose, every 3–4 weeks for six doses) or orally (2 mg/kg/day for 3–6 months).

Plasma exchange (five to seven sessions of daily plasmapheresis) is recommended in patients with severe GN, dialysis-dependent kidney failure, or life-threatening pulmonary hemorrhage. After 4–6 months of induction therapy, the maintenance therapy is instituted with tapering doses of prednisolone and azathioprine or mycophenolate mofetil for 3–5 years. Other agents used in the patient's refractory to standard therapy include IV immunoglobulins and rituximab. The overall kidney survival is 50%.

REFERENCES/SOURCES

- Srivastava RN, Bagga A (Eds). Pediatric Nephrology (Chapter 8), 6th edition. New Delhi: Jaypee Brothers Medical Publishers; 2016.
- Vasculitis syndromes. In: Kliegman RM, St Geme III JW (Eds). Nelson Textbook of Pediatrics, 21st edition. Amsterdam: Elsevier; 2019.

19. A preterm baby born at 32 weeks gestation is admitted to the neonatal intensive care unit (NICU). On Day 7, the baby developed gross hematuria. Antenatal ultrasounds were unremarkable. A peripherally inserted central catheter (PICC) was inserted into the right lower extremity on day 2 for vascular access. On examination, BP is 84/59 mm Hg (95th centile for age) a left-sided abdominal mass was palpable. Investigations reveal hemoglobin 9.3 g/dL, platelets 46,000/mm^3, sodium 121 mmol/L, blood urea 240 mg/dL, creatinine 2.3 mg/dL; coagulation profile was normal. Urinalysis demonstrated >50 RBCs per high power field. Which is the investigation of choice to reveal the etiology?

A. Ultrasonography of kidneys
B. Urine culture
C. Renal scintigraphy
D. Ultrasound Doppler of kidney vessels

EXPLANATION

A diagnosis of renal vein thrombosis (RVT) is suggested in the case above. The absence of Doppler venous flow and enlargement of the left kidney is diagnostic of RVT.

Key: D

BOOST YOUR KNOWLEDGE

Renal vein thrombosis is the most common vascular condition in the neonatal kidney, and the renal vein is the most common site of spontaneous (noncatheter-associated) thrombosis in neonates. It can be antenatally or postnatally diagnosed, most commonly unilateral (left is the most common), and more often occurs in males. It usually presents within the first week of life. Gross hematuria, palpable flank mass, and thrombocytopenia form the typical clinical triad; however, not all affected neonates have the complete triad. RVT may also be associated with anemia, acute kidney injury, electrolyte disturbances, and hypertension. Prenatal risk factors for RVT include maternal diabetes and chorioamnionitis. Risk factors after delivery include sepsis, dehydration, polycythemia, indwelling central venous lines (i.e., umbilical venous catheters or lower limb peripherally inserted central catheter (PICC)], prothrombotic conditions, and congenital heart disease.

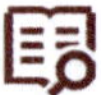

REFERENCE/SOURCE

- Vascular diseases associated with hematuria. In: Kliegman RM, St Geme III JW (Eds). Nelson Textbook of Pediatrics, 21st edition. Amsterdam: Elsevier; 2019.

20. A 12-year-old boy presented to the emergency with abdominal pain and gross hematuria for 2 days. There was a history of recurrent seizures since infancy requiring two anticonvulsants. He had delayed speech development, blurred vision, and poor school performance. Examination revealed hypopigmented macules on the trunk and left thigh, and multiple small, pinkish, erythematous papules on the face. Abdominal examination showed bilateral palpable kidneys, but no kidney angle tenderness. All of the following are expected on CT of the abdomen, *except:*

A. Enlarged kidneys
B. Multiple cysts in both kidneys
C. Rounded well-marginated echogenic mass arising from the kidney with mixed hyperdense and fatty tissue elements
D. Calcifications in kidney parenchyma

EXPLANATION

The classic kidney lesion of tuberous sclerosis is angiomyolipomas as described in option C, which occur in 50–80% of patients and often are bilateral and multiple. The dearth of macroscopic fat in CT in angiomyolipoma is a classic feature. Kidney cysts are the second most common kidney lesions and can be present with angiomyolipoma. Large kidney cysts can be present at birth. The incidence of renal cell carcinoma is $<5\%$. Calcifications are a feature of renal cell carcinoma.

Key: D

BOOST YOUR KNOWLEDGE

Angiomyolipomas, the most common benign solid tumors of the kidney, are composed of vascular, smooth muscle, and fatty tissue elements. They are an important component of the tuberous sclerosis complex, which includes developmental delay, facial angiofibromas, and lung cysts. Most children with angiomyolipoma are asymptomatic. Rarely are pain or hematuria are the presenting symptoms. Proteinuria can develop.

They can rupture on occasion to cause severe hemorrhage. Embolization followed by corticosteroids to alleviate postembolization syndrome is a first-line therapy for angiomyolipomas presenting with acute hemorrhage. Nephrectomy should be avoided as a way of maintaining kidney function because lesions can be numerous and bilateral. For asymptomatic, growing angiomyolipomas measuring larger than 3 cm in diameter, a mammalian target of rapamycin (mTOR) inhibitor, everolimus, is approved for treatment by the United States Food and Drug Administration (US-FDA).

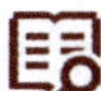

REFERENCE/SOURCE

- Neurocutaneous syndromes. In: Kliegman RM, St Geme III JW (Eds). Nelson Textbook of Pediatrics, 21st edition. Amsterdam: Elsevier; 2019.

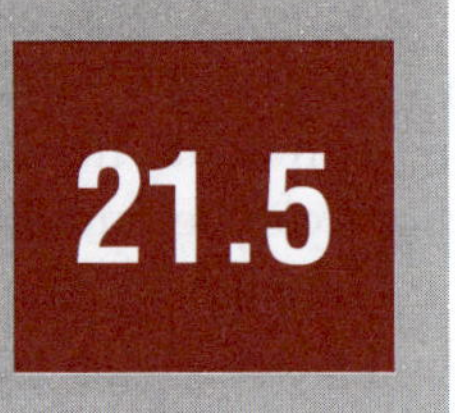

Proteinuria and Nephrotic Syndrome

Sriram Krishnamurthy

1. A 2-year-old boy is brought for evaluation of anasarca. He is found to have urine albumin 4+ by dipstick, serum albumin 2.2 g/dL, and serum cholesterol 450 mg/dL. Hemoglobin is 15 g/dL. Urinalysis reveals 2 red blood cells/high power field (RBCs/HPF) in a centrifuged urine specimen. There are no features of infection. Mantoux test is negative. Which of the following should be done next?

A. Initiate treatment with diuretics for anasarca management
B. Initiate treatment with prednisolone
C. Initiate treatment with prednisolone and diuretics
D. Wait for urine culture report, and then initiate treatment with prednisolone and diuretics

EXPLANATION

The child satisfies the definition of nephrotic syndrome (urine albumin 3+ or 4+, serum albumin <3 g/dL, and serum cholesterol 200 mg/dL). There is hemoconcentration (hemoglobin 15 g/dL) indicating low intravascular volume. One should avoid diuretics in this situation since they may worsen the already low intravascular volume, and instead, should encourage good fluid intake. Urine culture is indicated only in the presence of symptoms and signs of urinary tract infection. Prednisolone is the treatment of choice in nephrotic syndrome.

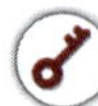

Key: B

BOOST YOUR KNOWLEDGE

Nephrotic syndrome is commonly encountered in children and is characterized by massive proteinuria (>1 g/m^2/day), hypoalbuminemia (serum albumin <3 g/dL), and edema. Recent guidelines have changed the serum albumin cut-off to <3 g/dL from the earlier value of <2.5 g/dL.

Nephrotic syndrome is commonly known to have a relapsing-remitting course. In most (85–90%) children with idiopathic nephrotic syndrome, the disease is sensitive to therapy with oral corticosteroids, and is termed steroid-sensitive nephrotic syndrome (SSNS). The prognosis in these cases is favorable. The remaining 10–15% of children do not respond to a 6-week course of daily corticosteroids and are labeled steroid-resistant nephrotic syndrome (SRNS).

REFERENCES/SOURCES

- Erkan E. Nephrotic syndrome. In: Kliegman RM, St Geme JW III, Blum NJ, Shah SS, Tasker RC, Wilson KM (Eds). Nelson Textbook of Pediatrics, 21st edition. Amsterdam: Elsevier; 2020. p. 2752.
- Sinha A, Bagga A, Banerjee S, Mishra K, Mehta A, Agarwal I, et al; Expert Group of Indian Society of Pediatric Nephrology. Steroid Sensitive Nephrotic Syndrome: Revised Guidelines. Indian Pediatr. 2021;58(5):461-81.

2. A 3-year-old girl is found to have urine albumin 2+ by dipstick persistently for the last 3 months. There is no microscopic hematuria. Which of the following statements is *true*?

A. Urine albumin 2+ indicates approximately 100 mg/dL albumin in the urine
B. Urine dipstick for protein testing picks up a variety of proteins in the urine including albumin, retinol binding proteins, beta-2 microglobulin, etc.
C. Urine spot protein:creatinine ratio is likely to be >2 in this case
D. Serum C3 is likely to be low in this case

EXPLANATION

Urine dipstick for protein is interpreted based on concentration of albumin in the sample, which is graded as follows: Trace (15 mg/dL); 1+ (30 mg/dL); 2+ (100 mg/dL); 3+ (300 mg/dL); and 4+ (2,000 mg/dL). Urine spot protein creatinine ratio >2 corresponds to 3+ or 4+ on dipstick. Serum C3 is usually low when there is microscopic or macroscopic hematuria.

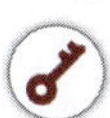

Key: A

BOOST YOUR KNOWLEDGE

A frequently used screening method for detection of proteinuria is urinary dipstick, which primarily detects albumin, leaving low-molecular-weight (LMW) proteins undetected. A color reaction between urinary albumin and tetrabromophenol blue produces various green hues based on the concentration of albumin in the sample, which is graded as follows: Trace (15 mg/dL); 1+ (30 mg/dL); 2+ (100 mg/dL); 3+ (300 mg/dL); and 4+ (2,000 mg/dL). Prior use of furosemide can produce false negative albuminuria since urine protein is being tested in diluted urine.

REFERENCES/SOURCES

- Flores FX. Clinical evaluation of the child with proteinuria. In: Kliegman RM, St Geme JW III, Blum NJ, Shah SS, Tasker RC, Wilson KM (Eds). Nelson Textbook of Pediatrics, 21st edition. Amsterdam: Elsevier; 2020. p. 2749.
- Sinha A, Bagga A, Banerjee S, Mishra K, Mehta A, Agarwal I, et al; Expert Group of Indian Society of Pediatric Nephrology. Steroid Sensitive Nephrotic Syndrome: Revised Guidelines. Indian Pediatr. 2021;58(5):461-81.

3. Which of the following tubular disorders is characterized by nephrotic range proteinuria and LMW proteinuria?

A. Distal renal tubular acidosis
B. Bartter syndrome
C. Gitelman syndrome
D. Dent disease

EXPLANATION

Tubular disorders generally have low grade proteinuria. However, Dent disease is an exception in that it is known to have significant amount of excretion of low molecular proteinuria (beta-2 microglobulins, retinol binding proteins, etc.). This manifests as nephrotic range proteinuria on 24-hour urine collection (>1 g/m^2 per day) or urine protein : creatinine ratio of >2. However, urine albumin by dipstick continues to be 1+ or 2+ since it detects only albumin. Bartter syndrome, Gitelman syndrome, and distal renal tubular disorders are not characterized by nephrotic range proteinuria.

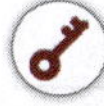

Key: D

BOOST YOUR KNOWLEDGE

Dent's disease is an X-linked recessive renal tubular disorder characterized by manifestations of proximal tubule dysfunction, including LMW proteinuria (often nephrotic range proteinuria), hypercalciuria, nephrolithiasis, nephrocalcinosis, hypophosphatemic rickets, and progressive renal failure. These features are generally found in males only, and may be present in early childhood, whereas female carriers may show a milder phenotype. The disease is caused by mutations in either the *CLCN5* (Dent disease 1) or *OCRL1* (Dent disease 2) genes.

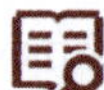

REFERENCE/SOURCE

- Kliegman RM, St Geme JW III, Blum NJ, Shah SS, Tasker RC, Wilson KM. Nelson Textbook of Pediatrics, 21st edition. Amsterdam: Elsevier; 2020. p. 2769.

4. A 6-year-old boy presents with nephrotic syndrome that is unresponsive to 6 weeks of treatment with steroids. He also has persistent microscopic hematuria and bilateral sensorineural hearing loss. He has never received any diuretics or ototoxic drugs. Kidney biopsy reveals focal segmental glomerulosclerosis (FSGS). Family history of recurrent hematuria, deafness on pure tone audiometry and chronic kidney disease is present in the mother. What is the most likely diagnosis?

A. Nail patella syndrome
B. Kearns–Sayre syndrome
C. Alport syndrome (AS)
D. Pierson syndrome

EXPLANATION

The clinical phenotype described earlier is most consistent with X-linked Alport syndrome (XLAS) since the mother too as similar complaints. AS can present with persistent microscopic hematuria, recurrent hematuria, nephrotic syndrome (that is steroid unresponsive) or chronic kidney disease. Kearns–Sayre syndrome is a mitochondrial disorder while Pierson syndrome is a congenital nephrotic syndrome with microcoria. Nail patella syndrome has abnormalities in nails, patella, and can have nephrotic syndrome, but deafness is not known.

Key: C

BOOST YOUR KNOWLEDGE

Alport syndrome is a progressive disorder of the glomerular basement membrane (GBM), accompanied by cochlear and ocular involvement. Three distinct genetic subtypes of AS include XLAS caused due to mutations in *COL4A5* gene, autosomal recessive Alport syndrome (ARAS) due to homozygous or compound heterozygous variations in *COL4A3* or *COL4A4* genes and autosomal dominant Alport syndrome (ADAS) due to heterozygous variations in *COL4A3* or *COL4A4* genes. The hallmark presentation of AS is microscopic hematuria. Intermittent gross hematuria is also occasionally described. Proteinuria, however, is often seen in late childhood or adolescence, with progression of the kidney disease from microscopic hematuria to microalbuminuria, overt proteinuria, or end-stage kidney disease (ESKD).

Alport syndrome children exhibit audiological abnormalities typically by late childhood as high tone (2,000–8,000 Hz range) hearing loss. Hearing impairment in AS is usually progressive; hence a hearing aid is advised upon identification. Ocular abnormalities manifest much later during second and third decade in 13–25% of AS patients. These specific manifestations include anterior lenticonus, dot and fleck maculopathy, or posterior polymorphous dystrophy; however, visual impairment is rarely seen.

REFERENCE/SOURCE

- Kliegman RM, St Geme JW III, Blum NJ, Shah SS, Tasker RC, Wilson KM. Nelson Textbook of Pediatrics, 21st edition. Amsterdam: Elsevier; 2020. p. 2721.

5. Congenital nephrotic syndrome due to diffuse mesangial sclerosis (DMS) can occur due to mutations involving which of the following genes?

A. *NPHS1*
B. *LMX1B*
C. *WT1*
D. *NPHS2*

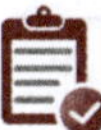

EXPLANATION

Congenital nephrotic syndrome is termed when nephrotic syndrome has onset before 3 months of age. It has two varieties: Finnish variety of congenital nephrotic syndrome and DMS. The former is caused by mutations in *NPHS1* gene, while the latter is due to mutations in *WT1, LAMB2,* and *PLCE1* genes.

LMX1B mutations lead to nail patella syndrome, while NPHS2 mutations (leading to structural defect in podocin) cause SRNS.

Key: C

BOOST YOUR KNOWLEDGE

Diffuse mesangial sclerosis is one of the rare causes of nephrotic syndrome in infantile and childhood period. It is characterized by progressive sclerosis of the mesangial matrix. Electron microscopy shows mesangial collagen fibrils along with wavy and split basement membranes. Genetic forms of nephropathy including DMS are usually resistant to immunosuppressive therapy and rapidly progress to ESKD. Genetic mutation in genes *WT1, LAMB2* and *PLCE1* are found in in DMS.

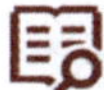

REFERENCE/SOURCE

- Erkan F. Nephrotic syndrome. In: Kliegman RM, St Geme JW III, Blum NJ, Shah SS, Tasker RC, Wilson KM (Eds). Nelson Textbook of Pediatrics, 21st edition. Amsterdam: Elsevier; 2020. p. 2760.

6. A 5-year-old girl is recently diagnosed with nephrotic syndrome and has persistent proteinuria despite 6 weeks of daily prednisolone (2 mg/kg/day). Which of the following statements is correct?

A. A trial of levamisole should be given
B. A kidney biopsy should be done
C. She requires genetic evaluation by next generation sequencing
D. Daily prednisolone should be continued for 4 more weeks (2 mg/kg/day)

EXPLANATION

This is a case of SRNS (nonresponse to daily steroids at 6 weeks). All cases of SRNS need kidney biopsy that may show FSGS, minimal change disease (MCD), or mesangioproliferative glomerulonephritis (MesPGN). Genetic testing by next-generation sequencing is required only in SRNS when it is infantile-onset, or when it is postinfancy with calcineurin inhibitor resistance, or in the presence of familial or syndromic features. Levamisole is not a drug for SRNS. It is used only in frequently relapsing nephrotic syndrome (FRNS) and steroid-dependent nephrotic syndrome (SDNS).

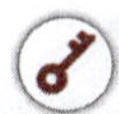

Key: B

BOOST YOUR KNOWLEDGE

While most of the children who presented with primary nephrotic syndrome respond to steroid treatment, 10–20% of these children do not achieve remission despite receiving second- or third-line of treatment, and more than half of the patients progress to end-stage renal disease (ESRD) within 10 years. Calcineurin inhibitors, such as cyclosporine and tacrolimus, are used as the first line of treatment. A significant number of patients with SRNS progress to ESRD if remission is not achieved.

REFERENCE/SOURCE

- Vasudevan A, Thergaonkar R, Mantan M, Sharma J, Khandelwal P, Hari P, et al; Expert Group of The Indian Society of Pediatric Nephrology. Consensus Guidelines on Management of Steroid-Resistant Nephrotic Syndrome. Indian Pediatr. 2021;58(7):650-66.

7. Kidney biopsy is indicated before starting which of the following drugs for nephrotic syndrome?

A. Mycophenolate mofetil (MMF)
B. Oral cyclophosphamide
C. Cyclosporine
D. Levamisole

EXPLANATION

A kidney biopsy should be performed before starting a course of a calcineurin inhibitor because it may cause interstitial fibrosis. MMF, cyclophosphamide, and levamisole are not nephrotoxic.

Key: C

BOOST YOUR KNOWLEDGE

Cyclosporine is a calcineurin inhibitor used at a dose of 4–6 mg/kg/day for FRNS and SDNS; as well as SRNS. Adverse effects include nephrotoxicity, hypertension, hyperkalemia, gum hypertrophy, hirsutism, acne, and hypomagnesemia. The drug dose should be titrated to attain blood trough levels of 80–120 ng/mL.

REFERENCES/SOURCES

- Erkan E. Nephrotic syndrome. In: Kliegman RM, St Geme JW III, Blum NJ, Shah SS, Tasker RC, Wilson KM (Eds). Nelson Textbook of Pediatrics, 21st edition. Amsterdam: Elsevier; 2020. p. 2752.
- Sinha A, Bagga A, Banerjee S, Mishra K, Mehta A, Agarwal I, et al; Expert Group of Indian Society of Pediatric Nephrology. Steroid Sensitive Nephrotic Syndrome: Revised Guidelines. Indian Pediatr. 2021;58(5):461-81.

8. Which of the following adverse effects can occur with the usage of tacrolimus for nephrotic syndrome in children?

A. Gum hypertrophy
B. Hirsutism
C. Hypermagnesemia
D. Diabetes mellitus

EXPLANATION

Adverse effects of tacrolimus include nephrotoxicity, hypertension, hyperkalemia, diabetes mellitus, headache, seizures, and hypomagnesemia. Adverse effects of cyclosporine include gum hypertrophy, hirsutism, acne, nephrotoxicity, hypertension, hyperkalemia, and hypomagnesemia.

Key: D

BOOST YOUR KNOWLEDGE

Tacrolimus is a calcineurin inhibitor used at a dose of 0.1–0.2 mg/kg/day for FRNS and SDNS; as well as SRNS. Adverse effects include nephrotoxicity, hypertension, hyperkalemia, diabetes mellitus, headache, seizures, and hypomagnesemia. The drug dose should be titrated to attain blood trough levels of 5–8 ng/mL.

REFERENCES/SOURCES

- Erkan E. Nephrotic syndrome. In: Kliegman RM, St Geme JW III, Blum NJ, Shah SS, Tasker RC, Wilson KM (Eds). Nelson Textbook of Pediatrics, 21st edition. Amsterdam: Elsevier; 2020. p. 2752.
- Sinha A, Bagga A, Banerjee S, Mishra K, Mehta A, Agarwal I, et al; Expert Group of Indian Society of Pediatric Nephrology. Steroid Sensitive Nephrotic Syndrome: Revised Guidelines. Indian Pediatr. 2021;58(5):461-81.
- Vasudevan A, Thergaonkar R, Mantan M, Sharma J, Khandelwal P, Hari P, et al; Expert Group of the Indian Society of Pediatric Nephrology. Consensus Guidelines on Management of Steroid-resistant Nephrotic Syndrome. Indian Pediatr. 2021;58(7): 650-66.

9. A 7-year-old boy presents with hematuria and proteinuria 3+. Serum creatinine is 1.2 mg/dL. There was history of palpable purpura over the buttocks and lower limbs along with abdominal pain and joint pains 2 months ago, which resolved with prednisolone. There were immunoglobulin A (IgA) deposits on the skin biopsy specimen at that time. Serum C3 is normal. What should be done in this child next?

A. Kidney biopsy
B. Reassurance that the hematuria and proteinuria will gradually resolve
C. Start immediately on enalapril for proteinuria management
D. Send urine culture and start on antibiotics

EXPLANATION

The clinical features of this case are consistent with Henoch–Schönlein purpura (HSP) (IgA vasculitis). The presence of hematuria and proteinuria in this case indicates the occurrence of nephritis as a complication. Kidney biopsy is required to stage the HSP nephritis. Enalapril is used in HSP nephritis, however, serum creatinine is high in this case and we should wait for creatinine to improve before enalapril can be considered. Urine culture has no role in a child without symptoms of urinary tract infection.

Key: A

BOOST YOUR KNOWLEDGE

Henoch–Schönlein purpura is the one of most common types of systemic vasculitis in childhood. Glomerulonephritis (HSPN) occurs in 30–50% of HSP patients, mostly in a mild form but a small percentage of patients present with nephrotic syndrome or renal failure. HSPN is caused by the glomerular deposition of immunoglobulin A1 (IgA1)-containing immune complexes in the mesangium, the subepithelial, and the subendothelial space. HSPN might lead to chronic renal disease and end-stage renal failure, thereby justifying immunosuppressive treatment. Long-term renal outcome correlates to the severity of the initial clinical presentation and the extent of renal biopsy changes, both of which are used to decide upon a possible treatment.

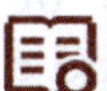

REFERENCE/SOURCE

- Kliegman RM, St Geme JW III, Blum NJ, Shah SS, Tasker RC, Wilson KM. Nelson Textbook of Pediatrics, 21st edition. Amsterdam: Elsevier; 2020. p. 2731.

10. A 1-year-old girl has been recently diagnosed to have megaloblastic anemia due to B_{12} deficiency and is responding well to parenteral B_{12} injections. She is referred for evaluation of persistent 2+ proteinuria. Serum creatinine is 0.25 mg/dL, and there is no edema or hematuria. She is normotensive. What is the likely possibility in this child?

A. Pearson marrow pancreas syndrome
B. Cobalamin C deficiency
C. Celiac disease
D. Imerslund–Gräsbeck syndrome (IGS)

EXPLANATION

Imerslund–Gräsbeck syndrome or selective vitamin B_{12} (cobalamin) malabsorption with proteinuria is a rare autosomal recessive disorder characterized by vitamin B_{12} deficiency commonly resulting in megaloblastic anemia, which is responsive to parenteral vitamin B_{12} therapy and appears in childhood. Other manifestations include failure to thrive and grow, infections and neurological damage. Mild proteinuria (with no signs of kidney disease) is present in about half of the patients.

Cobalamin C deficiency is a different disorder leading to atypical hemolytic uremic syndrome (HUS). Celiac disease and Pearson marrow-pancreas syndrome do not cause proteinuria.

Key: D

BOOST YOUR KNOWLEDGE

Imerslund–Gräsbeck syndrome is a rare autosomal recessive disorder characterized by proteinuria and selective malabsorption of cobalamin. Deficiency of cobalamin can lead to megaloblastic anemia, or pancytopenia. A biallelic mutation either in genes coding the proteins cubulin or amnionless cause IGS. Both these proteins act as a receptor for intrinsic factor-vitamin B_{12} complexes in the intestine. Cubulin is also an albumin binding protein important for renal tubular protein reabsorption. This explains the vitamin B_{12} deficiency and proteinuria. Because of absence of glomerular damage in kidney biopsies progressive kidney disease is not usual.

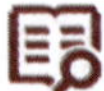

REFERENCE/SOURCE

- Kliegman RM, St Geme JW III, Blum NJ, Shah SS, Tasker RC, Wilson KM. Nelson Textbook of Pediatrics, 21st edition. Amsterdam: Elsevier; 2020. p. 2520.

11. A 1-month-old baby presents with edema all over the body. Urine albumin is 4+, serum albumin 2.1 g/dL. There is hepatosplenomegaly and a reddish rash all over the body. X-ray humerus reveals metaphysitis. What is the most likely diagnosis?

A. NPHS1 homozygous mutation
B. Congenital syphilis (CS)
C. Neonatal lupus
D. PLCE1 homozygous mutation

EXPLANATION

The clinical features of the child (rash, hepatosplenomegaly, congenital nephrotic syndrome, and metaphysitis) are overall consistent with CS. NPHS1 homozygous mutation causes Finnish variety of congenital nephrotic syndrome. Metaphysitis is not a feature of neonatal lupus and herpes simplex. PLCE1 mutations cause DMS.

Key: B

BOOST YOUR KNOWLEDGE

Congenital syphilis is caused by transmission of the spirochete *Treponema pallidum* from the mother to the fetus, resulting in a multitude of clinical presentations ranging from asymptomatic, premature birth, and a wide array of clinical signs and symptoms to stillbirth. Some infants with early CS are asymptomatic at birth. Clinical manifestations of early CS might include rhinitis ("snuffles"), hepatosplenomegaly, skin rash with desquamation, chorioretinitis, and pigmentary chorioretinopathy (salt and pepper type), glaucoma, cataracts, interstitial keratitis, optic neuritis, periostitis and cortical demineralization of metaphysis and diaphysis areas of long bones, anemia, and thrombocytopenia. Renal involvement varies in CS ranges from mild transient proteinuria to frank congenital nephrotic syndrome.

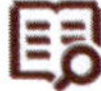

REFERENCE/SOURCE

- Kliegman RM, St Geme JW III, Blum NJ, Shah SS, Tasker RC, Wilson KM. Nelson Textbook of Pediatrics, 21st edition. Amsterdam: Elsevier; 2020. p. 1598.

12. Which of the following laboratory tests should be done 2–3 monthly when a child is receiving MMF for SDNS?

A. Serum sodium
B. Serum potassium
C. Serum creatinine
D. Complete blood counts

EXPLANATION

Mycophenolate mofetil is a selective and reversible inhibitor of inosine monophosphate dehydrogenase used in patients with nephrotic syndrome as a steroid sparing agent. It can cause bone marrow suppression. The drug is not nephrotoxic.

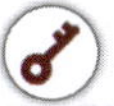 **Key: D**

 **BOOST YOUR KNOWLEDGE**

For children with FRNS or SDNS, MMF has been recommended as a steroid-sparing drug. MMF is administered at a dose of 800–1,200 mg/m^2/day (maximum 2 g/day) twice daily. The most common adverse effects are gastrointestinal, such as diarrhea, nausea, abdominal pain, and vomiting. Occasional infections, leukopenia, thrombocytopenia, and lymphocytopenia are reported.

 **REFERENCE/SOURCE**

- Erkan E. Nephrotic syndrome. In: Kliegman RM, St Geme JW III, Blum NJ, Shah SS, Tasker RC, Wilson KM (Eds). Nelson Textbook of Pediatrics, 21st edition. Amsterdam: Elsevier; 2020. p. 2752.

13. Which of the following genetic mutations is the most likely etiology in an infant with atypical HUS having urine albumin 4+, serum albumin 1.8 g/dL, and serum cholesterol 520 mg/dL?

A. CFH mutation
B. CFI mutation
C. THBD mutation
D. DGKE mutation

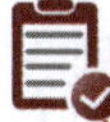 **EXPLANATION**

DGKE mutations can cause atypical HUS (aHUS), usually in infancy. In addition, chronic proteinuria is the characteristic feature of DGKE nephropathy. Almost all patients have proteinuria (predominantly nephrotic range, leading to nephrotic syndrome) at the onset of disease. Mutations in CFH, CFI, and THBD cause aHUS, but do not cause nephrotic syndrome usually.

 **Key: D**

 **BOOST YOUR KNOWLEDGE**

Atypical HUS is a rare systemic syndrome characterized by microangiopathic hemolytic anemia, thrombocytopenia, and acute kidney injury. In most cases, alternative complement pathway dysregulation is the identifying cause, including genes such as *CFH, CFI,* and *THBD* genes. These do not cause nephrotic syndrome commonly.

Recently, other genetic causes have been identified, including a mutation in the *diacylglycerol kinase epsilon (DGKE)* gene, which theoretically affect the coagulation pathway and does not affect the complement pathway. The common features of aHUS, microscopic hematuria, and hypertension along with the distinctive finding of nephrotic syndrome are seen in children with DGKE-HUS that presents most commonly in infancy.

 **REFERENCE/SOURCE**

- Kliegman RM, St Geme JW III, Blum NJ, Shah SS, Tasker RC, Wilson KM. Nelson Textbook of Pediatrics, 21st edition. Amsterdam: Elsevier; 2020. p. 2529.

14. An adolescent boy is referred for evaluation of urine albumin 2+. He has serum creatinine of 0.42 mg/dL, and blood pressure is normal, with serum albumin 4.1 g/dL. Urinalysis contains no RBCs. Evaluation reveals that evening albumin is high (urine protein creatinine ratio 0.5) but first morning sample after waking up from sleep has no proteinuria. What is the likely diagnosis?

A. Dent disease
B. Orthostatic proteinuria
C. Fabry disease
D. Overflow proteinuria

EXPLANATION

Orthostatic proteinuria is type of proteinuria that is usually observed while supine but disappears while standing. Children with orthostatic proteinuria usually have Up/Uc <1. Dent disease is a nephrotic range proteinuria with hypercalciuria/nephrocalcinosis and hypophosphatemic rickets. Fabry disease (alpha-galactose deficiency) can have proteinuria, but it has other features such as angiokeratoma, paresthesia of hands and feet, and cardiomyopathy. Overflow proteinuria occurs when the plasma concentration of certain small proteins exceeds the capacity of the tubules to reabsorb the filtered protein. Examples include the presence of immunoglobulin light chains in the urine in multiple myeloma, hemoglobinuria in intravascular hemolysis, myoglobinuria in rhabdomyolysis, and amylasuria in acute pancreatitis.

Key: B

BOOST YOUR KNOWLEDGE

Orthostatic proteinuria accounts for up to 60% of all cases of asymptomatic proteinuria reported in children, with an even higher incidence in adolescents. Variations in the quantity of daily protein excretion have been observed. If all laboratory tests (such as blood urea, serum creatinine, serum albumin, and serum cholesterol) and clinical findings (such as blood pressure, and growth) are normal except for persistently elevated protein excretion, the possibility of orthostatic proteinuria should be investigated, particularly if the child is older than 6 years of age. This is best done by using the *orthostatic test*.

The child is instructed to urinate just before going to bed at night and to discard the urine. He or she must remain supine all night and urinate the next morning immediately after arising. This urine sample is kept separate and labeled "supine" or "recumbent". Additional urine samples are then collected and pooled during the next 12–16 hours, while the patient maintains normal daily activity. The final sample should preferably be collected in the evening, just before the patient goes to bed; this pooled sample should be labeled "active" urine. The duration of collection time for the latter sample can be shortened to 12 hours or less. In patients with orthostatic proteinuria, the supine sample will be free of protein, but the evening sample will contain protein. Children with orthostatic proteinuria usually have Up/Uc <1. Yearly follow-up is recommended for children diagnosed with this condition.

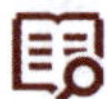

REFERENCE/SOURCE

- Kliegman RM, St Geme JW III, Blum NJ, Shah SS, Tasker RC, Wilson KM. Nelson Textbook of Pediatrics, 21st edition. Amsterdam: Elsevier; 2020. p. 2750.

15. On a 24-hour urine specimen, nephrotic range proteinuria is defined in children as:

A. >1 $g/m^2/24$ h
B. >3.5 $g/m^2/24$ h
C. >3 $g/m^2/24$ h
D. >2.5 $g/m^2/24$ h

EXPLANATION

Proteinuria of >1,000 $mg/m^2/day$ (or >40 $mg/m^2/h$) is known as nephrotic range proteinuria in children. In adults, nephrotic range proteinuria is defined as ≥3.5 g/day.

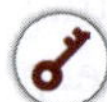

Key: A

BOOST YOUR KNOWLEDGE

On a 24-hour urine sample, a value >100 $mg/m^2/day$ (or >4 $mg/m^2/h$) is considered proteinuria. Proteinuria of >1,000 $mg/m^2/day$ (or >40 $mg/m^2/h$) is known as nephrotic range proteinuria. On a spot urine sample, proteinuria is defined as urinary protein/creatinine ratio (Up/Uc) of >0.2 mg protein/mg creatinine.

Nephrotic range proteinuria is defined as Up/Uc >2. On dipstick analysis of the first morning urine sample, a value >1+ on multiple occasions is abnormal and needs to be investigated. Nephrotic range proteinuria is manifested by 3+ or 4+ proteinuria on dipstick testing.

While the spot and 24-hour samples estimate total proteinuria (including albumin and other tubular proteins like beta-2 microglobulin), the dipstick usually estimates albuminuria only. Albuminuria is defined as urine albumin/creatinine ratio >30 mg/g; a value 30–300 mg/g is considered microalbuminuria. The dipstick protein usually remains negative unless albuminuria is >300 mg/g creatinine.

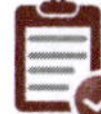

REFERENCES/SOURCES

- Kliegman RM, St Geme JW III, Blum NJ, Shah SS, Tasker RC, Wilson KM. Nelson Textbook of Pediatrics, 21st edition. Amsterdam: Elsevier; 2020. p. 2752.
- Sinha A, Bagga A, Banerjee S, Mishra K, Mehta A, Agarwal I, et al; Expert Group of Indian Society of Pediatric Nephrology. Steroid Sensitive Nephrotic Syndrome: Revised Guidelines. Indian Pediatr. 2021;58(5):461-81.

16. Which of the following antihypertensive drugs is also an antiproteinuric drug?

A. Amlodipine
B. Atenolol
C. Minoxidil
D. Losartan

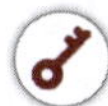

EXPLANATION

Losartan (an angiotensin receptor blocker) is an antiproteinuric drug. Amlodipine, atenolol. and minoxidil do not reduce proteinuria.

Key: D

BOOST YOUR KNOWLEDGE

In patients with glomerular proteinuria, therapy with an angiotensin-converting enzyme (ACE) inhibitor or angiotensin receptor blockers can bring about a significant reduction in proteinuria. ACE inhibitors and angiotensin receptor blockers have an established antiproteinuric effect which is, to some extent, independent of hypertension control. The mechanism of their antiproteinuric effect is by selective vasodilatation of the efferent arteriole which lowers the filtration pressure and hence, the amount of albumin in the ultrafiltrate.

REFERENCE/SOURCE

- Kliegman RM, St Geme JW III, Blum NJ, Shah SS, Tasker RC, Wilson KM. Nelson Textbook of Pediatrics, 21st edition. Amsterdam: Elsevier; 2020. pp. 2749, 2752.

17. Which of the following is *true* about SRNS in children?

A. Levamisole is one of the drugs used for management of SRNS
B. Biopsy may reveal FSGS
C. Enalapril is not ordinarily recommended in SRNS
D. A minority of children with SRNS will progress to advanced chronic kidney disease in 10 years

EXPLANATION

Steroid-resistant nephrotic syndrome in children requires a kidney biopsy, which shows FSGS, MCD, or MesPGN. Enalapril is recommended in SRNS as supportive care. A significant proportion of children with SRNS will progress to advanced chronic kidney disease in 10 years. Levamisole is not recommended for SRNS but is used in FRNS and SDNS.

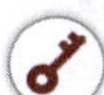

Key: B

BOOST YOUR KNOWLEDGE

While most of the children who presented with primary nephrotic syndrome respond to steroid treatment, 10–20% of these children do not achieve remission despite receiving second- or third-line of treatment, and more than half of the patients progress to ESRD within 10 years. Calcineurin inhibitors, such as cyclosporine and tacrolimus, are used as the first-line of treatment. A significant number of patients with SRNS progress to ESRD if remission is not achieved. SRNS in children requires a kidney biopsy, which shows FSGS, MCD, or MesPGN. Enalapril is recommended in SRNS as supportive care. A significant proportion of children with SRNS will progress to advanced chronic kidney disease in 10 years.

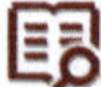

REFERENCES/SOURCES

- Kliegman RM, St Geme JW III, Blum NJ, Shah SS, Tasker RC, Wilson KM. Nelson Textbook of Pediatrics, 21st edition. Amsterdam: Elsevier; 2020. pp. 2749, 2752.
- Vasudevan A, Thergaonkar R, Mantan M, Sharma J, Khandelwal P, Hari P, et al; Expert Group of the Indian Society of Pediatric Nephrology. Consensus Guidelines on Management of Steroid-resistant Nephrotic Syndrome. Indian Pediatr. 2021;58(7): 650-66.

18. Steroid-dependent nephrotic syndrome is defined as:

A. Four relapses in a 12-month period
B. Three relapses in any 6 months
C. Two relapses within first 6 months of disease onset
D. Two consecutive relapses while on alternate day prednisolone or within 14 days of its discontinuation

EXPLANATION

Steroid-dependent nephrotic syndrome is defined as two consecutive relapses while on alternate day prednisolone or within 14 days of its discontinuation. The other three choices in the MCQ refer to the definition of FRNS.

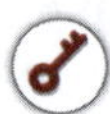

Key: D

BOOST YOUR KNOWLEDGE

Frequently relapsing nephrotic syndrome is defined as 2 or more relapses within the first 6 months of initial therapy, ≥3 relapses in any 6 months; or ≥4 relapses in 1 year. SDNS is defined as 2 consecutive relapses while on alternate day prednisolone or within 14 days of its discontinuation.

If the definition of FRNS or SDNS is satisfied, then, after treatment of the relapse, the prednisolone is not discontinued, but tapered by 0.25 mg/kg every 4 weeks and brought down to <0.5–0.7 mg/kg on alternate days, so that remission is maintained. This minimum dosage of prednisolone on every alternate day is administered to maintain remission for a period 9–18 months, along with calcium and vitamin D supplements to prevent osteoporosis.

If, on the contrary, the prednisolone threshold, to maintain remission, is >0.5–0.7 mg/kg or if features of corticosteroid toxicity are seen (cataract, glaucoma, short stature, obesity, etc.), additional use of the following immunomodulators is suggested, that would act as steroid-sparing agents: Levamisole, oral cyclophosphamide, MMF, cyclosporine or tacrolimus.

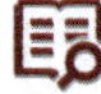

REFERENCE/SOURCE

- Sinha A, Bagga A, Banerjee S, Mishra K, Mehta A, Agarwal I, et al; Expert Group of Indian Society of Pediatric Nephrology. Steroid Sensitive Nephrotic Syndrome: Revised Guidelines. Indian Pediatr. 2021;58(5):461-81.

19. Which of the following vaccinations is recommended in an 18-month-old child with nephrotic syndrome?

A. Pneumococcal conjugate vaccine 13-valent (PCV13)
B. Pneumococcal polysaccharide vaccine 23-valent
C. PCV13 followed by pneumococcal polysaccharide vaccine 23-valent 4–8 weeks later
D. PCV10

EXPLANATION

Only the PCV13 is immunogenic below 2 years of age. The pneumococcal polysaccharide vaccine 23-valent is not immunogenic below 2 years of age. PCV13 is preferred over PCV10.

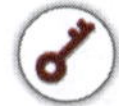

Key: A

BOOST YOUR KNOWLEDGE

Children with nephrotic syndrome are prone to pneumococcal infections because of loss of opsonins in the urine, making invasion by microorganisms with capsular polysaccharide more likely. The availability of safe and immunogenic vaccines has reduced the risk of pneumococcal infections in patients with relapsing nephrotic syndrome. Two categories of vaccines are available. The polysaccharide vaccine (PPSV23) is poorly immunogenic in patients younger than 2 years and does not induce immunological memory. Conjugate vaccines (PCV13) induce superior and sustained antibody responses and immune memory even in young infants. Even in children >2 years of age, PPSV23 alone should not be used to vaccinate children. In these children, PCV13 should be given first followed by PPSV23 4–8 weeks later.

REFERENCES/SOURCES

- Kliegman RM, St Geme JW III, Blum NJ, Shah SS, Tasker RC, Wilson KM. Nelson Textbook of Pediatrics, 21st edition. Amsterdam: Elsevier; 2020. pp. 1439, 2759.
- Sinha A, Bagga A, Banerjee S, Mishra K, Mehta A, Agarwal I, et al; Expert Group of Indian Society of Pediatric Nephrology. Steroid Sensitive Nephrotic Syndrome: Revised Guidelines. Indian Pediatr. 2021;58(5):461-81.

20. A 15-year-old girl, a known case of systemic lupus erythematosus, presents with periorbital edema. Urinalysis reveals 4+ proteinuria, but there are no RBCs in the urine. Urine protein:creatinine ratio is 8.5. Serum creatinine is 0.51 mg/dL. Blood pressure is 110/70 mm Hg. What class of lupus nephritis is the kidney biopsy likely to reveal?

A. Class 3 lupus nephritis
B. Class 4 lupus nephritis
C. Class 5 lupus nephritis
D. Class 6 lupus nephritis

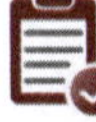

EXPLANATION

- Class 3 and Class 4 lupus nephritis present with microscopic or macroscopic hematuria. Class 6 lupus nephritis has reduced estimated glomerular filtration rate. Class 5 lupus nephritis usually has subnephrotic or nephrotic range proteinuria without hematuria.

Key: C

BOOST YOUR KNOWLEDGE

- Class 1 lupus nephritis is minimal mesangial lupus nephritis, in which glomeruli appear normal on light microscopy.
- Class 2 is proliferative mesangial lupus nephritis since mesangial proliferation is seen on light microscopy unlike class 1.

- Class 3 is focal proliferative lupus nephritis.
- Class 4 is diffuse proliferative lupus nephritis.
- Class 5 is membranous LN, in which immune complex deposits are in the mesangial and subepithelial space. Capillary loops are thickened. In this class, nephrotic range proteinuria occurs.
- Class 6 is advanced sclerosing lupus nephritis in which more than 90% of the glomeruli are sclerosed.

REFERENCES/SOURCES

- Musa R, Brent LH, Qurie A. Lupus Nephritis. Treasure Island (FL): StatPearls Publishing; 2023.
- Sadun RE, Ardoin SP, Schanberg LE. Systemic lupus erythematosus. In: Kliegman RM, St Geme JW III, Blum NJ, Shah SS, Tasker RC, Wilson KM (Eds). Nelson Textbook of Pediatrics, 21st edition. Amsterdam: Elsevier; 2020. p. 1274.

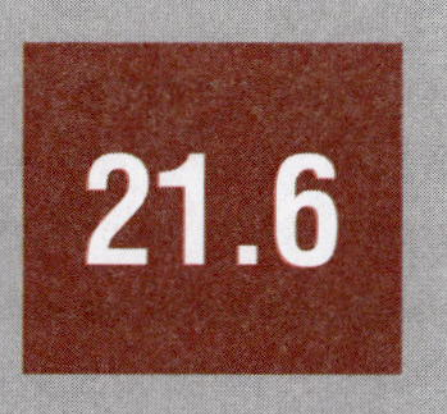

Enuresis and Voiding Disorders

Girish C Bhatt

1. A 7-year-old boy presented with nocturnal enuresis along with imperative sensations of urge from last 2 to 3 years. On further asking history, the parents informed that the child typically has a Vincent's curtsey. There is no history of constipation or recurrent urinary tract infection (UTI). Which of the following condition correctly labels this child?

A. Transient detrusor-sphincter discoordination
B. Stress incontinence
C. Detrusor overactivity
D. Giggle incontinence

EXPLANATION

The key features in the clinical settings are enuresis in a male child associated with urgency and holding maneuvers. Let us analyze the various terminologies in the given Table.

	Clinical features	*Management*
Transient detrusor discoordination	• Age <1 year • Interrupted voiding • May present with complications such as UTI	• Transient phenomena • Restores with toilet training
Stress incontinence	• Associated with increased intravesical pressure during laughing and running, coughing, etc.	• Standard urotherapy • Pelvic floor rehabilitation
Detrusor overactivity	• Urinary frequency • Urgency • Urge incontinence • Holding maneuvers	• Anticholinergic drugs • Standard urotherapy • Neuromodulation
Giggle incontinence	• Usually found in girls • Associated with laughing and giggling • May amount to complete bladder emptying	• Standard urotherapy • Pelvic floor rehabilitation

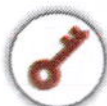

Key: C

BOOST YOUR KNOWLEDGE

One of the vital causes of bladder bowel dysfunction is constipation that should be always kept in mind while taking a detailed history.

REFERENCE/SOURCE

- Geary DF, Schaefer F. Comprehensive Pediatric Nephrology, 1st edition. Amsterdam, Netherlands: Elsevier; 2008. pp. 593-5.

2. Which of the following is *true* about monosymptomatic nocturnal enuresis?

A. The child can have bedwetting during daytime when he is sleeping
B. The child has frequency of micturition more than 12 times/day
C. The child usually has a history of constipation
D. History of holding maneuvers is present

EXPLANATION

In a child with monosymptomatic enuresis (ME), the daytime symptoms are not present. Let us review the various definitions:

Monosymptomatic enuresis refers to presence of enuresis without symptoms of lower urinary tract symptoms (LUTS), such as frequency, urgency, holding maneuvers, and daytime incontinence. ME is divided into primary monosymptomatic enuresis (PME) in which the child has never achieved night-time dryness, and secondary enuresis that occurs after a dry period of at least 6 months. Presence of constipation suggests nonmonosymptomatic enuresis (NME).

Enuresis in a child with LUTS is termed as NME or polysymptomatic enuresis.

Key: A

BOOST YOUR KNOWLEDGE

Dysfunctional voiding (DV) score is a validated scoring system used for the assessment of voiding disorder. The International Continence Society (ICS) defines DV as intermittent and/or fluctuating flow rate due to involuntary intermittent contractions of the periurethral striated muscle during voiding in neurologically normal individuals.

REFERENCE/SOURCE

- Gupta P, Menon PSN, Lodha R, Ramji S. PG Textbook of Pediatrics, 3rd edition. New Delhi: Jaypee Brothers Medical Publishers; 2022. pp. 2500-4.

3. A 10-year-old child presented with bedwetting during night. There were no symptoms suggestive of LUTS and previous history of UTI. The child never achieved dryness by night. The primary healthcare physician asked for a voiding diary with the following information:

Time	*Urine*	*Fluid intake*
7.00 AM	200 mL	200 mL
11.00 AM	200 mL	200 mL
1.00 PM	150 mL	300 mL
5.00 PM	150 mL	200 mL
8.00 PM	150 mL	300 mL
12.00 AM	300 mL (diaper weight)	
6.00 AM	250 mL	

Initially the child was put on behavior therapy and fluid-methods but did not achieve remission. The child is now planned for other therapies. Which would be the most appropriate therapy for this child?

A. Oxybutynin
B. Alarm therapy
C. Desmopressin
D. Imipramine

EXPLANATION

- The clinical clues are night-time bedwetting; child has not achieved dryness by night-time; no LUTS. All clinical features suggest that the child is having primary monosymptomatic nocturnal enuresis. The voiding diary shows night-time polyuria as the patient is having night-time—urine output >130% of bladder capacity, defined as night-time polyuria.
- The bladder capacity is defined as 30 + (age in years × 30). So, for this patient the bladder capacity will by 330 mL, and 550 mL is 166% of expected bladder capacity.
- For calculation of nocturnal urine volume, the last voided urine before sleep is excluded, and the first voided urine in the morning along with overnight urine volume is included (300 mL + 250 mL in this patient). In children with enuresis night urine volume is measured by the diaper weight.
- Desmopressin is most efficacious in children with nocturnal polyuria, defined as nocturnal urine production >130% of expected bladder capacity for age and normal bladder reservoir function.

Key: C

BOOST YOUR KNOWLEDGE

The bladder capacity is defined as 30 + (age in years × 30). So, for this patient the bladder capacity will by 330 mL, and 550 mL is 166% of expected bladder capacity.

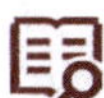

REFERENCE/SOURCE

- Gupta P, Menon PSN, Lodha R, Ramji S. PG Textbook of Pediatrics, 3rd edition. New Delhi: Jaypee Brothers Medical Publishers; 2022. pp. 2500-4.

4. A 9-year-old child presented with bedwetting during night. There were no symptoms suggestive of LUTS and previous history of UTI. The child never achieved dryness by night. The primary healthcare physician asked for a voiding diary with the following information:

Time	*Urine*	*Fluid intake*
7.00 AM	200 mL	200 mL
11.00 AM	150 mL	300 mL
1.00 PM	150 mL	200 mL
5.00 PM	150 mL	200 mL
8.00 PM	150 mL	300 mL
12.00 AM	150 mL (diaper weight)	
6.00 AM	220 mL	

Initially, the child was put on behavior therapy and fluid-methods but did not achieve remission. The child is now planned for other therapies. Which would be the most appropriate therapy for this child?

A. Oxybutynin
B. Alarm therapy
C. Desmopressin
D. Imipramine

EXPLANATION

The clinical clues are night-time bedwetting; child has not achieved dryness by night-time; no LUTS. All clinical features suggest that the child is having primary monosymptomatic nocturnal enuresis. The voiding diary does not show nocturnal polyuria and hence alarm therapy would be more appropriate in this setting.

Key: B

BOOST YOUR KNOWLEDGE

Enuresis alarms are not immediately effective and may take some time to show the desired results. The parents should be counseled as alarm therapy requires long-term commitment. Studies have shown that approximately one-third of the children will discontinue alarm therapy due to reasons such as irritation of skin, disturbance of other family members, and/or failure to wake the child.

REFERENCE/SOURCE

- Gupta P, Menon PSN, Lodha R, Ramji S. PG Textbook of Pediatrics, 3rd edition. New Delhi: Jaypee Brothers Medical Publishers; 2022. pp. 2500-4.

5. An 11-year-old child presented with bedwetting during daytime and night-time. The child also had symptoms of urgency and frequency. There was no history of recurrent UTI. The voiding diary of the child is shown in the given table. Which will be the most appropriate therapy for this child?

Time	*Urine*	*Fluid intake*
7.00 AM	70 mL	100 mL
11.00 AM	80 mL	300 mL
12.00 PM	112 mL	200 mL
2.00 PM	90 mL	200 mL
4.00 PM	100 mL	
6.00 PM	100 mL	200 mL
8.00 PM	200 mL	100 mL
10.00 PM	170 mL	200 mL
12.00 AM	180 mL (diaper weight)	
3.00 AM	200 mL (diaper weight)	
6.00 AM	140 mL	

A. Desmopressin plus imipramine
B. Amitriptyline plus oxybutynin
C. Desmopressin plus oxybutynin
D. Desmopressin plus alarm therapy

EXPLANATION

The typical clinical findings are suggestive of NME as the child is having increased frequency of micturition. The normal frequency of micturition ranges from four to eight times a day. As this child is having increased frequency (11 times/day with low-capacity bladder), hence anticholinergic with desmopressin would be the most appropriate answer.

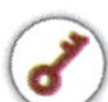

Key: C

BOOST YOUR KNOWLEDGE

Let us review the common management of nocturnal enuresis in the given Table:

Treatment modality/ drugs	*Dosage*	*Advantages*	*Disadvantages/adverse effects*
Education/fluid intake/ motivation		Initial treatment of choice for younger children (5–7 years) with good long-term success rate	Not useful for sleepovers/ immediate relief
Alarm therapy		Good success rate, lower number of relapses on discontinuation	Dropout rates are high and hence requires motivated child and family
Desmopressin	• *Oral solid form:* 0.2–0.4 mg 1 hour before bedtime • *Melt form:* 120–240 µg 30–60 minutes before bedtime	Choice of therapy for sleepovers/ overnight camps. High initial response rate	Abdominal discomfort, nausea, headache, epistaxis, hyponatremia
Anticholinergics: • Oxybutynin • Tolterodine • Propiverine	• 5–10 mg • 2–4 mg • 0.4–0.8 mg/kg	Monotherapy is not recommended for NME. Useful in patients with daytime urgency or frequency	Flushing, blurred vision, constipation, tremor, decreased salivation, and decreased ability to sweat
Tricyclic antidepressant (TCAs): • Imipramine	• 10–25 mg (6–12 years) • 10–50 mg (≥12 years)	Reserved for refractory enuresis	Irritability, dry mouth, decreased appetite, headaches, sleep disturbances, gastrointestinal (GI) upsets. Overdose can cause cardiac conduction disturbances and myocardial depression

REFERENCE/SOURCE

- Gupta P, Menon PSN, Lodha R, Ramji S. PG Textbook of Pediatrics, 3rd edition. New Delhi: Jaypee Brothers Medical Publishers; 2022. pp. 2503.

6. Which of the following statements defines the refractory enuresis?

A. <40% improvement in symptoms
B. <80% improvement in symptoms
C. <70% improvement in symptoms
D. <50% improvement in symptoms

EXPLANATION

Refractory enuresis is defined as no response or <50% improvement in the symptoms with the active symptoms. PME can be managed by a pediatrician, but children with refractory enuresis, recurrent or relapsing enuresis, and ME are referred to a healthcare provider specialized in the management of these conditions. The possible causes of refractory enuresis may include overactive bladder, underlying medical disorders, bladder bowel dysfunction, obstructive sleep apnea (OSA), or social and emotional factors.

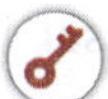

Key: D

BOOST YOUR KNOWLEDGE

The possible causes of refractory enuresis may include overactive bladder, underlying medical disorders, bladder bowel dysfunction, OSA, or social and emotional factors.

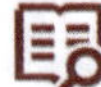

REFERENCE/SOURCE

- Gupta P, Menon PSN, Lodha R, Ramji S. PG Textbook of Pediatrics, 3rd edition. New Delhi: Jaypee Brothers Medical Publishers; 2022. pp. 2504.

7. A 12-year-old child was started on desmopressin by the physician for monosymptomatic nocturnal enuresis. The child responded to the treatment. Which of the following statement is *not true*?

A. The child should be evaluated for response at 2–3 weeks
B. The therapy should be continued for a period of 12 weeks
C. Desmopressin should be discontinued at 12 weeks
D. Behavioral therapy should be continued with desmopressin therapy

EXPLANATION

Here, for treatment of nocturnal enuresis, the child was put on desmopressin therapy and child responded well to the treatment, hence desmopressin should be continued for a period of 12 weeks. Reevaluation of the child is warranted at 2–3 weeks and behavioral therapy should always be a part of the pharmacological intervention.

After a total duration of 12 weeks, there should not be an abrupt discontinuation of the desmopressin. Studies have shown that structured tapering of desmopressin should be done to prevent relapses.

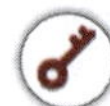

Key: C

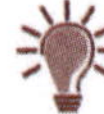

BOOST YOUR KNOWLEDGE

The subgroup analysis of the meta-analysis has shown that decreasing the dose is more beneficial as compared to increasing the duration of dose as a tapering strategy.

REFERENCES/SOURCES

- Chua ME, Silangcruz JM, Chang SJ, Williams K, Saunders M, Lopes RI, et al. Desmopressin withdrawal strategy for pediatric enuresis: a meta-analysis. Pediatrics. 2016;138(1):e20160495.
- Gupta P, Menon PSN, Lodha R, Ramji S. PG Textbook of Pediatrics, 3rd edition. New Delhi: Jaypee Brothers Medical Publishers; 2022. pp. 2504.

8. Which of the following is *not true* about desmopressin therapy for nocturnal enuresis?

A. Therapy should be stopped during fever or dehydration
B. Routine monitoring of electrolytes is indicated while child is on desmopressin
C. Nasal desmopressin can be given for nocturnal enuresis if oral formulation is unavailable
D. Fluid should be restricted after desmopressin due to risk of hyponatremia

EXPLANATION

While the patient is put on desmopressin, the following points should be kept in mind:

- Therapy with desmopressin should be stopped during episodes of electrolyte imbalance such as fever, recurrent vomiting, and diarrhea.
- There is no need for monitoring of electrolytes in these patients as there are negligible chances of electrolyte imbalance with low dose desmopressin.
- At present, nasal desmopressin is not recommended due to higher chances of hyponatremia with nasal formulations.
- As there is a risk of dilutional hyponatremia, only 240 mL of fluids should be taken 1 hour before and 8 hours after administration of desmopressin.

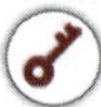

Key: C

BOOST YOUR KNOWLEDGE

The post-marketing surveillance of use of nasal desmopressin for nocturnal enuresis have shown high risk of hyponatremia and hence, nasal desmopressin is no more used for treatment of nocturnal enuresis.

REFERENCE/SOURCE

- Gupta P, Menon PSN, Lodha R, Ramji S. PG Textbook of Pediatrics, 3rd edition. New Delhi: Jaypee Brothers Medical Publishers; 2022. pp. 2504.

9. Which of the following is *not true* about anticholinergic drugs for the treatment of nocturnal enuresis?

A. Anticholinergics are indicated in children having daytime urgency or frequency
B. Monotherapy with anticholinergics is not recommended in cases of ME
C. The medication is contraindicated in patients with underactive bladder, interrupted voiding pattern, urinary retention
D. Mirabegron and solifenacin are approved for use in children >1 years of age

EXPLANATION

Anticholinergics suppress the detrusor overactivity. Oxybutynin, tolterodine, and propiverine are the anticholinergic drugs used for treatment of nocturnal enuresis.

- Anticholinergics are indicated in children having daytime urgency or frequency.
- Monotherapy with anticholinergics is not recommended in cases of ME. In such children, anticholinergic therapy may be used in combination with desmopressin to increase bladder capacity during sleep time.
- The initial dose of oxybutynin is 5 mg two to three times a day along with timed voiding (child is asked to void in a fixed time and asked to record in voiding diary). If no side effects are observed the dose is increased to 10 mg. A trial of stopping the medication is attempted after the child is free of symptoms of overactive bladder for a period of 4 months. If the symptoms of urgency or incontinence recur, the medication is restarted.
- Side effects are related to the anticholinergic action of the drug and include flushing, blurred vision, constipation, tremor, decreased salivation, and decreased ability to sweat.
- The medication is contraindicated in patients with underactive bladder, interrupted voiding pattern, urinary retention, or high postvoid residual volume.
- Mirabegron and solifenacin are newer anticholinergics approved for use in children >3 years and 2 years, respectively.

Key: D

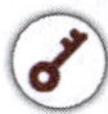

BOOST YOUR KNOWLEDGE

Monotherapy with anticholinergics is not recommended in cases of ME. In such children, anticholinergic therapy may be used in combination with desmopressin to increase bladder capacity during sleep time.

REFERENCE/SOURCE

- Gupta P, Menon PSN, Lodha R, Ramji S. PG Textbook of Pediatrics, 3rd edition. New Delhi: Jaypee Brothers Medical Publishers; 2022. pp. 2504.

10. **A 5-year-old child presented with continuous dribbling of urine since birth. Her imaging is shown in given Figure.**

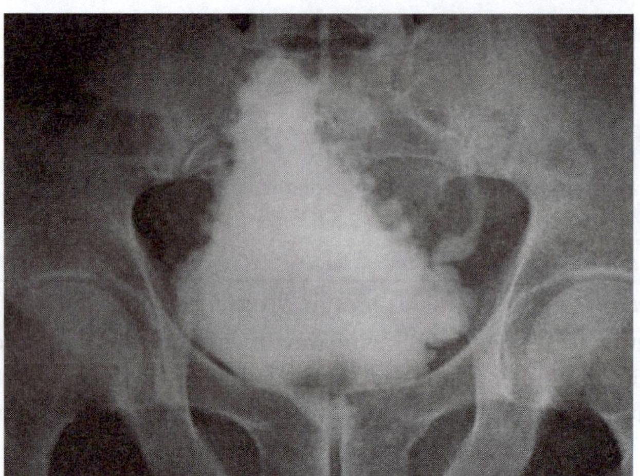

What is the imaging pattern and imaging modality?

A. Cobra-head pattern in intravenous urography (IVU)
B. Christmas-tree pattern in micturating cystourethrogram
C. Inverted funnel pattern in CT urography
D. Funnel pattern in micturating cystourethrography

EXPLANATION

The child presented with continuous dribbling since birth. The given image of the micturating cystourethrogram shows the Christmas-tree appearance typical of neurogenic bladder. Cobra-head pattern is seen in IVU in patients with ureterocele.

Key: B

BOOST YOUR KNOWLEDGE

Cobra-head pattern is seen in IVU in patients with ureterocele and not in micturating cystourethrogram.

REFERENCE/SOURCE

- Niinan G. Neurogenic bladder. In: Sinha CK, Davenport M (Eds). Handbook of Pediatric Surgery. London: Springer: 2010.

11. **In question 10, the most probable disorder present in this child is:**

A. Overactive bladder
B. Neurogenic bladder
C. Hinman syndrome
D. Ureterocele

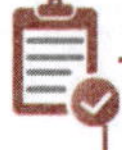

EXPLANATION

The child presented with continuous dribbling since birth. The given image of the micturating cystourethrogram shows the Christmas-tree appearance typical of neurogenic bladder.

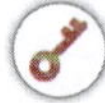

Key: B

BOOST YOUR KNOWLEDGE

The various patterns seen in micturating cystourethrogram are Christmas-tree pattern in neurogenic bladder, spinning top urethra in functional discoordination in voiding, or bladder instability.

REFERENCE/SOURCE

- Niinan G. Neurogenic bladder. In: Sinha CK, Davenport M (Eds). Handbook of Pediatric Surgery. London: Springer; 2010.

12. Nocturnal polyuria is defined as night-time voided volume of:

A. >80% of the expected bladder capacity
B. >90% of the expected bladder capacity
C. >100% of the expected bladder capacity
D. >130% of the expected bladder capacity

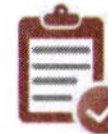

EXPLANATION

Nocturnal polyuria is defined as night-time urine volume of >130% of the expected bladder capacity. To calculate this last voided urine before sleep is excluded, and the first voided urine in the morning and overnight urine volume are included. In children with enuresis night urine volume is measured by the diaper weight.

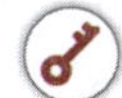

Key: D

BOOST YOUR KNOWLEDGE

The bladder capacity is defined as 30 + (age in years × 30) and this formula is valid till the adult value (approximately 400 mL) is reached.

REFERENCE/SOURCE

- Gupta P, Menon PSN, Lodha R, Ramji S. PG Textbook of Pediatrics, 3rd edition. New Delhi: Jaypee Brothers Medical Publishers; 2022. pp. 250.

13. Polyuria in a child is defined as:

A. Urine output >1 L/m^2 in 24 hours
B. Urine output >1.5 L/m^2 in 24 hours
C. Urine output >1.75 L/m^2 in 24 hours
D. Urine output >2 L/m^2 in 24 hours

EXPLANATION

Polyuria is defined as 24-hour urinary volume of 2 L/m^2.

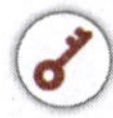

Key: D

BOOST YOUR KNOWLEDGE

Polyuria is commonly seen in conditions such as diabetes mellitus, diabetes insipidus, hypercalcemia, and primary polydipsia. In a child presenting with enuresis, it is important to quantify urine output to rule out polyuria, usually associated with these conditions.

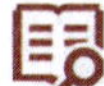

REFERENCE/SOURCE

- Gupta P, Menon PSN, Lodha R, Ramji S. PG Textbook of Pediatrics, 3rd edition. New Delhi: Jaypee Brothers Medical Publishers; 2022. pp. 2501.

14. Bristol chart is used to classify:

A. Bladder
B. Stool
C. Overactive bladder
D. Underactive bladder

EXPLANATION

A 7-day bowel diary based on the Bristol stool form scale is recommended to rule out bowel dysfunction, due to its high prevalence in children with voiding disorders. Constipation is present in almost two-thirds of children with voiding disorders, which further worsens bladder functioning.

Key: B

BOOST YOUR KNOWLEDGE

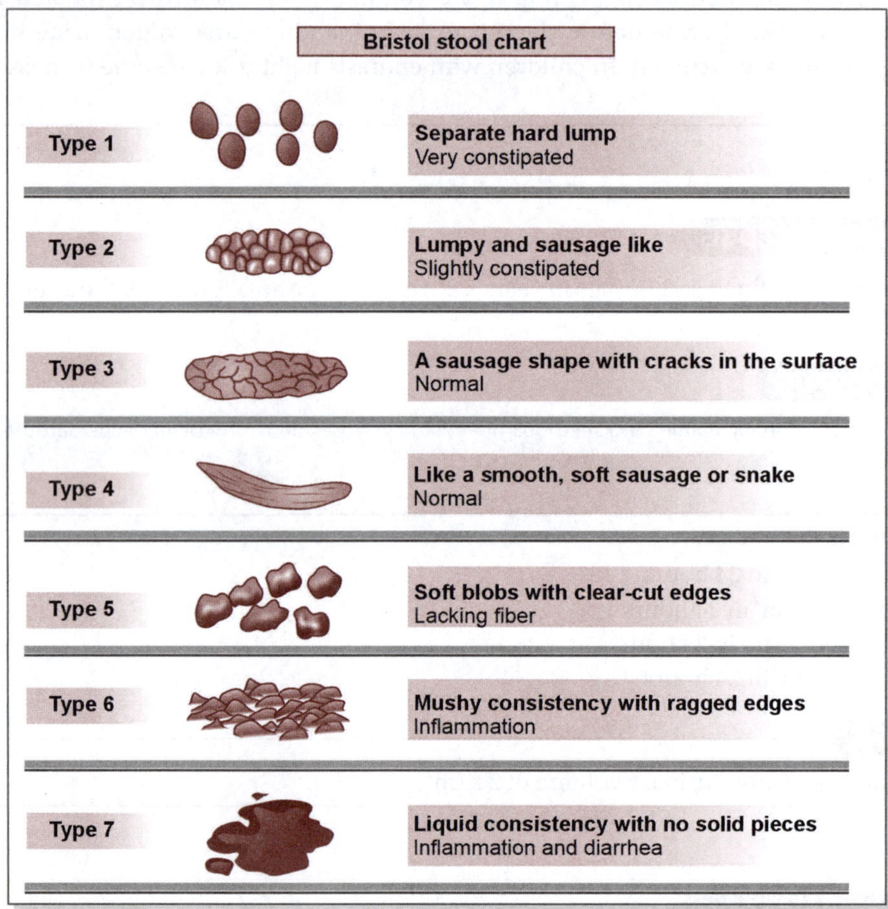

REFERENCE/SOURCE

- Gupta P, Menon PSN, Lodha R, Ramji S. PG Textbook of Pediatrics, 3rd edition. New Delhi: Jaypee Brothers Medical Publishers; 2022. pp. 2569.

15. A 8-year-old child presented with increased frequency of micturition, urgency, and intermittent incontinence. His voiding diary also showed a normal capacity bladder with increased frequency. On ultrasonography, the rectal diameter is 35 mm and Bristol chart showed type 2 pattern of stool. What is the most appropriate intervention for this child?

A. Start polyethylene glycol (PEG)
B. Start amitriptyline
C. Start imipramine
D. Start melt form of desmopressin

EXPLANATION

The key clinical features are NME, urgency, and increased frequency. The rectal diameter is >25 mm, and the Bristol chart showed type 2 (hard) stools. The most important intervention in this condition will be to start laxatives (PEG) for the treatment of constipation. Laxative use appears to be beneficial in children with bladder and bowel dysfunction (BBD). In one observational study of 46 patients with BBD and daytime urinary incontinence, PEG without electrolytes resulted in an overall increase in frequency of bowel movements and improved urinary continence.

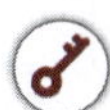

Key: A

BOOST YOUR KNOWLEDGE

Imipramine is usually used in cases of refractory enuresis when other interventions fail.

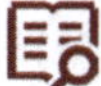

REFERENCES/SOURCES

- Erickson BA, Austin JC, Cooper CS, Boyt MA. Polyethylene glycol 3350 for constipation in children with dysfunctional elimination. J Urol. 2003;170(4 Pt 2):1518-20.
- Pashankar DS, Bishop WP. Efficacy and optimal dose of daily polyethylene glycol 3350 for treatment of constipation and encopresis in children. J Pediatr. 2001;139(3):428-32.

16. A tower-shaped curve in uroflowmetry is suggestive of the following disorder:

A. Overactive bladder
B. Sphincter overactive
C. Underactive bladders
D. Normal voiding pattern

EXPLANATION

The precise shape of the flow curve is determined by the detrusor contractility, by the presence of any abdominal straining, and by the bladder outlet. Tower-shaped curve is produced by explosive voiding contraction that is seen in an overactive bladder.

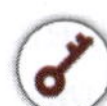

Key: A

BOOST YOUR KNOWLEDGE

Other curves that can be seen in different conditions are:

- *Bell-shaped:* Seen in normal voiding and a smooth increase and a subsequent decrease in flow rate should be observed.
- *Plateau-shaped:* This is seen in an outlet obstruction.
- *Staccato-pattern:* This is seen in sphincter overactivity during voiding with peaks and trough throughout the voiding.
- *Interrupted flow:* This condition is seen in underactive bladder.

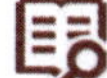

REFERENCE/SOURCE

- Geary DF, Schaefer F. Comprehensive Pediatric Nephrology, 1st edition. Amsterdam, Netherlands: Elsevier; 2008. pp. 595.

17. Observe the following uroflowmetry study. What does the point A indicate?

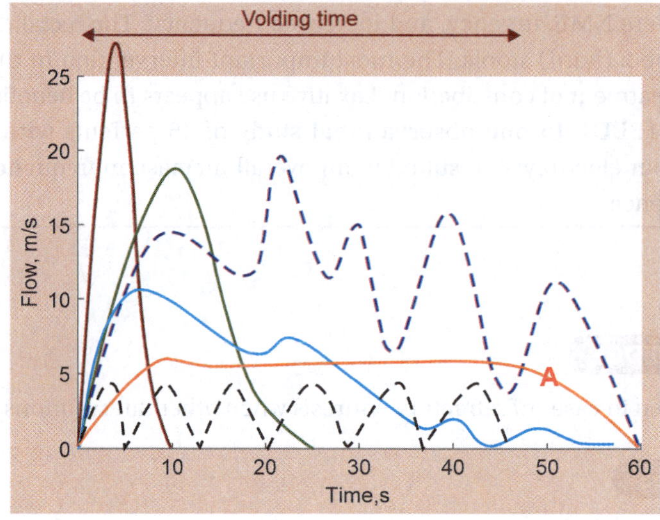

A. Overactive bladder
B. Urethral stricture
C. Underactive bladders
D. Normal voiding pattern

EXPLANATION

The following uroflow curve types are associated with specific voiding dynamics: (1) The bell-shaped curve which is normal, (2) the tower-shaped curve, which is either normal or indicative of detrusor overactivity, (3) the staccato curve which indicates DV, (4) the plateau curve which raises the suspicion of anatomical outflow obstruction as indicated by A, and (5) the intermittent curve which is typical of detrusor underactivity.

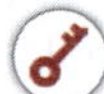

Key: B

BOOST YOUR KNOWLEDGE

For children old enough to void on command, the use of *flowmetry* is beneficial, especially for those with suspected voiding problems (e.g., weak stream or the need to strain to void) or with recurrent UTIs secondary to incomplete bladder emptying or therapy-resistant incontinence. To calculate flowmetry, a child will void on a toilet that measures the flow rate, and immediately afterward, the amount of residual urine still in the bladder is assessed via an ultrasound device.

REFERENCE/SOURCE

- Nevéus T, Estrada CR, Austin PF. Bladder disorders. In: Emma F, Goldstein S., Bagga A, Bates CM, Shroff R (Eds). Pediatric Nephrology, 8th edition. Switzerland: Springer Nature; 2022.

18. In a toilet-trained child, the significant postvoid residual urine is:

A. 10 mL
B. 20 mL
C. 50 mL
D. 150 mL

EXPLANATION

Residual urine volume >20 mL is considered as pathological and needs further evaluation for various bladder conditions.

Key: B

BOOST YOUR KNOWLEDGE

Postvoid residual urine volume should be measured during the first 5 minutes after micturition and ideally <1 minute after micturition. Postvoid residual urine volume >20 mL on more than one occasion is considered abnormal.

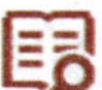

REFERENCE/SOURCE

- Nevéus T, Estrada CR, Austin PF. Bladder disorders. In: Emma F, Goldstein SL, Bagga A, Bates CM, Shroff R (Eds). Pediatric Nephrology. Switzerland: Springer Nature; 2022.

CHAPTER

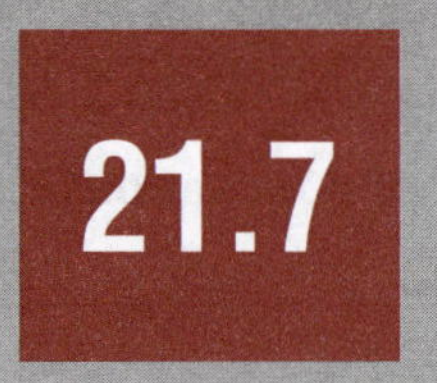

Acute Kidney Injury

Priyanka Khandelwal

1. A 5-year-old boy has been admitted with a 5-day history of fever, loose stools, and poor oral acceptance. On examination, pulses are well felt, heart rate is 110 beats/minute and blood pressure (BP) is 90/60 mm Hg. Serum creatinine at admission is 1.0 mg/dL (previously 0.4 mg/dL, 3 months ago). Urine output in the next 6 hours is 80 mL. He weighs 20 kg and is 100 cm tall. Using the Kidney Disease: Improving Global Outcomes (KDIGO) classification criteria, which stage of acute kidney injury (AKI) will he be classified into?

A. Stage 1 by KDIGO serum creatinine criteria
B. Stage 1 by KDIGO serum creatinine and urine output criteria
C. Stage 2 by KDIGO serum creatinine criteria
D. Stage 2 by KDIGO serum creatinine and urine output criteria

EXPLANATION

The KDIGO consensus classification was proposed in 2012, where AKI is defined by increase in serum creatinine ≥1.5-fold in the prior 7 days or decrease in urine output <0.5 mL/kg/h for 6–12 hours. AKI stage 2 is a serum creatinine increase of 2.0–2.9 times over the baseline. The child in the present question satisfies the definition of AKI using the serum creatinine criteria only and is classified as stage 2 AKI. His urine output in last 6 hours is 0.7 mL/kg/hour and does not meet the definition of AKI.

Key: C

BOOST YOUR KNOWLEDGE

Acute kidney injury definitions

Class/ stage*	*pRIFLE*		*AKIN*		*KDIGO*	
	Estimated CCl	*Urine output*	*SCr*	*Urine output*	*SCr*	*Urine output*
Risk/I	eCCl decreased by ≥25%	<0.5 mL/kg/h for ≥8 hours	SCr ≥0.3 mg/dL or 150–200% in ≤48 hours	<0.5 mL/kg/h for 8 hours	SCr ≥0.3 mg/dL in 48 h or 1.5–1.9 times in 7 days	<0.5 mL/kg/h for 6–12 hours
Injury/II	eCCl decreased by ≥50%	<0.5 mL/kg/h for ≥16 hours	SCr increase >200–300%	<0.5 mL/kg/h for 16 hours	SCr increase 2.0–2.9 times	<0.5 mL/kg/h for >12 hours
Failure/III	eCCl decreased by ≥75% or eCCl <35 mL/min/ 1.73 m^2	<0.3 mL/kg/h for 24 hours or anuria for 12 hours	SCr increase >300% or SCr ≥4 mg/dL	<0.5 mL/kg/h for 24 hours or <0.3 mL/kg/h for 12 hours	SCr increase ≥3.0 times or SCr ≥4.0 mg/dL or eCCl <35 mL/min/ 1.73 m^2 or need for dialysis	<0.3 mL/kg/h for 24 hours or anuria for 12 hours

*Class risk, injury and failure (pRIFLE) correspond to stage 1, 2 and 3 (AKIN and KDIGO), respectively
(AKIN: Acute Kidney Injury Network; eCCl: estimated creatinine clearance; KDIGO: Kidney Disease: Improving Global Outcomes; pRIFLE: pediatric version of the RIFLE criteria (Risk, Injury, Failure, and 2 outcome criteria, Loss and End-Stage Kidney Disease); SCr: serum creatinine)

The KDIGO consensus classification, proposed in 2012, defined AKI by increase in serum creatinine >0.3 mg/dL within 48 hours or ≥1.5-fold increase in the prior 7 days, or decrease in urine output <0.5 mL/kg/h for 6–12 hours. The degree of creatinine rise from its baseline, or the severity and duration of oliguria is used for staging (Table). Table also shows two other AKI classification used in children (pRIFLE and AKIN). The very first step for a standardized definition of AKI was taken by the Acute Dialysis Quality Initiative (ADQI) in 2004 when they proposed the RIFLE criteria, later modified for use in children (pRIFLE). pRIFLE criteria used estimated creatinine clearance based on Schwartz formula (instead of absolute changes in creatinine levels). Later, even small rise of serum creatinine by 0.3 mg/dL was shown to be independently associated with adverse outcomes in adults; therefore, the AKIN included this threshold. Presently, there is a general consensus for use of KDIGO classification as the standard for defining and staging pediatric AKI.

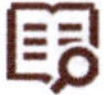

REFERENCES/SOURCES

- Kidney Disease: Improving Global Outcomes (KDIGO) Acute Kidney Injury Work Group. KDIGO clinical practice guideline for acute kidney injury. Kidney Inter Suppl. 2012;2:1-138.
- Kliegman RM, St Geme JW, Blum NJ, Shah SS, Tasker RC, Wilson KM. Renal failure. In: Kliegman RM, St Geme JW, Blum NJ, Shah SS, Tasker RC, Wilson KM (Eds). Nelson Textbook of Pediatrics, 21st edition. Amsterdam, Netherlands: Elsevier; 2019. pp. 2769-79.

2. Biomarkers under investigation for early diagnosis of AKI include plasma neutrophil gelatinase-associated lipocalin (NGAL), cystatin C levels and kidney injury molecule-1 (KIM-1). Which of the following properties are characteristic of serum creatinine, compared to these biomarkers?

A. Serum creatinine is an accurate marker of kidney injury
B. Creatinine is independent of muscle mass, metabolic state, and age
C. Baseline levels of serum creatinine are achieved by day 7 in neonates
D. Serum creatinine is affected by the volume status

EXPLANATION

The level of creatinine has significant drawbacks when used as a diagnostic marker for AKI since it is an insensitive and delayed measure of decreased kidney function. It is a marker of kidney function (functional marker), not kidney injury (damage marker); plasma NGAL and KIM-1 are biomarkers of structural kidney injury (option A). Limitations of creatinine as a marker are the influence of factors including muscle mass, age and metabolic state, etc. on creatinine concentration (option B). Fluid overload might put patients at risk of being underdiagnosed with AKI or lead to underestimation of its severity as serum creatinine is influenced by the volume of distribution (option D). Correction of serum creatinine for the degree of fluid overload may refine the diagnosis of AKI. At birth, creatinine reflects maternal levels. Postnatally, it may often peak in the first few days then a steady state is attained; the peak levels and time to steady state is influenced by gestational age. Preterm infants have a higher peak and slow decline (option C).

Key: D

BOOST YOUR KNOWLEDGE

Multiple biomarkers of structural injury have been identified, among which NGAL and a combination of tissue inhibitor of metalloproteinases-2 (TIMP-2) and insulin-like growth factor-binding protein 7 (Nephrocheck) are in clinical use. The combination of functional and damage biomarkers categorizes patients into four subsets and allows earlier diagnosis of AKI: (1) *No AKI:* Those with normal functional markers and negative damage markers, (2) *Subclinical AKI:* Elevation in kidney injury biomarkers (damage markers) in the absence of changes in functional markers (serum creatinine and urine output), (3) *Functional AKI:* Patients with a change in functional markers without an elevation in kidney injury biomarkers; usually having "prerenal" or fluid responsive AKI, (4) *Established AKI:* Patients who have a change in functional markers as well as elevation of injury markers.

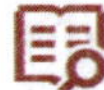

REFERENCES/SOURCES

- Khandelwal P, McLean N, Menon S. Update on Pediatric Acute Kidney Injury. Pediatr Clin North Am. 2022;69(6):1219-38.
- Kliegman RM, St Geme JW, Blum NJ, Shah SS, Tasker RC, Wilson KM. Renal failure. In: Kliegman RM, St Geme JW, Blum NJ, Shah SS, Tasker RC, Wilson KM (Eds). Nelson Textbook of Pediatrics, 21st edition. Amsterdam, Netherlands: Elsevier; 2019. pp. 2769-79.

3. The 0by25 initiative of the International Society of Nephrology (ISN) aims at:

A. Reducing preventable deaths due to AKI
B. Delivery of equitable care for chronic kidney disease (CKD) secondary to AKI
C. Establishing and maintaining hospital services in low-resource area for the care of AKI, including facilities for acute peritoneal dialysis (PD)
D. Development of climate resilient kidney care systems

EXPLANATION

The ISN 0by25 initiative aims to eliminate or at least reduce avoidable AKI-related deaths around the world by 2025 (option A). A complementary initiative to 0by25, the "Closing the Gaps" initiative addresses issues regarding gaps in clinical care delivery, research, and advocacy of CKD and provides a "blueprint" for bridging inequality in CKD (option B). Saving Young Lives, another ISN initiative, works in low-resource areas to help establish and maintain hospital services for the care of AKI, including facilities for acute PD. It focuses on providing training and educational activities in the community to improve awareness and equip local health practitioners to prevent and identify cases needing hospital care (option C). ISNs Green K initiative calls on the development of climate resilient kidney care systems that function through accountable, sustainable low carbon healthcare, and propose a pathway to achieve this goal through a global, collaborative, and multidisciplinary working group (option D).

Key: A

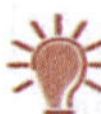

BOOST YOUR KNOWLEDGE

Two key points of the 0by25 initiative were essential for the initiative: Defining preventable death from AKI and promoting local recommendations for AKI care considering the healthcare infrastructure and socioeconomic conditions. As most studies on AKI are derived from developed countries and mainly focus on intensive care unit (ICU) populations, the 0by25 initiative developed two projects to assess how AKI contributes to the global burden of health loss: The Global AKI Snapshot (GSN) study, a multinational cross-sectional project that included all patients with AKI who presented to the participating physicians on a given index day in 2014, and the Pilot study, a prospective cohort of patients with high risk for community-acquired AKI in three different countries.

REFERENCES/SOURCES

- International Society of Nephrology. Initiatives. [online] Available from https://www.theisn.org/initiatives/. [Last accessed July, 2024].
- Mehta RL, Cerdá J, Burdmann EA, Tonelli M, García-García G, Jha V, et al. International Society of Nephrology's 0by25 initiative for acute kidney injury (zero preventable deaths by 2025): a human right case for nephrology. Lancet. 2015;385:2616-43.

4. A 4-year-old girl, a follow-up of kidney transplant (baseline serum creatinine 1.5 mg/dL), is admitted to the pediatric intensive care unit (PICU) with sepsis. She is mechanically ventilated and has oxygen saturation (SpO_2) of 90%. Arterial BP is 70/30 mm Hg on vasopressin, dopamine, and norepinephrine infusions. Central venous pressure is 35 mm Hg. Her weight is increased by 2.5 kg from baseline and chest X-ray demonstrates bilateral pulmonary edema. Serum creatinine is 3.5 mg/dL, sodium 135 mEq/L, potassium 4.5 mEq/L, bicarbonate 12 mEq/L, blood urea nitrogen (BUN) 70 mg/dL, and glucose 80 mg/dL. She has been administered furosemide bolus at 2 mg/kg followed by infusion, despite which she is anuric. Which intervention is *most* appropriate in this setting?

A. Give another intravenous (IV) bolus of furosemide 60 mg and increase the infusion to 15 mg/h
B. Start a nesiritide infusion
C. Initiate continuous venovenous hemofiltration (CVVH)
D. Initiate slow continuous ultrafiltration (SCUF)

EXPLANATION

The patient in this scenario has established severe AKI. Initiation of kidney replacement therapy (KRT) with CVVH is the most appropriate therapy for this hemodynamically unstable patient with AKI, diuretic refractory oliguria, and severe volume overload. Volume overload is contributing to pulmonary dysfunction, and possibly even to right-sided cardiac dysfunction and shock. The role of diuretics in established AKI is limited and it is highly unlikely that diuresis can correct volume overload in a timely fashion, particularly in someone refractory to furosemide infusion of 5–15 mg/h. Nesiritide is of no proven benefit and may aggravate hypotension. SCUF will not correct metabolic acidosis or provide therapy for evolving azotemia; only ultrafiltration or fluid removal is addressed by SCUF.

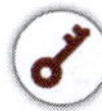

Key: C

BOOST YOUR KNOWLEDGE

Continuous renal replacement therapy (CRRT) is an extracorporeal therapy in which fluid, electrolytes, and small- and medium-sized solutes are continuously removed from the blood. CRRT is useful in critically ill hemodynamic unstable patients, with concomitant sepsis, or multiorgan failure. The pump-driven CRRT circuit continuously passes the patient's blood across a highly permeable filter. Based on the mechanism of solute clearance, CRRT is of three types: CVVH employs convective clearance of urea, creatinine, phosphorus, and other molecules in the blood that flows across the filter along with a large volume of fluid driven by pump-assisted pressure. A replacement fluid is infused intravenously, having an electrolyte composition to that of blood, to replenish the intravascular volume. Continuous venovenous hemodialysis (CVVHD) uses the principle of diffusion by circulating dialysate in a countercurrent direction on the ultrafiltrate side of the membrane. No replacement fluid is used. Continuous venovenous hemodiafiltration (CVVHDF) employs both replacement fluid and dialysate, offering the most effective solute removal of all forms of CRRT.

REFERENCES/SOURCES

- Kliegman RM, St Geme JW, Blum NJ, Shah SS, Tasker RC, Wilson KM. Renal failure. In: Kliegman RM, St Geme JW, Blum NJ, Shah SS, Tasker RC, Wilson KM (Eds). Nelson Textbook of Pediatrics, 21st edition. Amsterdam, Netherlands: Elsevier; 2019. pp. 2769-79.
- Management of pediatric acute kidney injury. In: Geary DF, Schaefer F (Eds). Pediatric Kidney Disease, 2nd edition. Berlin: Springer; 2017. p. 1251.

5. Which of the following statements is true about the use of loop diuretics in AKI in critically ill children?

A. Should be prescribed in all patients with oliguric AKI
B. Reduces the duration of AKI
C. A bolus IV dose helps identify patients at risk of severe AKI
D. Use of an IV infusion reduces the severity of AKI

EXPLANATION

A significant dose of furosemide (2–5 mg/kg IV) may be given in a patient with AKI, with adequate intravascular volume with anuria or severe oliguria. There is data to show that a furosemide trial (a single high dose as bolus with observation for response) may help to identify patients at risk of severe AKI. It is important to note that administration of furosemide and subsequent diuresis results in conversion of AKI from oliguric to nonoliguric and will not alter the course of the renal injury itself, including severity and duration of AKI. Indiscriminate use of furosemide is associated with risk of further AKI as well as drug-related toxicity such as hearing loss.

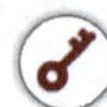

Key: C

BOOST YOUR KNOWLEDGE

A furosemide challenge is commonly used in a patient with AKI in the clinical setting. Chawla and colleagues described a standardized furosemide stress test (FST) in adult patients, wherein a dose of furosemide (1 mg/kg in loop diuretic naïve and 1.5 mg/kg in those who have previously received a loop diuretic) was administered and a urine output <200 mL in 2 hours after furosemide administration predicted progression to AKI stage 3 with a specificity of 84.1% and a sensitivity of 87.1%. It has since been used to improve risk stratification for more accurate assessment of the risk of severe AKI. In recent years, FST has also been used in pediatric patients, especially in patients after cardiac surgery.

REFERENCES/SOURCES

- Chawla LS, Davison DL, Brasha-Mitchell E, Koyner JL, Arthur JM, Shaw AD, et al. Development and standardization of a furosemide stress test to predict the severity of acute kidney injury. Crit Care. 2013;17:R207.
- Kliegman RM, St Geme JW, Blum NJ, Shah SS, Tasker RC, Wilson KM. Renal failure. In: Kliegman RM, St Geme JW, Blum NJ, Shah SS, Tasker RC, Wilson KM (Eds). Nelson Textbook of Pediatrics, 21st edition. Amsterdam, Netherlands: Elsevier; 2019. pp. 2769-79.
- Management of pediatric acute kidney injury. In: Geary DF, Schaefer F (Eds). Pediatric Kidney Disease, 2nd edition. Berlin: Springer; 2017. pp. 1251.

6. A 3-year-old boy is admitted to the pediatric ward for the past 24 hours with a history of bloody diarrhea for 5 days. Today, he is lethargic and sleepy but arousable and able to follow commands as appropriate. He has not passed urine for the last 18 hours. On examination, he looks pale and clammy and is peripherally cool. His temperature is 35.8°C and heart rate is 168 beats/minute, his respiratory rate is 37 breaths/minute and his capillary refill time is 3 seconds. What is the next best step in management?

A. 10 mL/kg 0.9% saline
B. Urgent urea, creatinine, and electrolytes
C. IV antibiotics
D. Urgent complete blood count and peripheral smear

EXPLANATION

The clinical presentation of the patient is suggestive of hemolytic uremic syndrome (HUS) and hypovolemic shock. Anuria >12 hours indicates AKI as a manifestation of HUS, perhaps with a prerenal component due to hypovolemia. The immediate management of this patient should be fluid resuscitation. Hypovolemia should be treated by volume expansion with 10 mL/kg of 0.9% sodium chloride. Antibiotics do not have a role in the management of HUS due to Shiga toxin-producing organisms (likely etiology here); volume resuscitation takes precedence. Fluid resuscitation should take precedence over diagnostic tests such as blood counts, urea, creatinine, and electrolytes; these investigations will be eventually required to make a diagnosis of HUS and confirm the presence of AKI.

Key: A

BOOST YOUR KNOWLEDGE

Hemolytic uremic syndrome, the triad of microangiopathic hemolytic anemia, thrombocytopenia, and AKI, is the leading cause of severe AKI requiring KRT in children. Worldwide, the most common cause of AKI is gastrointestinal infection following Shiga toxin-producing *Escherichia coli* HUS (STEC-HUS). There is no specific treatment for STEC-HUS; management focuses on best supportive therapy of AKI. Epidemiologic studies have shown an association between dehydration (hematocrit >23%) at presentation and adverse outcomes including neurological complications, oliguric AKI and need for KRT. Prompt volume expansion with isotonic fluids, given till the day of onset of AKI, is therefore recommended in patients with STEC infection; monitoring for fluid overload is important in patients with established AKI.

REFERENCES/SOURCES

- Bagga A, Khandelwal P, Mishra K, Thergaonkar R, Vasudevan A, Sharma J, et al; Indian Society of Pediatric Nephrology. Hemolytic uremic syndrome in a developing country: Consensus guidelines. Pediatr Nephrol. 2019;34:1465-82.
- Topjian AA, Raymond TT, Atkins D, Chan M, Duff JP, Joyner BL Jr, et al. Part 4: Pediatric basic and advanced life support: 2020 AHA Guidelines for Cardiopulmonary Resuscitation and Emergency Cardiovascular Care. Circulation. 2020;142(suppl 2): S469-523.

7. Following the management instituted in Question 7, the clinical state of the patient improves. His behavior becomes more communicative, and his observations become normal. His blood results are the following: Sodium 130 mEq/L, potassium 5.4 mEq/L, urea 114 mg/dL, creatinine 5.1 mg/dL, hemoglobin 8.2 g/dL, platelets 65,000/mm^3, and total leukocyte count 45,800/mm^3. Which of the following is the most appropriate fluid and electrolyte fluid and electrolyte management regimen?

A. 0.9% saline 5% dextrose at 400 mL/m^2 per day + ongoing losses
B. 0.9% saline 5% dextrose at 100% maintenance
C. 0.45% saline 5% dextrose at 400 mL/m^2 per day + ongoing losses
D. Allow normal fluid intake but monitor intake and output carefully

EXPLANATION

The patient in this scenario is in the oliguric phase of AKI, in which restriction of fluids to 400 mL/m^2 per day (insensible losses) and replacement of ongoing losses should be instituted. The figure of 400 mL/m^2 per day need not be strictly adhered to and should be determined based on the clinical state of the patient. In case of fluid overload, further fluid restriction might be necessary. Full maintenance or normal fluid intake might be dangerous in an anuric child with stage 3 AKI, since he is already expected to be fluid overloaded. 0.9% saline is the intravenous fluid (IVF) of choice in this patient with low serum sodium since the tonicity is within physiologic range and the risk of hyponatremia is minimal.

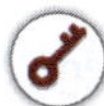

Key: A

BOOST YOUR KNOWLEDGE

Maintenance IVFs are used to provide critical supportive care for children who are acutely ill. Concerns about the use of hypotonic fluids are a high incidence of hyponatremia; isotonic IVFs have been shown to prevent the development of hyponatremia. The current American Academic of Pediatrics guideline recommend isotonic fluids (0.9% normal saline) for all children in surgical (postoperative) and medical acute care settings, including critical care and the general inpatient ward. Recently, trials in adults and observational studies in children have shown isotonic-balanced solutions (crystalloids that have a sodium, potassium, and chloride content closer to that of extracellular fluid) to be associated with lower incidence of hyperchloremia and AKI when use for fluid resuscitation in the acute care setting compared to 0.9% saline; however, clear evidence of superiority of balanced solutions are lacking.

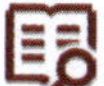

REFERENCES/SOURCES

- Feld LG, Neuspiel DR, Foster BA, Leu MG, Garber MD, Austin K, et al; Subcommittee on Fluid and Electrolyte Therapy. Clinical Practice Guideline: Maintenance Intravenous Fluids in Children. Pediatrics. 2018;142(6):e20183083.
- Kliegman RM, St Geme JW, Blum NJ, Shah SS, Tasker RC, Wilson KM. Renal failure. In: Kliegman RM, St Geme JW, Blum NJ, Shah SS, Tasker RC, Wilson KM (Eds). Nelson Textbook of Pediatrics, 21st edition. Amsterdam, Netherlands: Elsevier; 2019. pp. 2769-79.

8. A prospective multi-center quality improvement initiative [Nephrotoxic Injury Negated by Just in Time Action (NINJA)] showed reduction of which of the following?

A. PD-associated peritonitis rates
B. Nephrotoxic medication-associated AKI
C. Catheter-related bloodstream infection (CRBSI) rates in patents on hemodialysis
D. Complications associated with AKI

EXPLANATION

The NINJA program is a prospective quality improvement project that works to reduce nephrotoxic medication-associated AKI among noncritically ill hospitalized children. Since initiation, it was successful in reducing the number of AKI days per 100 days by 42% in its first year and has been successfully replicated across nine pediatric institutions. While audit of infectious complications due to PD and hemodialysis (peritonitis and CRBSI, respectively) is extremely important, with various quality improvement projects targeting to reduce these respective rates, this was not the focus of NINJA initiative.

Key: B

BOOST YOUR KNOWLEDGE

Nephrotoxic medication-associated AKI affects 19–31% of children who receive an IV aminoglycoside. The AKI rate doubles when children receive three or more nephrotoxic medications on the same day. It has been shown that nephrotoxic medication associated AKI goes unrecognized. Treatment of AKI is not yet available, so prevention continues to be the most effective approach. There is an opportunity to mitigate severity and prevent the occurrence of AKI if children at increased risk are identified early and nephrotoxins are used judiciously. With the widespread use of electronic medical records (EMRs), clinical decision support systems that include electronic alerts (e-alerts) have been used to improve recognition of patients with AKI. These systems may be used to either identify patients at risk for AKI or to detect patients already with AKI. NINJA's program triggered to alert the healthcare team of increasing nephrotoxic medication burden, and therefore improved recognition of the risk of AKI.

REFERENCE/SOURCE

- Goldstein SL, Dahale D, Kirkendall ES, Mottes T, Kaplan H, Muething S, et al. A prospective multi-center quality improvement initiative (NINJA) indicates a reduction in nephrotoxic acute kidney injury in hospitalized children. Kidney Int. 2020;97(3):580-8.

9. A 6-year-old girl weighing 20 kg is admitted to the PICU with dengue shock syndrome. After 48 hours of stay, during which multiple fluid boluses were given and dose of inotropes increased to achieve normal BP, she is noted to be puffy and oliguric. Which of the following is an evidence-based indication for initiating KRT in this child?

A. Weight gain of 4 kg since admission
B. Doubling of serum creatinine since admission
C. Fall in urine output to below 10 mL per hour for 6 hours
D. No change in urine output despite therapy with 20 mg IV furosemide

EXPLANATION

Overall, evidence suggests >10–20% fluid overload may represent a critical threshold at which outcomes are adversely affected and targeted interventions, including KRT, should be considered. Other indications for initiation of KRT in pediatric AKI have traditionally been those used for end-stage kidney disease including metabolic/electrolyte abnormalities refractory to medical therapy, pulmonary edema, and/or symptomatic uremia. Evidence-based recommendations on these indications are lacking. Response to furosemide challenge is used to predict the risk of severe AKI, is not an indication for KRT (option D).

Key: A

BOOST YOUR KNOWLEDGE

Fluid overload occurs in 10–80% patients in the ICU due to systemic inflammation, capillary leak, disordered fluid homeostasis, and AKI. It is an independent but modifiable predictor of mortality. Fluid overload can be calculated using the cumulative fluid balance or based on daily weights:

- Percent fluid overload (%FO) = [Daily input (liters) – Daily output (liters) × 100]/ICU admission weight (kilograms)
- Percent fluid overload (%FO) = [Daily weight – ICU admission weight × 100]/ICU admission weight (kilograms)

There is also a concern that fluid overload might put patients at risk of being underdiagnosed with AKI or lead to underestimation of its severity, as serum creatinine is influenced by the volume of distribution and correction of serum creatinine for the degree of fluid overload (by the following formula) may refine the diagnosis of AKI:

Corrected creatinine = serum creatinine (1 + net fluid balance/total body water)

where, total body water = 0.6 × weight (in kilograms)

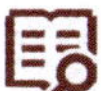

REFERENCES/SOURCES

- Khandelwal P, McLean N, Menon S. Update on Pediatric Acute Kidney Injury. Pediatr Clin North Am. 2022;69(6):1219-38.
- Kidney Disease: Improving Global Outcomes (KDIGO) Acute Kidney Injury Work Group. KDIGO clinical practice guideline for acute kidney injury. Kidney Inter Suppl. 2012;2:1-138.
- Kliegman RM, St Geme JW, Blum NJ, Shah SS, Tasker RC, Wilson KM. Renal failure. In: Kliegman RM, St Geme JW, Blum NJ, Shah SS, Tasker RC, Wilson KM (Eds). Nelson Textbook of Pediatrics, 21st edition. Amsterdam, Netherlands: Elsevier; 2019. pp. 2769-79.

10. An 11-year-old is admitted to the PICU one week following allogenic stem transplantation with septic shock. She is intubated and mechanically ventilated, maintaining a saturation of 96% on fraction of inspired oxygen (FiO_2) of 0.4. She required hemodynamic support with continuous infusion of epinephrine initially but is now hemodynamically stable without inotropic support. Her urine output was 600 mL/day on day one, which fell to 60 mL/day and a net positive balance of 10% is calculated. Investigations show creatinine of 2.7 mg/dL, sodium 134 mEq/L, potassium 4.7 mEq/L, and bicarbonate 22 mEq/L. Which of the following is correct regarding timing of initiation of KRT for this child?

A. KRT initiated within the first 24 hours after onset of oliguria reduces mortality risk
B. KRT should be delayed till the appearance of metabolic or electrolyte abnormalities
C. Delaying KRT till urea >140 mg/dL is associated with increased mortality
D. There is insufficient data from clinical trials in children to guide the optimal timing of KRT

EXPLANATION

While clinical trials have been conducted to address the question of timing of KRT, similar randomized trials are lacking in children.

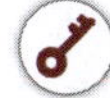

Key: D

BOOST YOUR KNOWLEDGE

Over the last 5 years, six randomized controlled trials have been published to address the optimal timing of KRT initiation in adults. Most of these trials defined early versus delayed approaches for KRT start based on AKI severity according to KDIGO staging and AKI-associated complications. The Early versus Late Initiation of Renal Replacement Therapy in Critical Ill Patients with Acute Kidney Injury (ELAIN) study showed a survival benefit with early versus late KRT, whereas the AKIKI, IDEAL-ICU, FST, and STARRT-AKI did not replicate these findings. More recently, the AKIKI2 trial showed that a more delayed approach is associated with worse outcomes.

These studies have questioned the need for earlier initiation of therapy, despite one study showing a benefit in survival. A delayed approach could translate into a potentially reduced burden of dialysis dependence in addition to saving health resources. However, it is important to note that the threshold of fluid overload for initiation of KRT in the STARRT-AKI trail was 3–7%, compared to 10–20% in previous retrospective studies. Therefore, the definition of "early" and "late" start of KRT with respect to fluid overload thresholds has evolved, with recognition of fluid overload having an important impact on outcomes.

REFERENCES/SOURCES

- Bouchard J, Mehta RL. Timing of kidney support therapy in acute kidney injury: what are we waiting for? Am J Kidney Dis. 2022;79(3):417-26.
- Kidney Disease: Improving Global Outcomes (KDIGO) Acute Kidney Injury Work Group. KDIGO clinical practice guideline for acute kidney injury. Kidney Inter Suppl. 2012;2:1-138.

11. A 7-year-old child presents with dark urine like "black tea", followed by swelling of the eyelids associated with malaise, anorexia, and weakness. She has no relevant medical history, although her mother reports her having an infection at the site of ear piercing 4 weeks ago for which she was prescribed some antibiotics. She took 2 days of these but stopped because the infection cleared. Her urinalysis is as follows: Protein 3+, blood 3+, nitrites negative, and leukocytes 1+. Kidney function tests revealed blood creatinine of 2.0 mg/dL. What is the most likely cause of AKI in the child?

A. Poststreptococcal glomerulonephritis (PSGN)
B. Membranoproliferative glomerulonephritis (MPGN)
C. Alkaptonuria
D. Acute intermittent porphyria

EXPLANATION

Acute glomerulonephritis (GN) is characterized by abrupt onset of variable degrees of hematuria (active urinary sediment; dysmorphic red blood cells and red blood cell casts), proteinuria (usually subnephrotic range; urine protein <1 g/m^2/day), oliguria, edema, hypertension, and AKI. PSGN is delayed sequelae of infection caused by nephritogenic strains of *Streptococcus pyogenes*, occurring 1–2 weeks after pharyngitis and 3–6 weeks following skin infection. PSGN is the most common type of acute GN in children, especially from developing countries. MPGN has variable clinical presentation and may present with AGN; it is much less common than PSGN. Alkaptonuria and porphyria are both associated with dark urine but are not associated with AGN or AKI.

Key: A

BOOST YOUR KNOWLEDGE

Etiology of acute glomerulonephritis

Condition	***Features to differentiate from PSGN***
Postinfectious: Streptococci (PSGN), staphylococci, pneumococci, meningococci, *Leptospira,* infection of shunts, bacterial endocarditis, hepatitis B or C, and human immunodeficiency virus (HIV)	Impetigo, pharyngitis, endocarditis, shunts, and abscess; PSGN usually self-limiting
Systemic vasculitis: IgA vasculitis and antineutrophilic cytoplasmic antibody (ANCA)-associated vasculitis	Systemic features, normal complement levels
Others: C3 glomerulopathy, immune complex MPGN, IgA nephropathy, systemic lupus erythematosus, and hereditary nephritis	Persistent hypocomplementemia, unresolving nephritic syndrome, synpharyngitic presentation; normal C3, systemic features, persistent hypocomplementemia, family history, and normal C3

REFERENCE/SOURCE

- Uthup S, Khandelwal P, Reddy SK. Acute glomerulonephritis (acute nephritic syndrome). Mumbai, India: Indian Academy of Pediatrics; 2022.

12. A 2-year-old child presents with a history of poor urine output over the past 2 days. Other than diarrhea about a week ago, he has no other significant history. His older sister is also admitted to another hospital with bloody diarrhea. On examination, he is alert, afebrile, and vital signs are stable. Which one of the following tests would be most useful for establishing the cause of his AKI?

A. Stool culture
B. Clotting screen
C. Blood film
D. Ultrasound kidney, ureter, and bladder

EXPLANATION

In developed countries, the leading cause of severe AKI is in children is HUS due to STEC infection. In developing countries, infectious etiologies, especially tropical infections and sepsis, are the leading causes of AKI. The history and physical examination (and a common contaminated source of infection since the sibling is simultaneously affected) points to the possibility of HUS. The diagnosis of HUS is clinical based on demonstration of fragmented red blood cells on the blood film (option C). While stool culture is required for classification of HUS, this is not required initially to recognize and diagnose HUS (option A). Ultrasonography (USG) of kidneys and bladder are required when obstructive etiologies are suspected.

Key: C

BOOST YOUR KNOWLEDGE

The clinical diagnosis of HUS is based on the presence of: (1) Microangiopathic hemolytic anemia: hemoglobin <10 g/dL and fragmented red cells on peripheral smear (schistocytes ≥2%) with either increased lactate dehydrogenase or undetectable haptoglobin; (2) Thrombocytopenia (platelets <150,000/μL), and (3) AKI (rise in creatinine by 50% over baseline). Sepsis and disseminated intravascular coagulation (DIC) must be excluded. STEC-HUS is clinically suspected in children older than 6 months, with history of bloody diarrhea 2–3 weeks prior to onset of HUS, and/or temporally associated with a STEC outbreak. The diagnosis of STEC-HUS is by stool (or rectal swab) culture and testing for Shiga toxin by detection of either virulence genes on fecal extracts or cultures by polymerase chain reaction (PCR) or detecting free fecal Shiga toxin by enzyme immunoassay (EIA). Fecal diagnostics might be falsely negative after the first 7–10 days of illness due to short lasting excretion of STEC in stool (isolation rate is ~90% within 6 days) and if antibiotics have been administered. Serum immunoglobulin M (IgM) antibodies to serogroup specific *E. coli* lipopolysaccharide [by enzyme-linked immunosorbent assay (ELISA)] suggest recent infection and is important for diagnosis in patients with delayed presentation.

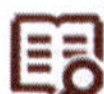

REFERENCES/SOURCES

- Bagga A, Khandelwal P, Mishra K, Thergaonkar R, Vasudevan A, Sharma J, et al; Indian Society of Pediatric Nephrology. Hemolytic uremic syndrome in a developing country: Consensus guidelines. Pediatr Nephrol. 2019;34:1465-82.
- Kliegman RM, St Geme JW, Blum NJ, Shah SS, Tasker RC, Wilson KM. Renal failure. In: Kliegman RM, St Geme JW, Blum NJ, Shah SS, Tasker RC, Wilson KM (Eds). Nelson Textbook of Pediatrics, 21st edition. Amsterdam, Netherlands: Elsevier; 2019. pp. 2769-79.

13. Which of the following statements are true about dialysis for AKI in the neonatal period?

A. Prophylactic use of a single dose of IV vancomycin given 60 minutes prior insertion of PD catheter decreases the rate of peritonitis
B. Peritonitis is defined as presence of >100 cells/mm and with 50% neutrophils in the PD fluid
C. Longer dwell times in PD are used for rapid urea, fluid, and potassium clearance
D. Cardio-Renal Pediatric Dialysis Emergency Machine (CARPEDIEM) and Newcastle Infant Dialysis and Ultrafiltration System (NIDUS) are neonatal hemodialysis machines

EXPLANATION

The International Society for PD has formulated guidelines for AKI. A prophylactic use of a single dose of IV vancomycin given 60 minutes prior to PD catheter insertion is recommended to decrease the rate of peritonitis, the most common complication of acute PD. Peritonitis, as defined by these guidelines, is the presence of >100 cells/mm *or* with 50% neutrophils in the PD fluid. Higher the fill volume and shorter dwell times are associated with greater ultrafiltration and clearance; shorter dwell time is used for rapid urea, fluid, and potassium clearance. Longer dwell times may be needed for phosphate clearance, especially in chronic PD. Hemodialysis machines are not developed for use in neonates. CRRT machines with accurate blood flow rates with minimal ultrafiltration error include the CARPEDIEM used between 2.0 and 9.9 kg, NIDUS in infants weighing between 0.8 and 8 kg and Aquadex used in children weighing between 2.7 and 12.4 kg.

Key: A

BOOST YOUR KNOWLEDGE

Peritoneal dialysis is the preferred mode of kidney replacement in neonates chiefly due to its technical simplicity, lack of hemodynamic compromise, and requirement of vascular access. The recently convened Acute Disease Quality Initiative (ADQI) conference for neonatal AKI recommended cuffed catheters (Tenckhoff catheters made of silicone polymer of methyl silicate) for prolonged PD due to its low risk of infection and visceral injury. PD works on the following principle: The two purposes of kidney replacement are dialysis (removal of solutes) and ultrafiltration (removal of water). Dialysis occurs by removal of plasma solutes by diffusion down their concentration gradient across the peritoneal lining that serves as a semipermeable membrane. Instillation of hypertonic dialysate into the peritoneal cavity creates a transmembrane osmotic gradient that allows removal of fluid by ultrafiltration. Therefore, PD allows slow continuous exchange of fluid and solutes.

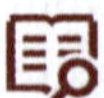

REFERENCES/SOURCES

- Nourse P, Cullis B, Finkelstein F, Numanoglu A, Warady B, Antwi S, et al. ISPD guidelines for peritoneal dialysis in acute kidney injury: 2020 Update (paediatrics). Perit Dial Int. 2021;41:139-57.
- Peritoneal dialysis. In: Agarwal R, Deorari A, Paul VK, Shankar J, Sachdeva A (Eds). AIIMS Protocols in Neonatology, 3rd edition. CBS Publishers; 2024.

14. A 3-month-old girl weighing 5 kg has septicemia, multiorgan dysfunction, AKI, and anuria. Tests show creatinine 2.0 mg/dL, sodium 132 mEq/L, potassium 6.4 mEq/L, pH 7.15, and bicarbonate 15 mEq/L. At initiation of PD, which of the following components of prescription are correct?

A. Dwell volume 150 mL
B. Dialysate dextrose concentration 3%
C. Dialysate potassium 4 mEq/L
D. Dwell time 60 minutes

EXPLANATION

The initial dwell volume recommended is 30 mL/kg, increased gradually up to 30–50 mL/kg. The dialysate fluid contains 1.7% dextrose as osmotic agents with lactate/bicarbonate as base. If higher gradient is required as in case of fluid overload 3% dextrose solution can be used. If patient becomes hypokalemic during the procedure, 3–4 mEq/L of potassium is added to dialysate fluid. Initial dwell times are 15–30 minutes, shorter cycles are the norm initially to increase clearance of solutes.

Key: A

BOOST YOUR KNOWLEDGE

Components of PD prescription include dialysate type and composition, number of exchanges, fill volume, inflow, dwell, and outflow times, and ultrafiltration volume.

Composition of PD fluid:
Osmotic agent: Dextrose 1.4–3.9 g/dL
Base:
- Lactate 35–40 mEq/L or bicarbonate 34 mEq/L
- Sodium 132–134 mEq/L, calcium 1.25–1.75 mM/L,
- Magnesium 0.25–0.75 mM/L, chloride 95–103.5 mEq/L

Lactate free and bicarbonate-based solutions are more biocompatible and are available commercially or may be made in house. Patients with liver failure may be unable to metabolize lactate quickly, and benefit with the use of such fluids. While limited evidence shows that even low fill volumes (10 mL/kg) with rapid exchanges can achieve adequate ultrafiltration and clearance, higher the fill volume, greater is the ultrafiltration and clearance.

The dwell time is determined by fluid balance and biochemical abnormalities; shorter dwell time is used for rapid urea, fluid, and potassium clearance. Complete drainage of effluent during outflow should be ensured to avoid elevated intra-abdominal pressure. Heparin 250–1,000 U/L should be added if hemorrhagic effluent is present to avoid catheter-related clotting.

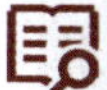

REFERENCES/SOURCES

- Fischbach M, Warady BA. Peritoneal dialysis prescription in children: bedside principles for optimal practice. Pediatr Nephrol. 2009;24:1633-42.
- Nourse P, Cullis B, Finkelstein F, Numanoglu A, Warady B, Antwi S, et al. ISPD guidelines for peritoneal dialysis in acute kidney injury: 2020 Update. Perit Dial Int. 2021;41:139-57.

15. Baby A in the neonatal ICU is a 3-day-old born by assisted vaginal delivery at 41 weeks of gestation and had poor Apgar scores at birth (1 at 1 minute and 3 at 5 minutes) with need for intubation. A diagnosis of hypoxic ischemic encephalopathy was made and presently he is undergoing therapeutic hypothermia. Serum creatinine was 0.9 mg/dL on day 1 and is now 2.1 mg/dL. His urine output has decreased in the last 12 hours, and his weight is up 800 g in the last 24 hours. Randomized trials in the neonatal age-group provides evidence for use of which of the following medications in this baby?

A. Low dose dopamine
B. Diuretics
C. Theophylline
D. Fenoldopam

EXPLANATION

A meta-analysis of randomized controlled trials suggests that prophylactic therapy with adenosine receptor antagonist, theophylline, reduces the incidence of severe renal dysfunction in term neonates with severe birth asphyxia. A single dose of theophylline (5–8 mg/kg) is recommended in neonates with severe perinatal asphyxia for preventing AKI as per the KDIGO guidelines.

Key: C

BOOST YOUR KNOWLEDGE

Studies have suggested that adenosine receptor antagonists (such as theophylline and caffeine) may inhibit renal vasoconstriction and therefore prevent AKI when given shortly after birth. Cautious use of theophylline is required due to its potential negative long-term neurologic implications. Caffeine has shown to decrease incidence and severity of AKI in preterm neonates. There is moderate quality evidence of decreased severity of AKI with acetaminophen and/or paracetamol use. Dopamine or fenoldopam have shown conflicting results in clinical studies and are not recommended for prevention or therapy of AKI. Data from the AWAKEN study found that diuretic administration was associated with a decreased risk of early-onset AKI in neonates, adequate evidence for recommending diuretics routinely is lacking given reports of rise in creatinine with diuretic use.

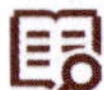

REFERENCES/SOURCES

- Kidney Disease: Improving Global Outcomes (KDIGO) Acute Kidney Injury Work Group. KDIGO clinical practice guideline for acute kidney injury. Kidney Inter Suppl. 2012;2:1-138.
- Starr MC, Menon S. Neonatal acute kidney injury: a case-based approach. Pediatr Nephrol. 2021;36:3607-19.

16. A 2-month-old boy is brought with complaints oliguria since birth. He was born at term by normal vaginal delivery at home. Mother did not seek antenatal care during pregnancy, and birth weight is unknown. Investigations show serum creatinine 2.5 mg/dL, sodium 132 mEq/L, and potassium 5.7 mEq/L. Ultrasound performed is shown in given Figures. What is the most likely diagnosis?

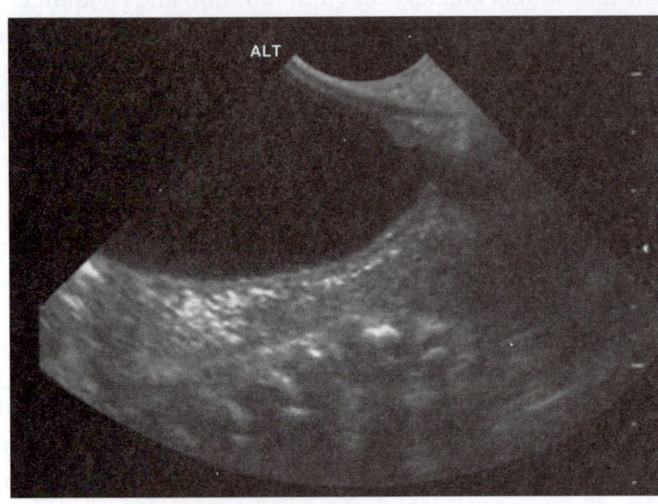

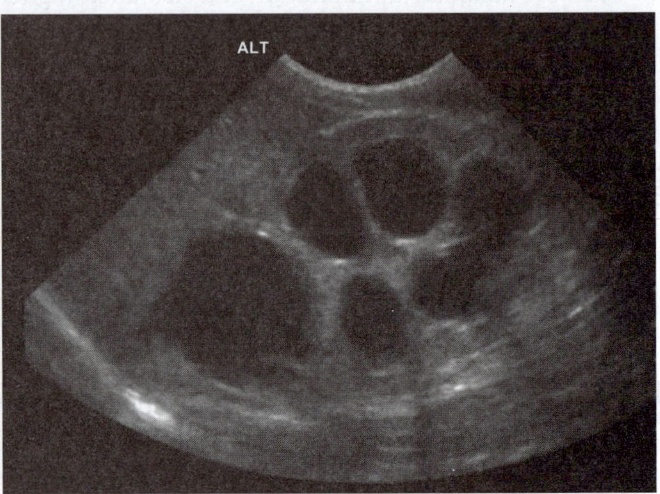

A. Neurogenic bladder with AKI
B. Cystic kidney disease
C. Renal tubular dysgenesis
D. Posterior urethral valve (PUV)

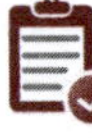

EXPLANATION

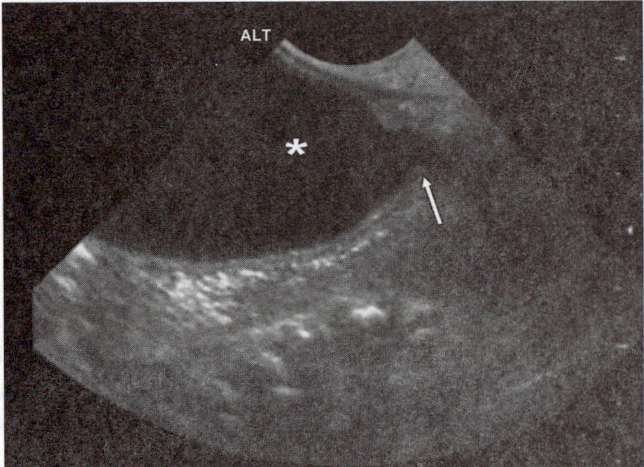

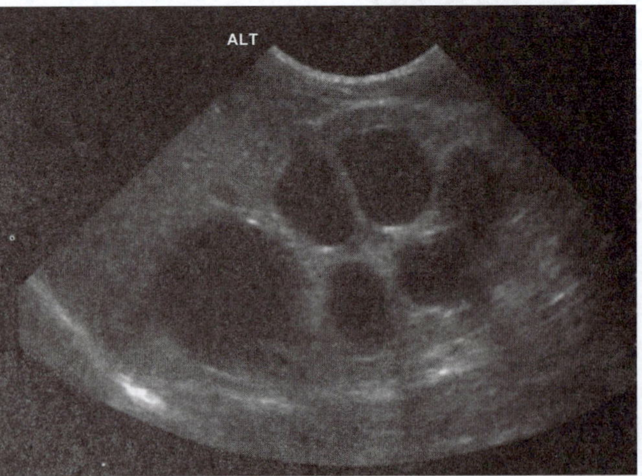

The first image shows distended bladder (*) with classic keyhole sign due to the presence of PUVs (arrow) distally. Presence of dilated renal calyces is seen on the second image, due to severe obstructive hydroureteronephrosis.

Key: D

BOOST YOUR KNOWLEDGE

Posterior urethral valve is the most common cause of severe obstructive uropathy in children. Affected males are often diagnosed prenatally with ultrasound showing bilateral hydronephrosis, a distended bladder, with or without oligohydramnios. In the male neonate, PUVs are suspected when there is a palpably distended bladder, and the urinary stream is weak. If the obstruction is severe and goes unrecognized during the neonatal period, infants can present later in life with AKI or urinary tract infection (UTI). With lesser degrees of obstruction, children present later in life with difficulty in achieving diurnal urinary continence or with UTI. Diagnosis is by ultrasound and micturating cystourethrography; management is valve ablation. About 30% progress to CKD.

REFERENCE/SOURCE

- Kliegman RM, St Geme JW, Blum NJ, Shah SS, Tasker RC, Wilson KM. Renal failure. In: Kliegman RM, St Geme JW, Blum NJ, Shah SS, Tasker RC, Wilson KM (Eds). Nelson Textbook of Pediatrics, 21st edition. Amsterdam, Netherlands: Elsevier; 2019. pp. 2769-79.

17. In a 6-year-old boy, which of the following indices indicates hypovolemia and prerenal AKI, as opposed to intrinsic acute tubular necrosis (ATN)?

A. Fractional excretion of sodium (FENA) 2.5%
B. Renal failure index (RFI) of 2
C. Urine specific gravity 1.010
D. Urine sodium 5 mEq/L

EXPLANATION

Urinary indices may be useful in differentiating prerenal AKI from intrinsic AKI.

Parameters to differentiate prerenal from intrinsic renal failure

Parameters	*Prerenal*	*Intrinsic renal*
Urinary Na	≤20 mEq/L	>40 mEq/L (>50 in newborn)
RFI*	Low <1	High ≥1 (>4 in newborn)
Urine osmolarity	>500 mOsm/kg	<350 mOsm/kg
Specific gravity	>1.020	< 1.010
FENA%$	≤1 (<2.5% in newborn)	>2 (>3–10 in newborn)

*RFI: $\frac{\text{Urinary Na} \times \text{Serum creatinine}}{\text{Urine creatinine}}$

$FENA%: $\frac{\text{Urinary Na} \times \text{Serum creatinine} \times 100}{\text{Serum sodium} \times \text{Urine creatinine}}$

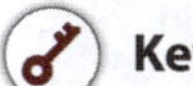

Key: D

BOOST YOUR KNOWLEDGE

For measuring urinary indices, the important prerequisite is that the urine sample for measuring indices must be obtained prior to fluid and diuretic challenge. The sensitivity and specificity of urine sodium of <20 mEq/L in differentiating prerenal azotemia from ATN are 90% and 82%, respectively. The sensitivity and specificity of FENA of <1% in differentiating prerenal azotemia from ATN are 96% and 95%, respectively. The FENA may be <1% in ATN secondary to radiocontrast material or rhabdomyolysis.

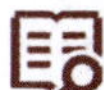

REFERENCE/SOURCE

- Kliegman RM, St Geme JW, Blum NJ, Shah SS, Tasker RC, Wilson KM. Renal failure. In: Kliegman RM, St Geme JW, Blum NJ, Shah SS, Tasker RC, Wilson KM (Eds). Nelson Textbook of Pediatrics, 21st edition. Amsterdam, Netherlands: Elsevier; 2019. pp. 2769-79.

18. A 7-year-old premorbid normal girl was admitted to the PICU with rhabdomyolysis following multiple bee stings. She had severe AKI requiring dialysis for 5 days, and multiorgan dysfunction. Duration of PICU stay was 8 days. She has now made a complete recovery and is planned for discharge. At hospital discharge her creatinine is 0.5 mg/dL, BP is 100/70 mm Hg and urine dipstick shows 2+ proteinuria. What is the most appropriate time to assess her for CKD following discharge?

A. 1 month
B. 3 months
C. 1 year
D. 3–5 years

EXPLANATION

The association between AKI and CKD has been clearly established in recent years. Proteinuria, hypertension, and reduced estimated glomerular filtration rate (eGFR) are common following AKI. Children who develop AKI need long-term observation and monitoring. The KDIGO guidelines suggest that AKI survivors should be reevaluated 3 months after the event to assess for resolution of AKI, the development of new onset CKD, and (if applicable) progression of preexisting CKD. The intensity and level of post-AKI care may depend on the severity of AKI, recovery, or lack of recovery of kidney function and other comorbidities.

Key: B

BOOST YOUR KNOWLEDGE

Recognizing that the duration of AKI also predicts adverse outcomes, the ADQI in 2017 proposed that the definition of AKI be limited to 7 days and acute kidney disease (AKD) be used for persistence of deranged kidney function beyond this period till the CKD criterion of 90 days. CKD is defined at a eGFR of <60 mL/min/1.73 m^2 or even higher with evidence of kidney injury/damage, as long as either criterion is present at least 3 months after the AKI event. The KDIGO has recently harmonized the definition of AKD to include abnormalities of kidney function and/or structure with a duration of 3 months or less that may or may not include prior AKI.

REFERENCES/SOURCES

- Kidney Disease: Improving Global Outcomes (KDIGO) Acute Kidney Injury Work Group. KDIGO clinical practice guideline for acute kidney injury. Kidney Inter Suppl. 2012;2:1-138.
- Lameire NH, Levin A, Kellum JA, Cheung M, Jadoul M, Winkelmayer WC, et al. Harmonizing acute and chronic kidney disease definition and classification: report of a Kidney Disease: Improving Global Outcomes (KDIGO) Consensus Conference. Kidney Int. 2021;100:516-26.

19. You are called to manage an 8-year-old boy with multisystem organ failure with AKI in the setting of disseminated staphylococcal sepsis and meningitis. His BP is 87/50 mm Hg with a heart rate of 96 beats/minute with continuous infusion of dopamine. He is mechanically ventilated and has SpO_2 of 93% while receiving FiO_2 of 0.6. His urine output is <5 mL/h. Laboratory data include a creatinine of 4.3 mg/dL, BUN of 92 mg/dL, potassium of 5.3 mEq/L, and a bicarbonate of 19 mEq/L. You decide to begin KRT. Which if the following regarding modality selection in this patient is correct?

A. CRRT is associated with improved survival compared to extended daily dialysis (EDD)
B. Sustained low-efficiency daily dialysis (SLEDD) avoids the need for systemic anticoagulation
C. Dialysis disequilibrium syndrome (DDS) is commonly associated with CVVHD
D. Sustained low-efficiency daily dialysis with filtration (SLEDD-f) includes faster clearance of small solutes and fluid removal compared to CVVHDF

EXPLANATION

Randomized trials in adults do not show a survival advantage of CRRTs over extended hemodialysis techniques such as SLEDD and SLEDD-f; studies in children are limited (option A). While extended hemodialysis techniques have lower heparin requirement than CRRT, systemic anticoagulation is required (option B). DDS is result of rapid changes in osmolarity inducing water shifts from the extracellular to the intracellular compartment. It is encountered during or immediately after hemodialysis associated with rapid clearance of solutes. Slow, continuous, modes of dialysis such as CRRT (including CVVHD) and PD are not associated with DDS (option C). SLEDD-f is aimed at improving clearance of middle molecular inflammatory mediators of the systemic inflammatory response associated with sepsis. Advantages of SLEDD-f over CVVHDF include faster clearance of small solutes and fluid removal.

Key: D

BOOST YOUR KNOWLEDGE

Extended hemodialysis techniques, also known as hybrid therapies, utilize intermittent hemodialysis machine technology while providing the slower solute and fluid removal for use in hemodynamically unstable patients with AKI. The terms for these modalities include SLEDD or EDD or slow continuous dialysis (SCD) and may be performed for 6–18 hours daily. These modalities allow flexible therapeutic schedules so that patients are accessible and can be mobilized for other medical treatments. Hybrid therapies have a high diffusive capacity for solutes; hypophosphatemia and metabolic alkalosis are common complications in a critically ill patient.

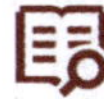

REFERENCE/SOURCE

- Management of pediatric acute kidney injury. In: Geary DF, Schaefer F (Eds). Pediatric Kidney Disease, 2nd edition. Berlin: Springer; 2017. p. 1251.

20. A 4-year-old boy presents with altered sensorium and AKI following ingestion of a paracetamol-containing cough syrup. Blood gas shows high anion gap metabolic acidosis, urine examination shows calcium oxalate crystals. Ingestion of which of the following agents is responsible for these clinical manifestations?

A. Paracetamol
B. Ethylene glycol
C. Propylene glycol
D. Oxalate

EXPLANATION

Ethylene glycol poisoning is an important cause of AKI in young children. The absorbed ethylene glycol is converted into four toxic substances by alcohol dehydrogenase, i.e., glycolaldehyde, glycolate, glyoxylate, and oxalate. Glycolaldehyde can hinder numerous aspects of cellular metabolism while also exacerbating cellular damage. The formation of oxalic acid and calcium oxalate monohydrate crystals, which can cause cerebral edema and kidney failure, related to tubular system blockade and injury, can be seen within 8–24 hours of consumption of a lethal dose. If untreated, death from multiorgan failure typically occurs within 24–36 hours of glycol ingestion.

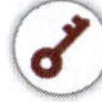

Key: B

BOOST YOUR KNOWLEDGE

Spurious ethylene glycol-containing syrups have been identified as a cause of several cases of pediatric AKI and deaths worldwide. Ethylene glycol is an odorless, water-miscible organic compound with a sweetish taste. Active pharmaceutical compounds, like paracetamol, are non-water soluble and require nontoxic solvents, such as glycerol and propylene glycol, to provide a liquid base and act as preservatives, thickeners, and sweetening agents. Manufacturers illegally replace glycerol and propylene glycol with toxic diethylene glycol and ethylene glycol, thereby leading to poisoning. Treatment involves concurrent hemodialysis with fomepizole (alcohol dehydrogenase inhibitor) administered over 4 hours.

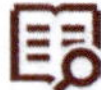

REFERENCES/SOURCES

- Theobald JL, Kostic MA. Poisoning. In: Kliegman RM, St Geme JW, Blum NJ, Shah SS, Tasker RC, Wilson KM (Eds). Nelson Textbook of Pediatrics, 21st edition. Amsterdam, Netherlands: Elsevier; 2019. pp. 490-510.
- Umar TP, Jain N, Azis H. Endemic rise in cases of acute kidney injury in children in Indonesia and Gambia: what is the likely culprit and why? Kidney Int. 2023;103(3):444-7.

21. Which one of the following statements is *not* an evidence-based recommendation for nutritional management in children with AKI?

A. Restriction of protein to below the suggested dietary intake (SDI) is the first step in critically ill children with persistently rising BUN levels
B. Oral feeding, including breastfeeding, is the preferred method of providing nutrition
C. In noncritically ill children, the initial prescription for protein intake should approximate the SDI for euvolemic weight
D. Protein prescription needs to be further increased to account for dialysis losses

EXPLANATION

Oral or enteral feeding is the preferred route of nutrition and is associated with decreased mortality in critically ill patients with AKI. Early initiation (within 48 hours of admission) of supplemental or exclusive enteral tube feeding should be considered when oral feeding does not meet nutritional requirements. In the setting of limited evidence, for noncritically ill children, the SDI guide protein recommendations. It is important to provide adequate protein in AKI to account for frequent catabolism and muscle wasting. Restriction of protein which would cause worsening malnutrition and is not recommended, lowering protein intake to lower range of SDI is useful for patients with persistently elevated BUN. The Kidney Disease Outcomes Quality Initiative (KDOQI) workgroup recommended additional 0.1 g/kg/day protein to account for dialysis-related protein losses in children; these losses are maximum in case of CRRT.

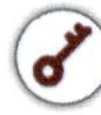

Key: A

BOOST YOUR KNOWLEDGE

The Pediatric Renal Nutrition Taskforce (PRNT), an international team of pediatric renal dietitians and pediatric nephrologists, has developed clinical practice recommendations for the nutritional management of children with AKI. Apart for the recommendations for protein intake (as mentioned earlier), recommendations for energy requirements are: For noncritically ill children, the initial prescription for energy intake should approximate SDI based on euvolemic weight, not measured weight. In the acute phase of critical illness, energy requirements should not exceed the resting energy expenditure. In the stable phase and recovery phase of critical illness, the energy prescription must account for energy debt, physical activity, rehabilitation, and growth. Modify the energy prescription to account for dialysis-related net gain or loss of energy. In critical illness, consider an increased percentage of energy intake from fat to reflect changes in beta-oxidation when parenterally fed. The reader is requested to refer to the following source for complete recommendations.

REFERENCE/SOURCE

- Vega MRW, Cerminara D, Desloovere A, Paglialonga F, Renken-Terhaerdt J, Walle JV, et al. Nutritional management of children with acute kidney injury-clinical practice recommendations from the Pediatric Renal Nutrition Taskforce. Pediatr Nephrol. 2023;38: 3559-80.

CHAPTER

21.8 Hemolytic Uremic Syndrome

Aditi Sinha

1. The adjacent diagram shows an important pathway in innate immunity. Dysregulation of which of the pathways is implicated in the pathogenesis of atypical hemolytic uremic syndrome (aHUS)?

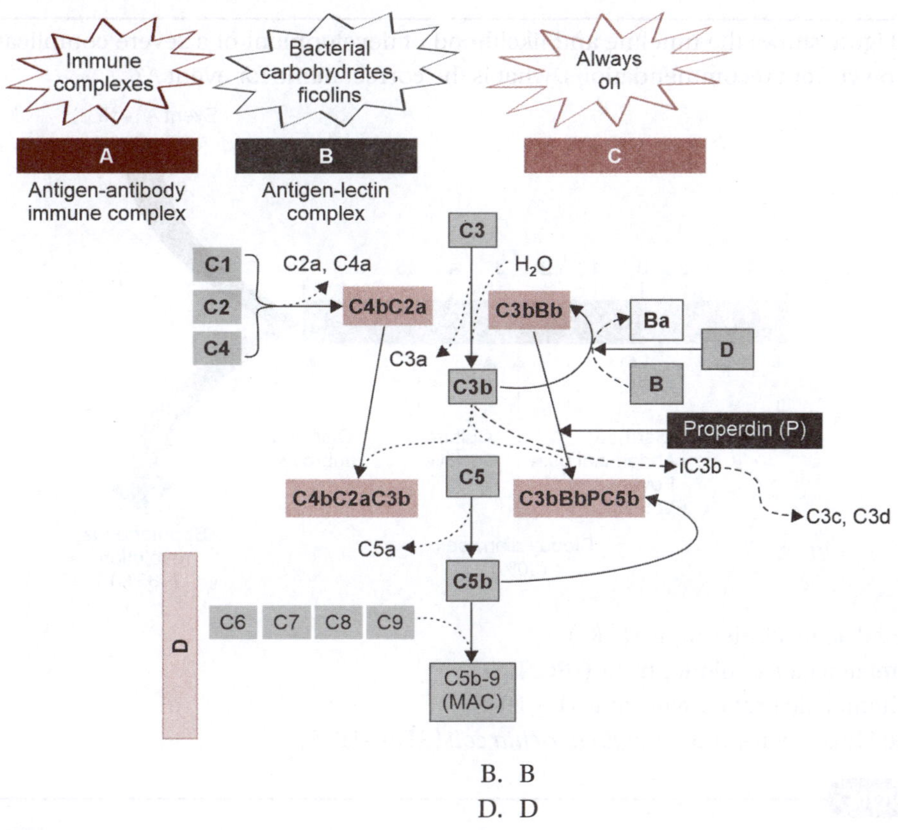

A. A
B. B
C. C
D. D

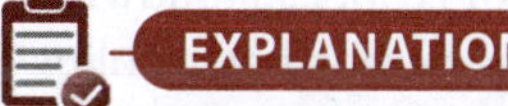

EXPLANATION

The diagram represents the complement system, also known as complement cascade, which is a part of the innate immune system. Three biochemical pathways activate the complement system, as shown in the diagram: (A) The classical complement pathway, (B) the lectin pathway, and (C) the alternative complement pathway. The three pathways converge to lead to terminal pathway activation, indicated as "D". The alternative pathway accounts for most of the terminal pathway activation, and its dysregulation leads to uncontrolled complement activation, leading to aHUS.

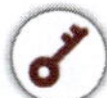

Key: C

BOOST YOUR KNOWLEDGE

The complement system enhances or "complements" the ability of antibodies and phagocytic cells to clear microbes and damaged cells from an organism, promote inflammation, and attack the pathogen's cell membrane. Therapeutic efforts in controlling disease in aHUS have revolved around the inhibition of the alternate complement pathway or terminal pathway activation.

REFERENCES/SOURCES

- Abbas AK, Lichtman AH, Pillai S. Cellular and Molecular Immunology, 10th edition. Philadelphia: Saunders/Elsevier; 2021. pp. 287-311.
- Bagga A, Khandelwal P, Mishra K, Thergaonkar R, Vasudevan A, Sharma J, et al; Indian Society of Pediatric Nephrology. Hemolytic uremic syndrome in a developing country: Consensus guidelines. Pediatr Nephrol. 2019;34:1465-82.
- Emma F, Goldstein SL, Bagga A, Bates CM, Shroff R. Pediatric Nephrology, 8th edition. Switzerland: Springer Nature; 2022. pp. 595-636.
- Kliegman RM, St Geme JW, Blum NJ, Shah SS, Tasker RC, Wilson KM. Nelson Textbook of Pediatrics, 21st edition. Philadelphia: Elsevier; 2019. pp. 2731-5.

2. The adjacent Figure shows the timeline and likelihood of development of a severe complication of an infectious illness. Based on current recommendations, what is the correct name for event A?

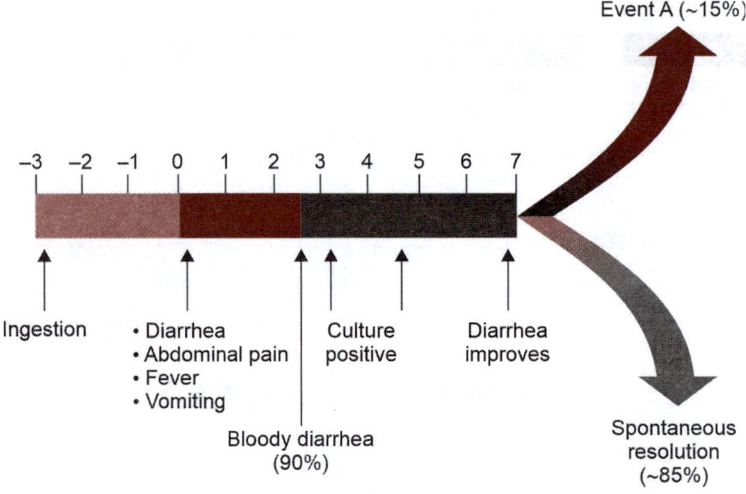

A. Sepsis related acute kidney injury (AKI)
B. Infection-related glomerulonephritis (IRGN)
C. Diarrheal hemolytic uremic syndrome (D+ HUS)
D. HUS due to Shiga toxin-producing *Escherichia coli* (STEC-HUS)

EXPLANATION

The Figure indicates the timeline and likelihood of development of the most common cause of HUS, i.e., following infection with certain strains of *E. coli* bacteria that make a toxin called Shiga toxin and causes hemorrhagic colitis leading to bloody diarrhea. Since these strains are called Shiga toxin-producing *E. coli* (STEC), this form of HUS is called STEC-HUS. The terms used in the past, like typical or diarrhea + HUS are no longer used because diarrhea can be a prodromal illness in "aHUS" as well, and the term "STEC" is specific in indicating the causative organism.

The term "sepsis-related AKI" refers to acute tubular necrosis in the context of any severe systemic infection. IRGN refers to immune complex-mediated glomerulonephritis (GN) which is most commonly poststreptococcal, though *Staphylococcus* and other infections are also implicated.

Key: D

BOOST YOUR KNOWLEDGE

The STEC-HUS is usually caused by enterohemorrhagic *E. coli* (EHEC), of which *E. coli* O157:H7 is the most common serotype. Recently, other serotypes have become more prevalent. In India, *Shigella dysenteriae* type 1 was described as being the most common cause of STEC-HUS, but this organism is rarely reported in North or East India recently.

REFERENCES/SOURCES

- Bagga A, Khandelwal P, Mishra K, Thergaonkar R, Vasudevan A, Sharma J, et al; Indian Society of Pediatric Nephrology. Hemolytic uremic syndrome in a developing country: Consensus guidelines. Pediatr Nephrol. 2019;34:1465-82.
- Emma F, Goldstein SL, Bagga A, Bates CM, Shroff R. Pediatric Nephrology, 8th edition. Switzerland: Springer Nature; 2022. pp. 595-636.
- Kliegman RM, St Geme JW, Blum NJ, Shah SS, Tasker RC, Wilson KM. Nelson Textbook of Pediatrics, 21st edition. Philadelphia: Elsevier; 2019. pp. 2731-5.

3. A 10-year-old boy presenting with acute onset of pallor, puffiness, and reduced urine output. Evaluation indicates hemoglobin of 6 g/dL, total leukocyte count 8,000/mm^3, platelet count 80,000/mm^3, urea 120 mg/dL, creatinine 4.0 mg/dL, sodium 135 mEq/L, and potassium 5.5 mEq/L. Peripheral smear and urinalysis are shown as images (A) and (B), respectively. Urine dipstick shows 3+ proteinuria.

Which of the following antibodies are the most likely cause of disease in this patient?

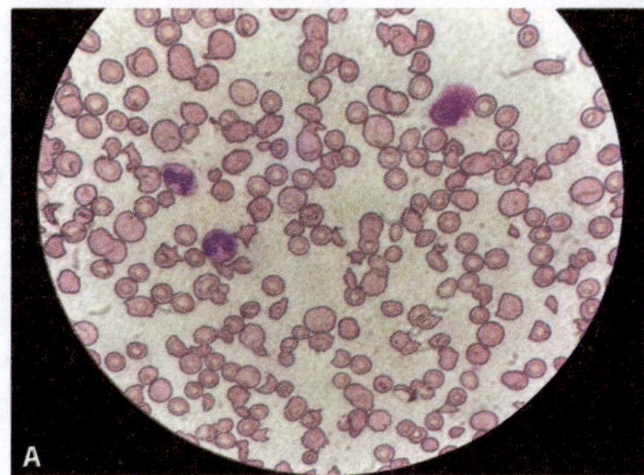

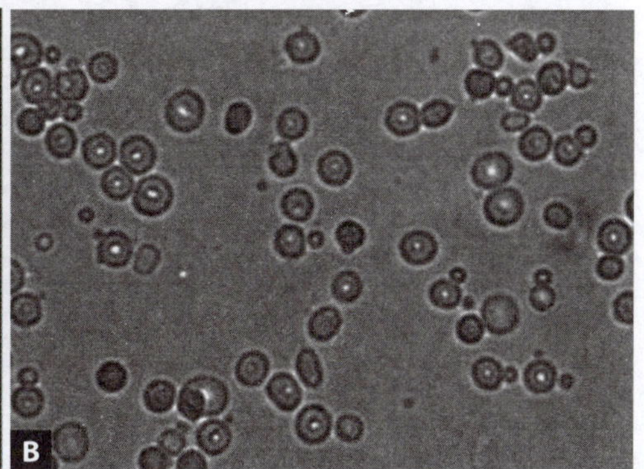

A. Antistreptolysin O antibodies
B. Antineutrophil cytoplasmic antibodies
C. Antibodies to complement factor H (FH)
D. Antibodies to double-stranded deoxyribonucleic acid (DNA)

EXPLANATION

The clinical scenario mentions a child with anemia, thrombocytopenia, and AKI. The image (A) shows the presence of schistocytes that are broken red blood cells (RBCs) passing through narrowed vessels. Image (B) shows hematuria with very little dysmorphic RBCs. The most likely etiology is HUS. At the given age, aHUS is more likely than STEC-associated HUS which is seen predominantly in 6 months to 3 years of age. Among the aHUS, 50% is caused by antibodies to factor-H which is the main regulator of complement system.

- Proteinuria and hematuria may also be seen in acute GN, but urinalysis in GN would show red cell casts as well as more frequently dysmorphic RBCs. Further, microangiopathic anemia and thrombocytopenia is present only in HUS.
- Antineutrophil cytoplasmic antibody (ANCA)-associated vasculitis and GN do not have microangiopathic hemolytic anemia and thrombocytopenia.
- Systemic lupus erythematosus (SLE) may also present with features of anemia, thrombocytopenia, and features of GN. However, patients with SLE typically show DCT positive hemolytic anemia rather than microangiopathic anemia. SLE is uncommon in boys, and other features of SLE are lacking.

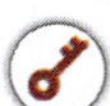

Key: C

BOOST YOUR KNOWLEDGE

Antibodies to FH disrupt the regulation of complement by FH, thereby allowing the alternate complement pathway to go unchecked. Early initiation of plasma exchanges along with immunosuppression is associated with favorable response. Relapse rates are higher in the initial 2 years necessitating maintenance immunosuppression. Complement inhibitors are useful, especially in disease refractory to plasma exchanges, but the high cost and unavailability is a major hindrance.

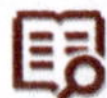

REFERENCES/SOURCES

- Abbas AK, Lichtman AH, Pillai S. Cellular and Molecular Immunology, 10th edition. Philadelphia: Saunders/Elsevier; 2021. pp. 287-311.
- Bagga A, Khandelwal P, Mishra K, Thergaonkar R, Vasudevan A, Sharma J, et al; Indian Society of Pediatric Nephrology. Hemolytic uremic syndrome in a developing country: Consensus guidelines. Pediatr Nephrol. 2019;34:1465-82.
- Emma F, Goldstein SL, Bagga A, Bates CM, Shroff R. Pediatric Nephrology, 8th edition. Switzerland: Springer Nature; 2022. pp. 595-636.

4. The adjacent image shows the alternate complement pathway and regulation of the complement cascade. Which of the depicted proteins is most commonly deficient or aberrant in patients with aHUS?

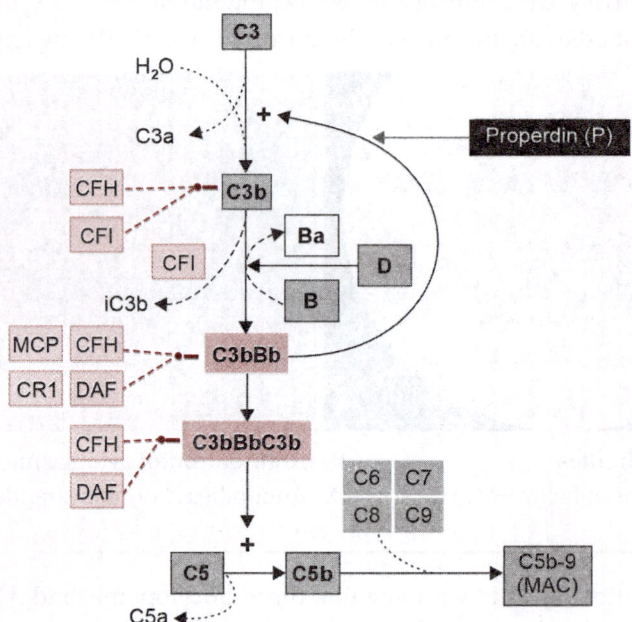

A. Complement factor B (FB)
B. Complement factor D
C. Complement FH
D. Complement factor I (FI)

EXPLANATION

Atypical HUS is caused predominantly by defects in alternate complement pathway. FH is the master regulator of the alternate complement pathway and keeps this "always active" pathway in check. Autoantibodies to FH are the most common cause of aHUS, particularly in school-going age group of children. Other causes include genetic variants in *FH* (20–30%), *CD46* (10–15%) and other complement genes. Genetic variants in *FH* may produce FH deficiency or may produce a dysfunctional protein.

Key: C

BOOST YOUR KNOWLEDGE

The complement system regulates several proteins. FH is the most important regulator of the alternative pathway and acts both in solution and on the cell surface. FH accelerates the decay of the C3 convertase (C3bBb), and functions as a cofactor for FI in cleaving C3b and C4b components. Properdin (P) is the only positive regulator of the alternative pathway: It stabilizes the C3 convertase (C3bBb) and promotes its association with further C3b molecules. The C1-inhibitor (C1-inh) is a negative regulator of all three pathways. It competes with FB to limit activation of the alternative pathway, inhibits C1r and C1s to prevent classical pathway activation, and inactivates MASP-1 and MASP-2 to prevent lectin pathway activation. Other proteins regulate complement activity further downstream. CD46 [membrane cofactor protein (MCP)], CD55 [decay-accelerating factor (DAF)], and CD59 (protectin) are expressed widely on host cell membranes and protect the cell from complement deposition. C8 binding protein (C8bp), clustering, and vitronectin (or S protein) are soluble proteins which prevent the complete assembly of the MAC.

REFERENCES/SOURCES

- Abbas AK, Lichtman AH, Pillai S. Cellular and Molecular Immunology, 10th edition. Philadelphia: Saunders/Elsevier; 2021. pp. 287-311.
- Bagga A, Khandelwal P, Mishra K, Thergaonkar R, Vasudevan A, Sharma J, et al; Indian Society of Pediatric Nephrology. Hemolytic uremic syndrome in a developing country: Consensus guidelines. Pediatr Nephrol. 2019;34:1465-82.
- Kindt TJ, Goldsby RA, Osborne BA, Kuby J. Kuby Immunology, 6th edition. New York: WH Freeman; 2007. pp. 168-88.
- Michael M, Bagga A, Sartain SE, Smith RJH. Hemolytic uremic syndrome. Lancet. 2022;400:1722-40.
- Shrivastava RN, Bagga A. Pediatric Nephrology, 6th edition. New Delhi: Jaypee Brothers Medical Publishers; 2016. pp. 259-66.

5. Eculizumab is the standard of care for patients with aHUS secondary to pathogenic variations in complement regulatory genes. Which of the following symbols in the adjacent image indicates the site of action of this monoclonal antibody?

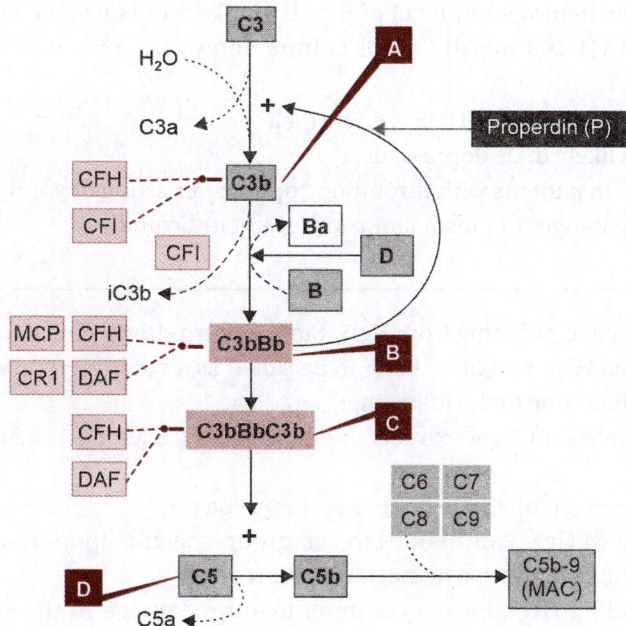

A. A
B. B
C. C
D. D

EXPLANATION

Given the current understanding about the pathophysiology of aHUS, complement blockade has become the gold standard for the treatment of aHUS. Eculizumab, a monoclonal humanized anti-C5 antibody, prevents C5 cleavage, and formation of both C5a and C5b-9. Thus, eculizumab therapy can reduce anaphylatoxin-induced inflammation and limit C5b-9 prothrombotic consequences of complement activation.

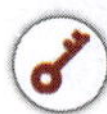

Key: D

BOOST YOUR KNOWLEDGE

Ravulizumab, a long-acting analogue of eculizumab, has been tested both in paroxysmal nocturnal hematuria and in aHUS and has been proven to effectively manage the disease while requiring less frequent infusions both in adults with aHUS and in children previously treated with eculizumab. Anti-C5 treatment (eculizumab and ravulizumab) or other complement-inhibiting agents that are under investigation are not disease modifying strategies, as they do not remove the underlying complement dysregulation in patients with aHUS. In most forms of aHUS due to alternative pathway of complement dysregulation, stopping this treatment involves a variable degree of risk of disease recurrence.

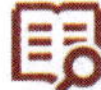

REFERENCES/SOURCES

- Bagga A, Khandelwal P, Mishra K, Thergaonkar R, Vasudevan A, Sharma J, et al; Indian Society of Pediatric Nephrology. Hemolytic uremic syndrome in a developing country: Consensus guidelines. Pediatr Nephrol. 2019;34:1465-82.
- Michael M, Bagga A, Sartain SE, Smith RJH. Hemolytic uremic syndrome. Lancet. 2022;400:1722-40.
- Shrivastava RN, Bagga A. Pediatric Nephrology, 6th edition. New Delhi: Jaypee Brothers Medical Publishers; 2016. pp. 259-66.

6. A 2-year-old boy presents with fever and bloody diarrhea for 3 days, followed 5 days later by oliguanuria and edema. Investigations show hemoglobin level of 6 g/dL, leukocyte count 34,000/mm^3, platelets 80,000/mm^3, creatinine 2.1 mg/dL and C3 100 mg/dL. Stool culture shows the presence of *Shigella* spp. Which of the following statements is true?

A. A diagnosis of Shiga toxin-associated HUS is confirmed
B. Complement C3 level is likely to be depressed
C. Eculizumab is indicated in patients with thrombocytopenia persisting beyond 10-days
D. Therapy with plasma exchanges or plasma infusions is not indicated

EXPLANATION

The clinical scenario is of a child suffering from HUS. Stool culture shows growth of *Shigella spp.* This makes the diagnosis of STEC-associated HUS probable. For it to be called as a confirmed case, apart from the positive stool culture, there should be at least one of the following:

- Detection of virulence genes on fecal extracts or cultures [*stx1, stx2*, and *eae* by polymerase chain reaction (PCR)]
- Free fecal Shiga toxin (detected on tissue culture or immunoassay)
- Serum immunoglobulin M (IgM) antibodies to serogroup specific lipopolysaccharide [by enzyme-linked immunosorbent assay (ELISA), passive hemagglutination assay]

All types of TMA, including HUS, have a common feature: damage to the endothelial cells that line the small blood vessels. In the form of HUS that is linked to diarrhea, some bacteria can make either Shiga toxin or a very similar toxin called Shiga-like verotoxin. These toxins can pass from the lining of the large intestine into the blood, where they attach to endothelial cells in the kidney and other organs, and harm them directly. Shiga toxin can also activate platelets to make them more aggregatory. RBCs get damaged as they squeeze through the thrombotic microvasculature, leading to a severe anemia that is not caused by immune reactions and has a negative direct Coombs test. Because there is no activation of complement in these cases and no production of antibodies, complement levels are usually normal and complement inhibitors do not play a role in management. Plasma exchanges and infusions are required for complement-mediated TMA and are not indicated in STEC-associated HUS.

 **Key: D**

BOOST YOUR KNOWLEDGE

The STEC encode two main variants of Shiga toxins (*Stx*), namely *Stx1* and *Stx2*, in the *Stx1* and *Stx2* genes. *Stx* consists of a single active A subunit (30 kDa) and five binding B subunits (each 7 kDa). Most STEC O157 strains carry *Stx2*, which is more pathogenic than *Stx1* and has a higher likelihood of causing HUS. *Stx* binds to enterocytes after bacterial colonization of the colon and translocates across the brush border into the bloodstream. The B subunit pentamer of the toxin attaches to Gb3 and TLR4 on the surface of blood cells, activating neutrophils, monocytes, platelets, and erythrocytes, and triggering the formation of microvesicles that carry the toxin internally and externally. Microvesicles have activated complement components C3b and C9 and tissue factor on their surface. The main pathogenic process in STEC-HUS is the delivery of *Stx* or *Stx*-bearing microvesicles to endothelial cells expressing Gb3, followed by docking and release of toxin by microvesicles. The A1 subunit of the toxin depurinates adenosine in a highly preserved region of the 28s ribosomal subunit of 60s ribosomal ribonucleic acid (RNA), disrupting its binding to transfer RNA (tRNA), inhibiting protein synthesis, and causing cell death. Other cytotoxic mechanisms involve enhanced production of chemokines (through the SDF-1–CXCR4–CXCR7 pathway) and adhesion molecules. *Stx* mobilizes P-selectin on the cell surface, which promotes C3 activation and the formation of alternative pathway C3 convertase (C3bBb) on the cell surface. The anaphylatoxin C3a binds to its endothelial receptor (C3aR), enhancing P-selectin expression and thrombomodulin cleavage with thrombus formation. Shiga toxin also attaches to ultra-large von Willebrand factor multimers and inhibits their breakdown by ADAMTS13, leading to more thrombosis. High free hemoglobin levels during hemolysis worsen endothelial damage by causing oxidative stress and a prothrombotic state. There is increasing evidence of alternative complement pathway activation in STEC-HUS, with some patients showing complement degradation products, soluble C5b-9 (sC5b-9), and complement-decorated microvesicles. In vitro, *Stx* interacts with short consensus repeats 6–8 and 18–20 of FH, reducing its complement regulatory function. Children with STEC-HUS and low C3 levels have a higher risk of neurological complications and severe clinical outcomes. The mechanisms of neurological manifestations are uncertain and involve the combination of *Stx*-mediated vascular injury and endothelial dysfunction, neural cell inflammation due to cytokine secretion, and direct binding of *Stx* to neural cells.

REFERENCES/SOURCES

- Bagga A, Khandelwal P, Mishra K, Thergaonkar R, Vasudevan A, Sharma J, et al; Indian Society of Pediatric Nephrology. Hemolytic uremic syndrome in a developing country: Consensus guidelines. Pediatr Nephrol. 2019;34:1465-82.
- Michael M, Bagga A, Sartain SE, Smith RJH. Hemolytic uremic syndrome. Lancet. 2022;400:1722-40.
- Shrivastava RN, Bagga A. Pediatric Nephrology, 6th edition. New Delhi: Jaypee Brothers Medical Publishers; 2016. pp. 259-66.

7. According to the Indian guidelines on the management of HUS, plasma exchanges are considered in all of the following scenarios, *except*:

A. Shiga toxin associated HUS with severe neurologic or cardiac involvement
B. aHUS due to *CFH* mutation
C. aHUS with anti-FH antibody
D. Pneumococcal-associated HUS

EXPLANATION

Plasma exchange is the main treatment modality for aHUS. The removal of antibodies and replenishment of normal complement helps in attaining remission in HUS affected with complement dysregulation. Apart from complement-mediated thrombotic microangiopathy (TMA), anecdotal reports suggest some benefit in STEC-HUS with severe systemic involvement. There is evidence of complement activation in STEC-HUS which may explain the reported benefit. Pneumococcal-associated HUS is reported to be exacerbated due to plasma exchanges and exchanges have conventionally been considered contraindicated.

Key: D

BOOST YOUR KNOWLEDGE

Pneumococcal neuraminidase removes terminal *N*-acetylneuraminic acid (sialic acid) from glycoproteins on erythrocytes, glomerular endothelial cells, renal epithelial cells, and platelets, revealing the normally concealed Thomsen–Friedenreich (T) antigen. Existing IgM antibodies bind to exposed T antigen on these cells, triggering a series of events that lead to *Streptococcus pneumoniae*-associated HUS (Sp-HUS). A high bacterial burden causes increased production of neuraminidase (which hydrolyzes glycosidic bonds of neuraminic acid), increasing the likelihood of Sp-HUS. It has been proposed that complement is involved in the pathogenesis of Sp-HUS, but the exact mechanisms are unknown. Two recent studies detected genetic defects of complement proteins that might cause Sp-HUS, while another study suggested that the loss of cell surface-binding sites for FH happens due to desialylation. Some pneumococcal serotypes (serotypes 2 and 3) directly interact with FH and impair its function, resulting in acquired complement dysregulation. Sp-HUS is managed supportively as previously mentioned. Pneumococcal infection should be treated with extended-spectrum cephalosporin and vancomycin in critically ill children with probable invasive pneumococcal disease. Due to the possibility of anti-T antigen antibodies in blood products, dextran washing of peripheral RBCs before transfusion is advised, and plasma-containing blood products such as fresh frozen plasma are usually avoided. Successful use of plasmapheresis specifically with albumin to remove the anti-T antigen antibodies has been reported; however, there is little systematic evidence that it improves outcomes. Due to evidence of complement activation, there are few reports of eculizumab use to treat severe cases of Sp-HUS, with improvement in platelet counts and subjective improvement in neuroirritability. More evidence from controlled trials is necessary before eculizumab can become standard therapy. Improved awareness of Sp-HUS could help to modify therapy appropriately and improve outcomes. Long-term follow-up of renal function is indicated to detect late-onset end-stage renal disease. A sustained pneumococcal vaccination program and vigilance for replacement serotypes is the key to sustain reduction in Sp-HUS cases worldwide.

REFERENCES/SOURCES

- Bagga A, Khandelwal P, Mishra K, Thergaonkar R, Vasudevan A, Sharma J, et al; Indian Society of Pediatric Nephrology. Hemolytic uremic syndrome in a developing country: Consensus guidelines. Pediatr Nephrol. 2019;34:1465-82.
- Michael M, Bagga A, Sartain SE, Smith RJH. Hemolytic uremic syndrome. Lancet. 2022;400:1722-40.
- Srivastava RN, Bagga A. Pediatric Nephrology, 6th edition. New Delhi: Jaypee Brothers Medical Publishers; 2016. pp. 259-66.

8. Which of the following genetic variations is almost always present in patients with anti-FH antibody associated HUS?

A. Heterozygous pathogenic missense variants in *CFH*
B. Homozygous pathogenic missense variants in *CFHR1*
C. Homozygous deletion of exons 19 or 20 of *CFH*
D. Homozygous deletion of *CFHR1*

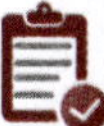

EXPLANATION

The gene of complement FH is closely associated with genes of complement FH-related protein 1 through 5. Anti-FH-associated aHUS is associated with an 84 kb homozygous deletion of the *CFHR1* gene, present in ~10% healthy individuals across the world.

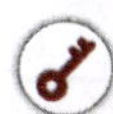

Key: D

BOOST YOUR KNOWLEDGE

Homozygous deletion in CHFR1 is present in 80–90% of patients in anti-FH-mediated HUS. Multiplex ligation-dependent probe amplification (MLPA) or end-point PCR is useful in confirming the deletion, but not required in clinical practice. Detection of deletion helps confirm antibody mediated disease, in patients with: (1) low antibody titers, especially if received plasma exchange before screening; (2) onset of illness <3 years of age; and (3) atypical presentation.

REFERENCES/SOURCES

- Bagga A, Khandelwal P, Mishra K, Thergaonkar R, Vasudevan A, Sharma J, et al; Indian Society of Pediatric Nephrology. Hemolytic uremic syndrome in a developing country: Consensus guidelines. Pediatr Nephrol. 2019;34:1465-82.
- Michael M, Bagga A, Sartain SE, Smith RJH. Hemolytic uremic syndrome. Lancet. 2022;400:1722-40.
- Shrivastava RN, Bagga A. Pediatric Nephrology, 6th edition. New Delhi: Jaypee Brothers Medical Publishers; 2016. pp. 259-66.

9. Pathogenic variations in complement regulatory genes cause aHUS which often recurs after transplantation. Which of the following genes is an *exception*, in causing aHUS that is unlikely to recur after transplantation?

A. *CFH*
B. *MCP*
C. *CFB*
D. *C3*

EXPLANATION

Genetic variants in the complement genes lead to deficient or aberrant complement proteins. Even after kidney transplantation, the production from liver may be deficient or aberrant. This explains the risk of recurrence in the transplanted kidney. The highest risk of recurrence is with genetic variants of *CFH* (80–90%) and *CFB* (up to 100%). The lowest risk of recurrence is seen with *CD46* or *MCP* genetic variant (15–20%).

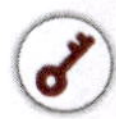

Key: B

BOOST YOUR KNOWLEDGE

Patients with aHUS have variable risk of allograft recurrence. Donors and recipients need thorough assessment and peritransplant care. Recipients should be screened for mutations in relevant genes and for anti-FH antibodies. Patients with alternate pathway dysregulation have a high risk of recurrence, while those with STEC-HUS and defects in membrane bound (CD46) and intracellular (DGKE) proteins have a low risk. Families should be advised about the recurrence risk, based on the presence and type of mutations and the level of anti-FH antibodies.

Live-related donation should be avoided in patients with high recurrence risk. Such patients need either combined liver kidney transplantation or eculizumab treatment (peri- and posttransplant), at a suitable center. Patients with high levels of anti-FH antibodies and no other defects are managed by PEX before and after transplantation, and use of rituximab.

Patients should be followed up for recurrence after transplantation. If HUS recurrence is verified, all efforts should be made to obtain and initiate therapy with eculizumab.

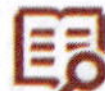

REFERENCE/SOURCES

- Bagga A, Khandelwal P, Mishra K, Thergaonkar R, Vasudevan A, Sharma J, et al; Indian Society of Pediatric Nephrology. Hemolytic uremic syndrome in a developing country: Consensus guidelines. Pediatr Nephrol. 2019;34:1465-82.
- Michael M, Bagga A, Sartain SE, Smith RJH. Hemolytic uremic syndrome. Lancet. 2022;400:1722-40.
- Shrivastava RN, Bagga A. Pediatric Nephrology, 6th edition. New Delhi: Jaypee Brothers Medical Publishers; 2016. pp. 259-66.

10. Which of the following statements is true regarding aHUS associated with DGKE variants?

A. Nephrotic range proteinuria is usually present
B. Complement C3 is decreased in the majority of cases
C. Patients typically present beyond 3–5 years of age
D. Hematological remission is rapidly achieved upon initiating plasma exchanges

EXPLANATION

DGKE variants are associated with aHUS in children usually <2 years of age. There is evidence of glomerular involvement without evidence of TMA on histopathology. The exact pathological basis for TMA remains unknown. Nephrotic range proteinuria is due to the active glomerular involvement.

Key: A

BOOST YOUR KNOWLEDGE

First reported in 2013, DGKE-associated aHUS is one of the most common forms of aHUS diagnosed in children <2 years old. Patients with this condition experience TMA recurrences until 5 years of age (usually triggered by infection), have increasingly worse hypertension and proteinuria with age, and develop ESKD between the ages of 10 and 25 years. The clinical features do not improve with eculizumab, and there are no documented cases of posttransplant aHUS recurrence. There are now >60 patients diagnosed with this ultra-rare condition: Patients with DGKE nephropathy account for ~4–5% of all aHUS patients. Patients with recessive pathogenic genotypes show almost complete deficiency of DGKE activity. While most patients have clear loss-of function *DGKE* variants (nonsense, frameshift, and splice site), about ~30% have missense *DGKE* variants. About 5–10% of patients with clearly pathogenic *DGKE* genotypes present with an active glomerulopathy, but without findings of TMA, a phenomenon that remains unexplained. While the exact pathophysiology remains elusive, it appears that DGKE deficiency causes endothelial cell activation, perhaps by interfering with prostaglandin E2 production or signaling by vascular endothelial factor receptor-2.

REFERENCES/SOURCES

- Bagga A, Khandelwal P, Mishra K, Thergaonkar R, Vasudevan A, Sharma J, et al; Indian Society of Pediatric Nephrology. Hemolytic uremic syndrome in a developing country: Consensus guidelines. Pediatr Nephrol. 2019;34:1465-82.
- Emma F, Goldstein SL, Bagga A, Bates CM, Shroff R. Pediatric Nephrology, 8th edition. Switzerland: Springer Nature; 2022. pp. 595-636.
- Michael M, Bagga A, Sartain SE, Smith RJH. Hemolytic uremic syndrome. Lancet. 2022;400:1722-40.
- Shrivastava RN, Bagga A. Pediatric Nephrology, 6th edition. New Delhi: Jaypee Brothers Medical Publishers; 2016. pp. 259-66.

11. Which of the following are true of anti-FH antibody associated HUS?

A. The condition most commonly affects children in the preschool or toddler age group
B. The condition is rarely reported outside South Asia
C. Therapy with plasma exchanges and immunosuppression induces remission satisfactorily in the majority of patients
D. Relapses usually occur beyond 5 years of disease onset

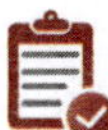

EXPLANATION

Anti-FH antibody associated aHUS is the most common etiology of aHUS in school-going children world-wide. Aim of therapy for patients with anti-FH-associated HUS is reduction of antibody titers. The American Society for Apheresis assigns level I category to anti-FH-associated HUS, implying that PEX is a primary therapeutic intervention. Since antibodies are chiefly IgG, 5–7 PEX achieve 80% reduction in antibody titers. Prompt initiation and continued PEX for at least 3–5 weeks, is advised. Blockade of the complement pathway by eculizumab is effective in inducing hematological remission but has limited impact on antibody titers.

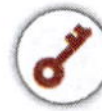

Key: C

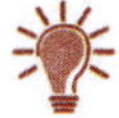

BOOST YOUR KNOWLEDGE

The Indian Society of Pediatric Nephrology (ISPN) advises the use of PEX with immunosuppression for management of these patients. Eculizumab therapy should be considered in patients who are resistant to PEX, have life-threatening features, or have concomitant defect (s) in complement regulation. Many centers in the developed world start empiric therapy with eculizumab, awaiting anti-FH antibody results. When high levels of anti-FH antibodies are found, there is debate whether eculizumab therapy should be maintained, or switched by PEX and immunosuppression. Eculizumab treatment does not influence antibody production and immunosuppression might be needed. Eculizumab has been used in 18 patients with anti-FH-associated disease, either after failing PEX or as first-line therapy. Since relapses were rare, the effectiveness of concurrent immunosuppression in lowering antibody levels and the relapse risk could not be established. Prospective studies are needed to determine the comparative effectiveness of eculizumab to PEX and immunosuppression in these patients.

REFERENCES/SOURCES

- Bagga A, Khandelwal P, Mishra K, Thergaonkar R, Vasudevan A, Sharma J, et al; Indian Society of Pediatric Nephrology. Hemolytic uremic syndrome in a developing country: Consensus guidelines. Pediatr Nephrol. 2019;34:1465-82.
- Emma F, Goldstein SL, Bagga A, Bates CM, Shroff R. Pediatric Nephrology, 8th edition. Switzerland: Springer Nature; 2022. pp. 595-636.
- Michael M, Bagga A, Sartain SE, Smith RJH. Hemolytic uremic syndrome. Lancet. 2022;400:1722-40.
- Schwartz J, Padmanabhan A, Aqui N, Balogun RA, Connelly-Smith L, Delaney M, et al. (2016) Guidelines on the use of therapeutic apheresis in clinical practice-evidence-based approach from the writing committee of the American Society for Apheresis: the seventh special issue. J Clin Apher. 2016;31:149-62.
- Shrivastava RN, Bagga A. Pediatric Nephrology, 6th edition. New Delhi: Jaypee Brothers Medical Publishers; 2016. pp. 259-66.

12. Which of the following is true of eculizumab?

A. It is a recombinant humanized monoclonal antibody against the complement protein C5
B. Therapy in aHUS comprises of a single subcutaneous age-appropriate dose, followed by surveillance for relapses
C. Therapy specifically increases the risk of life-threatening gram-negative infections
D. The medication has become readily available at low cost due to availability of biosimilars

EXPLANATION

Given the current understanding about the pathophysiology of aHUS, complement blockade has become the gold standard for the treatment of aHUS.

Key: A

BOOST YOUR KNOWLEDGE

Eculizumab, a monoclonal humanized anti-C5 antibody, prevents C5 cleavage and formation of both C5a and C5b-9. Thus, eculizumab therapy can reduce anaphylatoxin-induced inflammation and limit C5b-9 prothrombotic consequences of complement activation.

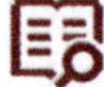

REFERENCES/SOURCES

- Bagga A, Khandelwal P, Mishra K, Thergaonkar R, Vasudevan A, Sharma J, et al; Indian Society of Pediatric Nephrology. Hemolytic uremic syndrome in a developing country: Consensus guidelines. Pediatr Nephrol. 2019;34:1465-82.
- Khursigara MR, Benoit S, Patriquin CJ, Lemaire M, Licht C. Thrombotic thrombocytopenic purpura, atypical hemolytic uremic syndrome, and spectrum of thrombotic microangiopathy. In: Emma F, Goldstein S, Bagga A, Bates CM, Shroff R (Eds). Pediatric Nephrology. Berlin, Heidelberg: Springer; 2022.

13. Which of the following is the longer acting congener of eculizumab?

A. Avacopan
B. Elizaria
C. Zilucoplan
D. Ravulizumab

EXPLANATION

Avacopan or CCX-168 is a small molecule antagonist of the complement component C5aR1, which is shown to induce remission in ANCA-associated vasculitis. It is not yet shown to be effective in aHUS. Elizaria, a cyclic peptide targeting C5, is the first biosimilar for eculizumab, marketed by a Russian pharmaceutical company. Dosing frequency in aHUS is derived from studies of equivalence in paroxysmal nocturnal hemoglobinuria (PNH) and is fairly similar to that for eculizumab. Zilucoplan is another targeted peptide inhibitor of C5 and is approved for the treatment of generalized myasthenia gravis in adult patients who are antiacetylcholine receptor positive. It is administered once daily as a subcutaneous injection. Ravulizumab is a monoclonal antibody that binds to inhibits C5, similar to eculizumab, and is approved for the treatment of PNH and aHUS. It was engineered from eculizumab to have a longer-lasting effect.

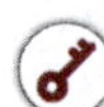

Key: D

BOOST YOUR KNOWLEDGE

The re-engineering of ravulizumab (Ultomiris®) from eculizumab (Soliris®) by Alexion Pharmaceuticals Inc., improved the pharmacokinetic properties considerably, with ravulizumab having a fourfold longer t½ (51.8 days) than eculizumab (11.3 days). This was achieved by incorporating two structural changes to eculizumab aimed at extending its terminal elimination t½.

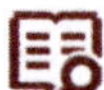

REFERENCES/SOURCES

- Anliker-Ort M, Dingemanse J, van den Anker J, Kaufmann P. Treatment of rare inflammatory kidney diseases: Drugs targeting the terminal complement pathway. Front Immunol. 2020;11:599417.
- Emma F, Goldstein SL, Bagga A, Bates CM, Shroff R. Pediatric Nephrology, 8th edition. Switzerland: Springer Nature; 2022. pp. 595-636.
- Michael M, Bagga A, Sartain SE, Smith RJH. Hemolytic uremic syndrome. Lancet. 2022;400:1722-40.
- Shrivastava RN, Bagga A. Pediatric Nephrology, 6th edition. New Delhi: Jaypee Brothers Medical Publishers; 2016. pp. 259-66.
- Syed YY. Ravulizumab: A review in atypical haemolytic uraemic syndrome. Drugs. 2021;81:587-94.

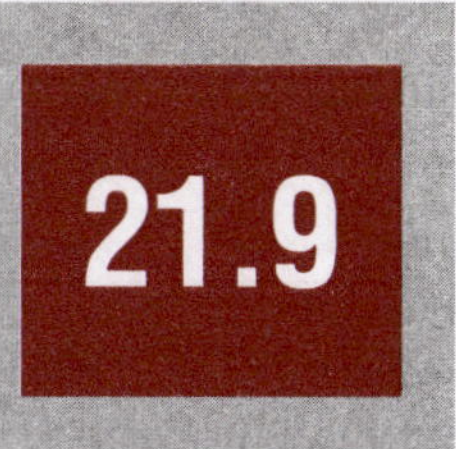

CHAPTER 21.9 Hemolytic Uremic Syndrome

Bobbity Deepthi

1. Which of the following is a long-acting C5 inhibitor used in atypical hemolytic uremic syndrome (aHUS)?

A. Eculizumab
B. Ravulizumab
C. Ruplizumab
D. Avacopan

EXPLANATION

Eculizumab and ravulizumab inhibit the cleavage of C5 into C5a and C5b. Ravulizumab was engineered from eculizumab to have a longer half-life, resulting in an infusion rate of every 8 weeks instead of every 2 weeks with eculizumab. Avacopan is an antagonist of the C5a receptor involved in inflammation pathways. Crovalimab is another long-acting C5 inhibitor that could be administered subcutaneously. Ruplizumab is a humanized monoclonal antibody against CD154 used in rheumatological disorders like systemic lupus erythematosus (SLE) and lupus nephritis.

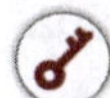

Key: B

BOOST YOUR KNOWLEDGE

- *Eculizumab:* The outcome of aHUS from large cohorts managed with plasma therapy alone is unsatisfactory, with 30–50% of patients progressing to kidney failure at 1–5 years follow-up. Complement blockade with eculizumab has emerged as a specific therapy for aHUS with inherited defects in complement regulation. Hematological remission is expected at a median of 7–8 days. Eculizumab is not indicated for therapy of noncomplement disorders, e.g., DGKE or MMACHC mutations. The discontinuation of treatment results in relapses of varying percentages, depending on the specific genetic mutation causing aHUS.
- Ravulizumab is a newer medication showing promise in aHUS treatment; it achieves complete thrombotic microangiopathy (TMA) response in a significant portion of patients (53.6%) and improves renal function and allows dialysis weaning in some patients (58%). The safety profile appears similar to eculizumab but needs confirmation in larger studies.

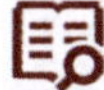

REFERENCES/SOURCES

- Bagga A, Khandelwal P, Mishra K, Thergaonkar R, Vasudevan A, Sharma J, et al. Hemolytic uremic syndrome in a developing country: Consensus guidelines. Pediatr Nephrol. 2019;34(8):1465-82.
- Werion A, Rondeau E. Application of C5 inhibitors in glomerular diseases in 2021. Kidney Res Clin Pract. 2022;41(4):412-21.

2. A 3-year-old boy presented to the emergency room (ER) with complaints of bloody diarrhea for the last 5 days following ingestion of goat's milk. For the last 2 days, parents noticed progressive pallor, decreased urine output, and edema. On examination, the child was noted to have pallor, hypertension, and edema. Biochemical investigations revealed Hb 5.5 g/dL, total leukocyte count 40,000/µL, differential count N76L23, and platelet count 60,000/µL. Peripheral smear showed 5% schistocytes with lactate dehydrogenase (LDH) 3,400 IU/L, urea 87 mg/dL, and serum creatinine 1.6 mg/dL. Which of the following is the most appropriate next step in the management of this child?

A. Immediate hemodialysis
B. Initiate plasma exchange (PEX)
C. Optimize volume status
D. Start eculizumab

EXPLANATION

It is a case of Shiga toxin-producing *Escherichia coli*-associated hemolytic uremic syndrome (STEC-HUS). Most children with STEC-HUS recover with appropriate supportive care and management of acute kidney injury (AKI). Supportive management of volume deficit or excess, anemia, hypertension, and electrolyte abnormalities is the mainstay of treatment of established HUS. Antibiotic therapy is not indicated for STEC-HUS and has been associated with worse outcomes in some studies. Often, in diarrhea-associated HUS, by the time, the child presents with signs of HUS, the diarrheal illness is resolving, and stool cultures may actually be negative. Judicious volume expansion early during HUS has been demonstrated to attenuate the degree of kidney impairment.

Key: C

BOOST YOUR KNOWLEDGE

Shiga toxin-producing *Escherichia coli*-associated hemolytic uremic syndrome is dominant in the age group younger than 5 years of age. *E. coli* serotype O157:H7 is the most common pathogen associated with STEC-HUS (90%). Cattle are the largest reservoir for STEC, in which it may cause bloody diarrhea but usually by a commensal organism. Transmission of STEC commonly occurs through ingestion of contaminated food products (beef, fruit, and produce washed in contaminated water), visits to dairy farms and petting zoos, and exposure to airborne organisms. Signs of gastrointestinal (GI) illness, characterized by abdominal pain, vomiting, and bloody diarrhea, precede the onset of STEC-HUS. A diarrheal prodrome is noted in 85–95% of patients with STEC-induced HUS and usually lasts 3–4 days. HUS evolves in 5–7 days after onset of diarrheal prodrome. Anorexia, weakness, pallor, and jaundice are the presenting manifestations in many children with HUS. Oliguria or hematuria may be the initial recognition of HUS by many parents. Neurologic manifestations can occur in 30% of patients with STEC-HUS.

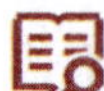

REFERENCE/SOURCE

- Kher K, Schnaper HW, Greenbaum LA (Eds). Clinical Pediatric Nephrology, 3rd edition. CRC Press: Taylor and Francis Group; 2020.

3. A 10-year-old boy presented with complaints of progressive pallor for 6 days and 2 episodes of generalized seizures. On examination, the child was found to have pallor and stage 2 hypertension (BP 170/100 mm Hg). Laboratory investigations showed a hemoglobin of 5.2 g/dL and platelet count 12,400/µL. Peripheral smear shows 5% schistocytes, LDH 2,456 IU/L, blood urea 158 mg/dL, serum creatinine 2.6 mg/dL, sodium 138 mEq/L, potassium 5.9 mEq/L (refractory), and antifactor H (FH) antibodies 2,400. Which of the following is the most appropriate next step?

A. Initiate prompt PEX and hemodialysis
B. Initiate prompt plasma infusions
C. Initiate prompt hemodialysis
D. Initiate prompt blood transfusion

EXPLANATION

The child has a clinical picture of microangiopathic hemolytic anemia, thrombocytopenia, and AKI. It is a case of anti-FH-associated HUS. The ongoing hemolysis with hemoglobin of 5.2 g/dL and refractory hyperkalemia needs initiation of hemodialysis with blood transfusion. The aim of therapy for patients with anti-FH-associated HUS is the reduction of antibody titers. The American Society for Apheresis assigns level I category to anti-FH-associated HUS, implying that PEX is a primary therapeutic intervention. Prompt initiation and continued PEX for at least 3–5 weeks are advised. The blockade of the complement pathway by eculizumab is effective in inducing hematological remission but has a limited impact on antibody titers.

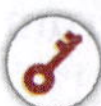

Key: A

BOOST YOUR KNOWLEDGE

Atypical hemolytic uremic syndrome with anti-FH antibodies needs to be initiated on prompt PEX. PEX is performed within 24 hours of diagnosis, daily for 5–7 cycles, and later tapered slowly over the next 3–5 weeks. Induction therapy with oral corticosteroids and intravenous (IV) cyclophosphamide is combined with PEX. Immunosuppression inhibits further production of antibodies, especially following PEX, with improved short- and medium-term outcomes. Antibody titers are monitored closely between days 7 and 28 and then every 3–6 months. Elevated titer (>1,500 AU/mL) during the first 12–24 months is associated with an increased risk of relapse. Relapses follow minor infectious illnesses in the initial 2 years. Therapy with azathioprine or mycophenolate mofetil and tapering doses of prednisolone is useful in significant reduction of this risk. Standard recommendations should be followed for AKI with attention to fluid and electrolytes, avoiding radiocontrast and nephrotoxic agents, and timely institution of dialysis. Blood transfusion is recommended for patients with hemoglobin <6 g/dL or hemodynamic instability.

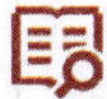

REFERENCE/SOURCE

- Bagga A, Khandelwal P, Mishra K, Thergaonkar R, Vasudevan A, Sharma J, et al. Hemolytic uremic syndrome in a developing country: Consensus guidelines. Pediatr Nephrol. 2019;34(8):1465-82.

4. Which of the following genetic abnormalities is most likely to be present in an 8-year-old child with atypical hemolytic syndrome and FH autoantibodies?

A. *CFHR1* deletion
B. CFI heterozygous mutation
C. MMACHC deletion
D. *DGKE* mutation

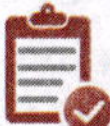

EXPLANATION

Anti-FH antibody-associated illness constitutes ~50% of pediatric patients with aHUS in India, chiefly affecting children between the ages of 5 and 15 years. Anti-FH-associated aHUS is associated with an 84 kb homozygous deletion of the *CFHR1* gene in almost 85% patients.

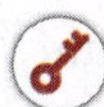

Key: A

BOOST YOUR KNOWLEDGE

Next-generation sequencing (NGS) allows rapid and simultaneous sequencing of large gene panels. Screening for the following genes using an NGS panel: *CFH, CFI, CFB, C3, CD46, THBD, CFHR1–5,* and *DGKE,* and multiplex ligation-dependent probe amplification (MLPA) for rearrangements of CFH-CFHR5 by MLPA is recommended in patients with suspected aHUS to guide regarding prognosis, risk of relapses, transplantation, and genetic counseling. Homozygosity for risk haplotypes of CFH and MCP has been shown to increase disease penetrance and severity.

Atypical HUS is characterized by dysregulation of the alternative complement pathway, resulting in endothelial damage and microvascular thrombosis. About 20–40% of patients have a pathogenic variant in genes encoding regulatory proteins of factors of the alternative complement pathway (FH, factor I, CD46, factor B, C3, and thrombomodulin) or rearrangements of genes encoding FH-related protein.

In contrast, patients with anti-FH antibodies show significant genetic abnormalities in a very small proportion of patients (3%), apart from the homozygous deletion of *CFHR1/3*. Therefore, there is a limited role for genetic testing for significant complement variants in patients with anti-FH-associated aHUS. *Genetic screening is advised with*: (1) Early age of onset, (2) relapsing course, (3) family history of HUS, (4) illness that is refractory to therapy with PEX, and (5) prior to renal transplantation. Detection of *CFHR1* deletion in patients with anti-FH antibodies helps confirm the antibody-mediated disease, in patients with: (1) low antibody titers, especially if received PEX before screening; (2) onset of illness <3 years of age; and (3) atypical presentation.

REFERENCE/SOURCE

- Bagga A, Khandelwal P, Mishra K, Thergaonkar R, Vasudevan A, Sharma J, et al. Hemolytic uremic syndrome in a developing country: Consensus guidelines. Pediatr Nephrol. 2019;34(8):1465-82.

5. Which of the following types of HUS exhibits a positive peanut agglutination test?

A. Shiga-toxin-associated HUS
B. Pneumococcal HUS
C. Anti-FH antibody-associated HUS
D. Complement factor I-associated HUS

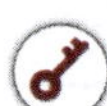

EXPLANATION

Fluorescein-labeled peanut agglutinin *(Arachis hypogaea)* has a high affinity for the normally unexposed Thomsen–Friedenreich (TF) antigen. *Pneumococcus* secretes neuraminidase, which cleaves n-acetyl neuraminic acid in the cell surface exposing the cryptic T-cell (TF antigen). TF antigen is present on RBCs, platelets, and glomerular endothelial cells. Naturally occurring immunoglobulin M (IgM) antibodies against T-antigen react with the exposed T-antigen to initiate cellular damage and hemolysis, and hence resulting in pneumococcal HUS.

Key: B

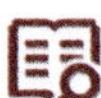

BOOST YOUR KNOWLEDGE

An atypical form of HUS caused by invasive *Streptococcus pneumoniae* is called pneumococcal HUS and constitutes 5% of all HUS. Many of these patients suffer from significant *S. pneumoniae* systemic disease and may have concurrent disseminated intravascular coagulopathy (DIC). HUS develops 3–13 (mostly 7–9) days after the onset of pneumococcal-related symptoms. Serotype 14 earlier and 19A now are most implicated. Compared to STEC-HUS, P-HUS has longer oligoanuria and a more frequent need for acute dialysis, longer hospital stays, longer duration of thrombocytopenia, and more red blood cell and platelet transfusions. Acute mortality is highest in patients with *S. pneumoniae* meningitis complicated by HUS. Management includes supportive care with appropriate antimicrobial therapy, fluid resuscitation, blood products, and kidney replacement therapy, if indicated. PEX is not routinely recommended.

REFERENCES/SOURCES

- Loupiac A, Elayan A, Cailliez M, Adra AL, Decramer S, Thouret MC, et al. Diagnosis of *Streptococcus pneumoniae*-associated hemolytic uremic syndrome. Pediatr Infect Dis J. 2013;32:1045-9.
- Spinale JM, Ruebner RL, Kaplan BS, Copelovitch L. Update on *Streptococcus pneumoniae*-associated hemolytic uremic syndrome. Curr Opin Pediatr. 2013;25:203-20.
- Thrombotic microangiopathies. In: Kher K, Schnaper HW, Greenbaum LA (Eds). Clinical Pediatric Nephrology, 3rd edition. CRC Press: Taylor and Francis Group; 2020.

6. What is the percentage of reduction in antibodies expected after performing five PEXs for anti-FH antibody positive?

A. 20%
B. 40%
C. 60%
D. 80%

EXPLANATION

Plasma exchange is a recommended treatment for anti-FH antibody HUS. Three exchanges reduce up to 74% after three exchanges, five up to 80–84%, and seven exchanges up to 88%.

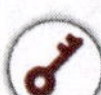

Key: D

 BOOST YOUR KNOWLEDGE

In the absence of eculizumab in developing countries, prompt PEX is recommended to be done daily till hematological remission (defined as platelets 100,000/μL, schistocytes <2%, LDH less than upper limit of normal on 2 consecutive days) and tapered over 4–6 weeks. PEX is done daily with 1.5 times plasma volume (60–75 mL/kg) per session for 5 days or until hematological remission, whichever is later, followed by alternate days at 40 mL/kg for 2 weeks; twice a week for 2–3 weeks. PEX is preferred to plasma infusions for initial therapy since large volumes of plasma can be infused even in patients with oliguria. PEX also enables the removal of dysfunctional proteins and antibodies, which might be present in a proportion of children with aHUS.

 REFERENCE/SOURCE

- Bagga A, Khandelwal P, Mishra K, Thergaonkar R, Vasudevan A, Sharma J, et al. Hemolytic uremic syndrome in a developing country: Consensus guidelines. Pediatr Nephrol. 2019;34(8):1465-82.

7. Which of the following factors is associated with favorable outcomes in aHUS kidney transplant patients?

A. FH (CFH) mutations
B. Factor I (CFI) mutations
C. C3 mutations
D. Membrane co-factor (MCP) mutations

 EXPLANATION

The mutations of FH and factor I have been associated with a high incidence of graft failure (>80%), often due to early graft thrombosis or HUS recurrence within 2 years of transplantation. Graft outcomes are more favorable in all patients who carry MCP mutations.

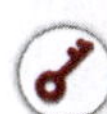 **Key: D**

 BOOST YOUR KNOWLEDGE

Patients with aHUS show a variable risk of recurrent disease in the allograft. Donors and recipients need careful evaluation and peritransplant management. The screening of recipients for mutations in relevant genes and for anti-FH antibodies is recommended. While the risk of recurrence is high in patients with dysregulation of the alternate pathway, those with STEC-HUS and abnormalities in membrane-anchored (CD46) and intracellular (DGKE) proteins have low risk. Families should be counseled about the risk of recurrence, based on the presence and type of mutations and titer of anti-FH antibodies. Live-related donation should be avoided in patients at high risk of disease recurrence. Such patients require either combined liver kidney transplantation or therapy with eculizumab (peri- and post-transplant), at an appropriate center. Patients with high titer of anti-FH antibodies and no additional defects are managed by PEX prior to and following transplantation and the use of rituximab.

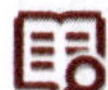 REFERENCE/SOURCE

- Bagga A, Khandelwal P, Mishra K, Thergaonkar R, Vasudevan A, Sharma J, et al. Hemolytic uremic syndrome in a developing country: Consensus guidelines. Pediatr Nephrol. 2019;34(8):1465-82.

8. Which of the following variants of complement regulatory proteins causing aHUS is most likely to present before 2 years of age?

A. *CD46* mutations
B. Factor I mutations
C. Complement FH antibodies
D. Diacylglycerol kinase ε *(DGKE)*

EXPLANATION

Mutations in DGKE encoding an intracellular protein with no direct role in the complement cascade are described in 4–5% of patients with HUS, characteristically presenting below 2 years of age. Patients with *CD46* mutations usually present beyond 1 year of age and older children. Heterozygous *CFH* and *CFI* variants can present at any age, while homozygous variants have an earlier age of onset.

Key: A

BOOST YOUR KNOWLEDGE

Diacylglycerol kinase ε nephropathy is extremely rare with an estimated annual incidence of 0.009 per million in the United Kingdom. Its prevalence as a cause of pediatric TMA ranges from 2 to 27% in various cohorts. A review of the largest cohort of 44 patients with DGKE nephropathy showed that patients, chiefly below 2 years of age, presented with clinical and histological features of TMA, and developed a progressive proteinuric nephropathy with 20% requiring dialysis or transplant within 10 years of diagnosis. A subgroup may show nephrotic syndrome and membranoproliferative pattern of glomerulonephritis (MPGN) injury. Recognition of the disorder is important to avoid therapy with complement inhibitors or immunosuppressive agents. The precise mechanisms underlying podocyte and endothelial damage in DGKE deficiency are not clear. It is proposed that DGKE deficiency might result in the activation of protein kinase C, resulting in a prothrombotic state and platelet activation, activation of podocyte calcium channels with actin-cytoskeletal rearrangements, and reduced expression of vascular endothelial growth factor receptor with downregulation of the decay-accelerating factor.

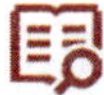

REFERENCE/SOURCE

- Khandelwal P, Thangaraju S, Krishnamurthy S, Ohri A, Pais P, Mathew G, et al. Clinical features and outcomes of patients with diacylglycerol kinase epsilon nephropathy: a nationwide experience. Pediatr Nephrol. 2023;38(9):3009-16.

9. A 10-year-old boy presented with complaints of progressive pallor, palpitations, and seizures. His parents also reported easy fatiguability, gingival bleeding, and dark reddish-brown urine. On examination, he was afebrile, had tachycardia (120 beats/min), and had a BP of 110/70 mm Hg. Laboratory investigations showed a hemoglobin of 4.1 g/dL, platelet count 10,000/μL, and high reticulocyte count 18.2%. Peripheral smear shows 8% schistocytes, LDH 1,886 IU/L, blood urea 28 mg/dL, serum creatinine 0.9 mg/dL, sodium 138 mEq/L, potassium 3.9 mEq/L, and anti-FH antibody 120 AU/L. Which of the following investigations would you consider next for making a diagnosis?

A. ADAMTS13 activity
B. Homocysteine levels
C. CD46 flow cytometry
D. Next-generation sequencing

EXPLANATION

In the presence of microangiopathic hemolytic anemia with severe thrombocytopenia, neurological features, and mildly deranged kidney functions, thrombotic thrombocytopenic purpura (TTP) is the most likely diagnosis. ADAMTS13 activity will help establish diagnosis. However, as anti-FH antibodies are the most common cause of atypical HUS, one should always rule out the possibility which was done in the above-described scenario. Anti-FH antibody levels <150 AU/L are normal.

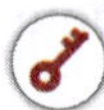

Key: A

BOOST YOUR KNOWLEDGE

Thrombotic thrombocytopenic purpura is an uncommon but life-threatening form of TMA that rarely occurs in children. The clinical manifestations and some of the laboratory features of TTP can, at times, be indistinguishable from those of HUS. The differentiation may be complicated further by the fact that neurologic and other organ dysfunction also can be encountered in children with HUS. The classic pentad of TTP has features of systemic illness, microangiopathic hemolytic anemia, thrombocytopenia, AKI, and neurologic involvement. Classic (antibody-mediated) TTP is seen in older adolescents and adults and affects females more than males. At presentation, the clinical pentad noted here is not observed universally and may be seen in only 40–50% of cases. The triad of microangiopathic hemolytic anemia, thrombocytopenia, and neurologic manifestations, on the other hand, is the most common manifestation and is seen in 80–90% of patients. AKI requiring kidney replacement therapy evolves quickly in 40–75% of cases. Thrombocytopenia-related petechial manifestations can be seen.

REFERENCE/SOURCE

- Kher K, Schnaper HW, Greenbaum LA (Eds). Clinical Pediatric Nephrology, 3rd edition. CRC Press: Taylor and Francis Group; 2020.

10. A 4-year-old male presented with vomiting, lethargy, hypotonia, and seizures. On examination, the child was found to have pallor, stage 2 hypertension, and periorbital edema. Laboratory investigations revealed hemoglobin 4.6 g/dL, total leukocyte count 2,400 WBC/μL, and platelet count 70,000/μL. Peripheral smear reveals megaloblastic anemia. Serum homocysteine levels were 200 μM/L, with normal serum B_{12} and folate levels. Which among the following is the mainstay of treatment for the above case?

A. Parenteral hydroxocobalamin
B. Oral hydroxocobalamin
C. Oral cyanocobalamin
D. Oral betaine

EXPLANATION

The above described is cobalamin deficiency-associated HUS. The mainstay of treatment is administration of parenteral hydroxocobalamin at a dose of 1 mg/kg/day. The treatment goals are reducing homocysteine levels to below 40–60 μM/L. Oral hydroxocobalamin and cyanocobalamin are ineffective. Based on the biochemical reasoning, adjunctive therapies like betaine and folate may be used, though they are not stand-alone mainstay therapies. Folate reduces homocysteine levels, while betaine has a synergistic action with hydroxocobalamin and helps in methylating homocysteine to methionine.

Key: A

BOOST YOUR KNOWLEDGE

Cobalamin deficiency is a rare disorder and constitutes a minor proportion of HUS. It has two recognized forms including classical early onset type with infantile presentation and late-onset milder mutations. HUS is, however, associated more commonly in 50% cases in the late-onset variety. Elevated homocysteine levels with normal levels of B_{12} and folate are a hallmark for the diagnosis of this variety of HUS. Samples of total homocysteine should be collected before PEX is initiated. The diagnosis of this entity is confirmed by homozygous or compound heterozygous mutations in the *MMACHC* gene. Amino acid and organic acid chromatography reveals elevated levels of plasma and urine methylmalonic acid. While TMA is most commonly seen, tubulointerstitial nephritis and proximal renal tubular acidosis are also reported in cobalamin deficiency.

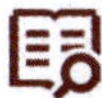

REFERENCE/SOURCE

- Iyengar AA, Uthup S, Sudha E (Eds). Nammalwar's Principles and Practice of Pediatric Nephrology, 3rd edition. New Delhi: Jaypee Brothers Medical Publishers; 2023.

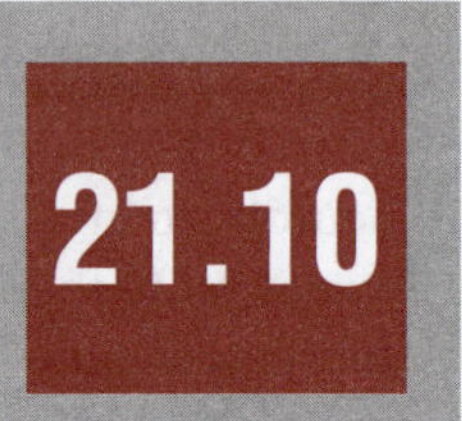

CHAPTER 21.10 Chronic Kidney Disease and End-Stage Kidney Disease

OP Mishra

1. A 13-year-old boy with steroid-dependent nephrotic syndrome (NS) was initially treated with alternate days prednisolone therapy followed by levamisole. Following failure of levamisole due to multiple relapses and steroid-dependent course, he was administered mycophenolate mofetil, which also failed to maintain remission. The patient was categorized as "difficult-to-treat disease." What would be the next line of management of this patient?

A. Oral cyclophosphamide for 8 weeks
B. Kidney biopsy, followed by tacrolimus for 12–24 months
C. Kidney biopsy, followed by rituximab infusions, 2 doses at 1 week interval
D. Ramipril 6 mg/m^2 daily and low dose alternate days prednisolone

EXPLANATION

The child satisfies the definition of "Difficult to treat nephrotic syndrome" as per the revised Indian Society of Pediatric Nephrology (ISPN) guidelines, 2021. Here, the child has received two steroid-sparing drugs besides prednisolone. However, the patient continued to have relapses of disease.

Key: B

BOOST YOUR KNOWLEDGE

As per the revised ISPN Guidelines, 2021, this new category of relapsing NS has been classified *(Patients who relapse despite therapy with two or more steroid-sparing agents).* These patients are considered for use of calcineurin inhibitors (cyclosporine 4–6 mg/kg/day or tacrolimus 0.1–0.2 mg/kg/day) for 2–3 years along with initial prednisolone in gradual tapering doses over 6 months. Before starting this regimen, kidney biopsy is required to know the initial histopathological lesion. Plasma levels of cyclosporine or tacrolimus are also needed to avoid drug-induced nephrotoxicity. Cyclophosphamide is best avoided in peripubertal boys due to risk of gonadal toxicity.

REFERENCE/SOURCE

- Sinha A, Bagga A, Banerjee S, Mishra K, Mehta A, Agarwal I, et al; Expert Group of Indian Society of Pediatric Nephrology. Steroid Sensitive Nephrotic Syndrome: Revised Guidelines. Indian Pediatr. 2021;58(5):461-81.

2. A 4-year-old unvaccinated child with frequent relapsing NS is in remission while receiving oral prednisolone (10 mg every alternate day). What would be the immunization schedule of Pneumococcal vaccine for this patient?

A. Two doses of pneumococcal conjugate vaccine (PCV13), 8 weeks interval
B. Single dose of pneumococcal polysaccharide vaccine (PPSV23)
C. Two doses of PPSV23, 8 weeks interval
D. One dose of PCV13, followed by PPSV23 8 weeks later

EXPLANATION

Infections are the chief complication in patients with steroid-sensitive NS. Most common pathogen responsible for peritonitis, sepsis, and pneumonia in these patients is *Streptococcus pneumoniae*. To prevent infection, pneumococcal vaccine (PCV13/10) is recommended in these patients.

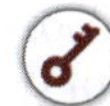

Key: D

BOOST YOUR KNOWLEDGE

As per the revised ISPN guidelines, 2021, in any unimmunized child having NS, PCV13/10, one dose is recommended followed by PPSV23 vaccine given 8 weeks later. These patients are more prone to infection with *Streptococcus pneumoniae* because of the use of immunosuppressive drugs, anasarca, and urinary losses of IgG and complement. Both PCV7/10/13 and PPSV23 elicit satisfactory serological response, even when given during relapse or while on immunosuppressive agents. However, the guideline suggests administration of vaccine during remission, and while on low or no immunosuppression.

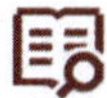

REFERENCES/SOURCES

- Erkan E. Nephrotic syndrome. In: Kliegman RM, St Geme III JW, Blum NJ, Shah SS, Tasker RC, Wilson KM (Eds). Nelson Textbook of Pediatrics, 21st edition. Elsevier; 2019. pp. 2752-60.
- Sinha A, Bagga A, Banerjee S, Mishra K, Mehta A, Agarwal I, et al; Expert Group of Indian Society of Pediatric Nephrology. Steroid Sensitive Nephrotic Syndrome: Revised Guidelines. Indian Pediatr. 2021;58(5):461-81.

3. A 3-month-old boy presented with anasarca for 2 weeks, decreased urine output, and cryptorchidism. Investigations showed early morning urine-protein-to-creatinine ratio 5.5 mg/mg, serum albumin 1.6 g/dL, and cholesterol 210 mg/dL. The recommended plan of management of this patient is:

A. Kidney biopsy followed by calcineurin inhibitor and prednisolone
B. Genetic analysis, IV albumin infusions, furosemide, and angiotensin-converting enzyme (ACE) inhibitor
C. IV albumin infusions and furosemide
D. Bilateral nephrectomy, followed by dialysis

EXPLANATION

This child is having onset of edema and biochemical features of NS. This is congenital NS (onset <3 months) with gonadal abnormalities. Genetic analysis can establish presence of genetic mutations such as *WT1* mutation, commonly associated with gonadal dysgenesis. Kidney biopsy is not recommended in congenital NS. Patients with congenital NS are steroid resistant and are managed with albumin infusions, diuretics, and ACE inhibitors (enalapril/ramipril) as an antiproteinuric drug.

Key: B

BOOST YOUR KNOWLEDGE

As per the revised ISPN guidelines, 2021, for management of steroid-resistant nephrotic syndrome (SRNS), about 70–80% patients with congenital nephrotic syndrome have a genetic cause; mutations in *NPHS1, NPHS2, WT1, LAMB2,* and *PLCE1* account for approximately 90% cases. Exome sequencing using an extended *SRNS* gene panel is recommended. The role of kidney biopsy is limited and may be considered if a genetic diagnosis is not established. Patients with *WT1* variants are monitored by ultrasonography for development of Wilms tumor every 3–6 months till the age of 7 years.

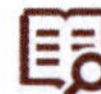

REFERENCE/SOURCE

- Vasudevan A, Thergaonkar R, Mantan M, Sharma J, Khandelwal P, Hari P, et al; Expert Group of The Indian Society of Pediatric Nephrology. Consensus Guidelines on Management of Steroid-Resistant Nephrotic Syndrome. Indian Pediatr. 2021;58(7):650-66.

4. An 11-year-old girl with chronic kidney disease (CKD) with estimated glomerular filtration rate (eGFR) of 25 mL/min/1.73 m^2 is on oral iron, vitamin B_{12}, folic acid, and recombinant human erythropoietin (rhEPO) therapy (50 IU/kg, three times in a week). What would be the target hemoglobin level in this patient?

A. 9–10 g/dL
B. 10–11 g/dL
C. 11–12 g/dL
D. 12–13 g/dL

EXPLANATION

As per the Kidney Disease Improving Global Outcomes (KDIGO) Clinical Practice Guidelines of anemia in CKD, oral iron, folic acid, and erythropoietin-stimulating agent (ESA) therapy are required to maintain target hemoglobin level between 11 and 12 g/L to avoid hypoxia, growth retardation, effort intolerance, and cardiovascular dysfunction. In addition, this also leads to improvement in quality of life, school performance, and avoidance of blood transfusion.

Key: C

BOOST YOUR KNOWLEDGE

Anemia in CKD is multifactorial, chiefly due to decreased nutritional intake because of diminished appetite, loss of blood due to repeated blood sampling, hemodialysis, bone marrow suppression due to uremia, and decreased erythropoietin synthesis by the kidney. Diagnosis is based on hemoglobin, serum iron, ferritin, transferrin saturation, B_{12}, and folic acid levels. These patients need screening for anemia in stage 3-5 CKD. In all pediatric CKD patients with anemia not on iron or ESA, oral iron (parenteral in CKD G5D) therapy is recommended if transferrin saturation is ≤20% and serum ferritin is ≤100 ng/mL.

REFERENCE/SOURCE

- Kidney Disease Improving Global Outcomes (KDIGO) Anemia Work Group. KDIGO Clinical Practice Guideline on Anemia in Chronic Kidney Disease. Kidney Int Suppl. 2012;2:279-335.

5. The most useful therapy for anti-FH antibody associated hemolytic uremic syndrome is:

A. Plasma infusions and prednisolone
B. Plasma exchanges and prednisolone
C. Plasma exchanges and mycophenolate mofetil
D. Plasma infusions and eculizumab therapy

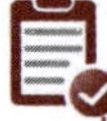

EXPLANATION

For anti-FH antibody associated HUS, the treatment of choice is plasma exchange for removal of anti-FH antibody and immunosuppressant (prednisolone) to decrease production of that antibody.

Key: B

BOOST YOUR KNOWLEDGE

HUS is characterized by:

- Microangiopathic hemolysis characterized by anemia (hemoglobin <10 g/dL), fragmented red cells on peripheral smear (schistocytes ≥2%) and either high lactate dehydrogenase >450 IU/L or undetectable haptoglobin

- Thrombocytopenia (platelets <150,000/µL)
- Acute kidney injury (AKI; rise in creatinine by 50% over baseline)

The approach to a patient with HUS is shown in Flowchart here.

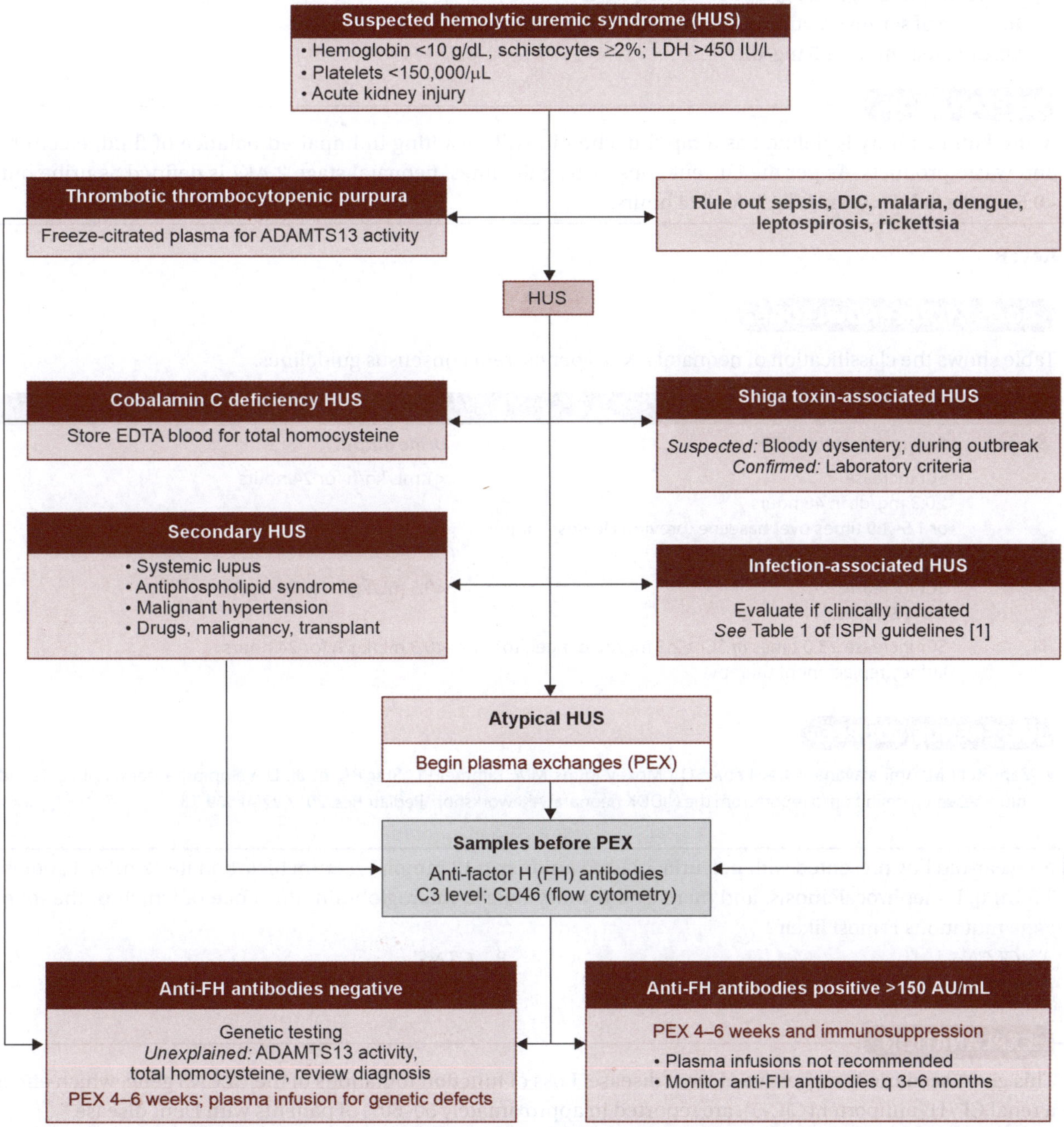

Suspected hemolytic uremic syndrome (HUS)
- Hemoglobin <10 g/dL, schistocytes ≥2%; LDH >450 IU/L
- Platelets <150,000/µL
- Acute kidney injury

Thrombotic thrombocytopenic purpura
Freeze-citrated plasma for ADAMTS13 activity

Rule out sepsis, DIC, malaria, dengue, leptospirosis, rickettsia

HUS

Cobalamin C deficiency HUS
Store EDTA blood for total homocysteine

Shiga toxin-associated HUS
Suspected: Bloody dysentery; during outbreak
Confirmed: Laboratory criteria

Secondary HUS
- Systemic lupus
- Antiphospholipid syndrome
- Malignant hypertension
- Drugs, malignancy, transplant

Infection-associated HUS
Evaluate if clinically indicated
See Table 1 of ISPN guidelines [1]

Atypical HUS
Begin plasma exchanges (PEX)

Samples before PEX
Anti-factor H (FH) antibodies
C3 level; CD46 (flow cytometry)

Anti-FH antibodies negative
Genetic testing
Unexplained: ADAMTS13 activity, total homocysteine, review diagnosis
PEX 4–6 weeks; plasma infusion for genetic defects

Anti-FH antibodies positive >150 AU/mL
PEX 4–6 weeks and immunosuppression
- Plasma infusions not recommended
- Monitor anti-FH antibodies q 3–6 months

(DIC: disseminated intravascular coagulation; EDTA: ethylenediaminetetraacetic acid; ISPN: Indian Society of Pediatric Nephrology; LDH: lactate dehydrogenase)

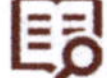

REFERENCE/SOURCE

- Bagga A, Khandelwal P, Mishra K, Thergaonkar R, Vasudevan A, Sharma J, et al; Indian Society of Pediatric Nephrology. Hemolytic uremic syndrome in a developing country: Consensus guidelines. Pediatr Nephrol. 2019;34(8):1465-82.

6. A male term neonate, weight 3 kg, had suffered from birth asphyxia. Which of the following criteria classifies him as stage 2 AKI on Day 5 of life?

A. Urine output ≤1 mL/kg/h but >0.5 mL/kg/h
B. Urine output ≤0.5 mL/kg/h but >0.3 mL/kg/h
C. Increase of serum creatinine ≥0.3 mg/dL from baseline
D. Serum creatinine ≥2.5 mg/dL

EXPLANATION

Acute kidney injury is defined as a rapid decline in GFR resulting in impaired balance of fluid, electrolytes, and waste products. As per the current consensus guidelines, neonatal stage 2 AKI is defined as urine output <0.5 mL/kg/h but >0.3 mL/kg/h for ≥24 hours.

Key: B

BOOST YOUR KNOWLEDGE

Table shows the classification of neonatal AKI as per current consensus guidelines.

Neonatal modifications		
Stage	***Serum creatinine (SCr)***	***Urine output***
I	SCr increase ≥0.3 mg/dL in 48 hours *or* 1.5–1.9 times over baseline (previous lowest value) in 7 days	<1 mL/kg/h for 24 hours
II	SCr increase 2.0–2.9 times	<0.5 mL/kg/h for 24 hours
III	SCr increase ≥3.0 times *or* SCr ≥2.5 mg/dL *or* need for kidney replacement therapy	<0.3 mL/kg/h for 24 hours

REFERENCE/SOURCE

- Zappitelli M, Ambalavanan N, Askenazi DJ, Moxey-Mims MM, Kimmel PL, Star RA, et al. Developing a neonatal acute kidney injury research definition: a report from the NIDDK neonatal AKI workshop. Pediatr Res. 2017;82(4):569-73.

7. A 2-year-old boy presented with polyuria, plasma anion gap 12 mmol/L, serum bicarbonate 12 mEq/L, potassium 2.5 mEq/L, nephrocalcinosis, and increased urinary beta-2-microglobulin. Presence of which of the following gene mutations is most likely?

A. *CLCN5*
B. *CTNS*
C. *GLUT2*
D. *FAH*

EXPLANATION

This given scenario is suggestive of Dent disease. Loss of function mutations of the *CLCN5* gene, which encodes a renal Cl^-/H^+ antiporter (ClC-5), are reported in approximately 50–60% of patients with Dent disease.

Key: A

BOOST YOUR KNOWLEDGE

Dent disease 1 is caused by mutations in the chloride channel encoded by the gene, *CLCN5*. The original term for this disorder was X-linked hypercalciuric nephrolithiasis; it is proximal tubulopathy with characteristic abnormalities that include low molecular weight proteinuria, hypercalciuria, and other features of Fanconi syndrome, such as glycosuria, aminoaciduria, and phosphaturia.

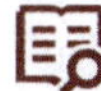

REFERENCES/SOURCES

- Devarajan P. Renal failure. In: Kliegman RM, St Geme III JW, Blum NJ, Shah SS, Tasker RC, Wilson KM (Eds). Nelson Textbook of Pediatrics, 21st edition. Elsevier; 2019. p. 2769.
- Mansour-Hendili L, Blanchard A, Le Pottier N, Roncelin I, Lourdel S, Treard C, et al. Mutation Update of the CLCN5 Gene Responsible for Dent Disease 1. Hum Mutat. 2015;36(8):743-52.

8. A patient of AKI is undergoing peritoneal dialysis (PD). After a few cycles, poor ultrafiltration is noted, but there is no peritoneal leakage. Which of the followings step will *NOT* improve ultrafiltration?

A. Increasing glucose concentration in PD fluid
B. Increasing dwell time
C. Increasing fill volume
D. Consideration of continuous flow PD technique

EXPLANATION

After few cycles of exchanges in PD, gradually diminished osmolar gradient occurs between plasma and dialysate solution and less efficient ultrafiltration is found and increasing the dwell time beyond 30–60 minutes will not improve the ultrafiltration.

Key: B

BOOST YOUR KNOWLEDGE

In PD, the usual time set for inflow of PD fluid (manual PD) is 5–10 minutes, dwell time (the period of the exchange when the dialysis solution remains in the peritoneal cavity) is for 30–60 minutes, and outflow time (manual PD) is 10–20 minutes during which PD fluid is drained out from the peritoneal cavity. If ultrafiltrate is not adequate (amount of fluid drained is lesser than the amount of fluid instilled inside the peritoneal cavity) and there is no pericatheter leak, the amount of ultrafiltrate can be increased by increasing dextrose concentration in PD fluid by using 2.5% fluid (usually 1.5%) or increasing fill volume to 30–40 mL/kg (usually 10–20 mL/kg) or by special procedures such as continuous flow PD.

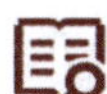

REFERENCE/SOURCE

- Nourse P, Cullis B, Finkelstein F, Numanoglu A, Warady B, Antwi S, et al. ISPD guidelines for peritoneal dialysis in acute kidney injury: 2020 Update (Paediatrics). Perit Dial Int. 2021;41(2):139-57.

9. A child with AKI on peritoneal dialysis, potassium should be added to the PD fluid once serum potassium level reaches:

A. 2 mEq/L
B. 2.5 mEq/L
C. 4 mEq/L
D. 5 mEq/L

EXPLANATION

According to ISPD guidelines 2020, once potassium levels in the serum fall below 4 mEq/L, potassium should be added to dialysate (using strict sterile technique to prevent infection) or alternatively oral or intravenous potassium should be given to maintain potassium levels at ≥4 mEq/L.

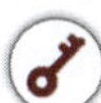

Key: C

BOOST YOUR KNOWLEDGE

Peritoneal dialysis has been effectively used to treat AKI. Losses of potassium can be high in acute PD; such removal may cause serious potassium depletion and cardiovascular instability. Large studies on PD in AKI patients demonstrated that serum potassium control was obtained after a 24-hour session of high-volume PD, and when serum potassium was <4 mmol/L, potassium (K) 3–4 mmol/L was added to dialysis solutions to avoid hypokalemia.

REFERENCE/SOURCE

- Nourse P, Cullis B, Finkelstein F, Numanoglu A, Warady B, Antwi S, et al. ISPD guidelines for peritoneal dialysis in acute kidney injury: 2020 Update (Paediatrics). Perit Dial Int. 2021;41(2):139-57.

10. Which of the following drugs has shown efficacy to slow down the growth of cysts and disease progression in autosomal dominant polycystic kidney disease (ADPKD)?

A. Metformin
B. Indomethacin
C. Tolvaptan
D. Bosutinib

EXPLANATION

Tolvaptan, a selective antagonist of the arginine vasopressin receptor type 2, is the first approved treatment that targets a mechanism directly contributing to cyst development and growth. Tolvaptan slowed kidney function decline in patients at risk of rapid ADPKD progression.

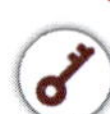

Key: C

BOOST YOUR KNOWLEDGE

Autosomal dominant polycystic kidney disease is the fourth leading cause of kidney failure, accounting for 5–10% of cases globally. Tolvaptan slowed kidney function decline in patients at risk of rapid ADPKD progression in two pivotal trials, the 3-year Tolvaptan Efficacy and Safety in Management of Autosomal Dominant Polycystic Kidney Disease and Its Outcomes (TEMPO) 3:4 trial (NCT00428948) and the 1-year Replicating Evidence of Preserved Renal Function: an Investigation of Tolvaptan Safety and Efficacy in Autosomal Dominant Polycystic Kidney Disease (REPRISE) trial (NCT02160145).

REFERENCE/SOURCE

- Torres VE, Chapman AB, Devuyst O, Gansevoort RT, Perrone RD, Lee J, et al. Multicenter study of long-term safety of tolvaptan in later-stage autosomal dominant polycystic kidney disease. Clin J Am Soc Nephrol. 2020;16(1):48-58.

11. The risk of recurrent urinary tract infection in a child with phimosis and high-grade vesicoureteral reflux (VUR) is 30%. After circumcision, it reduced to 10%. The number needed to treat (NNT) would be:

A. 5
B. 10
C. 15
D. 20

EXPLANATION

NNT is defined as the inverse of the absolute risk reduction.

NNT = 1/Absolute risk reduction

So in this case NNT = 1/30%–10%

= 1/20% or 100/20

= 5

Key: A

BOOST YOUR KNOWLEDGE

The NNT or number needed to treat for an additional beneficial outcome (NNTB) is an epidemiological measure used in communicating the effectiveness of a healthcare intervention, typically a treatment with medication. The NNT is the average number of patients who need to be treated to prevent one additional bad outcome (e.g., the number of patients that need to be treated for one of them to benefit compared with a control in a clinical trial).

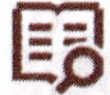

REFERENCE/SOURCE

- Hutton JL. Number needed to treat: properties and problems. Journal of the Royal Statistical Society: Series A (Statistics in Society). 2000;163(3):381-402.

12. A 6-month-old boy presented with two episodes of febrile urinary tract infections. What is the abnormality shown in voiding cystourethrogram (VCUG)?

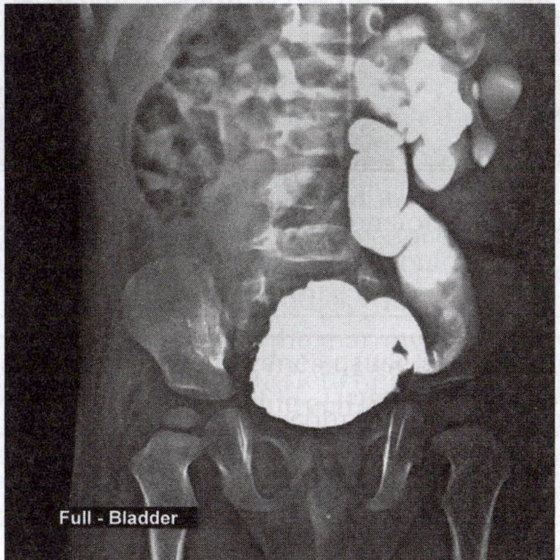

A. Unilateral grade V VUR
B. Unilateral grade V VUR with irregular bladder
C. Irregular urinary bladder
D. Irregular urinary bladder with contralateral nonvisualized kidney

EXPLANATION

In this VCUG, there is unilateral severely dilated and tortuous ureter and dilated pelvicalyceal system with loss of fornices and papillary impression, suggesting unilateral grade V VUR along with irregular bladder.

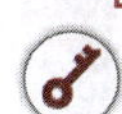

Key: B

BOOST YOUR KNOWLEDGE

Vesicoureteral reflux grading divides VUR according to the height of reflux up the ureters and degree of dilatation of the ureters:

- *Grade 1:* Reflux only into the nondilated ureter
- *Grade 2:* Reflux into the ureter and the renal pelvis without dilatation
- *Grade 3:* Reflux with mildly dilated ureter and pelvicalyceal system
- *Grade 4:* Reflux with the tortuous and moderately dilated ureter with blunting of renal fornices. The papillary impression is preserved.
- *Grade 5:* Reflux with the tortuous and severely dilated ureter, dilatation of pelvicalyceal with loss of fornices, and papillary impression.

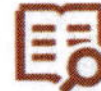

REFERENCE/SOURCE

- Darge K, Troeger J. Vesicoureteral reflux grading in contrast-enhanced voiding urosonography. Eur J Radiol. 2002;43(2):122-8.

13. Identify the abnormality present in this DMSA scan done for a child with febrile urinary tract infection.

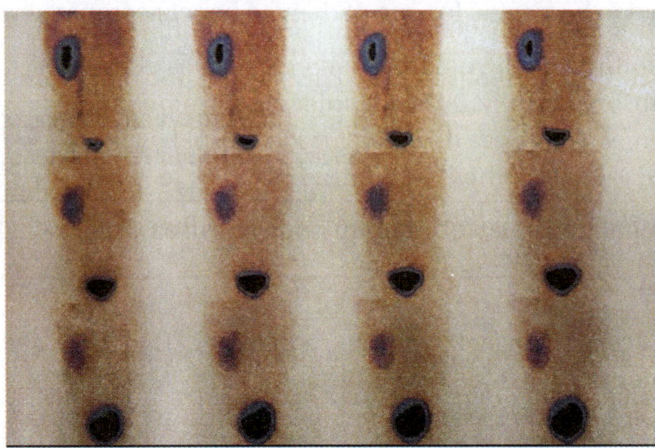

A. Normal scan
B. Unilateral nonexcretory kidney
C. Bilateral detection of radioisotope
D. Radioisotope in urinary bladder only

EXPLANATION

There is radioisotope uptake as visualized on the left kidney with intact excretory function but no uptake in the right kidney and no excretion through the ureter.

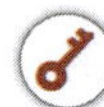

Key: B

BOOST YOUR KNOWLEDGE

A DMSA (dimercaptosuccinic acid) renal scan is a diagnostic imaging that evaluates the function, size, shape, and position of the kidneys and detects scarring caused by frequent infections. Technetium-99m DMSA is a radioisotope that is injected through an IV prior to the scan. It is taken up by the kidneys. A special camera, called a gamma camera, is used to take pictures of the kidneys and show how the kidneys are working. The DMSA renal scan can help assessment of pyelonephritis, differential renal function in the left and right kidneys, renal ectopia, infarction, hypertension, horseshoe kidney, AKI, and multicystic dysplastic kidneys.

REFERENCE/SOURCE

- Ataei N, Madani A, Habibi R, Khorasani M. Evaluation of acute pyelonephritis with DMSA scans in children presenting after the age of 5 years. Pediatric Nephrol. 2005;20(10):1439-44.

14. A 14-day-old baby boy was born to a primigravida and has been admitted in neonatal intensive care unit (NICU) for severe birth asphyxia. On Day 7, he developed decreased activity, oliguria, and facial puffiness. Investigations revealed total leukocyte counts 16,000/mm^3, polymorphs 72%, positive C-reactive protein (CRP), blood urea 215 mg/dL, serum creatinine 7.6 mg/dL, K 6.1 mEq/L, and Na 123 mEq/L. The most appropriate plan of management includes:

A. Salbutamol nebulization and IV calcium gluconate
B. Antibiotics therapy + salbutamol nebulization
C. Antibiotic therapy + aminophylline and calcium gluconate infusions
D. Antibiotics therapy + IV calcium gluconate + PD

EXPLANATION

In this case, the neonate is having severe birth asphyxia, late onset sepsis with stage 3 AKI, hyperkalemia, and hyponatremia. Therefore, the most appropriate therapy would be IV antibiotics for sepsis, IV calcium gluconate for hyperkalemia (membrane stabilization), and PD dialysis for correction of acidosis and electrolyte disturbances during severe AKI.

Key: D

BOOST YOUR KNOWLEDGE

In neonates with severe birth asphyxia and sepsis, AKI can occur due to acute tubular necrosis, resulting in azotemia, metabolic acidosis, and hyperkalemia. During acidosis, the myocardium is unduly sensitive to hyperkalemia, predisposing to arrythmia. Therefore, IV calcium gluconate is administered for membrane stabilization of cardiac myocytes. Peritoneal dialysis is done to correct acidosis and hyperkalemia and reduce blood urea, and it is the preferred mode of therapy in neonates with hemodynamic instability in regions where access to neonatal extracorporeal therapies is limited. Antibiotics are given in modified doses as per eGFR.

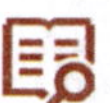

REFERENCE/SOURCE

- Mishra OP, Prasad R, Deepthi B, Krishnamurthy S, Sharma S, Bhardwaj A, et al. Disorders of kidneys and urinary tract. In: Gupta P (Ed). UG Textbook of Pediatrics, 1st edition. New Delhi: Jaypee Brothers Medical Publishers; 2023. pp. 729-34.

15. A 17-year-old girl presented with history of generalized edema for 25 days and decreased urine output for 10 days. On examination, she had mild pallor, blood pressure (BP) of 132/88 mm Hg, and no rashes over body. Investigations showed hemoglobin 9 g/dL, total leukocyte counts 7,500/mm^3, polymorphs 65%, lymphocytes 35%, creatinine 6.0 mg/dL, and normal C3 and C4 levels. Kidney biopsy revealed pauci-immune-crescentic glomerulonephritis (GN) with acute tubular injury and 15/26 glomeruli with global sclerosis. The appropriate treatment protocol includes:

A. Immunosuppression (IV cyclophosphamide + methylprednisolone) only
B. Immunosuppression (IV cyclophosphamide + methylprednisolone) + hemodialysis
C. Immunosuppression (IV cyclophosphamide + methylprednisolone) + plasmapheresis
D. Immunosuppression (IV cyclophosphamide + methylprednisolone) + hemodialysis + IV rituximab infusion (375 mg/m^2)

EXPLANATION

This is a case of pauci-immune vasculitis with crescentic GN. Antineutrophil cytoplasmic antibody (ANCA) levels are usually positive. According to the KDIGO guideline 2021, initial protocol for induction includes IV methylprednisone (30 mg/kg/day for 3 days followed by oral prednisone with IV cyclophosphamide or IV rituximab). Randomized trials have shown a beneficial effect of plasmapheresis for severe kidney involvement (serum creatinine >5.7 mg/dL).

Key: C

BOOST YOUR KNOWLEDGE

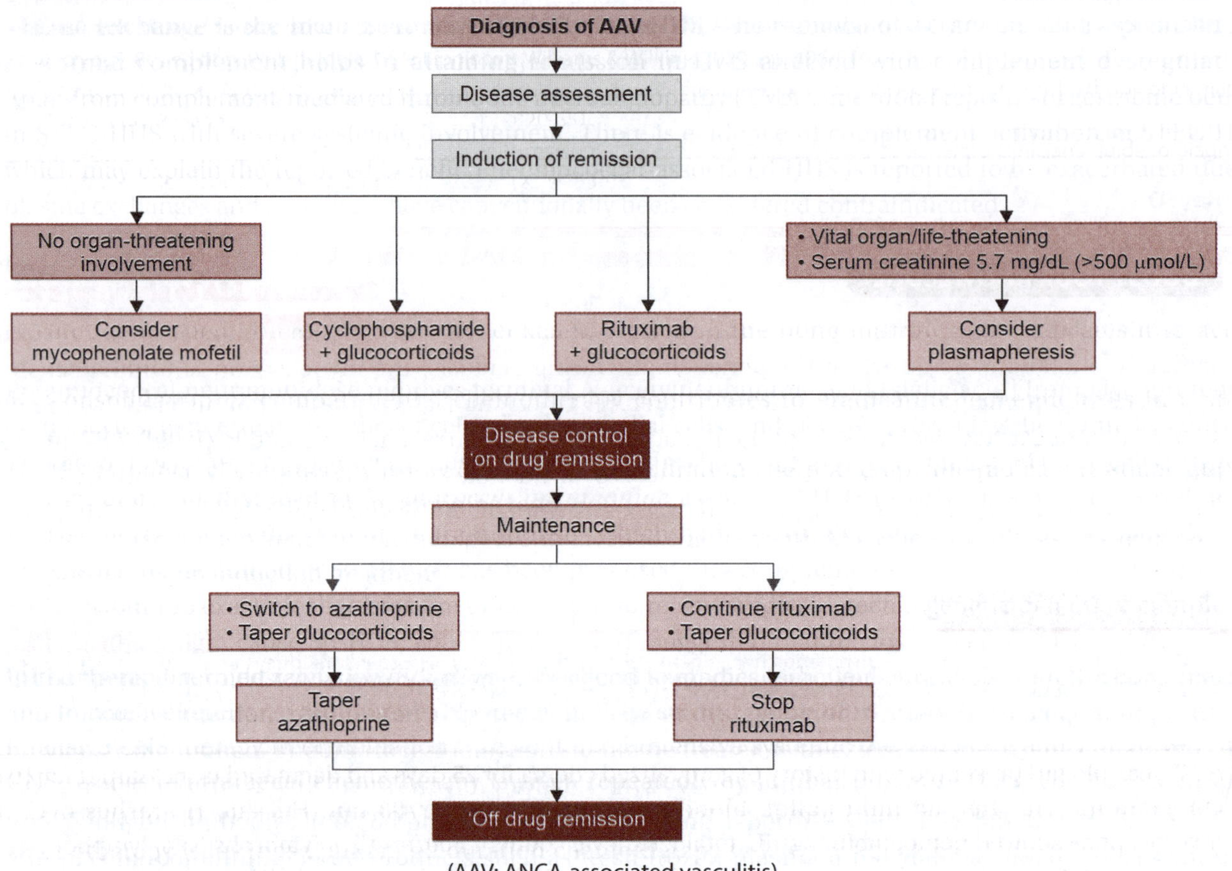

(AAV: ANCA-associated vasculitis)

REFERENCE/SOURCE

- Casal Moura M, Gauckler P, Anders HJ, Bruchfeld A, Fernandez-Juarez GM, Floege J, et al. Management of antineutrophil cytoplasmic antibody-associated vasculitis with glomerulonephritis as proposed by the ACR 2021, EULAR 2022 and KDIGO 2021 guidelines/recommendations. Nephrol Dial Transplant. 2023;38(11):2637-51.

16. A 4-year-old boy was evaluated for recurrent hematuria. Urinalysis showed 50–75 red blood cells (RBCs)/hpf and proteinuria Dipstick ++. Mother had blood in her urine since childhood but has been told that she has a benign disorder and no definite diagnosis was made. On further enquiry, it was found that father of the mother died of uremia. Pedigree chart is shown below. What is the mode of inheritance?

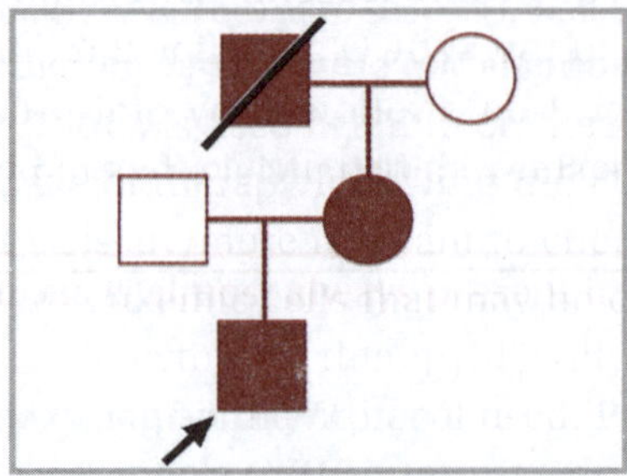

A. X- linked
B. Digenic
C. Autosomal recessive
D. Autosomal dominant

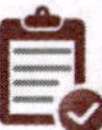

EXPLANATION

X-linked inheritance shows the pattern of inheritance from maternal grandfather to their grandchildren via mother [disease is probably Alport syndrome (AS)].

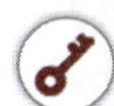

Key: A

BOOST YOUR KNOWLEDGE

Approximately 85% of patients with AS have X-linked inheritance caused by a mutation in the *COL4A5* gene encoding the α5 chain of type IV collagen. Autosomal recessive forms of AS in approximately 15% of patients are caused by mutations in the *COL4A3* and *COL4A4* genes on chromosome 2 encoding the α3 and α4 chains, respectively, of type IV collagen. An autosomal dominant form of AS linked to the *COL4A3-COL4A4* gene locus occurs in 5% of cases.

REFERENCE/SOURCE

- Flores FX. Isolated glomerular diseases associated with recurrent gross hematuria. In: Kliegman RM, St Geme III JW, Blum NJ, Shah SS, Tasker RC, Wilson KM (Eds). Nelson Textbook of Pediatrics, 21st edition. Elsevier; 2019. pp. 2721-2.

17. Which of the following is the confirmatory test to establish the diagnosis of Alport disease?

A. Kidney biopsy
B. Genetic testing
C. Brainstem-evoked response audiometry
D. Presence of RBCs and acanthocytes in urine

EXPLANATION

Recent expert guidelines recommend genetic testing for the diagnosis of AS. Here, we describe current best practice and likely future developments. In individuals with suspected AS, all three *COL4A5, COL4A3*, and *COL4A4* genes should be examined for pathogenic variants, probably by high throughput-targeted next generation sequencing (NGS) technologies.

Key: B

BOOST YOUR KNOWLEDGE

Alport syndrome is a genetic and hereditary disease, caused by mutations in the type IV collagen genes *COL4A3*, *COL4A4*, and *COL4A5*, which affect the glomerular basement membrane of the kidney. In recent years, diagnosis is based on DNA sequencing technologies such as NGS. The results make it possible to know the causative mutation, located in *COL4A* genes, and other possible variants that may be modifying the phenotype. The use of Sanger sequencing, at the diagnostic level, has been restricted to carry out segregation studies.

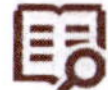

REFERENCE/SOURCE

- Savige J, Ariani F, Mari F, Bruttini M, Renieri A, Gross O, et al. Expert consensus guidelines for the genetic diagnosis of Alport syndrome. Pediatr Nephrol. 2019;34(7):1175-89.

18. A 10-year-old child presented with 7-day history of edema, oliguria, and red-colored urine. On examination, the patient had BP of 124/90 mm Hg and no rashes, arthralgia, or arthritis. Total leukocyte counts 7,600/mm^3, polymorphs 40%, lymphocytes 45%, and eosinophils 15%. Serum C3, C4, ASO, and IgA levels were normal, but peripheral ANCA (p-ANCA) was positive. The probable diagnosis is:

A. IgA nephropathy
B. Wegner Granulomatosis
C. Churg-Strauss syndrome (CSS)
D. Goodpasture syndrome

EXPLANATION

Acute GN with eosinophilia and p-ANCA positive with normal complements suggestive of eosinophilic granulomatosis with polyangiitis also known as CSS.

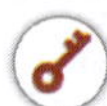

Key: C

BOOST YOUR KNOWLEDGE

Churg–Strauss syndrome is a small vessel necrotizing granulomatous (allergic granulomatosis) vasculitis associated with a history of refractory asthma and peripheral eosinophilia. ANCA test result is positive in 50–70% of cases of CSS, and myeloperoxidase (MPO)-ANCAs are more common than PR3-ANCAs.

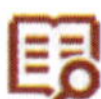

REFERENCE/SOURCE

- Sivaraman V, Fels EC, Ardoin SP. Vasculitis syndromes. In: Kliegman RM, St Geme III JW, Blum NJ, Shah SS, Tasker RC, Wilson KM (Eds). Nelson Textbook of Pediatrics, 21st edition. Elsevier; 2019. pp. 1324-6.

19. A patient presented with normal anion gap metabolic acidosis, blood urea 22 mg/dL, serum creatinine 0.6 mg/dL, urine pH <5.5, and fractional excretion of bicarbonate of 5–10%. What is the most likely diagnosis?

A. Type 1 renal tubular acidosis (RTA)
B. Type 2 RTA
C. Type 4 RTA
D. Mixed RTA

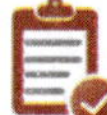

EXPLANATION

Normal anion gap metabolic acidosis with normal renal function suggestive of RTA. Urinary pH <5.5 excludes type 1 RTA (distal). Fractional bicarbonate excretion is 5–10%, which indicates type 4 RTA.

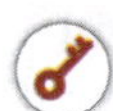

Key: C

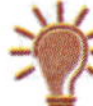

BOOST YOUR KNOWLEDGE

Renal tubular acidosis is a disease state characterized by a nonanion gap (hyperchloremic) metabolic acidosis in the setting of a normal or near-normal GFR. There are four main types: proximal (type II) RTA, classic distal (type I) RTA, hyperkalemic (type IV) RTA, and a combined proximal and distal (type III). Proximal RTA results from impaired bicarbonate reabsorption and distal RTA from failure to secrete acid.

Contrasting features and diagnostic studies in renal tubular acidosis

	Type of renal tubular acidosis (RTA)		
Finding	***Proximal RTA***	***Classic distal***	***Generalized distal dysfunction***
Plasma [K^+]	Low	Low	High
Urine pH with acidosis	<5.5	>5.5	<5.5 or >5.5
Urine net charge	Negative	Positive	Positive
Fanconi lesion	Present with acquired proximal renal tubular acidosis (pRTA)	Absent	Absent
Fractional bicarbonate excretion	>10–15% during alkali therapy	2–5%	5–10%
U-B P_{CO_2}	Normal	Low	Low
Response to therapy	Least responsive	Responsive	Less responsive
Associated features	Fanconi syndrome	Nephrocalcinosis/ hyperglobulinemia	Renal insufficiency

REFERENCE/SOURCE

- Dixon BP. Renal tubular acidosis. In: Kliegman RM, St Geme III JW, Blum NJ, Shah SS, Tasker RC, Wilson KM (Eds). Nelson Textbook of Pediatrics, 21st edition. Elsevier; 2019. pp. 2761-5.

20. Which of the following drugs is recommended to prevent AKI in a neonate with severe birth asphyxia and hypoxemic ischemic encephalopathy?

A. Aminophylline
B. Atrasentan
C. Sildenafil
D. Finerenone

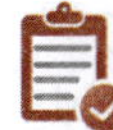

EXPLANATION

Neonates with hypoxic-ischemic encephalopathy (HIE) frequently develop AKI. Aminophylline has been shown to reduce severe renal dysfunction in neonates after perinatal asphyxia.

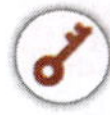

Key: A

BOOST YOUR KNOWLEDGE

The major role of adenosine in mediating renal vasoconstriction in hypoxemia is supported by the fact that administering theophylline, which is a nonspecific antagonist of adenosine cell surface receptors, could prevent the hypoxemia-induced decrease in GFR.

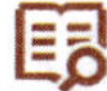

REFERENCE/SOURCE

- Saboute M, Balasi J, Tajalli S, Hajipour M, Heshmat S, Khalesi N, et al. Effect of aminophylline in preventing renal dysfunction among neonates with prenatal asphyxia: a clinical trial. Arch Iran Med. 2020;23(5):312-8.

21. A 12-year-old boy is having BP of 124/82 mm Hg, which is ≥90th percentile for the corresponding height. What is his definition of category as per revised American Academy of Pediatrics (AAP) Clinical Practice Guidelines for Hypertension 2017?

A. Normal BP
B. Elevated BP
C. Stage 1 hypertension
D. Stage 2 hypertension

EXPLANATION

According to AAP Clinical Practice Guideline for hypertension 2017, BP is classified as age- and height-specific percentiles for children <13 years of age, and absolute levels of BP for adolescents to make these cut-offs more consistent with adult definitions. In this patient, absolute levels of BP (124/82 mm Hg) would be used to classify him as elevated BP.

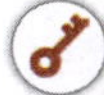

Key: B

BOOST YOUR KNOWLEDGE

The updated 2017 AAP classification of hypertension is given here.

Updated definitions of BP categories and stages	
For children aged 1 to <13 years	***For children aged >13 years***
Normal BP: <90th percentile	*Normal BP:* <120/<80 mm Hg
Elevated BP: ≥90th percentile to <95th percentile or 120/80 mm Hg to <95th percentile (whichever is lower)	*Elevated BP:* 120/<80 to 129/<80 mm Hg

Contd...

Contd...

For children aged 1 to <13 years	*For children aged >13 years*
Stage 1 hypertension (HTN): ≥95th percentile to <95th percentile + 12 mm Hg, or 130/80 to 139/89 mm Hg (whichever is lower)	*Stage 1 HTN:* 130/80 to 139/89 mm Hg
Stage 2 HTN: ≥95th percentile + 12 mm Hg, or ≥140/90 mm Hg (whichever is lower)	*Stage 2 HTN:* ≥140/90 mm Hg

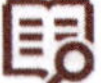

REFERENCE/SOURCE

- Flynn JT, Kaelber DC, Baker-Smith CM, Blowey D, Carroll AE, Daniels SR, et al; Subcommittee on Screening and Management of High Blood Pressure in Children. Clinical practice guideline for screening and management of high blood pressure in children and adolescents. Pediatrics. 2017;140(3):e20171904.

22. A 7-year-old girl is having normal BP in office setting, but BP at 97th percentile on ambulatory BP monitoring. Which of the following categories will she belong to as per the 2022 recommendations on classification of ambulatory hypertension?

A. Elevated BP
B. Masked hypertension
C. White coat hypertension (WCH)
D. Ambulatory hypertension

EXPLANATION

Masked hypertension is diagnosed if the office BP reading is normal but the out-of-office BP reading by either home BP monitoring or by ambulatory BP monitoring (ABPM) is increased.

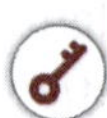

Key: B

BOOST YOUR KNOWLEDGE

Masked hypertension tends to occur in 10–30% of the normal population. Masked hypertension could be missed if out-of-clinic BP level is not evaluated. Home BP monitoring may emerge as a complementary prevention and treatment strategy in clinical practice and could help reduce the public health burden of cardiovascular disease. Table shows classification of ambulatory hypertension as per AHA 2022 guidelines:

Revised classification for ambulatory blood pressure studies in pediatric patients

	*Clinic systolic or diastolic blood pressure**		*Mean ambulatory systolic or diastolic blood pressure*	
Category	*<13 years of age*	*≥13 years of age*	*<13 years of age*	*≥13 years of age*
Normal blood pressure	<95th percentile	<130/80	<95th percentile OR adolescent cut points*	<125/75 mm Hg 24 hours AND <130/80 mm Hg wake AND <110/65 mm Hg sleep
White-coat hypertension	≥95th percentile	≥130/80		
Masked hypertension	<95th percentile	<130/80	≥95th percentile OR adolescent cut points*	≥125/75 mm Hg 24 hours OR ≥130/80 mm Hg wake OR ≥110/65 mm Hg sleep
Ambulatory hypertension	≥95th percentile	≥130/80		

*Including 24 hours, wake, and sleep blood pressure.

REFERENCE/SOURCE

- Flynn JT, Urbina EM, Brady TM, Baker-Smith C, Daniels SR, Hayman LL, et al; on behalf of the Atherosclerosis, Hypertension, and Obesity in the Young Committee of the American Heart Association Council on Lifelong Congenital Heart Disease and Heart Health in the Young; Ambulatory blood pressure monitoring in children and adolescents: 2022 update: a scientific statement from the American Heart Association. Hypertension. 2022;79(7):e114-e124.

23. A male neonate is having anteroposterior renal pelvis diameter (APRPD) of 16 mm with peripheral calyceal dilatation detected at Day 4 of postnatal life. He will be classified into which of the following risk categories as per urinary tract dilatation (UTD) classification?

A. No risk
B. Low risk
C. Intermediate risk
D. High risk

EXPLANATION

In this case scenario, APRPD is >15 mm and only dilatation of peripheral calyces without parenchymal involvement is detected. According to UTD classification system for postnatal UTD, it falls into the intermediate risk group.

Key: C

BOOST YOUR KNOWLEDGE

Urinary tract dilatation is detected postnatally (denoted as P), we recommend stratification of risk into three groups: Low-risk (UTD P1), intermediate-risk (UTD P2), and high-risk (UTD P3) groups.

Postnatal presentation		
>48 hours APRPD 10 to <15 mm	>48 hours APRPD ≥15 mm	>48 hours APRPD ≥15 mm
↓	↓	↓
Central calyceal dilation	Peripheral calyceal dilation	Peripheral calyceal dilation
Parenchymal thickness normal	Parenchymal thickness normal	Parenchymal thickness abnormal
Parenchymal appearance normal	Parenchymal appearance normal	Parenchymal appearance abnormal
Ureters normal	Ureters abnormal	Ureters abnormal
Bladder normal	Bladder normal	Bladder abnormal
↓	↓	↓
UTD P1: Low risk	*UTD P2:* Intermediate risk	*UTD P3:* High risk

(APRPD: anterior-posterior renal pelvis diameter)

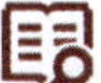

REFERENCE/SOURCE

- Nguyen HT, Benson CB, Bromley B, Campbell JB, Chow J, Coleman B, et al. Multidisciplinary consensus on the classification of prenatal and postnatal urinary tract dilation (UTD classification system). J Pediatr Urol. 2014;10(6):982-98.

24. Which of the following is an interleukin-2 (IL-2) receptor antagonist used in pediatric kidney transplant for immunosuppression?

A. Basiliximab
B. Alemtuzumab
C. Ofatumumab
D. Eculizumab

EXPLANATION

Basiliximab is a chimeric anti-IL-2 receptor (also known as CD25) monoclonal antibody. Basiliximab is a glycoprotein produced by recombinant technology. It is used to prevent acute kidney transplantation rejection. Basiliximab is used for induction in immunologically low-risk children. Among the other choices, alemtuzumab is an anti-CD52 inhibitor, ofatumumab is a fully humanized anti-CD20 inhibitor, and eculizumab blocks complement C5.

Key: A

BOOST YOUR KNOWLEDGE

Basiliximab, a chimeric (human/murine) monoclonal antibody, is indicated for the prevention of acute organ rejection in adult and pediatric kidney transplant recipients in combination with other immunosuppressive agents. Basiliximab reduces acute rejection without increasing the incidence of adverse events, including infection and malignancy, in kidney transplant recipients when combined with standard dual or triple immunotherapy.

REFERENCE/SOURCE

- Balani SS, Jensen CJ, Kouri AM, Kizilbash SJ. Induction and maintenance immunosuppression in pediatric kidney transplantation: Advances and controversies. Pediatr Transplant. 2021;25(7):e14077.

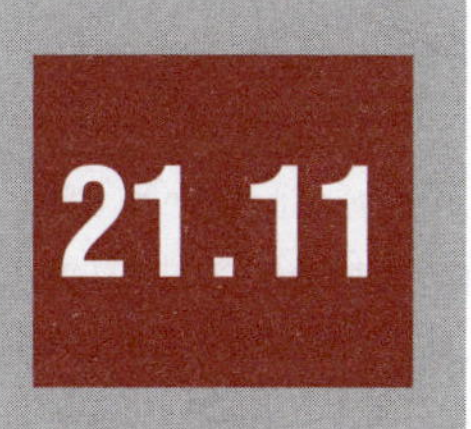

CHAPTER 21.11 Hypertension

Mukta Mantan

1. At what age is screening for blood pressure (BP) recommended to be started in children?

A. 3 years
B. 5 years
C. 8 years
D. 12 years

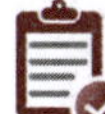

EXPLANATION

The AAP Clinical Practice Guidelines for Screening and Measurement of High Blood Pressure in Children and Adolescents published in 2017 recommend annual measurement of BP in children ≥3 years of age for screening of hypertension.

Key: A

BOOST YOUR KNOWLEDGE

Hypertension is less common in the pediatric age group compared to adults. Overall, 1–5% of children suffer from this condition. Therefore, it is recommended to screen children beyond 3 years if they do not have any comorbidity. However, it is recommended to monitor for hypertension even before 3 years in patients with underlying heart disease, chronic kidney disease (CKD), history of nursery stay, small-for-gestational age (SGA) babies, or history of neonatal acute kidney injury (AKI).

REFERENCES/SOURCES

- Flynn JT, Kaelber DC, Baker-Smith CM, Blowey D, Carroll AE, Daniels SR, et al. Clinical practice guideline for screening and management of high blood pressure in children and adolescents. Pediatrics. 2017;140(3):e20171904.
- Lande MB. Systemic hypertension. In: Kliegman R, Nelson WE (Eds). Nelson Textbook of Pediatrics, 19th edition. Philadelphia, PA: Elsevier/Saunders; 2011. pp. 1639-47.

2. A 5-year-old child needs BP measurement. What is the most appropriate cuff size for this patient?

A. A cuff length that is 75% of the arm length
B. A cuff length that is 65% of the arm length
C. A cuff width that is 40% of mid-upper arm circumference (MUAC)
D. A cuff width that is 60% of MUAC

EXPLANATION

The AAP Clinical Practice Guidelines for Screening and Measurement of High Blood Pressure in Children and Adolescents published in 2017 recommend that the size of the bladder cuff should be approximately 40% of the MUAC.

Key: C

BOOST YOUR KNOWLEDGE

Inappropriate bladder size can lead to errors in BP recording. A small cuff size will overestimate while a large cuff size will underestimate BP. The current guidelines mention that the bladder size of the cuff should be at least 40% of MUAC and the relationship between width and length should be 1:2, i.e., the bladder cuff length should be 80% of the MUAC.

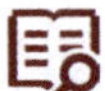

REFERENCES/SOURCES

- Flynn JT, Kaelber DC, Baker-Smith CM, Blowey D, Carroll AE, Daniels SR, et al. Clinical practice guideline for screening and management of high blood pressure in children and adolescents. Pediatrics. 2017;140(3):e20171904.
- Lande MB. Systemic hypertension. In: Kliegman R, Nelson WE (Eds). Nelson Textbook of Pediatrics, 19th edition. Philadelphia, PA: Elsevier/Saunders; 2011. pp. 1639-47.

3. A 10-year-old obese boy is being evaluated for hypertension. His office BP is elevated; however, the continuous ambulatory BP record shows normal BP. He should be categorized as which of the following?

A. Masked hypertension
B. White-coat hypertension
C. Elevated BP
D. Normotensive

EXPLANATION

He is normotensive with a continous ambulatory blood pressure monitoring (CABPM) record. White-coat hypertension is defined as increased BP at office visits, while normal BP is recorded on ambulatory blood pressure monitoring. As the CABPM records 24 hours BP, there is no likelihood of hypertension being missed.

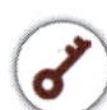

Key: B

BOOST YOUR KNOWLEDGE

Obesity is a major risk factor for hypertension, especially in adolescents. Obesity and stress among school-going children are emerging as important causes of borderline or raised recordings in older and adolescent children. CABPM monitoring has emerged as an important tool to identify hypertension and differentiate it from white-coat hypertension (WCH). Elevated BP is defined as BP between 90th and 95th centile (previously known as prehypertension), while masked hypertension is when the office BP recordings are normal, but the CABPM recordings show hypertension.

REFERENCE/SOURCE

- Flynn JT, Urbina EM, Brady TM, Baker-Smith C, Daniels SR, Hayman LL, et al. Ambulatory blood pressure monitoring in children and adolescents: 2022 update: a scientific statement from the American Heart Association. Hypertension. 2022;79(7):e114-24.

4. A 14-year-old overweight boy undergoes continuous ambulatory BP monitoring. Which of the following parameters is diagnostic of hypertension in the CABPM record?

A. Loss of nocturnal dipping
B. BP loads >25%
C. BP loads >50%
D. Ambulatory BP >130/80 mm Hg in the awake state

EXPLANATION

The parameters of BP loads and nocturnal dipping have been removed in the most recent guidelines in interpretation of CABPM in children and adolescents. BP loads mean the number of readings that are above the 95th centile in daytime and night-time. Usually, a load of >25% is taken as hypertension. The fall in pressure, called the "dip", is defined as the difference between daytime mean systolic pressure and night-time mean systolic pressure expressed as a percentage of the daytime value; 10–20% is considered a normal dip. A dip <10% has been considered as predicting an adverse cardiovascular event/left ventricular hypertrophy (LVH).

Key: D

BOOST YOUR KNOWLEDGE

Classification of BP according to the new CABPM monitoring guidelines

	*Clinic systolic or diastolic blood pressure**		*Mean ambulatory systolic or diastolic blood pressure*	
Category	***<13 years of age***	***≥13 years of age***	***<13 years of age***	***≥13 years of age***
Normal blood pressure	<95th percentile	<130/80	<95th percentile OR adolescent cut points*	<125/75 mm Hg 24 hour AND <130/80 mm Hg wake AND <110/65 mm Hg sleep
White-coat hypertension (WCH)	≥95th percentile	≥130/80		
Masked hypertension	<95th percentile	<130/80	≥95th percentile OR adolescent cut points*	≥125/75 mm Hg 24 hour OR ≥130/80 mm Hg wake OR ≥110/65 mm Hg sleep
Ambulatory hypertension	≥95th percentile	≥130/80		

*Including 24 hours, wake, and sleep blood pressure.

REFERENCE/SOURCE

- American Heart Association. (2022). Ambulatory Blood Pressure Monitoring in Children and Adolescents: 2022 Update: A Scientific Statement from the American Heart Association. https://www.ahajournals.org/doi/full/10.1161/HYP.0000000000000215 [Last accessed July, 2024].

5. Which of the following mechanisms is *not* a cause of hypertension associated with obesity in children?

A. Hyperinsulinemia and hyperleptinemia
B. Renin–angiotensin–aldosterone system (RAAS) activation
C. Hypothyroidism
D. Endothelial dysfunction

EXPLANATION

The correct answer is hypothyroidism which may be associated with obesity but is not directly responsible for the causative mechanisms of hypertension.

Key: C

BOOST YOUR KNOWLEDGE

The mechanisms through which obesity causes hypertension are complex and include sympathetic nervous system overactivation, stimulation of the renin–angiotensin–aldosterone system, alterations in adipose-derived cytokines, insulin resistance, and structural and functional renal changes. Endothelial dysfunction is also one of the mechanisms. However, hypothyroidism does not occur in all obese patients and is not a direct causative for hypertension (occurs in 12–15% of obese children and adolescents).

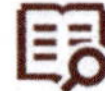

REFERENCE/SOURCE

- Yamaguchi I, Flynn JT. Pathophysiology of pediatric hypertension. In: Avner ED, Harmon WE, Niaudet P, Yoshikawa N, Emma F, Goldstein SL (Eds). Pediatric Nephrology, 7th edition. Berlin Heidelberg: Springer; 2015. pp. 1951-96.

6. What is the most likely mechanism for the occurrence of white-coat hypertension in children?

A. RAAS activation
B. Sympathetic nervous system overactivity
C. Endothelial dysfunction
D. Genetic influences

EXPLANATION

Mechanisms like RAAS activation, endothelial dysfunction, and genetic influences are more likely to cause hypertension than white-coat hypertension. The correct answer is sympathetic nervous system over activity which is the proposed mechanism for white-coat hypertension. It is a part of the "flight or fight response" mediated by the sympathetic nervous system.

Key: B

BOOST YOUR KNOWLEDGE

Long-term studies have shown that patients with white-coat hypertension do not develop LVH and other target organ damage. Hence, it is important to identify it and for patient reassurance.

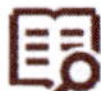

REFERENCE/SOURCE

- Yamaguchi I, Flynn JT. Pathophysiology of pediatric hypertension. In: Avner ED, Harmon WE, Niaudet P, Yoshikawa N, Emma F, Goldstein SL (Eds). Pediatric Nephrology, 7th edition. Berlin Heidelberg: Springer; 2015. pp. 1951-96.

7. A 5-year-old child presents with stage 2 hypertension. His blood investigation reveals a normal kidney function test (KFT), a blood pH of 7.5, HCO_3 of 28 mEq/L, serum sodium of 140 mEq/L, and serum K of 2.8 mEq/L. Which of the following is an *unlikely* diagnosis in this child?

A. Liddle's syndrome
B. Familial hyperaldosteronism type 1
C. Bartter syndrome
D. Familial hyperaldosteronism type 2

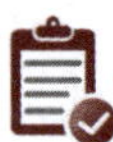

EXPLANATION

Familial hyperaldosteronism 1 and 2 can cause alkalosis and hypokalemia. Bartter syndrome is associated with alkalosis and hypokalemia but has polyuria and hypotension instead of hypertension. Liddle's syndrome is an autosomal dominant disorder characterized by severe hypertension, metabolic alkalosis, and hypokalemia with low renin and aldosterone levels.

Key: C

BOOST YOUR KNOWLEDGE

Activating mutations in the β- or γ-subunit of the epithelial Na channel (ENaC) are responsible for elevated renal sodium reabsorption in Liddle's syndrome.

REFERENCE/SOURCE

- Yamaguchi I, Flynn JT. Pathophysiology of pediatric hypertension. In: Avner ED, Harmon WE, Niaudet P, Yoshikawa N, Emma F, Goldstein SL (Eds). Pediatric Nephrology, 7th edition. Berlin Heidelberg: Springer; 2015. pp. 1951-96.

8. A 5-year-old girl presents with a hypertensive emergency. On evaluation, her KFT shows urea 20 mg/dL, serum creatinine 0.4 mg/dL, serum Na/K 135, and 4.2 mEq/L, respectively. On ultrasound [kidney, ureter, and bladder (KUB)], the right kidney is 5.5 × 4 cm, and the left kidney (LK) is 7 × 4.5 cm in size with normal corticomedullary differentiation of both kidneys. Which radiological investigation will help the most in identifying the underlying cause of hypertension?

A. Intravenous pyelogram (IVP)
B. Micturating cystourethrogram (MCUG)
C. Contrast-enhanced computed tomography (CECT) Abdomen
D. Magnetic resonance (MR) angiography

EXPLANATION

This child has normal kidney functions; however, the ultrasound is showing asymmetrical kidneys though they have normal corticomedullary differentiation. In unilateral renal artery stenosis, the kidney on the side of vascular obstruction shrinks in size over a period of time.

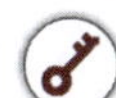

Key: D

BOOST YOUR KNOWLEDGE

The best investigation to identify renal artery stenosis with almost 99% sensitivity is MR angiography of the abdominal aorta and renal arteries. A computed tomography (CT) angiography can also be used if MR is not available. A CECT abdomen will not detect the vascular abnormality and will only confirm the small size of the kidney, which is evident in the sonography itself. An MCUG is primarily used for detecting lower urinary tract structural abnormalities like posterior urethral valves, neurogenic bladder, vesicoureteric reflux, etc. An IVP is a dynamic scan that tells about the functioning and drainage of each kidney and is hardly done these days as has been replaced by functional nuclear scans like DTPA (diethylenetriamine pentaacetic acid) that are exposed to lower radiation compared to traditional IVP.

REFERENCE/SOURCE

- Lande MB. Systemic hypertension. In: Kliegman R, Nelson WE (Eds). Nelson Textbook of Pediatrics, 19th edition. Philadelphia, PA: Elsevier/Saunders; 2011. pp. 1639-47.

9. A 6-year-old child presents with generalized swelling, cola-colored urine, and hypertension. On evaluation, her antistreptolysin O (ASO) is 400 IU/L and C3 is 30 mg/dL. Her KFT shows urea of 125 mg/dL, serum creatinine of 3.5 mg/dL, serum Na 140 mEq/L, and K 5.8 mEq/L. Which of the following antihypertensives should be avoided in this child?

A. Amlodipine
B. Enalapril
C. Labetalol
D. Nitroprusside

EXPLANATION

Both angiotensin-converting enzyme (ACE) and angiotensin receptor blockers (ARBs) should be avoided in AKI as they can worsen kidney functions and hyperkalemia.

Key: B

BOOST YOUR KNOWLEDGE

Angiotensin-converting enzyme inhibitors like enalapril, lisinopril, and ramipril should be considered as the first-line drugs in patients with renal parenchymal diseases like chronic glomerulonephritis, lupus, and CKD (stages 1–3).

Patients with transient hypertension like poststreptococcal glomerulonephritis can be managed with diuretics like frusemide (2–6 mg/kg/day) alone. If the hypertension is not controlled by these drugs, calcium channel blockers like amlodipine (0.1–0.5 mg/kg/day) or beta-blockers like atenolol (1–2 mg/kg/day) can be added. If the patient has a hypertensive emergency, intravenous (IV) sodium nitroprusside or IV labetalol infusion at doses of 0.5–5 μg/kg/min for the first 48–72 hours can be given, and further control can be done with the abovementioned drugs.

REFERENCE/SOURCE

- Lande MB. Systemic hypertension. In: Kliegman R, Nelson WE (Eds). Nelson Textbook of Pediatrics, 19th edition. Philadelphia, PA: Elsevier/Saunders; 2011. pp. 1639-47.

10. A 14-year-old obese child has a BP of 125/80 mm Hg. His weight is 80 kg, and his height is 160 cm. As per 2017 AAP Clinical Practice Guidelines, his BP will be categorized as which of the following?

A. Normal BP
B. Hypertension stage 1
C. Hypertension stage 2
D. Elevated BP

EXPLANATION

This child has BP between 120–129 and 80–85 mm Hg that categorizes him into the elevated BP group. The AAP Clinical Practice Guidelines for Screening and Measurement of High Blood Pressure in Children and Adolescents published in 2017 recommend BP categories as below 13 years and above 13 years. In the <13 years category age, gender and height-based BP charts need to be referred. However, for >13 years, the definition is the same as used for adults.

Key: D

BOOST YOUR KNOWLEDGE

Classification of BP in children according to the new guidelines is as follows:

Classification	*Children aged 1–12 years (percentile based)*	*Adolescents >13 years (mm Hg based)*
Normotensive	<90th percentile	<120/<80 mm Hg
Elevated BP (previously called prehypertension)	≥90th percentile to <95th percentile or 120/80 mm Hg to <95th percentile (whichever is lower)	120/<80–129/<80 mm Hg
Stage 1 hypertension	≥90th percentile to <95th percentile + 12 mm Hg or 130/80 to 139/89 mm Hg (whichever is lower)	130/80–139/89 mm Hg
Stage 2 hypertension	≥95th percentile + 12 mm Hg, or ≥140/90 mm Hg (whichever is lower)	≥140/90 mm Hg

REFERENCE/SOURCE

- Flynn JT, Kaelber DC, Baker-Smith CM, Blowey D, Carroll AE, Daniels SR, et al. Clinical practice guideline for screening and management of high blood pressure in children and adolescents. Pediatrics. 2017;140(3):e20171904.

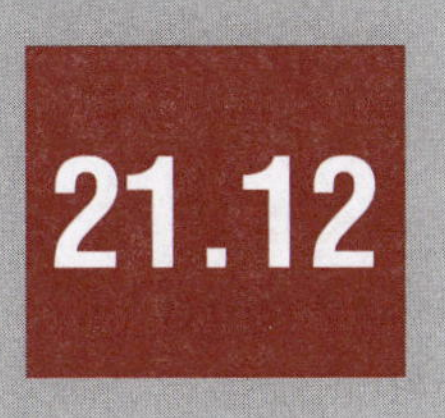

Renal Tubular Disorders

Rajiv Sinha

1. Which of the following is the most common cause of proximal renal tubular acidosis (RTA) in children?

A. Tyrosinemia
B. Cystinosis
C. Cystinuria
D. Malignancy

EXPLANATION

Unlike adults where malignancy is a common cause of proximal RTA, in children it is usually an underlying genetic disease. Among these cystinosis is the most common.

Key: B

BOOST YOUR KNOWLEDGE

Cystinosis, the most common etiology of Fanconi syndrome in children, presents in infancy in ~90% of patients. It is a storage disorder with a lysosomal accumulation of cystine in all organ systems, especially in the kidneys, cornea, thyroid, pancreas, muscle, peripheral nerves, bone marrow, and gonads.

Biallelic loss of function variants in the *CTNS* gene causes this autosomal recessive disorder. *CTNS* encodes for cystinosin, a transmembrane lysosomal protein that actively exports cystine from the lysosome to the cytoplasm. Consequently, cystinosin deficiency causes cystine to accumulate form cystine crystals within the acidic pH of lysosomes in virtually all organ systems.

One should note that cystinuria is not a cause of proximal RTA. It leads to urolithiasis from excess of cysteine in the urine.

REFERENCES/SOURCES

- Bagga A, Sinha A. Renal Tubular Acidosis. Indian J Pediatr. 2020;87(9):733-44.
- van't Hoff WG, Bockenhauer D, Kleta R. Fanconi syndrome. In: Geary DF, Schaefer F (Eds). Comprehensive Pediatric Nephrology, 1st edition. Philadelphia: Mosby; 2018. pp. 433-49.

2. A 3-year-old girl presented with failure to thrive (weight and height < third centile) along with a history of polyuria and polydipsia. The initial work-up is shown below. Which type of RTA is she having?

Blood, urea, and nitrogen (BUN)	11 mg/dL
Creatinine	0.4 mg/dL (eGFR = 93.4 mL/min/1.73 m^2)
Calcium	9.3 mg/dL
Phosphate	1.6 mg/dL
Alkaline phosphatase	1261 U/L
Sodium	136 mmol/L

Contd...

Contd...

Potassium	2.5 mmol/L
Chloride	111 mmol/L
Venous blood gas (VBG)	pH—7.19; HCO_3^- 13 mEq/L, PCO_2—37.9 mm Hg
Urine electrolyte (mmol/L)	Spot urine: Na—39, K—19.5, Cl—52
Urinalysis	pH—5.3, protein-trace, sugar ++, specific gravity—1005
X-ray wrist	Consistent with rickets
Ultrasound Kidney ureter bladder	Bilateral moderate hydronephrosis

A. Type 1
B. Type 2
C. Type 3
D. Type 4

EXPLANATION

The child is having metabolic acidosis (pH 7.19 with HCO_3^- 13). Metabolic acidosis is of normal anion gap (sodium + potassium – chloride + bicarbonate, i.e., 136 + 2.5 – 111 + 13 = 14.5). The urine anion gap (UAG) is positive (Na + K - Cl = 39 + 19.5 – 52 = +6.5, reinforcing the likely diagnosis of RTA. Hypokalemia along with glycosuria and proteinuria suggests proximal RTA and this diagnosis is further reinforced by the fact that urine pH is <5.5. A formal urinary acidification test could be useful in further confirming the diagnosis of proximal RTA (type 2 RTA).

Key: B

BOOST YOUR KNOWLEDGE

Hydronephrosis is not uncommon in children with significant polyuria and is thought to be secondary to high urinary volume rather than due to any obstructive etiology.

Steps for diagnosis and characterization of renal tubular acidosis (RTA)

Step	***Remarks***
Plasma anion gap, calculated as: $Na^+ - (Cl^- + HCO_3^-)$	Normal 8–12 mEq/L in patients with RTA and diarrhea
UAG estimates urine ammonium excretion and is calculated as: $Na^+ + K^+ - Cl^-$	• UAG = 80 – Urinary ammonium excretion • UAG is positive in RTA. Extrarenal bicarbonate losses (diarrhea) cause increased ammonium excretion causing negative UAG
• Urine pH is measured on the freshly voided specimens with a pH meter • The furosemide test involves the administration of furosemide 1 mg/kg with fludrocortisone (1 mg), either simultaneously or 2 hours before testing. Urine pH is checked hourly for a maximum of 6 hours	• pH >5.5 during metabolic acidosis suggests distal RTA; value <5.5 suggests proximal RTA • The furosemide test assesses the ability to lower urine pH maximally provided distal sodium delivery is adequate, especially in patients without metabolic acidosis. In patients with distal RTA, the urine pH remains >5.3
• Bicarbonate loading with oral or intravenous sodium bicarbonate till urine pH >7.5 and blood bicarbonate >22 mEq/L, to estimate: – Fractional excretion of bicarbonate ($FEHCO_3$)* – Urine to blood pCO_2 gradient (U-B CO_2)[†]	• $FEHCO_3$ >15% suggests proximal RTA. The level is normal in distal RTA (<5%) • Urine pCO_2 reflects distal H^+ secretion. U-B CO_2 <10 mm Hg suggests distal RTA. The level is normal in proximal RTA (>20 mm Hg)
• *Additional evaluation:* – Calculation of fractional excretion of phosphate[‡] on a timed (6- and 12-hours) void, to estimate tubular reabsorption of phosphate (TRP)[§] and tubular maximum reabsorption of phosphate corrected for GFR (TmP/GFR)	• About 88–95% of phosphate is reabsorbed in the proximal tubule. The threshold for urinary phosphate excretion is expressed as TmP/GFR, derived using the Bijvoet nomogram to index for plasma phosphorus and kidney function. TmP/GFR <2.8 reflects phosphaturia

Contd...

Contd…

Step	Remarks
– Urinary aminoacidogram, beta-2-micrglobin, glucose – 24-hour urine calcium, ultrasound for nephrocalcinosis, hearing assessment – Slit lamp examination for cysteine crystals	• Markers of proximal tubular dysfunction • Patients with distal RTA may have hypercalciuria (urine calcium >4 mg/kg/day), nephrocalcinosis, and hearing loss • Corneal cystine crystals, a diagnostic marker of cystinosis, are found in patients older than 2-years
• Clinical exome sequencing for variations in implicated genes	Genetic studies enable diagnosis, prognostication, and prenatal diagnosis

$$^{*}FEHCO_3\,(\%) = \frac{\text{Urine bicarbonate} \times \text{serum creatinine} \times 100}{\text{Serum bicarbonate} \times \text{urine creatinine}}$$

$$^{\dagger}\text{U-B } CO_2 = \text{urine } pCO_2 - \text{blood } pCO_2$$

$$^{\ddagger}FEPO_4\,(\%) = \frac{\text{Urine phosphate} \times \text{plasma creatinine} \times 100}{\text{Plasma phosphate} \times \text{urine creatinine}}$$

$$^{\S}TRP\,(\%) = 100 - FEPO_4\,(\%)$$

Differentiating between the different types of renal tubular acidosis (RTA)

		Distal RTA		
	Proximal RTA	***Classic***	***Hyperkalimic (voltage-dependent)***	***Type IV RTA***
Plasma K	Normal/low	Low	High	High
Urine pH	<5.3	>5.3	>5.3	<5.3
UAG	Positive	Positive	Positive	Positive
Fractional excretion of HCO_3	>10–15%	<5%	<5%	>5–10%
U-B P CO_2	>20	<20	<20	>20
Urine calcium	Normal	High	High/normal	Normal/low
Other tubular defects	Usually, present	Absent	Absent	Absent
Nephrocalcinosis	Absent	Present	Present/absent	Absent
Rickets	Usually, present	Usually, present	Uncommon	Absent

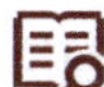

REFERENCES/SOURCES

- Bagga A, Sinha A. Renal Tubular Acidosis. Indian J Pediatr. 2020;87(9):733-44.
- Bianchetti MG, Bettinelli A. Differential diagnosis and management of fluid, electrolyte, and acid–base disorders. In: Geary DF, Schaefer F (Eds). Comprehensive Pediatric Nephrology, 1st edition. Philadelphia: Mosby; 2018. pp. 395-431.
- Khandelwal P, Bagga A. Renal Tubular Disorders. In: Ramchandran P, Gupta A, Gupta P, Menon PSN (Eds). IAP Recent Advances in Pediatrics, 2nd edition. New Delhi: Jaypee Brothers Medical Publishers; 2022.
- van't Hoff WG, Bockenhauer D, Kleta R. Fanconi syndrome. In: Geary DF, Schaefer F (Eds). Comprehensive Pediatric Nephrology, 1st edition. Philadelphia: Mosby; 2018. pp. 433-49.

3. Which of the following is relatively uncommon in Fanconi syndrome/proximal RTA?

A. Glycosuria
B. Aminoaciduria
C. Nephrocalcinosis
D. Proteinuria

EXPLANATION

The hallmark of proximal tubulopathy is the loss of glucose along with amino acids and tubular protein in the urine. They usually have high urinary citrate levels and hence nephrocalcinosis is uncommon in it. Dent/Lowe syndrome despite proximal RTA may have nephrocalcinosis.

Key: C

BOOST YOUR KNOWLEDGE

Hypocitraturia is common in distal RTA and is one of the reasons for nephrocalcinosis.

REFERENCES/SOURCES

- Bagga A, Sinha A. Renal Tubular Acidosis. Indian J Pediatr. 2020;87(9):733-44.
- Bianchetti MG, Bettinelli A. Differential diagnosis and management of fluid, electrolyte, and acid–base disorders. In: Geary DF, Schaefer F (Eds). Comprehensive Pediatric Nephrology, 1st edition. Philadelphia: Mosby; 2018. pp. 395-431.
- van't Hoff WG, Bockenhauer D, Kleta R. Fanconi syndrome. In: Geary DF, Schaefer F (Eds). Comprehensive Pediatric Nephrology, 1st edition. Philadelphia: Mosby; 2018. pp. 433-49.

4. Which extra renal manifestation is usually not commonly seen in distal RTA?

A. Hemolytic anemia
B. Sensorineural deafness
C. Amelogenesis imperfecta
D. Photophobia

EXPLANATION

Hemolytic anemia, sensorineural deafness, and amelogenesis imperfecta are found in certain variants of distal renal tubular acidosis (dRTA).

Key: D

BOOST YOUR KNOWLEDGE

Photophobia is due to corneal crystal deposition in cystinosis and is uncommon in dRTA. The genetic causes of dRTA with extrarenal manifestations are shown here:

Etiology	*Gene, protein*	*Additional features*
Distal RTA	*SCL4A1*, anion exchanger 1 (Cl^-/HCO_3^- exchanger)	Hemolytic anemia
	ATP6V1B1, H^+-ATPase (B1 subunit); Forkhead transcription factor 11 (*FOXI1*)	Early onset deafness
	ATP6V0A4, H^+-adenosine triphosphatase (ATPase) (A4 subunit)	Normal hearing or delayed hearing loss
	WDR72, tryptophan-aspartate repeat domain 72	Amelogenesis imperfecta

REFERENCES/SOURCES

- Bianchetti MG, Bettinelli A. Differential diagnosis and management of fluid, electrolyte, and acid–base disorders. In: Geary DF, Schaefer F (Eds). Comprehensive Pediatric Nephrology, 1st edition. Philadelphia: Mosby; 2018. pp. 395-431.
- Khandelwal P, Bagga A. Renal Tubular Disorders. In: Ramchandran P, Gupta A, Gupta P, Menon PSN (Eds). IAP Recent Advances in Pediatrics, 2nd edition. New Delhi: Jaypee Brothers Medical Publishers; 2022.
- van't Hoff WG, Bockenhauer D, Kleta R. Fanconi syndrome. In: Geary DF, Schaefer F (Eds). Comprehensive Pediatric Nephrology, 1st edition. Philadelphia: Mosby; 2018. pp. 433-49.

5. Which of the following genes is *not* associated with Bartter syndrome?

A. *SLC12A1* coding for Na–K–Cl cotransporter (NKCC2) protein channel
B. *KCNJ1* coding for renal outer medullary potassium channel (ROMK) protein channel
C. *CLCKNB* coding for chloride channel Kb (ClC-Kb) protein channel
D. *SLC12A3* coding for sodium-chloride cotransporter (NCC) protein channel

EXPLANATION

SLC12A3 codes for the NCC protein channel, i.e., NCC and its dysfunction leads to Gitelman syndrome.

Key: D

BOOST YOUR KNOWLEDGE

Different genotypes of Bartter syndrome

Type	Inheritance	Gene	Affected protein
BS type 1	Autosomal recessive	*SLC12A1*	NKCC2
BS type 2	Autosomal recessive	*KCNJ1*	ROMK
BS type 3	Autosomal recessive	*CLCNKB*	CLC-Kb
BS type 4	Autosomal recessive	*BSND, CLCKNB + CLCKNA*	Barttin protein or CLC-Kb and Ka combined
BS type 5	X-Linked recessive	*MAGED2*	MAGED2

Clinical/biochemical differentiation between various subtypes of Bartter syndrome

Characteristic	BS type 1	BS type 2	BS type 3	BS type 4	BS type 5
Polyhydramnios	Present	Present	Absent	Present	Present
Leading symptoms	Polyuria, hypochloremia, alkalosis, and hypokalemia	Polyuria, hypochloremia, alkalosis, and transient neonatal hyperkalemia	Hypokalemia, hypochloremia, alkalosis, and failure to thrive	Polyuria, hypochloremia, alkalosis, and hypokalemia	Polyuria, hypochloremia, alkalosis, and hypokalemia Often transient
Calcium phosphate	High	High	Variable	Variable	High
Nephrocalcinosis	Present	Present	Rare	Rare	Sometime
Plasma chloride/ sodium	Normal	Normal	Decreased	Decreased	Increased
Hypomagnesemia	Absent	Absent	+/–	+/–	Absent
Deafness	Absent	Absent	Absent	Present	Absent

REFERENCES/SOURCES

- Konrad M, Nijenhuis T, Ariceta G, Bertholet-Thomas A, Calo LA, Capasso G, et al. Diagnosis and management of Bartter syndrome: executive summary of the consensus and recommendations from the European Rare Kidney Disease Reference Network Working Group for Tubular Disorders. Kidney Int. 2021;99(2):324-35.
- Waldegger S. Bartter, Gitelman, and related syndromes. In: Geary DF, Schaefer F (Eds). Comprehensive Pediatric Nephrology, 1st edition. Philadelphia: Mosby; 2018. pp. 451-9.

6. Which of the following type of Bartter syndrome is associated with sensorineural deafness?

A. Type 1 defect in *SLC12A1* gene coding for NKCC2 protein channel
B. Type 2 *KCNJ1* coding for ROMK protein channel
C. Type 3 *CLCNKB* coding for CLC-Kb protein channel
D. Type 4 *BSND* coding for Barttin protein channel

EXPLANATION

Barttin defect is invariably associated with sensorineural deafness.

Key: D

BOOST YOUR KNOWLEDGE

The marginal cells of the *stria vascularis* contribute to the endolymph formation by apical potassium secretion. Transcellular potassium transport is mediated by the furosemide-sensitive NKCC1, ensuring basolateral potassium entry into the marginal cells. Voltage-dependent potassium channels mediate apical potassium secretion into the endolymph. The proper function of NKCC1 requires basolateral recycling of chloride. Deafness associated with Barttin deficiency suggests that this recycling is enabled by the ClCK/Barttin channel complex.

REFERENCES/SOURCES

- Konrad M, Nijenhuis T, Ariceta G, Bertholet-Thomas A, Calo LA, Capasso G, et al. Diagnosis and management of Bartter syndrome: executive summary of the consensus and recommendations from the European Rare Kidney Disease Reference Network Working Group for Tubular Disorders. Kidney Int. 2021;99(2):324-35.
- Waldegger S. Bartter, Gitelman, and related syndromes. In: Geary DF, Schaefer F (Eds). Comprehensive Pediatric Nephrology, 1st edition. Philadelphia: Mosby; 2018. pp. 451-9.

7. Bartter syndrome is classically associated with hypokalemia. Which type of Bartter syndrome is associated with transient neonatal hyperkalemia?

A. Type 1 defect in *SLC12A1* coding for NKCC2 protein channel
B. Type 2 *KCNJ1* coding for ROMK protein channel
C. Type 3 *CLCNKB* coding for CLC-Kb protein channel
D. Type 4 *BSND* coding for Barttin protein channel

EXPLANATION

Mutation in *KCNJ1* coding ROMK exhibits transient hyperkalemia in the first days of life.

Key: B

BOOST YOUR KNOWLEDGE

The simultaneous appearance of hyperkalemia and hyponatremia resembles the clinical picture of mineralocorticoid deficiency (which, however, shows low aldosterone levels) or that of pseudohypoaldosteronism type I (PHA-I) (high aldosterone levels). Several cases of PHA-I which classically present with hyperkalemia have turned out to be a misdiagnosis with subsequent genetic analysis revealing ROMK mutations as the underlying defect. The severity of initial hyperkalemia decreases with gestational age. Hyperkalemia may be attributed to the additional role of ROMK in the cortical collecting duct (CCD) where it participates in the process of potassium secretion.

REFERENCES/SOURCES

- Konrad M, Nijenhuis T, Ariceta G, Bertholet-Thomas A, Calo LA, Capasso G, et al. Diagnosis and management of Bartter syndrome: executive summary of the consensus and recommendations from the European Rare Kidney Disease Reference Network Working Group for Tubular Disorders. Kidney Int. 2021;99(2):324-35.
- Waldegger S. Bartter, Gitelman, and related syndromes. In: Geary DF, Schaefer F (Eds). Comprehensive Pediatric Nephrology, 1st edition. Philadelphia: Mosby; 2018. pp. 451-9.

8. Pattern recognition is important in tubular disorders. Which of the following patterns are wrongly matched with the likely disease?

A. Failure to thrive, polyuria, glycosuria, hypophosphatemia, and hypokalemia with normal anion gap metabolic acidosis—proximal RTA
B. Failure to thrive with polyuria, hypercalciuria, and hypokalemia with metabolic alkalosis—Bartter syndrome

C. Failure to thrive, hyperkalemia, hyponatremia, normal anion gap metabolic acidosis—type 4 RTA
D. Failure to thrive, hypokalemia, metabolic alkalosis with hypotension—Gordon syndrome

EXPLANATION

Pseudohypoaldosteronism type II (also called *Gordon syndrome or familial hyperkalemia*) is an autosomal-dominant form of hypertension associated with hyperkalemia, normal glomerular filtration rate, and occasionally increased renal salt reabsorption and acidemia.

Key: D

BOOST YOUR KNOWLEDGE

Biochemical fingerprint for tubulopathy

	Proximal tubule Classical representative tubulopathy: Type 2 proximal RTA	*Thick ascending loop of Henle Classical representative tubulopathy: Bartter syndrome*	*Distal convoluted tubule Classical representative tubulopathy: Gitelman syndrome*	*Collecting ducts Classical representative tubulopathy: Type 4 RTA*
Plasma sodium	Normal	Normal	Normal	Low-normal
Plasma potassium	Low	Low	Low	High
Plasma bicarbonate	Low	High	High	Low
Plasma magnesium	Normal	Low-normal	Low	Normal
Plasma phosphate	Low	Normal	Normal	Normal
Urine potassium	High	High	High	Low
Urine calcium	High	High	Low	Low
Tubular proteins	High	Normal	Normal	Normal

REFERENCES/SOURCES

- Bianchetti MG, Bettinelli A. Differential diagnosis and management of fluid, electrolyte, and acid–base disorders. In: Geary DF, Schaefer F (Eds). Comprehensive Pediatric Nephrology, 1st edition. Philadelphia: Mosby; 2018. pp. 395-431.
- van't Hoff WG, Bockenhauer D, Kleta R. Fanconi syndrome. In: Geary DF, Schaefer F (Eds). Comprehensive Pediatric Nephrology, 1st edition. Philadelphia: Mosby; 2018. pp. 433-49.
- Waldegger S. Bartter, Gitelman, and related syndromes. In: Geary DF, Schaefer F (Eds). Comprehensive Pediatric Nephrology, 1st edition. Philadelphia: Mosby; 2018. pp. 451-9.

9. A 7-year-old girl was referred to pediatric nephrology for incidental hypertension. Her clinic blood pressure was 140/90, sodium 137 mmol/L, potassium 2.2 mmol/L, chloride 100 mmol/L, bicarbonate 35 mmol/L, urinary Na 18, and urinary chloride 128. She had a past history of recurrent urinary tract infections and her father had died from a Stroke at 45 years after being on antihypertensive medication since 19 years of age. Ultrasound and Doppler of kidneys were normal and echocardiography showed mild left ventricular hypertrophy. Plasma renin activity (PRA) was 0.01 ng/mL/h (N—0.5-3 ng/mL/h) and aldosterone <10 pg/mL (N—5-90 ng/dL). The urinary steroid profile was normal. Which is the most likely underlying etiology for her hypertension?

A. Renal artery stenosis
B. Familial hyperaldosteronism
C. Liddle syndrome
D. Gordon syndrome

EXPLANATION

Among the four options Gordon and Liddle syndrome has low PRA but the presence of hypokalemia goes in favor of Liddle syndrome whereas Gordon syndrome usually has hyperkalemia. Renin artery stenosis is renin-mediated hypertension with high PRA levels. Familial hyperaldosteronism is associated with very high levels of aldosterone (with comparatively low renin levels).

Key: C

BOOST YOUR KNOWLEDGE

Differential diagnosis of low PRA hypertension

	Physiology	*Genetics*
Steroidogenic enzyme defects:		
Steroid 11β-hydroxylase deficiency	• High serum androgens/urine 17 ketosteroids; elevated DOC and 11-deoxycortiso • Low PRA and aldosterone	*CYP11B1* mutation (encodes cytochrome P45011β/18 of zona fasciculata); impairs synthesis of cortisol and zona fasciculata 17 deoxysteroids
Steroid 11α-hydroxylase/17,20-lyase deficiency	• Low serum/urinary 17-hydroxysteroids; decreased cortisol, high corticosterone (B), and DOC in plasma; serum androgens and estrogens very low; serum gonadotropins very high • Low PRA and aldosterone	*CYP17* mutation (encodes cytochrome P450C17) impairs cortisol and sex steroid production
Hyperaldosteronism:		
Primary aldosteronism/adrenocortical hyperplasia	• Normal 18-OH/aldosterone ratio • High aldosterone but low PRA	Genetics yet to be determined. Very rare in children
Glucocorticoid remediable aldosteronism (GRA)	High Aldosterone and low PRA. Plasma and urinary aldo responsive to adrenocorticotropic hormone (ACTH); as well as dexamethasone suppressible within 48 hours	Unequal crossing over between the *CYP11B1* and *CYP11B2* genes generates a chimeric product that is ACTH-sensitive and produces aldosterone
Syndrome of apparent mineralocorticoid excess	High aldosterone and low PRA. hydroxysteroid 11-beta dehydrogenase 2 (HSD11B2) deficiency allows excess cortisol stimulation at the mineralocorticoid receptor (MR)	Type 2 11β-OHSD mutations
Nonsteroidal defects:		
Liddle's syndrome	Low aldosterone and PRA with normal or low potassium. Abnormality in epithelial sodium transporter, epithelial sodium channel (ENaC)	Hyperactive ENaC reabsorbs sodium at elevated levels, resulting in volume expansion and hypertension
Pseudohypoaldosteronism II—Gordon syndrome	Normal aldosterone but low PRA with high potassium	Mutations in regulatory proteins for the NCC channel allow for unchecked activity, causing subsequent electrolyte and fluid overabsorption

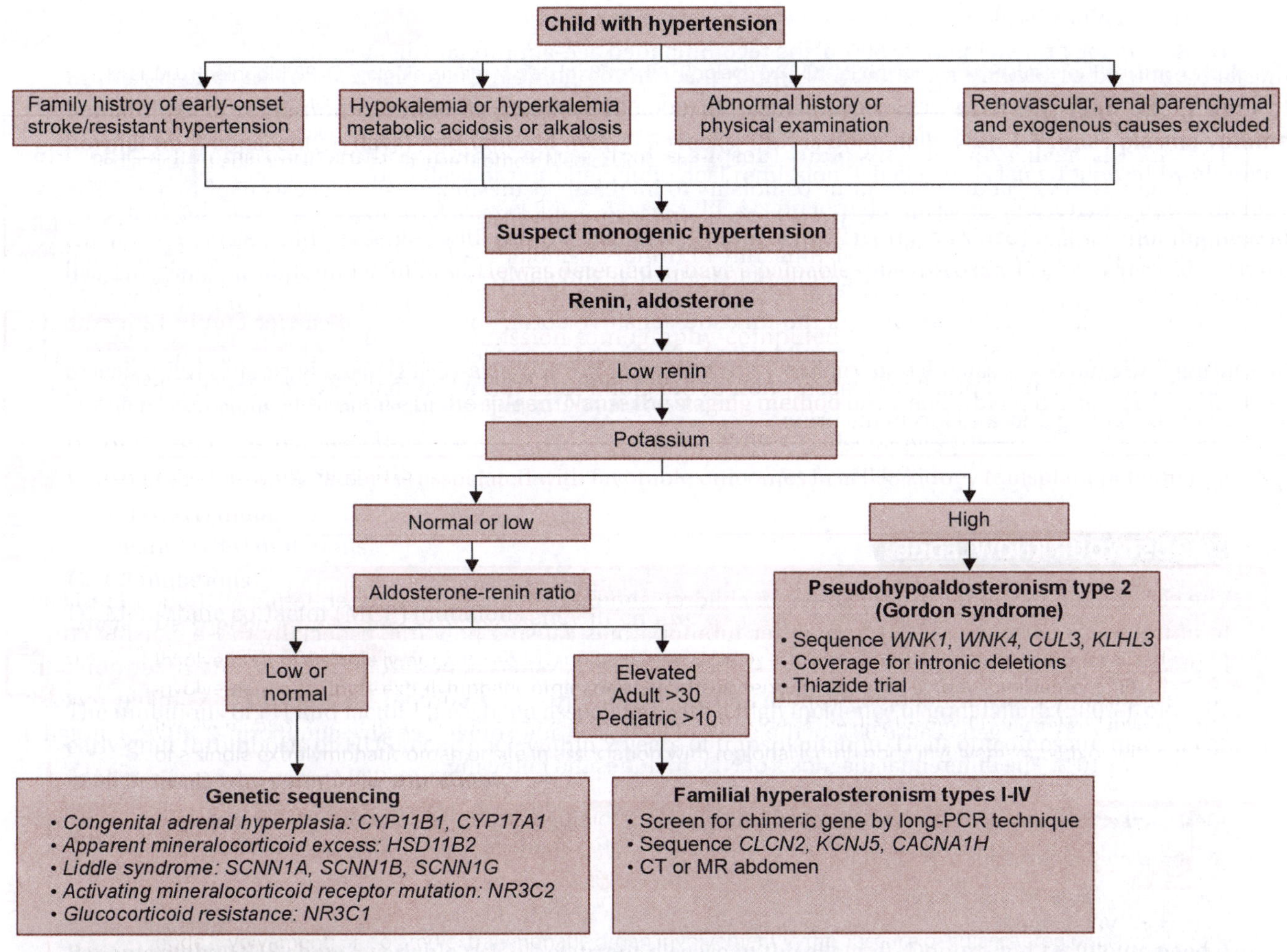

REFERENCES/SOURCES

- Ingelfinger JR. Etiology of childhood hypertension. In: Geary DF, Schaefer F (Eds). Comprehensive Pediatric Nephrology, 1st edition. Philadelphia: Mosby; 2018. pp. 665-75.
- Raina R, Krishnappa V, Das A, Amin H, Radhakrishnan Y, Nair NR, et al. Overview of monogenic or mendelian forms of hypertension. Front Pediatr. 2019;7:263.

10. A 13-month-old boy presents with polyuria, polydipsia, and failure to thrive. His electrolytes were Na 160 mmol/L, K 3.9 mmol/L, chloride 112 mmol/L, bicarbonate 24 mmol/L, creatinine 0.6 mg/dL. He underwent a paired serum and urine osmolality test followed by a desmopressin challenge test as detailed in the table below. Which of the following can be useful in his management?

Biochemistry	*Predesmopressin*	*Postdesmopressin*
Serum sodium, mmol/L	160	163
Urine sodium, mmol/L	16	14
Plasma osmolality, mOsm/kg	305	298
Urine osmolality, mOsm/kg	144	138

A. Initiation of desmopressin to reduce polyuria
B. Fluid restriction—which will reduce polyuria

C. Hydrochlorothiazide
D. Restricting protein intake to 50% of the recommended age-appropriate dietary intake

EXPLANATION

The child is having diabetes insipidus (despite a high serum sodium and plasma osmolality—the urine osmolality is low). Failure of the urine osmolality to increase postdesmopressin suggests nephrogenic diabetes insipidus (NDI). Desmopressin hence is unlikely to work. Fluid restriction will further worsen hypernatremia. Although protein does contribute significantly to urinary osmolar load, restricting it in an infant will hamper growth. Hydrochlorothiazide has been shown to be useful in NDI. It is postulated that hydrochlorothiazide decreases salt reabsorption through the thiazide-sensitive cotransporter solute carrier family 12 member 3 (*SLC12A3*) in the distal tubule. The resultant loss of sodium in urine leads to a reduction in plasma volume with subsequent enhanced proximal reabsorption of the glomerular filtrate so that less water would be presented to the collecting duct and lost in the urine.

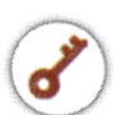

Key: C

BOOST YOUR KNOWLEDGE

The clinical and biochemical assessment in children should be focused on differentiating NDI due to resistance to antidiuretic hormone, ADH) from other tubulopathies causing polyuria, especially those causing chronic hypokalemia or hypercalciuria, structural kidney diseases (dysplasia, nephronophthisis) and other nonkidney causes, such as central diabetes insipidus, diabetes mellitus, and adrenal insufficiency. X-linked recessive defects in the *AVPR2* gene cause 90% of the cases of NDI, and autosomal recessive aquaporin-2 (*AQP2*) mutations account for 10%. The differential diagnosis of NDI includes the following:

Basic defect	***Acquired etiology***	***Hereditary etiology***
Central diabetes insipidus:		
Deficiency in arginine vasopressin disorder (AVP) synthesis or secretion	• Cranial trauma • Cranial neoplasia • Cranial vascular malformation • Cranial granuloma/infectious • Inflammatory or autoimmune • Drug or toxin exposure	• Rare • Autosomal dominant/autosomal recessive *AVP* mutations
NDI:		
Reduced renal sensitivity to antidiuretic effect of physiological AVP levels	• Drug exposure • Hypercalemia or hypokalemia • Infiltrating lesions • Vascular disorders	• X-linked: *AVPR2* mutations • *Autosomal recessive or* dominant: *AQP2* mutations
Primary polydipsia:		
Excessive fluid intake at a diminished set point	• Psychosis • Compulsive water drinker	

REFERENCES/SOURCES

- Bockenhauer D, Bichet DG. Pathophysiology, diagnosis and management of nephrogenic diabetes insipidus. Nat Rev Nephrol. 2015;11(10):576-88.
- Böckenhauer D. Diabetes insipidus. In: Geary DF, Schaefer F (Eds). Comprehensive Pediatric Nephrology, 1st edition. Philadelphia: Mosby; 2018. pp. 489-98.
- Christ-Crain M, Bichet DG, Fenske WK, Goldman MB, Rittig S, Verbalis JG, Verkman AS. Diabetes insipidus. Nat Rev Dis Primers. 2019;5(1):54.

11. Which of the following is wrongly matched?

A. A 6-month-old girl with recurrent episodes of fever, and a history of polyhydramnios. Her weight and length are on the 0.4th and 10th centile, blood pressure is 80/60 mm Hg
Investigations: pH 7.47, bicarbonate 32 mEq/L, Na 135 mEq/L, K 2.1 mEq/L, Cl 80 mEq/L, creatinine 0.6 mg/dL, Urine Na 40 mEq/L, and K 50 mEq/L—*Bartter syndrome.*

B. 18-month-old boy, with 6-month history of polyuria and polydipsia. Swollen wrist and knee, photophobia, and blood pressure 100/80 on examination
Investigations: pH 7.25, HCO_3 18 mEq/L, Na 130 mEq/L, K 2.7 mEq/L, creatinine 0.8 mg/dL, calcium 10.2 mg/dL, phosphate 2.3 mg/dL, serum alkaline phosphatase (SAP) 2030 IU/L, thyroid-stimulating hormone (TSH) raised, T3 low. Urine dipstick proteinuria 3+—*cystinosis*

C. A 2-year-old boy with failure to thrive, bilateral congenital cataract, global developmental delay, and hypotonia
Investigations: Na 135 mEq/L, K 3.2 mEq/L, Cr 0.6 mg/dL, phosphate 3.0 mg/dL, calcium 10.1 mg/dL, pH 7.29, HCO_3 15 mEq/L, CL 108 mEq/L, Urine pH 5.5, glucose positive—*Lowe syndrome*

D. A 2-year-old presented with chronic diarrhea and a recurrent history of pneumonia. His weight is on the 0.4th centile and height 25th centile. Blood pressure is 90/60
Investigations: pH 7.47, pCO_2 40 mm Hg, HCO_3 30 mmol/L. Urine Na 3 mmol/L, urine chloride 7 mmol/L. Serum Na 135 mmol/L, K 2.7 mmol/L, creatinine 0.2 mg/dL, magnesium 1.4 mmol/L—*EAST syndrome*

EXPLANATION

Scenario (d) has hypokalemic metabolic alkalosis but unlike Bartter/Gitelman/EAST syndrome there is no urinary loss of chloride (<15–20 mEq/L) which makes these disorders unlikely. The case favors a diagnosis of pseudo-Bartter syndrome most probably secondary to cystic fibrosis. Hence the child should be worked up for cystic fibrosis.

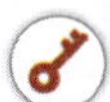

Key: D

BOOST YOUR KNOWLEDGE

Approach to a child with metabolic alkalosis and hypokalemia:

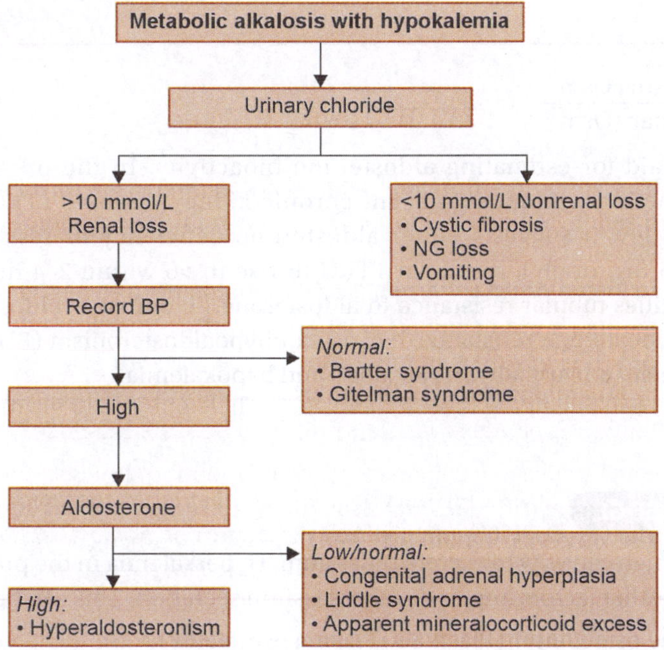

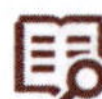

REFERENCES/SOURCES

- Bagga A, Sinha A. Renal Tubular Acidosis. Indian J Pediatr. 2020;87(9):733-44.
- Chapters 27, 28, 29, 43. In: Geary DF, Schaefer F (Eds). Comprehensive Pediatric Nephrology, 1st edition. Philadelphia: Mosby; 2018.

12. **An 11-month-old girl presented with failure to thrive (birth weight 2.6 kg; current weight 3.9 kg). She was admitted twice for respiratory tract infection. Her biochemical work-up is given below. The transtubular potassium gradient (TTKG) calculated for hyperkalemia was 1.2. Which one of the following statements related to TTKG is correct?**

Biochemical	*Plasma*	*Urine*	*Remarks*
Sodium (Na), mmol/L	126	70	
Potassium (K), mmol/L	8.0	8	
Chloride (Cl), mmol/L	109	65	
Bicarbonate (HCO_3), mEq/L	16		
Anion gap (Na + K – Cl + HCO_3)	15	33	
Osmolality (Osm), mOsm/Kg	234	290	
Renin, ng/mL/h	0.9		(normal 2.9–24)
Aldosterone, pg/mL	92,000		(30–160)

A. $\text{TTKG} = \dfrac{\text{Urinary Na} \times \text{Plasma Osm}}{\text{Plasma K} \times \text{Urinary Osm}}$

B. $\text{TTKG} = \dfrac{\text{Urinary K} \times \text{Urinary Osm}}{\text{Plasma K} \times \text{Plasma Osm}}$

C. Values <7 among persons with hyperkalemia imply impaired potassium secretion either due to aldosterone deficiency or resistance.

D. The most likely underlying diagnosis for the child is: Primary hyperaldosteronism

EXPLANATION

$$\text{TTKG} = \frac{\text{Urinary K} \times \text{Plasma Osm}}{\text{Plasma K} \times \text{Urinary Osm}}$$

TTKG is an important aid for estimating aldosterone bioactivity. In the presence of hyperkalemia and appropriate tubular function without significant chronic kidney disease, TTKG is usually >10. If despite hyperkalemia, TTKG is low it suggests either aldosterone deficiency or resistance. Fludrocortisone, in physiological dose (0.05 mg, orally), results in TTKG to rise to >6 within 2–4 hours in hypoaldosteronism. The absence of this signifies tubular resistance to aldosterone. In our case, aldosterone is already very high, and this points toward aldosterone resistance, i.e., pseudohypoaldosteronism (PHA). Option D is wrong as in primary hyperaldosteronism one usually gets alkalosis and hypokalemia.

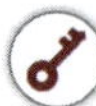

Key: C

BOOST YOUR KNOWLEDGE

The kidneys have a very high capacity to excrete potassium. Hyperkalemia in the presence of good urinary output develops virtually only if other factors impair distal potassium secretion. This can be estimated using TTKG:

TTKG = (Urine K/Urine osmolality)/(Plasma K/Plasma osmolality)

TTKG in normal persons is generally in the range of 6–12. Hypokalemia would result in potassium conservation by the kidney and TTKG will be <2. If TTKG in the presence of hypokalemia is >2 it indicates renal loss. During hyperkalemia, the expected TTKG is >10 and a value <7 would indicate aldosterone resistance or aldosterone deficiency.

REFERENCES/SOURCES

- Bagga A, Sinha A. Renal Tubular Acidosis. Indian J Pediatr. 2020;87(9):733-44.
- Bianchetti MG, Bettinelli A. Differential diagnosis and management of fluid, electrolyte, and acid–base disorders. In: Geary DF, Schaefer F (Eds). Comprehensive Pediatric Nephrology, 1st edition. Philadelphia: Mosby; 2018. pp. 395-431.
- Tubular disease. In: Rees L, Brogan P, Bockenhauer D, Webb W (Eds). Pediatric Nephrology, 2nd edition. Oxford, Oxford University Press; 2012.

CHAPTER

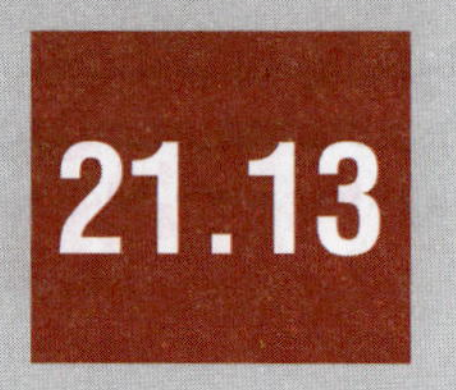

21.13 Lupus Nephritis, Renal Calculi, Alport Syndrome, and Related Disorders

Manish Kumar

1. According to the 2019 European League Against Rheumatism (EULAR)/American College of Rheumatology (ACR) classification criteria, which of the following is an entry criterion for the diagnosis of systemic lupus erythematosus (SLE)?

A. Fever with a rash
B. Anti-double-stranded deoxyribonucleic acid (dsDNA) antibody
C. Antinuclear antibody (ANA) titer of ≥1:80 by immunofluorescence (IF) assay
D. ANA titer of ≥1:160 by IF assay

EXPLANATION

Systemic lupus erythematous classification has evolved over time from ACR 1997 to Systemic Lupus International Collaborating Clinics (SLICC) 2012 to finally ACR/EULAR 2019 classification system. ACR 1997 required 4/11 criteria, out of which at least one should be clinical or immunological criteria. SLICC 2012 required 4 criteria, at least one clinical and one immunological criterion, or kidney biopsy-proven nephritis and positive ANA. ACR/EULAR criteria required an ANA titer of 1:80 or higher by IF; plus, a score of ≥10 points on clinical and immunological criteria.

Key: C

BOOST YOUR KNOWLEDGE

Fever as a constitutional symptom is present in up to 50% of cases, with mucocutaneous involvement in up to 90% of cases. Approximately half of the children with SLE develop kidney involvement at one time of their disease course, with 80–90% developing lupus nephritis (LN) within 1 year of diagnosis of SLE. Though ANA is used as a screening test for SLE, diagnosis is confirmed with more specific autoantibodies, such as anti-dsDNA, associated with homogenous, and peripheral ANA patterns on IF. Antismith antibody, specific for SLE, though poorly sensitive, is associated with speckled ANA pattern on IF. Other immunological criteria for SLE diagnosis are low C3 and/or C4 and the presence of antiphospholipid antibodies.

REFERENCE/SOURCE

- Lupus nephritis. In: Emma F, Goldstein SL, Bagga A, Bates CM, Shroff R (Eds). Pediatric Nephrology, 8th edition. Switzerland AG: Springer Nature; 2022. pp. 507-31.

2. Each of the following diseases is associated with the presence of a specific autoantibody:

a. SLE	1. Lupus anticoagulant
b. Antiphospholipid syndrome	2. Antifactor H antibody
c. Membranous nephropathy	3. Antiphospholipase A2 receptor (PLA2R) antibody
d. Atypical hemolytic uremic syndrome	4. Antismith antibody

Select the correct matching option from below:

A. a-1, b-3, c-3, d-2
B. a-1, b-3, c-4, d-2
C. a-4, b-3, c-1, d-2
D. a-4, b-1, c-3, d-2

EXPLANATION

Antismith antibody is a specific autoantibody for SLE. Antiphospholipid syndrome is characterized by the presence of any of the three autoantibodies, namely lupus anticoagulant, anticardiolipin, and anti-β2 glycoprotein-I antibodies. Primary membranous nephropathy is characterized by the presence of anti-PLA2R antibody (anti-PLA2R antibody) and antifactor H antibodies are present in up to 50% of cases of the atypical hemolytic uremic syndrome.

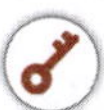

Key: D

BOOST YOUR KNOWLEDGE

Antiphospholipid antibodies are detected in up to 30% of cases of childhood SLE. The presence of at least one antiphospholipid antibody in patients with SLE increases the risk of arterial, venous, or small-vessel thrombosis in any tissue or organ.

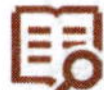

REFERENCE/SOURCE

- Autoantibodies and kidney diseases. In: Emma F, Goldstein SL, Bagga A, Bates CM, Shroff R (Eds). Pediatric Nephrology, 8th edition. Switzerland AG: Springer Nature; 2022. pp. 541-58.

3. A 10-year-old boy presents with a history of fever, generalized swelling, and decreased urine output for 7 days. On examination, pedal edema+ and blood pressure (BP) were 130/86 mm Hg. Laboratory tests reveal urine protein 4+, 30–40 red blood cells (RBCs)/high power field (HPF), serum albumin—2.5 g/dL, creatinine—0.4 mg/dL, C3—76 mg/dL and ANA/dsDNA-reactive. Kidney biopsy shows diffuse thickening of the glomerular capillary wall, "full house" IF pattern, and subepithelial immune deposits. Which of the following is the most likely histopathological classification of LN?

A. Class II
B. Class III
C. Class IV
D. Class V

EXPLANATION

In class II LN, there is mesangial hypercellularity with immune complex deposits. Class III and class IV LN are characterized by endocapillary proliferation with subendothelial immune complex deposition, whereas class V LN, also known as membranous nephritis, is characterized by diffuse thickening of the GBM and subepithelial immune complex deposition. So, the correct answer is "D".

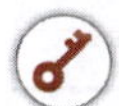

Key: D

BOOST YOUR KNOWLEDGE

Kidney biopsy is indicated in cases with nephrotic syndrome where it is associated with hypertension, hematuria, or any systemic signs, such as rash and arthritis. In the above-mentioned case, kidney biopsy is suggestive of LN. Classification of LN is based on the recommendations of the International Society of Nephrology (ISN)/Renal Pathology Society (RPS) revised in 2018. Class I and II are also termed as nonproliferative LN, whereas classes III and IV are termed as proliferative glomerulonephritis (GN). In class I LN, glomeruli are histologically normal with mesangial immune complex deposition, whereas in class II glomerulonephritis, there is a mild mesangial hypercellularity with immune complex deposition. In class III or focal LN, a type of proliferative glomerulonephritis, <50% of glomeruli are involved, whereas, in class IV LN, >50% of glomeruli are affected. There is marked endocapillary proliferation, with subendothelial immune deposits, resulting in characteristic "wire-loop" lesions.

REFERENCE/SOURCE

- Lupus nephritis. In: Emma F, Goldstein SL, Bagga A, Bates CM, Shroff R (Eds). Pediatric Nephrology, 8th edition. Switzerland AG: Springer Nature; 2022. pp. 507-31.

4. An 8-year-old boy presenting with initial steroid-resistant nephrotic syndrome shows features of membranous glomerulonephritis on kidney biopsy. Which of the following investigations is least helpful in further evaluation of this child?

A. Hepatitis B virus serology
B. Anti-PLA2R antibody
C. ANA/anti-ds DNA antibody
D. Antineutrophilic cytoplasmic antibody (ANCA)

EXPLANATION

Histopathology findings of membranous glomerulonephritis are seen in primary membranous glomerulonephritis due to anti-PLA2R antibody, or secondary causes of membranous nephropathy due to hepatitis B infection or LN class V. LN is associated with the presence of ANA/anti-dsDNA autoantibodies. ANCA serology is not helpful in cases with membranous glomerulonephritis. So, the correct answer is option "D".

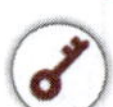

Key: D

BOOST YOUR KNOWLEDGE

Antineutrophil cytoplasmic antibodies, based upon the IF staining pattern, cytoplasmic (C-ANCA) or perinuclear (P-ANCA), are autoantibodies against the cytoplasmic antigens expressed in the primary granules of neutrophils. These are associated with a group of disorders characterized by necrotizing inflammation of small to medium blood vessels, called ANCA-associated vasculitides. P-ANCA corroborates to antimyeloperoxidase (anti-MPO) antibody on enzyme-linked immunosorbent assay (ELISA) and is associated with necrotizing small vessel vasculitis, whereas C-ANCA corroborates to antiproteinase 3 (anti-PR-3) antibody and is associated with granulomatosis polyangiitis. Anti-GBM antibody disease or Goodpasture syndrome may be associated with the coexistence of anti-GBM antibody and ANCA in up to one-third of cases, where the histopathology finding is crescentic glomerulonephritis with linear deposits of immune complex in GBM.

REFERENCE/SOURCE

- Membranous nephropathy. In: Emma F, Goldstein SL, Bagga A, Bates CM, Shroff R (Eds). Pediatric Nephrology, 8th edition. Switzerland AG: Springer Nature; 2022. pp. 412-30.

5. A 10-year-old girl diagnosed with a case of SLE 1 year ago, now presents with generalized swelling and nephrotic range proteinuria. Kidney biopsy shows normal glomeruli on light microscopy, absence of immune deposits on IF, and diffuse foot process effacement on electron microscopy in >70% of glomeruli. Which of the following is the most likely diagnosis?

A. Minimal change disease (MCD)
B. Class I LN
C. Lupus podocytopathy
D. Class V LN

EXPLANATION

Nephrotic syndrome in LN is particularly a feature of proliferative glomerulonephritis or membranous nephropathy. However, in a group of patients with SLE presenting as nephrotic syndrome with normal glomeruli or mild mesangial proliferation in light microscopy and diffuse foot process effacement without immune deposits in the capillary wall is suggestive of lupus podocytopathy. Normal glomeruli in light microscopy can be a feature of class I LN, but it is associated with mesangial immune complex deposits. MCD is not a histopathological classification term for LN. Class V LN often presents as nephrotic syndrome, but normal glomeruli and absence of immune complex deposits are not a feature. So, the correct answer is "C".

Key: C

BOOST YOUR KNOWLEDGE

Lupus podocytopathy is a distinct entity of LN and has been reported in up to 1% of cases with adult-onset SLE, and rarely in children. These patients present as nephrotic syndrome with either MCD, mild mesangial proliferation, or focal segmental glomerular sclerosis (FSGS) on histology with extensive glomerular foot processes effacement on electron microscopy (typically >70%) with no or minimal immune deposits confined to the mesangium. In contrast to the FSGS pattern, patients with MCD pattern on histology respond well to corticosteroid therapy, with an overall response rate of 95% at 12 weeks and a complete response of 75%. Therapy for lupus podocytopathy includes low-dose steroids and a steroid-sparing agent like mycophenolate mofetil (MMF).

REFERENCE/SOURCE

- Lupus nephritis. In: Emma F, Goldstein SL, Bagga A, Bates CM, Shroff R (Eds). Pediatric Nephrology, 8th edition. Switzerland AG: Springer Nature; 2022. pp. 507-31.

6. A 1-month-old girl is admitted with an erythematous confluent macular rash over her face. On examination, she is clinically stable, with a heart rate (HR)—62 beats/min and moderate hepatosplenomegaly. Blood investigations—hemoglobin (Hb) 13 g/dL, platelets—92,000/mm^3. Which of the following investigations in the baby and mother will be most appropriate to confirm the diagnosis?

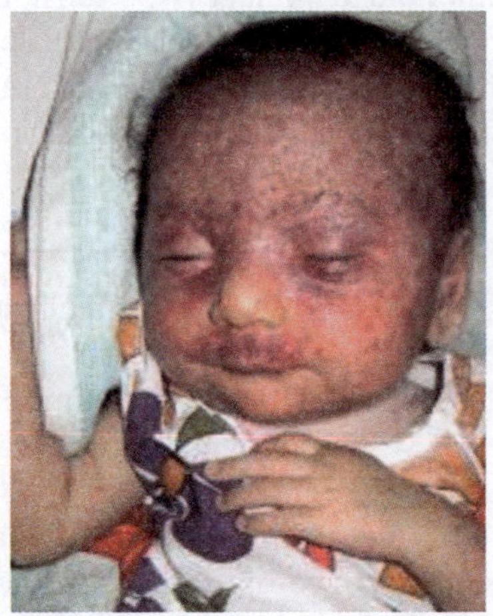

A. ANA with anti-dsDNA autoantibodies
B. ANA with anti–Sjögren's-syndrome-related antigen A (anti-Ro/SSA) and anti-La/SSB antibodies
C. Venereal disease research laboratory (VDRL)
D. TORCH (toxoplasmosis, rubella cytomegalovirus, herpes simplex, and human immunodeficiency virus) serology

EXPLANATION

The presence of an erythematous rash chiefly over the scalp and periorbital areas, along with hepatosplenomegaly, thrombocytopenia, and bradycardia, suggestive of congenital heart block in the aforementioned case raises the suspicion of neonatal lupus erythematosus. This may be confirmed by testing the child and mother for ANA and autoantibodies specific to neonatal lupus, anti-Ro, and anti-La antibodies; electrocardiography is required to confirm congenital heart block.

Venereal disease research laboratory and TORCH serology are advised in suspected cases with intrauterine infections; such as syphilis and the TORCH group of organisms but congenital heart block, which is very specific for neonatal lupus, is not a feature in TORCH infections.

Key: B

BOOST YOUR KNOWLEDGE

Neonatal lupus occurs in up to 2% of babies of mothers with anti-SSA (Ro) and ani-SSB (La) antibodies irrespective of maternal history of autoimmune disease. The rash spontaneously resolves as maternal autoantibodies clear by 6–8 months of age. However, congenital heart block is associated with significant mortality in 20–30% of neonates, with up to two-thirds of surviving neonates requiring pacemaker implantation.

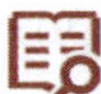

REFERENCE/SOURCE

- Lupus nephritis. In: Emma F, Goldstein SL, Bagga A, Bates CM, Shroff R (Eds). Pediatric Nephrology, 8th edition. Switzerland AG: Springer Nature; 2022. pp. 507-31.

7. A 10-year-old previously healthy girl presents with fever, erythematous rash over both the lower limbs, dark-colored urine, and oliguria for 7 days. On examination, she appears puffy with mild pedal edema, respiratory rate—20/min, BP—150/96 mm Hg, chest bilateral clear, and no hepatomegaly. Urinalysis- protein 3+, 30-40 RBCs/HPF, granular and RBC casts+. Blood test; Hb—8 g/dL, platelets—100,000/mm^3, C3—36 mg/dL, ANA/dsDNA—positive, creatinine—1.4 mg/dL, potassium—4.2 mEq/L, and albumin—2.8 g/dL. Kidney biopsy is suggestive of class IV LN. Which of the following statements regarding the treatment of this child is most appropriate?

A. Angiotensin convertase enzyme inhibitors to manage hypertension
B. Urgent hemodialysis with plasmapheresis to treat kidney failure and removal of autoantibodies
C. A short course of intravenous methylprednisolone, followed by oral steroids is recommended
D. A short course of intravenous methylprednisolone, followed by oral glucocorticoids and either intravenous cyclophosphamide or oral MMF is recommended

EXPLANATION

- Kidney biopsy findings are suggestive of class IV LN, a type of proliferative glomerulonephritis, requiring prompt and aggressive immunosuppression.
- *Kidney Disease:* Improving Global Outcomes (KDIGO) recommends treatment with glucocorticoids plus intravenous cyclophosphamide or oral MMF as induction therapy in class III/IV LN based on evidence from randomized controlled trials in adults.
- The use of angiotensin convertase enzyme inhibitors for the management of hypertension in acute kidney injury should be cautious due to concerns of compromising glomerular filtration rate (GFR) and worsening hyperkalemia.
- There are no indications for urgent hemodialysis in this case (e.g., fluid overload, hyperkalemia, etc.) and hypertension can be managed with antihypertensive agents. The efficacy of plasmapheresis in LN is equivocal, and its use is reserved for refractory LN.

Key: D

BOOST YOUR KNOWLEDGE

The KDIGO guidelines (2024) recommend that patients with active Class III or IV LN, with or without a membranous component, be treated initially with glucocorticoids plus any one of the following: (1) MMF, (2) low-dose intravenous cyclophosphamide, (3) belimumab and either MMF or low-dose intravenous cyclophosphamide, or (4) MMF and a calcineurin inhibitor (CNI) when kidney function is not severely impaired [i.e., estimated glomerular filtration rate (eGFR) >45 mL/min/1.73 m^2]. These recommendations are based on a 1B level of evidence for all of the above therapies.

Acute kidney injury in association with gross hematuria, oliguria, and nephrotic range proteinuria is suggestive of rapidly proliferative glomerulonephritis (RPGN), and the presence of fever and rash point toward kidney manifestation of a systemic disease. Kidney biopsy should be performed urgently in these cases. Important differentials may be LN, immunoglobulin A vasculitis nephritis (IgAVN), or ANCA-associated vasculitis (AAV). Low C3 in the aforementioned case rules out the possibility of IgAVN or AAV.

Patients with RPGN require aggressive immunosuppression with a combination of IV or oral glucocorticoids and cyclophosphamide as an induction therapy followed by a tapering dose of prednisolone and MMF as maintenance therapy.

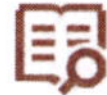

REFERENCE/SOURCE

- Kidney Disease: Improving Global Outcomes (KDIGO) Glomerular Diseases Work Group. KDIGO 2024 Clinical Practice Guideline for the Management of Glomerular Diseases. Kidney Int Suppl. 2024;105(1):S1-S669.

8. According to KDIGO clinical practice guidelines which of the following statements regarding response to therapy in children with LN is true?

A. Complete response is normal serum creatinine and reduction in proteinuria <300 mg/m^2/day in 24 hours of urine collection within 6–12 months of starting therapy

B. Complete response is the normalization of serological parameters such as anti-dsDNA and C3 level within 6 months of starting therapy

C. Partial response is the normalization of serum creatinine but the persistence of nephrotic range proteinuria after 6–12 months of starting therapy

D. Refractory LN is failure to achieve complete or partial response within 3 months from the start of immunosuppressive therapy

EXPLANATION

Serological parameters such as ANA and anti-dsDNA or C3 have no role in the monitoring of SLE or LN. Persistence of nephrotic range proteinuria after 6–12 months of therapy, even with normalization of serum creatinine value is considered as no response or refractory LN. To label, the response to treatment as refractory the child must have received treatment for at least for 6–12 months. So, the correct response is "A".

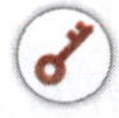

Key: A

BOOST YOUR KNOWLEDGE

Response to therapy in lupus is assessed by improvement in serum creatinine and decrease in proteinuria. KDIGO defines the complete response to therapy in LN as stabilization or improvement of kidney function (within 10–15% of baseline) and decline in proteinuria as <0.5 g/1.73m^2/day or <300 mg/m^2/day in a 24-hour urine collection within 6–12 months of starting therapy but could take >12 months. Partial remission is defined as a decrease in serum creatinine, but not to normal, plus a ≥50% decrease in proteinuria within 6–12 months of starting therapy. Refractory LN is defined as the absence of partial or complete remission within 6–12 months of starting therapy.

The workgroup suggests that if the patient shows continuous improvement allowing 18–24 months to achieve a complete response is a reasonable option.

REFERENCES/SOURCES

- Kidney Disease: Improving Global Outcomes (KDIGO) Glomerular Diseases Work Group. KDIGO 2024 Clinical Practice Guideline for the Management of Glomerular Diseases. Kidney Int Suppl. 2024;105(1):S1-S669.
- Lupus nephritis. In: Emma F, Goldstein SL, Bagga A, Bates CM, Shroff R (Eds). Pediatric Nephrology, 8th edition. Switzerland AG: Springer Nature; 2022. pp. 507-31.

9. A 9-year-old boy presents with a history of recurrent gross hematuria for the last 1 year, each episode associated with an upper respiratory tract infection. On examination, no edema or rash, and BP is normal. Urinalysis—full field isomorphic RBCs, protein-trace. Blood examination: Creatinine—0.4 mg/dL, calcium—9 mg/dL, C3—96 mg/dL. USG of the kidney tract showed normal-sized bilateral kidneys with no evidence of calculi. Which of the following is the most probable diagnosis?

A. IgA nephropathy
B. Idiopathic hypercalciuria
C. Alport syndrome (AS)
D. Thin basement membrane disease nephropathy

EXPLANATION

All of the aforementioned conditions may cause recurrent gross hematuria. Isomorphic RBCs in urinalysis suggest nonglomerular hematuria. Only idiopathic hypercalciuria is a cause of non-glomerular hematuria, whereas the rest of the three results in glomerular hematuria with dysmorphic RBCs in urinalysis. Also, urine protein in nonglomerular hematuria rarely exceeds 1+/2+. So, the correct answer is "B".

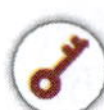

Key: B

BOOST YOUR KNOWLEDGE

A 24-hour urine calcium estimation is a part of the evaluation of patients with isolated hematuria, especially in those with a family history of kidney stones. Hypercalciuria is defined as calcium excretion of >4 mg/kg/day in 24-hour urine collection or >0.2 in spot urine sample. Idiopathic hypercalciuria is urinary calcium overexcretion despite normal serum calcium and in the absence of any secondary cause and is the most common risk factor for kidney stones causing 50–80% of pediatric kidney stones. Mechanisms of hypercalciuria include (1) primary increase in intestinal absorption of calcium, type I absorptive hypercalciuria (not vitamin D mediated) or type II absorptive hypercalciuria (excess of 1,25-(OH_2) vitamin D_3-mediated), (2) decrease in renal calcium reabsorption (type III absorptive hypercalciuria) and (3) increase in bone resorption (resorptive hypercalciuria).

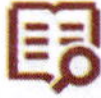

REFERENCE/SOURCE

- Urinary stone disease and nephrocalcinisis. In: Emma F, Goldstein SL, Bagga A, Bates CM, Shroff R (Eds). Pediatric Nephrology, 8th edition. Switzerland AG: Springer Nature; 2022. pp. 1296-316.

10. Which of the following statements regarding the management of recurrent kidney stones due to hypercalciuria is NOT true?

A. Dietary sodium restriction to 2–3 mEq/kg/day
B. Dietary calcium restriction to less than the recommended daily allowance (RDA)
C. Hydrochlorothiazide
D. Potassium citrate

EXPLANATION

- High dietary sodium intake increases urinary calcium excretion by inhibiting tubular calcium reabsorption, so dietary sodium restriction is advised to decrease hypercalciuria.
- Adequate amount of dietary calcium binds intestinal oxalate and prevents its increased intestinal absorption and thus reduces hyperoxaluria, which is an important risk factor for nephrolithiasis. Bone mineral density is reduced in patients with idiopathic hypercalciuria, so dietary calcium at RDA is suggested for the treatment of hypercalciuria. So, dietary calcium restriction is not recommended in nephrolithiasis.
- The use of hydrochlorothiazide is debated, with some centers preferring its use in the presence of refractory hypercalciuria.
- Potassium citrate corrects the underlying hypocitraturia, an important risk factor for nephrolithiasis in children with distal renal tubular acidosis. It also prevents crystallization of urinary calcium by increasing the urinary pH and thus decreasing the risk of recurrence of renal calculi.

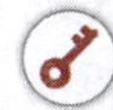

Key: B

BOOST YOUR KNOWLEDGE

Ensuring a high fluid intake and avoiding episodes of dehydration are the most important aspects of the management of idiopathic hypercalciuria. Dietary advice includes avoiding a meat-based diet and moderate salt restriction. Animal protein in diet increases the acid load, causing bone resorption and thus increasing hypercalciuria.

REFERENCE/SOURCE

- Urinary stone disease and nephrocalcinosis. In: Emma F, Goldstein SL, Bagga A, Bates CM, Shroff R (Eds). Pediatric Nephrology, 8th edition. Switzerland AG: Springer Nature; 2022. pp. 1296-316.

11. An adolescent girl presents to the emergency room with severe colicky pain abdomen and vomiting. Ultrasonography revealed a 4 mm hyperechoic lesion at the right pelviureteric junction, without any urinary tract dilatation. Which of the following treatment options is most appropriate?

A. Observation and conservative treatment
B. Extracorporeal shockwave lithotripsy (ESWL)
C. Percutaneous nephrolithotomy (PCNL)
D. Medical expulsive therapy (MET)

EXPLANATION

In up to 50% of cases, renal and ureteral calculi <5 mm sizes can pass spontaneously, so most cases with smaller size renal calculi can be managed by watchful waiting. As the child is clinically stable and it is a case of non-obstructing renal calculus, there is no need for emergency surgery in any form. MET is useful in cases with ureteric calculi only. As the stone is situated higher up in the renal pelvis, MET will not be the right choice of therapy for this patient. So, the correct answer is "A".

Key: A

BOOST YOUR KNOWLEDGE

Extracorporeal shockwave lithotripsy is an important mode of surgical management of upper tract renal calculi up to 15 mm in diameter, although a significant number of cases require repeated treatments and there is a risk of parenchymal damage.

Except for larger stones (>15 mm), open pyelolithotomy is rarely required and has been replaced by minimally invasive endoscopic techniques nowadays.

Medical expulsive therapy, a well-established therapy in adults with ureteric calculi of <5 mm diameter, where α blockers (doxazosin and tamsulosin) or calcium channel blockers are used to relax ureteral smooth muscles for easy passage of ureteric stones. Two recent studies in children have proved MET beneficial in children, with tamsulosin reported to have 3.3 times the odds for spontaneous stone passage.

REFERENCES/SOURCES

- Hernandez JD, Ellison JS, Lendvay TS. Current Trends, Evaluation, and Management of Pediatric Nephrolithiasis. JAMA Pediatr. 2015;169(10):964-70.
- Urinary stone disease and nephrocalcinisis. In: Emma F, Goldstein SL, Bagga A, Bates CM, Shroff R (Eds). Pediatric Nephrology, 8th edition. Switzerland AG: Springer Nature; 2022. pp. 1296-316.

12. A 7-year-old boy presents with a history of recurrent episodes of pain abdomen, gross hematuria, and bowing deformity of the legs. Ultrasonography kidney and urinary tract revealed bilateral multiple renal calculi with nephrocalcinosis. His maternal uncle had a history of renal stones and required dialysis 5 years ago. Urinalysis shows calcium oxalate crystals and urine protein 2+. Spot urine calcium:creatinine—0.8, $FePO_4$—25%, tubular maximum reabsorption of phosphate (TmP)/GFR—1.7 mg/dL. Serum creatinine—0.4 mg/dL, calcium—8.8 mg/dL, and phosphorous—2.1 mg/dL. Which of the following is the most probable diagnosis?

A. Cystinuria
B. Dent disease
C. Primary hyperoxaluria type I (PHI)
D. Hereditary hypophosphatemic rickets with hypercalciuria (HHRH)

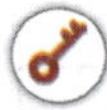

EXPLANATION

- Urine microscopic examination in cystinuria shows typical flat hexagonal cystine crystals.
- Dent disease, an X-linked tubular disorder, is characterized by low molecular weight proteinuria, hypercalciuria, renal calculi, nephrocalcinosis, hypophosphatemia, rickets, and progressive kidney failure. In the above case, the history of renal stones in maternal uncle requiring dialysis favors X-linked inheritance.
- Rickets is not a usual clinical manifestation in primary hyperoxaluria. Urine microscopy may show calcium oxalate crystals, but hypercalciuria, phosphaturia, hypophosphatemia, and proteinuria are characteristically absent.
- In HHRH, rickets and hypercalciuria are two important features, but proteinuria is not seen.

Key: B

BOOST YOUR KNOWLEDGE

Cystinuria is an autosomal recessive condition, characterized by excessive urinary excretion of cystine and dibasic amino acids ornithine, lysine, and arginine. Cystine stone formation occurs due to low urine solubility of cystine.

Dent disease is an X-linked proximal tubulopathy, seen in males only. In 60% of cases, it results from inactivating mutation of *CLCN5* genes and is termed Dent disease type I. The remaining cases with Dent disease phenotype result from *OCRL1* gene mutation and are termed dent disease type II.

Primary hyperoxaluria is an autosomal recessive disease, due to *AGXT* gene mutation, resulting in recurrent kidney stones, nephrocalcinosis, and ultimately kidney failure.

Hereditary hypophosphatemic rickets with hypercalciuria is an autosomal recessive tubular disorder due to the loss of function of NaPi2c (proximal tubule type IIc sodium-phosphate cotransporter) transporter in the proximal tubule resulting from mutation in *SLC34A3* gene mutation.

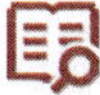

REFERENCE/SOURCE

- Pediatric Fanconi syndrome. In: Emma F, Goldstein SL, Bagga A, Bates CM, Shroff R (Eds). Pediatric Nephrology, 8th edition. Switzerland AG: Springer Nature; 2022. pp. 850-70.

13. All of the following are predisposing factors for renal calculi formation, *except:*

A. Hypercalciuria
B. Hyperuricosuria
C. Hypercitraturia
D. Cystinuria

EXPLANATION

Urinary citrate is the most important chelator of calcium in the urine and prevents stone formation by binding it with urinary phosphate and oxalate. So, hypocitraturia, and not hypercitraturia is a risk factor for renal calculi.

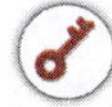

Key: C

BOOST YOUR KNOWLEDGE

Idiopathic hypercalciuria is the most common risk factor for kidney stones, accounting for 50–60% of pediatric kidney stone-related diseases. Other causes of hypercalciuria; such as hyperparathyroidism, vitamin D toxicity, and distal renal tubular acidosis should be excluded before labeling hypercalciuria as "idiopathic".

Hyperuricosuria accounts for 4–27% of all pediatric kidney stones and is a risk factor for both calcium oxalate and uric acid stone formation. The diagnosis of uric acid stone prompts the physician to look for an inherited disorder such as hypoxanthine-guanine-phosphoribosyl transferase (HPRT) enzyme deficiency and secondary causes of hyperuricemia leading to hyperuricosuria, such as tumor lysis syndrome. Alkalization of urine with bicarbonate or citrate aiming for urine PH between 6 and 7 helps in preventing the precipitation of uric acid crystals.

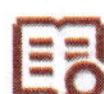

REFERENCE/SOURCE

- Urinary stone disease and nephrocalcinosis. In: Emma F, Goldstein SL, Bagga A, Bates CM, Shroff R (Eds). Pediatric Nephrology, 8th edition. Switzerland AG: Springer Nature; 2022. pp. 1296-316.

14. Which of the following statement is correct regarding primary hyperoxaluria type I?

A. Reduced alanine-glyoxylate aminotransferase (AGT) activity in kidney tissues
B. Intensive hemodialysis followed by kidney transplantation is the treatment of choice
C. Burosumab is the recently approved drug for this disease
D. Lumasiran is the recently approved drug for this disease

EXPLANATION

- PH1 is an autosomal recessive condition, resulting from a mutation of the *AGXT* gene, which causes reduced activity of peroxisomal enzyme AGT activity in the liver and not in the kidney.
- Intensive hemodialysis is required in cases with PH1, but kidney transplantation alone is not recommended as reduced enzyme activity is in the liver and not the kidney, so dual liver-kidney transplant, either simultaneous or sequential, is the treatment of choice in these cases.
- Burosumab is an approved drug from X-linked hypophosphatemic rickets.
- Lumasiran is an approved drug for PHI.

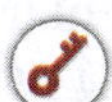

Key: D

BOOST YOUR KNOWLEDGE

Primary hyperoxalurias are a group of autosomal recessive disorders of glyoxylate metabolism in the liver characterized by increased excretion of urinary oxalate. PHI is the most severe form of primary hyperoxaluria presenting as recurrent kidney stone formation, nephrocalcinosis, and end-stage kidney failure in late childhood or early adult life.

Diagnosis is suspected in cases of kidney stones with increased plasma oxalate and hyperoxaluria. In the later stages when kidneys become unable to excrete all oxalate load, oxalate gets deposited in the bones, eyes, blood vessels, skin, muscles, and heart. Confirmation of diagnosis is done by sequencing of *AGXT* gene.

Hydration is the mainstay of supportive therapy. Only 15% of oxalate is derived from the diet and the remainder is from the metabolism of glyoxylate ascorbic acid, so dietary restriction is not of much importance in its management. Oral pyridoxine (5–20 mg/kg/day) treatment is helpful in selected cases by reducing urinary oxalate excretion.

REFERENCES/SOURCES

- Groothoff JW, Metry E, Deesker L, Garrelfs S, Acquaviva C, Almardini R, et al. Clinical practice recommendations for primary hyperoxaluria: an expert consensus statement from ERKNet and OxalEurope. Nat Rev Nephrol. 2023;19(3):194-211.
- Hyperoxaluria. In: Emma F, Goldstein SL, Bagga A, Bates CM, Shroff R (Eds). Pediatric Nephrology, 8th edition. Switzerland AG: Springer Nature; 2022. pp. 832-43.

15. Which of the following statement regarding Alport syndrome is *true*?

A. It results from variants in genes encoding α1, α2, and α3 chains of type IV collagen
B. Only boys manifest the disease and girls are always carriers
C. Autosomal recessive Alport syndrome (ARAS) results from variants in *COL4A3*
D. Diffuse thinning of GBM in the absence of characteristic basket weave appearance completely rules out the diagnosis of Alport syndrome

EXPLANATION

- Alport syndrome results from genetic variants in *COL4A3*, *COL4A4*, and *COL4A5* encoding α3, α4, and α5 chains of type IV collagen respectively, a component of GBM in the kidney.
- The mode of inheritance is X-linked in 80% of cases, autosomal recessive in 15%, and autosomal dominant in 5% of cases of Alport syndrome. So, both sexes may manifest clinical features of Alport syndrome depending on the mode of inheritance.
- X-linked Alport syndrome (XLAS) is caused by an abnormality in the *COL4A5* gene, whereas autosomal recessive and autosomal dominant Alport syndrome is caused by an abnormality in the *COL4A3 or COL4A4* gene.
- Extensive thinning of the glomerular basement, a frequent finding in benign familial hematuria, can be the only finding of GBM in the early stages of Alport syndrome. This will be even more suggestive of Alport syndrome in the presence of hearing loss, ocular abnormalities, and a family history of kidney failure.

So, the correct answer is "C".

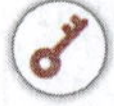

Key: C

BOOST YOUR KNOWLEDGE

Alport syndrome is an inherited nephropathy characterized by glomerular hematuria with a variable rate of progression to chronic kidney disease, bilateral high-pitched sensorineural hearing loss, and specific ocular findings like anterior lenticonus and retinal flecks. It is caused by mutation in three genes: (1) *COL4A3*, (2) *COL4A4*, and (3) *COL4A5* encoding α3, α4, and α5 chains of type IV collagen, components of GBM, cochlea, eyes, and

Bowman capsules. These three α chains are arranged as triple helical structures in GBM. Mutation in any of the three genes results in defective α chain formation and disorganized triple helical structure.

REFERENCE/SOURCE

- Inherited diseases of the glomerular basement membrane. In: Emma F, Goldstein SL, Bagga A, Bates CM, Shroff R (Eds). Pediatric Nephrology, 8th edition. Switzerland AG: Springer Nature; 2022. pp. 328-45.

16. A 6-year-old girl is detected with microscopic hematuria during urinalysis for pain abdomen. There is no history of fever, dysuria, or gross hematuria. One year later, she is asymptomatic, normotensive, urinalysis—20–30 dysmorphic RBCs/HPF and protein 1+. Blood investigations; creatinine—0.4 mg/dL, C3—92 mg/dL, ANA—nonreactive. Her maternal grandfather died of kidney failure 5 years ago. Hearing and eye evaluation are normal. Which of the following statement is most appropriate regarding the next step of evaluation of this child?

A. Urinalysis of parents and siblings for microscopic hematuria
B. No need for further evaluation as the child is asymptomatic
C. Annual hearing and eye evaluation till 10 years of age
D. Kidney biopsy, only if there is gross hematuria or kidney function deterioration

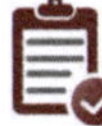

EXPLANATION

Screening of family members for microscopic hematuria is one of the initial steps in the evaluation of children with asymptomatic microscopic hematuria toward working up for hereditary nephritis. A family history of death due to kidney failure further points toward hereditary nephritis.

In the presence of a family history of kidney failure or death due to kidney diseases, children with even asymptomatic glomerular microscopic hematuria should undergo annual follow-up for hearing assessment and urinalysis for the appearance of proteinuria.

Approximately, 30% of males with X-linked Alport syndrome and 20% of children with autosomal recessive Alport syndrome develop hearing loss by 10 years of age. So, annual hearing evaluation needs to be continued beyond 10 years of age, as the majority develop sensorineural deafness beyond 10 years of age.

Kidney biopsy with electron microscopy examination is useful for differential diagnosis in patients with persistent microscopic hematuria if the child develops proteinuria even in the absence of gross hematuria or kidney function deterioration.

Key: A

BOOST YOUR KNOWLEDGE

Persistent glomerular hematuria (gross or microscopic) for >3 months (confirmed by urinalysis on at least 2 occasions) is the primary feature of Alport syndrome. To confirm the diagnosis of Alport syndrome, the patient must have one or more secondary features; such as a significant genetic variant in the type IV collagen gene, abnormal expression of type IV collagen α chain on immunostaining of kidney biopsy specimen and specific abnormalities of GBM on electron microscopy sample of kidney biopsy specimen; like diffuse thickening and thinning of GBM, lamellation and basket weave appearance of GBM. The patient may have accessory features of Alport syndrome, namely the family history of kidney disease, bilateral sensorineural deafness, ocular abnormalities, such as lenticonus, retinal flecks, and diffuse leiomyomatosis.

REFERENCES/SOURCES

- Inherited diseases of the glomerular basement membrane. In: Emma F, Goldstein SL, Bagga A, Bates CM, Shroff R (Eds). Pediatric Nephrology, 8th edition. Switzerland AG: Springer Nature; 2022. pp. 328-45.
- Nozu K, Nakanishi K, Abe Y, Udagawa T, Okada S, Okamoto T, et al. A review of clinical characteristics and genetic backgrounds in Alport syndrome. Clin Exp Nephrol. 2019;23(2):158-68.

17. A 12-year-old boy presents as a case of initial steroid-resistant nephrotic syndrome. No history of gross hematuria, rash, or joint pain. On examination, pedal edema+, BP—130/80 mm Hg. Urinalysis—protein 3+, 8–10 dysmorphic RBCs/HPF. Serum creatinine—0.6 mg/dL, albumin—2.6 g/dL, C3—120 mg/dL and ANA—negative. Kidney biopsy is suggestive of focal and segmental glomerulosclerosis with diffuse thinning of GBM. No family history of kidney diseases. Genetic study reveals pathogenic *COL4A5* gene variant. Which of the following statement regarding the management of this child is *not* correct?

A. Parental and sibling screening for *COL4A5* genetic variants
B. Immunosuppression with CNI is the mainstay of therapy
C. Hearing assessment for high-frequency deafness
D. Eye evaluation for retinal flecks

EXPLANATION

Genetic screening of family members is important for early identification of at-risk patients.

There is no role of immunosuppression, so these drugs should not be started or discontinued once the diagnosis of Alport syndrome is confirmed either with a kidney biopsy or genetic test.

Hearing and eye evaluation should always be performed in cases with steroid-resistant nephrotic syndrome with microscopic hematuria and strong suspicion of Alport syndrome. Bilateral high-frequency deafness may be present in up to 80% of cases of Alport syndrome.

Specific ocular abnormalities include anterior lenticonus, posterior subcapsular cataract, posterior polymorphous dystrophy, and retinal flecks.

So, the correct answer is "B".

Key: B

BOOST YOUR KNOWLEDGE

The onset of nephrotic syndrome at an adolescent age with the presence of hypertension and microscopic hematuria should always raise the suspicion of secondary causes of nephrotic syndrome. With normal C3 and ANA, the probability of LN is less likely. However, viral markers for hepatitis B virus (HBV) and hepatitis C virus (HCV) should also be performed in all cases of steroid-resistant nephrotic syndrome. Kidney biopsy in Alport syndrome may show features of MCD or FSGS with occasional foamy cells in the interstitium. Diffuse thinning of GBM may be the only electron microscopic finding in the early stages of Alport syndrome. However, lamellated GBM with basket weave appearance is characteristic of Alport syndrome.

Despite kidney biopsy reports being suggestive of Alport syndrome, genetic study should always be performed as knowing the type of genetic mutation and mode of inheritance will help to diagnose and ascertain the severity of disease in other family members and also to determine the affected status of potential living-related kidney donors.

Angiotensin-converting enzyme (ACE) inhibitor is the only established treatment at present in reducing the progression of disease and delaying the need for kidney replacement therapy.

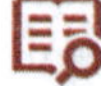

REFERENCE/SOURCE

- Inherited diseases of the glomerular basement membrane. In: Emma F, Goldstein SL, Bagga A, Bates CM, Shroff R (Eds). Pediatric Nephrology, 8th edition. Switzerland AG: Springer Nature; 2022. pp. 328-45.

18. An 8-year-old boy has been referred for persistent microscopic hematuria for 6 months, which was detected during a routine urine examination for pain abdomen. On examination, he has no edema, normotensive, and normal hearing and eye evaluation. Urinalysis—8-10 dysmorphic RBCs/HPF, protein—traces. There is no history of kidney disease in the family. Which of the following statement is *true* regarding the management of this child?

A. No further evaluation as the child is asymptomatic
B. Urinalysis of the parents and siblings
C. Annual hearing and eye evaluation
D. Both B and C

EXPLANATION

Asymptomatic persistent microscopic hematuria, with dysmorphic RBCs, may be a feature of an underlying glomerular disorder and these children should be kept under regular follow-up for the development of hypertension and proteinuria. These children need to be evaluated for proteinuria at least annually or early in the presence of any febrile illness. The onset of proteinuria is suggestive of the progression of the underlying disease and an indication of kidney biopsy. Family members should always be subjected to urinalysis, as the presence of hematuria in either of the parents or siblings may be indicative of hereditary nephritis.

Hearing and eye manifestation may be absent in the early stage of Alport syndrome, so these children should undergo annual audiological examination and eye evaluation.

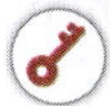

Key: D

BOOST YOUR KNOWLEDGE

Persistent microscopic hematuria, even in the absence of symptoms, requires detailed evaluation. The presence of isomorphic RBCs may be indicative of hypercalciuria. Microscopic hematuria with dysmorphic RBCs may be an early feature of Alport syndrome, IgA nephropathy, or C3 glomerulopathy.

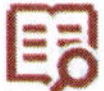

REFERENCE/SOURCE

- Inherited diseases of the glomerular basement membrane. In: Emma F, Goldstein SL, Bagga A, Bates CM, Shroff R (Eds). Pediatric Nephrology, 8th edition. Switzerland AG: Springer Nature; 2022. pp. 328-45.

19. A 15-year-old boy referred to as a case of steroid-resistant nephrotic syndrome, has been diagnosed with Alport syndrome on kidney biopsy. Immunostaining for the α5 component of type IV collagen shows negative expression on GBM, but positive on Bowman's capsule. Both the parents are healthy. Hearing evaluation shows bilateral sensorineural deafness. What is the most likely mode of inheritance?

A. X-linked dominant
B. Autosomal recessive
C. X-linked recessive
D. Autosomal dominant

EXPLANATION

About 85% of cases of Alport syndrome result from X-linked inheritance, with males always manifesting the disease and females with milder clinical symptoms, such as microscopic hematuria. However, 15% of cases show autosomal mode of inheritance, where males and females present with similar clinical severity.

X-linked Alport syndrome results from mutation of the *COL4A5* gene encoding the α5 chain of collagen IV of GBM. As the α5 chain is present in GBM and Bowman's capsule both, children with X-linked Alport syndrome are completely negative for α5 staining. Whereas, cases with autosomal recessive inheritance show mutation in *COL4A4* and *COL4A3* genes encoding α4 and α3 chains, respectively. As Bowman's capsule has α5α5α6 chain, immunostaining shows positivity on Bowman's capsule and negative on GBM. Based on the immunostaining pattern, the aforementioned case has an autosomal recessive mode of inheritance with a mutation in the *COL4A4/COL4A3* gene.

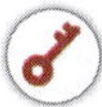

Key: B

BOOST YOUR KNOWLEDGE

Routine IF in Alport syndrome is normal or shows nonspecific immune-complex deposition. As the disease results from abnormal expression of α3α4α5 chain and α5α5α6 chain in GBM and Bowman's capsule respectively, specific immunostaining for α5 chain will help in differentiating Alport syndrome due to

X-linked inheritance or autosomal recessive inheritance. X-linked Alport syndrome results from *COL4A5* gene mutation resulting in the complete absence of immunostaining for α5 chain in both basement membrane and Bowman's capsule, whereas in autosomal recessive Alport syndrome resulting from *COL4A3* or *COL4A4* gene mutation immunostaining for α5 chain in GBM is absent, but immunostaining for α5 chain in Bowman's capsule is present as expression of α5α5α6 chain is preserved.

REFERENCE/SOURCE

- Inherited diseases of the glomerular basement membrane. In: Emma F, Goldstein SL, Bagga A, Bates CM, Shroff R (Eds). Pediatric Nephrology, 8th edition. Switzerland AG: Springer Nature; 2022. pp. 328-45.

20. Which of the following is the correct statement regarding current recommendations for the start of treatment with angiotensin convertase enzyme inhibitors in Alport syndrome?

A. Males with X-linked Alport syndrome—at the time of diagnosis
B. Males with X-linked Alport syndrome—at the onset of microalbuminuria
C. Females with X-linked Alport syndrome—at the time of diagnosis
D. Patients of either sex with autosomal recessive Alport syndrome—at the onset of microalbuminuria

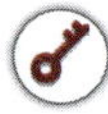

EXPLANATION

Earlier, ACE inhibitors were recommended as first-line therapy in patients with Alport syndrome with overt proteinuria or at the onset of microalbuminuria. However, results of the EARLY PRO-TECT trial of ramipril treatment in pediatric Alport syndrome showed a significant delay in the start of kidney replacement therapy in those who were started on ramipril early at diagnosis.

As males and females with an autosomal recessive mode of inheritance have similar disease severity and risk of progression to kidney failure, in contrast to X-linked inheritance where males only have severe disease manifestation and females have a mild clinical presentation, patients with an autosomal recessive mode of inheritance, irrespective of gender, are treated similar to the males with X-linked inheritance, i.e., at the time of diagnosis.

Key: A

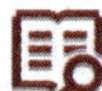

BOOST YOUR KNOWLEDGE

Treatment protocols for the treatment of Alport syndrome have been revised based on the result of the EARLY PRO-TECT trial.

REFERENCE/SOURCE

- Kashtan CE, Gross O. Clinical practice recommendations for the diagnosis and management of Alport syndrome in children, adolescents, and young adults—an update for 2020. Pediatr Nephrol. 2021;36(3):711-9.

SECTION 22

Neurology

CHAPTER

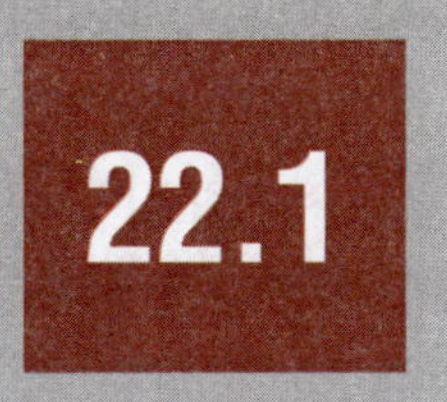

Localization in Neurological Disorders

Vishal Sondhi

1. A patient has a contusion of the foot and describes the pain as well localized to the dorsum of the foot and "pricking and sharp." Which of the following fibers are responsible for sharp, localized pain?

A. A-alpha fibers
B. A-beta fibers
C. A-delta fibers
D. A-gamma fibers

EXPLANATION

The various types of neurons involved in the peripheral nervous system are as:

Fiber type(s)	***Name***	***Subtype***	***Diameter (mm)***	***Conduction velocity (m/s)***
Myelinated somatic afferent/efferent:				
Cutaneous afferent	A	β δ	6–12 1–5	35–75 5–30
Muscle afferent	A	α β δ	12–21 6–12 1–5	80–120 35–75 5–30
Muscle efferent Anterior horn cells (α and γ motor neurons)	A	6–12	35–75	
Myelinated autonomic efferent:				
Preganglionic efferent	B		3	3–15
Unmyelinated somatic/autonomic afferent/efferent:				
Postganglionic efferent	C		0.2–1.5	1–2
Afferent to dorsal root ganglion (pain)	C		0.2–1.5	1–2
Sensory receptor	***Fiber type***			
Hair follicle	Aβ			
Skin follicle	Aβ			
Muscle spindle	Aa			
Joint receptor	Aβ			
Pain, temperature	Aδ, C			

Thus, A-delta fibers carry pain and temperature.

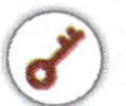

Key: C

BOOST YOUR KNOWLEDGE

The strict definition of the peripheral nervous system includes that part of the nervous system in which the Schwann cell is the major supporting cell, as opposed to the central nervous system in which the glial cells are the major support cells. Not all human peripheral nerve fibers are myelinated. Unmyelinated fibers, which conduct very slowly (typically 0.2–1.5 m/s), primarily mediate pain, temperature, and autonomic functions. Schwann cells also support these "unmyelinated" fibers; however, one Schwann cell typically surrounds several unmyelinated fibers but without the formation of concentric spirals of myelin.

REFERENCES/SOURCES

- Baron R. Mechanisms of disease: neuropathic pain—a clinical perspective. Nat Clin Pract Neurol. 2006;2(2):95-106.
- Preston DC, Shapiro BE (Eds). Electromyography and Neuromuscular Disorders: Clinical–Electrophysiologic Correlations, 3rd edition. Elsevier; 2013. p. 17.

2. A 12-year-old boy is brought to the emergency department with left-sided weakness. The patient is not on any medications, and there is no relevant medical history. On examination, he is lethargic but oriented. His cranial nerve evaluation reveals hemianopia and facial weakness with sparing of the upper half of the face. He has left hemiparesis and hyperreflexia. His sensory evaluation reveals hemisensory loss. Which of the following best explains these symptoms?

A. Anterior choroidal artery territory infarction
B. Medial posterior choroidal artery territory infarction
C. Lenticulostriate artery territory infarction
D. Medial striate artery territory infarction

EXPLANATION

Facial weakness may result from an upper or lower motor neuron (LMN) lesion. Muscles of the upper half of the face, which have bilateral cortical innervation, are not affected in supranuclear lesions. Thus, if there is an upper motor neuron (UMN) type of facial paresis (involvement of the lower half of the face with sparing of muscles of the upper half such as frontalis and orbicularis oculi) on the same side of hemiplegia, the lesion is localizable above upper pons; likely sites being motor cortex, corona radiata, or internal capsule. Hemianopia can occur due to the involvement of the optic tract, lateral geniculate body, or optic radiations in the internal capsule. The place in neuroanatomy where corticospinal, corticobulbar, and optic radiations fibers converge is the posterior limb of the internal capsule, which is supplied by the anterior choroidal artery.

Key: A

BOOST YOUR KNOWLEDGE

The blood supply of the internal capsule is shown here.

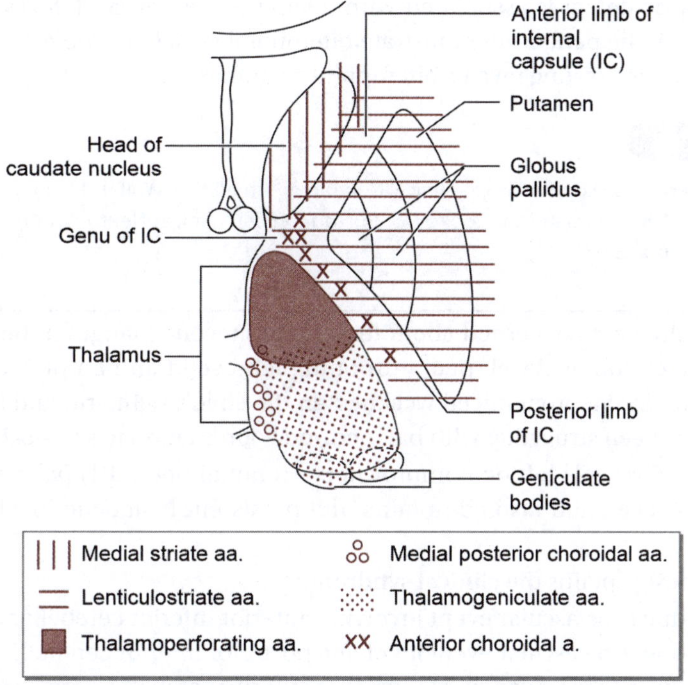

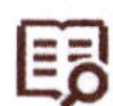

REFERENCES/SOURCES

- Brazis PW, Masdeu JC, Biller J (Eds). Localization in Clinical Neurology, 7th edition. Wolters Kluwer; 2016. pp. 11-2.
- Haines DE, Mihailoff GA (Eds). Fundamental Neuroscience for Basic and Clinical Applications, 5th edition. Elsevier; 2018. pp. 225-41.

3. A 9-year-old child is brought with complaints of visual difficulties. The child's parents report that over the past few months, they have observed a significant decline in their child's vision. The child now frequently stumbles into objects and has difficulty navigating her surroundings. The parents also mention that their child has developed unusual behavioral changes, such as excessive thirst and urination. Examination reveals that the child has bilateral temporal hemianopia. The rest of the neurological examination is normal. Which of the following best explains the findings?

A. Craniopharyngioma impinging on optic radiations
B. Craniopharyngioma impinging on the optic chiasma
C. Temporal lobe dysembryoplastic neuroepithelial tumor (DNET) impinging on the optic chiasma
D. Temporal lobe DNET impinging on optic radiations

EXPLANATION

The most important for lesion localization in visual field defects is to note whether the field defect is monocular, in which case the lesion usually affects the retina or the optic nerve, or binocular, in which case the lesion is localized to or beyond the optic chiasma. Bitemporal field defects are most often due to a compressive mass lesion affecting the optic chiasma such as pituitary tumors. Rarely, processes that cause rapidly developing hydrocephalus may result in bitemporal defects, perhaps through dilatation of the optic recess of the third ventricle.

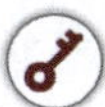

Key: B

BOOST YOUR KNOWLEDGE

Clinically, three chiasmatic syndromes may be recognized: (1) The anterior chiasm or junctional syndrome in which a unilateral optic defect is associated with a superior temporal defect in the other eye; (2) body of chiasm syndrome in which the patients demonstrate bitemporal visual field defects; and (3) the posterior chiasm syndrome in which visual field testing reveals bitemporal scotomas.

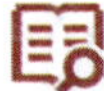

REFERENCES/SOURCES

- Brazis PW, Masdeu JC, Biller J (Eds). Localization in Clinical Neurology, 7th edition. Wolters Kluwer; 2016. pp. 157-9.
- Walsh FB, Hoyt WF, Miller NR, Newman NM, Cooke DB. Burton F (Eds). Clinical Neuro-Ophthalmology, 5th edition. Lippincott Williams and Wilkins; 1998. pp. 237-386.

4. Parents of a 7-year-old child are concerned about their child's recent changes in behavior and physical abilities. Over the past week, the child has developed a drooping left eyelid and an outward deviation of the left eye. Additionally, they have noticed a pronounced weakness in the child's right arm and leg. The child's schoolteacher mentioned that they have been struggling with balance and coordination in physical education class.

Neurological examination reveals left oculomotor nerve (cranial nerve III) palsy with ptosis, strabismus, and right-sided hemiparesis. The child also complains of a persistent headache localized to the right side of the head.

Which of the following best explains the clinical syndrome?

A. Midbrain infarction due to a vascular event involving anterior inferior cerebellar artery
B. Midbrain infarction due to a vascular event involving posterior inferior cerebellar artery
C. Midbrain infarction due to a vascular event involving anterior cerebral artery
D. Midbrain infarction due to a vascular event involving posterior cerebral artery

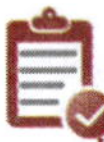

EXPLANATION

The child has a lesion involving the third cranial nerve and corticospinal tracts. Lesions can affect the third nerve in the brainstem (nucleus or fascicular portion), in the subarachnoid space, in the cavernous sinus, at the superior orbital fissure, or in the orbit. A brainstem lesion such as an infarction may damage the pyramidal fibers and fascicle of CN III, causing an ipsilateral oculomotor paresis with pupillary involvement and a contralateral hemiparesis including the lower portion of the face, also known as Weber syndrome. The most common etiology of Weber syndrome is infarction involving the posterior cerebral artery.

Key: D

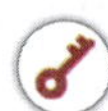

BOOST YOUR KNOWLEDGE

Weber syndrome is contralateral hemiparesis with ipsilateral oculomotor palsy that does not spare the pupil. A lesion in the ventromedial portion of the midbrain leads to Weber syndrome. The midbrain receives its blood supply from the paramedian mesencephalic branches (basilar), peduncular perforating branches (posterior cerebral artery), as well as from the superior cerebellar artery, and the choroidal arteries. It most commonly results from the occlusion of a branch of the posterior cerebral artery. Less common etiologies include hemorrhage, aneurysms, tumors, and demyelinating diseases.

REFERENCES/SOURCES

- Brazis PW, Masdeu JC, Biller J (Eds). Localization in Clinical Neurology, 7th edition. Wolters Kluwer; 2016. p. 12.
- Zimmerman EE, Misulis KE. Brainstem and cranial nerves. In: Zimmerman EE, Samuels MA, Kirshner HS, Misulis KE (Eds). Neurologic Localization and Diagnosis. Elsevier; 2022. pp. 89-106.

5. A 14-year-old child is brought with complaints of recent visual and coordination difficulties. The parents report that over the past several weeks, their child has developed a noticeable inability to move their right eye inward toward the nose when looking to the left. On examination, when asked to follow your finger with their eyes from right to left, the right eye remains stationary or deviates outward (abduction), while the left eye moves smoothly to the left. Which of the following best explains the clinical features?

A. Lesion involving right III cranial nerve nucleus
B. Lesion involving right III cranial nerve in the cavernous sinus
C. Lesion involving right medial longitudinal fasciculus
D. Lesion involving left medial longitudinal fasciculus

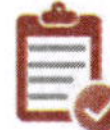

EXPLANATION

The scenario described in the question is of internuclear ophthalmoplegia. Internuclear ophthalmoplegia is defined as the lack of adduction of the ipsilateral eye with preserved abduction of the contralateral eye with nystagmus. It is the result of a lesion affecting the medial longitudinal fasciculus (MLF)—a paired, highly specialized, and heavily myelinated nerve bundle traveling in a craniocaudal direction near the midline within the tegmentum of the midbrain and dorsal pons.

Key: C

BOOST YOUR KNOWLEDGE

Functionally, the MLF carries excitatory and inhibitory axonal nerves between the paramedian pontine reticular formation (PPRF) and cranial nerves III, IV, and VI during activation of the frontal eye fields in the cerebral cortex. This allows for agonist and antagonist extraocular muscle movement for saccadic eye movement (horizontal eye movement allowing for the change in fixation point) and smooth pursuit (eye movement allowing for following a moving object). In addition, vestibular-ocular nerve fibers traveling from cranial nerve VIII, which include both a semicircular and otolith-mediated oculomotor reflex, also run within the MLF to help coordinate balance and linear acceleration, respectively.

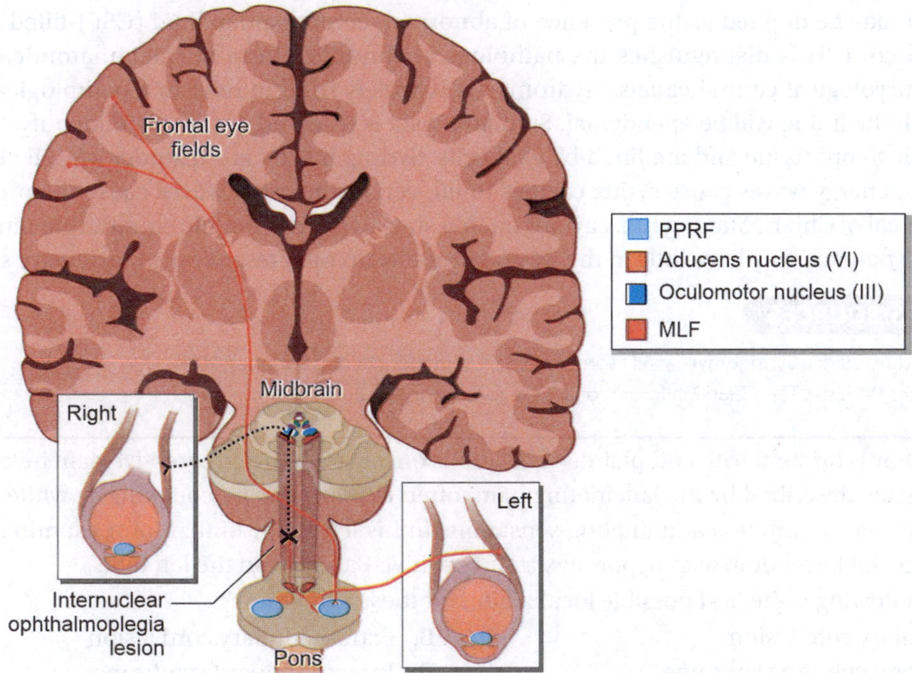

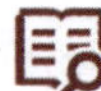

REFERENCES/SOURCES

- Fiester P, Baig SA, Patel J, Rao D. An anatomic, imaging, and clinical review of the medial longitudinal fasciculus. J Clin Imaging Sci. 2020;10:83.
- Lee S-H, Kim JM, Kim J-S. Update on the medial longitudinal fasciculus syndrome. Neurol Sci. 2022;43(6):3533-40.

6. A 13-year-old child is brought with complaints of insidious onset and gradually progressive numbness, tingling sensations, and weakness primarily affecting the upper limbs. On examination, the child exhibits pronounced weakness and muscle atrophy in the upper limbs, particularly in the hands and arms. Fine motor tasks such as buttoning clothes and writing have become increasingly difficult. Deep tendon reflexes are diminished (hyporeflexia) in the affected upper limbs, while they appear normal in the lower limbs.

Sensory examination reveals thermoanesthesia and analgesia in a "suspended" bilateral distribution, with reservation of touch and proprioception. Which of the following lesions can best explain these symptoms?

A. Syringomyelia
B. Subacute combined degeneration of the spinal cord
C. Spinal subdural hematoma
D. Spinal epidural abscess

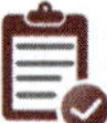

EXPLANATION

Syringomyelia is a term applied to a fluid-filled cavity (syrinx) present within the spinal cord. It is thought to be produced by various conditions that create pressure gradients that force spinal fluid from the fourth ventricle into the central spinal canal. Signs and symptoms of syringomyelia are classically characterized by a dissociative loss of pain and temperature sensations (maintenance of touch and position) along a cape-like distribution to the lower neck, shoulder, and upper arms. Occipital headaches, upper neck pain, and Lhermitte's phenomenon (electrical sensations descending down the back and arms) can occur. Upper-extremity asymmetric muscle weakness and atrophy can be found with decreased deep tendon reflexes, and the lower extremities may exhibit muscle spasticity.

Key: A

BOOST YOUR KNOWLEDGE

Syringomyelia may be defined as the presence of abnormal, cerebrospinal fluid (CSF)-filled cavities within the mature spinal cord. This distinguishes the pathological condition from normal anatomical variants such as persisting embryological central canals. Hydromyelia is widely used to refer to a pathologically dilated central canal, in which the lining will be ependymal. Syringomyelia is reserved, by some, to identify cavities that dissect into surrounding cord tissue and are lined by glial cells. Syringomyelia is a disorder of CSF circulation. Regular, systolic arterial energy waves cause syrinx cavities to fill; venous pressure waves cause the pressure dissociation headaches typical of Chiari. Many syrinx cavities enter a state of hydrodynamic equilibrium and may be managed conservatively; patients may have little in the way of disability, in the presence of an extensive syrinx cavity.

REFERENCES/SOURCES

- Flint G, Rusbridge C (Eds). Syringomyelia: A Disorder of CSF Circulation. Berlin: Springer; 2014.
- Tubbs RS, Oakes WJ (Eds). The Chiari Malformations. New York: Springer; 2013.

7. A 12-year-old boy is brought with complaints of insidious onset, gradually progressive pain involving the left lower limb. It is typically described by the lancinating pain, often exacerbated by coughing or while straining at stools. Examination reveals numbness and tingling sensations in his left lower limb. Motor examination demonstrates weakness of the left lower limb with hyporeflexia and positive Babinski on the left foot.

Which of the following is the best possible localization for these symptoms?

A. Intramedullary cord lesion
B. Extramedullary cord lesion
C. Posterolateral column syndrome
D. Brown–Séquard syndrome

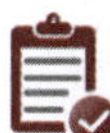

EXPLANATION

The differentiating features between intramedullary and extramedullary lesions are listed here.

Symptoms/signs	***Intramedullary lesions***	***Extramedullary lesions***
Radicular pain	Unusual	Common, occurs early
Vertebral pain	Unusual	Common
Funicular pain	Common	Less common
UMN signs	Yes, late	Yes, early
LMN signs	Prominent and diffuse	Segmental, if present
Paresthesia progression	Descending progression	Ascending
Sphincter abnormalities	Early with caudal lesions (conus/cauda equina)	Late
Trophic changes	Common	Unusual

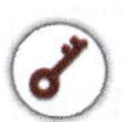

Key: B

BOOST YOUR KNOWLEDGE

The spinal canal can be divided into the extradural, intradural-extramedullary, and intramedullary compartments. Each compartment contains unique anatomic and histologic structures, greatly informing and simplifying the differential diagnosis of lesions in each compartment. Extrinsic causes of myelopathy or cauda equina symptoms can occur in the intradural-extramedullary and extradural compartments. The intramedullary compartment includes the parenchyma (spinal cord and conus).

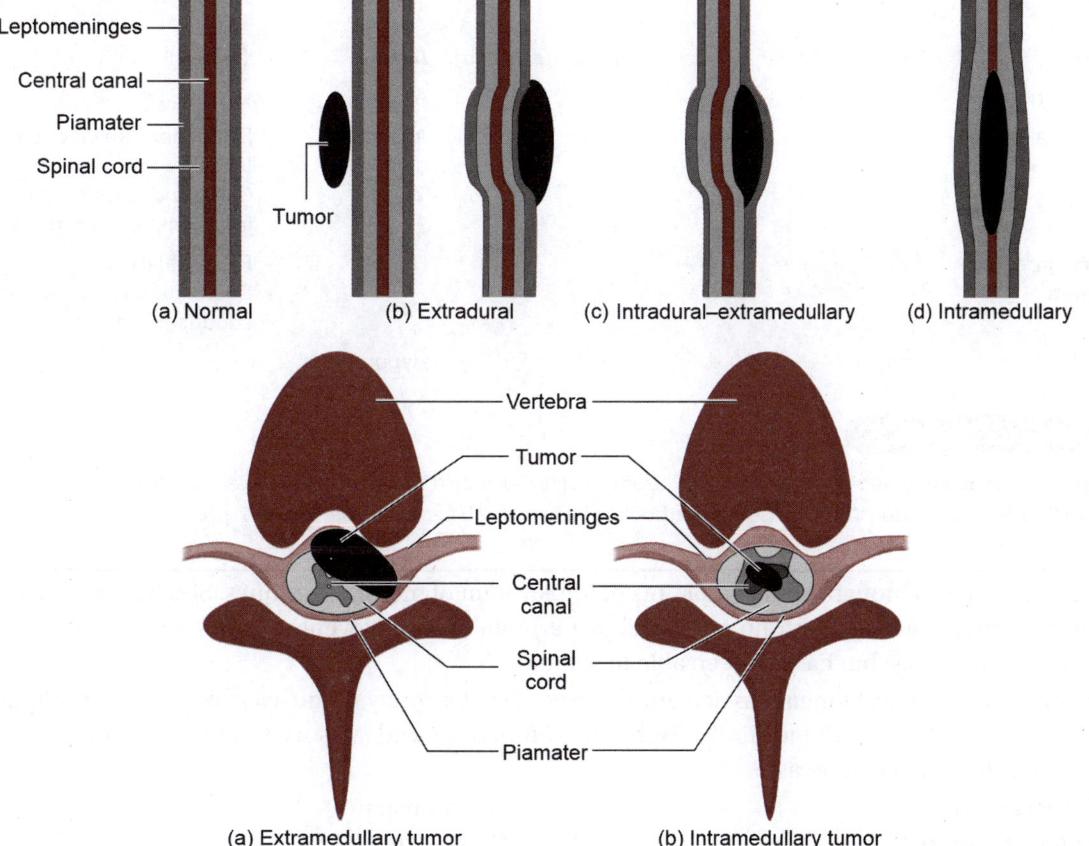

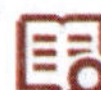

REFERENCES/SOURCES

- Brazis PW, Masdeu JC, Biller J (Eds). Localization in Clinical Neurology, 7th edition. Wolters Kluwer; 2016. p. 119.
- Diehn FE, Krecke KN. Neuroimaging of spinal cord and cauda equina disorders. Continuum (Minneap Minn). 2021;27(1):225-63.

8. A 7-year-old child is brought with complaints of ptosis and diplopia. On examination, the pupils are bilaterally equal and reactive to light. The child has ptosis and diplopia, which worsens later in the day. In addition, the child has abnormalities of saccadic eye movements and quick phases of nystagmus. Where would you localize the lesion?

A. Superior division third cranial nerve palsy
B. Palsy involving III, IV, and VI cranial nerve
C. Neuromuscular junction
D. Muscle

EXPLANATION

The child has fatiguability as confirmed by worsening of symptoms later in the day, with involvement of extraocular muscles and sparing of pupillary muscle. The fatigable weakness is a hallmark of the neuromuscular junction involvement. This is typically seen in myasthenia.

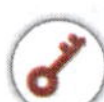

Key: C

BOOST YOUR KNOWLEDGE

The differentiation between different categories of LMN lesions is shown here.

	Weakness					
Locus	***Face***	***Arms***	***Legs***	***Proximal–distal***	***DTR***	***Other***
Anterior horn cell	Late	++++	++++	≥	Absent	Fasciculations
Peripheral nerve	0	+++	+++	<	Absent to decreased	• Fibrillations on electromyography (EMG) • Glove and stocking sensory impairment if mixed neuropathy
Neuromuscular junction	+++	+++	+++	=	Normal	• Fatiguability • Decremental response on nerve conduction studies
Muscles	Variable	++	+	>	Hyporeflexia	

REFERENCE/SOURCE

- Sarnat HB. Evaluation and investigation of neuromuscular disorders (Table 625-1). In: Kliegman RM, St Geme III JW, Blum NJ, Shah SS, Tasker RC, Wilson KM (Eds). Nelson Textbook of Pediatrics, 21st edition. Elsevier; 2019. pp. 3245-54.

9. A 2-year-old child is brought with complaints of impairment of motor milestones. She was born of a third-degree consanguineous marriage with no antenatal or perinatal adverse events. The child attained sitting between 8 and 10 months of age but has not been able to stand.

On examination, she has tongue fasciculations, generalized atrophy of muscles, weakness of muscles (proximal > distal), and areflexia in all four limbs. Her mental functions and sensory examination are normal. Where do you localize the lesion in this case?

A. Cerebral cortex
B. Brainstem
C. Anterior horn cell
D. Muscle

EXPLANATION

The lesion described in question is an LMN lesion. The child has atrophy of muscles, weakness, and areflexia, all of which can be present in LMN lesions. UMN lesion will classically have hyperreflexia and spasticity. In general, myopathies follow a proximal distribution of weakness and muscle wasting (with the notable exception of myotonic muscular dystrophy); neuropathies are generally distal in distribution (with the notable exception of juvenile spinal muscular atrophy). Muscle fasciculation, often best seen in the tongue, is a sign of denervation. Within the LMN, the presence of fasciculations localizes the lesion to anterior horn cells.

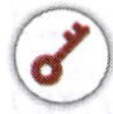

Key: C

BOOST YOUR KNOWLEDGE

The LMN consists of the anterior horn cell, root, nerve, neuromuscular junction, and muscle. A lesion in the anterior horn cell is typically characterized by fasciculations and polyminimyoclonus. Root and nerve lesions are characterized by pain and sensory and motor findings. The neuropathies typically have a glove and stocking pattern of sensory impairments. Fatiguability and preserved deep reflexes are the hallmarks of neuromuscular junction involvement. Muscle diseases will have a proximal weakness with hyporeflexia.

REFERENCE/SOURCE

- Sarnat HB. Evaluation and investigation of neuromuscular disorders (Table 625-1). In: Kliegman RM, St Geme III JW, Blum NJ, Shah SS, Tasker RC, Wilson KM (Eds). Nelson Textbook of Pediatrics, 21st edition. Elsevier; 2019. pp. 3245-54.

10. **A 16-year-old teenager is brought with complaints of difficulty with rapid movements. On examination, the child has a muscular body with well-chiseled muscles, though he denies going to the gymnasium. The teenager demonstrates noticeable muscle stiffness, particularly in the hands and lower limbs. When asked to perform rapid movements like gripping a pen and leaving it or walking quickly and stopping and again walking, there is a delay in initiating these actions. Where do you localize the lesion?**

A. Muscle
B. Myoneural junction
C. Nerve
D. Anterior horn cell

EXPLANATION

Delay in releasing a pen suggests a delay in the relaxation of muscle after contraction. This is the hallmark of myotonia. Myotonia is, by definition, the impairment of relaxation of skeletal muscles after voluntary contraction or electrical stimulation. Many etiologies result in myotonia, including dystrophic and nondystrophic myotonias.

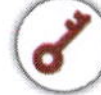

Key: A

BOOST YOUR KNOWLEDGE

The four main categories of inherited muscle diseases are: (1) Muscular dystrophies, (2) congenital myopathies, (3) muscle ion-channel disorders (also called channelopathies), and (4) metabolic myopathies.

REFERENCE/SOURCE

- Bharucha-Goebel DX. Muscular dystrophies. In: Kliegman RM, St Geme III JW, Blum NJ, Shah SS, Tasker RC, Wilson KM (Eds). Nelson Textbook of Pediatrics, 21st edition. Elsevier; 2019. pp. 3280-94.

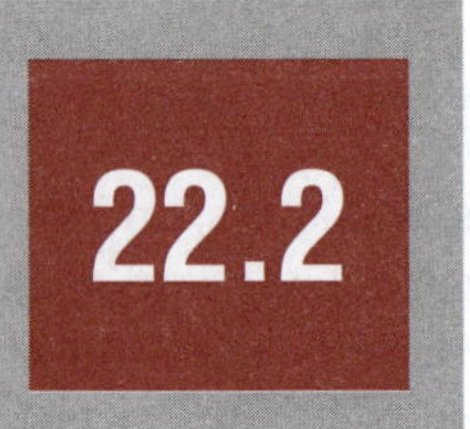

Neurological Investigations

Suvasini Sharma

1. A 9-month-old developmentally normal infant presents with a history of first episode of brief generalized tonic-clonic seizure with fever. Which of the following investigations is *not* indicated?

A. Complete blood count
B. Lumbar puncture
C. Electroencephalography (EEG)
D. Serum calcium levels

EXPLANATION

A febrile seizure is defined as a seizure occurring with fever in a child from 6 months to 5 years of age without any evidence of central nervous system (CNS) infection or dyselectrolytemia and without any prior history of afebrile seizures. A febrile seizure is said to be simple, if it is brief (<15 minutes in duration), single, and generalized. The child mentioned in the question has presented with the first episode of simple febrile seizure. In this situation, fever work-up including complete blood count, and other fever-related investigations as per clinical indication are recommended. Serum calcium levels are usually recommended, as children with rickets and hypocalcemia can present with seizures in this age group. In infants <12 months of age, a lumbar puncture to rule out meningitis should be considered in all children with the first episode of febrile seizures, especially if they have not received immunization against *Streptococcal pneumoniae* and *Haemophilus influenzae* type B. EEG and magnetic resonance imaging (MRI) are not indicated in simple febrile seizures, as there is a very low risk of development of epilepsy in this group.

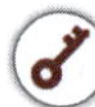

Key: C

BOOST YOUR KNOWLEDGE

Complex febrile seizures are said to occur when a febrile seizure has any of the following characteristics:

- Prolonged (>15 minutes duration)
- Focal
- >1 seizure occurring in 24 hours
- Investigations are individualized in these patients, but generally MRI and EEG are usually performed in these patients. However, the prognostic significance of the abnormalities seen in EEG and MRI to predict future epilepsy is unclear.

REFERENCE/SOURCE

- Kaushik JS, Sondhi V, Yoganathan S, Dubey R, Sharma S, Vinayan KP, et al. Association of Child Neurology (AOCN) Consensus Statement on the diagnosis and management of Febrile seizures. Indian Pediatr. 2022;59(4):300-6.

2. A 5-day-old girl baby, born full term, weighed 3.5 kg, cried immediately at birth, was well till Day 3 and developed lethargy, poor feeding, and vomiting on Day 4 of life. The serum bilirubin and blood sugar were normal. The cranial ultrasound was normal. Urine ketones were negative. The sepsis screen was negative, and there was no metabolic acidosis. The serum ammonia levels were 350 mmol/L. What is the likely diagnosis?

A. Organic acidemia
B. Nonketotic hyperglycinemia
C. Fatty acid oxidation defect
D. Urea cycle defect

EXPLANATION

Common causes of encephalopathy in neonates include sepsis/meningitis, hypoxic-ischemic injury, hypoglycemia, bilirubin encephalopathy, intracranial hemorrhage, and inborn errors of metabolism (IEM). The baby in question was a term baby appropriate for gestational age with no immediate perinatal concerns and is hence unlikely to have hypoxic-ischemic brain injury. Hypoglycemia was absent. Sepsis must be considered in this situation, but the sepsis screen was negative. A normal cranial ultrasound and normal serum bilirubin level ruled out intracranial bleeding and bilirubin encephalopathy, respectively. Hence inborn error of metabolism is a strong possibility. The next step is to do the basic metabolic investigations to classify the category of metabolic disorders. *This includes four basic investigations:* (1) Arterial/venous blood gas to look for acidosis, (2) blood ammonia levels, (3) urine ketones, and (4) serum lactate, in addition to blood sugar.

Table explains the categorization of IEM based on simple metabolic screening tests:

Categorization of neonatal IEM using metabolic screening tests

Acidosis	*Ketosis*	*↑Lactate*	*↑Ammonia*	*Hypoglycemia*	*Diagnosis*
+/–	+	–	+/–	+/–	Maple syrup urine disease
++	++	–	+	+/–	Organic aciduria
+	+/–	++	–	+/–	Lactic acidosis (caused by abnormal oxidative metabolism in mitochondrial disorders, glycogen storage disorders, and disorders of gluconeogenesis)
–	–	–	++	–	Urea cycle defects
+/–	–	+/–	+/–	+	Fatty acid oxidation disorders
–	–	–	–		Nonketotic hyperglycinemia, sulfite oxidase deficiency, peroxisomal disorders, phenylketonuria, and galactosemia

As per the Table, the baby in question fits into the urea cycle defect.

Key: D

BOOST YOUR KNOWLEDGE

The next steps for diagnosing the type of urea cycle defect include testing for plasma citrulline levels and urinary orotic acid levels (*See* Flowchart).

Approach to the patient with suspected urea cycle defect and hyperammonemia:

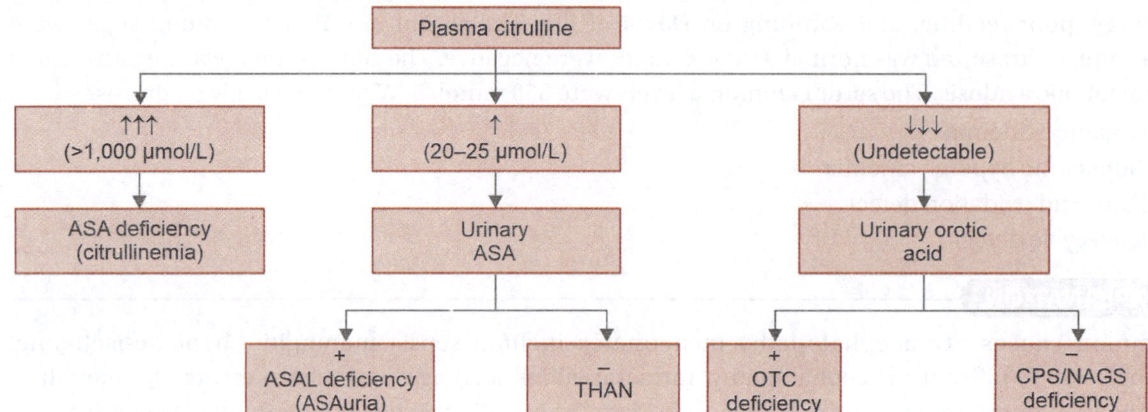

(ASA: argininosuccinic acid; ASAL: argininosuccinic acid lyase; CPS: carbamoylphosphate synthetase I; NAGS: N-acetylglutamate synthetase; OTC: ornithine transcarbamoylase; THAN: transient hyperammonemia of newborn)

Genetic testing in the form of whole-exome sequencing is also recommended to confirm the diagnosis and help with genetic counseling, especially for future pregnancies.

REFERENCE/SOURCE

- Sharma S, Arushi GS. Inborn Errors of Metabolism. AIIMS NICU Protocols 2023 *(In press).*

3. A 6-month-old baby presents with a history of episodes of sudden flexion of the head and upper body occurring in clusters, noted since the last 2 weeks. These episodes occur chiefly when the baby wakes up from sleep. The birth and perinatal period were uneventful, and the child gained developmental milestones in an age-appropriate manner. Since the onset of these movements, the parents have noticed reduced eye contact, reduced smiling, and irritability. On examination, he was noted to have leaf-shaped hypopigmented macules on the back. Neurological examination revealed no abnormalities. An EEG was obtained, which showed chaotic high-voltage activity intermixed with spikes and sharp wave discharges from bilateral brain regions. What will be the treatment of choice?

A. Vigabatrin
B. Sodium valproate
C. Adrenocorticotropic hormone
D. Prednisolone

EXPLANATION

The child in question was presented with infantile spasms. Infantile spasms are a type of seizure, typically seen in young children, characterized by flexion/extension of the head and trunk with stiffening, occurring in clusters, and usually related to the sleep-wake cycle. Infantile epileptic spasms syndrome is a type of developmental and epileptic encephalopathy characterized by the presence of infantile spasms, and EEG showing epileptiform abnormalities, typically hypsarrhythmia. Hypsarrhythmia is the EEG appearance of chaotic high-voltage activity with intermixed spike and sharp wave discharges from multifocal brain regions. The infant in question had a clear history suggestive of infantile spasms, and EEG concurrent with hypsarrhythmia. The term West syndrome was previously used to describe the trial of infantile spasms, developmental delay/regression, and EEG findings of hypsarrhythmia. The presence of cutaneous findings supports the possibility of tuberous sclerosis as etiology.

Etiology of Infantile Epileptic Spasms Syndrome (West Syndrome)

Prenatal:

- Brain malformations, e.g., lissencephaly
- Genetic epileptic encephalopathies, e.g., STXBP1

- Neurocutaneous syndromes, e.g., tuberous sclerosis
- Chromosomal abnormalities, e.g., Down syndrome
- Intrauterine infections, e.g., TORCH

Perinatal:
- Perinatal hypoxia
- Neonatal hypoglycemia
- Neonatal meningitis
- Perinatal stroke
- Neonatal intracranial hemorrhage

Postnatal:
- CNS infections
- Traumatic brain injury
- Near drowning

The etiology of infantile epileptic spasm syndrome is varied and includes prenatal, perinatal, and postnatal causes as shown given Box. The treatment of choice is hormonal therapy, which includes adrenocorticotropic hormone or oral corticosteroids, for all cases other than tuberous sclerosis complex, and vigabatrin should be the first choice for tuberous sclerosis complex.

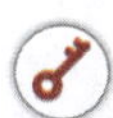

Key: A

BOOST YOUR KNOWLEDGE

Vigabatrin is recommended as first-line monotherapy in tuberous sclerosis complex-related infantile spasms or focal seizures in children <1 year of age. Initiating treatment at an early age, at or prior to the clinical onset of seizures, may improve the long-term outcome of epilepsy and neurodevelopment. Vigabatrin treatment may be initiated presymptomatically in the presence of focal spike-wave discharges on EEG.

REFERENCE/SOURCE

- Sharma S, Kaushik JS, Srivastava K, Goswami JN, Sahu JK, Vinayan KP, et al. Association of Child Neurology (AOCN)—Indian Epilepsy Society (IES) Consensus Guidelines for the Diagnosis and Management of West Syndrome. Indian Pediatr. 2021;58(1):54-66.

4. A 5-year-old boy was presented with acute onset ascending paralysis of all four limbs. On examination, there is hypotonia and areflexia. A nerve conduction study was obtained. Which of the following findings suggests the presence of an acute inflammatory demyelinating polyneuropathy (AIDP) variant of Guillain-Barré syndrome?

A. Reduced compound muscle action potential (CMAP) amplitude
B. Absent sensory nerve action potentials
C. Presence of conduction block
D. Reduced distal latency

EXPLANATION

The demyelinating variant (AIDP) of Guillain-Barré syndrome has the following electrophysiological characteristics:
- Prolonged distal latency
- Reduced conduction velocity
- Presence of conduction block or temporal dispersion
- Prolonged F-wave latency or absent F-waves

The acute motor axonal (AMAN) variant is characterized by the presence of reduced CMAP amplitudes with preserved conduction velocity and distal latency with normal sensory nerve action potentials.

The acute motor and sensory axonal neuropathy (AMSAN) variant is characterized by the reduced CMAP amplitudes with preserved conduction velocity and distal latency and reduced sensory nerve action potential amplitude.

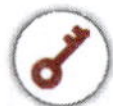 **Key: C**

BOOST YOUR KNOWLEDGE

Nerve conduction studies can be normal in the first week of illness. In such cases, treatment should be started on clinical diagnosis, and the study should be repeated after 1 week. The earliest nerve conduction abnormality to occur is the prolonged F-wave latency or absent F-waves. This is because F-waves assess the proximal nerve segments, which are usually affected early in Guillain-Barré syndrome.

REFERENCE/SOURCE

- Rabie M, Ashwal S, Nevo Y. Inflammatory neuropathies. In: Swaiman KF, Ashwal S, Ferriero DM, Schor NF, Finkel RS, Gropman AL, et al. (Eds). Swaiman's Pediatric Neurology: Principles and Practice, 6th edition. Elsevier; 2017. pp. 1086-91.

5. Which of the following statements regarding glucose transporter 1 deficiency syndrome (Glut1DS) is *correct*?

A. It usually presents with acute flaccid paralysis and dizziness
B. The MRI of the brain shows abnormalities in the occipital lobe
C. The cerebral spinal fluid (CSF) to blood sugar ratio is <0.8
D. It results from a mutation in the *SLC2A1* gene

EXPLANATION

Glucose transporter 1 deficiency syndrome is a brain energy failure disorder, resulting from impaired glucose transport into the brain caused by pathogenic variants in the *SLC2A1* gene. Clinical features include infantile-onset epilepsy, movement disorders, ataxia, microcephaly, developmental delay, learning difficulties, and dysarthria. The diagnosis is confirmed on lumbar puncture by low CSF glucose levels with normal or low CSF lactate after a 4–6 hours fasting period in the absence of hypoglycemia and other causes of hypoglycorrhachia. Typically, CSF glucose levels are <40 mg/dL, and a low ratio of CSF : Blood glucose ratio (<0.6) is noted. The MRI of the brain is usually normal or may show nonspecific changes such as delayed myelination.

 **Key: D**

BOOST YOUR KNOWLEDGE

The ketogenic diet is an effective treatment for this condition as it provides alternative sources of energy substrate in the form of ketone bodies that the brain preferentially utilizes. In older children, adolescents, and adults, less restrictive variants such as the modified Atkins diet and the low glycemic index treatment may be used. Triheptanoin, an anaplerotic agent that replenishes the Krebs cycle metabolites, has been found useful in reducing the nonepileptic paroxysmal manifestations and normalizing the brain bioenergetics profile in patients with GLUT1DS. Drugs that impair GLUT1 function, e.g., caffeine, phenobarbital, diazepam, chloral hydrate, and tricyclic antidepressants, are best avoided.

REFERENCE/SOURCE

- Sharma S, Prasad AN. Inborn errors of metabolism and epilepsy: current understanding, diagnosis, and treatment approaches. Int J Mol Sci. 2017;18(7):1384.

6. All of the following statements regarding traumatic lumbar puncture are true, *except*:

A. It increases in an artificial rise in WBC count
B. The increase in WBC is approximately one WBC per 100 RBCs in the CSF
C. If a traumatic tap occurs, CSF should be collected in three consecutive tubes to look to differentiate between intracranial hemorrhage and traumatic lumbar puncture
D. In patients with abnormal hemogram, a correction factor should be applied to predict the WBC in CSF

EXPLANATION

Traumatic tap results in an artificial increase in WBC count by approximately one WBC for every 700 RBCs in the CSF. In patients with an abnormal hemogram, the direct calculation is corrected by the observed plasma ratio: predicted WBC (CSF) = RBC (CSF) × [WBC (plasma)/RBC (plasma)]. If a traumatic tap occurs, CSF is collected in three consecutive tubes, and cell count is measured. If the number of RBCs is relatively constant, then it is assumed that the presence of blood is due to intracranial hemorrhage. A falling count suggests a traumatic tap. This three-tube method, however, is not always reliable.

Key: B

BOOST YOUR KNOWLEDGE

Traumatic lumbar puncture has been reported in 10–30% of lumbar punctures in children, with higher rates in neonates. A thinner bore needle (such as the use of a 25G needle in neonates instead of 22G) can reduce the rates of traumatic lumbar puncture.

REFERENCES/SOURCES

- Choudhary A. Cerebrospinal fluid and neurophysiology. In: Gupta P, Menon PSN, Ramji S, Lodha R (Eds). PG Textbook of Pediatrics, 3rd edition. New Delhi: Jaypee Brothers Medical Publishers; 2022. pp. 2395-401.
- Nigrovic LE, Kuppermann N, Neuman MI. Risk factors for traumatic or unsuccessful lumbar punctures in children. Ann Emerg Med. 2007;49(6):762-71.

7. Repetitive nerve stimulation tests are used for the diagnosis of:

A. Peripheral neuropathies
B. Myasthenia gravis
C. Congenital myopathy
D. Myotonic dystrophy

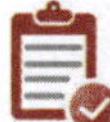

EXPLANATION

A repetitive nerve stimulation test is performed for the diagnosis of a disorder of neuromuscular transmission. The classic abnormality is the documentation of a decremental response of the CMAP to repetitive stimulation of a motor nerve. The percentage of decrease in amplitude and area is calculated between the first CMAP produced by a train of stimuli and each successive one. A decrement of greater than 10% is considered a positive study.

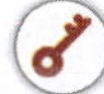

Key: B

BOOST YOUR KNOWLEDGE

The decrement is attributable to the failure of some muscle fibers to reach the threshold and contract when several volleys of acetylcholine vesicles are released at the neuromuscular junction.

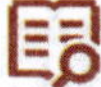

REFERENCE/SOURCE

- Silvestri NJ, Barohn RJ, Wolfe GI. Acquired disorders of the neuromuscular junction. In: Swaiman KF, Ashwal S, Ferriero DM, Schor NF, Finkel RS, Gropman AL, et al. (Eds). Swaiman's Pediatric Neurology: Principles and Practice, 6th edition. Elsevier; 2017. pp. 1098-105.

8. A 7-year-old girl is brought with a history of proximal muscle weakness for the last 3 months. Note the clinical photographs.

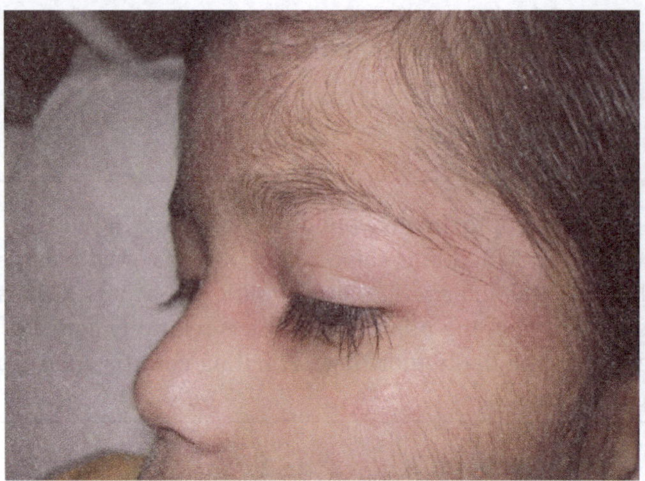
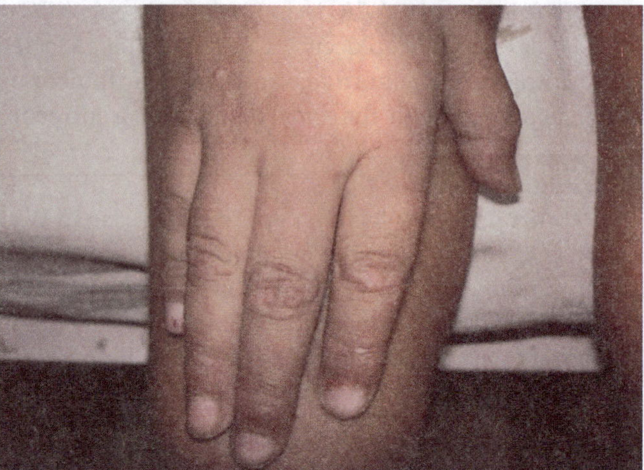

Which of the following statements regarding this condition is *true*?

A. Steroids are contraindicated as children may have underlying immunodeficiency
B. The risk of malignancy is increased
C. Electrocardiogram (ECG) abnormalities are noted in 50% of affected children
D. There is complete sparing of distal muscle strength

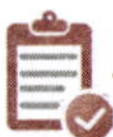

EXPLANATION

This child has juvenile dermatomyositis as seen by the periorbital heliotrope rash and Gottron's papules over the knuckles. Weakness typically affects the neck flexors and shoulder and pelvic girdles first. Distal weakness is usually present, though as severe as proximal muscles. Complete sparing of the distal strength should lead the clinician to seek an alternative diagnosis, most frequently, dystrophy. About 50% of the affected children have ECG abnormalities including conduction defects and dysrhythmias. In contrast to adult dermatomyositis patients, children do not have an increased incidence of malignancy. Corticosteroids are the most effective therapeutic options.

Key: C

BOOST YOUR KNOWLEDGE

Subcutaneous calcifications are noted in 30–70% of childhood cases. Apart from ECG abnormalities, cardiac involvement can occur in the form of pericarditis, myocarditis, and congestive cardiac failure. Lung involvement can occur in the form of interstitial lung disease or bronchiolitis obliterans. Dysphagia and delayed gastric emptying are common.

REFERENCE/SOURCE

- Amato A, Kissel JT. Inflammatory myopathies. In: Swaiman KF, Ashwal S, Ferriero DM, Schor NF, Finkel RS, Gropman AL, et al. (Eds). Swaiman's Pediatric Neurology: Principles and Practice, 6th edition. Elsevier; 2017. pp. 1041-7.

9. A 2-year-old premorbidly normal boy was brought with complaints of falls while walking and increasing stiffness of limbs for 18 months of age. He has had a mild cognitive decline for the last 1 month. There is no history of seizures, vision, or hearing problems. The head size is normal. On examination, the tone is increased with absent reflexes and extensor plantar responses. Note the MRI image. What is the likely diagnosis?

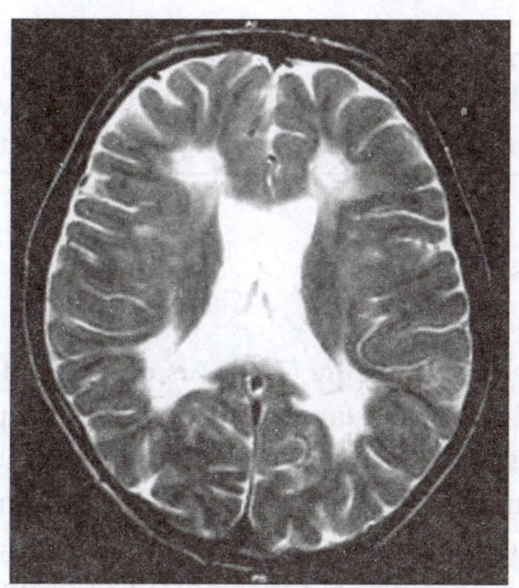

A. Metachromatic leukodystrophy
B. Tay-Sachs disease
C. Adrenoleukodystrophy
D. Neuronal ceroid lipofuscinosis

EXPLANATION

This premorbidly normal child with progressive neuroregression has a neurodegenerative disorder. By clinical phenotype, it is likely to be a white matter disorder, as he developed gait difficulty and stiffness in limbs early in the course of the illness. In white matter disorders, motor problems like gait difficulties and stiffness occur early while seizures and cognitive decline occur late in the illness, as shown in Table here.

Differentiating features	***White matter disorders***	***Gray matter disorders***
Seizures	Late, rare	Early, severe
Cognitive functions	Initially normal	Progressive dementia
Peripheral neuropathy	Early demyelination	Late, axonal loss
Spasticity	Early, severe	Later, progressive
Reflexes	Absent (neuropathy) or exaggerated (long tracts)	Normal or exaggerated

The further approach depends on the head size and the presence of peripheral nervous system (PNS) involvement. (*See* Flowchart)

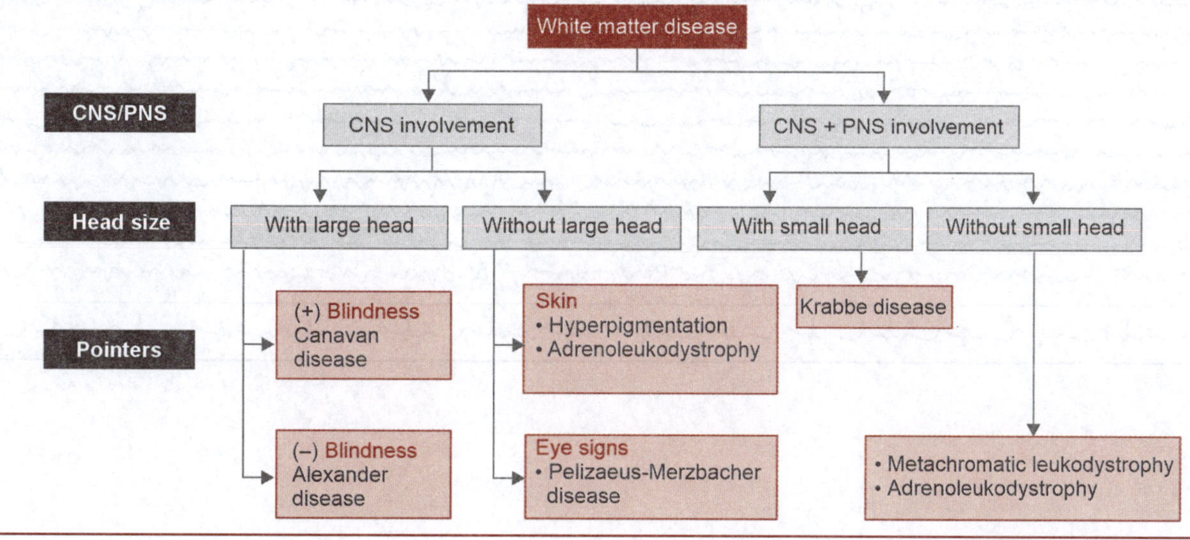

The patient in question has a normal head size and features of PNS involvement, i.e., absent deep tendon reflexes. Hence, the clinical possibilty is metachromatic leukodystrophy. This is further strengthened by the MRI appearance of periventricular white matter signal abnormalities with sparing of the subcortical U fibers.

Key: A

BOOST YOUR KNOWLEDGE

The diagnosis of metachromatic leukodystrophy (MLD) is confirmed by enzyme testing for the arylsulfatase enzyme levels, which are decreased by molecular genetic testing. This presentation is late-infantile MLD, which is the most common clinical presentation of MLD. A close differential would be late infantile Krabbe disease, which is rare, as Krabbe disease more commonly has an early infantile presentation. Infants with Krabbe disease also have microcephaly. The MRI appearance in Krabbe also demonstrates periventricular white matter involvement, like MLD, but in addition, there is involvement of brainstem tracts, especially the corticospinal tracts, and the dentate nuclei.

REFERENCE/SOURCE

- Sankhyan N. Neurodegenerative disorders. In: Gupta P, Menon PSN, Ramji S, Lodha R (Eds). PG Textbook of Pediatrics, 3rd edition. New Delhi: Jaypee Brothers Medical Publishers; 2022. pp. 2566-74.

10. A 9-year-old premorbidly normal boy was presented with two episodes of seizures in sleep. The seizures were associated with drooling and twitching of the mouth with twisting of the mouth to one side. He appeared as if he was trying to speak, but unable to. The MRI was normal. See EEG images below.

EEG in Drowsiness

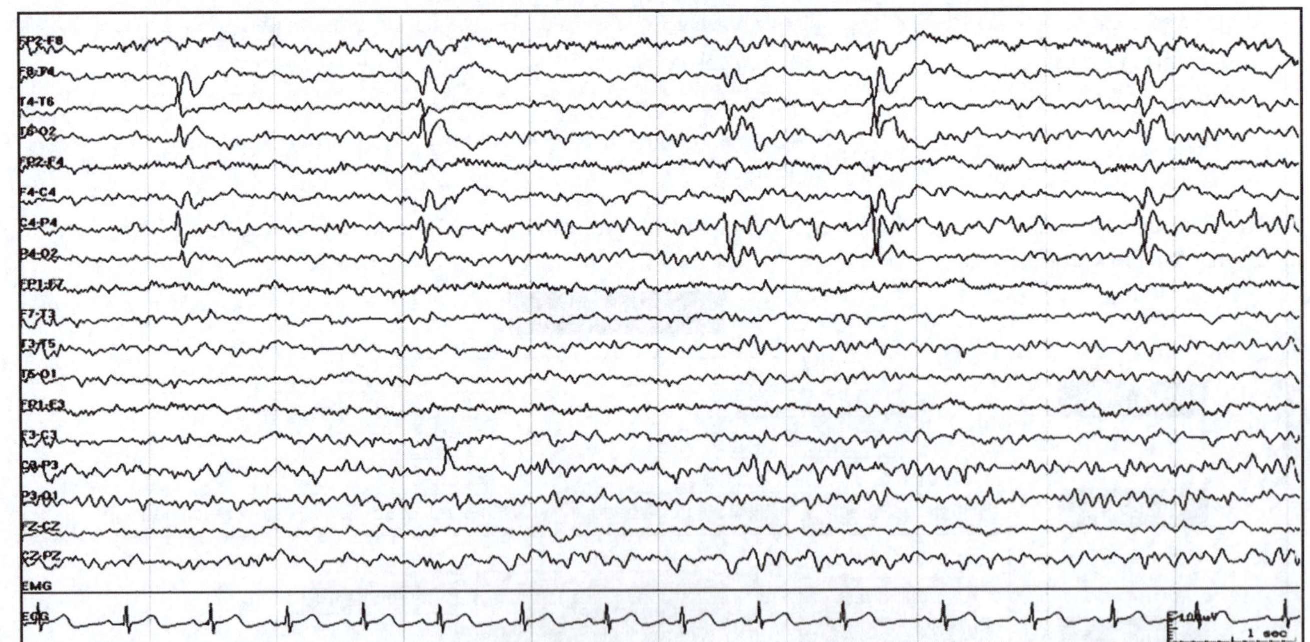

EEG in Stage 2 Sleep

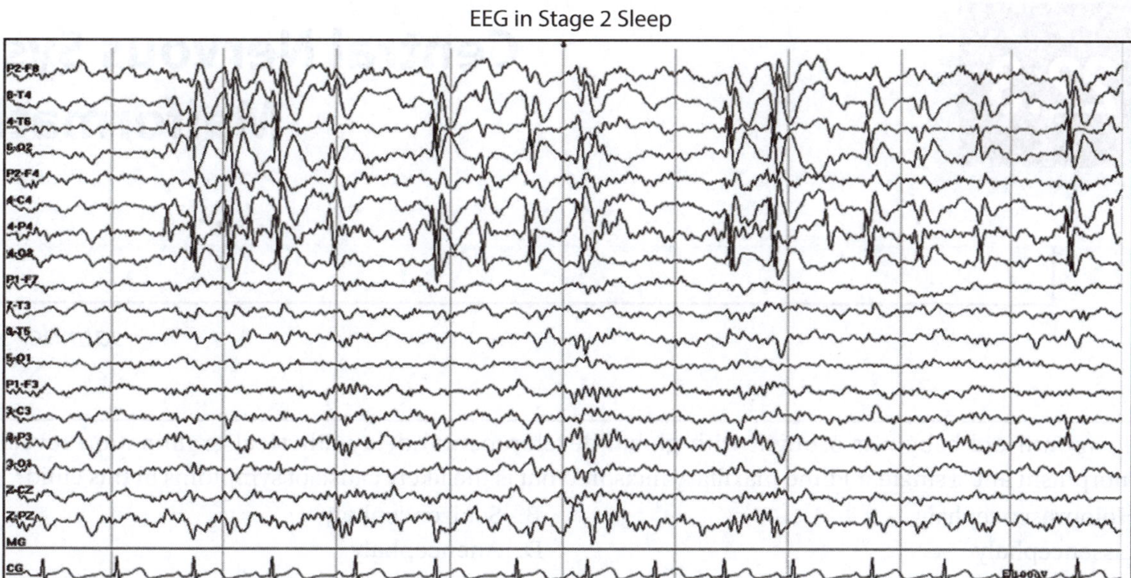

What is the likely diagnosis?

A. Childhood absence epilepsy
B. Self-limited epilepsy with centrotemporal spikes (SeLECTS)
C. Nocturnal frontal lobe epilepsy
D. Self-limited epilepsy with autonomic seizures

EXPLANATION

This child has SeLECTS, an electroclinical syndrome, earlier called benign childhood epilepsy with centrotemporal spikes (BECTS) or benign rolandic epilepsy. This is the most common and most characteristic form of self-limited epilepsy in children. It occurs in neurodevelopmentally normal children between 5 and 12 years of age. The nocturnal seizures are characterized by unilateral facial sensorimotor symptoms (30%), oropharyngolaryngeal manifestations (53%), speech arrest (40%), and hypersalivation (30%). The EEG is a diagnostic and shows focal spike-wave discharges arising from the central and temporal leads, which markedly increase in sleep. Childhood absence epilepsy is characterized by absence seizures (vacant stares with an abrupt onset and offset when awake) and EEG showing generalized 3 Hz spike-wave discharges. Nocturnal frontal lobe epilepsy also presents with nocturnal seizures, but these seizures are very brief, and the patient shows a lot of movement during the seizure (hypermotor). The EEG shows frontal spikes, or may be normal. Self-limited epilepsy with autonomic seizures presents in young children (3–6 years of age) with seizures in sleep with predominant autonomic symptoms, especially vomiting and pallor.

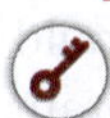

Key: B

BOOST YOUR KNOWLEDGE

The absence of obvious interictal neurologic or mental impairment is one of the main features of SeLECTS. However, several minor cognitive and behavioral problems can occur. Language, executive function, attention, memory, and behavior problems have been noted. The treatment of choice is sodium valproate or levetiracetam. Carbamazepine should be avoided, as it can precipitate the occurrence of continuous spike-wave discharges in sleep (CSWS), which can sometimes occur in these children.

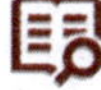

REFERENCE/SOURCE

- Specchio N, Wirrell EC, Scheffer IE, Nabbout R, Riney K, Samia P, et al. International League Against Epilepsy classification and definition of epilepsy syndromes with onset in childhood: Position paper by the ILAE Task Force on Nosology and Definitions. Epilepsia. 2022;63(6):1398-442.

CHAPTER 22.3

Central Nervous System Malformations

Jatinder S Goraya

1. An 11-month-old baby was brought with global developmental delay. Physical examination revealed facial dysmorphism and a single midline maxillary incisor. What is the likely cause of symptoms in this child?

A. Holoprosencephaly
B. Schizencephaly
C. Lissencephaly
D. Anencephaly

EXPLANATION

Almost all the brain malformations mentioned here present with developmental delay. Midline facial defects hypotelorism, flattened nasal bridge, median cleft lip and palate, or a single median maxillary central incisor suggest the possibility of holoprosencephaly. Miller–Dieker syndrome has characteristic facial feature and is associated with lissencephaly. Anencephaly is a brain malformation that is easily recognizable from visual inspection.

Key: A

BOOST YOUR KNOWLEDGE

Brain malformations are a common cause of neurological dysfunction in children. Onset of clinical manifestations depends on the type and severity of the malformation. Some are part of a clinically recognizable syndromes such as trisomy 13, trisomy 18, Smith–Lemli–Opitz syndrome, Zellweger syndrome (list is extensive), while other are diagnosed only on neuroimaging. Other than developmental delay, other signs and symptoms associated with brain malformation include neonatal seizures, infantile spasms and other neonatal and infantile epileptic encephalopathies, focal epilepsies, cognitive and language deficits, behavioral disorders, specific learning disorders, motor deficits, spasticity, ataxia, and movement disorders. Diagnosis is by neuroimaging, and brain magnetic resonance imaging (MRI) is the first choice. Genetic testing should be done if available. Family should be counseled regarding prenatal diagnosis in future pregnancies. There is no specific treatment for this brain malformation.

REFERENCES/SOURCES

- Gupta P, Menon PSN, Ramji S, Lodha R. Chapter: Brain malformations. PG Textbook of Pediatrics, 2nd edition. New Delhi: Jaypee Brothers Medical Publishers; 2018. p. 2426
- Tekendo-Ngongang C, Muenke M, Kruszka P. Holoprosencephaly Overview. 2000. In: Adam MP, Feldman J, Mirzaa GM, Pagon RA, Wallace SE, Bean LJH, et al. (Eds). GeneReviews® [Internet]. Seattle (WA): University of Washington, Seattle; 1993-2023.

2. Which of the following non-neurological complications are often associated with holoprosencephaly?

A. Cardiac defects
B. Renal anomalies
C. Endocrinological dysfunction
D. Limb deformities

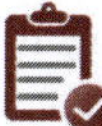

EXPLANATION

Holoprosencephaly (HPE), being the defect of failure to divide in midline, hypothalamic/pituitary dysfunctions are common. Diabetes insipidus is the most frequent abnormality, and less commonly growth hormone deficiency, hypocortisolism, and hypothyroidism are seen. Other anomalies such as renal, cardiac or limb abnormalities are not a feature of holoprosencephaly. Endocrinological deficiencies are also seen in children with septo-optic dysplasia.

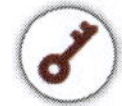

Key: C

BOOST YOUR KNOWLEDGE

Holoprosencephaly is classified as—alobar, semilobar, lobar, midline interhemispheric and recently described septopreoptic types. In addition to nonseparation of cerebral hemispheres, there is variable degree of nonseparation of hypothalamic, thalamic, lentiform, and caudate nuclei. The alobar HPE is the most severe, showing almost complete absence of separation of the cerebral hemispheres with characteristic midline single ventricle (a crescent-shaped monoventricle). Lobar HPE is the mildest form, and here the lack of separation is restricted to the most rostral and ventral parts of the cerebral hemispheres. Dysmorphism characterized by midline facial anomalies frequently accompany HPE.

REFERENCES/SOURCES

- Gupta P, Menon PSN, Ramji S, Lodha R. Chapter: Brain malformations. PG Textbook of Pediatrics, 2nd edition. New Delhi: Jaypee Brothers Medical Publishers; 2018. p. 2426.
- Ramakrishnan S, Gupta V. Holoprosencephaly. In: StatPearls. Treasure Island (FL): StatPearls Publishing; 2023.
- Tekendo-Ngongang C, Muenke M, Kruszka P. Holoprosencephaly Overview. 2000. In: Adam MP, Feldman J, Mirzaa GM, Pagon RA, Wallace SE, Bean LJH, et al. (Eds). GeneReviews®. Seattle (WA): University of Washington, Seattle; 1993-2023.

3. A 7-month-old girl with developmental delay presented with frequent episodes of sudden body flexion for 2 weeks. These episodes occurred commonly when she woke up from sleep, and she will continue to have multiple episodes at a time lasting 5–10 minutes. She would often cry during these episodes. Her electroencephalogram (EEG) showed hypsarrhythmia. Ophthalmological examination revealed lacunae in the retina. Brain MRI of this patient is likely to reveal:

A. Lissencephaly
B. Schizencephaly
C. Cortical tubers
D. Agenesis of corpus callosum

EXPLANATION

Occurrence of developmental delay, infantile spasms and hypsarrhythmia on EEG defines West syndrome. Its occurrence in a girl who has retinal lacunae points to Aicardi syndrome which is associated with agenesis of corpus callosum.

Key: D

BOOST YOUR KNOWLEDGE

Aicardi syndrome is a rare genetic neurological disorder with an X-linked dominant transmission that occurs almost exclusively in females. It is characterized by the occurrence of triad of infantile spasms, retinal lacunae and agenesis of corpus callosum. Infantile spasms begin during infancy and often evolve into other types of seizures which are generally refractory to treatment. Affected children have microcephaly, moderate-to-severe psychomotor retardation, and intellectual disability. Dysmorphism affecting face and extremities is common. Vertebral anomalies such as hemivertebrae, block vertebrae, fused vertebrae, and missing ribs are common and can cause scoliosis. In eyes, in addition to chorioretinal lacunae, microphthalmia and optic nerve coloboma may be noted. Agenesis of corpus callosum may have other associated brain abnormalities such as polymicrogyria, periventricular and subcortical heterotopias, and third ventricular or choroid plexus cysts.

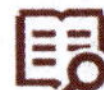

REFERENCES/SOURCES

- Gupta P, Menon PSN, Ramji S, Lodha R. Chapter: Brain malformations. PG Textbook of Pediatrics, 2nd edition. New Delhi: Jaypee Brothers Medical Publishers; 2018. p. 2426.
- Sutton VR, Van den Veyver IB. Aicardi Syndrome. In: Adam MP, Feldman J, Mirzaa GM, Pagon RA, Wallace SE, Bean LJH, et al. (Eds). GeneReviews®. Seattle (WA): University of Washington, Seattle; 1993-2023.

4. This infant presented with poor vision. Though he was born normally, he had neonatal seizures secondary to hypoglycemia during the neonatal period. Physical examination was unremarkable except for small looking penis. Ophthalmological examination revealed poor vision, nystagmus, and hypoplastic optic nerve heads. What is the most important finding on brain MRI?

A. Absent septum pellucidum
B. Septum cavum pellucidum
C. Arnold–Chiari malformation
D. Dandy–Walker malformation

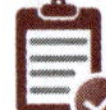

EXPLANATION

Clinical presentation of poor vision, nystagmus, and small optic head (suggesting optic nerve hypoplasia) are seen in children with septo-optic dysplasia (SOD) or de Morsier syndrome. SOD is associated with midline brain abnormalities and pituitary dysfunction. *Absence of septum pellucidum* is the characteristic neuroimaging finding.

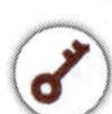

Key: A

BOOST YOUR KNOWLEDGE

Septo-optic dysplasia, previously called de Morsier syndrome is a rare disorder of brain developmental and comprises optic nerve hypoplasia, pituitary abnormalities, and absent septum pellucidum. Most cases are sporadic but familial transmission (both autosomal recessive and autosomal dominant) are known. Mutations in *HESX1*, *SOX2*, *SOX3* and *OTX2* have been found in small number of patients. In others, environmental factors such as alcohol and drug abuse, young maternal age may be implicated.

Majority of the patients come to attention through neonatal seizures secondary to hypoglycemia, poor vision, developmental delay, other endocrinal dysfunction such as hypothyroidism, diabetes insipidus, precocious puberty, obesity, thermoregulatory disturbances. Microphallus may be an important clinical pointer.

Neuroimaging with brain MRI reveals characteristic absence of septum pellucidum and/or corpus callosum. Treatment is symptomatic. Hormonal deficiencies are monitored and treated with specific hormone replacements.

REFERENCE/SOURCE

- Gupta P, Menon PSN, Ramji S, Lodha R. Chapter: Brain malformations. PG Textbook of Pediatrics, 2nd edition. New Delhi: Jaypee Brothers Medical Publishers; 2018. p. 2426.

5. Inborn errors of metabolism are rarely causative of brain malformations. Which of the following inborn errors of metabolism is associated with brain malformation?

A. Homocystinuria
B. Zellweger syndrome
C. Tyrosinemia
D. Alkaptonuria

EXPLANATION

Homocystinuria, tyrosinemia, and alkaptonuria are aminoacidopathies and do not affect brain in-utero. Homocystinuria can cause brain lesions in the after-birth period. Tyrosinemia may cause CNS involvement secondary to decompensation or liver dysfunction. Alkaptonuria does not involve brain. Zellweger syndrome, a peroxisomal disorder, on the other hand is associated with brain malformations and other brain parenchymal changes during intrauterine life. Polymicrogyria and germinolytic cysts in the caudothalamic region are typical neuroimaging findings associated with Zellweger syndrome.

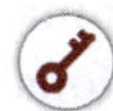

Key: B

BOOST YOUR KNOWLEDGE

Zellweger syndrome is a rare and devastating genetic disorder, belonging to a group of inherited metabolic disorders known as peroxisome biogenesis disorders. This autosomal recessive disorder involving biallelic pathogenic variants in *PEX* gene disrupts the normal functioning of peroxisomes, cellular organelles critical for various metabolic processes, particularly the breakdown of fatty acids and the detoxification of harmful substances. Zellweger spectrum disorder (ZSD) actually is a phenotypic continuum ranging from severe-to-mild and included all the previously described phenotypes of Zellweger syndrome, neonatal adrenoleukodystrophy, and infantile Refsum disease. The term "ZSD" is now used to refer to all individuals with a defect in one of the ZSD-PEX genes irrespective of the clinical phenotype.

Infants born with Zellweger syndrome typically present a grim clinical picture, including distinctive facial features, poor muscle tone, seizures, hearing and vision impairments, and liver dysfunction. Brain MRI reveals cerebral atrophy, white matter changes, germinolytic cysts, and neuronal migration abnormalities, particularly perisylvian polymicrogyria. The prognosis for individuals with Zellweger syndrome is extremely poor, with most not surviving beyond the first year of life.

REFERENCES/SOURCES

- Gupta P, Menon PSN, Ramji S, Lodha R. Chapter: Brain malformations. PG Textbook of Pediatrics, 2nd edition. New Delhi: Jaypee Brothers Medical Publishers; 2018. p. 2426.
- Steinberg SJ, Raymond GV, Braverman NE, Moser AB. Zellweger Spectrum Disorder. 2003 Dec 12 [Updated 2020 Oct 29]. In: Adam MP, Feldman J, Mirzaa GM, Pagon RA, Wallace SE, Bean LJH, et al. (Eds). GeneReviews®. Seattle (WA): University of Washington, Seattle; 1993-2023.

6. An 11-year-old girl came to OPD with posterior headaches, made worsened by bending forward, sneezing or coughing. Brain MRI revealed downward displacement of cerebellar tonsils into spinal canal by 7 mm. An additional finding was noted in the visible cervical cord; it is likely to be:

A. Spinal cord infarction
B. Extradural hematoma
C. Syringomyelia
D. Myelomeningocele

EXPLANATION

This patient has Arnold-Chiari malformation type 1 (ACM-1) and typical headaches associated with it. Spinal cord infarction is an exceedingly rare occurrence and is not associated with ACM. Extradural hematoma will be unlikely in the absence of trauma or a bleeding disorder. Myelomeningocele will be obvious from clinical examination. Syringomyelia is a common complication of ACM-1.

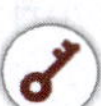

Key: C

BOOST YOUR KNOWLEDGE

Named after the Austrian pathologist Hans Chiari, Arnold-Chiari malformations, or Chiari malformations, are a group of congenital neurological disorders characterized by abnormal brain development in the region of the cerebellum. Chiari malformations are categorized into four types. In type I, the most common type, the cerebellar tonsils extend into the upper spinal canal, potentially obstructing the flow of cerebrospinal fluid and causing a variety of symptoms, including headaches, neck pain, balance problems, and in some cases, difficulty swallowing or breathing. Syringomyelia and hydrocephalus are known complications. Types II, III, and IV are rarer and involve more severe abnormalities, often associated with other congenital conditions such as spina bifida. Early diagnosis and intervention are crucial in managing Chiari malformations, as they can lead to serious complications if left untreated. Treatment typically involves surgical intervention to relieve pressure on the brain and improve cerebrospinal fluid (CSF) flow.

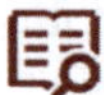

REFERENCES/SOURCES

- Gupta P, Menon PSN, Ramji S, Lodha R. Chapter: Brain malformations. PG Textbook of Pediatrics, 2nd edition. New Delhi: Jaypee Brothers Medical Publishers; 2018. p. 2426.
- Hidalgo JA, Tork CA, Varacallo M. Arnold-Chiari Malformation. In: StatPearls. Treasure Island (FL): StatPearls Publishing; 2023.

7. Hypoplasia and upward rotation of the cerebellar vermis, cystic dilatation of the fourth ventricle, and an enlarged posterior fossa on brain MRI in a child with developmental delay are suggestive of:

A. Ponto-cerebellar hypoplasia
B. Dandy-Walker malformation
C. Joubert syndrome
D. Zellweger syndrome

EXPLANATION

Pontocerebellar hypoplasias are a group of heterogeneous disorders characterized by the presence of an abnormally small cerebellum and brain stem. Dandy-Walker malformation (DWM) is characterized by small sized and abnormally placed cerebellar vermis, cystic enlargement of the 4th ventricle and enlargement of the posterior fossa as is evident in the case described. Joubert syndrome has abnormal development of the cerebellar vermis and the brainstem which produces characteristic molar tooth sign on brain MRI. Zellweger syndrome is on the other hand has malformations of cortical development and posterior fossa structures are usually normal.

Key: B

BOOST YOUR KNOWLEDGE

Dandy-Walker malformation is a rare congenital brain anomaly that primarily affects the cerebellum and its surrounding structures. Its epidemiology suggests an incidence of approximately one in 25,000 live births. While the exact cause remains unclear, there appears to be a genetic component as DWM can occur sporadically or be associated with genetic syndromes such as Meckel-Gruber syndrome. It often presents in early childhood or infancy, though it can go undetected until later in life. Clinically, DWM manifests with a range of neurological and developmental abnormalities. Infants with DWM may have an enlarged head due to the accumulation of cerebrospinal fluid (hydrocephalus). Other common symptoms include poor coordination, muscle weakness, and difficulties with balance and fine motor skills. Intellectual and developmental delays are also common, and some individuals may experience seizures. DWM can be identified through prenatal imaging, such as ultrasound or fetal MRI, or diagnosed postnatally using neuroimaging techniques such as CT scans or MRI. Management typically involves treating associated complications, such as hydrocephalus, with shunt placement or other surgical interventions. Multidisciplinary care teams, including neurologists, neurosurgeons, and genetic counselors, work together to provide supportive care and interventions to improve the quality of life for individuals with DWM.

REFERENCES/SOURCES

- Gupta P, Menon PSN, Ramji S, Lodha R. Chapter: Brain malformations. PG Textbook of Pediatrics, 2nd edition. New Delhi: Jaypee Brothers Medical Publishers; 2018. p. 2426.
- Zamora EA, Ahmad T. Dandy-Walker Malformation. In: StatPearls. Treasure Island (FL): StatPearls Publishing; 2023.

8. A 3-month-old girl presented with floppiness, and lack of developmental. She looks dysmorphic with broad forehead. Brain MRI showed bilateral perisylvian polymicrogyria and germinolytic cysts. What is the likely diagnosis?

A. Joubert syndrome
B. Tay-Sachs disease
C. Canavan disease
D. Zellweger syndrome

EXPLANATION

Joubert syndrome can present clinically with floppiness and developmental delay and affected children can look dysmorphic but neuroimaging changes (abnormal development of the cerebellar vermis and the brainstem producing molar tooth sign) allow diagnosis. Tay-Sachs disease causes brain parenchymal changes (cerebral atrophy, white matter, and basal ganglia signal abnormalities) on MRI but is not associated with brain malformations. Similarly, Canavan disease produces leukodystrophy but not associated with brain malformations. Zellweger syndrome has malformations of cortical development such as perisylvian polymicrogyria and germinolytic cysts.

Key: D

BOOST YOUR KNOWLEDGE

See Booster for Question 5.

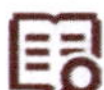

REFERENCES/SOURCES

- Gupta P, Menon PSN, Ramji S, Lodha R. Chapter: Brain malformations. PG Textbook of Pediatrics, 2nd edition. New Delhi: Jaypee Brothers Medical Publishers; 2018. p. 2426.
- Steinberg SJ, Raymond GV, Braverman NE, Moser AB. Zellweger Spectrum Disorder. 2003. In: Adam MP, Feldman J, Mirzaa GM, Pagon RA, Wallace SE, Bean LJH, et al. (Eds). GeneReviews®. Seattle (WA): University of Washington, Seattle; 1993-2023.

9. What category of disorders does the patient mentioned above (Question No. 8) belong to?

A. Peroxisomal disorders
B. Mitochondrial disorders
C. Lysosomal disorders
D. Channelopathy

EXPLANATION

Peroxisomal disorders, also called peroxisomal biogenesis disorders, are rare genetic disorders characterized by the dysfunction or absence of peroxisomes, cellular organelles involved in the metabolism of fatty acids, detoxification, and synthesis of biomolecules. Mitochondrial disorders on the other hand result from the dysfunction in the mitochondria, the energy producing organelles in the cells. Lysosomal disorders, also called lysosomal storage disorders (LSDs), result from the malfunction of lysosomes, the cellular organelles responsible for breakdown and recycling of various substances within the cells. Lysosomes contain several important enzymes. Channelopathies are genetic disorders resulting from abnormal functioning of various ion channels and result in various paroxysmal disorders.

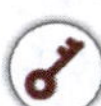

Key: A

BOOST YOUR KNOWLEDGE

There are several types of peroxisomal disorders:

- *Zellweger spectrum disorders* include Zellweger syndrome, neonatal adrenoleukodystrophy, and infantile Refsum disease. Individuals with ZSD have severe impairments in peroxisome function, leading to a wide range of symptoms, including developmental delays, neurological abnormalities, liver dysfunction, and vision problems. ZSDs are typically diagnosed in infancy or early childhood.
- *X-linked adrenoleukodystrophy (X-ALD)* is one of the most well-known peroxisomal disorders. It primarily affects males and is characterized by the accumulation of very long-chain fatty acids in the body. Symptoms can vary widely and may include progressive neurological deterioration, adrenal gland dysfunction, and behavioral changes.
- *Rhizomelic chondrodysplasia punctata (RCDP)* is a rare peroxisomal disorder that primarily affects bone development and leads to skeletal abnormalities, growth retardation, and facial dysmorphism. Individuals with RCDP often have joint contractures and cataracts.
- *Peroxisomal acyl-CoA oxidase deficiency:* This disorder affects the breakdown of fatty acids and can lead to a range of symptoms, including muscle weakness, vision problems, and developmental delays.

REFERENCES/SOURCES

- Gupta P, Menon PSN, Ramji S, Lodha R. Chapter: Brain malformations. PG Textbook of Pediatrics, 2nd edition. New Delhi: Jaypee Brothers Medical Publishers; 2018. p. 2426.
- Steinberg SJ, Raymond GV, Braverman NE, Moser AB. Zellweger Spectrum Disorder. 2003. In: Adam MP, Feldman J, Mirzaa GM, Pagon RA, Wallace SE, Bean LJH, et al. (Eds). GeneReviews®. Seattle (WA): University of Washington, Seattle; 1993-2023.

10. Combination of dysmorphism, lissencephaly, and 17p13.3 del, defines which syndrome?

A. Miller–Dieker syndrome
B. Dandy–Walker syndrome
C. Walker–Warburg syndrome
D. Fukuyama muscular dystrophy

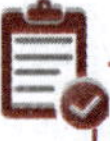

EXPLANATION

Miller–Dieker syndrome, characterized by facial dysmorphism, microcephaly, and classical lissencephaly on brain MRI is caused by 17p13.3 del. Dandy–Walker malformation typically is not associated with lissencephaly, although brain stem and cerebellar abnormalities are associated with certain types of lissencephaly syndromes caused by mutations in other genes. Walker–Warburg syndrome and Fukuyama muscular dystrophy are types of congenital muscular dystrophy associated with type of lissencephaly called cobblestone lissencephaly. In addition, there are variable ocular abnormalities and muscle weakness with raised creatine phosphokinase (CPK). Both the latter disorders are caused by specific gene mutations.

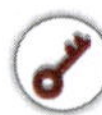

Key: A

BOOST YOUR KNOWLEDGE

Miller–Dieker syndrome (MDS) is a rare and severe genetic disorder characterized by brain malformations, intellectual disabilities, and distinct facial features. This condition is primarily caused by a deletion of genetic material on the short arm of chromosome 17 (17p13.3) which includes the *LIS1* gene. MDS is associated with a condition known as lissencephaly, where the brain lacks the normal folds and grooves, resulting in a smooth appearance. This abnormal brain development leads to significant intellectual and developmental delays, as well as seizures. Additionally, individuals with MDS often exhibit distinctive facial features, including a high forehead, a prominent nasal bridge, and a small jaw. Severity of symptoms can vary among affected individuals, but most face lifelong challenges related to motor and cognitive development.

Management typically involves supportive care, including physical therapy and antiepileptic medications to control seizures. Due to its genetic basis, genetic counseling is important for families at risk of having a child with MDS, and prenatal testing may be available to diagnose the condition early in pregnancy.

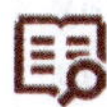

REFERENCES/SOURCES

- Brock S, Dobyns WB, Jansen A. PAFAH1B1-related Lissencephaly/Subcortical Band Heterotopia. 2009. In: Adam MP, Feldman J, Mirzaa GM, Pagon RA, Wallace SE, Bean LJH, et al. (Eds). GeneReviews®. Seattle (WA): University of Washington, Seattle; 1993-2023.
- Gupta P, Menon PSN, Ramji S, Lodha R. Chapter: Brain malformations. PG Textbook of Pediatrics, 2nd edition. New Delhi: Jaypee Brothers Medical Publishers; 2018. p. 2426.

11. Which of the following genes is *NOT* associated with X-linked lissencephaly?

A. *ARX* B. *LIS1*
C. *LARGE* D. *TUBA1A*

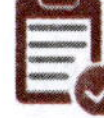

EXPLANATION

Aristaless-related homeobox (*ARX*) gene causes X-linked lissencephaly with abnormal genitalia (XALG). *LIS1* gene mutations are associated with classic lissencephaly and is not X-linked. Mutations in *TUBA1A* are associated with lissencephaly and other related brain malformations. Mutations in *LARGE* gene are associated with congenital muscular dystrophy which are autosomal disorders.

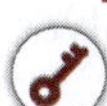

Key: A

BOOST YOUR KNOWLEDGE

X-linked lissencephaly, also known as "X-linked lissencephaly with abnormal genitalia (XALG)" is a rare genetic disorder that affects brain development and causes intellectual disabilities. Key characteristics and features of X-linked lissencephaly include lissencephaly, abnormal genitalia, hypotonia, developmental delay, moderate-to-severe intellectual disability and epilepsy. Seizures can be difficult to control. Some individuals with XLAG may exhibit behavioral problems or psychiatric issues, such as mood disorders or autism spectrum disorders. The severity of X-linked lissencephaly can vary among affected individuals, even within the same family. Some individuals may have more profound disabilities than others.

Mutations in genes such as *ARX* are commonly associated with XLAG. There is currently no cure for X-linked lissencephaly, and treatment mainly focuses on managing symptoms and providing supportive care. This may include anticonvulsant medications to control seizures, physical therapy to improve motor skills, and educational and behavioral interventions to help individuals with intellectual disabilities reach their fullest potential. Genetic counseling is often recommended for families with a history of X-linked lissencephaly to assess the risk of passing the condition to future generations.

REFERENCES/SOURCES

- Gupta P, Menon PSN, Ramji S, Lodha R. Chapter: Brain malformations. PG Textbook of Pediatrics, 2nd edition. New Delhi: Jaypee Brothers Medical Publishers; 2018. p. 2426.
- Uyanik G, Aigner L, Martin P, Gross C, Neumann D, Marschner-Schäfer H, et al. ARX mutations in X-linked lissencephaly with abnormal genitalia. Neurology. 2003;61(2):232-5.

12. Which of the followings is a neuronal migration disorder?

A. Holoprosencephaly
B. Periventricular nodular heterotopia
C. Septo-optic dysplasia
D. Agenesis of corpus callosum

EXPLANATION

Brain malformation results from failure of the forebrain or prosencephalon to divide in the midline into two distinct cerebral hemispheres. Periventricular neuronal heterotopia refers to the presence of masses of gray matter at an abnormal location in the brain and results from arrested neural migration. Septo-optic dysplasia and agenesis of corpus callosum are forebrain malformation involving midline brain structures.

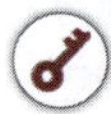

Key: B

BOOST YOUR KNOWLEDGE

Neuronal migration disorders are a group of rare neurological disorders that affect the migration of neurons in the developing brain. During fetal development, neurons need to migrate from their place of origin to their destination in the cortex. Many genetic influences are involved in the process. Any disruption in this migration process can lead to a range of neurological and cognitive impairments. These disorders can be caused by genetic mutations or environmental factors and typically manifest in early childhood. They are often associated with epilepsy, intellectual disability, and developmental delays. There are several subtypes of neuronal migration disorders, including lissencephaly, polymicrogyria, and heterotopia, each with distinct characteristics.

Lissencephaly, characterized by a smooth brain surface due to incomplete gyration, often results in severe intellectual and motor impairments. Polymicrogyria, on the other hand, is marked by excessive, small gyri and can lead to a range of neurological symptoms, including seizures and speech difficulties. Heterotopia involves clusters of neurons that fail to migrate to their proper location and can result in epilepsy and cognitive deficits.

Treatment options for neuronal migration disorders are limited and primarily focus on managing symptoms, such as seizures, with medications. Early intervention and supportive therapies, such as physical and occupational therapy, can help improve the quality of life for affected individuals.

REFERENCES/SOURCES

- Gupta P, Menon PSN, Ramji S, Lodha R. Chapter: Brain malformations. PG Textbook of Pediatrics, 2nd edition. New Delhi: Jaypee Brothers Medical Publishers; 2018. p. 2426.
- Spalice A, Parisi P, Nicita F, Pizzardi G, Del Balzo F, Iannetti P. Neuronal migration disorders: clinical, neuroradiologic and genetics aspects. Acta Paediatr. 2009;98(3):421-33.

13. A 2-year-old boy was brought with developmental delay and epilepsy. On examination, he has hemiparesis on right side. Which brain malformation is likely to be causative of these symptoms?

A. Schizencephaly
B. Lissencephaly
C. Pontocerebellar hypoplasia
D. Arnold-Chiari malformation

EXPLANATION

While typical of schizencephaly, hemiplegia can be seen with other brain malformation such as polymicrogyria, focal cortical dysplasia affecting the motor cortex. Lissencephaly typical causes bilateral motor deficits. Pontocerebellar hypoplasia is more likely to have developmental delay, hypotonia, and ataxia as the dominant symptom and Arnold Chiari malformations are not associated with epilepsy or hemiplegia. Its symptoms are more likely to be headaches, and if at all motor signs are bilateral.

Key: A

BOOST YOUR KNOWLEDGE

Schizencephaly is a rare congenital brain malformation characterized by abnormal clefts or cleft-like openings in the cerebral hemispheres of the brain. These clefts can extend from the brain's surface to deeper structures and are typically lined with abnormal gray matter. Schizencephaly is thought to result from disruptions in the early stages of brain development, particularly during neuronal migration. There are two main types of schizencephaly—open-lip and closed-lip. Open-lip schizencephaly features a visible gap or cleft in the brain tissue, often associated with more severe neurological symptoms. In contrast, closed-lip schizencephaly presents with a cleft that is covered by a thin layer of brain tissue, making it less apparent on imaging but still causing neurological issues. Common symptoms of schizencephaly include varying degrees of motor impairment (hemiparesis in unilateral cases), developmental delays, intellectual disability, and epilepsy. Diagnosis typically involves neuroimaging studies such as MRI or CT scans, and if available genetic studies. Treatment for schizencephaly is symptomatic and may involve therapies such as physical, occupational, and speech therapy to address motor and communication difficulties. Medications are often prescribed to manage seizures.

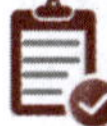

REFERENCES/SOURCES

- Gupta P, Menon PSN, Ramji S, Lodha R. Chapter: Brain malformations. PG Textbook of Pediatrics, 2nd edition. New Delhi: Jaypee Brothers Medical Publishers; 2018. p. 2426.
- Veerapaneni P, Veerapaneni KD, Yadala S. Schizencephaly. In: StatPearls. Treasure Island (FL): StatPearls Publishing; 2023.

14. What brain malformation is expected on brain MRI in an infant with developmental delay, hypotonia, poor vision, and elevated creatine phosphokinase?

A. Lissencephaly
B. Schizencephaly
C. Holoprosencephaly
D. Septo-optic dysplasia

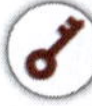

EXPLANATION

Lissencephaly specifically does not cause visual impairment but is often associated with other abnormalities that can result in visual failure. For example, children with congenital muscular dystrophy have cobblestone lissencephaly, ocular abnormalities causing poor vision, and elevated CPK. Schizencephaly can cause developmental delay but no visual failure (unless cleft is in the unlikely position of occipital region) or elevated CPK. Similarly, holoprosencephaly causes developmental delay, but no specific visual dysfunction. Such patients have normal CPK. Septo-optic dysplasia can cause developmental delay, visual dysfunction due to optic nerve hypoplasia, but have normal CPK.

Key: A

BOOST YOUR KNOWLEDGE

Congenital muscular dystrophy (CMD) is a group of rare genetic disorders characterized by muscle weakness and wasting that typically manifests from birth or early infancy. It is caused by mutations in various genes that are essential for muscle structure and function. CMD can vary in severity and clinical presentation, but common features include delayed motor milestones, muscle stiffness, joint contractures, and respiratory difficulties. There are several subtypes of CMD, each associated with specific genetic mutations. Some of the well-known subtypes include laminin alpha-2 (merosin)-deficient CMD, collagen VI-related CMD, and SEPN1-related CMD. These subtypes can have distinct clinical features and prognosis.

Congenital muscular dystrophy can be associated with various syndromes. Some common syndromes that can be associated with CMD are Walker–Warburg syndrome (WWS). WWS is a severe form of CMD often associated with brain and eye abnormalities. It is characterized by muscle weakness, structural brain malformations, and eye defects, such as congenital glaucoma and retinal abnormalities. Muscle-eye-brain (MEB) disease is another severe form of CMD with brain and eye involvement. It shares similarities with WWS but may have a slightly better prognosis. Fukuyama congenital muscular dystrophy (FCMD) is a CMD subtype predominantly found in Japan. It is characterized by muscle weakness, structural brain abnormalities, and intellectual disability. Eye problems, such as glaucoma and retinal abnormalities, can also be present.

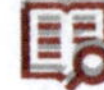

REFERENCES/SOURCES

- Gupta P, Menon PSN, Ramji S, Lodha R. Chapter: Brain malformations. PG Textbook of Pediatrics, 2nd edition. New Delhi: Jaypee Brothers Medical Publishers; 2018. p. 2426.
- Pasrija D, Tadi P. Congenital muscular dystrophy. In: StatPearls. Treasure Island (FL): StatPearls Publishing; 2023.

15. Which of the following disorders is not associated with polymicrogyria on brain MRI?

A. Zellweger syndrome spectrum
B. *GPR56* gene mutation
C. Aicardi syndrome
D. Menkes disease

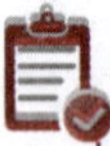

EXPLANATION

Polymicrogyria is a common brain malformation in children with Zellweger syndrome spectrum, *GPR56* gene mutation, and Aicardi syndrome. In Menkes disease children have cerebral atrophy and white matter changes but no brain malformations on brain MRI.

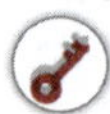

Key: D

BOOST YOUR KNOWLEDGE

Polymicrogyria (PMG) is a rare neurological disorder characterized by abnormal development of the cerebral cortex, the outer layer of the brain responsible for complex cognitive functions. In PMG, the cortex has too many (poly-) small (micro-), irregularly formed folds (gyria). PMG is typically present from birth but may not become apparent until early childhood. The exact cause of PMG is not well understood, but it is believed to result from a combination of genetic and environmental factors. Some cases of PMG may be linked to genetic mutations, while others may be associated with prenatal factors such as maternal infections or drug exposure. Common symptoms may include seizures (often difficult to control), developmental delay, cognitive impairment, speech and language impairments, and swallowing difficulties. Diagnosis of PMG typically involves brain imaging studies, such as MRI, which can reveal the characteristic brain abnormalities, and genetic testing to identify underlying mutations. Treatment approaches for PMG primarily focus on managing symptoms and may include antiepileptic medications to control seizures, physical and occupational therapy to improve motor skills, and speech therapy for communication difficulties. In some cases, surgery may be considered to address severe seizures that do not respond to medication.

REFERENCES/SOURCES

- Gupta P, Menon PSN, Ramji S, Lodha R. Chapter: Brain malformations. PG Textbook of Pediatrics, 2nd edition. New Delhi: Jaypee Brothers Medical Publishers; 2018. p. 2426.
- Stutterd CA, Dobyns WB, Jansen A, Mirzaa G, Leventer RJ. Polymicrogyria Overview. 2005. In: Adam MP, Feldman J, Mirzaa GM, Pagon RA, Wallace SE, Bean LJH, et al. (Eds). GeneReviews®. Seattle (WA): University of Washington, Seattle; 1993-2023.

16. An infant with developmental delay, microcephaly, and infantile spasms has ambiguous genitalia. What is the most likely neuroimaging diagnosis?

A. Lissencephaly
B. Agenesis of corpus callosum
C. Focal cortical dysplasia
D. Absent septum pellucidum

EXPLANATION

Developmental delay, microcephaly, and infantile spasms in an infant point to underlying lissencephaly. The disorder is known as X-linked lissencephaly and abnormal genitalia (XALG). Combination of developmental delay and infantile spasms in a female child with retinal lacunae is suggestive of Aicardi syndrome and is associated with agenesis of corpus callosum. Focal cortical dysplasia can cause infantile spasms but presence of ambiguous genitalia is odd. Absent septum pellucidum is suggestive of septo-optic dysplasia which can cause developmental delay and micropenis (but not specifically ambiguous genitalia). Infantile spasms are unusual in this condition.

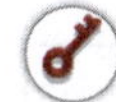

Key: A

BOOST YOUR KNOWLEDGE

See Booster for Question 11.

REFERENCES/SOURCES

- Bonneau D, Toutain A, Laquerrière A, Marret S, Saugier-Veber P, Barthez MA, et al. X-linked lissencephaly with absent corpus callosum and ambiguous genitalia (XLAG): clinical, magnetic resonance imaging, and neuropathological findings. Ann Neurol. 2002;51(3):340-9.
- Gupta P, Menon PSN, Ramji S, Lodha R. Chapter: Brain malformations. PG Textbook of Pediatrics, 2nd edition. New Delhi: Jaypee Brothers Medical Publishers; 2018. p. 2426.

17. In the case described above (Question No. 16), what is the likely gene mutation?

A. *ARX* B. *LIS1*
C. *DCX* D. *RELN*

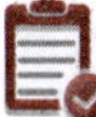

EXPLANATION

Mutations in all these genes, namely *ARX, LIS1, DCX,* and *RELN* are associated with lissencephaly. Only *ARX* mutation is associated with abnormal genitalia.

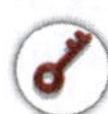

Key: A

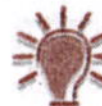

BOOST YOUR KNOWLEDGE

Lissencephaly is a rare and severe brain malformation disorder characterized by the smooth appearance of the brain surface due to a lack of normal convolutions (gyri and sulci). It is primarily caused by genetic mutations that disrupt the normal development of the cerebral cortex. Key characteristics of common specific mutations associated with lissencephaly are:

- *LIS1 (PAFAH1B1)* mutations are one of the most common genetic causes of lissencephaly. Affected individuals typically have a classic form of lissencephaly called "type 1" lissencephaly.
- *DCX* (doublecortin) mutations are another common genetic cause of lissencephaly. Affected individuals often have a milder form of lissencephaly known as "X-linked lissencephaly" or "subcortical band heterotopia" (SBH).
- *TUBA1A* (alpha-tubulin) mutations are associated with a rare subtype of lissencephaly. Affected individuals may exhibit a spectrum of brain malformations, including classic lissencephaly.
- *RELN* (reelin) mutations can lead to a condition known as "lissencephaly with cerebellar hypoplasia" (LCH). Individuals with LCH have lissencephaly as well as underdeveloped cerebellums.
- Aristaless-related homeobox mutations in the *ARX* gene are associated with a wide range of brain malformations, including lissencephaly.

REFERENCES/SOURCES

- Bonneau D, Toutain A, Laquerrière A, Marret S, Saugier-Veber P, Barthez MA, et al. X-linked lissencephaly with absent corpus callosum and ambiguous genitalia (XLAG): clinical, magnetic resonance imaging, and neuropathological findings. Ann Neurol. 2002;51(3):340-9.
- Gupta P, Menon PSN, Ramji S, Lodha R. Chapter: Brain malformations. PG Textbook of Pediatrics, 2nd edition. New Delhi: Jaypee Brothers Medical Publishers; 2018. p. 2426.

18. Refractory epilepsy secondary to which brain malformation is treated by resective surgery?

A. Closed lip unilateral schizencephaly
B. Focal cortical dysplasia
C. Cobblestone lissencephaly
D. Subcortical bad heterotopia

EXPLANATION

Brain malformations are permanent alterations in the brain structure and are not amenable to any treatment. Drug refractory epilepsy is a common feature of most of them. Only focal cortical dysplasia is amenable to respective surgery.

Key: B

BOOST YOUR KNOWLEDGE

Focal cortical dysplasias (FCDs) are a group of complex developmental brain disorders characterized by abnormal growth and organization of neurons in localized areas of the cerebral cortex. These dysplasias represent a leading cause of intractable epilepsy, particularly in children and young adults.

Focal cortical dysplasias are often classified into various subtypes (FCD I to FCD III) based on histopathological criteria. FCD type II is further divided into subtypes IIA, IIB, and IIC. Each subtype exhibits distinct histological characteristics, making accurate diagnosis and classification critical for treatment planning.

While the exact causes of FCDs remain unclear, genetic, and environmental factors are believed to contribute. Mutations in certain genes (such as *DEPDC5, NPRL2, TSC1*, and *TSC2*) related to brain development have been associated with FCDs.

Management of FCDs typically involves a multidisciplinary approach, including neurological evaluation, neuroimaging (such as MRI), and EEG monitoring to pinpoint the location and extent of the dysplasia. Treatment options may include medications, surgical resection, or other advanced techniques such as laser interstitial thermal therapy (LITT) or neurostimulation.

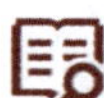

REFERENCES/SOURCES

- Gupta P, Menon PSN, Ramji S, Lodha R. Chapter: Brain malformations. PG Textbook of Pediatrics, 2nd edition. New Delhi: Jaypee Brothers Medical Publishers; 2018. p. 2426.
- Najm IM, Sarnat HB, Blümcke I. Review: The International Consensus Classification of Focal Cortical Dysplasia: a critical update 2018. Neuropathol Appl Neurobiol. 2018;44(1):18-31.

19. Which intrauterine infection is commonly associated with brain malformations?

A. Toxoplasmosis
B. Cytomegalovirus
C. Syphilis
D. Rubella

EXPLANATION

All these disorders involve brain but brain malformations are seen only with cytomegalovirus (CMV). Toxoplasmosis causes hydrocephalus and intracranial calcifications. Congenital syphilis can cause meningitis while congenital rubella causes encephalitic presentation.

Key: C

BOOST YOUR KNOWLEDGE

Congenital cytomegalovirus (CMV) infection can have a range of neurological and developmental consequences in affected infants. It can lead to a variety of brain abnormalities and developmental disorders.

Congenital cytomegalovirus infection during pregnancy can result in microcephaly, resulting in intellectual disabilities and developmental delays. Lissencephaly has often been associated with congenital CMV.

Periventricular calcification in the brain is another characteristic of congenital CMV infection in the fetus. In addition, white matter abnormalities with anterior temporal lobe cysts are seen. CMV is a leading cause of sensorineural hearing loss in infants.

Similarly, vision impairments from damage to the brain, optic nerves, and retina can occur in affected infants. It is important to note that not all infants born to mothers with CMV infection will develop these complications, and the severity of the outcomes can vary widely. Timely diagnosis, early intervention, and medical management can help mitigate some of the neurological and developmental challenges associated with congenital CMV infection.

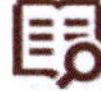

REFERENCES/SOURCES

- Akpan US, Pillarisetty LS. Congenital cytomegalovirus infection. In: StatPearls. Treasure Island (FL): StatPearls Publishing; 2023.
- Gupta P, Menon PSN, Ramji S, Lodha R. Chapter: Brain malformations. PG Textbook of Pediatrics, 2nd edition. New Delhi: Jaypee Brothers Medical Publishers; 2018. p. 2426.

20. A 14-year-old girl presents with a history of recurrent focal seizures, often characterized by altered consciousness and unusual sensations. Imaging studies of her brain reveal clusters of gray matter nodules located along the lateral ventricles, separated from the cerebral cortex. What condition is most likely responsible for these findings?

A. Lissencephaly
B. Periventricular heterotopia (PVNH)
C. Chiari malformation type I
D. Polymicrogyria

EXPLANATION

Location of clusters of gray matter nodules in the periventricular location is characteristic of periventricular heterotopia. Lissencephaly is associated with thickened cortex and reduced umbers of gyri on neuroimaging. The cortex has too many (poly-) small (micro-), irregularly formed folds (gyria). Chiari malformation type 1 is not associated with brain malformation but can have associated hydrocephalus.

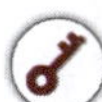

Key: B

BOOST YOUR KNOWLEDGE

See Booster for Question 15.

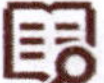

REFERENCES/SOURCES

- Gupta P, Menon PSN, Ramji S, Lodha R. Chapter: Brain malformations. PG Textbook of Pediatrics, 2nd edition. New Delhi: Jaypee Brothers Medical Publishers; 2018. p. 2426.
- Stutterd CA, Dobyns WB, Jansen A, Mirzaa G, Leventer RJ. Polymicrogyria Overview. 2005. In: Adam MP, Feldman J, Mirzaa GM, Pagon RA, Wallace SE, Bean LJH, et al. (Eds). GeneReviews®. Seattle (WA): University of Washington, Seattle; 1993-2023.

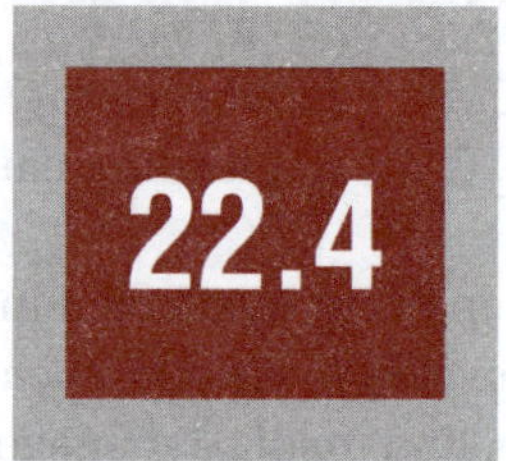

CHAPTER 22.4

Seizure Disorders including Antiepileptic Drugs and Febrile Seizures

Mahesh Kamate

1. A 4-month-old male baby developed one episode of febrile seizure (FS). Four months later, the child had a febrile status epilepticus (FSE) involving the right half of the face and the right upper and lower limbs. He started walking at 18 months. He was noticed to have ataxia at 2 years of age. The most possible etiology in this child could be:

A. *KCNQ2* mutation
B. *SCN1B* mutation
C. *PRRT2* mutation
D. *SCN1A* mutation

EXPLANATION

SCN1A mutation presents with early onset (less than one year) FS (usually hemiclonic) that are more prolonged and are known to be associated with gait abnormalities such as (ataxic gait and crouch gait) and movement disorders later in life.

Key: D

BOOST YOUR KNOWLEDGE

- Epileptic disorders which are also associated with movement disorders include *SCN1A, PRRT2, SCN8A, SLC2A1, KCNT1, SCN2A, GRIN1, STXBP1,* and *CACNA1A*.
- *SCN1A* is the most common cause of Dravet syndrome. Other causes include *SCN2A, SCN8A, SCN1B, PCDH19, HCN1, GABRA1, GABRB3, GABRG2.*
- Diseases that can be associated with *SCN1A* mutation include Dravet syndrome, genetic epilepsy with febrile seizures plus (GEFS+) spectrum disorders, West syndrome, Doose syndrome, epilepsy of infancy with migratory focal seizures, Lennox–Gastaut syndrome, and Rett syndrome.
- Characteristic features of Dravet syndrome include:
  - Typical onset between 1 and 18 months
  - Recurrent generalized tonic–clonic or hemiconvulsive seizures (often prolonged but may be shorter).
  - Myoclonic seizures are typically seen by age 2 years. Obtundation status, focal dyscognitive seizures, and atypical absences are also typical but usually occur after age 2 years. Typical absences and epileptic spasms are atypical.
  - Hyperthermia, which may be associated with vaccination, triggers seizures in most patients; other triggers may include flashing lights, visual patterns, bathing, eating, and overexertion.
  - Normal development and neurological examination at the onset
  - Normal MRI and nonspecific electroencephalogram (EEG) findings at onset. Later may show generalized atrophy or hippocampal sclerosis.
  - Persisting seizures, which include focal and/or generalized convulsive seizures, and, in many cases, myoclonic, focal, atypical absence, and tonic seizures. Recurrent status epilepticus (SE) and obtundation status become less frequent with time and may not be seen in adolescence and young adulthood.

- Intellectual disability, which is typically evident by the age of 18–60 months.
- Abnormalities on neurological examination, which are typically evident by age 3–4 years and include crouched gait, hypotonia, incoordination, and impaired dexterity.

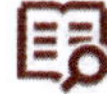

REFERENCES/SOURCES

- Kliegman RM, St Geme III JW (Eds). Nelson Textbook of Pediatrics, 21st edition. Amsterdam: Elsevier; 2019. p. 3093.
- Swaiman KF, Ashwal S, Ferriero DM, Schor NF, Finkel RS, Gropman AL, et al (Eds). Swaiman's Paediatric Neurology, 6th edition. Amsterdam: Elsevier; 2017. p. 567.

2. A 12-month-old girl presented with clusters of left versive and focal clonic seizures from the age of 3 months. Birth and developmental history are normal. Magnetic resonance imaging (MRI) brain is normal, and the EEG shows few focal epileptiform discharges. The most likely cause for her condition could be:

A. *CDKL5* mutation
B. *PRRT2* mutation
C. *SCN1A* mutation
D. *GABRA* mutation

EXPLANATION

Proline-rich transmembrane protein 2 (PRRT2) is the most common cause of self-limiting epilepsy in infancy.

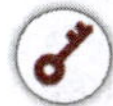

Key: B

BOOST YOUR KNOWLEDGE

- Pathogenic variants in PRRT2 are the most common genetic etiology of self-limiting epilepsy in infancy.
- Familial cases show autosomal dominant inheritance, with incomplete penetrance
- Patients with PRRT2 pathogenic variants may develop paroxysmal kinesigenic dyskinesia/dystonia beginning from childhood to adult life.
- Focal seizures are mandatory for diagnosis, and occur with behavioral arrest, cyanosis, staring with impaired awareness, automatisms, head/eye version, and clonic movements.
- Seizures are brief (<3 minutes) but can be frequent (e.g., 5–10/day over 1–3 days at onset).
- Other genes rarely associated with this syndrome include *SCN8A*, in which a movement disorder is also observed. Infantile onset is also seen in patients with pathogenic variants in *SCN2A*.
- Genetic etiology can be identified in about 80% of cases.

REFERENCES/SOURCES

- Kliegman RM, St Geme III JW (Eds). Nelson Textbook of Pediatrics, 21st edition. Amsterdam: Elsevier; 2019. p. 3093.
- Swaiman KF, Ashwal S, Ferriero DM, Schor NF, Finkel RS, Gropman AL, et al (Eds). Swaiman's Paediatric Neurology, 6th edition. Amsterdam: Elsevier; 2017. p. 514.

3. An 8-year-old girl presented with the second episode of deviation of eyes and mouth to right with clonic jerking of right upper-limb lasting for 5 minutes associated with drooling of saliva, 2 hours after sleeping. EEG shows centrotemporal spikes during the sleep phase. The next course of action should be:

A. Get magnetic resonance imaging of the brain
B. Start her on levetiracetam
C. Refer for presurgical workup
D. Watch for further seizures

EXPLANATION

The semiology described is that of SeLECTS (Self-limited epilepsy with centrotemporal spikes, earlier known as benign Rolandic epilepsy). MRI is not mandatory for diagnosis. EEG should include sleep records as epileptiform discharges are seen more during sleep. The majority of them have less than five seizures that are very brief and occur mostly during sleep. Hence, this self-limited epilepsy can be managed with reassurance, midazolam nasal spray.

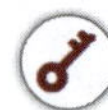 **Key: D**

 **BOOST YOUR KNOWLEDGE**

- SeLECTS is a self-limited epilepsy syndrome, formerly known as benign Rolandic epilepsy or benign epilepsy with centrotemporal spikes, which begins in children in their early school years.
- Seizures are often brief and typically involve focal clonic or tonic activity of the throat/tongue and one side of the lower face, which may then evolve into focal to bilateral (B/L) tonic–clonic seizures.
- This epilepsy syndrome occurs in children who are otherwise neurologically and cognitively normal, and imaging studies, if done, show no causal lesion.
- The EEG shows a normal background with high-amplitude centrotemporal sharp-and-slow-wave complexes, which are activated in drowsiness and sleep.
- Seizures cease by puberty.

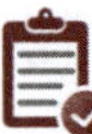 **REFERENCES/SOURCES**

- Kliegman RM, St Geme III JW (Eds). Nelson Textbook of Pediatrics, 21st edition. Amsterdam: Elsevier; 2019. p. 3096.
- Swaiman KF, Ashwal S, Ferriero DM, Schor NF, Finkel RS, Gropman AL, et al (Eds). Swaiman's Paediatric Neurology, 6th edition. Amsterdam: Elsevier; 2017. p. 572.
- Zuberi SM, Wirrell E, Yozawitz E, Wilmshurst JM, Specchio N, Riney K, et al. ILAE classification and definition of epilepsy syndromes with onset in neonates and infants: Position statement by the ILAE Task Force on Nosology and Definitions. Epilepsia. 2022;63(6): 1349-97.

4. A 6-month-old girl had multiple episodes of head drop with flexion of both upper limbs occurring soon after waking up. Screening for tuberous sclerosis was negative. Her EEG showed features of modified hypsarrhythmia. The treatment of choice for her would be:

A. Vigabatrin
B. Perampanel
C. Valproic acid
D. Corticosteroids like prednisolone

EXPLANATION

The treatment of choice for epileptic spasms is hormonal therapy (steroids) and in case of epileptic spasms in a case of tuberous sclerosis, vigabatrin. When either one fails, the next best treatment would be the other (i.e., vigabatrin if steroids fail and steroids if vigabatrin fails). Both adrenocorticotropic hormone (ACTH) and prednisolone are equally efficacious, and prednisolone is easy to administer.

 **Key: D**

 **BOOST YOUR KNOWLEDGE**

- *Modified hypsarrhythmia*:
  - Increased interhemispheric synchronization
  - Asymmetric hypsarrhythmia
  - Hypsarrhythmia with a consistent focus on abnormal discharge
  - Hypsarrhythmia with episodes of attenuation (burst suppression pattern)
  - Pauci-epileptiform (high voltage slow activity with little sharp/spike wave)
- *High-dose ACTH:* 150 U/m^2/body surface area (BSA) or 6 U/kg intramuscular (IM) OD for 2 weeks to assess therapeutic response.
- High-dose prednisolone (4 mg/kg/day) is recommended. This treatment should be given for 2 weeks to assess the response.
- If there is clinical spasms cessation → EEG to look for resolution of hypsarrhythmia. If there is EEG resolution as well (electroclinical cessation) → first-line drug (ACTH/prednisone) should be tapered off over 2–4 weeks.

- *Vigabatrin:* Start at 50 mg/kg/day and hiked by 50 mg/kg every 3–7 days intervals as tolerated to a max dose of 150 mg/kg/day (maximum within 14 days) or cessation of clinical and electrophysiological spasm has been achieved, whichever is earlier.

REFERENCES/SOURCES

- Kliegman RM, St Geme III JW (Eds). Nelson Textbook of Pediatrics, 21st edition. Amsterdam: Elsevier; 2019. p. 3103.
- Sharma S, Kaushik JS, Srivastava K, Goswami JN, Sahu JK, Vinayan KP, et al. Association of Child Neurology (AOCN)–Indian Epilepsy Society (IES) Consensus Guidelines for the Diagnosis and Management of West Syndrome. Indian Pediatr. 2021;58(1):54-66.
- Swaiman KF, Ashwal S, Ferriero DM, Schor NF, Finkel RS, Gropman AL, et al (Eds). Swaiman's Paediatric Neurology, 6th edition. Amsterdam: Elsevier; 2017. p. 566.

5. **As per the FEBSTAT (consequences of prolonged FS in childhood) study, which infection is likely to be associated with FSE?**

A. Human herpesvirus 6A (HHV-6A)
B. Human herpesvirus 6B (HHV-6B)
C. Varicella-zoster virus (VZV)
D. Herpes simplex virus 1 (HSV-1)

EXPLANATION

Human herpesvirus 6B (more frequently) and human herpesvirus 7 (HHV7) are associated with FSE. Together they account for one-third (30%) of the FSE. They are associated with an increased risk of hippocampal injury and subsequent temporal lobe epilepsy.

Key: B

BOOST YOUR KNOWLEDGE

Febrile seizures are the single most common seizure type and occur in 2–5% of children younger than age 5 years with a peak incidence in the second year of life. The majority are brief, generalized convulsions or simple FS, which are thought to be benign. A small proportion of FS are prolonged and 5–8% of cases meet the criteria for SE. FSE accounts for 5% of FS but 25% of all childhood SE and >70% of SE in the second year of life. FSE is associated with a substantially increased risk of epilepsy and temporal lobe epilepsy. There is evidence of acute hippocampal injury following FSE. HHV-6 and HHV-7 are closely related B-herpesviruses that are universally acquired in early childhood. HHV-6B is a common cause of both febrile illnesses and of FS, whereas HHV-6A has been associated with reactivated infection later in life, predominantly in the central nervous system, often as a result of immunologic suppression. HHV-7 primary infection is most often asymptomatic, but like HHV-6, can present with fever and, in this setting, has an even higher association with FS.

REFERENCES/SOURCES

- Epstein LG, Shinnar S, Hesdorffer DC, Nordli DR, Hamidullah A, Benn EK, et al. Human herpesvirus 6 and 7 in febrile status epilepticus: The FEBSTAT study. Epilepsia. 2012;53(9):1481-8.
- Kliegman RM, St Geme III JW (Eds). Nelson Textbook of Pediatrics, 21st edition. Amsterdam: Elsevier; 2019. p. 3093.
- Swaiman KF, Ashwal S, Ferriero DM, Schor NF, Finkel RS, Gropman AL, et al (Eds). Swaiman's Paediatric Neurology, 6th edition. Amsterdam: Elsevier; 2017. p. 520.

6. **A 10-year-old boy came with a history of myoclonic jerks for the past 1 month. His EEG was as shown below. What could be the likely diagnosis?**

A. Herpes simplex encephalitis
B. N-methyl D-aspartate receptor antibody-associated encephalitis
C. Subacute sclerosing panencephalitis (SSPE)
D. Progressive multifocal leukoencephalopathy

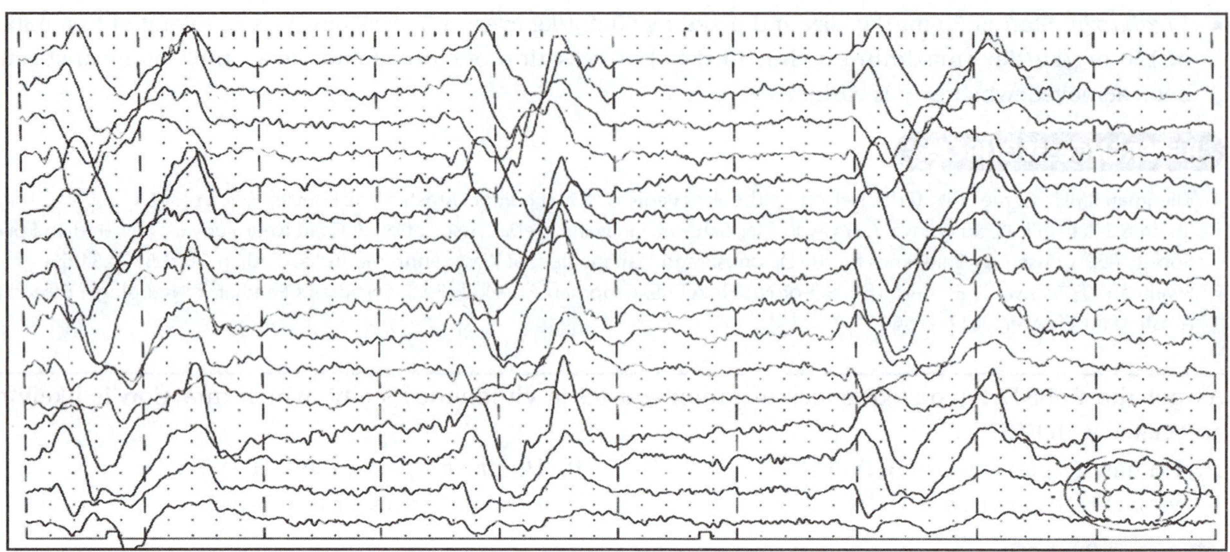

EXPLANATION

Typical EEG finding in SSPE—suppression burst pattern (Radermecker complexes)—periodic high amplitude delta waves that repeat every 4–7 seconds (long interval periodic epileptiform discharges).

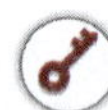

Key: C

BOOST YOUR KNOWLEDGE

Clinical Stages of Subacute Sclerosis Panencephalitis—Jabbour

Stage	*Clinical manifestations*
Stage I	Personality changes, failure in school, and strange behavior
Stage II	Massive, repetitive, and frequent myoclonic jerks, seizures, and dementia
Stage III	Rigidity, extrapyramidal symptoms, and progressive unresponsiveness
Stage IV	Coma, vegetative state, autonomic failure, and akinetic mutism

Short interval periodic epileptiform discharges when they occur every <4 seconds are seen in hypoxic encephalopathy, hepatic encephalopathy, toxin/drug exposure, and slow viral diseases.

REFERENCES/SOURCES

- Kliegman RM, St Geme III JW (Eds). Nelson Textbook of Pediatrics, 21st edition. Amsterdam: Elsevier; 2019. p. 1674.
- Swaiman KF, Ashwal S, Ferriero DM, Schor NF, Finkel RS, Gropman AL, et al (Eds). Swaiman's Paediatric Neurology, 6th edition. Amsterdam: Elsevier; 2017. p. 903.

7. Which of the following drugs acts on the slow sodium channel?

A. Lacosamide
B. Lamotrigine
C. Perampanel
D. Levetiracetam

EXPLANATION

The mechanism of action of lacosamide is different from other antiseizure medications acting on the sodium channel such as phenytoin, and carbamazepine, as it acts on the slow sodium channel.

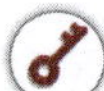

Key: A

BOOST YOUR KNOWLEDGE

Lacosamide causes slow inactivation of voltage-gated sodium channels. In patients with epilepsy, sustained depolarization occurs with prolonged high-frequency trains of repetitive firing. In this scenario, the pore of the sodium channel undergoes a structural rearrangement, i.e., a slow inactivated state. Lacosamide enhances this transition of voltage-gated sodium channels (VGSCs) into a slow inactivated state. Conventional sodium channel-blocking antiseizure medications protect against seizures primarily interacting with the fast inactivated state of VGSCs. Lacosamide does not affect normal synaptic transmission. Side effects noted in 50% and include somnolence, behavior changes, headache, and dizziness. Use of >1 sodium channel blockers is associated with increased side effects.

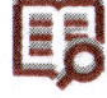

REFERENCES/SOURCES

- Kliegman RM, St Geme III JW (Eds). Nelson Textbook of Pediatrics, 21st edition. Amsterdam: Elsevier; 2019. p. 3102.
- Swaiman KF, Ashwal S, Ferriero DM, Schor NF, Finkel RS, Gropman AL, et al (Eds). Swaiman's Paediatric Neurology, 6th edition. Amsterdam: Elsevier; 2017. p. 511.

8. **A 3-month-old baby had abnormal movements of the head and a few weeks later was noted to have early morning seizures. On examination, the child had abnormal rapid multidirectional eye movements with head movement in the same direction and cerebrospinal fluid (CSF) glucose 30 mg/dL. The whole exome sequencing was ordered. The causative mutation and treatment could be:**

A. *SLC6A5* mutation, ketogenic diet
B. *SLC2A1* mutation, modified Atkins diet
C. *SCN1A* mutation, valproic acid
D. *SCN8A* mutation, phenytoin

EXPLANATION

SLC2A1 mutations cause glucose transporter type 1 (GLUT-1) deficiency and usually presents with seizures in the first 4 months of life, and can be associated with abnormal movements or postures, ataxia, lethargy, confusion, alternating hemiparesis, and sleep disturbances. It responds well to a ketogenic diet. Modified Atkin's diet is a modification of the ketogenic diet.

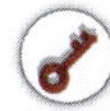

Key: B

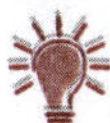

BOOST YOUR KNOWLEDGE

Precision therapies for some epileptic conditions include:
GLUT1 (SLC2A1): Ketogenic diet, KCNT1—quinidine, specific diet for phenylketonuria and maple syrup urine disease, pyridoxine, and pyridoxal phosphate for pyridoxine-dependent epilepsies, avoiding sodium channel blockers in Dravet syndrome, sodium channel blockers for *SCN8A, SCN2A, and KCNQ2* gene-related epilepsy, folinic acid for primary cerebral folate deficiency.

REFERENCES/SOURCES

- Kliegman RM, St Geme III JW (Eds). Nelson Textbook of Pediatrics, 21st edition. Amsterdam: Elsevier; 2019. p. 3099, 3109, 3127.
- Swaiman KF, Ashwal S, Ferriero DM, Schor NF, Finkel RS, Gropman AL, et al (Eds). Swaiman's Paediatric Neurology, 6th edition. Amsterdam: Elsevier; 2017. p. 597.

9. **A 4-year-old girl who was normal till 8 months of life, had regression of motor and language milestones. She had hand flapping, deceleration of head growth, and a history of seizures. What could be the diagnosis?**

A. Landau–Kleffner syndrome
B. Neuronal ceroid lipofuscinoses (NCLs)
C. Methyl CpG binding protein 2 (MECP2) mutation
D. Lennox–Gastaut syndrome

EXPLANATION

Methyl CpG binding protein 2 mutation causes Rett's syndrome, which is inherited by X-linked mode, primarily affects females and presents with normal development followed by regression of language milestones, stereotypical hand gestures, seizures, deceleration of head growth, and autistic features.

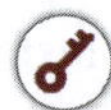

Key: C

BOOST YOUR KNOWLEDGE

Stereotypies are non-goal-directed movement patterns or vocalizations that are repeated continuously for a period in the same form and on multiple occasions and which are typically distractible.

Rett syndrome has an X-linked dominant mode of inheritance and affects females. It is usually caused by de novo mutation. A natural course is that of regression followed by stabilization or recovery. There is a partial or complete loss of hand skills and acquired speech. The stereotypic hand movements include hand wringing, flapping, clapping, squeezing, tapping, mouthing, rubbing, or washing automatisms. They have acquired microcephaly and seizures are commonly seen. MRI can show atrophy.

REFERENCES/SOURCES

- Kliegman RM, St Geme III JW (Eds). Nelson Textbook of Pediatrics, 21st edition. Amsterdam: Elsevier; 2019. p. 3193.
- Swaiman KF, Ashwal S, Ferriero DM, Schor NF, Finkel RS, Gropman AL, et al (Eds). Swaiman's Paediatric Neurology, 6th edition. Amsterdam: Elsevier; 2017. p. 244.

10. A 3-day-old male baby did not cry after birth and required admission to the neonatal intensive care unit (NICU). The baby started developing intractable seizures from the second day of life that were not responding to phenytoin, phenobarbitone, and levetiracetam. Mother had appreciated some rapid fetal movements in the last trimester. The possible cause and treatment would be:

A. Pyridoxamine-5'-phosphate oxidase (PNPO) deficiency, pyridoxine
B. GLUT1 deficiency, glucose
C. Hypoxic ischemic encephalopathy, midazolam
D. Hypoglycemia, dextrose

EXPLANATION

Pyridoxamine-5'-phosphate oxidase deficiency causes pyridoxine-dependent epilepsy, which responds dramatically to pyridoxal phosphate. It can present with delayed crying after birth and seizures within the first few days of life. Life-long treatment is required.

Key: A

BOOST YOUR KNOWLEDGE

Pyridoxine-dependent epilepsies are caused by genetic-metabolic defects within the lysine degradation pathway. Seizures are resistant to standard antiseizure medications. Seizure control can be achieved in almost all cases with pyridoxine and pyridoxal-5'-phosphate. Lysine reduction therapies including a lysine-restricted diet and L-arginine therapy may provide additional benefits in terms of seizure control and cognitive outcome. Seizures may manifest antenatally as excessive fetal movements and typically present in the first hours to days of life. EEG in neonates with severe encephalopathy before Rx can show a burst-suppression pattern. Genes affected: *ALDH7A1* and *PNPO*.

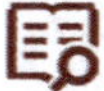

REFERENCES/SOURCES

- Kliegman RM, St Geme III JW (Eds). Nelson Textbook of Pediatrics, 21st edition. Amsterdam: Elsevier; 2019. p. 3115.
- Swaiman KF, Ashwal S, Ferriero DM, Schor NF, Finkel RS, Gropman AL, et al (Eds). Swaiman's Paediatric Neurology, 6th edition. Amsterdam: Elsevier; 2017. p. 375.
- Zuberi SM, Wirrell E, Yozawitz E, Wilmshurst JM, Specchio N, Riney K, et al. ILAE classification and definition of epilepsy syndromes with onset in neonates and infants: Position statement by the ILAE Task Force on Nosology and Definitions. Epilepsia. 2022;63(6): 1349-97.

11. Deep brain stimulation (DBS) for epilepsy is given to which thalamic nucleus?

A. Anterior nucleus
B. Medial nucleus
C. Lateral nucleus
D. Posterolateral nucleus

EXPLANATION

The rationale for anterior nucleus stimulation is based partly on its role as the primary relay nucleus of the limbic system—it receives major projection from the mammillary bodies of the thalamus and projects fibers to areas of the cortex such as the cingulum, amygdala, hippocampus, orbitofrontal cortex, and hypothalamus.

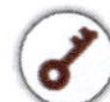

Key: A

BOOST YOUR KNOWLEDGE

The conditions for which DBS has been tried including:

- Dystonia
- Epilepsy
- Essential tremor
- Obsessive-compulsive disorder
- Parkinson's disease

It is an elective surgical procedure in which electrodes are implanted into certain areas in the brain, which generate electrical impulses that control abnormal brain activity. Stimulation is controlled by a programmable generator placed under the skin in the upper chest. Risks associated with DBS include brain hemorrhage, stroke, infection, device malfunction, lack of benefit for certain symptoms, and headache.

REFERENCES/SOURCES

- Kliegman RM, St Geme III JW (Eds). Nelson Textbook of Pediatrics, 21st edition. Amsterdam: Elsevier; 2019. p. 3160.
- Swaiman KF, Ashwal S, Ferriero DM, Schor NF, Finkel RS, Gropman AL, et al (Eds). Swaiman's Paediatric Neurology, 6th edition. Amsterdam: Elsevier; 2017. p. 627.

12. Which of the following genes is associated with fever-associated seizures and epilepsy?

A. Protein protocadherin-19 (*PCDH19*)-related epilepsy
B. Glutamate ionotropic receptor NMDA type subunit 2A (*GRIN2A*)-related epilepsy
C. Proline-rich transmembrane protein 2 (PRRT2)-related epilepsy
D. KCNQ3-related epilepsy

EXPLANATION

Protein protocadherin-19 mutation associated with seizures triggered by elevation in body temperature.

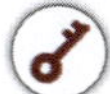

Key: A

BOOST YOUR KNOWLEDGE

- *PCDH19* clustering epilepsy is an X-linked disease, seen predominantly in females, caused by pathogenic variants in the *PCDH19* gene. Few males are reported. Although the *PCDH19* gene is located on Xq22, this condition has an unusual X-linked mode of inheritance sparing transmitting males. Only heterozygous females and mosaic males are affected due to presumed cellular interference.
- Epilepsy onset is often during the first year of life (mostly during the first 3 years).
- The most characteristic feature is clusters of seizures often induced by fever.
- Intellectual disability and psychiatric symptoms in two-thirds of cases.
- The severity of the phenotype seems to be correlated with the age of epilepsy onset.
- After the first decade, a decrease in the frequency of the seizure clusters generally occurs regardless of the treatment, and remission of seizures may occur in at least one quarter, usually in adolescence to midadulthood.
- Signs of intellectual disability and autism spectrum disorder, affecting up to 70%, emerge during the second year of life and often become the most relevant symptoms after the first decade.
- Behavioral disorders, with prominent hyperactivity and possible psychosis in up to 25% of women, are often problematic in adolescents and adults.

REFERENCE/SOURCE

- Swaiman KF, Ashwal S, Ferriero DM, Schor NF, Finkel RS, Gropman AL, et al (Eds). Swaiman's Paediatric Neurology, 6th edition. Amsterdam: Elsevier; 2017. p. 567.

13. Which of the following is the correct composition for a ketogenic diet?

A. 90% fat, 4% carbohydrates, and 6% protein
B. 85% fat, 68% carbohydrates, and 9% protein
C. 4080 fat, 9% carbohydrates, and 11% protein
D. 75% fat, 12% carbohydrates, and 13% protein

EXPLANATION

Diet	Regular	Ketogenic	Modified Atkins	Low glycemic index
Fat	30	90	60	60
Carbohydrate	50	4	10	10
Protein	20	6	30	30

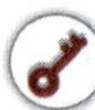

Key: A

BOOST YOUR KNOWLEDGE

- Mechanisms of action of the ketogenic diet include increasing synaptic levels of gamma-aminobutyric acid (GABA), direct anticonvulsant action of acetone and acetoacetate, reducing reactive oxygen species, creating a positive bioenergetic balance, and thus stabilization of resting membrane potential.
- Contraindications to the ketogenic diet include pyruvate carboxylase deficiency, porphyria, fatty acid oxidation defects, and carnitine deficiency.
- *Complications of the ketogenic diet include:*
  - *Short-term*—dehydration, vomiting, diarrhea, constipation, hypoglycemia, and refusal to eat
  - *Long-term*—renal calculi, growth failure, fracture, anemia, recurrent infection, metabolic derangements (hyperuricemia, hypocalcemia, acidosis, hypercholesterolemia, and reduced amino acids), prolonged QT interval, irritability, lethargy, and refusal to eat

REFERENCES/SOURCES

- Kliegman RM, St Geme III JW (Eds). Nelson Textbook of Pediatrics, 21st edition. Amsterdam: Elsevier; 2019. p. 3109.
- Swaiman KF, Ashwal S, Ferriero DM, Schor NF, Finkel RS, Gropman AL, et al (Eds). Swaiman's Paediatric Neurology, 6th edition. Amsterdam: Elsevier; 2017. p. 625.

14. Which of the following is a risk factor for sudden unexpected death in a person with epilepsy; sudden unexpected death in epilepsy (SUDEP)?

A. Myoclonic seizures
B. Epileptic spasms
C. Clonic seizures
D. Tonic-clonic seizures

EXPLANATION

Occurrence and frequency of tonic-clonic seizures (primary generalized tonic-clonic seizures or focal to bilateral tonic-clonic seizures) are associated with a high risk of SUDEP.

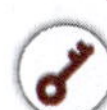

Key: D

BOOST YOUR KNOWLEDGE

SUDEP is defined as a sudden, unexpected death in a person with epilepsy, with or without evidence of a seizure preceding the death, in which there is no evidence of other disease, injury, or drowning that caused the death. The incidence of sudden death in people with epilepsy is 20 times higher than in the general population. SUDEP is the most common epilepsy-related cause of death in them. The overall risk is 1 per thousand person-years. Optimizing seizure control, especially of tonic-clonic seizures—is the most important measure to reduce the risk of SUDEP. Sleep supervision or monitoring devices may be considered.

REFERENCES/SOURCES

- Kliegman RM, St Geme III JW (Eds). Nelson Textbook of Pediatrics, 21st edition. Amsterdam: Elsevier; 2019.
- Swaiman KF, Ashwal S, Ferriero DM, Schor NF, Finkel RS, Gropman AL, et al (Eds). Swaiman's Paediatric Neurology, 6th edition. Amsterdam: Elsevier; 2017. p. 644.

15. A 16-year-old girl developed behavior change and poor scholastic performance. She presented to you with generalized tonic + focal seizures and was treated on multiple antiseizure medications. EEG is shown below. What is a likely diagnosis?

A. SSPE
B. N-methyl-D-aspartate receptor (NMDAR) encephalitis
C. Psychogenic nonepileptic seizure (PNES)
D. Pediatric acute-onset neuropsychiatric syndrome (PANS)

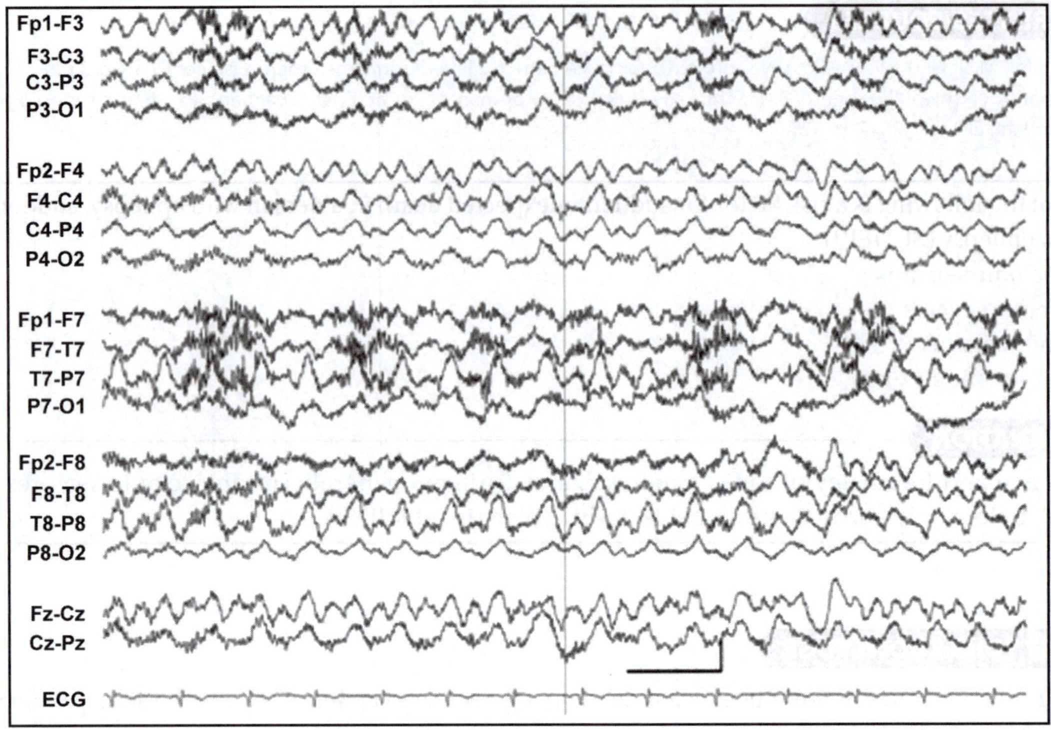

EXPLANATION

Electroencephalogram in NMDAR encephalitis is characterized by rhythmic 1–3 Hz delta activity with superimposed 20–30 Hz beta activity (extreme delta brush).

Key: B

BOOST YOUR KNOWLEDGE

- N-methyl-D-aspartate receptor encephalitis (NMDARE) is a serious, yet potentially reversible autoimmune neuropsychiatric disorder associated with immunoglobulin G (IgG) auto-ab against the NR1 subunit of the NMDAR.
- NMDARE accounts for 4% of all encephalitis.
- *Three clinical phenotypes are described*:
  1. Classic form
  2. Psychiatric form (associated with good outcomes)
  3. Catatonia-predominant form (associated with poor outcome)
- Atypical forms have also been described with children presenting with dominant autistic regression, catatonia and neuroleptic malignant syndrome, and gait disorder
- Management includes intravenous (IV) methylprednisolone pulse therapy, intravenous immunoglobulin (IVIG), and plasma exchange as first-line therapies. Second-line management includes rituximab, cyclophosphamide, and other immunomodulatory agents.

Probable Anti-NMDA Receptor Encephalitis

Diagnosis can be made when all three of the following criteria have been met:

1. *Rapid onset (<3 months) of at least four of the six following major groups of symptoms*:
   i. Abnormal (psychiatric) behavior or cognitive dysfunction
   ii. Speech dysfunction (pressured speech, verbal reduction, and mutism)

iii. Seizures
iv. Movement disorders, dyskinesias, or rigidity/abnormal postures
v. Decreased level of consciousness
vi. Autonomic dysfunction or central hypoventilation

2. *At least one of the following laboratory study results*:
   i. Abnormal EEG (focal or different use slow or disorganized activity, epileptic activity, or extreme delta brush)
   ii. CSF with pleocytosis or oligoclonal bands
3. Reasonable exclusion of other disorders

Note: Diagnosis can also made in the presence of three of the above groups of symptoms accompanied by a systemic teratoma.

Definite anti-NMDA Receptor Encephalitis

Diagnosis can be made in the presence of one or more of the six major groups of symptoms, and IgG anti-GluN1(NR1 submit of NMDAR) antibodies, after reasonable exclusion of other disorders.

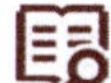

REFERENCES/SOURCES

- Kliegman RM, St Geme III JW (Eds). Nelson Textbook of Pediatrics, 21st edition. Amsterdam: Elsevier; 2019. p. 3182.
- Swaiman KF, Ashwal S, Ferriero DM, Schor NF, Finkel RS, Gropman AL, et al (Eds). Swaiman's Paediatric Neurology, 6th edition. Amsterdam: Elsevier; 2017. p. 931.

16. A 3-year-old boy was brought with it a history of regression of milestones, and generalized tonic-clonic and myoclonic seizures. Then, he developed ataxia and vision impairment. What specific activation procedure would you advise for doing an EEG?

A. Hyperventilation
B. Sleep deprivation and sleep
C. Photic stimulation at 1–3 Hz
D. Photic stimulation at 14–16 Hz

EXPLANATION

The disease here appears to be NCL. Low-frequency photic stimulation shows characteristic giant occipital polyspikes.

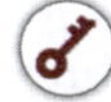

Key: C

BOOST YOUR KNOWLEDGE

- Also known as Batten disease, ceroid lipofuscinosis.
- The NCLs are a group of neurodegenerative lysosomal storage disorders, resulting in excess accumulation of lipopigments (lipofuscin).
- They were originally classified by age at onset: the infantile-onset form (Finnish form), late infantile-onset form, juvenile-onset form, and adult-onset form.
- NCLs are now classified according to the underlying pathogenic gene and age at onset. The diagnosis is based on genetic testing, assays of enzyme activity, electron microscopy of lymphocytes or tissue for nonclassical presentations
- Ceroid lipofuscinosis type 2 (CLN2; previously known as NCL type 2, the classic late infantile-onset form) is the most prevalent NCL. A new onset of epilepsy in a child aged 2–4 years, with a history of early language delay, should prompt consideration of CLN2. Multiple seizure types can occur, including febrile, tonic-clonic, absence, myoclonic, atonic, and focal (with or without focal to the bilateral tonic-clonic) seizures.

Myoclonic seizures may not be present at onset. Delayed speech development is often recognized before the onset of seizures. Disease progression is often rapid, with loss of mobility and language by the age of 4–5 years. Further regression occurs, with loss of vision occurring over the next few years. Patients die between the ages of 8 and 12 years.

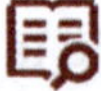

REFERENCES/SOURCES

- Kliegman RM, St Geme III JW (Eds). Nelson Textbook of Pediatrics, 21st edition. Amsterdam: Elsevier; 2019. p. 3190.
- Swaiman KF, Ashwal S, Ferriero DM, Schor NF, Finkel RS, Gropman AL, et al (Eds). Swaiman's Paediatric Neurology, 6th edition. Amsterdam: Elsevier; 2017. p. 390.

17. Identify the gene which was first reported to be associated with GEFS+ syndrome.

A. *SCN1A*
B. *SCN1B*
C. *SCN2A*
D. *SCN8A*

EXPLANATION

SCN1B mutations were first reported in a large family with GEFS+. *SCN1B*—first gene identified but not the most common gene. Subsequently, SCN1A, SCN2A, and other sodium channel mutations, GABRG2, and GABRD (mutations in GABA-A subunit genes) have been found. SCN1A pathogenic variants were identified in ~10% of GEFS+ families. Nonsense and truncated mutations often lead to Dravet syndrome.

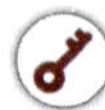

Key: B

BOOST YOUR KNOWLEDGE

- GEFS+ spectrum was described initially as an autosomal dominant familial epilepsy with variable penetrance.
- It includes a spectrum of epilepsy phenotypes: epilepsy with myoclonic atonic seizures, Dravet syndrome, idiopathic and other genetic generalized epilepsy syndromes, and focal epilepsies.
- Heterogeneous phenotypes are usually in the same family.
- FS is the hallmark of GEFS+ and occurs in many affected family members.
- GEFS+ has heterogeneous genetic etiologies, with pathogenic variants in several genes identified.
- The most common phenotype in GEFS+ is classical FS, the next most common phenotype is febrile seizures plus (FS+). FS+ has several different presentations: Most common—typical FS continues beyond the age of 6 years, the typical age at which most FS stops. FS+ continues beyond the age of 6 years, the typical age at which most fs stop.

REFERENCE/SOURCE

- Swaiman KF, Ashwal S, Ferriero DM, Schor NF, Finkel RS, Gropman AL, et al (Eds). Swaiman's Paediatric Neurology, 6th edition. Amsterdam: Elsevier; 2017. p. 407.

18. Following is the EEG of a 7-year-old boy. Which of the following drugs is best suited for this condition?

A. Oxcarbazepine
B. Carbamazepine
C. Valproate
D. Eslicarbazepine

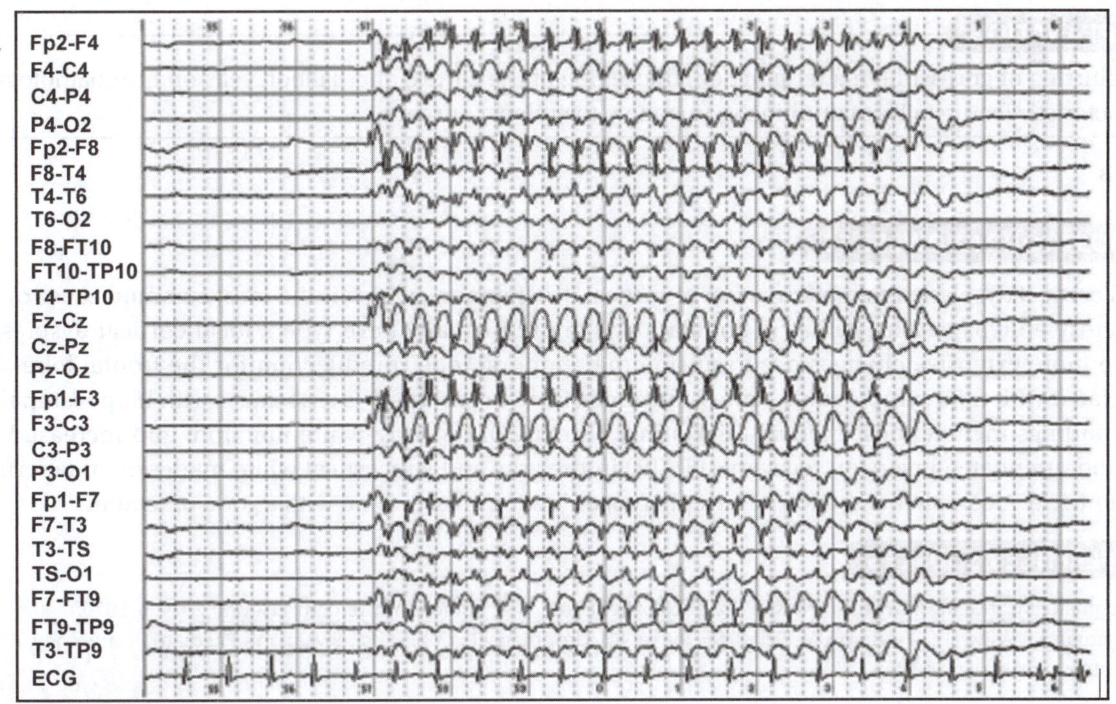

EXPLANATION

This EEG shows the classic 3 Hz spike-and-wave pattern of absence seizures. The treatment should be ethosuximide or valproic acid. Zonisamide can also be used. However, drugs such as carbamazepine and oxcarbazepine can worsen absence seizures and cause absence SE, and hence, should be avoided.

Key: C

BOOST YOUR KNOWLEDGE

- Childhood absence epilepsy (CAE) occurs in an otherwise normal child with daily absence seizures associated with 2.5–4-Hz generalized spike-wave at seizure onset.
- Absence seizures are provoked by hyperventilation.
- Neurological examination, development, and cognition are normal. Attention deficit hyperactivity disorder (ADHD) and learning difficulties may occur.
- Epilepsy remits in 60% of children, often within 2 years of onset or by early adolescence.
- The age at onset is typically 4–10 years. Suspect juvenile absence epilepsy when onset is >10 years.
- Occipital intermittent rhythmic delta activity (OIRDA) occurs in 30% of children with CAE.

REFERENCE/SOURCE

- Kliegman RM, St Geme III JW (Eds). Nelson Textbook of Pediatrics, 21st edition. Amsterdam: Elsevier; 2019. p. 3097, 3102.

19. A 6-year-old girl presented with refractory left focal seizures. Neuroimaging reveals focal cortical dysplasia. Which of the following is a feature of this condition?

A. Sharply delineated focal lesion in the cortex
B. Blurring of gray-white matter junction
C. Neuronal migration abnormality
D. Cystic changes in the gray matter

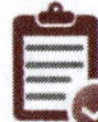

EXPLANATION

The blurring of gray-white matter junction, thickening of the cortex, and balloon cells on histopathology are the characteristic features. This condition is amenable to epilepsy surgery.

Key: B

BOOST YOUR KNOWLEDGE

Focal cortical dysplasia is a malformation of cortical development, which is the most common cause of medically refractory epilepsy in the pediatric population. Children usually have type 2 focal cortical dysplasia (FCD), where more extensive changes occur outside the temporal lobe (predilection for the frontal lobe). Type 1 is associated with mild symptomatic expression and is late onset. Type 3 is associated with hippocampal sclerosis. MRI findings include focal cortical thickening, blurring of the gray-white junction, and increased signal on T2/fluid-attenuated inversion recovery (FLAIR) in the gray and subcortical white matter often tapering toward the ventricle. A complete resection of the epileptogenic zone is associated with a good outcome.

REFERENCES/SOURCES

- Kliegman RM, St Geme III JW (Eds). Nelson Textbook of Pediatrics, 21st edition. Amsterdam: Elsevier; 2019. p. 3070.
- Swaiman KF, Ashwal S, Ferriero DM, Schor NF, Finkel RS, Gropman AL, et al (Eds). Swaiman's Paediatric Neurology, 6th edition. Amsterdam: Elsevier; 2017. p. 583.

20. A 2-month-old infant is brought to the out-patient department (OPD) with complaints of a cluster of jerky movements of both upper and lower limbs which occur two to three times a day once she sleeps. She was born with no perinatal complications, feeds well, and normal neurological examination. Parents were worried as their cousin's child was diagnosed with epilepsy. What is the most likely diagnosis?

A. Myoclonic epilepsy of infancy
B. Shuddering attacks
C. Benign neonatal sleep myoclonus
D. West syndrome

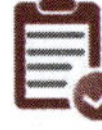

EXPLANATION

Benign neonatal sleep myoclonus is characterized by repetitive myoclonic jerks occurring during sleep mainly in the nonrapid eye movement (NREM) stage in neurologically normal newborns.

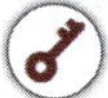

Key: C

BOOST YOUR KNOWLEDGE

- *Myoclonus:* Sudden brief involuntary 'jerks' of a single muscle or group
- Conditions causing physiological myoclonus include hypnagogic myoclonus, benign sleep myoclonus of infancy, hiccups, physiological startle, and anxiety.
- Secondary or symptomatic myoclonus occurs with hypoxia, infection, drugs, metabolic, neurodegenerative conditions, and toxins.

REFERENCES/SOURCES

- Kliegman RM, St Geme III JW (Eds). Nelson Textbook of Pediatrics, 21st edition. Amsterdam: Elsevier; 2019. p. 3127.
- Swaiman KF, Ashwal S, Ferriero DM, Schor NF, Finkel RS, Gropman AL, et al (Eds). Swaiman's Paediatric Neurology, 6th edition. Amsterdam: Elsevier; 2017. p. 724.

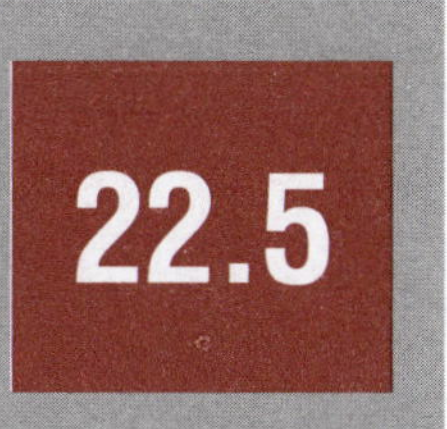

CHAPTER 22.5

Central Nervous System Infections (Meningitis, Encephalitis, Brain Abscess, Neurocysticercosis, and Tuberculoma)

Lokesh Saini

1. A 5-year-old girl presented to the emergency with history of fever, vomiting, and headache for the past 20 days and seizures for 4 days. On examination, she opened her eyes spontaneously, was following motor commands and was oriented and talking relevantly. There was left lateral gaze palsy with inability to close left eyelid and weakness of left upper and lower limbs. Last seizure was 6 hours back. She had a history of contact with an active case of pulmonary tuberculosis in the family. According to the modified Medical Research Council, what is the stage of tubercular meningitis (TBM)?

A. I B. II
C. III D. IV

EXPLANATION

Glasgow Coma Scale (GCS) of the child is E4V5M6 (E4-opening eyes spontaneously, V5-relevant talking, oriented, and M6-obeying motor commands). However, left side 6th and 7th cranial nerve palsy is evidenced by left lateral gaze palsy and inability to close left eyelid. Associated there is left hemiparesis. Thus, she has TBM stage II according to modified Medical Research Council (MRC) scale.

Key: B

BOOST YOUR KNOWLEDGE

Severity of TBM (modified MRC scale):

Stage I	Alert and oriented without focal neurological deficits
Stage II	GCS 10–14 with or without focal neurological deficits or GCS 15 with focal neurological deficits
Stage III	GCS <10 with or without focal neurological deficits

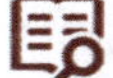

REFERENCES/SOURCES

- Gupta P, Menon PSN, Ramji S, Lodha R. PG Textbook of Pediatrics, 3rd edition. New Delhi: Jaypee Brothers Medical Publishers; 2022.
- Van Toorn R, Springer P, Laubscher JA, Schoeman JF. Value of different staging system for predicting neurological outcome in childhood tuberculous meningitis. Int J Tuberc Lung Dis. 2012;16:628-32.

2. A 10-year-old boy with normal development presented with a history of fever, headache for 12 days, and abnormal behavior for the past 7 days. There was also a history of facial rash with no photosensitivity present for the last 2 years. On examination, there were no focal deficits. Mini-mental state examination (MMSE) score was 7. Cerebrospinal fluid (CSF) examination was done with the following results—sugar 62 mg/dL, protein 67 mg/dL, WBC 24/mm^3 (lymphocytes 95%). CT head shows hypodensities in bilateral temporal areas (right > left) as well as the basi-frontal regions near the cingulate gyrus.

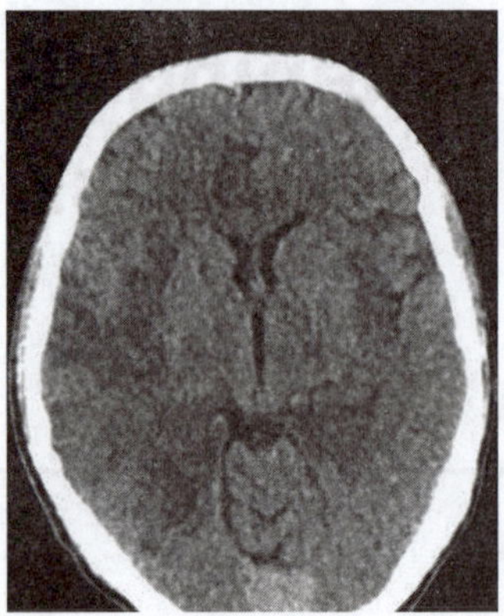

What is the possible diagnosis?

A. NMDA (anti-N-methyl-d-aspartate) encephalitis
B. HSV (herpes simplex virus) encephalitis
C. CNS (central nervous system) vasculitis
D. SLE (systemic lupus erythematosus) associated CNS dysfunction

EXPLANATION

On the basis of the given history of an adolescent boy with a history of fever, headache, and altered behavior; the first differential diagnosis is acute herpes viral encephalitis or autoimmune (NMDAR) encephalitis. Another confusing point here is skin rash present for 2 years but since there is no photosensitivity, it is irrelevant to the recent case scenario.

Cerebrospinal fluid examination clears the doubt between the two main differential diagnoses. A greater number of cells with mildly elevated proteins point towards acute viral infection, which is confirmed by CT scan findings. Thus, our diagnosis would be HSV encephalitis.

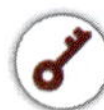

Key: B

BOOST YOUR KNOWLEDGE

Autoimmune encephalitis usually has elevated proteins without CSF leukocytosis. While an infectious illness of the nervous system will have both elevated proteins as well as cells. Neuroimaging in herpes shows specific predilection for the temporal regions causing edema and magnetic resonance imaging (MRI) showing T2 hyperintensities with diffusion restriction. Electroencephalogram (EEG) characteristically shows PLEDs (periodic lateralized epileptiform discharges) in herpes encephalitis.

REFERENCES/SOURCES

- Kliegman RM, St Geme III JW. Nelson Textbook of Pediatrics, 21st edition. Elsevier; 2019.
- Tedyanto EH, Susilawathi NM, Suryapraba Indradewi AAA. Herpes simplex virus encephalitis: a literature review. Romanian J Neurol. 2022.

3. A 4-year-old boy with history of right ear discharge for past 2 years, presented now with history of fever, headache, and vomiting for past 2 weeks. He had a history of recurrent hospitalizations due to respiratory illness since 6 months of age. On examination, child had altered sensorium with low grade fever, BP 144/90, PR 62/minute. MRI was suggestive of an irregular lesion with T2 hypointense rim with diffusion restriction and blooming seen on the border of the lesion on susceptibility weighted image. The most likely diagnosis could be:

A. Bacterial abscess
B. Tuberculous meningitis
C. Fungal abscess
D. Tuberculoma

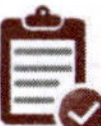

EXPLANATION

In the given case scenario with history of recurrent chest infections requiring hospitalization, the given history of low-grade fever, with headache and vomiting against a background of right ear discharge, the given case scenario supports the possibility of a brain abscess likely fungal given the background of possible immunodeficiency state and imaging showing blooming (bleed), the likely diagnosis if fungal abscess.

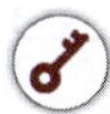

Key: C

BOOST YOUR KNOWLEDGE

- The development of fungal abscesses is dependent on the patient's immune system and fungal virulence factors. The major contributing factors for decreased host immunity include immunodeficiencies either primary or secondary to chemotherapies and diseases such as human immunodeficiency virus (HIV) infections. Common routes of spread of infection are hematogenous dissemination from a distant focus such as lung, through direct implantation after trauma, or secondary to the local extension from sinonasal, orbital, or spinal infections.
- The most common fungi are *Cryptococcus* and *Candida*. Due to their small size, they can access the microcirculation and can cause diffuse leptomeningitis or manifest as parenchymal granulomas or abscesses. *Aspergillus* and *Mucor* due to their larger size cannot access the meningeal microcirculation and cause a more focal disease. They cause cerebritis, abscess formation, or involvement of larger vessels resulting in vasculitis, vascular occlusion, cerebral infarctions, or formation of mycotic aneurysms.
- The goals of treatment are: (1) relief of mass effect when present, (2) identification of a pathologic agent by specimen culture, (3) control and eradication of infection, (4) minimization of loss of neurologic function, and (5) systemic supportive care.
- Antifungal agents in general have poor penetration across the blood-brain barrier, and medical therapy alone is not helpful for fungal brain abscesses. Antifungal agents are selected based upon the offending agent.
- *Candida albicans* infection is treated with amphotericin B, fluconazole, or caspofungin. Cryptococcal infections require amphotericin B and flucytosine, though fluconazole can be used as an alternative. Liposomal amphotericin B has increased permeability across the blood-brain barrier and has been used to treat *Aspergillus* nonsurgically; however, *Aspergillus fumigatus* (*A. fumigatus*) and *Mucormycosis* species abscesses are still best treated with surgery followed by antifungal therapy. Prophylaxis with anticonvulsants is recommended for all patients with brain abscesses.
- An aggressive diagnostic approach and timely initiation of antifungal therapy is imperative to reduce morbidity and mortality.

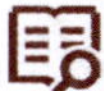

REFERENCES/SOURCES

- Feraco P, Donner D, Gagliardo C, Leonardi I, Piccinini S, Del Poggio A, et al. Cerebral abscesses imaging: a practical approach. J Popul Ther Clin Pharmacol. 2020;27(3):e11-24.
- Kliegman RM, St Geme III JW. Nelson Textbook of Pediatrics, 21st edition. Elsevier; 2019.

4. A 12-year-old girl with normal development presented with history of two episodes of right focal seizures for last 1 month. These episodes occurred during awake state with no associated autonomic features. On MRI, there were two ring enhancing lesions seen in the left temporal lobe and cerebellum. These lesions were hypointense on T2W image with T1W image showing hyperintense rim. Magnetic resonance spectroscopy (MRS) showed lipid peak. What is the diagnosis?

A. Neurocysticercosis
B. Tuberculoma
C. Fungal abscess
D. Toxoplasmosis

EXPLANATION

The given case scenario of an adolescent with a history of two unprovoked focal seizures occurring in awake state supports the diagnosis of most likely a structural cause of epilepsy. The two most common lesions are neurocysticercosis and tuberculoma. On neuroimaging the lesions are seen both in supratentorial as well as infratentorial regions with hyperintense rim of the ring enhancing lesion seen on T1W image point toward the diagnosis of tuberculoma. Further history of contact and other systemic symptoms should be thought of.

Key: B

BOOST YOUR KNOWLEDGE

Difference between tuberculoma and parenchymal neurocysticercosis (NCC):

Features	***Tuberculoma***	***NCC***
Size and site	>20 mm, supratentorial, and infratentorial	<20 mm, supratentorial (gray-white junction)
Perilesional edema and midline shift	Moderate-to-severe edema, midline shift present	Mild edema, midline shift less common
MRI T1	Hyperintense rim present	No hyperintense rim seen
MRI T2	No scolex visualized	Hypointense T2 eccentric scolex seen
MRI fluid-attenuated inversion recovery (FLAIR)	No/incomplete suppression on FLAIR	Complete suppression on FLAIR
MRS	Lipid peak present	Multiple amino-acid peak seen

(MRI: magnetic resonance imaging; MRS: Magnetic resonance spectroscopy)

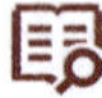

REFERENCES/SOURCES

- Barkovich AJ, Raybaud C. Diagnostic Imaging Pediatric Neuroradiology, 6th edition. Philadelphia: Wolters Kluwer; 2019. Section 1: Infection/inflammation.
- Hanumaiah R, Patwari S. Diagnostic dilemma in differentiating tuberculomas and NCC on neuroimaging. Educational exhibit. ECR 2017.

5. A 4-year-old malnourished boy presented to the emergency room (ER) with complaints of fever, vomiting, and lethargy for past 16 days. There was a history of falling from bed 3 days prior to the onset of symptoms. On examination, the child had signs of raised intracranial pressure (ICP) with anisocoria. CSF examination revealed 240 WBC/mm^3 with 85% lymphocytes, protein 780 mg/dL, sugar 20 mg/dL, and nil RBCs. An emergency CT revealed the following:

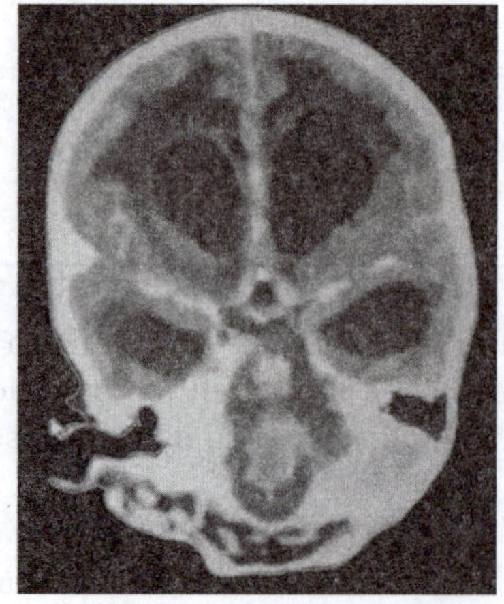

What is the most likely diagnosis?

A. Intraventricular hemorrhage
B. ICSOL (intracranial space occupying lesion) with hydrocephalus
C. Tubercular meningitis
D. Acute meningoencephalitis

EXPLANATION

The child has a history of symptoms since past 2 weeks. The history of fall is just a distracter added. CSF done was suggestive of TBM and neuroimaging shows gross hydrocephalus with periventricular ooze with basal exudates seen on the CT scan. These findings corroborate with TBM.

- There is no visible hyperdensity in the ventricles, so there is no evidence of intracerebral (IC) bleed.
- This is not ICSOL as no mass lesion appreciable in the posterior fossa.
- Acute meningoencephalitis could be another differential diagnosis, however, the presence of gross hydrocephalus with basal exudates points toward the diagnosis of TBM.

Key: C

BOOST YOUR KNOWLEDGE

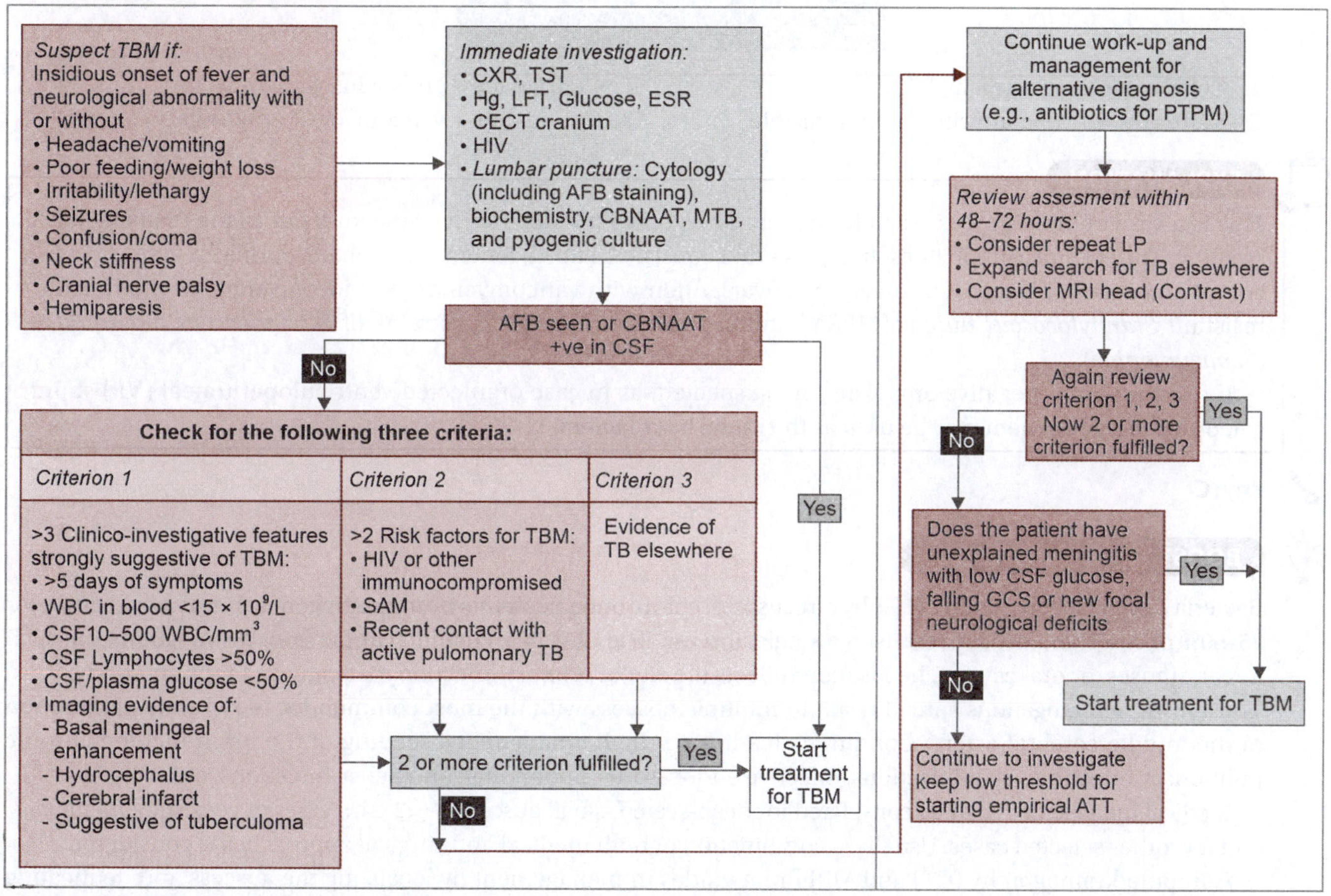

Suspect TBM if:
Insidious onset of fever and neurological abnormality with or without
- Headache/vomiting
- Poor feeding/weight loss
- Irritability/lethargy
- Seizures
- Confusion/coma
- Neck stiffness
- Cranial nerve palsy
- Hemiparesis

→ *Immediate investigation:*
- CXR, TST
- Hg, LFT, Glucose, ESR
- CECT cranium
- HIV
- *Lumbar puncture:* Cytology (including AFB staining), biochemistry, CBNAAT, MTB, and pyogenic culture

→ AFB seen or CBNAAT +ve in CSF
- Yes → Start treatment for TBM
- No → **Check for the following three criteria:**

Criterion 1	Criterion 2	Criterion 3
>3 Clinico-investigative features strongly suggestive of TBM: • >5 days of symptoms • WBC in blood <15 × 10^9/L • CSF10–500 WBC/mm^3 • CSF Lymphocytes >50% • CSF/plasma glucose <50% • Imaging evidence of: - Basal meningeal enhancement - Hydrocephalus - Cerebral infarct - Suggestive of tuberculoma	>2 Risk factors for TBM: • HIV or other immunocompromised • SAM • Recent contact with active pulomonary TB	Evidence of TB elsewhere

→ 2 or more criterion fulfilled?
- Yes → Start treatment for TBM
- No → Continue work-up and management for alternative diagnosis (e.g., antibiotics for PTPM)

→ *Review assessment within 48–72 hours:*
- Consider repeat LP
- Expand search for TB elsewhere
- Consider MRI head (Contrast)

→ Again review criterion 1, 2, 3 Now 2 or more criterion fulfilled?
- Yes → Start treatment for TBM
- No → Does the patient have unexplained meningitis with low CSF glucose, falling GCS or new focal neurological deficits
  - Yes → Start treatment for TBM
  - No → Continue to investigate keep low threshold for starting empirical ATT

(AFB: acid-fast bacilli; ATT: anti-tubercular treatment; CBNAAT: cartridge-based nucleic acid amplification test; CSF: cerebrospinal fluid; CXR: chest X-ray; ESR: erythrocyte sedimentation rate; GCS: Glasgow coma scale; LP: lumbar puncture; PTPM: partially treated pyogenic meningitis; SAM: severe acute malnutrition; TST: tuberculin skin test)

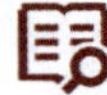

REFERENCE/SOURCE

- Indian Academy of Pediatrics. RNTCP Updated Pediatric TB Guidelines 2019. Indian Pediatr. 2019;56:692.

6. A 1-year-old boy with insignificant perinatal history and normal development presented with a history of fever, vomiting for 10 days, and four episodes of right focal seizures. Examination revealed swelling over the left temporal region without any other focal neurological deficits. MRI brain is shown. Which of the following will be the most appropriate empirical antimicrobial regime for this condition?

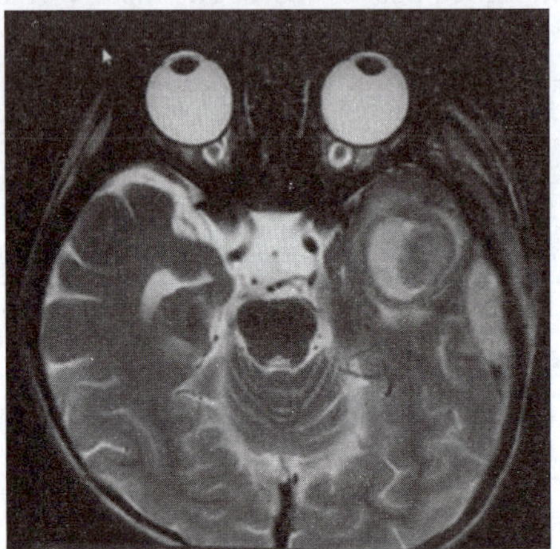

A. Ceftriaxone + gentamicin
B. Ceftriaxone + amikacin + vancomycin
C. Ceftriaxone + vancomycin + metronidazole
D. Ceftriaxone + vancomycin + antifungals

EXPLANATION

This is a case of brain abscess seen in the temporal lobe extending in the subcutaneous planes causing facial swelling. The empirical antibiotics therapy should consist of a third-generation cephalosporin (for gram-negative cover) and metronidazole (for anaerobic cover), often with vancomycin to provide coverage for methicillin-resistant *Staphylococcus aureus* (MRSA) and cephalosporin resistant strains of *Streptococcus pneumoniae* (*S. pneumoniae*).

If resistant gram-negative organisms are suspected, as in case of infected ventriculoperitoneal (VP) shunt, cefepime, or meropenem may be used as the initial beta-lactam.

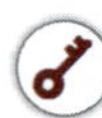

Key: C

BOOST YOUR KNOWLEDGE

Bacteria can invade the brain either by direct spread or through hematogenous seeding. Direct spread accounts for 25–50% of cases and usually results in a single abscess. The direct inoculation can be from a contiguous site such as ear, sinuses, or oral cavity. The location reflects the site of primary infection that spreads to the cerebral cortex. Those with hematogenous spread result in multiple abscess with the most common location in the distribution of the middle cerebral artery. Conditions leading to the hematogenous seeding of the brain include chronic pulmonary infections, skin infections, infective endocarditis, abdominal, and pelvic infections, etc.

Medical management can be considered for deep-seated, small abscesses (<2 cm), cases of coexisting meningitis, and few other selected cases. Usually, a combination of both medical and surgical approaches is considered.

Computed tomography (CT) and MRI brain guides in management by localizing the abscess and delineating details including dimensions and several abscesses. Usually, large abscesses (>2 cm) are considered for aspiration or excision based on the surgical skills of the operator. The approach for multiple abscesses includes a long course (4–8 weeks) of high-dose antibiotics with or without aspirations, based on weekly CT scanning.

The selection of an antibiotic regimen should be wisely made based on microorganisms isolated from blood or CSF. Certain antibiotics are unable to cross the blood-brain barrier and are not useful in treating brain abscess; these antibiotics include first-generation cephalosporins, aminoglycosides, and tetracyclines.

With the advent of antimicrobials and imaging studies such as CT scanning and MRI, the mortality rate has reduced from 5 to 10%. Rupture of a brain abscess, however, is more fatal. The long-term neurological sequelae after the infection are dependent on the early diagnosis and administration of antibiotics.

REFERENCES/SOURCES

- Bokhari MR, Mesfin FB. Brain abscess. In: StatPearls. Treasure Island (FL): StatPearls Publishing; 2023.
- Kliegman RM, St Geme III JW. Nelson Textbook of Pediatrics, 21st edition. Elsevier; 2019.
- Mameli C, Genoni T, Madia C, Donedo C, Penagini F, Zuccotti G. Brain abscess in pediatric age: a review. Childs Nerv Syst. 2019;35(7):1117-28.

7. An 11-year-old boy presented with first episode of unprovoked right focal seizures. On examination, there was no focal deficit and no signs of raised ICP. MRI brain revealed a single ring enhancing lesion in the left parietal region suggestive of NCC. Which of the following is the first choice of anti-epileptic drug?

A. Lacosamide
B. Oxcarbazepine
C. Phenytoin
D. Levetiracetam

EXPLANATION

The anti-seizure medication (ASM) for focal epilepsy includes carbamazepine, oxcarbazepine, and lacosamide. Other drugs include brivaracetam, levetiracetam, valproate, phenytoin among others.

In cases of NCC, the ASM of first choice include oxcarbazepine or carbamazepine. Other ASM recommended are levetiracetam or phenytoin.

Key: B

BOOST YOUR KNOWLEDGE

Diagnosis of NCC should be based on clinical history and neuroimaging. Contrast-enhanced magnetic resonance imaging of the brain is the modality of choice. For single enhancing lesion, albendazole therapy for 10–14 days is recommended. In the case of NCC presenting with symptoms other than seizures, there appears to be no role for routine anti-seizure medication prophylaxis. For a single ring-enhancing lesion, 6 months of anti-seizure medication is sufficient if the lesion resolves on follow-up. Those with persistent lesions, calcification, or multiple lesions, require a longer treatment duration of at least 24 months.

REFERENCE/SOURCE

- Sankhyan N, Kadwa RA, Kamate M, Kannan L, Kumar A, Passi GR, et al. Management of neurocysticercosis in children: Association of Child Neurology Consensus Guidelines. Indian Pediatr. 2021;58:871-80.

8. Computed tomography head is *not* recommended in which of the following neurological deficits associated with meningitis?

A. Right lateral gaze palsy
B. Right absent pupillary reflex
C. Right hemiparesis
D. Left eye adduction palsy

EXPLANATION

The clinical features of bacterial meningitis can be subtle, variable, and nonspecific or absent in the pediatric population. Neuroimaging is not essential for the diagnosis or management of patients with acute bacterial meningitis.

The Infectious Diseases Society of America (IDSA) guidelines recommend that infants and children with the following should have a cranial CT scan done:

- History of central nervous system disease (CSF shunts, hydrocephalus, head trauma, post neurosurgery, and space-occupying lesions)
- Immunocompromised
- Papilledema
- Focal neurological deficits (except palsy of abducens or facial nerve)

Key: A

BOOST YOUR KNOWLEDGE

- *Lateral gaze palsy* is an inability to produce horizontal, conjugate eye movements in one or both directions.
- Lesions of the cranial nerve VI (abducens) nucleus in the pons (cause ipsilateral, horizontal gaze palsy by disrupting motor neurons that innervate the ipsilateral lateral rectus muscle by way of cranial nerve VI, and interneurons that connect to the contralateral cranial nerve III nucleus in the midbrain, via the *medial longitudinal fasciculus*, to stimulate the medial rectus of the opposite eye).
- Lesions of the paramedian pontine reticular formation, adjacent to the abducens nucleus, (may cause lateral gaze palsy, particularly involving ipsilateral saccadic eye movements).
- Lesions of the frontal or parietal cortical eye fields (may also cause weakness of horizontal gaze (contralateral to frontal lesions and ipsilateral to parietal lesions) that becomes more subtle over time).
- *Absent pupillary reflex:* Optic nerve injury, oculomotor nerve damage, brainstem lesions, such as tumors, and medications such as barbiturates.
- *Right hemiparesis:* Stroke, brain damage due to trauma and head injuries, tumors.
- *Adduction palsy:* Mostly caused by internuclear ophthalmoplegia caused by demyelination disorders such as multiple sclerosis, cerebrovascular events, tumors, mass lesions, etc.

REFERENCES/SOURCES

- Alamarat Z, Hasbun R. Management of acute bacterial meningitis in children. Infect Drug Resist. 2020;13:4077-89.
- Tunkel ARHB, Kaplan SL, Kaufman BA, Roos KL, Scheld WM, Whitley RJ. Practice guidelines for the management of bacterial meningitis. Clin Infect Dis. 2004;39(9):1267-84.
- Wanson D. Meningitis. Pediatr Rev. 2015;36(12):514-26.

9. A 16-year-old male was diagnosed with HSV encephalitis, received IV acyclovir for 21 days. Now after 6 weeks patient is having abnormal behavior, excessive talkativeness, movement disorder, memory disturbance, and wandering spells. What is the next management of choice?

A. Repeat IV acyclovir
B. Start Immunotherapy
C. Send HSV, DNA, PCR, and start immunotherapy
D. Send HSV, DNA, PCR, and NMDAR antibodies

EXPLANATION

Latency between HSV encephalitis and NMDA encephalitis is significantly short in children. Secondary NMDA encephalitis should be ruled out during relapse of symptoms, presence of movement disorder, and psychiatric symptoms.

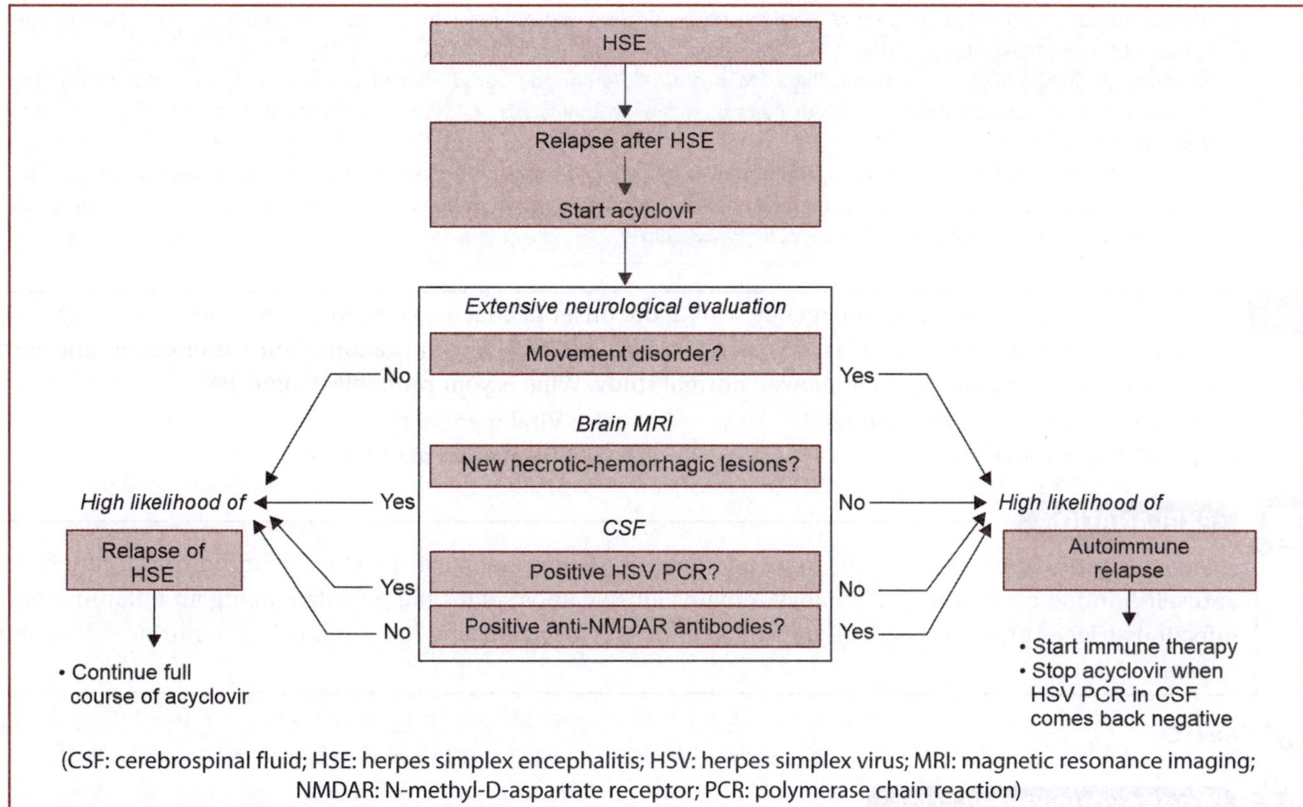

(CSF: cerebrospinal fluid; HSE: herpes simplex encephalitis; HSV: herpes simplex virus; MRI: magnetic resonance imaging; NMDAR: N-methyl-D-aspartate receptor; PCR: polymerase chain reaction)

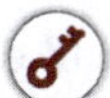

Key: D

BOOST YOUR KNOWLEDGE

- Herpes simplex type 1 (HSV1) encephalitis is a destructive and highly inflammatory encephalitis that predominantly affects temporal lobes and surrounding structures.
- After recovery from HSV infection approximately 20% of children with HSV1 encephalitis deteriorate with a "second phase" of encephalitis with clinical features typical of anti-NMDAR encephalitis, including florid movement disorders and encephalopathy, associated with the emergence of anti-NMDAR antibodies.
- Anti-NMDA receptor (NMDAR) encephalitis, is the most common autoimmune encephalitis which is defined by a characteristic clinical syndrome and the presence of CSF autoantibodies to the NR1 subunit of the NMDAR.
- If NMDARE is suspected, immunotherapy should be started promptly, even before antibody results are available, if alternative diagnoses have been reasonably excluded (i.e., infectious encephalitis).
- IV corticosteroids should be the first immunotherapy used (i.e., IV methylprednisolone). If IV corticosteroids are not available or are contraindicated, oral corticosteroids (prednisone, OP, or dexamethasone, DEX) should be used.

REFERENCES/SOURCES

- Armangue T, Leypoldt F, Málaga I, et al. Herpes simplex virus encephalitis is a trigger of brain autoimmunity. Ann Neurol. 2014;75: 317-23.
- Dale RC, Nosadini M. Infection-triggered autoimmunity: The case of herpes simplex virus type 1 and anti-NMDAR antibodies. Neurol Neuroimmunol Neuroinflamm. 2018;5(4):e471. doi: 10.1212/NXI.0000000000000471. PMID: 29904645; PMCID: PMC5999348

- Mohammad SS, Sinclair K, Pillai S, et al. Herpes simplex encephalitis relapse with chorea is associated with autoantibodies to N-methyl-D-aspartate receptor or dopamine-2 receptor. Mov Disord. 2014;29:117-22.
- Nosadini M, Mohammad SS, Corazza F, Ruga EM, Kothur K, Perilongo G, et al. Herpes simplex virus-induced anti-N-methyl-d-aspartate receptor encephalitis: a systematic literature review with analysis of 43 cases Review. Dev Med Child Neurol. 2017;59(8): 796-805.
- Nosadini M, Thomas T, Eyre M, Anlar B, Armangue T, Benseler SM, et al. International Consensus Recommendations for the Treatment of Pediatric NMDAR Antibody Encephalitis. Neurol Neuroimmunol Neuroinflamm. 2021;8(5):e1052. doi: 10.1212/NXI.0000000000001052. PMID: 34301820; PMCID: PMC8299516.

10. A 15-year-old boy presented to emergency with acute onset headache, vomiting, and positive meningeal signs. He had three similar episodes in last 1 year. CSF revealed 25 cells with predominant lymphocytes and normal sugar/protein. Neuroimaging done showed normal study. What is your probable diagnosis?

A. Partially treated bacterial meningitis
B. Viral meningitis
C. HaNDL syndrome
D. Tubercular meningitis

EXPLANATION

Headache and neurological deficits associated with CSF lymphocytosis (HaNDL syndrome) is a rare benign and self-limiting condition. The etiology remains elusive, most plausible postulate being an inflammatory or infectious trigger precipitating a migraine-like illness. This syndrome has a relapsing-remitting self-limiting course.

Key: C

BOOST YOUR KNOWLEDGE

Headache and neurological deficits associated with CSF lymphocytosis (HaNDL syndrome) is a migraine-like headache associated with aphasia, sensory, and motor deficits which are usually self-limiting. It is a rare self-limiting disease with single to multiple episodes. Although patients are usually symptomless between the episodes, the neurologic deficits can last up to 7 weeks. Though both HaNDL syndrome and meningitis can present with headache, vomiting, photophobia, and signs of raised ICP, there are a few differentiating features. There is no accompanying fever in HaNDL syndrome as is seen in cases of meningitis. Patients with meningitis on the other hand have a consistent course with toxic look and symptoms lasting until treated with appropriate antibiotics. There is no waxing or waning course in meningitis and the leukocytosis is predominantly neutrophilic in cases of meningitis. HaNDL syndrome on the other hand has an infectious trigger. The neurologic deficits are often different from one episode to the next due to the involvement of varying cortical regions.

REFERENCES/SOURCES

- Fiamingo G, Canavero I, Gastaldi M, Coloberti E, Buongarzone G, Ghiotto N, et al. HaNDL syndrome: a reversible cerebral vasoconstriction triggered by an infection? A case report and a case-based review. Eur J Med Res. 2022;27(1):196.
- Lay CL, Sun-Edelstein C. Syndrome of transient headache and neurologic deficits with cerebrospinal fluid lymphocytosis (HaNDL). UpToDate; 2022.
- Saini L, Kumar RM, Chakrabarty B, Gulati S. Recurrent headache in a five year old boy. Ann Indian Acad Neurol. 2016;19(1):143-5.

11. A 16-year-old boy presented with symptoms suggestive of brainstem encephalitis. CSF study showed polymorphonuclear leukocytosis and increased protein. What antibiotic combination would be rationale in this case?

A. Ceftriaxone + ampicillin + acyclovir
B. Ceftriaxone + acyclovir + vancomycin
C. Ceftriaxone + metronidazole + acyclovir
D. Ceftriaxone + doxycycline + acyclovir

EXPLANATION

Listerial brainstem encephalitis (mesenrhombencephalitis or rhombencephalitis) can be seen in healthy individual. It has high mortality, and serious sequelae are frequently reported in survivors. Early recognition and correct diagnosis, as well as the timely use of appropriate antibiotics, can reduce the severity of listerial infections. The trigeminal nerve is proposed as a pathway through which *Listeria monocytogenes* (*L. monocytogenes*) reaches the brainstem after entering damaged oropharyngeal mucosa or periodontal tissues, invade the brainstem along the vagus nerve after it infects enteric neurons in the walls of the gastrointestinal tract. Intravenous ampicillin (likely combined with one of the aminoglycosides) or penicillin has been proven to be effective for the treatment of listerial meningitis and brainstem encephalitis, with the former often considered as the first choice.

Key: A

BOOST YOUR KNOWLEDGE

Encephalitis involving the brainstem is relatively uncommon. The proposed etiologies of brainstem encephalitis (BE) include infectious and autoimmune causes. The existing knowledge of BE, or encephalitis in general, is usually directed toward infectious entities. Over the last decade, more attention has been paid toward the other possible causes of BE.

The diagnosis of BE can be challenging in most cases. Nonetheless, adjuvant serological markers, CSF examination, radiological evaluation, and histopathological confirmation of the diagnosis are of paramount importance. The utility of serological markers in cases of BE is to detect those antibodies that have been described to be of an autoimmune nature. Lumbar puncture for CSF chemistries (which include white blood cell counts, as well as protein and glucose levels) and the need to obtain cultures are essential to exclude infection. The role of brain imaging, CT, and MRI is helpful to narrow the differential diagnosis.

The treatment of BE is highly variable. If an infectious cause is suspected, specific antimicrobial, or empirical treatments are warranted. Ampicillin is usually the drug of choice in suspected cases of listeria; alternatives include trimethoprim-sulfamethoxazole, vancomycin, and linezolid. Cases of viral BE, specifically those caused by herpes, can be treated effectively with acyclovir. While the involvement of tuberculosis in BE is rarely encountered, the proper administration of anti-tuberculosis medications is essential. The treatment of BE attributable to an autoimmune cause includes steroid therapy, plasma exchange, and intravenous immunoglobulin. When no etiology is established for BE, treating it as an autoimmune condition can be effective. However, in clinical practice, treatment of BE is usually initiated empirically even without clinical or laboratory confirmation, as was observed in our case. In one study, it was found that CSF parameters (glucose and protein in particular) played a role in predicting outcomes. The patients with high CSF protein and glucose levels exhibited poor outcomes. The clinical outcomes in the infectious group are generally worse and they are also associated with higher mortality rates.

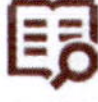

REFERENCES/SOURCES

- Bin Abdulqader SA, Alkhalidi HM, Ajlan AM. Brainstem encephalitis: a diagnostic dilemma. Neurosciences (Riyadh). 2018;23(2): 152-7.
- Tan IL, Mowry EM, Steele SU, Pardo CA, McArthur JC, Nath A, et al. Brainstem encephalitis: etiologies, treatment, and predictors of outcome. J Neurol. 2013;260(9):2312-9.
- Wei P, Bao R, Fan Y. Brainstem encephalitis caused by *Listeria monocytogenes*. Pathogens. 2020;9(9):715.

12. A 3-year-old child, second born of non-consanguineous marriage presented with fever, seizures, and altered sensorium for 2 days. On examination the child had deep encephalopathy with dystonia. The child has similar three episodes in the past. Elder sibling expired at 2 years of age due to similar illness. MRI brain showed the following finding. Which of the following would be the appropriate treatment for this child?

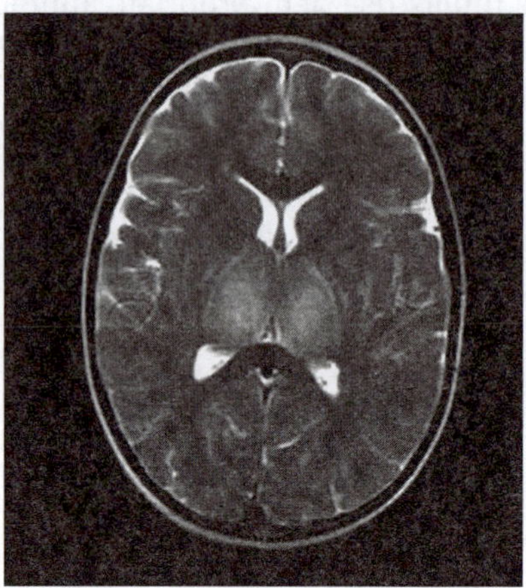

A. Mitochondrial cocktail
B. Plasmapheresis
C. Injection sodium bicarbonate + L-carnitine + thiamine + sodium benzoate
D. Injection methyl prednisolone

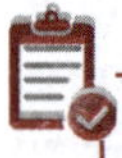

EXPLANATION

The given clinical scenario and the MRI image show the typical doughnut sign seen in ANE (acute necrotizing encephalopathy). The child had acute onset of deep encephalopathy that can be either due to meningo-encephalitis, drug toxicity, and metabolic disorders such as Leigh's disease or a parainfectious phenomenon secondary to viral infections such as dengue, influenza. However, the typical imaging finding points to the final diagnosis of ANE. This can be easily picked by in the CT scan easily available in the emergency settings that can show swollen and hypodense thalami.

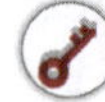

Key: D

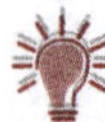

BOOST YOUR KNOWLEDGE

Acute necrotizing encephalopathy is a serious subtype of acute encephalopathy seen in children following a viral illness. The diagnostic criteria for this were proposed by Mizuguchi et al., which consist of: (1) encephalopathy preceded by viral febrile illness with rapid deterioration in the level of consciousness and convulsions, (2) absent cerebrospinal fluid (CSF) pleocytosis, (3) symmetric multifocal brain lesions, (4) elevation in serum aminotransferase levels, and (5) exclusion of similar diseases.

Genetic predisposition to this condition can be secondary to *RANBP2* gene mutation.

Acute necrotizing encephalopathy severity score:

Parameter	Score
Age >48 months	2
Shock at onset	3
Brainstem lesions	2
Platelet count <10 × 10*4/μL	1
CSF protein>60 mg/dL	1

Severity	*Points*
Low risk	0–1
Medium risk	2–4
High risk	5–9

REFERENCES/SOURCES

- Kliegman RM, St Geme III JW. Nelson Textbook of Pediatrics, 21st edition. Elsevier; 2019.
- Mizuguchi M. Acute necrotizing encephalopathy of childhood: a novel form of acute encephalopathy prevalent in Japan and Taiwan. Brain Dev. 1997;19:81-92.
- Yamamoto H, Okumura A, Natsume J, Kojima S, Mizuguchi M. A severity score for acute necrotizing encephalopathy. Brain Dev. 2015;37(3):322-7.

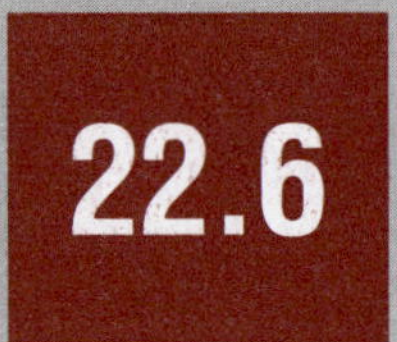

CHAPTER 22.6

Coma, Raised Intracranial Pressure, and Stroke

Rohit Khandelwal

1. A 3-year-old male child was brought to OPD with complaints of reduced movement of the right side of the body since the past 4 hours. No history of fever, seizures, loss of consciousness or trauma was there. As the duty doctor attending the child, which of the following investigations you would ask for to confirm the diagnosis?

A. Computed tomography (CT) brain
B. Diffusion-weighted magnetic resonance imaging (MRI)
C. MR angiogram
D. Routine blood investigations

EXPLANATION

Diagnosis: This 3-year-old child who presented with these above complaints could be a case of pediatric stroke—most probably secondary to arterial ischemic stroke.

Diffusion-weighted MRI (option B) demonstrates AIS from minutes to 7 days following the onset; MR angiography can confirm vascular occlusion and suggest possible arteriopathy. Diffusion-weighted MRI can also demonstrate Wallerian degeneration in the descending corticospinal tract, which correlates with chronic hemiparesis.

CT brain (option A)—does not demonstrate small infarcts.

MR angiogram (option C)—will only confirm vascular occlusion.

Routine blood test (option D)—will not confirm the diagnosis of cerebrovascular events.

Key: B

BOOST YOUR KNOWLEDGE

The diagnosis of stroke in children is frequently delayed. This is a consequence of subtle and nonspecific clinical presentations, poor awareness by primary care physicians, a complicated differential diagnosis and a high frequency (>50%) of negative initial brain CT scans in true AIS. The acute onset of a focal neurologic deficit in a child is stroke until proven otherwise. The most common focal presentation is hemiparesis, but acute visual, speech, sensory, or balance deficits also occur. Importantly, new-onset seizures, especially focal motor seizures, frequently herald stroke in children. Children with these presentations require urgent neuroimaging and consultation with a child neurologist because emergency interventions may be indicated. AIS is a clinical and radiographic diagnosis. Although CT imaging can demonstrate mature AIS and exclude hemorrhage, cerebral MRI is required to identify early and small infarcts. Arterial blood reaches the brain via the anterior (internal carotid) and posterior (vertebrobasilar) circulations, converging at the circle of Willis. Strokes most often involve the middle cerebral artery territory but can occur in any cerebral artery of any size. AIS is the focal brain infarction that results from occlusion of these arteries.

REFERENCE/SOURCE

- Dlamini N, deVeber GA. Pediatric stroke (Chapter 619). In: Kliegman RM, St Geme III JW, Blum NJ, Shah SS, Tasker RC, Wilson KM, et al (Eds). Nelson Textbook of Pediatrics, 21st edition. Elsevier; 2019. p. 12480.

2. **A 7-year-old boy is brought to the emergency department with severe headache, vomiting, and altered mental status. On examination, his BP—80/60 mm Hg, PR—70 bpm, RR—16 pm, with irregular breathing pattern. A CT scan of brain reveals a large brain tumor causing obstruction of cerebrospinal fluid flow and increased intracranial pressure (ICP). MRI brain imaging showed "uncal herniation". Which of the following is the most appropriate immediate management for this patient?**

A. Administer mannitol to decrease ICP
B. Perform a lumbar puncture to measure ICP
C. Administer 3% NS to decrease ICP
D. Perform a craniotomy to remove the brain tumor

EXPLANATION

- Mannitol (option A) is contraindicated in this child as the child is hypotensive (BP—80/60 mm Hg) and with renal failure and the child is hemodynamically unstable (BP—80/60 mm Hg, PR—70 bpm, with irregular breathing pattern)
- Administering 3% NS (option C) will cause fluid shift from neurons and interstitial compartment to the intravascular compartment resulting in brain shrinkage and lowering of ICP, additional advantage is the ability to maintain circulating volume and thus the cerebral perfusion pressure (CPP), even in a hemodynamically unstable child.
- Lumbar puncture (option B) though reduces ICP but is contraindicated in suspected brain herniation. Craniotomy (option D) to be planned later (not immediately) once the child is hemodynamically stable and his ICP is normal.

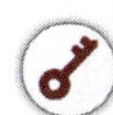

Key: C

BOOST YOUR KNOWLEDGE

The intracranial pressure (ICP) is derived from the volume of its components and the bony compliance. The perfusion pressure of the brain (CPP) is equal to the pressure of blood entering the cranium (mean arterial pressure, MAP) minus the ICP, in most cases. Increases in intracranial volume can result from swelling, masses, or increases in blood and cerebrospinal fluid (CSF) volumes. As these volumes increase, compensatory mechanisms decrease ICP by decreasing CSF volume (CSF is displaced into the spinal canal or absorbed by arachnoid villi), decreasing cerebral blood volume (venous blood return to the thorax is augmented), and/or increasing cranial volume (sutures pathologically expand or bone is remodeled). Once compensatory mechanisms are exhausted (the increase in cranial volume is too large), small increases in volume lead to large increases in ICP, or intracranial hypertension. As ICP continues to increase, brain ischemia can occur as CPP falls. Further increases in ICP can ultimately displace the brain downward into the foramen magnum—a process called cerebral herniation, which can become irreversible in minutes and may lead to severe disability or death.

REFERENCES/SOURCES

- Kliegman RM, St Geme III JW. Pediatric stroke (Chapter 619). Nelson Textbook of Pediatrics, 21st edition. Elsevier; 2019. p. 2653.
- Ranjith S. Manual of Paediatric Emergencies and Critical Care, 2nd edition. Paras Medical Publishers; 2010. p. 229.

3. **"Call-Fleming syndrome" can cause arterial ischemic stroke. What is the basic pathophysiology causing stroke in this syndrome?**

A. Vasospasm
B. Bleed
C. Embolus
D. Both A and C

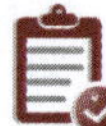

EXPLANATION

Call-Fleming syndrome is a part of reversible cerebral vasoconstriction syndrome (RCVS) group and is thought to be of idiopathic origin. It is classically described to be having multisegmental *focal vasospasms* in the cerebral arteries. It is characterized clinically by the sudden onset of severe headache, classically described as thunderclap headache, with or without associated neurological deficits. The importance of it lies in that it is a potentially reversible cause of this clinical presentation, unlike its other counterparts, aneurysmal subarachnoid hemorrhage (SAH) or vasculitis. It is not associated with bleeding or embolic phenomenon.

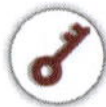

Key: A

BOOST YOUR KNOWLEDGE

Vasospasm as occurs in migraine, subarachnoid hemorrhage, or reversible cerebral vasoconstriction syndrome (sometimes called Call-Fleming syndrome) can cause AIS. Metabolic strokes are seen in organic acidemia, methylmalonic acidemia, propionic acidemia, isovaleric acidemia, glutaric aciduria type II, mitochondrial encephalomyopathies, MELAS (mitochondrial encephalopathy, myopathy, lactic acidosis, and stroke-like episodes), MERRF (myoclonus epilepsy with ragged red fibers), MERRF/MELAS overlap syndrome, and Kearns-Sayre syndrome.

Classification of cerebral vasculitis:

- Infectious vasculitides
- Bacterial, fungal, parasitic
- Spirochetal (syphilis, Lyme disease, leptospirosis)
- Viral, rickettsial, mycobacterial, free-living amebae, cysticercosis, and other helminths
- Necrotizing vasculitides
- Classic polyarteritis nodosa
- Wegener granulomatosis
- Allergic angiitis and granulomatosis (Churg–Strauss syndrome)
- Necrotizing systemic vasculitis overlap syndrome
- Lymphomatoid granulomatosis
- Vasculitis associated with collagen vascular disease
- Systemic lupus erythematosus
- Rheumatoid arthritis
- Scleroderma
- Sjögren syndrome
- Vasculitis associated with other systemic diseases
- Behçet disease
- Ulcerative colitis
- Sarcoidosis
- Relapsing polychondritis
- Kohlmeier–Degos disease
- Takayasu arteritis
- Hypersensitivity vasculitides
- Henoch–Schönlein purpura
- Drug-induced vasculitides
- Chemical vasculitides
- Essential mixed cryoglobulinemia
- Miscellaneous vasculitides
- Vasculitis associated with neoplasia
- Vasculitis associated with radiation
- Cogan syndrome
- Dermatomyositis–polymyositis
- X-linked lymphoproliferative syndrome
- Kawasaki disease
- Primary central nervous system vasculitis

Source: Modified from:

- Roach ES, Golomb MR, Adams R, Biller J, Daniels S, Deveber G, et al. Management of stroke in infants and children. Stroke. 2008;39: 2644-91. Table 5.
- Dlamini N, deVeber GA. Pediatric stroke (Chapter 619). In: Kliegman RM, St Geme III JW, Blum NJ, Shah SS, Tasker RC, Wilson KM, et al. (Eds). Nelson Textbook of Pediatrics, 21st edition. Elsevier; 2019. p. 12483.

REFERENCE/SOURCE

- Skandhan AK, Ramakrishnan KG, Anand R. Call-Fleming syndrome. Indian J Radiol Imaging. 2013;23(3):198-201.

4. Which of the following statements is true regarding hematologic conditions causing arterial ischemic stroke?

A. Prothrombotic states are associated with reduced incidence of stroke

B. Iron deficiency anemia is not a risk factor for stroke

C. There is a 400 fold increase in risk of stroke for children with sickle cell anemia
D. Medical management can reduce the risk of stroke in sickle cell anemia

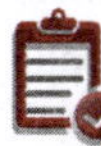

EXPLANATION

Hematologic disorders associated with AIS include sickle cell anemia, in which the stroke risk is increased 400-fold.

- Prothrombotic states (option A) are associated with increased (not reduced) incidence of stroke—hence option A is incorrect.
- Iron deficiency anemia (option B) is a risk factor for stroke.
- Medical management (option D) cannot reduce the risk of stroke in sickle cell anemia—only transfusion therapy will reduce incidence of stroke in sickle cell anemia.

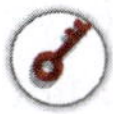

Key: C

BOOST YOUR KNOWLEDGE

Healthy red blood cells are round in shape, but a "sickled" red blood cell is crescent-shaped and stiff. Sickled cells tend to stick together, and they cannot move easily through the blood vessels. They can clump together and block blood vessels. This can lead to a clot forming and moving to the brain, causing a stroke. A stroke can also be due to damage to the blood vessels in the brain caused by SCD. SCD can sometimes lead to bleeding in the brain (hemorrhagic stroke).

Stroke syndrome is sickle cell disease include: (1) arterial ischemic stroke secondary to middle cerebral artery vasculopathy, (2) posterior reversible encephalopathy syndrome, (3) spontaneous intracerebral hemorrhage, (4) extracranial carotid occlusion in a teenager with previous ataxia presenting with stroke, (5) bilateral watershed infraction, and (6) straight sinus thrombosis.

REFERENCES/SOURCES

- Kirkham FJ, Lagunju IA. Epidemiology of stroke in sickle cell disease. J Clin Med. 2021;10(18):4232.
- Kliegman RM, St Geme III JW. Pediatric stroke (Chapter 619). Nelson Textbook of Pediatrics, 21st edition. Elsevier; 2019.

5. An otherwise healthy, 6-week-old baby presented with sudden onset of irritability followed by focal left-sided seizures. Plain CT scan of head demonstrates a large hyperdense lesion in the right parietal region with surrounding edema. What is the diagnosis in this child?

A. Hemorrhagic stroke
B. Cerebral sinovenous thrombosis
C. Disseminated intravascular coagulation
D. Periventricular leukomalacia

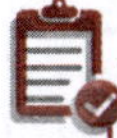

EXPLANATION

- The description is consistent with acute hemorrhage.
- DIC (option C) is unlikely as there are no generalized bleeding tendencies all over the body with multisystem involvement.
- *Periventricular leukomalacia PVL (option D):* The white matter necrosis often occurs in a characteristic distribution with the pattern being dorsal and lateral to the lateral ventricles and with the involvement of the centrum semiovale, the optic (trigone and occipital horns) and acoustic (temporal horn) radiations.

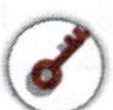

Key: A

BOOST YOUR KNOWLEDGE

Hemorrhagic stroke (HS) includes nontraumatic intracranial hemorrhage and is classified by the intracranial compartment containing the hemorrhage. Intraparenchymal bleeds may occur in any location, whereas intraventricular hemorrhage may be isolated or an extension of intraparenchymal hemorrhage.

Bleeding outside the brain may occur in the subarachnoid, subdural, or epidural spaces.

Clinical presentations vary according to location, cause, and rate of bleeding. Acute hemorrhages may feature instantaneous or thunderclap headache, loss of consciousness, and nuchal rigidity in addition to focal neurologic deficits and seizures. HS can be rapidly fatal. In bleeds associated with vascular malformations, pulsatile tinnitus, cranial bruit, macrocephaly, and high-output heart failure may be present.

The diagnosis relies on imaging, and CT scanning is highly sensitive to acute HS. However, lumbar puncture may be required to exclude subarachnoid hemorrhage. MRI is highly sensitive to even small amounts of both acute and chronic hemorrhage and offers improved diagnostic accuracy. Angiography by CT, MR, or conventional catheterization means is often required to exclude underlying vascular abnormalities (e.g., vascular malformations, aneurysms).

Management of acute childhood HS requires emergency neurosurgical intervention for a large or rapidly expanding hemorrhage. The same principles of neuroprotection for vulnerable brain suggested in the AIS sections also apply to HS. Reversal of anticoagulant therapy (with, for example, vitamin K, fresh frozen plasma) may be required, but the role of other medical interventions, such as factor VII, are unstudied in children. The recurrence risk for those with structural lesions is significant, and serial imaging may be required. Definitive repair or removal of vascular malformation may require a combined approach with interventional endovascular methods and neurosurgery. Outcomes from childhood HS are not well studied but likely depend on lesion size, location, and etiology. Compared with AIS, the HS mortality rate is higher, but long-term deficits are less common.

REFERENCE/SOURCE

- Kliegman RM, St Geme III JW. Pediatric stroke (Chapter 619). Nelson Textbook of Pediatrics, 21st edition. Elsevier; 2019.

6. A 5-year-old child was brought with complaints of weakness of the left lower limb for the past 2 hours. Similar episodes have happened in the past, but it has resolved spontaneously. In the emergency department, you notice some dystonic movements of the left leg. Intensity of the movements seems to reduce during sleep. Previous genetic testing showed positive result for ATP1A3. The most probable diagnosis in this case would be:

A. Moyamoya disease
B. Alternating hemiplegia of childhood
C. MELAS (mitochondrial encephalopathy lactic acidosis, and stroke-like episodes)
D. Transient ischemic attack

EXPLANATION

- Moyamoya disease is a progressive blood vessel disorder that causes stroke or recurrent transient ischemic attack (TIA), especially in children. It is associated with genetic causes and certain disease conditions such as Down syndrome, sickle cell anemia, and neurofibromatosis type 1. Treatment options include medication and surgery.
- Alternating hemiplegia of childhood (AHC) is an ultra-rare neurological disorder that causes transient episodes of hemiplegia (weakness or paralysis) in children. It typically presents before the age of 18 months and may cause cognitive and developmental delays or disability. Treatment options include medication and therapy.

- Mitochondrial encephalopathy, lactic acidosis, and stroke-like episodes syndrome is a rare disorder that affects many of the body's systems, particularly the brain and nervous system (encephalo-) and muscles (myopathy). The signs and symptoms of this disorder appear in childhood following a period of normal development. Treatment options include medication and surgery.
- Transient ischemic attack (TIA) is a temporary period of symptoms similar to those of a stroke. It occurs when the blood supply to part of the brain is briefly interrupted. Symptoms usually occur suddenly and are similar to those of stroke but do not last as long. Treatment options include medication, surgery, and self-care.

Key: B

BOOST YOUR KNOWLEDGE

Alternating hemiplegia of childhood:

- *Presentation and episodes:*
  - Alternating hemiplegia of childhood appears in late infancy.
  - It involves episodes of hemiplegia (paralysis) that switch sides in the body.
  - These episodes last from minutes to weeks and go away on their own.
- *Movements and patterns:*
  - Affected limb often shows choreoathetosis (twisting) and dystonic movements (contractions).
  - Symptoms improve during sleep but return upon waking.
- *Skin changes:*
  - Kids might suddenly get redness and warmth (flushing) or unusual paleness (pallor) of the skin.
  - These skin changes can happen with or without the hemiplegia episodes.
- *Developmental impact:*
  - Almost all affected children experience developmental delay and intellectual disability.
  - These issues usually worsen over time.
- *Neuroimaging:* Neuroimaging, including MRA, is used to rule out moyamoya disease (a similar condition).
- *Genetic link:* Alternating hemiplegia of childhood is caused by mutations in the *ATP1A3* gene.

REFERENCE/SOURCE

- Kliegman RM, St Geme III JW. Pediatric stroke (Chapter 619). Nelson Textbook of Pediatrics, 21st edition. Elsevier; 2019.

7. A 9-year-old girl presented with fever, ear discharge and progressive right-sided headache. She complained of double vision and papilledema on examination. CT venography demonstrates a large thrombus in the right transverse sinus that fails to opacify with contrast. What is the diagnosis?

A. CSVT
B. AIS
C. TIA
D. Vein of Galen malformation (VOGM)

EXPLANATION

- *Cerebral sinovenous thrombosis (CSVT)* is a rare condition that occurs when a blood clot forms in the veins that drain blood from the brain. It can cause symptoms such as headache, seizures, and weakness on one side of the body. Treatment options include medication and surgery.
- *Arterial ischemic stroke* (AIS) is a type of stroke that occurs when blood flow to the brain is blocked by a clot. Symptoms may include sudden weakness or numbness on one side of the body, difficulty speaking or understanding speech, and vision problems. Treatment options include medication and surgery.

- *Transient ischemic attack (TIA)* is a temporary period of symptoms similar to those of a stroke. It occurs when the blood supply to part of the brain is briefly interrupted. Symptoms usually occur suddenly and are similar to those of stroke but do not last as long. Treatment options include medication, surgery, and self-care.
- *Vein of Galen malformation (VOGM)* is a rare type of blood vessel abnormality inside the brain that develops before birth. It may be found during pregnancy or very soon after birth. This condition affects a large vein deep at the base of the brain and can cause symptoms such as high-output cardiac failure in the neonatal period. Treatment options include medication and surgery.

Key: A

BOOST YOUR KNOWLEDGE

Cerebral sinovenous thrombosis:

- Cerebral sinovenous thrombosis involves blockage of veins in the brain by blood clots.
- This can cause increased pressure inside the skull, brain swelling, and sometimes stroke or bleeding.
- *Symptoms and presentation:*
  - Symptoms of CSVT develop gradually and can be varied and not specific like in adult stroke (AIS).
  - Newborns might show signs such as encephalopathy (brain dysfunction) and seizures.
  - Older children might have symptoms similar to a condition called idiopathic intracranial hypertension, including headache, eye problems, and weakness on one side.
- *Common signs:* Seizures, drowsiness, and confusion are common signs of CSVT.
- *Diagnosis:*
  - Detecting CSVT needs strong suspicion and specific
  - Contrast CT venography or MR venography is needed to see clots in brain veins.
  - Magnetic resonance imaging is better than CT for seeing brain tissue clearly.

REFERENCE/SOURCE

- Kliegman RM, St Geme III JW. Pediatric stroke (Chapter 619). Nelson Textbook of Pediatrics, 21st edition. Elsevier; 2019.

8. Which of the following are the three indicators of brain death?

A. Absence of pupillary reflexes, hypoxia, hypercarbia
B. Absence of brainstem reflexes, flat EEG, hypercarbia
C. Absence of brainstem reflexes, irreversible coma, apnea
D. Apnea, lack of reflexes, coma

EXPLANATION

The three components for determining brain death are demonstration of coexisting irreversible coma with a known cause, absence of brainstem reflexes, and apnea.

Key: C

BOOST YOUR KNOWLEDGE

Brain death is a clinical and legal definition of death that refers to the permanent and irreversible cessation of all brain function. It is different from a coma or vegetative state, where the person may still have some brain function. Brain death is diagnosed by a qualified physician, typically a neurologist, who performs an extensive physical examination and documents brain death criteria. Before brain death is pronounced, three clinical criteria must be met—unresponsiveness, absence of reflexes, and apnea (inability to breathe without a ventilator). Brain death testing falls into three main categories—physical examination, apnea testing, and other testing (also known as ancillary testing). The physical examination is done to determine the level of responsiveness. If the examination shows a lack of responsiveness, the physical examination would proceed to check for certain reflexes. Someone who is brain dead will not have any brainstem reflexes.

REFERENCE/SOURCE

- Kliegman RM, St Geme III JW. Pediatric stroke (Chapter 619). Nelson Textbook of Pediatrics, 21st edition. Elsevier; 2019. p. 2675.

9. What are the two most widely used ancillary tests to certify brain death?

A. EEG, radionuclide cerebral blood flow studies
B. EEG, ECG
C. ECG, radionuclide cerebral blood flow studies
D. EEG, PET scan

EXPLANATION

The two most widely used ancillary tests are EEG and radionuclide CBF studies. Ancillary studies are not required for the diagnosis of brain death unless the clinical examination including the apnea test cannot be safely or reliably completed.

Electrocardiogram (ECG) and arterial blood gas (ABG) can be required additionally for documentation of brain death, but not as a part of ancillary tests to certify brain death.

Key: A

BOOST YOUR KNOWLEDGE

A valid electroencephalogram to support suspected brain death must be performed according to the American EEG Society standards and technical requirements, under conditions of normothermia and appropriate hemodynamics, and in the absence of drug levels sufficient to suppress the EEG response. An EEG that demonstrates electrocerebral silence over a 30-minute recording time under these conditions supports the diagnosis of brain death. Advantages of this study are its wide availability and low risk. Disadvantages include potential confounders, such as artifact in the tracing and the presence of suppressing levels of drugs such as barbiturates. A radionuclide cerebral blood flow study consists of intravenous (IV) injection of a radio-pharmaceutical agent followed by imaging of the brain to look for cerebral uptake. As with EEG, nuclear medicine scans are widely available and low risk. Unlike EEG, radionuclide CBF studies are not affected by drug levels. A study that shows absence of uptake in the brain demonstrates absence of CBF and is supportive of brain death. Four-vessel intracranial contrast angiography was previously used as the definitive ancillary test, but practical technical difficulties and risks have led to the use of nuclear medicine scans instead.

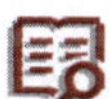

REFERENCE/SOURCE

- Kliegman RM, St Geme III JW. Pediatric stroke (Chapter 619). Nelson Textbook of Pediatrics, 21st edition. Elsevier; 2019. p. 2675.

10. Which of these following statements regarding cerebral autoregulation is true?

A. Cerebral blood flow is autoregulated at MAP of 10–50 mm Hg
B. Pressure autoregulation is mediated by changes in arteriolar diameter
C. When MAP and CPP falls, the vessels dilate
D. When MAP and CPP raises, the vessels constricts

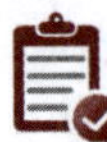

EXPLANATION

- Cerebral blood flow is autoregulated at MAP of 50–150 mm Hg
- Pressure autoregulation is mediated by changes in arteriolar diameter—true
- When MAP and CPP falls, the vessels constricts
- When MAP and CPP raises, the vessels dilates

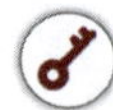

Key: B

BOOST YOUR KNOWLEDGE

Cerebral oxygen delivery is a function of brain blood flow and blood oxygen content, whereby cerebral blood flow (CBF) is dependent on cerebral perfusion pressure (CPP) and inversely proportional to cerebrovascular resistance (CVR). Another way to conceptualize blood flow to the brain is via the pressure gradient between the supplying arteries (mean arterial pressure, MAP) and the cerebral venous system, the latter being approximately equivalent to intracranial pressure (ICP).

$$\text{CBF} = \text{CPP}/\text{CVR} = (\text{MAP} - \text{ICP})/\text{CVR}$$

Vascular resistance within the brain reflects the smooth muscle tone of the vessels, which is partially influenced by mean arterial pressure (MAP). If CPP increases or decreases, the myogenic reflex will result in vasoconstriction or vasodilation, respectively. This assertion is the classical view of pressure-flow autoregulation. If intracranial pressure is stable, CPP is replaceable by MAP. In this manner, changes in brain blood flow can be measured for a range of blood pressures to determine autoregulation.

REFERENCES/SOURCES

- Ranjith S. Manual of Paediatric Emergencies and Critical Care, 2nd edition. Paras Medical Publishers; 2010. p. 227.
- Silverman A, Petersen NH. Physiology, cerebral autoregulation. In: StatPearls. Treasure Island (FL): StatPearls Publishing; 2023.

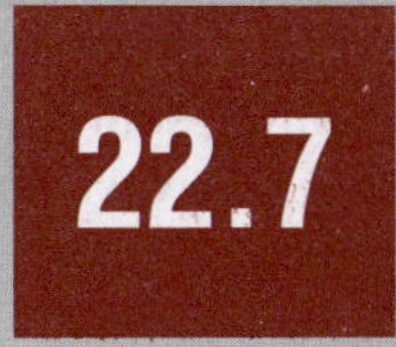

Ataxia and Movement Disorders

Kavita Srivastava

1. A 10-year-old boy is brought with progressive difficulty in walking since last 3 years. There is no failure to thrive or fatty stools. On examination, he has ataxia and other cerebellar signs such as dysdiadochokinesia, nystagmus, past pointing, and intention tremors. His eye examination is normal. He also has depressed deep tendon reflexes, loss of position, and vibration sense in lower limbs with pes cavus. Which of the following investigations is most likely to reveal the diagnosis?

A. Magnetic resonance imaging (MRI) brain
B. Lysosomal enzyme studies
C. Whole-exome sequencing
D. Polymerase chain reaction (PCR) for triplet repeats

EXPLANATION

With progressive difficulty in walking and presence of cerebellar signs, this is a likely case of progressive cerebellar ataxia. Common causes at this age would be ataxia telangiectasia, Friedreich ataxia, spinocerebellar ataxias, etc. Other causes like neuronal ceroid lipofuscinosis (NCL) will have refractory seizures. The loss of position and vibration sense and depressed deep tendon reflexes indicate posterior column affection. This narrows the differentials to Friedreich ataxia. Pes cavus is commonly associated with Friedreich ataxia. Absence of fatty stools (steatorrhea) and failure to thrive make abetalipoproteinemia unlikely.

Regarding the options, MRI brain is nonspecific for etiology and may show cerebellar atrophy with additional basal ganglia changes in mitochondrial etiology. Lysosomal storage disorder like NCL looks clinically unlikely. Whole-exome sequencing cannot pick up causes like Friedreich ataxia (which is due to GAA triplet nucleotide repeats picked up on PCR technique). For mitochondrial disorders, whole-exome and mitochondrial DNA sequencing is required. Hence, option D is the most likely correct answer.

Key: D

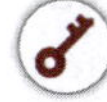

BOOST YOUR KNOWLEDGE

Friedreich ataxia is a progressive degenerative disorder of cerebellum, spinocerebellar tracts, and posterior columns of spinal cord. This causes sensory neuropathy leading to positive Romberg's sign, loss of joint position, and vibration with depressed reflexes, especially in lower limbs and pes cavus. The other complications associated with Friedreich ataxia are cardiomyopathy, diabetes mellitus, and scoliosis. The patients have homozygous expansion of GAA (trinucleotide) repeats in the noncoding region of the gene coding for mitochondrial protein frataxin. This leads to oxidative injury and excess iron deposition in mitochondria.

REFERENCE/SOURCE

- Nelson WE. Movement disorders. In: Kliegman R, Stanton B, St Geme JW, Schor NF, Behrman RE (Eds). Nelson Textbook of Pediatrics, 20th edition. Philadelphia: Elsevier; 2016. p. 2885.

2. A 7-year-old boy has been brought with abnormal movements since last 3 months. The movements are repetitive brief twitches of face, eye blinks, and shoulder, along with occasional throat clearing sounds. He can voluntarily suppress these movements for few seconds. These movements happen only in awake state and are increased during stressful periods. He feels embarrassed to attend school, though he is a bright student. Detailed neurological examination is normal. What should be the next step?

A. An awake and sleep EEG
B. 3 Tesla MRI brain with contrast
C. Immunotherapy like steroids
D. Behavioral and habit reversal therapy

EXPLANATION

The description of the movements—simple motor and vocal tics for duration of <1 year, fits in tic disorder. Tics can worsen on anxiety and can be suppressed temporarily on distraction and sleep. Electroencephalogram (EEG) and MRI are not indicated, unless the child has any other associated neurological symptoms. Psychoeducation and behavior therapy are the mainstay for management. The child should be screened for comorbidities such as obsessive compulsive disorder, attention deficit hyperactivity disorder (ADHD), etc. Medications like clonidine may be used, if the symptoms are distressing and limiting the activities of daily living, or associated with complex motor/vocal tics or Tourette's disorder.

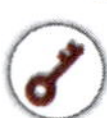

Key: D

BOOST YOUR KNOWLEDGE

Tics may be present in various neurological illnesses such as Wilson, Huntington, and other frontal brain lesions. However, these conditions will have other manifestations such as motor or cognitive dysfunction, chorea, dystonia, etc. Tourette disorder is characterized by both multiple types of motor and complex vocal tics, lasting for more than a year. Autoimmune mediated mechanisms have been proposed for tic associated with disorders such as PANDAS (Pediatric autoimmune neuropsychiatric disorder associated with streptococcal infection) and PANS (pediatric acute onset neuropsychiatric syndrome), where the role of preceding infection is not clear.

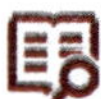

REFERENCE/SOURCE

- Nelson WE. Tic disorders. In: Kliegman R, Stanton B, St Geme JW, Schor NF, Behrman RE (Eds). Nelson Textbook of Pediatrics, 20th edition. Philadelphia: Elsevier; 2016. pp. 140-2.

3. A 5-year-old girl is brought with developmental delay followed by loss of ambulation and speech with cognitive deterioration since last 1 year. She had two episodes of focal clonic seizures in last 3 months. Her antenatal and perinatal history was normal. She is noted to have microcephaly, autistic features, and repetitive side-to-side head movements along with hand wringing and clapping in awake state. Parents have also noted cold hands, sleep disturbances, and irregular breathing. Considering the most likely diagnosis, which of the following best describes the movement disorder and the likely mode of inheritance?

A. Progressive myoclonus epilepsy—autosomal dominant
B. Tic disorder—autosomal recessive
C. Choreoathetosis—X-linked recessive
D. Stereotypic movements—X-linked dominant

EXPLANATION

Stereotypic movements are involuntary, patterned, repetitive, and rhythmic movements seen more frequently in children with autism and intellectual disability. This is a girl with regression of milestones, typical hand wringing stereotypies, and microcephaly. These features are suggestive of Rett syndrome, which has X-linked dominant inheritance.

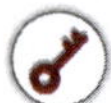

Key: D

BOOST YOUR KNOWLEDGE

Rett syndrome is a disorder of early brain development marked by developmental regression and slowing of brain growth. It mostly affects girls and is caused by mutations in *MECP2*, which is a transcription factor that silences transcription by binding to methylated CpG islands. The hallmark is loss of purposeful use of the hands, replaced by typical hand wringing stereotypies. The inheritance is X-linked dominant.

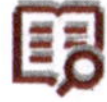

REFERENCE/SOURCE

- Nelson WE. Rett syndrome. In: Kliegman R, Stanton B, St Geme JW, Schor NF, Behrman RE (Eds). Nelson Textbook of Pediatrics, 20th edition. Philadelphia: Elsevier; 2016. pp. 2916-17.

4. A 10-year-old girl is brought with sudden onset of left-sided abnormal semi-purposive dance like movements which were continuous, irregular, jerky, and could not be suppressed voluntarily. The movements made it difficult to walk and perform voluntary movements. On examination, she had hypotonia, mild weakness of left side. Her cardiovascular (CVS) examination revealed a systolic murmur in pulmonary area. Echo was suggestive of 4 mm atrial septal defect. What would be the preferred modality to diagnose the lesion responsible for her symptoms?

A. MRI brain—plain and contrast
B. MRI brain—diffusion weighted
C. MRI brain—angiography
D. CT brain—plain and contrast

EXPLANATION

From the description of the movements, the child has hemichorea, hypotonia, and mild hemiparesis on left side. In view of acute onset of the event, the cause may be stroke or demyelination. The localization of lesion will be in basal ganglia, most likely caudate nucleus on the opposite (right) side. In view of underlying congenital heart defect, it is more likely to be a cardioembolic stroke. The radiological finding in acute stroke is diffusion restriction noted on diffusion-weighted sequence on MRI brain. CT scan is a poor modality to pick up early stroke, though it is a part of adult stroke protocol to rule out hemorrhage. As the small lenticulostriate vessels supply the basal ganglia, routine MR angiography cannot identify any vessel abnormalities/thrombus, etc. Hence, the correct answer is B.

Key: B

BOOST YOUR KNOWLEDGE

Chorea can be due to acquired or inherited causes. Sydenham chorea is the most common acquired chorea in childhood. Up to 20% of children with acute rheumatic fever may develop Sydenham chorea. It is usually symmetric, though may be asymmetric in 20%. Due to molecular mimicry, antibodies against the GlcNAc (N-acetyl beta D glucosamine epitope of streptococcal group A) cross react with intracellular beta-tubulin and extracellular lysoganglioside GM1 proteins in caudate-putamen. Increased dopamine release into the synapse causes the neurological manifestations of Sydenham chorea.

REFERENCE/SOURCE

- Nelson WE. Chapter 615.2. In: Kliegman R, Stanton B, St Geme JW, Schor NF, Behrman RE (Eds). Nelson Textbook of Pediatrics, 20th edition. Philadelphia: Elsevier; 2016. p. 3156.

5. An 8-month-old baby is brought with delayed development followed by regression of milestones, tremulous movements of head, limbs, and tongue. The mother also has a moderate degree of anemia. The baby shows moderate pallor (hemoglobin 6 g/dL) and reticular pigmentation of skin, hypotonia, and tremors. Which of the following is the most likely hematological finding?

A. Microcytic anemia, leukopenia, thrombocytopenia
B. Macrocytic anemia, leukopenia, thrombocytopenia
C. Macrocytic anemia, leukocytosis, thrombocytopenia
D. Microcytic anemia, leukopenia, thrombocytosis

EXPLANATION

The history and examination findings is suggestive of infantile tremor syndrome. The cause is attributed to vitamin B_{12} deficiency. The hematological manifestations of B_{12} deficiency include macrocytosis of red blood cell (RBC), hypersegmented neutrophils. If severe, there may be pancytopenia.

Key: B

BOOST YOUR KNOWLEDGE

Infantile tremor syndrome is seen in exclusively breastfed babies of pure vegan (thus vitamin B_{12} deficient) mothers. The babies may have prior developmental delay, but loss of milestones ensues as the condition progresses. Reticular pigmentation, knuckle pigmentation, hair changes are seen in most. The baby develops tremors, involving the whole body, including tongue and larynx giving rise to a goat like cry. The treatment involves parenteral administration of vitamin B_{12}.

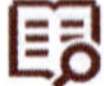

REFERENCE/SOURCE

- Nelson WE. Chapter: B_{12} deficiency. In: Kliegman R, Stanton B, St Geme JW, Schor NF, Behrman RE (Eds). Nelson Textbook of Pediatrics, 20th edition. Philadelphia: Elsevier; 2016.

6. A 6-year-old boy is brought with complaints of developmental delay and abnormal movements of head and eyes. There is no history of regression of milestones or seizures. Mother's brother is also affected with a similar illness. On examination, there is spasticity of all four limbs, titubation of head, ataxia, and nystagmus. There is no regression of milestones. MRI brain shows hypomyelination. The parents are planning another child. What is appropriate prenatal counseling in this situation?

A. 25% risk of having an affected son
B. 25% risk of having an affected daughter
C. 50% chance of disease irrespective of gender
D. The risk cannot be predicted

EXPLANATION

The clinical description and MRI findings fit the diagnosis of Pelizaeus–Merzbacher disease (PMD) or PMD like hypomyelinating leukodystrophy. It has X-linked recessive inheritance. As mother's brother is also affected, it indicates carrier state in the mother. Female carriers are mostly unaffected, or mildly affected. Female carriers have 25% risk of having an affected son, 25% risk of having a carrier daughter, and 50% chance of having a child who does not inherit the mutant gene.

Key: A

BOOST YOUR KNOWLEDGE

Pelizaeus–Merzbacher disease is caused by mutations in the *PLP1* gene, characterized by nystagmus, head nodding movements (titubation), and nystagmus. Development is usually delayed, and spasticity and ataxia eventually develop. MRI shows symmetrical changes of delayed myelination. Mutations in the same gene can be associated with familial spastic paraparesis.

REFERENCE/SOURCE

- Nelson WE. Patterns of genetic transmission (Chapter 80). In: Kliegman R, Stanton B, St Geme JW, Schor NF, Behrman RE (Eds). Nelson Textbook of Pediatrics, 21st edition; 2020. p. 595

7. A 12-year-old girl born of third-degree consanguineous marriage is brought with complaints of gradually progressive deterioration in handwriting, speech, and swallowing since last 2 years. Her birth, development history was normal, and she had good scholastic performance till 2 years back. Her paternal uncle was diagnosed with a similar illness and is on long-term treatment. On examination, she has a brownish discoloration of corneal rim, dysarthria, and dystonia of limbs. Which of the following is true regarding the suspected diagnosis?

A. Hepatic involvement is predominant in older age
B. Renal failure is the earliest manifestation
C. Hemolytic anemia may be early presentation
D. Eye involvement is visible since infancy

EXPLANATION

The combination of progressive dystonia causing difficulty in functioning and brownish corneal ring—Kayser–Fleischer ring (K-F ring) points to Wilson disease. In young patients, hemolytic anemia and hepatic involvement is more likely and may precede neurological manifestations by up to 10 years. Neurological manifestations are predominant manifestations after first decade. Eye involvement (K-F ring) is seen in up to 95% of those with brain affection.

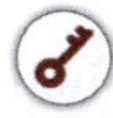

Key: C

BOOST YOUR KNOWLEDGE

Wilson disease is an autosomal recessive disorder associated with dysfunction of copper transporting ATPase. This leads to impaired copper excretion in bile and copper accumulation in hepatocytes. Later, the copper is redistributed to the eye, brain, and kidneys causing dysfunction of these organs. Treatment modalities include restriction of dietary copper, copper chelating agents such as penicillamine, trientine, and zinc. Liver transplantation is curative and should be considered in those with fulminant liver failure, decompensated cirrhosis, and progressive neurological disorder.

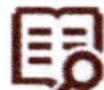

REFERENCE/SOURCE

- Nelson WE. Metabolic diseases of the liver (Chapter 357). In: Kliegman R, Stanton B, St Geme JW, Schor NF, Behrman RE (Eds). Nelson Textbook of Pediatrics, 20th edition. Philadelphia: Elsevier; 2016. pp. 1938-39.

8. An 8-month-old boy, born of third-degree consanguineous marriage was brought with severe encephalopathy. He had a brief febrile illness 1 week back, after which he had been lethargic, though no fever. On admission, he had poor Glasgow Coma Scale (GCS), deep sighing respiration for which he was ventilated. His cerebrospinal fluid (CSF) showed proteins of 20 mg/dL, sugar of 70 mg/dL, and 3 nucleated cells. His arterial blood gas (ABG) showed severe acidosis and blood, and CSF lactate levels were elevated. His MRI brain showed bilateral symmetrical basal ganglia hyperintensities with brainstem lesions. He remained admitted for almost a month. After discharge, he was quadriparetic with no eye contact and had severe dystonia affecting all four limbs with feeding difficulties and failure to thrive. Which of the following is the most likely diagnosis?

A. Tubercular meningitis
B. Leigh disease
C. Japanese B encephalitis
D. Glutaric aciduria

EXPLANATION

The infant developed a debilitating neurological disorder characterized by dystonia and loss of all milestones following a febrile infection. This raises a possibility of severe encephalitis, neurotransmitter disorder, neurometabolic disorder like glutaric aciduria, organic aciduria, fatty acid oxidation defect, biotin thiamine responsive basal ganglia disease, etc.

Out of the given four options, let us analyze the clinical and investigations data given in the following table:

S. No.	Findings in the case	Clinical—No fever at present, preceding febrile illness	CSF Normal protein cells	CSF Elevated lactate	MRI—Symmetrical basal ganglia hyperintensities with brainstem lesions
1.	Tubercular	–	–	–	–
2.	Leigh disease	++	++	+++	+++
3	Japanese encephalitis	–	+/–	–	+
4	Glutaric aciduria	++	+	–	Basal ganglia ++ Brainstem–

As we can see, only Leigh disease satisfies all the criteria.

Key: B

BOOST YOUR KNOWLEDGE

Mitochondrial disorders are genetic disorders with heterogeneous clinical presentations causing impaired energy production by affecting oxidative phosphorylation. They can present with variable combinations of organ affection such as brain, muscle, nerve, heart, ear, etc. They can be caused by mutations of nuclear DNA or mitochondrial DNA. The nuclear DNA mutations follow Mendelian (autosomal recessive) inheritance, while mitoDNA disorders have complex non-Mendelian inheritance. The manifestations will depend on heteroplasmy (ratio of wild to mutant mitoDNA in different tissues) and threshold effect. Mitochondrial encephalomyopathies include myoclonic epilepsy associated with ragged red fibers (MERRF), mitochondrial encephalomyopathy, lactic acidosis, and stroke-like episodes (MELAS), neurogenic weakness with ataxia and retinitis pigmentosa (NARP), Kearns-Sayre syndrome (KSS), Leigh syndrome, and Leber hereditary optic neuropathy (LHON).

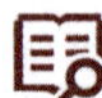

REFERENCE/SOURCE

- Nelson WE. Mitochondrial encephalomyopathies (Chapter 598.2). In: Kliegman R, Stanton B, St Geme JW, Schor NF, Behrman RE (Eds). Nelson Textbook of Pediatrics, 20th edition. Philadelphia: Elsevier; 2016.

9. A 1-year-old boy is brought with normal development till the age of 4 months followed by gradual regression of milestones. The child lost fixation on objects and has unusual excessive startle on even low volume sudden sounds. There is no dysmorphism or seizures. Fundus examination shows cherry red spot, there is hypotonia with brisk reflexes. There are no organomegaly or neurocutaneous markers. Which of the following is most likely to reveal the diagnosis?

A. Lysosomal enzyme studies in leukocytes
B. Magnetic resonance spectroscopy (MRS) of brain
C. Urine—Gas chromatography/mass spectrometry (GCMS)
D. Blood—Tandem mass spectrometry (TMS)

EXPLANATION

The clinical picture is suggestive of a slowly progressive neurodegenerative disorder, most likely storage disorder in view of cherry red spots. The hyperacusis and absence of organomegaly points to Tay–Sachs disease which is GM2 gangliosidosis. The other GM2 ganglioside Sandhoff's disease will have splenomegaly. Other early infantile causes to be considered would be GM1 gangliosidosis (will have organomegaly), neuronal ceroid lipofuscinosis (will have myoclonic seizures), etc. Dysmorphism, if present, may point to peroxisomal disorders like Zellweger syndrome (which may also have hepatomegaly).

Early onset leukodystrophies (such as Krabbe and Aicardi–Goutières) will usually have spasticity and dystonia. Other neurometabolic disorders presenting in early infancy such as organic acidemias, urea cycle defects, fatty acid oxidation defects, aminoacidopathies, etc., will present with metabolic crises, hence look unlikely.

Key: A

BOOST YOUR KNOWLEDGE

The following table presents the different features in neurodegenerative/neurometabolic disorders with early infantile onset.

S. No.	Disorder	Seizures	Dysmorphism	Cherry red spot	Organo-megaly	Metabolic crisis	Test of choice
1	Aminoacidopathies	+	–	–	–	+	GCMS/TMS
2	Organic acidemias	+	–	–	–	+	GCMS/TMS
3	Fatty acid oxidation defects	+	–	–	+	+	GCMS/TMS
4	Urea cycle defects	+	–	–	+/–	+	GCMS/TMS
5	Neurotransmitter disorders	++	– (fair skin)	–	–	+/–	Neurotransmitter study/ exome
6	GM1/GM2 gangliosidosis	+/–	–	++	++ except Tay–Sachs	–	Lysosomal enzyme study
7	Mucolipidosis	+	++	+/–	++	–	Lysosomal enzyme studies
8	Menkes	++	++	–	–	–	MRI, copper studies
9	Leukodystrophies*	–	–	+/–	–	–	Lysosomal enzyme studies
10	NCL (neuronal ceroid lipofuscinosis)	+++	–	–	–	–	Lysosomal enzyme studies

*In infancy—Krabbe, Aicardi–Goutières, etc.

REFERENCE/SOURCE

- Nelson WE. Chapter Metabolic disorders. In: Kliegman R, Stanton B, St Geme JW, Schor NF, Behrman RE (Eds). Nelson Textbook of Pediatrics, 20th edition. Philadelphia: Elsevier; 2016.

10. A 1-year-old baby with quadriparetic cerebral palsy is brought with repeated episodes of arching of whole body, mostly after feeding, and has been admitted twice in last 3 months for pneumonia. On examination, the child is malnourished, has severe spasticity of all four limbs with drooling. What is the most likely diagnosis?

A. Dystonic storm
B. Myoclonic seizures
C. Sandifer syndrome
D. Extensor spasms

EXPLANATION

The typical history of arching (opisthotonos posturing) happening after feeds is suggestive of gastroesophageal reflux disease (GERD), called Sandifer syndrome. Children with cerebral palsy are more prone to GERD. Dystonic storm will have persistent dystonic posturing and not intermittent after feeds. Myoclonic seizures and extensor spasms will have a very different semiology.

Key: C

BOOST YOUR KNOWLEDGE

Spastic quadriplegia is the most severe form of cerebral palsy (CP) with marked motor impairment of all four extremities. There is a higher chance of intellectual disability, seizures, visual, speech, and other impairments. Swallowing difficulties result from supranuclear bulbar palsy and result in repeated aspiration pneumonias. The most common MRI correlate is severe periventricular leukomalacia (PVL) and multicystic encephalomalacia.

REFERENCE/SOURCE

- Nelson WE. Encephalopathies (Chapter 598). In: Kliegman R, Stanton B, St Geme JW, Schor NF, Behrman RE (Eds). Nelson Textbook of Pediatrics, 20th edition. Philadelphia: Elsevier; 2016. p. 2897.

CHAPTER 22.8

Neurometabolic and Neurogenetic Disorders

Sangeetha Yoganathan

1. Which of the following is *true* about metachromatic leukodystrophy (MLD)?

A. It is an autosomal dominant disease
B. Cerebrospinal fluid (CSF) protein is always normal in late infantile and juvenile MLD
C. Subcortical U-fibers are involved in early MLD
D. Urinary sulfatide excretion is increased in all patients with MLD

EXPLANATION

Metachromatic leukodystrophy is an autosomal recessive disease caused by the deficiency of arylsulfatase A, encoded by the *ARSA* gene. Based on the age at onset of symptoms, MLD can be categorized into late infantile, juvenile, and adult variants. CSF protein is usually elevated in children with late infantile MLD and most patients with juvenile MLD. Urinary sulfatide excretion is increased in all patients with MLD. Demyelination predominantly involves the corpus callosum, periventricular area, and centrum semiovale. The arcuate fibers are relatively spared. The internal capsule, cerebral peduncles, and pyramidal tracts in the brainstem are also involved.

Key: D

BOOST YOUR KNOWLEDGE

Metachromatic leukodystrophy due to saposin B deficiency also has autosomal recessive inheritance, and it is caused by mutations in *PSAP* gene. Autosomal recessive inheritance is the usual mode of inheritance in many of the leukodystrophies, except adrenoleukodystrophy (ALD) and fewer mutations in Aicardi–Goutières syndrome. Urinary sulfatide excretion is increased in all patients with MLD but remains normal in pseudodeficiency. The predominance of subcortical U-fibers has been identified in patients with L-2-hydroxy glutaric aciduria, Kearns–Sayre syndrome, Canavan disease, propionic acidemia, and urea cycle disorders (UCDs).

2. An 11-month-old infant born to third-degree consanguineous parents was brought for the evaluation of regression of milestones from 6 months of age. Excessive irritability, unexplained pyrexia, and exaggerated startle responses were noticed since early infancy. Microcephaly, spasticity, extensor plantar responses, absent deep tendon reflexes, and dystonia were observed. Brain magnetic resonance imaging (MRI) revealed hyperintense signal changes involving periventricular white matter, corpus callosum, posterior limb of the internal capsule, pyramidal tract, and cerebellar white matter. What is the likely diagnosis in this patient?

A. Metachromatic leukodystrophy
B. Krabbe disease (KD)
C. Canavan disease
D. Alexander disease

EXPLANATION

Krabbe disease, also known as globoid cell leukodystrophy, is a progressive white matter disease caused by a deficiency of galactocerebrosidase enzyme. The type of KD includes early infantile or classic type, late-infantile, juvenile, and adolescent–adult. Classic-type KD progresses from stage I to stage III. Children with stage I disease exhibit hyperirritability and excessive startle responses. Pyrexial episodes occur without any signs of infection. In stage II, there is deterioration of motor and mental skills with the occurrence of pyramidal signs, dystonia, visual failure, optic atrophy, and seizures. In stage III, children progress to a vegetative stage. Brain MRI revealed hyperintense signal changes involving periventricular white matter, corpus callosum, posterior limb of the internal capsule, pyramidal tract, and cerebellar white matter. Computed tomography (CT) brain reveals hyperdense thalami.

Key: B

BOOST YOUR KNOWLEDGE

Krabbe disease is an autosomal recessive disorder, resulting from a deficiency of galactocerebrosidase, a lysosomal enzyme that catalyzes cerebroside degradation, and it is encoded by the *GALC* gene. Saposin A, a sphingolipid activator protein, is essential for the degradation of cerebroside by galactocerebrosidase. The predominance of periventricular white matter involvement has been identified in patients with MLD, KD, Sjögren–Larsson syndrome, periventricular leukomalacia, and leukoencephalopathy with brainstem and spinal cord involvement and lactate elevation (LBSL).

3. Which of the following enzyme deficiencies causes Hunter disease [mucopolysaccharidoses (MPS) type II]?

A. α-L-iduronidase
B. α-N-acetylglucosaminidase
C. Iduronate-2-sulfatase
D. Galactosamine-6-sulfatase

EXPLANATION

MPS type	*Enzyme deficiency*
MPS I or Hurler–Scheie disease	α-L-iduronidase
MPS II or Hunter disease	Iduronate-2-sulfatase
MPS IIIA or Sanfilippo A	Sulfamidase
MPS IIIB, Sanfilippo B	α-N-acetylglucosaminidase
MPS IIIC, Sanfilippo C	Acetyl-CoA: α-glucosaminide N-acetyltransferase
MPS IIID, Sanfilippo D	N-acetylglucosamine-6-sulfatase
MPS IVA, Morquio A	Galactosamine-6-sulfatase
MPS IVB, Morquio B	β-D-galactosidase
MPS VI, Maroteaux–Lamy	N-acetylgalactosamine-4-sulfatase
MPS VII, Sly disease	β-D-glucuronidase
MPS IX, Natowicz	Hyaluronoglucosaminidase

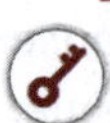

Key: C

BOOST YOUR KNOWLEDGE

Mucopolysaccharidoses are a group of inherited disorders caused by the deficiency of lysosomal enzymes that are involved in the degradation of glycosaminoglycans/mucopolysaccharides. MPS are classified into types and subtypes based on the underlying biochemical and genetic defect. All types of MPS have autosomal recessive inheritance, except Hunter disease, which has X-linked recessive inheritance. The clinical features vary depending on the enzyme deficiency and may often overlap. The common clinical manifestations include psychomotor retardation, coarse facies, hernias, hepatosplenomegaly, cardiac involvement, and dysostosis multiplex. Corneal clouding is absent in Hunter disease. Mild cognitive impairment and severe skeletal dysplasia are seen in MPS type IV. Hydrops fetalis is well described in MPS VII deficiency.

4. An 8-year-old boy was brought for the evaluation of recent onset hyperactivity and generalized diffuse hyperpigmentation. There were no perinatal risk factors, and his milestones were attained age appropriately. On examination, brisk deep tendon reflexes were observed, but there were no tone abnormalities. Brain MRI revealed symmetrical hyperintensity involving parieto-occipital white matter with contrast enhancement along the margins of white matter lesions. Which of the following is the likely diagnosis?

A. Refsum disease
B. ALD
C. Mucolipidosis
D. Mannosidosis

EXPLANATION

Adrenoleukodystrophy is an X-linked inherited disorder caused by mutation in *ABCD1* gene and has a wide phenotypic variability. The phenotypes include cerebral forms (childhood, adolescent, and adult onset), Addison disease, and adrenomyeloneuropathy (AMN). Affected boys remain normal till 4–8 years of age and then manifest with behavioral problems and scholastic deterioration. The scholastic performance deterioration may be attributed to loss of auditory discrimination, loss of spatial orientation, speech disturbances, and difficulty in writing. Seizures occur in one-third of cases and rapid clinical deterioration, resulting in vision loss, spastic quadriparesis, swallowing difficulty, and progression to a vegetative state. Brain MRI scan reveals involvement of parieto-occipital white matter (majority of cases) or frontal white matter lesions. Contrast enhancement along the leading edge of white matter lesions is observed.

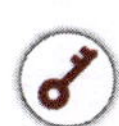

Key: B

BOOST YOUR KNOWLEDGE

Isolated or combined involvement of central or peripheral nervous system and adrenal cortex has been described in patients with ALD. The diagnosis of ALD is established by the biochemical detection of elevated very long-chain fatty acids and the identification of a hemizygous variant in *ABCD1* gene in males with suspected ALD. Affected males may manifest with isolated primary adrenal insufficiency, cerebral ALD with or without primary adrenocortical insufficiency, and AMN.

- The onset of symptoms in AMN occurs around 20–30 years of age, and these patients manifest with spasticity, gait disturbances, and bladder and bowel dysfunction.
- Primary adrenocortical insufficiency may manifest as early as 2 years of age to adulthood. Heterozygous females are at risk to develop primary adrenocortical insufficiency and AMN with advancing age.
- The predominance of parieto-occipital white matter involvement has been observed in patients with ALD, KD, certain peroxisomal disorders, and neonatal hypoglycemia.

5. Which of the following vitamins is used in the management of children with maple syrup urine disease (MSUD)?

A. Thiamine
B. Riboflavin
C. Niacin
D. Folic acid

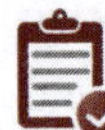

EXPLANATION

Maple syrup urine disease is an autosomal receive disorder caused by the defect in the branched-chain alpha-ketoacid dehydrogenase (BCKD) complex, an enzyme involved in the metabolism of branched-chain amino acids (leucine, isoleucine, and valine). Based on the clinical presentation and outcome, the phenotypes include classical, intermediate, intermittent, thiamine-responsive, and dihydrolipoyl dehydrogenase (E3)-deficient forms of MSUD. Enteral thiamine trial should be considered in children with MSUD to identify the thiamine-responsive variants.

Key: A

BOOST YOUR KNOWLEDGE

Vitamin responsive childhood neurological disorders include vitamin B_{12} deficiency-related infantile tremor syndrome, intracellular cobalamin metabolism defects, homocystinuria, cerebral folate deficiency, hereditary folate malabsorption, biotinidase deficiency, biotin-thiamine-responsive basal ganglia disease, pyridoxine-dependent epilepsy, PNPO deficiency, riboflavin transporter deficiency, aromatic amino acid decarboxylase deficiency, pyruvate dehydrogenase deficiency and ataxia with vitamin E deficiency.

Thiamine and biotin are used in the management of biotin-thiamine responsive basal ganglia disease. Biotin is used to treat children with biotinidase deficiency. Riboflavin is used in the management of children with riboflavin transporter deficiency. Folinic acid is used in the management of children with hereditary folate malabsorption and cerebral folate deficiency (CFD).

6. Which of the following is *false* regarding isochromosomes?

A. Isochromosomes are those chromosomes that are present as add-on to normal chromosome complement
B. In isochromosome, one arm is missing, and the other arm of chromosome is duplicated
C. Isochromosomes are formed due to misdivision through centromere in meiosis
D. Isochromosomes account for 15% of cases with Turner syndrome

EXPLANATION

An isochromosome refers to a chromosome with one arm missing, and the other arm is duplicated in a mirror-image fashion. The formation of an isochromosome occurs due to the misdivision of the centromere in meiosis II. The centromere divides transversely instead of longitudinal division. The most common isochromosome encountered in clinical practice consists of two long arms of the X chromosome. About 15% of cases with Turner syndrome occur due to isochromosomes.

Key: A

BOOST YOUR KNOWLEDGE

Chromosomal abnormalities may be structural or numerical. Aneuploidy is a numerical chromosomal abnormality due to variation from the normal diploid complement of chromosomes, while there is a presence of a complete extra set of chromosomes in polyploidy. Structural chromosomal abnormalities include deletion, duplication, inversion, insertion, marker and ring chromosomes, and isochromosomes.

7. A 3-year-old child has been referred to your center with a provisional clinical diagnosis of peroxisomal disorder. Which of the following biochemical patterns would suggest a diagnosis of Zellweger spectrum disorder (ZSD)?

A. Elevated very-long-chain fatty acid (VLCFA) level and elevated plasmalogens
B. Elevated VLCFA level and normal plasmalogens
C. Normal VLCFA level and abnormal plasmalogens
D. Normal VCLFA level and normal plasmalogens

EXPLANATION

Elevated VLCFA level and elevated plasmalogens	ZSD
Elevated VLCFA level and normal plasmalogens	ALD or other single-enzyme defect of beta oxidation
Normal VLCFA level and abnormal plasmalogens	Rhizomelic chondrodysplasia punctata or other single-enzyme defect of plasmalogen synthesis
Normal VLCFA level and elevated phytanic acid	Refsum disease

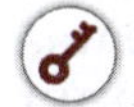

Key: A

BOOST YOUR KNOWLEDGE

Zellweger spectrum disorders are a heterogeneous group of disorders with an autosomal recessive inheritance caused by biallelic variants in one of the *PEX* genes. The clinical manifestations in neonates with ZSDs are distinctive facies, hypotonia, poor feeding, seizures, malformation of the brain, renal cysts, hepatic dysfunction, and chondrodysplasia punctata. Older children manifest with developmental delay, failure to thrive, vision and hearing impairment, hepatic dysfunction, adrenal insufficiency, ataxia, peripheral neuropathy, and leukodystrophy.

8. N-carbamylglutamate is used as a long-term alternative pathway treatment in which of the following UCDs?

A. Argininemia
B. Argininosuccinic acidemia
C. Citrullinemia
D. N-acetyl glutamate synthetase (NAGS) deficiency

EXPLANATION

Agents used in the treatment of UCDs are shown in Table:

N-carbamylglutamate	*NAGS deficiency*
Sodium phenylbutyrate/sodium benzoate	• Carbamoyl phosphate synthetase 1 (CPS1) or ornithine transcarbamylase (OTC) deficiency • Argininemia • Argininosuccinic acidemia • Citrullinemia
L-Arginine	Citrullinemia and argininosuccinic acidemia

Key: D

BOOST YOUR KNOWLEDGE

Urea cycle disorders (UCDs) occur due to deficiency in any one of the five catalytic enzymes that includes carbamoylphosphate synthetase I (CPS1), ornithine transcarbamylase (OTC), argininosuccinic acid synthetase 1 (ASS1), argininosuccinic acid lyase (ASL) or arginase; deficiency of one cofactor producing enzyme namely N-acetyl glutamate synthetase (NAGS). UCD may also occur due to defect in the two amino acid transporters that include ornithine translocase 1 (ORNT1) and citrin.

- Neonates with UCD exhibit a period of normalcy after birth followed by lethargy, poor feeding, vomiting, seizures, hypothermia, and hyperventilation.
- Children with later onset UCD exhibit chronic and episodic symptoms. These children manifest with psychomotor retardation, seizures, behavioral problems, learning problems, ataxia, and hepatomegaly. Episodic worsening may occur with increased dietary protein intake, intercurrent illness, surgery, trauma, or

initiation of valproate. Obvious precipitating factors may not be identified in many cases. Symptoms during episodic worsening include headache, vomiting, lethargy, irritability, confusion, agitation, hallucinations, dysarthria, ataxia, or stroke-like events.

Clinical phenotypes often overlap among the UCDs due to various enzyme deficiencies or transporter defects except for arginase deficiency. Children with arginase deficiency manifest with slowly progressive spastic diplegia to tetraplegia, psychomotor retardation, epilepsy, hyperactivity, ataxia, tremor, and choreoathetosis. Trichorrhexis nodosa is a specific clinical finding detected in children with UCD due to ASL deficiency. Protein aversion may be observed in children with UCD.

9. A 3-month-old infant was brought with a history of refractory seizures since the neonatal period. There was no response to multiple antiseizure medications, and a probability of pyridoxine-dependent epilepsy (PDE) was considered. Genetic testing identified a likely pathogenic variant in the *ALDH7A1* gene. Seizures were controlled after initiation of pyridoxine. Which of the following is *not* a finding in children with PDE?

A. Seizures beginning in the neonatal period or early infancy
B. Autosomal recessive disorder
C. Elevated alpha-aminoadipic semialdehyde (α-AASA) concentration in urine and/or plasma is a specific marker in PDE
D. Elevated pipecolic acid level in plasma and CSF

EXPLANATION

Pyridoxine-dependent epilepsy is an autosomal recessive disorder caused by mutations in the *ALDH7A1* gene. Children with PDE manifest with refractory seizures not controlled by antiseizure medications but respond to appropriate daily dosages of pyridoxine. Classical and atypical presentations may occur in children with PDE. Children with classical PDE usually have an onset of symptoms within the first few weeks or months of life, while children with atypical PDE have a later onset of symptoms in the late infantile age or till 3 years of age. α-AASA in urine and/or plasma is a nonspecific marker and may be observed in children with molybdenum cofactor deficiency or sulfite oxidase deficiency. Children with PDE are managed with dietary restriction of lysine, arginine supplementation, and supplementation of pyridoxine (30 mg/kg/day in divided doses).

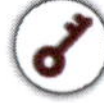

Key: C

BOOST YOUR KNOWLEDGE

Pyridoxine responsiveness occurs in antiquitin deficiency, PNPO deficiency, hyperprolinemia type II, severe neonatal hypophosphatasia, and severe forms of KCNQ2 deficiency.

10. Which of the following neurotransmitter disorders does not have elevated phenylalanine level?

A. 6-Pyruvoyltetrahydrobiopterin synthase deficiency
B. GTP cyclohydrolase deficiency (autosomal recessive)
C. Sepiapterin reductase deficiency
D. Dihydropteridine reductase deficiency

EXPLANATION

Elevated phenylalanine level is observed in patients with GTP cyclohydrolase deficiency (autosomal recessive inheritance), 6-Pyruvoyltetrahydrobiopterin synthase deficiency, dihydropteridine reductase deficiency, and primapterinuria.

Key: C

BOOST YOUR KNOWLEDGE

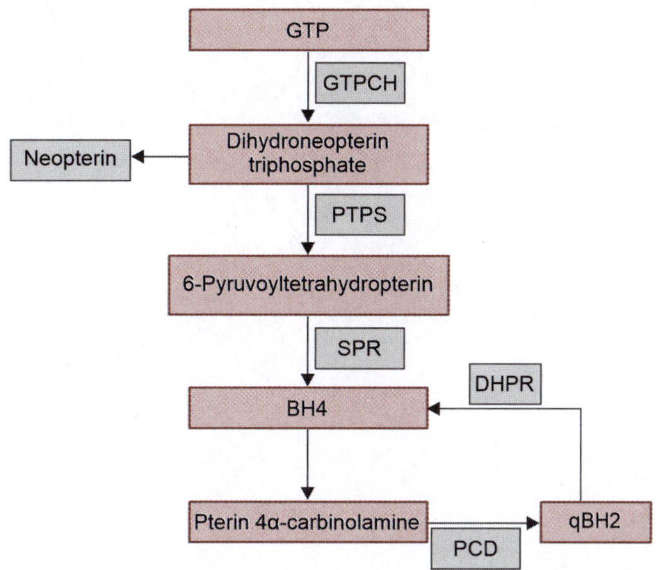

(BH4: tetrahydrobiopterin; DHPR: dihydropteridine reductase; GTP: guanosine triphosphate; GTPCH: GTP cyclohydrolase; PCD: pterin 4-α carbinolamine dehydratase; PTPS: 6-pyruvoyl-tetrahydrobiopterin synthase; qBH2: dihydrobiopterin quinoid; SPR: sepiapterin reductase)

Elevated phenylalanine level is not observed in children with SPR deficiency due to the presence of an alternate salvage pathway.

REFERENCES/SOURCES

- Ah Mew N, Simpson KL, Gropman AL, et al. Urea cycle disorders overview. In: Adam MP, Feldman J, Mirzaa GM, Pagon RA, Wallace SE, Bean LJH, et al. (Eds). GeneReviews® [Internet]. Seattle (WA): University of Washington, Seattle; 1993. [online] Available from: https://www.ncbi.nlm.nih.gov/books/NBK1217/ [Last accessed July, 2024].
- Opladen T, López-Laso E, Cortès-Saladelafont E, Pearson TS, Sivri HS, Yildiz Y, et al. International Working Group on Neurotransmitter related Disorders (iNTD). Consensus Guideline for the Diagnosis and Treatment of Tetrahydrobiopterin (BH4) Deficiencies. Orphanet J Rare Dis. 2020;15(1):126. doi: 10.1186/s13023-020-01379-8. Erratum in: Orphanet J Rare Dis. 2020;15(1):202. doi: 10.1186/s13023-020-01464-y. PMID: 32456656; PMCID: PMC7251883.
- Schiffmann R, van der Knaap MS. Invited article: an MRI-based approach to the diagnosis of white matter disorders. Neurology. 2009;72(8):750-9.
- Steinberg SJ, Raymond GV, Braverman NE, Moser AB. Zellweger spectrum disorder. In: Adam MP, Feldman J, Mirzaa GM, Pagon RA, Wallace SE, Bean LJH, et al. (Eds). GeneReviews® [Internet]. Seattle (WA): University of Washington, Seattle; 1993. [online] Available from https://www.ncbi.nlm.nih.gov/books/NBK1448/ [Last accessed July, 2024].
- Swaiman KF, Ashwal S, Ferriero DM, Schor NF, Finkel RS, Gropman AL, et al. (Eds). Swaiman's Pediatric Neurology: Principles and Practice, 6th edition. Elsevier; 2017.
- van der Knapp MS, Valk J. Magnetic resonance of myelination and myelin disorders, 3rd edition. Berlin Heidelberg: Springer-Verlag; 2005.

SECTION 23

Endocrinology

Section Editor: *Aashima Dabas*

CHAPTER

23.1

Growth Disorders

Aashima Dabas

1. Which of the following is correct regarding linear growth during infancy?

A. Growth is dependent on growth hormone (GH)
B. Growth is rapid and accelerating
C. Growth is greater in boys than girls
D. Growth is slower in babies born small for gestation than term healthy babies

EXPLANATION

Growth during infancy is chiefly determined by nutrition. Growth is maximum during infancy and accelerates till second year after which it begins to decelerate. Nutrition is a critical determinant with thyroid hormone and insulin-like growth factor 1 (IGF-1) that affect growth during infancy. Growth is similar in both genders during infancy; gender-wise differences are apparent during pubertal growth spurt. Babies with small for gestational age (SGA) show a catch-up growth that is greater than those with normal birth weight.

Key: B

BOOST YOUR KNOWLEDGE

The infancy-childhood-puberty (ICP) growth model explains the interplay of different hormones that determine growth in children. The growth in fetal period is governed by insulin (IGF-1 and IGF-2) and IGF-binding proteins (IGFBPs). The period during infancy records significant growth in weight and height under the effect of nutrition. The pace of growth during childhood remains steady till puberty when growth peaks under the effect of GH and sex steroids.

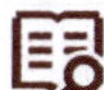

REFERENCES/SOURCES

- Sharma S. Growth: normal and abnormal. In: Gupta P, Menon PSN, Ramji S, Lodha R (Eds). PG Textbook of Pediatrics, 3rd edition. New Delhi: Jaypee Brothers Medical Publishers; 2022.
- Tse WY, Hindmarsh PC, Brook CG. The infancy-childhood-puberty model of growth: clinical aspects. Acta Paediatr Scand Suppl. 1989;356:38-45.

2. Which of these is the approximate rate of increase in length/height during 1–3 year of life?

A. 0.6–0.8 cm/month
B. 0.8–1.0 cm/month
C. 1.0–1.2 cm/month
D. 1.2–1.4 cm/month

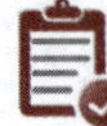

EXPLANATION

The peak growth velocity is seen soon after birth at 3.5 cm/months for the first 3 months, then 2 cm per months for 3–6 months, 1.5 cm/month between 6 and 9 months, and 1.2 cm/month between 9 and 12 months of age. Growth is thus maximum during infancy and gradually decelerates during toddler age group to reach a rate of 4–5 cm per year after the age of 4 years.

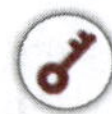

Key: B

BOOST YOUR KNOWLEDGE

The peak growth rate is seen during the first few months for increase in weight, length, and head circumference. The weight gain after birth should be interpreted with respect to birth weight of the child rather than reference standards alone. Children born SGA or large for gestational age (LGA) are expected to have catch-up and catch-down growth, respectively.

REFERENCE/SOURCE

- Sharma S. Growth: normal and abnormal. In: Gupta P, Menon PSN, Ramji S, Lodha R (Eds). PG Textbook of Pediatrics, 3rd edition. New Delhi: Jaypee Brothers Medical Publishers; 2022.

3. Which of these statements is the correct reason for the assertion stated below?

Assertion—Children with deficiency of IGF-1 are short

A. GH stimulates the secretion of IGF-1 from the liver
B. Children born SGA have low IGF-1 levels
C. IGF-1 acts in a paracrine manner on chondrocytes to promote growth
D. IGF-1 improves insulin sensitivity and increases protein synthesis

EXPLANATION

Growth hormone is released from the anterior pituitary gland that mediates growth through direct action on chondrocytes in long bones. It also acts indirectly to produce IGF-1 in the liver which is responsible for the linear growth through its paracrine action on the chondrocytes. IGF-1 also has other metabolic effects on the body. A deficiency of IGF-1 thus manifests as short stature. Children with SGA usually show a catch-up growth in first two years of life. SGA children who do not catch-up in growth need to be investigated and can be initiated on recombinant GH therapy irrespective of the GH levels. They usually have low IGF-1 levels.

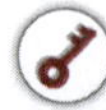

Key: C

BOOST YOUR KNOWLEDGE

The IGF-1 is a protein secreted from the liver in response to GH. It can be used as a screening test for growth hormone deficiency (GHD) where IGF-1 levels are low. However, the levels may also be low in poor nutritional states and in hepatic diseases. IGF-1 levels need to be interpreted according to age and gender and ideally as per local reference values.

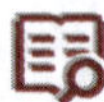

REFERENCE/SOURCE

- Sharma S. Growth: normal and abnormal. In: Gupta P, Menon PSN, Ramji S, Lodha R (Eds). PG Textbook of Pediatrics, 3rd edition. New Delhi: Jaypee Brothers Medical Publishers; 2022.

4. Choose the correct midparental height (MPH) for child A and B, respectively.

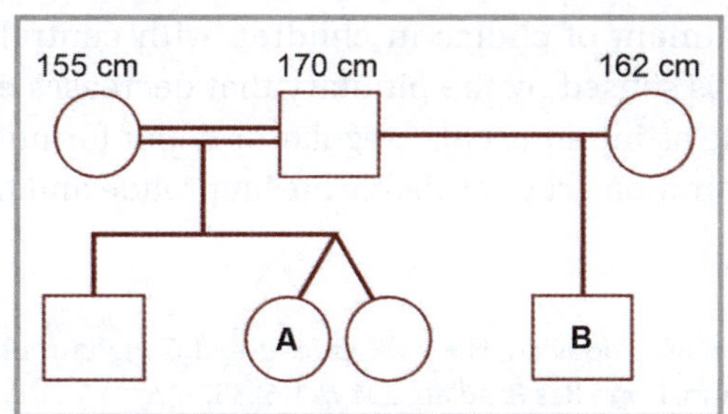

A. 156 cm, 169 cm
B. 156 cm, 172.5 cm
C. 159.5 cm, 169 cm
D. 169 cm, 172.5 cm

EXPLANATION

The pedigree shown here shows calculation of MPH of half-siblings. The MPH is calculated as follows:
Boy = (Father's height + Mother's height + 13)/2
Girl = (Father's height + Mother's height – 13)/2

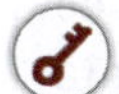

Key: B

BOOST YOUR KNOWLEDGE

The MPH helps us predict the growth potential of a child. Ideally, the final height of a child is within ±8.5 cm of the MPH (target height range). A child who falls short of target height range should be investigated for pathological short stature. The predicted adult height is a height predicted by the child's current skeletal age and chronological age.

REFERENCE/SOURCE

- Sharma S. Growth: normal and abnormal. In: Gupta P, Menon PSN, Ramji S, Lodha R (Eds). PG Textbook of Pediatrics, 3rd edition. New Delhi: Jaypee Brothers Medical Publishers; 2022.

5. Which of these is the most likely outcome of growth in a 7-year-old girl recently diagnosed with idiopathic central precocious puberty on gonadotropin-releasing hormone (GnRH) analogs—present height 124 cm (75th centile); MPH 155 cm (25th centile)?

A. Treatment with GnRH analogs will improve the height gain
B. Normal height velocity (HV) on treatment with GnRH analogs is reassuring
C. Final height will be within target height for MPH
D. Final height will be shorter than 75th centile

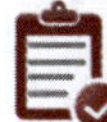

EXPLANATION

Children with central precocious puberty have an accelerated bone age and are taller for their age. The premature gain in height with an advanced bone age may gradually plateau early resulting in shorter final height. It usually falls short of the target height range. Treatment with GnRH in a 7-year-old girl will halt the progression of puberty and rate of increase in height.

Key: D

BOOST YOUR KNOWLEDGE

The GnRH analogs are the treatment of choice in children with central precocious puberty. A continuous exposure of GnRH as an analog is sensed by the pituitary that decreases endogenous gonadotropins and thus halts puberty. These are available as intramuscular regular or depot formulations and administered monthly or 3–6 monthly, respectively. The common drugs available are leuprolide and triptorelin.

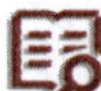

REFERENCES/SOURCES

- Krishna KB, Fuqua JS, Rogol AD, Klein KO, Popovic J, Houk CP, et al. Use of Gonadotropin-Releasing Hormone Analogs in Children: Update by an International Consortium. Horm Res Paediatr. 2019;91(6):357-72.
- Sharma S. Growth: normal and abnormal. In: Gupta P, Menon PSN, Ramji S, Lodha R (Eds). PG Textbook of Pediatrics, 3rd edition. New Delhi: Jaypee Brothers Medical Publishers; 2022.

6. Which of these statements are correct for the WHO-2006 growth charts?

A. They are based on longitudinal growth data from 0 to 5 years
B. Weight-for-age centiles represented are 3rd, 25th, 50th, 75th, and 97th
C. Body mass index (BMI) charts are available after 2 years of age
D. The charts contain standards for triceps and subscapular skinfold-for-age

EXPLANATION

The WHO-2006 growth charts were devised after collection of data from WHO Multicentre Growth Reference Study conducted across Brazil, Ghana, India, Norway, Oman, and the USA. The longitudinal growth data was collected from 0 to 2 years and cross-sectional data from 2 to 5 years onward. The growth observations for weight, height, head circumference, arm circumference, triceps, and subscapular skin fold thickness were obtained to generate gender specific charts using centile and standard deviation scores (SDS). The centiles are represented for 3rd, 15th, 50th, 85th, and 97th centile and SDS as −3, −2, 0, +2, +3, and also −1 and +1 in a few charts. The BMI charts are available from birth till 18 years of age.

Key: D

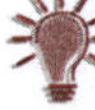

BOOST YOUR KNOWLEDGE

The WHO growth charts were based on babies delivered at term and are used as reference charts from birth to 5 years of age in Indian children. The growth of babies who are delivered preterm should be interpreted on Intergrowth-21st charts. These were based on data from >4,500 pregnancies who were serially monitored from early fetal period (9 weeks) till 2 years of age. The Intergrowth charts indicate the optimal fetal and newborn growth pattern and are recommended to interpret postnatal growth in preterm infants.

REFERENCES/SOURCES

- Papageorghiou AT, Kennedy SH, Salomon LJ, Altman DG, Ohuma EO, Stones W, et al. The INTERGROWTH-21st fetal growth standards: toward the global integration of pregnancy and pediatric care. Am J Obstet Gynecol. 2018;218(2S):S630-40.
- World Health Organization. Child growth standards. [online] Available from https://www.who.int/tools/child-growth-standards/standards. [Last accessed July, 2024].

7. Which of these is helpful in the diagnosis of constitutional delay in growth and puberty?

A. Total testosterone level
B. Beta-human chorionic gonadotropin (hCG) level
C. Inhibin-B level
D. Androstenedione level

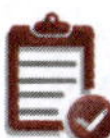

EXPLANATION

Constitutional delay of growth and puberty (CDGP) is a physiological state that manifests with short stature and delay in pubertal onset. The hormonal profile resembles a prepubertal stage with suppressed gonadotropins and low testosterone. The condition needs to be differentiated from hypogonadotropic hypogonadism (HH). Children with CDGP have a height that is in accordance to the bone age and pubertal stage. They mount a normal response on GnRH test. The random levels of testosterone, beta-hCG and androstenedione are not useful. Inhibin-B is released by the Sertoli cells of the testis in males, and in the granulosa cells of the ovary in females and exerts a negative feedback on follicle-stimulating hormone (FSH) levels. Children with CDGP have normal levels of inhibin B but those with HH have low levels.

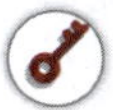

Key: C

BOOST YOUR KNOWLEDGE

Delayed puberty is defined as absence of sexual maturation—girls as absence of thelarche by age of 13 and boys as testicular volume below 4 mL by 14 years. Delayed puberty is classified as hypogonadotropic [low luteinizing hormone (LH) and FSH levels] or hypogonadotropic (high FSH and LH levels). CDGP remains the most common cause of delayed puberty in both boys and girls, and is more commonly seen in boys than girls. The diagnosis should be suspected in the absence of an underlying systemic disorder and presence of family history of delayed puberty. The bone age may show mild delay. Boys with CDGP can be treated with a short course of monthly testosterone (50–100 mg) to jump start the puberty.

REFERENCES/SOURCES

- Bozzola M, Bozzola E, Montalbano C, Stamati FA, Ferrara P, Villani A. Delayed puberty versus hypogonadism: a challenge for the pediatrician. Ann Pediatr Endocrinol Metab. 2018;23(2):57-61.
- Wehkalampi K, Widén E, Laine T, Palotie A, Dunkel L. Patterns of inheritance of constitutional delay of growth and puberty in families of adolescent girls and boys referred to specialist pediatric care. J Clin Endocrinol Metab. 2008;93:723-8.

8. Which of the centile cut-offs describes obesity for Indian children on the revised Indian Academy of Pediatrics (IAP) BMI chart in girls and boys, respectively?

A. 90th and 95th centile
B. 95th and 90th centile
C. 95th and 97th centile
D. 97th and 95th centile

EXPLANATION

The IAP BMI charts provide age-based cut-offs to indicate overweight and obesity as per a BMI ≥23 kg/m^2 and ≥27 kg/m^2 of adult reference. These references for overweight and obesity in terms of centiles in girls are ≥75th and 95th and ≥71st and 90th centile in boys.

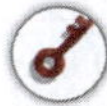

Key: B

BOOST YOUR KNOWLEDGE

The cut-offs to define overweight and obesity as per the WHO reference charts are different as per the age group. In younger children (0–5 years), BMI or weight for length/height >+2 SD indicates overweight and BMI or weight for length/height >+3 SD indicates obesity. The cut-offs for overweight and obesity in 5–18 years as per the WHO are BMI >+1 SDS or >85th centile, and BMI >+2 SDS or >97th centile, respectively.

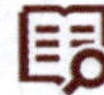

REFERENCE/SOURCE

- Sharma S. Growth: normal and abnormal. In: Gupta P, Menon PSN, Ramji S, Lodha R (Eds). PG Textbook of Pediatrics, 3rd edition. New Delhi: Jaypee Brothers Medical Publishers; 2022.

9. A 5-year old boy is brought with complaints of short stature [weight 16 kg, weight-for-age z-score (WAZ) –0.9 and height 89 cm, height-for-age Z-score (HAZ) –4.29], significantly short for parental heights. He has frontal bossing with short limb length (upper to lower segment ratio 1.4). Baseline hormonal workup showed a parathyroid hormone level of 15 pg/mL (normal range 10–60), thyroid-stimulating hormone (TSH) of 6.2 mU/L (normal range 0.5–4.5) with normal serum-free thyroxine. Which of the following tests are suggested for the diagnosis in this child?

A. Antithyroid peroxidase antibodies
B. GH stimulation test
C. Serum calcium and vitamin D level
D. Mutation analysis for *FGFR3*

EXPLANATION

There is significant disproportionate short stature in this child suggesting short limb dwarfism. This could be seen in rickets, hypothyroidism, or skeletal dysplasia most prominent being achondroplasia. A normal parathyroid hormone suggests against concurrent calcium or vitamin D deficiency seen in rickets. The mildly elevated TSH with a normal thyroxine level cannot justify hypothyroidism as a cause of short stature which negates the need to measure antithyroid peroxidase antibodies. A GH stimulation test may be noninformative in the presence of disproportionate short stature. Skeletal dysplasia like achondroplasia will require skeletal survey followed by confirmatory gene testing for *FGFR3* gene.

Key: D

BOOST YOUR KNOWLEDGE

Skeletal dysplasia is a rare genetic disorder that present with limb deformities and/or short stature. The location of shortening of bones can be classified as follows:

- Rhizomelic affects proximal part of long bones. Common examples are achondroplasia and spondyloepiphyseal punctata.
- Mesomelic affects the middle part of appendicular skeleton (such as radius and ulna). Examples like mesomelic dysplasia.
- Acromelic affects the distal portions of limbs such as hands and feet. Examples include acrodysostosis.
- Micromelic results from a generalized shortening of limb as seen in achondrogenesis.

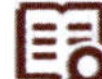

REFERENCES/SOURCES

- Sharma S. Growth: normal and abnormal. In: Gupta P, Menon PSN, Ramji S, Lodha R (Eds). PG Textbook of Pediatrics, 3rd edition. New Delhi: Jaypee Brothers Medical Publishers; 2022.
- Unger S, Ferreira CR, Mortier GR, Ali H, Bertola DR, Calder A, et al. Nosology of genetic skeletal disorders: 2023 revision. Am J Med Genet A. 2023;191(5):1164-209.

10. An 8-year old boy is evaluated for obesity (weight 35 kg at +1.66 Z score, height 114 cm at minus 2.05 Z score and BMI Z score +3.02). He was seen at 10 months as a floppy infant and feeding problems and required gastrostomy. Which of these examination findings will suggest a genetic cause of his obesity?

A. Acanthosis nigricans
B. Long slender fingers
C. Right retractile testis
D. Lumbar lordosis

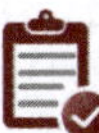

EXPLANATION

The most common form of obesity is constitutional that results from an imbalance in energy intake and expenditure. A few pointers in this child suggest pathological obesity such as history of floppiness and feeding difficulty after birth. The presence of acanthosis nigricans suggests insulin resistance and can be seen in any form of obesity. Retractile testis is a normal finding and does not require any management. Lumbar lordosis may be seen in children with obesity with increased abdominal circumference. Long slender fingers maybe associated with underlying genetic disorders such as Prader–Willi syndrome and Cohen syndrome.

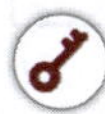

Key: B

BOOST YOUR KNOWLEDGE

Genetic causes of obesity include monogenic disorders with mutations in leptin, leptin receptor, proopiomelanocortin (POMC). The other group includes syndromic disorders such as Prader–Willi syndrome, Cohen syndrome, Bardet–Biedl syndrome, and Albright hereditary osteodystrophy.

REFERENCE/SOURCE

- Sharma S. Growth: normal and abnormal. In: Gupta P, Menon PSN, Ramji S, Lodha R (Eds). PG Textbook of Pediatrics, 3rd edition. New Delhi: Jaypee Brothers Medical Publishers; 2022.

11. Choose the correct statement for growth during adolescence.

A. Girls attain peak growth velocity just after menarche
B. Gonadarche coincides with the appearance of facial hair
C. Estrogen enhances GH secretion
D. Testosterone promotes growth of chondrocytes

EXPLANATION

The pubertal progression in boys and girls follows a respective sequential pattern. Girls develop thelarche as the first sign of puberty that is followed by pubarche and adrenarche. Menarche occurs approximately after 1.5–2 years of thelarche. The girls attain peak HV after thelarche between stages II and III of puberty and have minimum growth left after menarche. Boys develop increase in testicular size (gonadarche) as the first sign of puberty. They gradually develop pubarche and adrenarche but attain peak HV toward the end of puberty. The overall growth spurt is higher in boys than girls. The estrogens promote GH secretion in low doses as seen during initial phases of pubertal development, and promote epiphyseal fusion later. Testosterone does not have a growth promoting effect on chondrocytes.

Key: C

BOOST YOUR KNOWLEDGE

Normal pubertal development always follows the normal sequence in both boys and girls. This is important in investigating a child with growth and pubertal disorder.

REFERENCE/SOURCE

- Sharma S. Growth: normal and abnormal. In: Gupta P, Menon PSN, Ramji S, Lodha R (Eds). PG Textbook of Pediatrics, 3rd edition. New Delhi: Jaypee Brothers Medical Publishers; 2022.

12. Which of the following is an approved indication for use of recombinant GH?

A. Prader–Willi syndrome
B. Down syndrome
C. Congenital nephrotic syndrome
D. VACTERL

EXPLANATION

Growth hormone treatment was licensed for use in GHD initially. The indications were gradually expanded to treat children born SGA, idiopathic short stature of undetermined etiology, chronic renal disease, and Turner syndrome. Prader–Willi syndrome is an approved indication of GH even in the absence of short stature to improve body composition, muscle strength and quality of life.

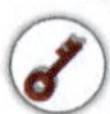

Key: A

BOOST YOUR KNOWLEDGE

The earliest GH derivatives for medicinal use were derived from cadaveric human pituitary. Its use was associated with iatrogenic Creutzfeldt–Jakob disease. The GH preparations now available are prepared by recombinant technology and are safe for use.

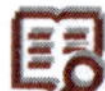

REFERENCE/SOURCE

- Danowitz M, Grimberg A. Clinical Indications for Growth Hormone Therapy. Adv Pediatr. 2022;69(1):203-17.

13. A 10-year old girl is being evaluated for tall stature (height 90th centile and MPH 25th centile). She is prepubertal, skeletal age 9.6 years with normal examination findings. Which of these dynamic function tests can be useful for further management?

A. Glucagon stimulation test
B. GnRH stimulation test
C. Insulin tolerance test
D. Glucose challenge test

EXPLANATION

Glucagon stimulation test is for pituitary GH reserve in suspected GHD. The GnRH stimulation test is performed in conditions of early or delayed puberty. Insulin tolerance test can test the pituitary function for cortisol and GH production. The glucose challenge test measures suppression of GH levels in those with excess GH levels.

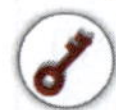

Key: D

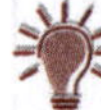

BOOST YOUR KNOWLEDGE

Tall stature is a less common condition. The causes include constitutional tall stature, hormonal excess, genetic disorders such as Marfan syndrome, overgrowth disorders, and metabolic conditions.

REFERENCE/SOURCE

- Goyal A, Jyotsna VP, Singh AKC, Gupta Y, Khadgawat R. Etiology and clinical profile of patients with tall stature: a single-center experience. Indian J Endocrinol Metab. 2020;24(5):428-33.

14. A 6-year-old boy with difficulty to control asthma is evaluated for growth (weight-for-age +1.20 Z score, height for age minus 1.98 Z score). He is on systemic and inhaled corticosteroids and frequent rescue beta-2 agonists. Which of the following statements is correct?

A. Use of beta-2 agonists increases the risk of hypothyroidism
B. Systemic corticosteroids decrease the production of IGF-1 levels

C. Inhaled corticosteroids do not affect linear growth
D. Steroid use results in advanced bone age and short stature

EXPLANATION

Children with systemic disorders like poorly controlled asthma can have short stature. This child also has a history of intake of corticosteroids that can further impact growth. Both inhaled and systemic glucocorticoids can affect growth, larger effect seen with oral than inhaled or topical steroids. Corticosteroids affect the chondrocytes in the growth plate, decrease GH secretion, and IGF-1 production. The bone age is delayed in conditions with excess steroids. Children with Cushing syndrome have higher weight but shorter height and delayed bone age. Beta-blockers are used in hyperthyroidism for their cardiac actions and do not have any risk of hypothyroidism.

Key: B

BOOST YOUR KNOWLEDGE

Normally, the weight and height follow a similar centile on the growth chart. Children with short stature with an underlying systemic cause have lower weight than height centile. Children with endocrinal or genetic disorder have lower height than weight. Children with constitutional obesity are usually tall, though the weight centile is higher than height centile. A child with obesity and short stature should be investigated for hypothyroidism, Cushing syndrome, or pathological causes of obesity.

REFERENCE/SOURCE

- Sharma S. Growth: normal and abnormal. In: Gupta P, Menon PSN, Ramji S, Lodha R (Eds). PG Textbook of Pediatrics, 3rd edition. New Delhi: Jaypee Brothers Medical Publishers; 2022.

15. Which of the following is a risk factor for childhood obesity?

A. Maternal valproate consumption
B. Exclusive breastfeeding till 6 months
C. Complementary feeding at 4 months
D. Dietary gluten introduction at 12 months

EXPLANATION

The nutrition in first 1,000 days of life (fetal period till first 2 years of life) plays an important role in determining later risk of childhood obesity. Exclusive breastfeeding and introduction of complementary feeding at 6 months are protective. Early timing of complementary feeding is associated with increased risk of obesity. The timing of dietary gluten introduction is associated with risk of celiac disease but not obesity. Maternal intake of valproate is associated with risk of fetal valproate spectrum disorder that presents with dysmorphism and congenital anomalies.

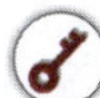

Key: C

BOOST YOUR KNOWLEDGE

Antenatal exposure like maternal hyperglycemia and maternal intake of cafeteria diets that are energy dense promote fetal growth and risk of later life obesity. In contrast, fetal growth restriction also increases the risk of obesity (fetal origin of adult diseases).

REFERENCES/SOURCES

- Calkins K, Devaskar SU. Fetal origins of adult disease. Curr Probl Pediatr Adolesc Health Care. 2011;41(6):158-76.
- Sharma S. Growth: normal and abnormal. In: Gupta P, Menon PSN, Ramji S, Lodha R (Eds). PG Textbook of Pediatrics, 3rd edition. New Delhi: Jaypee Brothers Medical Publishers; 2022.

16. A 12-year old girl presents with recent onset generalized weakness and weight gain. She is prepubertal and short. Baseline blood workup is normal. TSH is 65.3 IU/L. Serum tissue transglutaminase is normal. Bone age is delayed. What will be the next appropriate step in her management?

A. Plan a GH stimulation test
B. Start levothyroxine at 3 µg/kg/day
C. Measure urinary iodine
D. Order ultrasound of the neck for goiter

EXPLANATION

The case details mention recent onset weight gain. The TSH is clearly elevated suggesting a likely primary hypothyroidism. As part of workup of the cause of hypothyroidism, she should be clinically checked for goiter with a neck examination and systemic examination. She will benefit from measurement of total thyroxine levels and antithyroid peroxidase antibody. The measurement of urinary iodine is mainly reserved for epidemiological studies and is seldom useful in case management. A GH stimulation test is not indicated in the presence of hypothyroidism. She needs to be initiated on replacement thyroxine with further follow-up.

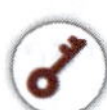

Key: B

BOOST YOUR KNOWLEDGE

Urine iodine excretion is an inexpensive and good screening tool for iodine deficiency at a population level. Urinary iodine level <100 µg/L is a marker of iodine deficiency in the area.

REFERENCE/SOURCE

- Pandav CS, Yadav K, Srivastava R, Pandav R, Karmarkar MG. Iodine deficiency disorders (IDD) control in India. Indian J Med Res. 2013;138:418-33.

17. Which of the following chromosomal pattern is associated with tall stature?

A. 47, XX +21
B. 47, XXY
C. 46, XX+ SHOX haploinsufficiency
D. 45, XO/46, XX

EXPLANATION

Tall stature is a less common endocrinal disorder. The causes of tall stature are familial, genetic syndromes such as Klinefelter syndrome, Marfan syndrome, Fragile X, and overgrowth syndromes (Sotos syndrome and Weaver syndrome). Children with Down syndrome and Turner syndrome are usually short.

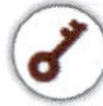

Key: B

BOOST YOUR KNOWLEDGE

The anthropometry of children with Down syndrome or Turner syndrome should be interpreted on syndrome specific gender-based charts.

REFERENCES/SOURCES

- CDC. Down syndrome. [online] Available from https://www.cdc.gov/birth-defects/about/down-syndrome.html. [Last accessed July, 2024].
- Pedsendo.org. Turner syndrome. [online] Available from https://pedsendo.org/wp-content/uploads/2020/07/Growth-Chart-Turner-syndrome.pdf. [Last accessed July, 2024].

18. A 12-year-old girl is brought for concerns of rapid weight gain. There are no other systemic complaints. Her anthropometry at 6 years of age (point A) recorded in school report was weight 15.5 kg and height 105 cm, MPH is 150 cm. She now (point B) weighs 48 kg and has height 138.5 cm, SMR-B2P2 and does not have acanthosis. Her thyroid function tests are normal. What will be the next step in management?

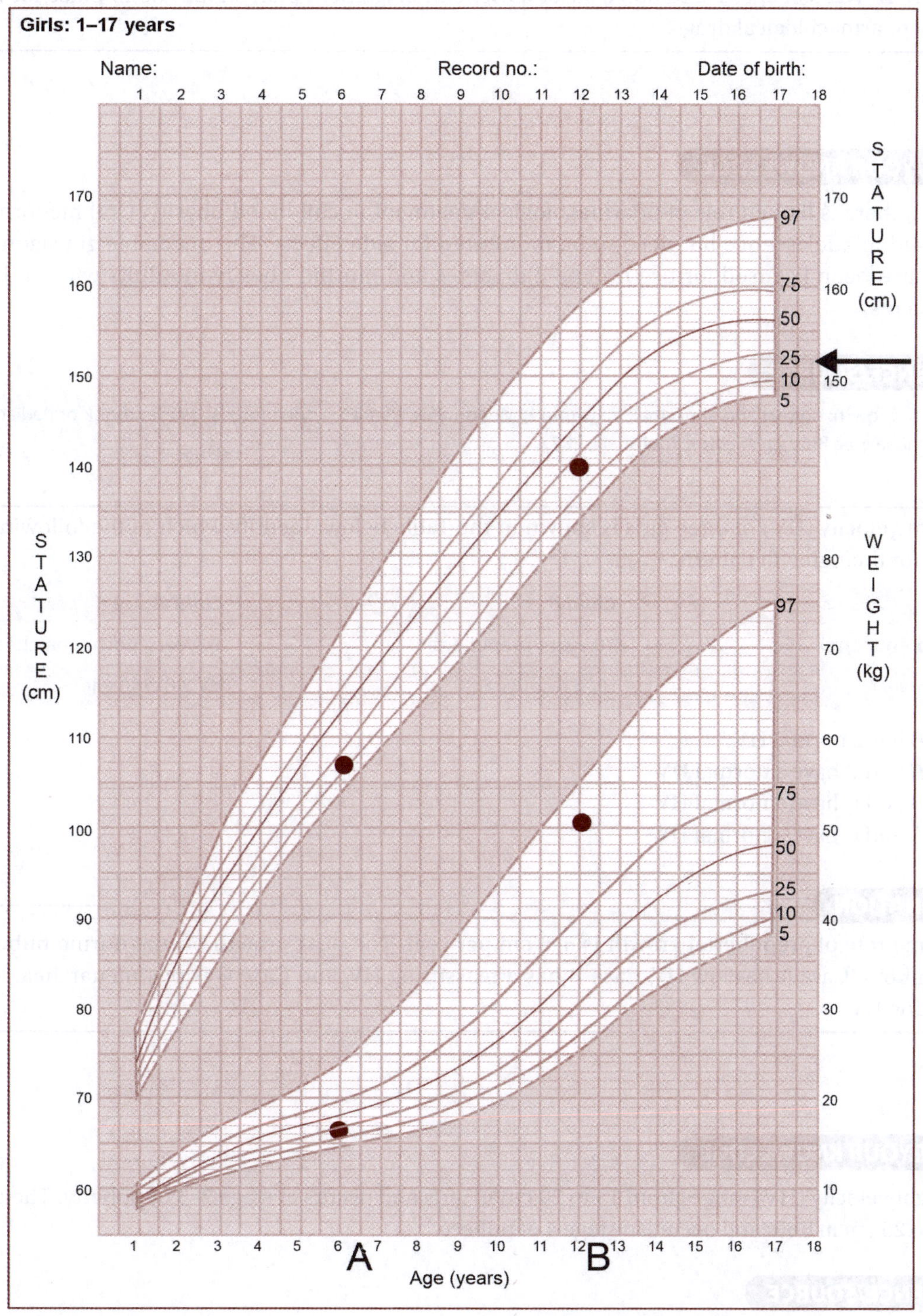

A. Start oral metformin
B. Strict lifestyle advice
C. Measure 8 AM cortisol
D. Perform GH stimulation test

EXPLANATION

The growth chart appended shows a trajectory suggestive of constitutional obesity. There is no height deceleration that would suggest against a Cushing syndrome or GHD. She does not have any acanthosis and is only 12 years of age. Therefore, a strict lifestyle management plan should be in place for her instead of use of any pharmacological drugs.

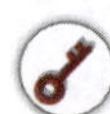

Key: B

BOOST YOUR KNOWLEDGE

At present, there is limited role of pharmacological treatment in childhood obesity. Oral metformin and orlistat can be used in adolescence but need to be monitored for side effects. The injectable glucagon-like peptide-1 analogs have been licensed for use in type 2 diabetes and morbid obesity in adults with limited experience in adolescents.

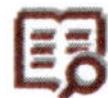

REFERENCE/SOURCE

- Sharma S. Growth: normal and abnormal. In: Gupta P, Menon PSN, Ramji S, Lodha R (Eds). PG Textbook of Pediatrics, 3rd edition. New Delhi: Jaypee Brothers Medical Publishers; 2022.

19. The height velocity (HV) of three girls is shown in the Table below. Identify which of the following is the correct response for their growth pattern.

Child A	*Child B*	*Child C*
5.6 year, prepubertal	10 years, prepubertal	14 years, postmenarcheal
HV 3.9 cm/year	HV 5.4 cm/year	HV 3.8 cm/year

A. Only B has a normal HV
B. Both A and B have a normal HV
C. Both B and C have a normal HV
D. Both A and C have a normal HV

EXPLANATION

The normal rate of prepubertal growth is 5–6 cm per year. The peak growth occurs during puberty, earlier in girls than boys. Case A has low HV, Case B has a reassuring HV, and Case C is postmenarcheal with a normal decelerating HV.

Key: C

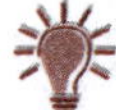

BOOST YOUR KNOWLEDGE

Peak height velocity (HV) ranges from 15 to 20 cm in girls and occurs at stage 2–3 of puberty. The peak HV ranges from 20 to 25 cm in boys and occurs in stage 4 of puberty.

REFERENCE/SOURCE

- Sharma S. Growth: normal and abnormal. In: Gupta P, Menon PSN, Ramji S, Lodha R (Eds). PG Textbook of Pediatrics, 3rd edition. New Delhi: Jaypee Brothers Medical Publishers; 2022.

20. An 8-year-old girl (birth weight 2.7 kg) is brought with poor growth since 3 years of age. There is history of blood transfusion 1 year back (hemoglobin 7.2 g%). She was diagnosed as Celiac disease and continues to be on gluten-free diet (GFD). Her present weight is 14 kg (–3.11), height 108 cm (–2.71) and does not show a catch-up. Bone age is 6 years and thyroid function is normal. Which of the following is the next step in management?

A. Reassure for catch-up growth over 12 months
B. Perform GH stimulation test
C. Measure serum tissue transglutaminase levels
D. Perform upper gastrointestinal (GI) endoscopy

EXPLANATION

An underlying systemic disease like celiac disease with poor control can cause short stature. The index child was started on GFD over last year. Ideally, her weight and height should have shown a good catch-up with adequate management of the underlying disease. As she has not shown a good catch-up, she needs to be investigated for the underlying cause. Measurement of serum tissue transglutaminase will indicate the compliance to GFD and control of Celiac disease. An upper GI endoscopy is an invasive test and can be avoided to check compliance to GFD. She does not require a GH stimulation test at present as children with GHD are usually not GH deficient but have low IGF-1 levels because of underlying poor nutrition.

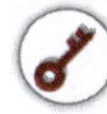

Key: C

BOOST YOUR KNOWLEDGE

Children with Celiac disease usually manifest with short stature. The causes include poor compliance to GFD that can cause anemia, hypoproteinemia, and micronutrient deficiencies that adversely affect growth. A small proportion may develop concomitant autoimmune conditions such as hypothyroidism and hepatitis that can adversely affect growth.

REFERENCES/SOURCES

- Husby S, Koletzko S, Korponay-Szabó I, Kurppa K, Mearin ML, Ribes-Koninckx C, et al. European Society Paediatric Gastroenterology, Hepatology and Nutrition Guidelines for Diagnosing Coeliac Disease 2020. J Pediatr Gastroenterol Nutr. 2020;70(1):141-56.
- Sharma S. Growth: normal and abnormal. In: Gupta P, Menon PSN, Ramji S, Lodha R (Eds). PG Textbook of Pediatrics, 3rd edition. New Delhi: Jaypee Brothers Medical Publishers; 2022.

CHAPTER

23.2 Thyroid Disorders

Tushar Godbole

1. A newborn baby, born by cesarean section to a primigravida without any history of thyroid disorders, is planned for discharge on Day 4. Baby is asymptomatic and feeding well, with no jaundice. What advice is correct?

A. Thyroid screening is only done for babies with history of maternal thyroid
B. Thyroid screening is recommended for this baby using thyroid-stimulating hormone (TSH) as the preferred test
C. High-risk babies such as small for gestational age (SGA), twins, and very low birth weight (VLBW) need thyroid screening soon after birth
D. Thyroid screening is not needed as the baby is asymptomatic

EXPLANATION

Congenital hypothyroid is a common disorder in India. It is one of the preventable causes of mental retardation if diagnosed early and treated on time. Congenital hypothyroid can happen in babies regardless of maternal thyroid status. Hence, universal newborn screening (NBS) is recommended for all babies. TSH-based testing is preferred in India. Either cord-blood or blood sample after 48–72 hours is preferred. High-risk babies such as SGA, twins, or premature babies have delayed TSH rise, hence TSH screening is done at a later date.

Key: B

BOOST YOUR KNOWLEDGE

Congenital hypothyroid is common in India than what is reported in the Western literature. Dysgenesis (congenital malformation) is the most common form, followed by dyshormonogenesis (genetic defect causing enzymatic block in the hormonogenesis pathway). Rarely, it could be a transient congenital hypothyroid caused by maternal drug exposure or maternal antibodies.

REFERENCES/SOURCES

- Desai MP, Sharma R, Riaz I, Sudhanshu S, Parikh R, Bhatia V. Newborn Screening Guidelines for Congenital Hypothyroidism in India: Recommendations of the Indian Society for Pediatric and Adolescent Endocrinology (ISPAE)—Part I: Screening and Confirmation of Diagnosis. Indian J Pediatr. 2018;85(6):440-7.
- Palani R. Hypothyroidism and thyroiditis. In: Gupta P, Menon PSN, Ramji S, Lodha R (Eds). PG Textbook of Pediatrics, 2nd edition. New Delhi: Jaypee Brothers Medical Publishers; 2018.

2. Which of the following is *not* a correct statement regarding the etiology of congenital hypothyroidism (CH)?

A. Most common cause is transplacental passage of maternal antibodies
B. Dyshormonogenesis can present as neonatal goiter
C. Maternal drug consumption can cause transient CH
D. Central hypothyroidism is much rare than the primary hypothyroidism

EXPLANATION

Most common cause of CH is dysgenesis (birth defect), and not maternal hypothyroid. Dyshormonogenesis causes accumulation of precursors of thyroid hormone due to chemical blockade, resulting in a goiter. This goiter can be detected antenatally, during neonatal period or sometimes during childhood. Fetal exposure to maternally consumed drugs such as carbimazole can cause transient but severe hypothyroid. Central hypothyroid, where TSH production is deficient, is much rare (1:15,000) as compared to primary congenital hypothyroid (1:1,200).

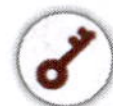

Key: A

BOOST YOUR KNOWLEDGE

Dysgenesis could be agenesis, hypoplasia, or ectopic gland such as lingual. Dyshormonogenesis is largely genetic and inherited autosomal recessively.

REFERENCES/SOURCES

- Desai MP, Sharma R, Riaz I, Sudhanshu S, Parikh R, Bhatia V. Newborn Screening Guidelines for Congenital Hypothyroidism in India: Recommendations of the Indian Society for Pediatric and Adolescent Endocrinology (ISPAE)—Part I: Screening and Confirmation of Diagnosis. Indian J Pediatr. 2018;85(6):440-7.
- Palani R. Hypothyroidism and thyroiditis. In: Gupta P, Menon PSN, Ramji S, Lodha R (Eds). PG Textbook of Pediatrics, 2nd edition. New Delhi: Jaypee Brothers Medical Publishers; 2018.

3. A NBS test was ordered for a neonate on Day 1 of life. All the parameters of the NBS were within normal limits, except TSH value that was 49 mIU/L. Which of the following is a correct statement?

A. A cut-off of TSH 20 at this day-of-life should be considered as screen positive
B. A TSH screen should not be performed on Day 1 of life
C. This baby needs immediate levothyroxine replacement to prevent mental retardation
D. A TSH below 20 can reliably rule out central hypothyroidism

EXPLANATION

There is a physiological TSH surge that starts within 30 minutes of birth and stays for first 72 hours of life. Hence NBS for congenital thyroid can be done by either cord-blood TSH or after 72 hours of life. It should not be done in first 24 hours. There is no defined cut-off at 24 hours of life. As per the Indian Society for Pediatric and Adolescent Endocrinology (ISPAE) guidelines, the cut-off for TSH screening between 24 and 48 hours is 34 mIU/L and 20 mIU/L for the cord-blood or 48–72 hours onward till 15 days of life. By TSH screening, one can only rule out primary congenital hypothyroid (problems with thyroid gland). Central hypothyroid cannot be picked up or ruled out by TSH screening. A screen positive should not be started on treatment, but should be confirmed by repeat venous sampling.

Key: B

BOOST YOUR KNOWLEDGE

Newborn screening is a cost-effective method of diagnosing and treating congenital conditions before they cause permanent damage. The idea is to treat the reports and not to wait for the symptoms. While cord blood is easy to procure without pricking the baby, samples collected after 72 hours could also be used for screening other feed-dependent diseases like phenylketonuria.

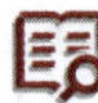

REFERENCES/SOURCES

- Desai MP, Sharma R, Riaz I, Sudhanshu S, Parikh R, Bhatia V. Newborn Screening Guidelines for Congenital Hypothyroidism in India: Recommendations of the Indian Society for Pediatric and Adolescent Endocrinology (ISPAE)—Part I: Screening and Confirmation of Diagnosis. Indian J Pediatr. 2018;85(6):440-7.
- Palani R. Hypothyroidism and thyroiditis. In: Gupta P, Menon PSN, Ramji S, Lodha R (Eds). PG Textbook of Pediatrics, 2nd edition. New Delhi: Jaypee Brothers Medical Publishers; 2018.

4. A 10-month-old infant is being evaluated for constipation. His growth and development are normal. A thyroid profile was ordered that showed a normal TSH with low total T3 and low total T4. The free T3 and free T4 levels were normal. Which of the statement best depicts the condition?

A. Constipation in this case is a strong predictor of hypothyroidism
B. A low total T4 with a normal TSH is an indicator of primary hypothyroidism
C. Urgent thyroid scan followed by treatment with levothyroxine is needed
D. This condition is likely to be X-linked inherited

EXPLANATION

Low total thyroid hormones and normal free thyroid hormones in an otherwise healthy child indicate thyroid-binding globulin (TBG) deficiency. TBG deficiency could be congenital or acquired due to liver or kidney disease. Congenital TBG deficiency (complete or partial) is X-linked inherited and a benign condition that does not need any further investigations or treatment as free thyroid hormones are within normal limits and are exerting their biologic action. As a result, TSH remains normal, indicating biochemical thyroid sufficiency. Constipation is the least consistent or reliable symptom of congenital hypothyroid, and could have many other reasons such as fiber-poor diet.

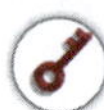

Key: D

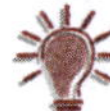

BOOST YOUR KNOWLEDGE

The manifestations of hypothyroidism such as constipation or dry skin are due to fall in the circulating free hormones. Total thyroid hormone is largely bound to TBG or albumin. In central hypothyroidism where the pituitary is at fault, the TSH may be normal, low or mildly elevated. It is the free hormone deficiency in central hypothyroid that cause the biochemical effects.

REFERENCES/SOURCES

- Kliegman RM, St Geme JW, Blum NJ, Shah SS, Tasker RC, Wilson KM. Nelson Textbook of Pediatrics, 21st edition. Philadelphia: Elsevier; 2019.
- Palani R. Hypothyroidism and thyroiditis. In: Gupta P, Menon PSN, Ramji S, Lodha R (Eds). PG Textbook of Pediatrics, 2nd edition. New Delhi: Jaypee Brothers Medical Publishers; 2018.

5. A 13-years-old girl is referred with slowing of growth from last 2 years. On examination, she has dry skin and goiter which is recent onset. Her thyroid profile shows a total T4 of 4.5 μg/dL (range 5–12) and TSH of >150 mIU/L (range 0.3–5.0). Which of the following will *not* be found in this patient?

A. Soft goiter
B. Family history of thyroid disease
C. High serum prolactin levels
D. Delay in bone age

EXPLANATION

Autoimmune hypothyroidism is the most common cause of acquired hypothyroidism. Common in girls than boys, they often have a history of affected blood relative. The goiter is firm, nontender with rubbery consistency. Long-standing cases have delayed bone age. Elevated prolactin levels are common in pubertal girls as the elevated thyrotropin-releasing hormone (TRH) also acts on prolactin. Some of them can also have galactorrhea.

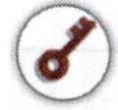

Key: **A**

BOOST YOUR KNOWLEDGE

Congenital hypothyroid such as dyshormonogenesis can sometimes present later, during childhood. Goiter in dyshormonogenesis is large, very soft to touch and nontender. It is a slow growing goiter that gets detected in childhood, but the severe varieties may present during the neonatal or antenatal age as well.

REFERENCES/SOURCES

- Kliegman RM, St Geme JW, Blum NJ, Shah SS, Tasker RC, Wilson KM. Nelson Textbook of Pediatrics, 21st edition. Philadelphia: Elsevier; 2019.
- Palani R. Hypothyroidism and thyroiditis. In: Gupta P, Menon PSN, Ramji S, Lodha R (Eds). PG Textbook of Pediatrics, 2nd edition. New Delhi: Jaypee Brothers Medical Publishers; 2018.

6. A neonate is born with a large goiter. Which of the following is *not* a correct statement?

A. Congenital goiter can present with respiratory distress necessitating urgent surgery
B. Maternal overtreatment with antithyroid drugs is a cause
C. Hearing test should be performed to rule out sensorineural deafness
D. Dysgenesis is a common cause of neonatal goiter

EXPLANATION

Neonatal goiter can happen due to block in fetal thyroid hormone genesis due to either enzymatic deficiency or exposure to maternally consumed antithyroid drugs. It is sometimes detected on antenatal fetal ultrasound or noticed during/immediately after the birth. Large goiters can sometimes cause difficult labor and respiratory distress due to neck position and sometimes need urgent surgery. Pendred syndrome, a cause of neonatal goiter has associated sensorineural deafness. Dyshormonogenesis (enzymatic block), not dysgenesis (birth defect), is a common cause of neonatal goiter. Dysgenesis (defective structural development of thyroid gland) can have absent or ectopic gland instead of goiter. Replacement with thyroxine is the treatment for neonatal goiter in all cases except neonatal Graves' disease.

Key: **D**

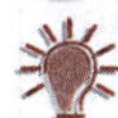

BOOST YOUR KNOWLEDGE

Pendred syndrome is caused by mutations in the *SLC26A4* gene. Although goiter in such cases can occur at birth, most of them get noticed later in life.

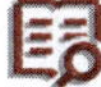

REFERENCES/SOURCES

- Kliegman RM, St Geme JW, Blum NJ, Shah SS, Tasker RC, Wilson KM. Nelson Textbook of Pediatrics, 21st edition. Philadelphia: Elsevier; 2019.
- Palani R. Hypothyroidism and thyroiditis. In: Gupta P, Menon PSN, Ramji S, Lodha R (Eds). PG Textbook of Pediatrics, 2nd edition. New Delhi: Jaypee Brothers Medical Publishers; 2018.

7. A neonate is diagnosed with congenital hypothyroid and is about to be started on levothyroxine supplementation. Which of the sentences best depicts the management?

A. Thyroid replacement is started at the lowest possible dose to prevent arrhythmias and tremors
B. Thyroxine is replaced in three divided doses, preferably before the feeding time
C. Avoid giving iron and calcium supplementations together with thyroxine
D. Watchful expectancy is mainstay, and treatment is given only when symptomatic

EXPLANATION

Congenital hypothyroid is a medical emergency and needs urgent treatment. Levothyroxine should be given at 10–15 µg/kg/day as a single dose dissolved in mother's milk. Lower the T4 levels, higher the initial dose (to protect brain). Lower starting doses are preferred in long-standing acquired hypothyroidism to prevent arrhythmias and tremors. As iron, protein, and soy protein may hamper with its absorption, when given concomitantly with thyroxine.

Key: C

BOOST YOUR KNOWLEDGE

On follow-up, the T4 has to be normalized by 2 weeks and TSH by 4 weeks. Later, the babies can be monitored every 2 monthly till 6 months, every 3 monthly till 3 years and 3–6 monthly thereafter till completion of growth and puberty. Low initial serum T4 levels are associated with poor cognitive functions.

REFERENCE/SOURCE

- Sudhanshu S, Riaz I, Sharma R, Desai MP, Parikh R, Bhatia V. Newborn Screening Guidelines for Congenital Hypothyroidism in India: Recommendations of the Indian Society for Pediatric and Adolescent Endocrinology (ISPAE)—Part II: Imaging, Treatment and Follow-up. Indian J Pediatr. 2018;85(6):448-53.

8. A 9-year-old girl comes to outpatient department (OPD) with recurrent off and on swelling in the thyroid region along with redness, fever, and pain. Examination shows a tender fluctuant thyroid swelling. Which of the following is the next *best* step in management?

A. Thyroid scan
B. Antibiotics and surgical drainage
C. Carbimazole and propranolol
D. Radioiodine ablation

EXPLANATION

Recurrent painful thyroid swelling is likely to be an abscess due to acute suppurative thyroiditis. Underlying pyriform sinus fistula and remnant of thyroglossal duct are likely causes. The causative organisms are often of a mixed flora. Ultrasound can show collected pus, but a CT scan after subsidence of the infection may visualize the underlying fistulous tract. Surgical drainage is preferred treatment for abscess, and removal of underlying fistulous tract prevents its recurrence. Radioiodine ablation is the treatment for hyperfunctioning gland such as Graves' disease, and has got no role in suppurative thyroiditis.

Key: B

BOOST YOUR KNOWLEDGE

Acute suppurative thyroiditis often happens after upper respiratory infection. Common causes are alpha-hemolytic streptococci, *Staphylococcus aureus* followed by gram negative and anaerobic organisms. Immunocompromised individuals can have mycobacterial, fungal, and other opportunists.

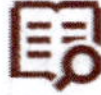

REFERENCE/SOURCE

- Kliegman RM, St Geme JW, Blum NJ, Shah SS, Tasker RC, Wilson KM. Nelson Textbook of Pediatrics, 21st edition. Philadelphia: Elsevier; 2019.

9. A neonate, born of consanguineous union, was screened positive for TSH on cord-blood. Repeat venipuncture on Day 7 showed a T4 value of 7 µg/dL and TSH of 56 mIU/L. Her elder sister also has CH. There are no other associated congenital malformations. What is the correct statement about her radioimaging?

A. Treatment should be deferred till starting of thyroid nuclear scan
B. Ultrasound of neck will show hypoplastic thyroid gland
C. Technetium scan will show reduced thyroid uptake
D. If scan is not done at diagnosis, it can be done at 3 years of age by stopping the tablets for 4 weeks

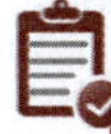

EXPLANATION

Congenital hypothyroidism is a medical emergency that needs early diagnosis and prompt treatment. Nonavailability of scan should not delay the beginning of therapy. Scan can be done until 7 days of starting tablets. If not done immediately, it can be done at third birthday after stopping the tablet for 4 weeks. With consanguineous union and sibling affection, the diagnosis is likely to be dyshormonogenesis (which is autosomal recessive). Dyshormonogenesis shall have enlarged gland that can be seen clinically, or on ultrasound. Technetium scan will show normal to high uptake. Low uptake is seen in hypoplasia. Transcription factor defects are also autosomal recessive causes of CH, but they are often associated with other anomalies such as cleft lip/palate, cardiac, or skeletal defects.

Key: D

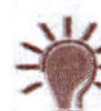

BOOST YOUR KNOWLEDGE

Drug-induced hypothyroid can happen if the pregnant female is being overtreated with antithyroid drugs like propylthiouracil or carbimazole.

REFERENCES/SOURCES

- Palani R. Hypothyroidism and thyroiditis. In: Gupta P, Menon PSN, Ramji S, Lodha R (Eds). PG Textbook of Pediatrics, 2nd edition. New Delhi: Jaypee Brothers Medical Publishers; 2018.
- Sudhanshu S, Riaz I, Sharma R, Desai MP, Parikh R, Bhatia V. Newborn Screening Guidelines for Congenital Hypothyroidism in India: Recommendations of the Indian Society for Pediatric and Adolescent Endocrinology (ISPAE)—Part II: Imaging, Treatment and Follow-up. Indian J Pediatr. 2018;85(6):448-53.

10. A 9-year-old girl has been recently noticed to have a grade II goiter during her routine OPD visit for minor ailments. The goiter is painless, without difficulty in deglutition. She has short stature but is otherwise healthy. Paternal aunt suffers from hypothyroidism. Which is of the statements is *correct*?

A. Despite best treatment, she is likely to remain very short
B. The condition is likely to be caused by T cell-mediated destruction
C. She is likely to have subnormal scholastic performance
D. Thyroid peroxidase (TPO) antibodies are negative

EXPLANATION

Chronic lymphocytic thyroiditis or autoimmune hypothyroid is the common form of thyroid disorder in children beyond infancy. Typically happens around the beginning of puberty, it is common in females. A family history is common. If onset is beyond 3 years of life, brain development and school performance are normal.

Although the destruction is T cell-mediated, antibody positivity is corollary and is a proof toward autoimmune origin. If detected on time and treated well, they can have a normal final height.

Key: B

BOOST YOUR KNOWLEDGE

Graves' disease and simple colloid goiter are other common causes of goiter in a child/adolescent.

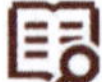

REFERENCES/SOURCES

- Kliegman RM, St Geme JW, Blum NJ, Shah SS, Tasker RC, Wilson KM. Nelson Textbook of Pediatrics, 21st edition. Philadelphia: Elsevier; 2019.
- Palani R. Hypothyroidism and thyroiditis. In: Gupta P, Menon PSN, Ramji S, Lodha R (Eds). PG Textbook of Pediatrics, 2nd edition. New Delhi: Jaypee Brothers Medical Publishers; 2018.

11. A 12-years-old boy has been diagnosed with a painless goiter. He has tachycardia, systolic hypertension, and has documented weight loss. Which of the following is a correct statement?

A. This condition is common in males
B. This thyroid condition is curable in many cases
C. The underlying pathology is T cell-mediated destruction of thyroid gland
D. Thyroid nuclear scan shows reduced uptake

EXPLANATION

This is an adolescent boy with symptoms of hyperthyroidism and painless goiter. Graves' disease being the most common cause, is antibody mediated. Along with many other thyroid disorders, Graves' disease is common in females. Being a hyperfunctioning gland, it shows up brightly on a nuclear scan (increased uptake). Around 30–40% have remission within 2 years of starting of antithyroid medications. Longer therapies achieve higher remission rates. Subacute thyroiditis is sudden onset, painful, and shows a reduced radiouptake on a nuclear scan.

Key: B

BOOST YOUR KNOWLEDGE

Graves' disease is a genetically mediated disorder that has human leukocyte antigen (HLA) predilection. Other autoimmune conditions such as type 1 diabetes mellitus (DM), Addison's disease, systemic lupus erythematosus, and genetic conditions such as Down's syndrome, and DiGeorge syndrome are associated with Graves' disease.

REFERENCES/SOURCES

- Kliegman RM, St Geme JW, Blum NJ, Shah SS, Tasker RC, Wilson KM. Nelson Textbook of Pediatrics, 21st edition. Philadelphia: Elsevier; 2019.
- Palani R. Hypothyroidism and thyroiditis. In: Gupta P, Menon PSN, Ramji S, Lodha R (Eds). PG Textbook of Pediatrics, 2nd edition. New Delhi: Jaypee Brothers Medical Publishers; 2018.

12. Which of the following statements is correct about radioactive elements and their role in managing thyroid disorders?

A. Technetium 99m pertechnetate is trapped and organified by thyroid gland
B. Iodine 131 (^{131}I) is used for thyroid scans due to its shorter half-life

C. Perchlorate discharge test is useful for diagnosis in suspected dyshormonogenesis
D. Iodine 123 (^{123}I) has got high radiation exposure and yield low quality scintigraphs

EXPLANATION

Nuclear isotopes are used for diagnosis of CH, thyroid nodules, and hyperthyroidism. Technetium 99m pertechnetate and ^{123}I are both having short half-lives, low radiation exposure, and high-quality imaging, thus making them suitable for diagnostic procedures. Technetium is easily available in India, while ^{123}I is not. Technetium is taken-up by the gland but not organified, hence perchlorate discharge is employed for diagnosis of organification defects in cases of dyshormonogenesis. ^{131}I is having longer half-life of 8 days and higher cytotoxic effect, making it suitable for radio-ablation as a therapy.

Key: C

BOOST YOUR KNOWLEDGE

Radio-ablation using ^{131}I is one of the therapies for Graves' disease. The contraindications being large goiters, presence of orbitopathy and age below 5 years.

REFERENCES/SOURCES

- Kliegman RM, St Geme JW, Blum NJ, Shah SS, Tasker RC, Wilson KM. Nelson Textbook of Pediatrics, 21st edition. Philadelphia: Elsevier; 2019.
- Palani R. Hypothyroidism and thyroiditis. In: Gupta P, Menon PSN, Ramji S, Lodha R (Eds). PG Textbook of Pediatrics, 2nd edition. New Delhi: Jaypee Brothers Medical Publishers; 2018.

13. A 13-year-old boy comes with a painless neck swelling of insidious onset. It is a nodular swelling with firm consistency; and moves with deglutition. Thyroid profile is normal. Which of the following statements is correct?

A. Ultrasound examination helps only if thyroid profile is abnormal
B. Fine-needle aspiration cytology (FNAC) is risky in thyroid swelling and should be avoided
C. Firm consistency with areas of calcifications is suggestive of autoimmune thyroid disorder
D. Papillary thyroid carcinoma (PTC) could be a differential diagnosis

EXPLANATION

Ultrasound is the first step in evaluating thyroid swelling with a normal thyroid profile. FNAC, particularly ultrasound guided, is recommended if the nodules are >1 cm is size. Goiter in autoimmune thyroid is diffuse. Nodular goiter with firm consistency, associated with lymph nodes, hoarse voice, and dysphagia should raise suspicion about malignancy. Cervical metastasis is common in thyroid malignancies.

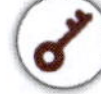

Key: D

BOOST YOUR KNOWLEDGE

Most of the thyroid nodules in pediatric age group are benign. PTC is most common thyroid malignancy in adolescents. Follicular and medullary being the second and third common.

REFERENCES/SOURCES

- Kliegman RM, St Geme JW, Blum NJ, Shah SS, Tasker RC, Wilson KM. Nelson Textbook of Pediatrics, 21st edition. Philadelphia: Elsevier; 2019.
- Palani R. Hypothyroidism and thyroiditis. In: Gupta P, Menon PSN, Ramji S, Lodha R (Eds). PG Textbook of Pediatrics, 2nd edition. New Delhi: Jaypee Brothers Medical Publishers; 2018.

14. A neonate is born to a mother with history of Graves' disease. She had undergone radioiodine ablation 2 years ago, and is on thyroid replacement since then. Her thyroid reports were normal throughout pregnancy. Which of the following statements is *correct*?

A. Neonate is likely to go into CH
B. Neonate is unlikely to suffer from neonatal Graves' disease because mother is a cured case
C. The neonate will present with macrocephaly and hypotonia
D. The possible thyroid disease in this neonate is likely to get better in 6–12 weeks

EXPLANATION

Mothers with Graves' disease can have persisting TSH receptor-stimulating antibodies (TRSAb) long after they have undergone radio-ablation or thyroidectomy. Typical symptoms of hyperthyroid start in the neonate soon after birth. If the mother is on antithyroid medicines, the symptoms appear after 3–5 days postdelivery. Rarely, if there are mixed (stimulating and blocking) antibodies, the presentation of neonatal Graves' disease may be delayed by a few weeks. Neonatal Graves' disease is a transient condition that gets better with washing off of the maternally acquired antibodies. Transient form of congenital hypothyroid may happen in children born to hypothyroid mothers, not Graves' disease.

Key: D

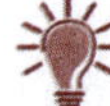

BOOST YOUR KNOWLEDGE

Neonatal Graves' disease can present with prematurity, intrauterine growth restriction (IUGR), goiter at birth, hyperthermia, periorbital edema, irritability, diarrhea, tachycardia, and heart failure. If not treated on time, some of them can have microcephaly due to premature suture closure.

REFERENCES/SOURCES

- Kliegman RM, St Geme JW, Blum NJ, Shah SS, Tasker RC, Wilson KM. Nelson Textbook of Pediatrics, 21st edition. Philadelphia: Elsevier; 2019.
- Palani R. Hypothyroidism and thyroiditis. In: Gupta P, Menon PSN, Ramji S, Lodha R (Eds). PG Textbook of Pediatrics, 2nd edition. New Delhi: Jaypee Brothers Medical Publishers; 2018.

15. A 10-year-old boy has been having pyrexia of unknown origin, diarrhea, palpitations, and weight loss over last 2 months. On examination, he has tachycardia, bounding pulse, mild goiter, and sweaty skin. Which of the following treatment is correct?

A. This is physiological (puberty) goiter. Blood culture for brucellosis needs to be ordered
B. Anti-TPO peroxidase antibody is likely to hint at the diagnosis
C. Longer duration of therapy is associated with higher remission rates
D. Propylthiouracil is preferred therapy, with duration around 2 years

EXPLANATION

This is classic depiction of pediatric Graves' disease. Puberty goiter is often felt on palpation in thin and otherwise healthy pubertal children. The antibody to be ordered is anti-TSH receptor antibody and not anti-TPO antibody. Drug therapy is initial preferred therapy with carbimazole or methimazole being the first choices. Propylthiouracil is hepatotoxic and not a preferred drug except for first trimester pregnancy. Longer duration is associated with higher remission rates. Studies have treated children with these drugs between 4 and 10 years.

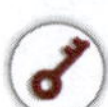

Key: C

BOOST YOUR KNOWLEDGE

Mild skin rash and itching is a common side effect of antithyroid drugs. Asymptomatic granulocytopenia is common with methimazole and is not a reason to discontinue medicines. Agranulocytosis is rare and can present with fever, oral ulcers, and pharyngitis. Cholestatic jaundice, glomerulonephritis, and lupus-like reaction are also reported with methimazole, while severe hepatitis and hepatic failure is reported with propylthiouracil.

REFERENCES/SOURCES

- Kliegman RM, St Geme JW, Blum NJ, Shah SS, Tasker RC, Wilson KM. Nelson Textbook of Pediatrics, 21st edition. Philadelphia: Elsevier; 2019.
- Palani R. Hypothyroidism and thyroiditis. In: Gupta P, Menon PSN, Ramji S, Lodha R (Eds). PG Textbook of Pediatrics, 2nd edition. New Delhi: Jaypee Brothers Medical Publishers; 2018.

16. **A 9-year-old boy was detected to have a thyroid swelling by the pediatrician during routine visit. On palpation, it was a single nodule in the left lobe of thyroid. Which of the following statement is *correct*?**

A. Parents need to be counseled that most pediatric thyroid nodules are benign

B. A solid hypoechoic nodule on ultrasound is low risk for malignancy

C. A solid-cystic lesion on ultrasound with diameter >2 cm does not need FNAC

D. A nodule with suppressed TSH does not need nuclear imaging

EXPLANATION

Unlike adults, most thyroid nodules in pediatric age are benign. They may be colloid swellings, adenomatous swellings or cysts. Thyroid function test and ultrasonography are the next tests to be ordered. A cystic lesion is low risk for malignancy, whereas solid lesions with hypoechoic areas are high risk. A cystic lesion with solid component >2 cm deserves FNAC. Lesions associated with firm consistency, pain, voice change, and history of neck radiation deserve FNAC regardless of their size.

Key: A

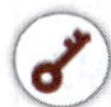

BOOST YOUR KNOWLEDGE

Ultrasound features such as solid lesions with irregular margins, calcifications, extrathyroidal extensions, or associated lymph nodes are high risk for malignancy.

REFERENCE/SOURCE

- Kliegman RM, St Geme JW, Blum NJ, Shah SS, Tasker RC, Wilson KM. Nelson Textbook of Pediatrics, 21st edition. Philadelphia: Elsevier; 2019.

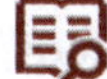

17. **A 15-years-old girl presented with sudden onset thyroid swelling that was firm on palpation. Ultrasound shows solid hypoechoic nodule with lymph nodes. Which of the following best depicts the condition?**

A. Medullary thyroid cancer is most likely pathology

B. Calcitonin and carcinoembryonic antigen (CEA) are biomarkers of follicular neoplasia

C. FNAC is likely to miss the diagnosis of papillary thyroid cancer

D. Recurrence after thyroidectomy is treated with radioiodine

EXPLANATION

Papillary thyroid cancer is the most common variety in children. Being a well-differentiated malignancy, the nuclear atypia is evident on FNAC, confirming the diagnosis. Surgery is the mainstay treatment but recurrence is common. Recurrence is amenable to radioiodine therapy. Medullary thyroid cancer is the third most common malignancy (follicular being second) and tumor markers such as calcitonin and CEA are used for diagnosis and monitoring of therapy.

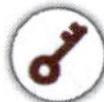

Key: D

BOOST YOUR KNOWLEDGE

Medullary thyroid cancer could be familial and as a part of the multiple endocrine neoplasia 2 (MEN2).

REFERENCE/SOURCE

- Kliegman RM, St Geme JW, Blum NJ, Shah SS, Tasker RC, Wilson KM. Nelson Textbook of Pediatrics, 21st edition. Philadelphia: Elsevier; 2019.

18. A 14-years-old girl was operated for thyroid nodule and histopathology has confirmed the diagnosis of PTC. Which of the following statements is *correct* about her condition?

A. PTC is a slow growing tumor and metastasis is very rare
B. Thyroid sparing surgeries such as lobectomy or local resection are preferred in growing age
C. Thyroglobulin antibody levels need to be monitored along with thyroglobulin on follow-up
D. Prognosis is poor, with 5-year survival rate <30%

EXPLANATION

Papillary thyroid carcinoma is the most common thyroid malignancy in pediatric age. Intrathyroidal spread is common, necessitating near-total thyroidectomy and not thyroid sparing surgeries. Local lymph node spread and pulmonary metastasis is common at diagnosis. Despite metastasis, they are amenable to radioiodine therapy and multiple sessions may be needed on long-term follow-up. Most PTCs have excellent prognosis and many are able to achieve cure, while others can live long with stable cancer burden. Thyroglobulin is a biochemical marker of residual tumor and needs to be monitored periodically. Thyroglobulin antibody may coexist and make thyroglobulin interpretation inaccurate. Hence, they need to be monitored together.

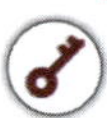

Key: C

BOOST YOUR KNOWLEDGE

Most of the thyroid tumor cells are well differentiated, and grow with TSH. Hence, patients are treated with a slightly higher dose of levothyroxine after surgery, with the idea of suppressing TSH. Levothyroxine replacement is stopped for some time before radiotherapy, so that the cancer cells respond to TSH and take up radioiodine.

REFERENCE/SOURCE

- Kliegman RM, St Geme JW, Blum NJ, Shah SS, Tasker RC, Wilson KM. Nelson Textbook of Pediatrics, 21st edition. Philadelphia: Elsevier; 2019.

19. An 8-year-old girl has presented with abdominal distention, constipation, dry skin, and pendular knee jerks. She is short, has breast development Tanner stage 2, no pubic or axillary hair, with irregular menses. Which of the following statement is correct about her condition?

A. Pelvic ultrasound is likely to show normal ovaries
B. Serum prolactin levels are normal
C. Serum sodium may be elevated
D. Serum cholesterol and triglycerides can be elevated

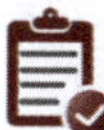

EXPLANATION

This is a clinical picture of long-standing hypothyroidism. With prolonged exposure to high levels of TSH, ovaries become enlarged and cystic. A peculiar condition called Van Wyk–Grumbach syndrome is seen due to specificity spillover and TSH acting on the follicle-stimulating hormone (FSH) receptors. This "pseudoprecocious puberty" is characterized by delayed bone age and precocious puberty with altered sequence of puberty. Hyponatremia (not hyper) and dyslipidemia are consistent features of long-standing hypothyroidism. Prolactin levels are often elevated in primary hypothyroidism as a result of elevated TRH acting on both thyrotrope and lactotrope cells.

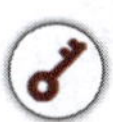

Key: D

BOOST YOUR KNOWLEDGE

Elevated creatine phosphokinase along with pseudohypertrophy and proximal myopathy can also happen in long-standing hypothyroidism.

REFERENCES/SOURCES

- Kliegman RM, St Geme JW, Blum NJ, Shah SS, Tasker RC, Wilson KM. Nelson Textbook of Pediatrics, 21st edition. Philadelphia: Elsevier; 2019.
- Palani R. Hypothyroidism and thyroiditis. In: Gupta P, Menon PSN, Ramji S, Lodha R (Eds). PG Textbook of Pediatrics, 2nd edition. New Delhi: Jaypee Brothers Medical Publishers; 2018.

CHAPTER

23.3 Diabetes Mellitus

Deepika Harit

1. A 6-year-old asymptomatic girl was asked to get screened for diabetes by the endocrinologist who is treating her sibling who was diagnosed with type 1 diabetes (T1D) years ago. Her investigations are as follows: Fasting blood glucose (FBG): 98 mg/dL, blood glucose (BG) after 2 hours of oral glucose tolerance test (OGTT): 148 mg/dL, insulin autoantibodies (IAAs): positive, islet cell antibodies (ICAs): positive, glutamic acid decarboxylase (GAD) antibody: negative, zinc transporter 8 autoantibody (ZnT8A): negative, and hemoglobin A1c (HbA1c): 5%. What is the interpretation of these tests?

A. Stage 1 diabetes
B. Stage 2 diabetes
C. Stage 3 diabetes
D. Stage 4 diabetes

EXPLANATION

The type 1 diabetes (T1D) staging has been divided into four stages depending on the presence/absence of clinical symptoms of diabetes, autoantibodies, and BG levels.

	Stage 1	*Stage 2*	*Stage 3*	*Stage 4*
Blood glucose	Normal	Abnormal [impaired glucose tolerance/ impaired fasting glucose (IGT/IFG)]	Abnormal	Long-standing T1D
Autoantibodies	≥2	≥2	≥2	
Clinical symptoms	Nil	Nil	Clinical diagnosis	

Key: B

BOOST YOUR KNOWLEDGE

Type 1 diabetes is an autoimmune disorder characterized by dysglycemia. Four antibodies are implicated in its pathogenesis: Antibody GAD, ICAs, insulinoma-associated-2 autoantibodies (IA-2A), which is more common in children than adults, ZnT8A. Antibodies are usually present even before the overt diabetes develops and thus screening of the siblings is recommended to know who is at risk. The risk of developing diabetes varies in different individuals, the more the number of antibodies present, the more is the lifetime risk of developing diabetes. Though very small percentage of people may not develop clinical diabetes ever despite the presence of autoantibodies. IAAs are usually the first to appear, followed by GAD antibody, and later IA2A and ZnT8A. The earliest antibodies are predominantly immunoglobulin G (IgG) class.

REFERENCES/SOURCES

- Besser REJ, Bell KJ, Couper JJ, Ziegler AG, Wherrett DK, Knip M, et al. ISPAD clinical practice consensus guidelines 2022: Stages of type 1 diabetes in children and adolescents. Pediatr Diabetes. 2022;23(8):1175-87.
- Kliegman RM, St Geme JW, Blum NJ, Shah SS, Tasker RC, Wilson KM. Nelson Textbook of Pediatrics, 21st edition. Philadelphia: Elsevier; 2019.

2. Which of the following drugs can be administered to the index 6-year-old girl in the Question 1?

A. Metformin
B. Corticosteroids
C. Teplizumab
D. Glargine

EXPLANATION

This child is in stage 2 T1D and recently teplizumab has been approved by the Food and Drug Administration (FDA) in this group of patients. Teplizumab is a 150 kD humanized monoclonal antibody (mAb) that binds to the epsilon chain of the CD3 protein (CD3ε), a cell surface antigen presents on T-lymphocytes.

Key: C

BOOST YOUR KNOWLEDGE

The US-FDA approved teplizumab injection to delay the onset of stage 3 T1D in adults and pediatric patients 8 years and older who currently have stage 2 T1D. This is the first disease-modifying therapy in humans that preserves beta cell function in patients with early, stage 2 disease who are at risk of developing stage 3 clinical T1D. It has been seen to delay the progression for up to 2 years.

Side effects of teplizumab include reversible lymphopenia and mild cytokine release. A decline in total lymphocyte count is generally observed over the first 5 days of dosing and begins to resolve on Day 6 despite continued dosing.

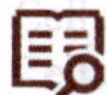

REFERENCE/SOURCE

- Hirsch JS. FDA approves teplizumab: a milestone in type 1 diabetes. Lancet Diabetes Endocrinol. 2023;11(1):18. doi: 10.1016/S2213-8587(22)00351-5. Epub 2022 Nov 24.

3. A 16-year-old boy with a body mass index (BMI) of 30 kg/m^2 has been diagnosed with type 2 diabetes 1 year ago. He has been under regular follow-up and compliant with the metformin therapy (1 g OD). However, he exercises infrequently and consumes a lot of junk food. There has been no improvement in the BMI over past 1 year and his recent HbA1c is 9.2%. What will be the appropriate approach to the management of this patient?

A. Continue same treatment and counsel for lifestyle modification
B. Increase the dose of metformin and lifestyle modification
C. Start the patient on pramlintide injections
D. Start the patient on insulin injections

EXPLANATION

With a HbA1c of >9%, patient must be started on Insulin injection like T1D patients. Once the BG is controlled, patients can be managed with lifestyle modifications and oral hypoglycemic agents.

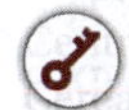

Key: D

BOOST YOUR KNOWLEDGE

Pramlintide is approved for use in the United States and is indicated for patients with type 1 or type 2 diabetes who take mealtime insulin. Pramlintide can be considered when despite efforts with optimized insulin treatment, patients who are ≥18 years old and are unable to achieve recommended glycemic targets. Pramlintide is an analog of islet amyloid polypeptide (IAPP), which is a peptide that is cosecreted with insulin by the beta cells and delays gastric emptying, suppresses glucagon, and possibly suppress food intake.

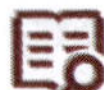

REFERENCE/SOURCE

- Kliegman RM, St Geme JW, Blum NJ, Shah SS, Tasker RC, Wilson KM. Nelson Textbook of Pediatrics, 21st edition. Philadelphia: Elsevier; 2019.

4. A 6-day-old girl is admitted in neonatal intensive care unit (NICU) with complaints of poor feeding, irritability, and dehydration. Investigations revealed hyperglycemia with glucosuria, there was no ketosis. The BG remained above 350 mg/dL despite complete rehydration. The patient started on insulin infusion with intravenous (IV) fluid therapy. What would be the best next approach?

A. Genetic testing should be done
B. Start the patient on oral glibenclamide
C. Counsel the patient that the child will require insulin lifelong injections
D. Start the patient on metformin

EXPLANATION

This patient has neonatal diabetes (ND) mellitus which could be either transient or permanent. All patients of ND should undergo genetic testing ASAP because approximately 50% of the neonates have K^+ channel mutation related to *KCNJ11* gene. Patients with K^+ channel mutation can be easily managed on oral sulfonylureas like glibenclamide.

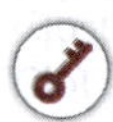

Key: A

BOOST YOUR KNOWLEDGE

Neonatal diabetes is transient in ~50% of the cases. All patients with ND will initially be managed on insulin and IV fluids during the active phase of diabetes. Once their BG is stabilized, insulin injections are started. A switch to glibenclamide is initiated depending on the genetic mutations. Doses of glibenclamide range from 0.4 to 1 mg/kg/day. It is recommended that all children developing diabetes before 6 months of age must get a genetic testing done. Some experts even recommend that all patients diagnosed with diabetes under 1 year of age should undergo genetic testing.

REFERENCE/SOURCE

- Kliegman RM, St Geme JW, Blum NJ, Shah SS, Tasker RC, Wilson KM. Nelson Textbook of Pediatrics, 21st edition. Philadelphia: Elsevier; 2019.

5. An 8-year-old child with T1D who is on multiple daily injections (MDIs) of glargine and lispro is not well. He is having fever, cough, cold, poor appetite, and frequent vomiting for past 16 hours. What should be the ideal approach to manage a child during sickness?

A. Check the BG frequently, stop insulin, and give insulin injections only when the child stops vomiting and starts eating
B. Check BG and urine ketones every 2–4 hourly and continue with the insulin injections as before
C. Check the BG and urinary/blood ketones frequently, continue glargine, and give correction doses of lispro every 1–2 hourly
D. Admit the patient for IV insulin therapy

EXPLANATION

Children with T1D can be easily managed at home during sick days. Whenever older children fall sick, they tend to develop hyperglycemia despite not eating anything (due to the release of counter regulatory hormones). Therefore, one must continue with the basal long-acting insulin as before. Ketones should be checked frequently at home (either in urine/blood).

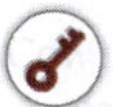 **Key: C**

 **BOOST YOUR KNOWLEDGE**

- *If the urinary ketones are nil-small:* Give rapid-acting insulin correction doses every 2 hours. If the BG is >250 mg/dL, check ketones in every other void.
- *If urinary ketones are moderate-large:* Give rapid acting insulin correction doses every 1 hour. If the BG is >250 mg/dL, check ketones in each void. If BG is >250 mg/dL, give plain fluids (sugar free). If BG is <250 mg/dL, give sugar-containing fluids.

REFERENCE/SOURCE

- Kliegman RM, St Geme JW, Blum NJ, Shah SS, Tasker RC, Wilson KM. Nelson Textbook of Pediatrics, 21st edition. Philadelphia: Elsevier; 2019.

6. A 2-year-old girl came to outpatient department (OPD) with a history of frequent urination, increased thirst, and weight loss for past 1 month. The mother has T1D and is well controlled on MDIs. The mother of the child is apprehensive and wants to know if her child has diabetes too? What investigation/s will you do to confirm the diagnosis?

A. FBG and postprandial BG by glucometer
B. HbA1c
C. OGTT
D. Fasting plasma glucose (FPG), postprandial plasma glucose, and HbA1c

 **EXPLANATION**

The T1D can be diagnosed if any of the following is abnormal: FPG, postprandial plasma glucose, and HbA1c. A formal plasma glucose measurement is required to confirm the diagnosis using an analyzer rather than a glucometer.

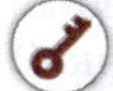 **Key: D**

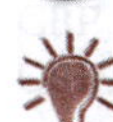 **BOOST YOUR KNOWLEDGE**

For diagnosis any of the following is required:

- Classic symptoms of diabetes or hyperglycemic crisis with plasma glucose concentration 200 mg/dL or
- FPG ≥7.0 mmol/L (≥126 mg/dL) or
- 2-hour postload glucose ≥11.1 mmol/L (≥200 mg/dL) during an OGTT or
- HbA1c ≥6.5%

The HbA1c value <6.5% does not exclude diabetes diagnosed using glucose tests. The role of HbA1c alone in diagnosis of T1D in children is unclear. HbA1c can be used as a diagnostic test for diabetes, in particular to test for prediabetes or type 2 diabetes in youth when done in standardized laboratories.

REFERENCE/SOURCE

- Libman I, Haynes A, Lyons S, Pradeep P, Rwagasor E, Tung JYL, et al. ISPAD Clinical Practice Consensus Guidelines 2022: Definition, epidemiology, and classification of diabetes in children and adolescents. Pediatr Diabetes. 2022;23(8):1160-74.

7. Which of the following is *not* a contraindication to high intensity exercise in a child with T1D?

A. Proliferative retinopathy
B. Urinary ketones ≥2+
C. Severe hypoglycemia in preceding 24 hours
D. Inability to wear continuous glucose monitoring (CGM)

EXPLANATION

Inability to wear CGM is not a contraindication to doing high intensity exercises in T1D. If a T1D person has proliferative retinopathy, he/she should not be doing high intensity exercise as it may worsen the retinopathy. If urine ketones are ≥2+, all forms of exercise need to be postponed until the ketones normalize. Exercise is also contraindicated if the child had episode of severe hypoglycemia within the previous 24 hours because antecedent severe hypoglycemia impairs the hormonal counter-regulatory response during exercise and increases the risk for recurrent hypoglycemia.

Key: D

BOOST YOUR KNOWLEDGE

Exercise is also contraindicated in the presence of injury or acute infection.

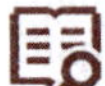

REFERENCE/SOURCE

- Adolfsson P, Taplin CE, Zaharieva DP, Pemberton J, Davis EA, Riddell MC, et al. ISPAD Clinical Practice Consensus Guidelines 2022: Exercise in children and adolescents with diabetes. Pediatr Diabetes. 2022;23(8):1341-72.

8. What is the ideal protein intake in a child with T1D?

A. 6–12% of recommended total energy
B. 15–25% of recommended total energy
C. 26–30% of recommended total energy
D. None of the above

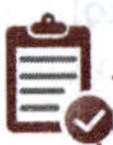

EXPLANATION

A person with T1D should consume protein in the recommended range. The International Society for Pediatric and Adolescent Diabetes (ISPAD) recommends a protein intake of 15–25%. Protein intake in excess of 25% may cause diabetic nephropathy and is therefore not recommended. The target is the lower end of the range.

Key: B

BOOST YOUR KNOWLEDGE

Macronutrients needs in T1D according to total daily energy intake are carbohydrate: 40–50% energy, moderate sucrose intake (up to 10% total energy), fat: 30–40% energy (<10% saturated and trans fatty acid), and protein: 15–25% of the total daily energy intake. Dietary patterns that restrict intake from one macronutrient may compromise growth and lead to nutritional deficiencies. Vegetable protein such as legumes should be encouraged. Recommended sources of animal protein include fish, lean cuts of meat and low-fat dairy products.

REFERENCE/SOURCE

- Annan SF, Higgins LA, Jelleryd E, Hannon T, Rose S, Salis S, et al. ISPAD Clinical Practice Consensus Guidelines 2022: Nutritional management in children and adolescents with diabetes. Pediatr Diabetes. 2022;23(8):1297-321.

9. What is the recommended target HbA1c for all children with diabetes?

A. <8%
B. <7%
C. <6%
D. <5%

EXPLANATION

The ISPAD recommends that all the patients with diabetes should have a target HbA1c of <7%.

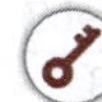

Key: B

BOOST YOUR KNOWLEDGE

It has been seen that at this target (<7%) the short- and the long-term complications are avoided. A level <6% may continue to yield risk reduction, but the relative gains are less. An HbA1c target of <6.5% is recommended in honeymoon phase and when using CGM or automated insulin delivery.

REFERENCE/SOURCE

- De Bock M, Codner E, Craig ME, Huynh T, Maahs DM, Mahmud FH, et al. ISPAD Clinical Practice Consensus Guidelines 2022: Glycemic targets and glucose monitoring for children, adolescents, and young people with diabetes. Pediatr Diabetes. 2022;23(8): 1270-76.

10. Which of the following tests is recommended to detect diabetic kidney disease (DKD) in children with diabetes?

A. Serum creatinine
B. Blood urea nitrogen (BUN)
C. Urine albumin-creatinine ratio (ACR) and serum creatinine
D. Ultrasonography of kidney, ureter, and bladder (KUB) region along with BUN

EXPLANATION

All the children having T1D with ≥2–5 years of diabetes and aged ≥11 years or puberty should be screened for DKD annually by doing urine ACR in the first morning sample preferably and serum creatinine to calculate eGFR. Doing only serum creatinine or BUN will not give any information on proteinuria.

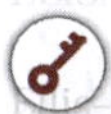

Key: C

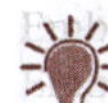

BOOST YOUR KNOWLEDGE

If ACR is >30 mg/g or >3 mg/mol; DKD is present. One must repeat two additional samples (first morning preferred) over 3–6 months. If 2/3 samples are ≥3 mg/mmol, the diagnosis of DKD is confirmed and the treatment should be started. It is also important to note that DKD can occur in the absence of increased albuminuria. As albuminuria is not the only indicator of DKD, evaluation of kidney function is also important. Estimated glomerular filtration rate (eGFR) should be monitored regularly to detect both declining kidney function and hyperfiltration.

REFERENCE/SOURCE

- Bjornstad P, Dart A, Donaghue KC, Dost A, Feldman EL, Tan GS, et al. ISPAD Clinical Practice Consensus Guidelines 2022: Microvascular and macrovascular complications in children and adolescents with diabetes. Pediatr Diabetes. 2022;23(8):1432-50.

11. Which of the following statements is true regarding dyslipidemia in children with T1D?

A. Screening for dyslipidemia should commence at 11 years of age
B. Nonfasting blood lipid profile is not valid for screening
C. High low-density lipoprotein cholesterol (LDL-C) is defined as values >150 mg/dL in children with diabetes
D. Statins should be started in the patients with LDL-C >200 mg/dL

EXPLANATION

The ISPAD recommends screening for dyslipidemia in all children with T1D at 11 years of age. All patients should be screened in nonfasting state.

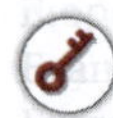

Key: A

BOOST YOUR KNOWLEDGE

Lipid profile should be done in fasting state only if it is deranged in non-fasting state or if the patient is already on treatment for dyslipidemia. A high LDL-C is defined as a value of >100 mg/dL and if it is high, the first approach should be to improve glycemic control, dietary restrictions, and increased physical activity. Only if after 6 months of this approach, the LDL-C remains high; start the patient on statins.

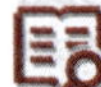

REFERENCE/SOURCE

- Bjornstad P, Dart A, Donaghue KC, Dost A, Feldman EL, Tan GS, et al. ISPAD Clinical Practice Consensus Guidelines 2022: Microvascular and macrovascular complications in children and adolescents with diabetes. Pediatr Diabetes. 2022;23(8):1432-50.

12. An 18-years-old boy with transfusion-dependent thalassemia (TDT) who is on insulin therapy for his T1D for past 2 years comes to you. His latest investigations show an HbA1c of 6.5%. He is doing self-monitored BG very infrequently (one test/1–2 days). He also has stage 3 DKD and nonproliferative diabetic retinopathy. His HbA1c values are always lower than 7% and yet, he is developing many complications. What could be a possible reason?

A. His HbA1c readings are spurious
B. Thalassemia is causing DKD and diabetic retinopathy despite good glycemic control
C. DKD and retinopathy may be a temporary phenomenon related to blood transfusion and chelation
D. HbA1c is not reliable in TDT

EXPLANATION

The HbA1c is not reliable in various diseases and states. In conditions with increased red blood cell (RBC) turnover, RBCs are exposed to elevated BG for a lesser duration, therefore, the HbA1c is falsely low despite elevated BG. In thalassemia patients, fructosamine and 1,5-anhydroglucitol (1,5-AG) are better to predict glycemic variability.

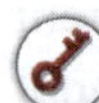

Key: D

BOOST YOUR KNOWLEDGE

- *Conditions with increased erythrocyte turnover resulting in lower HbA1c:* Recovery from iron, vitamin B_{12}, and folate deficiency; pregnancy—second trimester; chronic kidney disease—erythropoietin treatment and dialysis; acute blood loss; hemolysis [e.g., sickle cell trait/disease, thalassemia, and glucose-6-phosphate dehydrogenase (G6PD)]; cystic fibrosis; and chemotherapy.
- *Conditions with reduced erythrocyte turnover resulting in higher HbA1c:* Iron, vitamin B_{12}, and folate deficiency, pregnancy—third trimester, and CKD with uremia.

REFERENCE/SOURCE

- De Bock M, Codner E, Craig ME, Huynh T, Maahs DM, Mahmud FH, et al. ISPAD Clinical Practice Consensus Guidelines 2022: Glycemic targets and glucose monitoring for children, adolescents, and young people with diabetes. Pediatr Diabetes. 2022;23(8):1270-6.

13. **Which of the following investigation is not mandatory in a newly diagnosed T1D child?**

A. Tissue transglutaminase-IgA (tTG-IgA)
B. Thyroid profile
C. Blood pressure (BP)
D. Serum cortisol

EXPLANATION

Since T1D is an autoimmune condition, these patients are prone to develop few more autoimmune illnesses frequently. Therefore, all newly diagnosed must be screened for celiac disease (CD) and thyroid disorders. BP should be taken on all visits. Serum cortisol should be done only if there are features suggestive of Addison's disease.

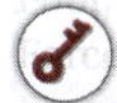

Key: D

BOOST YOUR KNOWLEDGE

Screening for CD is recommended during the initial year of diabetes diagnosis and at 2–5 years interval.

Other autoimmune conditions in T1D are juvenile idiopathic arthritis (JIA), autoimmune gastritis, and other gastrointestinal diseases (e.g., Crohn's disease, ulcerative colitis, and autoimmune hepatitis), although these are rare.

Addison's disease should be suspected in patients with frequent hypoglycemia, increased skin pigmentation, unexplained decrease in insulin requirements, lassitude, weight loss, hyponatremia, and hyperkalemia as well as severe or recurrent infections.

REFERENCE/SOURCE

- Fröhlich-Reiterer E, Elbarbary NS, Simmons K, Buckingham B, Humayun KN, Johannsen J, et al. ISPAD Clinical Practice Consensus Guidelines 2022: Other complications and associated conditions in children and adolescents with type 1 diabetes. Pediatr Diabetes. 2022;23(8):1451-67.

14. **Which of the following is true for maternally inherited diabetes mellitus and deafness?**

A. Inheritance is X-linked recessive
B. Metformin should not be given in this scenario
C. Diabetes presentation is acute and sudden
D. Presents early in first 5 years of life

EXPLANATION

Metformin should not be given in these patients as there is a theoretical risk of severe lactic acidosis.

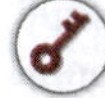

Key: B

BOOST YOUR KNOWLEDGE

Maternally inherited diabetes mellitus and deafness is mitochondrially inherited and therefore, is not X-linked recessive. It is caused by point mutation in m.3243A>G in the transfer ribonucleic acid (*tRNA*) leucine gene. This mutation is identical to the one seen in mitochondrial myopathy, encephalopathy, lactic acidosis, and stroke-like episodes (MELAS). In this disease, diabetes is insidious and only ~20% of the patients have acute presentations of T1D. The mean age of diagnosis is 37 years. Not all patients have deafness.

REFERENCE/SOURCE

- Zheng S, Wang J, Sun M, Wang P, Shi W, Zhang Z, Wang Z, Zhang H. The clinical and genetic characteristics of maternally inherited diabetes and deafness (MIDD) with mitochondrial m.3243A >G mutation: a 10-year follow-up observation study and literature review. Clin Case Rep. 2024(1);12(2):e8458. doi: 10.1002/ccr3.8458.

15. A 15-year-old child with T1D is on basal bolus regimen. His follow-up is infrequent, and he has poor glycemic control. On examination, he has chubby face and protuberant abdomen with palpable liver. His Sexual Maturity Rating (SMR) stage is 2 and he is <–3SDS in height for his age. He is also complaining of pain in the right side of upper abdomen. He wants to grow in his height, what would be the best approach?

A. Start growth hormone injections
B. Counsel him to achieve good glycemic control
C. Counsel that nothing can be done now to increase the height
D. Start on him on Mixtard injections

EXPLANATION

This patient appears to have developed Mauriac syndrome. It causes growth retardation and hepatomegaly in children with long-standing poor glycemic control. Most of the patients will start growing well, if they achieve and sustain good glycemic control. However, the final adult height may remain compromised in some.

Key: B

BOOST YOUR KNOWLEDGE

Mauriac syndrome is also known as glycogenic hepatopathy. Its pathogenesis is not well known, and it has been hypothesized that the glycogen synthase enzyme is activated in the presence of excessive glucose and insulin. This leads to glycogen formation and storage in the liver and hepatic enlargement and also deranged liver function test (LFT). The elevation in liver enzymes is reversible with optimal glucose control. Recovery to baseline may take about 2–4 weeks. There may be an increase in lactic acid also. Diagnosis can be confirmed by liver biopsy. Treatment is adequate insulin therapy to achieve good glucose control.

REFERENCE/SOURCE

- Fröhlich-Reiterer E, Elbarbary NS, Simmons K, Buckingham B, Humayun KN, Johannsen J, et al. ISPAD Clinical Practice Consensus Guidelines 2022: Other complications and associated conditions in children and adolescents with type 1 diabetes. Pediatr Diabetes. 2022;23(8):1451-67.

16. The blood investigations of a 9-year-old girl on routine testing shows following results as incidental findings: FPG: 95 mg/dL, 2 hour plasma glucose after glucose load: 146 mg/dL, and random BG: 169 mg/dL. What is your interpretation?

A. Diabetes
B. IFG
C. IGT
D. Normal BG

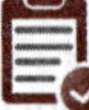

EXPLANATION

Impaired fasting glucose: FBG between 100 and 125 mg/dL, IGT: post 2 hours glucose load BG between 140 and 180 mg/dL.

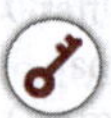

Key: C

BOOST YOUR KNOWLEDGE

The IGT and IFG are intermediate stages in the natural history of disordered carbohydrate metabolism between normal glucose homeostasis and diabetes. IFG and IGT should not be considered interchangeable, as both represent different abnormalities of glucose regulation or different stages in the progression of dysglycemia. IFG is a measure of disturbed carbohydrate metabolism in the basal state, whereas IGT is a dynamic measure of carbohydrate intolerance after a standardized glucose load. IFG and IGT are not clinical entities in their own right; individuals with IFG and/or IGT are referred to as having "prediabetes" indicating their relatively high risk.

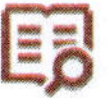

REFERENCES/SOURCES

- Kliegman RM, St Geme JW, Blum NJ, Shah SS, Tasker RC, Wilson KM. Nelson Textbook of Pediatrics, 21st edition. Philadelphia: Elsevier; 2019.
- Libman I, Haynes A, Lyons S, Pradeep P, Rwagasor E, Tung JYL, et al. ISPAD Clinical Practice Consensus Guidelines 2022: Definition, epidemiology, and classification of diabetes in children and adolescents. Pediatr Diabetes. 2022;23(8):1160-74.

17. A 5-year-old girl is being treated as having mild diabetic ketoacidosis (DKA). The patient responded well to the IV insulin and fluid therapy over the next 24 hours only. Later she was started on intensive basal bolus regimen with glargine and lispro. On Day 7 of admission, she developed swelling over the dorsum of hands and feet. Her BP, urine output, LFT, serum proteins, and kidney function tests (KFTs) were all normal. What is the likely diagnosis?

A. Insulin edema
B. Liver cell failure
C. Diabetes kidney disease
D. Refeeding syndrome

EXPLANATION

Insulin edema is a self-limiting edema which develops in newly diagnosed patients on intensive insulin therapy. The condition is usually self-limiting and resolves over the next 1–3 weeks. It improves on reducing the insulin dose.

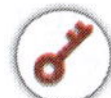

Key: A

BOOST YOUR KNOWLEDGE

Insulin edema is an uncommon side effect of Insulin therapy. It can vary from mild ankle swelling to severe edema and anasarca. This is frequently encountered either at the start of insulin therapy or after recent intensification of insulin therapy. It has been observed in both type 1 and type 2 diabetes. All the LFT, KFT, and serum proteins are normal in these patients and usually it is a diagnosis of exclusion. Poor glucose control and low BMI have been suggested as risk factors. There is no guideline for its management. It may respond to diuretic therapy/salt and fluid restriction.

REFERENCE/SOURCE

- Kliegman RM, St Geme JW, Blum NJ, Shah SS, Tasker RC, Wilson KM. Nelson Textbook of Pediatrics, 21st edition. Philadelphia: Elsevier; 2019.

18. Which of the following is *correct* regarding insulin?

A. It should be kept in direct contact with ice while carrying it during travel
B. When in use, it can be easily stored at room temperature (below 30°C) for up to 4 weeks
C. If insulin gets frozen accidentally, it can be used after thawing
D. Insulin can be given both intramuscular and subcutaneous

EXPLANATION

When not in use, store insulin at 2–8°C. However, when in use, it can be stored at up to 30°C for a period of 4 weeks. Insulin should not be used if it gets frozen and therefore, it should not be kept in direct contact with the ice. Freezing compromises the efficacy of insulin. Insulin is always given subcutaneously, and it should not be given intramuscularly.

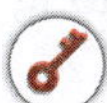

Key: B

BOOST YOUR KNOWLEDGE

The correct dose of insulin achieves good glycemic control, minimal hypoglycemia episodes, and optimal growth. The usual insulin dose range is 0.5–1 U/kg/day, during puberty the requirement may increase up to 1–2 U/kg/day. Insulin requirement can be 1–1.5 U/kg/day post-DKA and post-diagnosis. If insulin requirement is below 0.6 U/kg/day even 2–3 years post-diagnosis; one should suspect the possibility of monogenic diabetes. The ideal regime is the basal bolus regime, where 40% of the insulin is initiated as basal and the remaining as bolus doses before meals.

REFERENCE/SOURCE

- Cengiz E, Danne T, Ahmad T, Ayyavoo A, Beran D, Ethisham S, et al. ISPAD Clinical Practice Consensus Guidelines 2022: Insulin treatment in children and adolescents with diabetes. Pediatr Diabetes. 2022;23(8):1277-96.

19. Which of the following is *not* responsible for causing hypoglycemia in a T1D patient?

A. Excessive insulin
B. Exercise
C. Alcohol intake
D. Anaerobic exercise

EXPLANATION

The risk of hypoglycemia is increased during moderate-intensity exercise, immediately after as well as 7–11 hours after exercise. On the other hand, anaerobic exercises can lead to increase in BG levels. Alcohol causes hypoglycemia by inhibiting gluconeogenesis and hypoglycemia may occur if there is an inadequate intake of carbohydrates.

Key: D

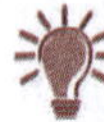

BOOST YOUR KNOWLEDGE

Insulin dose adjustments are mostly required for aerobic exercise, and less likely required for very high intensity or anaerobic exercise which is more commonly associated with elevated glucose levels.

REFERENCE/SOURCE

- Abraham MB, Karges B, Dovc K, Naranjo D, Arbelaez AM, Mbogo J, et al. ISPAD Clinical Practice Consensus Guidelines 2022: Assessment and management of hypoglycemia in children and adolescents with diabetes. Pediatr Diabetes. 2022;23(8):1322-40.
- Adolfsson P, Taplin CE, Zaharieva DP, Pemberton J, Davis EA, Riddell MC, et al. ISPAD Clinical Practice Consensus Guidelines 2022: Exercise in children and adolescents with diabetes. Pediatr Diabetes. 2022;23(8):1341-72.

20. Which of the following is *true* about diabetic neuropathy?

A. Manifestations are acute
B. Manifestations begin with motor involvement
C. Can affect the ninth and tenth cranial nerve
D. Can affect the autonomic nervous system

EXPLANATION

Diabetic neuropathy involves all three nerves, i.e., sensory, motor, and autonomic.

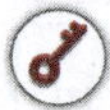

Key: D

BOOST YOUR KNOWLEDGE

Poor glycemic control can affect the somatic and autonomic nervous system. Diabetic neuropathy has a prevalence of up to 27% according to various studies. The most common risk factors include poor glycemic control and long duration of disease.

Sensorimotor neuropathy: It is the most common type of diabetic neuropathy. It is a polyneuropathy caused by diffuse damage to all peripheral nerve fibers (motor, sensory, and autonomic). The damage is insidious and progressive. It is characterized at first by sensory loss and later by mild loss of motor function in a "stocking and glove" pattern. Patients may complain of pins and needles sensation, numbness/tingling in limbs, loss of balance, pain and burning sensation in feet/hands, and muscle cramping or twitching. Neuropathy can result in complications such as muscle and joint disease, foot ulcers, claw toe deformity, callus/fissure formation, and Charcot joint. Focal neuropathies like carpal tunnel syndrome or peroneal nerve palsy are less common.

Screening involves evaluation of touch sensation, pressure vibration, and reflexes in the feet.

Autonomic neuropathy: It is rare in childhood and adolescence. This affects cardiovascular, urogenital, and gastrointestinal systems. Clinical features include vomiting, diarrhea, postural hypotension, sweating abnormalities, urinary incontinence, or incomplete voiding. It can also result in abnormal heart rate responses and prolonged QT intervals, which are associated with increased risk of sudden death.

The various tests to detect autonomic neuropathy include heart rate variability, at rest and its response to deep breathing, Valsalva maneuver, and postural changes in BP (orthostatic hypotension).

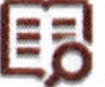

REFERENCE/SOURCE

- Fröhlich-Reiterer E, Elbarbary NS, Simmons K, Buckingham B, Humayun KN, Johannsen J, et al. ISPAD Clinical Practice Consensus Guidelines 2022: Other complications and associated conditions in children and adolescents with type 1 diabetes. Pediatr Diabetes. 2022;23(8):1451-67.

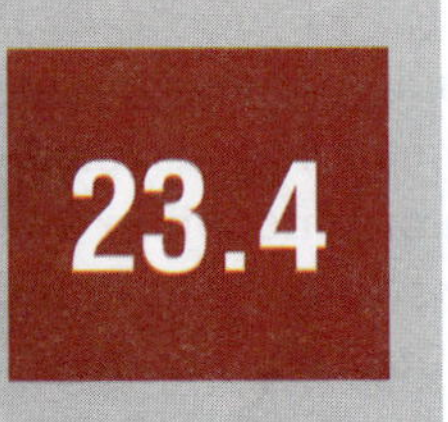

CHAPTER 23.4

Obesity, Diabetes Insipidus, and Hyperlipidemia

Aaradhana

1. A 12-year-old girl with exogenous obesity [body mass index (BMI) 29 kg/m^2] reported a raised serum thyroid-stimulating hormone (TSH) of 8.0 mIU/L and normal free T4 level. She does not have goiter. What should be the next step?

A. Start levothyroxine at a dose of 25 μg/day
B. Advise ultrasonography (USG) neck for thyroid gland enlargement
C. Reassure and repeat thyroid function at follow-up
D. Advise antithyroid peroxidase antibody levels in blood

EXPLANATION

Mild TSH elevation is commonly found in children with exogenous obesity, which is not the cause but the effect of obesity. Treatment with levothyroxine is required in presence of goiter, raised antithyroid peroxidase (anti-TPO) antibody levels, and serum TSH level >10 mIU/L.

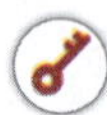

Key: C

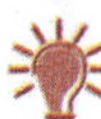

BOOST YOUR KNOWLEDGE

Obesity in children can be physiological (98%) or pathological (2%). Pathological causes of obesity include endocrine causes such as hypothyroidism, Cushing syndrome, pseudohypoparathyroidism, and growth hormone deficiency; syndromes such as Prader–Willi syndrome (PWS), Bardet–Biedl syndrome, Cohen syndrome, Carpenter syndrome; monogenic obesity due to mutations of MC4R, leptin R, POMC, and leptin deficiency; hypothalamic obesity due to intracranial tumors and infections; and drug-induced obesity due to valproate, carbamazepine, steroid, etc. Physiological obesity is also known as exogenous obesity or constitutional obesity, which occurs due to an imbalance between energy intake and energy expenditure. Management includes lifestyles measures such as healthy diet and physical activity.

REFERENCE/SOURCE

- Gahagan S. Overweight and obesity. In: Kliegman RM, St Geme III JW, Blum NJ, Shah SS, Tasker RC, Wilson KM (Eds). Nelson Textbook of Pediatrics, 21st edition. Elsevier; 2019. p. 349.

2. A 13-year-old boy with mild obesity underwent evaluation for complications of obesity. His fasting lipid profile was deranged in the form of total serum cholesterol 280 mg/dL, low-density lipoprotein cholesterol (LDL-C) 180 mg/dL, and serum triglyceride 200 mg/dL. He does not have family history of hyperlipidemia and premature cardiovascular disease. What should be the management?

A. Lifestyle modifications
B. Lifestyle modifications and statins
C. Lifestyle modifications and fibrates
D. Lifestyle modifications and statins and fibrates

EXPLANATION

The boy has exogenous obesity with dyslipidemia as a complication of obesity. Initial treatment of dyslipidemia includes lifestyle measures such as healthy diet, physical activity, and avoidance of screen exposure >1 hour a day. Persistent dyslipidemia even after 3–6 months of lifestyle measures warrants treatment with statins for elevated LDL-C and fibrates for raised triglyceride level of >400 mg/dL. Absence of family history in this case is against familial combined dyslipidemia, which is characterized by metabolic syndrome, dyslipidemia, and positive family history of dyslipidemia.

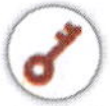

Key: A

BOOST YOUR KNOWLEDGE

The complications of obesity include dysglycemia, steatohepatitis, hypertension, dyslipidemia, and polycystic ovarian disease. Regular monitoring of the complications and appropriate management is a part of obesity management.

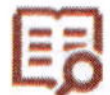

REFERENCE/SOURCE

- Gahagan S. Overweight and obesity. In: Kliegman RM, St Geme III JW, Blum NJ, Shah SS, Tasker RC, Wilson KM (Eds). Nelson Textbook of Pediatrics, 21st edition. Elsevier; 2019. p. 349.

3. **A 5-year-old developmentally normal girl presented with progressively increasing weight since the age of 6 months. She is shorter as compared to her peers and has excessive appetite and lack of satiety. Her blood pressure, thyroid profile, and liver function tests are normal. Her serum calcium, phosphorous, and alkaline phosphatase levels are within normal limits. What can be the most likely cause?**

A. Leptin deficiency
B. MC4R mutation
C. Pseudohypoparathyroidism
D. PWS

EXPLANATION

Leptin deficiency is characterized by early-onset obesity, hyperphagia, and short stature. Affected children are developmentally normal. Melanocortin receptor (MC4R) mutation causes growth acceleration resulting in tall stature of affected children. Pseudohypoparathyroidism is characterized by intellectual disability, hypocalcemia, hyperphosphatemia, and elevated serum TSH levels in addition to obesity. PWS is characterized by failure to thrive in the first year of life associated with feeding difficulties. Weight gain starts after 2–3 years of life. Children with PWS have dysmorphism and developmental delay.

Key: A

BOOST YOUR KNOWLEDGE

Monogenic obesity is rare and is characterized by early onset obesity and hyperphagia. The following are common forms of monogenic obesity:

Genetic defect	*Features*
Leptin deficiency/leptin receptor gene mutation	Recurrent infections, short stature, delayed puberty (hypogonadotropic hypogonadism)
MC4R mutation	Increased linear growth, hyperinsulinemia
Pro-opiomelanocortin (POMC) deficiency	Red hair, adrenal insufficiency due to adrenocorticotropic hormone (ACTH) deficiency
Proprotein convertase subtilisin/kexin type 1 (PCSK1) deficiency	Malabsorption due to small bowel enteropathy, hypothyroidism, ACTH deficiency, and diabetes insipidus

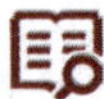

REFERENCE/SOURCE

- Gahagan S. Overweight and obesity. In: Kliegman RM, St Geme III JW, Blum NJ, Shah SS, Tasker RC, Wilson KM (Eds). Nelson Textbook of Pediatrics, 21st edition. Elsevier; 2019. p. 349.

4. The following is the growth chart plotting of an 8-year-old boy. What can be the likely cause of obesity in him?

A. Cushing syndrome
B. PWS
C. Constitutional obesity
D. Leptin deficiency

WHO 2006 and IAP 2015 Combined Boys Charts 0–18 Years

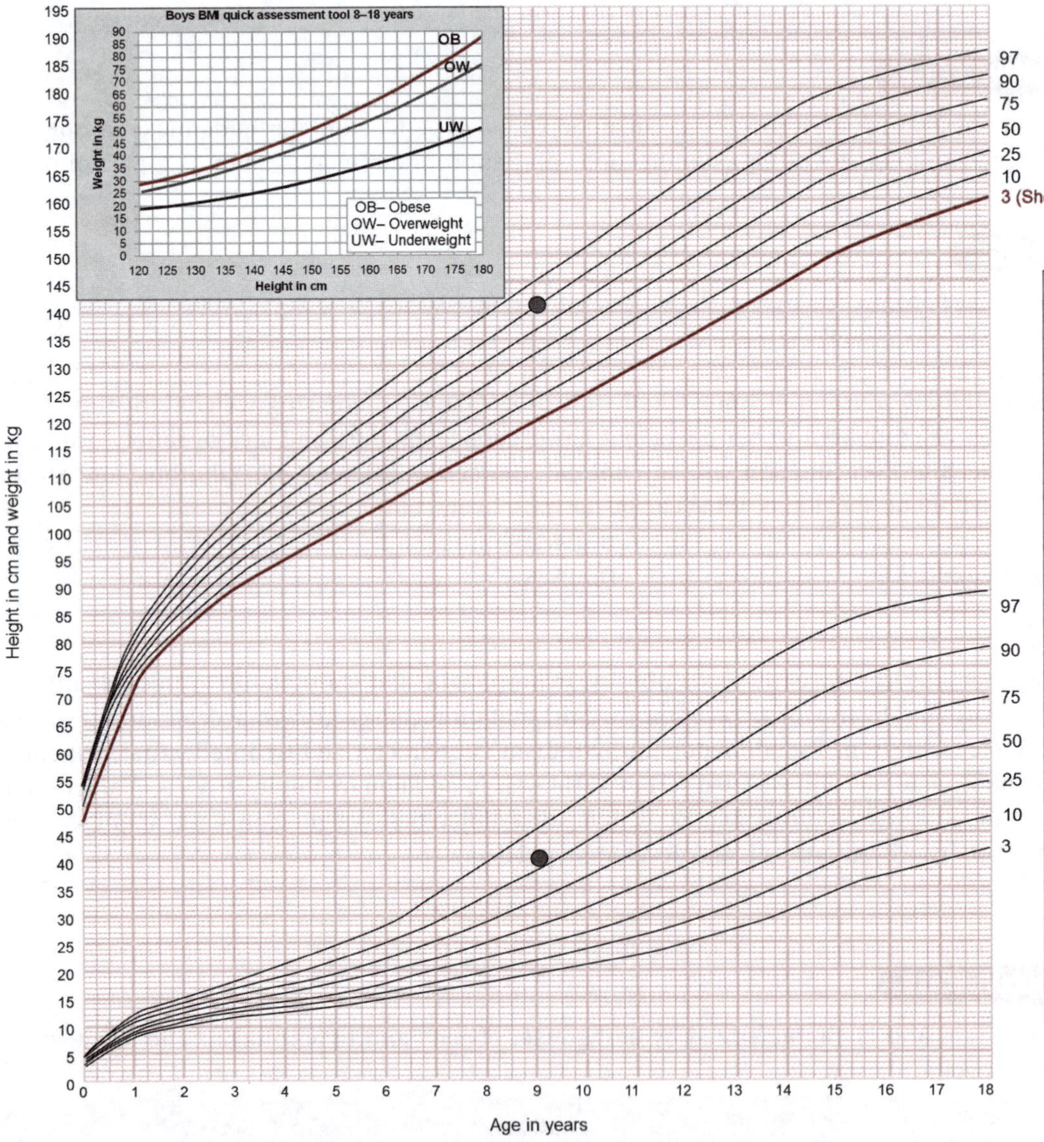

Boys BMI quick assessment tool 8–18 years

Weight in kg; Height in cm

OB– Obese
OW– Overweight
UW– Underweight

Height in cm and weight in kg

Age in years

Height percentiles: 97, 90, 75, 50, 25, 10, 3 (Short below this line)

Weight percentiles: 97, 90, 75, 50, 25, 10, 3

MPH Percentile Calculator

Father's height	MPH centile	Mother's height
150		137
151		138
152		139
153		140
154		141
155		142
156		143
157		144
158	3rd	145
159		146
160		147
161		148
162		149
163	10th	150
164		151
165		152
166		153
167		154
168	25th	155
169		156
170		157
171		158
172		159
173	50th	160
174		161
175		162
176		163
177		164
178	75th	165
179		166
180		167
181		168
182	90th	169
183		170
184		171
185		172
186		173
187	97th	174
188		175
189		176
190		177

Source:

Modified from:

1. WHO MGRS (Multicentre Growth Reference Study) 2006.
2. Revised IAP growth charts for height, weight and body mass index for 5 to 18 years old Indian children. V Khadilkar et al., from Indian Academy of Pediatrics, Growth Chart Committee, Indian Pediatrics, Jan 2015, Vol 52.
3. Khadilkar V, Lohiya N, Chiplonkar S, Khadilkar A. Body mass index quick screening tool for IAP 2015 growth chart (published online ahead of print, 2020 Jun 12). Indian Pediatr. 2020;5097475591600197.

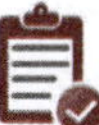

EXPLANATION

As shown in the growth chart, weight of the child lies on the 90th centile and height lies between 75th and 90th centile indicating that not only weight but also height has increased, which happens in constitutional obesity. While other causes such as Cushing syndrome, PWS, and leptin deficiency cause short stature (height <3rd centile).

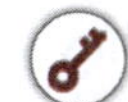

Key: C

BOOST YOUR KNOWLEDGE

Constitutional obesity is characterized by normal growth, puberty, and development. While endocrine, syndromic, and monogenic causes of obesity are characterized by short stature and developmental delay with few exceptions such as MC4R mutation, which causes tall stature.

REFERENCE/SOURCE

- Gahagan S. Overweight and obesity. In: Kliegman RM, St Geme III JW, Blum NJ, Shah SS, Taskèr RC, Wilson KM (Eds). Nelson Textbook of Pediatrics, 21st edition. Elsevier; 2019. p. 352.

5. A 12-year-old boy with a BMI of 30 kg/m^2 came to casualty with sudden onset pain in right hip and knee. He limps while walking. History of trauma and fever are absent. State the preliminary investigation to diagnose this condition.

A. Doppler USG lower limb
B. Magnetic resonance imaging (MRI) pelvis
C. X-ray spine
D. X-ray pelvis

EXPLANATION

The boy is obese. Sudden onset hip pain, knee pain, and limp are pointers toward slipped capital femoral epiphysis, which is an orthopedic complication of obesity. X-ray pelvis can establish the diagnosis.

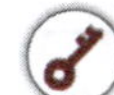

Key: D

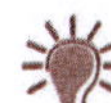

BOOST YOUR KNOWLEDGE

Orthopedic complications of obesity include Blount disease, slipped capital femoral epiphysis, and other musculoskeletal problems such as back pain, hip pain, knee pain, strains, and sprains. Blount disease (tibia vara) is characterized by severe bowing of tibia, limp, and pain in knees and is also diagnosed by radiographs.

REFERENCE/SOURCE

- Gahagan S. Overweight and obesity. In: Kliegman RM, St Geme III JW, Blum NJ, Shah SS, Tasker RC, Wilson KM (Eds). Nelson Textbook of Pediatrics, 21st edition. Elsevier; 2019. p. 352.

6. A 5-year-old girl is evaluated for obesity. She had feeding difficulties, hypotonia, and failure to thrive during infancy. Which of the following is the most likely genetic defect?

A. Maternal deletion of chromosome 15q
B. Paternal uniparental disomy of chromosome 11
C. Maternal uniparental disomy of chromosome 11
D. Paternal deletion of chromosome 15q

EXPLANATION

Hypotonia, failure to thrive, and feeding difficulties during infancy in an obese child are pointers toward PWS. One of the genetic defects causing PWS is paternal deletion of chromosome 15q. Maternal deletion of chromosome 15q causes Angelman syndrome. Paternal uniparental disomy of chromosome 11 leads to Beckwith-Wiedemann syndrome. Maternal uniparental disomy of chromosome 11 causes Russell-Silver syndrome.

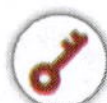 **Key: D**

 **BOOST YOUR KNOWLEDGE**

PWS is a disorder of genomic imprinting occurring due to lack of expression of paternally inherited genes on chromosome 15q11.2-q13 region. PWS is characterized by feeding difficulties, poor weight gain, and hypotonia during infancy followed by hyperphagia and rapid weight gain by 2–3 years of age. These children also have behavioral and cognitive dysfunction, developmental delay, and sleep disordered breathing. Dysmorphism includes almond-shaped eyes, strabismus, thin upper lip, and downturned mouth. Deletion of the paternally inherited 15q11.2-q13 region, uniparental disomy of the maternal chromosome 15q11.2-q13 region (UPD 15), an imprinting defect of the paternal chromosome 15q11.2-q13 region either due to an imprinting center deletion or epimutation. First tier test is DNA methylation study.

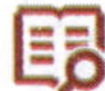 **REFERENCE/SOURCE**

- Bacino CA, Lee B. Uniparental disomy and imprinting. In: Kliegman RM, St Geme III JW, Blum NJ, Shah SS, Tasker RC, Wilson KM (Eds). Nelson Textbook of Pediatrics, 21st edition. Elsevier; 2019. p. 673.

7. The most common manifestations of autonomic nervous system (ANS) dysregulation in ROHHAD (rapid-onset obesity with hypothalamic dysfunction, hypoventilation, and autonomic dysregulation) patients are:

A. Ophthalmologic including pupillary dysfunction, strabismus, and alacrima
B. Gastrointestinal dysmotility like chronic constipation or chronic diarrhea
C. Impaired thermoregulation in the form of decreased body temperature
D. Decreased sensitivity to pain

 **EXPLANATION**

All of the above are manifestations of ANS dysregulation in ROHHAD patients but the most common are ophthalmologic.

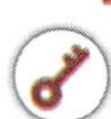 **Key: A**

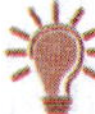 **BOOST YOUR KNOWLEDGE**

ROHHAD is a rare disease. Features of hypothalamic dysfunction include rapid-onset obesity, disordered water balance (hypernatremia, hyponatremia, adipsia, and polydipsia), growth hormone deficiency, hyperprolactinemia, central hypothyroidism, adrenal insufficiency, and delayed and precocious puberty. Sleep disordered breathing includes obstructive sleep apnea and central hypoventilation ultimately requiring mechanical ventilation. Other features include neural crest tumors, behavioral or psychologic disorders, and seizures.

 **REFERENCE/SOURCE**

- Barclay SF, Zhou A, Rand CM, Weese-Mayer DE. Rapid-onset obesity with hypothalamic dysfunction, hypoventilation, and autonomic dysregulation (ROHHAD). In: Kliegman RM, St Geme III JW, Blum NJ, Shah SS, Tasker RC, Wilson KM (Eds). Nelson Textbook of Pediatrics, 21st edition. Elsevier; 2019. p. 358.

8. In obesity due to *POMC* deficiency, which of the following medications can be most useful?

A. Orlistat
B. Setmelanotide
C. Lorcaserin
D. Leptin

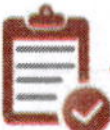

EXPLANATION

Orlistat is a pancreatic lipase inhibitor, which decreases absorption of fat. It is the only Food and Drug Administration (FDA)-approved medication for obesity in children aged 12 years and older. Lorcaserin is a selective serotonin 2c ($5HT_{2c}$) receptor agonist, which is an FDA-approved drug for adults with obesity. Setmelanotide is MC4R agonist and is useful in POMC deficiency. Leptin is used for leptin deficiency.

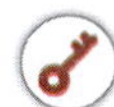

Key: B

BOOST YOUR KNOWLEDGE

Weight reduction through pharmacologic therapy in the pediatric age group is not studied well. Pharmacologic therapy includes: (1) medications that decrease calorie intake by decreasing appetite (anorexiants), (2) medications that reduce absorption of nutrients from intestine or renal tubules, and (3) medications that affect metabolism. Available medications result in modest weight loss even when combined with behavioral therapy.

REFERENCE/SOURCE

- Gahagan S. Overweight and obesity. In: Kliegman RM, St Geme III JW, Blum NJ, Shah SS, Tasker RC, Wilson KM (Eds). Nelson Textbook of Pediatrics, 21st edition. Elsevier; 2019. p. 356

9. Which of the following statements is true about sitosterolemia?

A. Caused by defect in LDL receptor-mediated endocytosis in the liver
B. Plasma triglyceride levels are severely elevated
C. Characterized by tendon xanthomas and macrothrombocytopenia
D. Treatment with β-Hydroxy β-methylglutaryl-coenyme A (HMG-CoA) reductase inhibitors is effective

EXPLANATION

Defect in LDL receptor-mediated endocytosis in the liver causes familial hypercholesterolemia (FH). In sitosterolemia, plasma cholesterol levels are severely elevated and not the triglycerides. Characterized by tendon xanthomas, hemolytic anemia, macrothrombocytopenia, and hemorrhage. Treatment with HMG-CoA reductase inhibitors is not effective. Cholesterol absorption inhibitors (ezetimibe) and bile acid sequestrants are effective.

Key: C

BOOST YOUR KNOWLEDGE

Sitosterolemia is a rare autosomal recessive disorder caused by mutations in the ATP binding cassette transporter system ABCG5 or ABCG8, which limits absorption of plant sterols in the intestine and promotes biliary excretion of small amounts adsorbed.

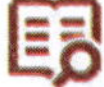

REFERENCE/SOURCE

- Pyles LA, Neal WA. Disorders of lipoprotein metabolism and transport. In: Kliegman RM, St Geme III JW, Blum NJ, Shah SS, Tasker RC, Wilson KM (Eds). Nelson Textbook of Pediatrics, 21st edition. Elsevier; 2019. pp. 757-8.

10. A 13-year-old boy presented with tonsillar hypertrophy of orange color, hepatosplenomegaly, intermittent peripheral neuropathy, and extremely low high-density lipoprotein (HDL) cholesterol levels. What is the likely diagnosis?

A. Smith-Lemli-Opitz syndrome (SLOS)
B. Tangier disease
C. Sitosterolemia
D. Wolman disease

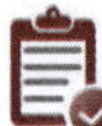

EXPLANATION

Tangier disease is caused by mutation in *ABCA1* that facilitates binding of cholesterol to apoA-1 resulting in accumulation of free cholesterol in reticuloendothelial system resulting in tonsillar hypertrophy and hepatosplenomegaly. Accumulation in Schwann cells causes peripheral neuropathy. HDL cholesterol (HDL-C) is low.

Key: B

BOOST YOUR KNOWLEDGE

Smith-Lemli-Opitz syndrome is characterized by craniofacial anomalies (microcephaly, blepharoptosis, anteverted nares, low set posterior rotated ears, cleft palate, and cataracts), skeletal anomalies (syndactyly of toes and polydactyly), genital anomalies (hypospadias, cryptorchidism, and ambiguous genitalia), developmental delay, and low plasma cholesterol.

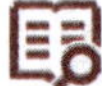

REFERENCE/SOURCE

- Pyles LA, Neal WA. Disorders of lipoprotein metabolism and transport. In: Kliegman RM, St Geme III JW, Blum NJ, Shah SS, Tasker RC, Wilson KM (Eds). Nelson Textbook of Pediatrics, 21st edition. Elsevier; 2019. pp. 760-1.

11. An 8-year-old boy presented with tendon xanthomas. His father is on medication for high lipid levels in blood and grandfather expired at 45 years of age with myocardial infarction. The index case has normal thyroid profile, blood sugar, and serum LDL-C of 800 mg/dL. What is the most likely genetic defect for this condition?

A. LDL receptor mutation
B. *apoE* gene mutation
C. *ABCG5* mutation
D. *apoC-II* gene mutation

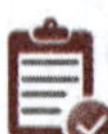

EXPLANATION

Low-density lipoprotein receptor mutation causes FH. *apoE* gene mutation causes familial dysbetalipoproteinemia. ATP-binding cassette transporter system (*ABCG5/ABCG8*) mutation causes sitosterolemia. *apoC-II* gene mutation causes familial chylomicronemia.

Key: A

BOOST YOUR KNOWLEDGE

Familial hypercholesterolemia (FH) is a monogenic codominant disorder, causing elevated LDL-C, tendon xanthomas, and premature cardiovascular disease. It is of two types—homozygous FH and heterozygous FH.

REFERENCE/SOURCE

- Pyles LA, Neal WA. Disorders of lipoprotein metabolism and transport. In: Kliegman RM, St Geme III JW, Blum NJ, Shah SS, Tasker RC, Wilson KM (Eds). Nelson Textbook of Pediatrics, 21st edition. Elsevier; 2019. p. 754.

12. A 7-year-old boy presents with tendon xanthomas. Father had myocardial infarction at the age of 40 years. Mother is also on statins. The index case has serum LDL-C 600 mg/dL. He was advised lifestyle interventions including low-fat diet and statin. The serum LDL-C level is 520 mg/dL after 2 months of maximum dose of statins. What should be the next line of management?

A. Plasmapheresis
B. Ezetimibe
C. Omega-3 fatty acids
D. Fibrates

EXPLANATION

Hypercholesterolemia, tendon xanthomas before 10 years of age, and history of premature cardiovascular disease in father are suggestive of FH in the boy. First line of treatment is lifestyle intervention and high potency statins. Second line of treatment includes ezetimibe, which reduces intestinal absorption of cholesterol from the intestine. Omega-3 fatty acids and fibrates are treatment options for hypertriglyceridemia.

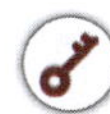

Key: B

BOOST YOUR KNOWLEDGE

Medications for hypercholesterolemia include:

Drugs	*Mechanism of action*
Statins	β-Hydroxy β-methylglutaryl-CoA (HMG-CoA) inhibitor limiting synthesis of cholesterol
Ezetimibe	ATP-binding cassette transporter system (ABCG5/8) inhibitor. Selectively blocks cholesterol absorption in the intestine
Bile acid sequestrant	Reduces absorption of cholesterol from the intestine
Lomitapide	Microsomal triglyceride transfer protein (MTP) inhibition. Reduces all apoB lipoproteins including LDL
Mipomersen	An antisense oligonucleotide that binds to the sequence that encodes apolipoprotein B (apoB) thus reducing synthesis of apoB and also of very low-density lipoprotein (VLDL) and LDL
Evolocumab	Proprotein convertase subtilisin/kexin type 9 (PCSK9) inhibitor. Boosts LDL-receptor (LDL-R) levels resulting in marked reduction in plasma LDL-C levels

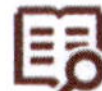

REFERENCE/SOURCE

- Pyles LA, Neal WA. Disorders of lipoprotein metabolism and transport. In: Kliegman RM, St Geme III JW, Blum NJ, Shah SS, Tasker RC, Wilson KM (Eds). Nelson Textbook of Pediatrics, 21st edition. Elsevier; 2019. p. 755.

13. A 6-month-old male baby presented with failure to thrive, anemia, and hepatosplenomegaly. During laboratory work-up, milky plasma was noticed. Refrigerator test showed creamy supernatant only. Serum triglyceride level was 4,000 mg/dL, HDL-C was low, and LDL-C was within normal limits. What should be the most effective management strategy for the boy to prevent pancreatitis?

A. High potency statins
B. Fibrates
C. Intensive dietary fat restriction
D. Fibrates + niacin

EXPLANATION

This boy has milky plasma with hypertriglyceridemia with low HDL-C and normal LDL-C, which is found in familial chylomicronemia (type I) and combined hypertriglyceridemia (type 5). Refrigerator test shows creamy supernatant only which occurs due to increased chylomicrons and is suggestive of familial chylomicronemia (type I). In type 5, both chylomicrons and VLDL are increased to give creamy supernatant due to increased chylomicrons and turbid infranatant due to increased VLDL. So, this boy most likely is having familial chylomicronemia. The most effective treatment is vigorous dietary restriction of fat along with supplementation of fat-soluble vitamins. Medium chain triglycerides may replace dietary fat. Fish oils are also beneficial. Other drugs such as fibrates and niacin are not much beneficial.

Key: C

BOOST YOUR KNOWLEDGE

Hypertriglyceridemia can occur due to primary and secondary causes. Secondary causes include diabetes, obesity, alcohol, renal failure, sepsis, Cushing syndrome, hepatitis, acquired immunodeficiency syndrome (AIDS), and drugs such as protease inhibitors, anabolic steroids, estrogen, beta-blockers, and thiazides. Primary causes are familial disorders of triglyceride-rich lipoproteins and include familial chylomicronemia (type I), familial hypertriglyceridemia (type IV), and combined hypertriglyceridemia (type V).

REFERENCE/SOURCE

- Pyles LA, Neal WA. Disorders of lipoprotein metabolism and transport. In: Kliegman RM, St Geme III JW, Blum NJ, Shah SS, Tasker RC, Wilson KM (Eds). Nelson Textbook of Pediatrics, 21st edition. Elsevier; 2019. pp. 758-9.

14. A 14-year-old girl is a known case of type 1 diabetes mellitus for 5 years. Her fasting lipid profile shows LDL-C 240 mg/dL, serum triglyceride 98 mg/dL, and HDL-C 60 mg/dL. She was started on CHILD-2 LDL diet and lifestyle changes. Six months later, her LDL-C is 170 mg/dL. What should be the next line of treatment?

A. Continue with lifestyle changes and CHILD-2 LDL diet
B. Continue with lifestyle changes and stop CHILD-2 LDL diet
C. Add statin to the ongoing treatment
D. Add fish oil to the ongoing treatment

EXPLANATION

Type 1 diabetes is a high-level risk factor. Even after 6-month trial of lifestyle interventions, LDL-C is >160 mg/dL, which is an indication to start statin therapy in the presence of one high-level risk factor.

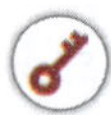

Key: C

BOOST YOUR KNOWLEDGE

Children with dyslipidemia are stratified into high- and moderate-level risk factors to guide the treatment. High level risk factors are: hypertension requiring drug therapy, obesity with BMI ≥ 97th centile, type 1 or 2 diabetes mellitus, chronic kidney disease, and Kawasaki disease with current aneurysms. Moderate-level risk factors include hypertension not requiring drug therapy, BMI ≥ 95th centile but <97th centile, Kawasaki disease with regressed aneurysms, human immunodeficiency virus (HIV) infection, nephrotic syndrome, and HDL-C <40 mg/dL. The initial treatment for dyslipidemia in a child begins with a 6-month trial of lifestyle interventions including physical activity and diet. If even after 6 months, the LDL-C is ≥160–189 mg/dL in presence of one high risk factor, statin therapy should be initiated.

REFERENCE/SOURCE

- Pyles LA, Neal WA. Disorders of lipoprotein metabolism and transport. In: Kliegman RM, St Geme III JW, Blum NJ, Shah SS, Tasker RC, Wilson KM (Eds). Nelson Textbook of Pediatrics, 21st edition. Elsevier; 2019. p. 762.

15. A 7-year-old boy is having polyuria and polydipsia. His serum sodium is 140 mmol/L, serum osmolality 290 mOsm/kg, and urine osmolality 350 mOsm/kg. What should be the next step?

A. Vasopressin challenge test
B. Start intranasal preparation of DDAVP
C. MRI of brain and hypothalamic pituitary region
D. Water deprivation test

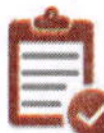

EXPLANATION

In a child with pathologic polyuria and polydipsia (exceeding 2 L/m^2/24 h), if serum osmolality is <300 mOsm/kg but >270 mOsm/kg, water deprivation test is indicated to establish the diagnosis of diabetes insipidus (DI). Vasopressin test helps to differentiate between central and nephrogenic DI (NDI). MRI of brain is done to find out the cause of central DI (CDI). DDAVP (desmopressin) is the treatment of CDI.

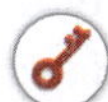

Key: D

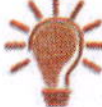

BOOST YOUR KNOWLEDGE

Diagnosis of DI is established if serum osmolality is >300 mOsm/kg and urine osmolality <300 mOsm/kg. DI is unlikely if serum osmolality is <270 mOsm/kg or urine osmolality >600 mOsm/kg.

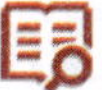

REFERENCE/SOURCE

- Breault DT, Majzoub JA. Diabetes insipidus. In: Kliegman RM, St Geme III JW, Blum NJ, Shah SS, Tasker RC, Wilson KM (Eds). Nelson Textbook of Pediatrics, 21st edition. Elsevier; 2019. p. 2888.

16. What is the triphasic response in the postneurosurgical setting?

A. CDI–SIADH (syndrome of inappropriate antidiuretic hormone secretion)–CDI
B. SIADH–CDI–SIADH
C. CDI–SIADH–primary polydipsia
D. CDI–SIADH–NDI

EXPLANATION

Triphasic response after a neurosurgical intervention includes transient DI–SIADH–permanent DI.

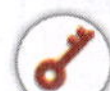

Key: A

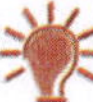

BOOST YOUR KNOWLEDGE

Initial transient DI phase results from local edema interfering with release of vasopressin and lasts for 12–48 hours. The second phase is SIADH resulting from release of vasopressin from dying neurons lasting for up to 10 days. The third phase is permanent DI resulting from destruction of >90% vasopressin neurons.

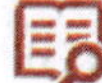

REFERENCE/SOURCE

- Breault DT, Majzoub JA. Diabetes insipidus. In: Kliegman RM, St Geme III JW, Blum NJ, Shah SS, Tasker RC, Wilson KM (Eds). Nelson Textbook of Pediatrics, 21st edition. Elsevier; 2019. p. 2888.

17. DIDMOAD occurs due to defect of which gene?

A. *HESX1*
B. *Neurophysin II*
C. *WFS1*
D. *Vasopressin V2* receptor

EXPLANATION

DIDMOAD syndrome, also known as Wolfram syndrome, is characterized by diabetes insipidus, diabetes mellitus, optic atrophy, and deafness. It occurs due to defect in *WFS1* gene. *HESX1* gene causes multiple pituitary hormone deficiencies including DI. *Neurophysin II* gene causes CDI. *Vasopressin 2* receptor gene mutation causes NDI.

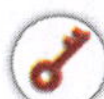

Key: C

BOOST YOUR KNOWLEDGE

Diabetes insipidus is of two types: CDI and NDI. CDI can be due to genetic defects in neurophysin II, *HESX1*, or *WFS1* genes; central nervous system (CNS) trauma and neurosurgery; CNS infiltration due to histiocytosis, tuberculosis, and sarcoidosis; CNS tumors such as germinomas, pinealomas, and craniopharyngiomas. NDI is due to genetic defects such as vasopressin 2 receptor defect (X-linked), aquaporin 2 defect (autosomal recessive), sodium potassium chloride channel defect in Bartter syndrome, ciliary abnormality in Bardet-Beidl syndrome; renal insult such as obstructive uropathy, cystinosis, sickle cell disease, and polycystic kidney disease; hypokalemia and hypercalcemia; drugs such as amphotericin B, ifosfamide, and lithium.

REFERENCE/SOURCE

- Breault DT, Majzoub JA. Diabetes insipidus. In: Kliegman RM, St Geme III JW, Blum NJ, Shah SS, Tasker RC, Wilson KM (Eds). Nelson Textbook of Pediatrics, 21st edition. Elsevier; 2019. p. 2888.

18. A 4-year-old girl has seborrheic dermatitis, anemia, hepatosplenomegaly, and polyuria. Her serum sodium is 154 mmol/L. Which of the following tests needs to be performed with caution?

A. Bone marrow aspiration
B. Contrast MRI brain
C. Water deprivation test
D. Arginine vasopressin (AVP) test

EXPLANATION

Polyuria with hypernatremia is a pointer toward DI. The next important test to confirm DI is urine osmolality. AVP test helps to differentiate between central and NDI and is the next phase of water deprivation test too. Contrast MRI is done in cases of CDI to locate the cause. This girl has seborrheic dermatitis, hepatosplenomegaly, and polyuria, which is likely due to Langerhans cell histiocytosis. Bone marrow aspiration will be required for confirmation. Water deprivation test aims to create hypernatremia in cases where DI is suspected but serum sodium is within normal range. In the presence of hypernatremia, water deprivation test may increase hypernatremia and may be life-threatening.

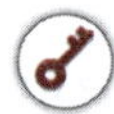

Key: C

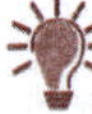

BOOST YOUR KNOWLEDGE

If serum sodium is within normal range and/or serum osmolality is <300 mOsm/kg, water deprivation test is done. The first phase of the water deprivation test is done till the end points are met (urine osmolality reaches 800 mOsm/kg or serum sodium >150 mEq/L and plasma osmolality >300 mOsm/kg or 3–5% weight loss or urine osmolality has stabilized). This phase establishes the diagnosis of DI. The second phase is desmopressin phase where urine osmolality is checked after giving subcutaneous vasopressin or intranasal desmopressin. This phase differentiates CDI and NDI. Rise of urine osmolality by >50% is CDI, <10% suggests NDI, and between 10 and 50% is compatible with partial CDI or partial NDI.

REFERENCES/SOURCES

- Breault DT, Majzoub JA. Diabetes insipidus. In: Kliegman RM, St Geme III JW, Blum NJ, Shah SS, Tasker RC, Wilson KM (Eds). Nelson Textbook of Pediatrics, 21st edition. Elsevier; 2019. p. 2888.
- Desai M, Menon PSN, Bhatia V (Eds). Pediatric Endocrine Disorders, 4th edition. Universities Press; 2023.

19. A 6-month-old boy had failure to thrive. He had serum sodium 168 mEq/L, urine osmolality of 200 mOsm/kg, which did not increase by vasopressin. Which of the following is not the treatment option for this boy?

A. Thiazide
B. DDAVP
C. Amiloride
D. Indomethacin

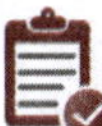

EXPLANATION

Failure to thrive with hypernatremia and decreased urine osmolality unresponsive to vasopressin in an infant are suggestive of NDI. Treatment of NDI includes thiazide diuretics, amiloride, and indomethacin. DDAVP is vasopressin analog used to treat CDI.

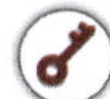

Key: B

BOOST YOUR KNOWLEDGE

Central DI occurs due to deficiency of AVP whereas NDI results from resistance to AVP. NDI is characterized by impaired urinary concentrating ability despite normal or elevated levels of AVP. There is no permanent cure. Management of NDI is challenging and includes increased fluid intake, reduction of salute load, thiazides, amiloride, and indomethacin.

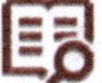

REFERENCE/SOURCE

- Breault DT, Majzoub JA. Diabetes insipidus. In: Kliegman RM, St Geme III JW, Blum NJ, Shah SS, Tasker RC, Wilson KM (Eds). Nelson Textbook of Pediatrics, 21st edition. Elsevier; 2019. p. 2888.

20. What instruction should be given to the patients on desmopressin for DI?

A. On days of fever, loose motions, and vomiting, desmopressin should be discontinued

B. Give the next dose of desmopressin only when the effect of the previous day's dose has finished, and the patient begins passing urine frequently for at least 2 hours

C. If the patient on desmopressin becomes lethargic or unconscious, give more fluids

D. Provide plenty of fluids to the patients on desmopressin

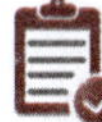

EXPLANATION

Desmopressin should be continued even on days of fever, loose motions, and vomiting. Extraoral fluids should be given according to the thirst. Allow diuresis before giving next dose to the patient. If a patient on desmopressin becomes lethargic, suspect hyponatremia and investigate and manage for the same. Patients on DDAVP should be provided fluids as per thirst only to avoid the risk of hyponatremia.

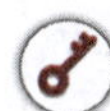

Key: B

BOOST YOUR KNOWLEDGE

Treatment of CDI is DDAVP. It is desmopressin acetate, a synthetic analog (1-deamino-8-D-arginine vasopressin). It is available in intravenous, oral, and nasal spray forms. For treatment of CDI, oral form is preferred to nasal sprays.

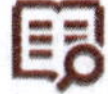

REFERENCE/SOURCE

- Breault DT, Majzoub JA. Diabetes insipidus. In: Kliegman RM, St Geme III JW, Blum NJ, Shah SS, Tasker RC, Wilson KM (Eds). Nelson Textbook of Pediatrics, 21st edition. Elsevier; 2019. p. 2888.

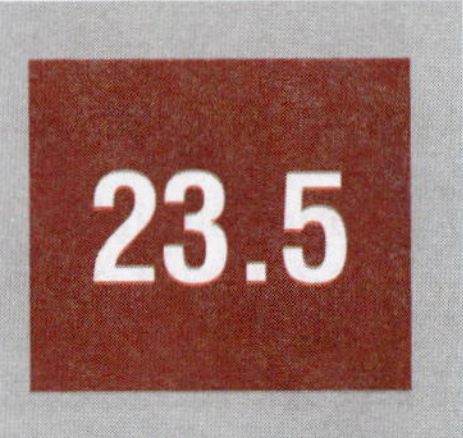

Pubertal Disorders

Ganesh Jevalikar

1. What Tanner stage of breast development is depicted in this clinical photograph?

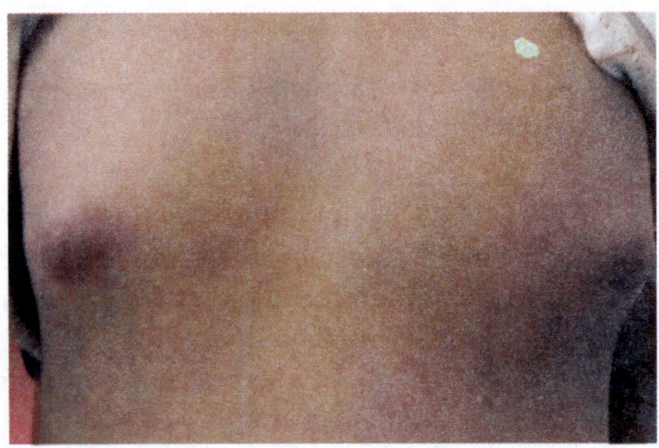

A. B2
B. B3
C. B4
D. B5

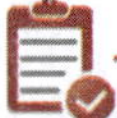

EXPLANATION

Pubertal assessment is done in clinical practice using Marshall and Tanner staging of breast and pubic hair development in girls and genital, penile, and pubic hairs staging in boys. The description of breast stages is described in the table below. In this clinical photograph, the nipple and areola can be seen forming a secondary mound above the contour of the breast. Hence, the most appropriate answer is stage B4.

Breast stage	*Description*
1	Preadolescent; elevation of papilla only
2	Breast bud stage; elevation of breast and papilla as a small mound, with enlargement of the areolar diameter
3	Further enlargement of the breast and areola, with no separation of their contours
4	Projection of the areola and papilla to form a secondary mound above the level of the breast
5	Mature stage; projection of papilla only, resulting from the recession of the areola to the general contour of the breast

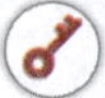

Key: C

BOOST YOUR KNOWLEDGE

In the initial stage of breast development, it may be difficult to distinguish between fat and glandular breast tissue. The examination of breast should include inspection as well as palpation at this stage. On palpation, with thumb and index finger, glandular breast tissue is felt as firm, rubbery, circular tissue underneath the nipple, and areola.

 REFERENCE/SOURCE

- Styne DM. Physiology and disorders of puberty. In: Melmed S, Auchus RJ, Goldfine AB, Koenig RJ, Rosen CJ (Eds). Williams Textbook of Endocrinology, 14th edition. Philadelphia, PA: Elsevier, Inc.; 2020. p. 1033.

2. An 8-year and 9-month-old girl presents with menarche. She is short for age and has little breast development. What is the most likely etiology of precocious puberty in her?

A. Ovarian cyst
B. Primary hypothyroidism
C. Exogenous estrogen exposure
D. Central precocious puberty

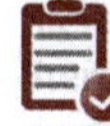 EXPLANATION

During the course of normal pubertal development, menarche is seen after 2–2.5 years of thelarche. Early menarche in the absence of little or no breast development suggests intermittent estrogen exposure usually because of conditions leading to peripheral precocious puberty. These include exogenous estrogen exposure, ovarian cyst, primary hypothyroidism, and McCune-Albright syndrome. Amongst these, primary hypothyroidism is the only condition where the child would be short. In all other conditions, estrogen-driven growth would lead to tall stature for age. The bone age is retarded in primary hypothyroidism unlike other causes of precocious puberty.

 **Key: B**

 BOOST YOUR KNOWLEDGE

The Van Wyk-Grumbach syndrome is sexual precocity associated with juvenile hypothyroidism. It is also associated with increased prolactin and galactorrhea. Neuroimaging may show sellar enlargement which can be mistaken for an intracranial tumor.

Per vaginal bleeding in the absence of any breast development can also be a result of trauma, foreign body or local tumors affecting vagina or cervix. In children with central precocious puberty secondary to cranial irradiation or intracranial tumors, concurrent growth hormone deficiency can lead to masking of rapid growth velocity.

 REFERENCE/SOURCE

- Rosenfield RL, Cooke DW, Radovick S. Puberty in the Female and its Disorders. In: Sperling MA, Majzoub JA, Menon RK, Stratakis CA (Eds). Sperling Pediatric Endocrinology, 5th edition. Philadelphia, PA; Elsevier, Inc.; 2021. p. 568-70.

3. Which of the following is the most common gene associated with idiopathic familial central precocious puberty (CPP)?

A. *MKRN3*
B. *Kisspeptin*
C. *KISS1R*
D. *DLK1*

EXPLANATION

Family history of precocity is common in cases of CPP. Recently the understanding of genetics of onset of puberty has improved and mutations in Kisspeptin and its receptor *KISS1R* were the first genetic causes identified in cases of precocious puberty. However, the most common genetic cause of PP appears to be loss of function mutations in makorin ring finger protein-3 (*MKRN-3*), which is maternally imprinted, and paternal allele is expressed. The gene in located in the region of chromosome 15q11-q13 (Prader-Willi critical region). *MKRN-3* appears to be an inhibitor of puberty in childhood and several families with mutations in this gene have now been described. Gain of function mutations of Kisspeptin and its receptor and loss of function on delta-like homolog1 (DLK1) also lead to familial central precocious puberty.

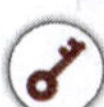 **Key: A**

BOOST YOUR KNOWLEDGE

The *MKRN-3* mutations follow a paternal pattern of inheritance as the maternal allele is silenced. Hence, an autosomal dominant pattern with paternal inheritance should give clue to this etiology in both boys and girls with precocity. A few patients have been described to have syndromic features such as esotropia, a high arched palate, dental abnormalities, clinodactyly, and hyperlordosis.

REFERENCE/SOURCE

- Valadares LP, Meireles CG, De Toledo IP, Santarem de Oliveira R, Gonçalves de Castro LC, Abreu AP, et al. *MKRN3* Mutations in Central Precocious Puberty: A Systematic Review and Meta-Analysis. J Endocr Soc. 2019;3(5):979-95.

4. An 18-year-old girl presents with primary amenorrhea. She has no systemic ailments and started breast development at the age of 11 years. On examination, she has normal BMI and has stage 5 breast development along with stage 5 pubic hairs. Her ultrasound reveals absence of uterus, what is her likely karyotype?

A. 45, X
B. 46, XX
C. 46, XY
D. 45, X/46, XY

EXPLANATION

Primary amenorrhea can result from deficiency of gonadotropins, gonadal failure, or abnormalities of Müllerian structures. Adult type of breast development in this girl suggests the estrogen production is normal. Lack of menstruation in such a case could be a result of acquired sex hormone deficiency, anovulation leading to progesterone deficiency or end organ defects. Absent uterus on ultrasound favors a diagnosis of Mayer–Rokitansky–Küster–Hauser (MRKH) syndrome in this case, hence the most likely karyotype in this case will be 46, XX. In cases with monosomy X, 46, XY gonadal dysgenesis as well as 45, X/46, XY mosaicism, complete breast development is unusual. In all these cases, the uterus is present. The only other condition which can have above features is 46, XY complete androgen insensitivity syndrome (CAIS), however stage 5 pubic hairs is not seen in CAIS.

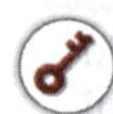

Key: B

BOOST YOUR KNOWLEDGE

Primary amenorrhea is defined as lack of menarche even after 5 years of breast development or beyond 15 years of age. The common differential diagnosis of amenorrhea despite complete breast development includes arrested puberty, Müllerian agenesis, complete androgen insensitivity, and polycystic ovary syndrome. In some conditions such as partial androgen insensitivity and some testosterone biosynthetic defects (17-hydroxylase deficiency, 17-β-hydroxysteroid dehydrogenase deficiency) some breast development can be seen.

REFERENCE/SOURCE

- Zacharin M, Banerjee I. Delayed puberty. In: Desai M, Menon PSN, Bhatia V, Seth A, (Eds). Pediatric Endocrine Disorders, 4th edition. Hyderabad, India: Universities Press; 2022. pp. 139-51.

5. A 10-month-old boy presents with onset of pubic hairs from 8 months of age. His height and weight are 85th centile, his testes are 1 mL each, he has Tanner stage 2 pubic hairs and stage 2 genital development. His bone age is 2 years. Biochemistry reveals serum LH < 0.07 IU/L and serum total testosterone of 75 ng/dL (N <20 ng/dL). His 17-hydroxyprogesterone (17-OHP) levels are 19.5 ng/mL (normal <2 ng/mL). What diagnosis is most likely in this child?

A. 3-B-HSD deficiency
B. 21-hydroxylase deficiency
C. 11-hydroxylase deficiency
D. Leydig cell tumor

EXPLANATION

The clinical presentation is suggestive of premature development of pubic hairs, thereby suggestive of androgen effect. The advanced bone age and prepubertal testicular volume indicates peripheral precocious puberty. In a male child the most common endogenous cause of precocious puberty is congenital adrenal hyperplasia due to 21-hydroxylase deficiency. However, usually the classic form of 21-hydroxylase deficiency has very high levels of 17-OHP, unlike in this case where there is only a modest elevation of this steroid. In such a case, 11-hydroxylase deficiency would be the most likely condition with modest elevation of 17-OHP. While elevated 17-OHP can be seen in 3-β-hydroxysteroid dehydrogenase deficiency, boys with this condition have undervirilization. A Leydig cell tumor can present with androgen excess, elevated testosterone and advanced bone age with small testicular volume but will not have elevated 17-OHP in this range.

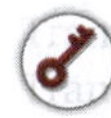

Key: C

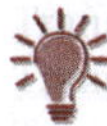

BOOST YOUR KNOWLEDGE

The 11-hydroxylase deficiency is an autosomal recessive condition due to mutations in *CYP11B1* gene and is the second most common cause of congenital adrenal hyperplasia. Affected girls present with atypical genitalia and symptoms of androgen excess, whereas affected males have normal genitalia. There is evidence of mineralocorticoid excess mediated by very high levels of 11-deoxycorticosterone (DOC) leading to hypertension with hypokalemia and metabolic alkalosis. However, blood pressure can be normal in infancy. The diagnosis is established with clinical findings, elevated 11-DOC and 11-deoxycortisol levels, and genetic studies showing mutations in *CYP11B1* gene.

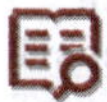

REFERENCE/SOURCE

- Auchus RJ. The uncommon forms of congenital adrenal hyperplasia. Curr Opin Endocrinol Diabetes Obes. 2022;29:263-70.

6. Which of the following statements is *false* regarding karyotype-phenotype correlations in Turner syndrome?

A. Structural cardiac anomalies are more common with monosomy X
B. Isochromosome Xq is associated with increased risk of autoimmune thyroid disease
C. Cognitive impairment is seen in ring chromosome
D. Presence of monosomy is associated with high risk of gonadoblastoma

EXPLANATION

Turner syndrome (TS) results from partial or total loss of one X chromosome material in women. There is significant phenotypic variability even with similar karyotype in women with TS, possibly resulting from variable loss of genes on X-chromosome, presence of mosaicism and additional genetic or epigenetic factors. However, some features have been reported with increased frequency in certain karyotypes. These include features such as webbing of neck, coarctation of aorta being more common with monosomy, increased risk of cognitive impairment in ring chromosome and increased autoimmune thyroid disease with isochromosome Xq. However, the increased risk of gonadoblastoma is directly associated with mosaicism with presence of Y-chromosome material.

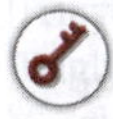

Key: D

BOOST YOUR KNOWLEDGE

Women with Turner syndrome with mosaic karyotypes account for nearly 50% of cases. The phenotype in these cases may not have cardinal clinical features. Due to the significant phenotypical variability, it is important to keep a high index of suspicion in all girls presenting with short stature or pubertal failure. The presence of

Y-cell line is associated with risk of gonadoblastoma in nearly 22–43% cases, hence a prophylactic gonadectomy is recommended in these cases.

REFERENCES/SOURCES

- Backelijauw P, Chernausek SD, Gravholt CH, Kruzska P. Turner syndrome. In: Sperling MA, Majzoub JA, Menon RK, Stratakis CA (Eds). Sperling Pediatric Endocrinology, 5th edition. Philadelphia, PA; Elsevier, Inc.; 2021. pp. 627-52.
- Kwon A, Hyun SE, Jung MK, Chae HW, Lee WJ, Kim TH, et al. Risk of gonadoblastoma development in patients with Turner Syndrome with Cryptic Y-chromosome material. Horm Cancer. 2017;8:166-73.

7. Which of the following is the most confirmatory to differentiate constitutional delay of growth and puberty (CDGP) versus isolated hypogonadotropic hypogonadism in a boy with delay in puberty?

A. Clinical follow-up
B. hCG stimulation test
C. GnRH stimulation test
D. Inhibin B

EXPLANATION

Constitutional delay of growth and puberty (CDGP) is the most common cause of delayed puberty in boys. However, it is a diagnosis of exclusion and needs to be differentiated from isolated hypogonadotropic hypogonadism (IHH) or other pathological conditions associated with delayed puberty. Several tests are used to differentiate these two conditions and include basal (8 AM) gonadotropins, testosterone, inhibin B, hCG stimulation test, and GnRH analog (GnRHa)-stimulated gonadotropin levels. However, none of these tests can be 100% diagnostic in the differential diagnosis and hence, a clinical follow-up showing progressive enlargement of testes either spontaneously or following a short course of testosterone treatment remains the gold standard for the diagnosis of CDGP versus IHH.

Key: A

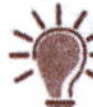

BOOST YOUR KNOWLEDGE

Clinical pointers to presence of IHH include micropenis, cryptorchidism, anosmia, mirror movements, dysmorphic features, deafness, renal anomalies, or coloboma. The height in IHH is typically normal during childhood and if untreated could be tall in adulthood with eunuchoid body proportions. The family history of delayed puberty is very common in CDGP and could be present on either side of the family.

REFERENCE/SOURCE

- Bozzola M, Bozzola E, Montalbano C, Stamati FA, Ferrara P, Villani A. Delayed puberty versus hypogonadism: a challenge for the pediatrician. Ann Pediatr Endocrinol Metab. 2018;23(2):57-61.

8. Which of the following is the most common site reported for germ cell tumors in Klinefelter syndrome?

A. Testis
B. Abdomen
C. Mediastinum
D. Central nervous system (CNS)

EXPLANATION

Klinefelter syndrome (KS) is a common condition usually presenting with hypogonadism, infertility, gynecomastia, relatively tall stature, and several other clinical features. People with KS have been reported to have increased risk of malignancies such as male breast cancer and germ cell tumors. The most reported site for germ cell tumors in mediastinum followed by CNS, testes, and abdomen.

Key: C

BOOST YOUR KNOWLEDGE

Klinefelter syndrome results from presence on an extra X-chromosome material in men. The most common karyotype is 47, XXY. Childhood presentations include cryptorchidism, relatively tall stature, difficulties in scholastic performance, behavioral issues, and gynecomastia. KS has been associated with conditions such as venous disease, autoimmune disorders, mild neurobehavioral deficit, diabetes mellitus, and osteoporosis. Extragonadal germ cell tumors commonly tend to occur in midline such as pineal region, mediastinum, retroperitoneum, and sacrococcygeal region. Mediastinal germ cell tumors (GCTs) are the most common site in KS and usually are diagnosed in the second decade of life. This could even be a presenting feature of KS. In a study, nearly one-third of men with mediastinal GCT were diagnosed to have KS.

REFERENCE/SOURCE

- Bonouvrie K, van der Werff Ten Bosch J, van den Akker M. Klinefelter syndrome and germ cell tumours: review of the literature. Int J Pediatr Endocrinol. 2020;2020:18.

9. Which of the following genes is known to be associated with precocious puberty as well as delayed puberty because of similar mutation?

A. *SF-1 (NR5A1)*
B. *DAX-1 (NR0B1)*
C. *Kisspeptin*
D. *MKRN3*

EXPLANATION

In a large pedigree, a mutation in NR0B1 (nuclear receptor subfamily 0, group B, member 1) encoding for DAX-1 was shown to be associated with precocious puberty and arrested/delayed puberty in different members of the same family. Mutations in NR5A1 encoding for transcription factor steroidogenic factor-1 (SF-1) are associated with hypogonadism and loss of function mutations of *MKRN3* gene are associated with precocious puberty. Kisspeptin (*KISS1* gene) mutations can cause precocious as well as delayed puberty, however the mutations causing those are different.

Key: A

BOOST YOUR KNOWLEDGE

X-lined adrenal hypoplasia congenita (AHC) is a rare disorder caused by mutations in the NR0B1 (nuclear receptor subfamily 0, group B, member 1) gene encoding for *DAX-1* (dosage-sensitive sex reversal adrenal hypoplasia congenita critical region on the X chromosome). Affected males may present with adrenal insufficiency at 6–8 weeks of life. Some may present with isolated delays of puberty. Primary gonadal insufficiency may also be present but is usually masked by the presence of hypogonadotropic hypogonadism.

REFERENCE/SOURCE

- Palmert MR, Chan YM, Dunkel L. Puberty and its disorders in the male. In: Sperling MA, Majzoub JA, Menon RK, Stratakis CA (Eds). Sperling Pediatric Endocrinology, 5th edition. Philadelphia, PA; Elsevier, Inc.; 2021. pp. 661-94.

10. Which of the following conditions causing peripheral precocious puberty is usually associated with symmetrical enlargement of testes?

A. Leydig cell tumor
B. Familial male-limited precocious puberty (FMPP)
C. Congenital adrenal hyperplasia (CAH)
D. McCune-Albright syndrome (MAS)

EXPLANATION

Examination of testicular volume and its symmetry gives valuable clues to etiology in boys with precocious puberty (PP). Typically, symmetrically enlarged testes indicate central PP. However, in some conditions causing peripheral PP symmetrical testicular enlargement can be present. FMPP (previously known as testotoxicosis) is a familial form of peripheral PP resulting from constitutive activation of LH/hCG receptor, which presents in boys between 1 and 4 years of age with rapid virilization, bone age acceleration, and symmetrical enlargement of testes. The pubertal changes are disproportionately more compared to the testicular volumes. In PP, due to Leydig cell tumor there is asymmetric enlargement of testes. Whereas children with CAH have PP with small size of testes unless there is a superimposed central PP. Precocious puberty is less common in boys with MAS compared to girls. hCG-producing tumors can present with bilateral symmetrical enlargement of testes.

Key: B

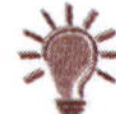

BOOST YOUR KNOWLEDGE

The gene for LH/hCG receptor is located on chromosome 2p21 and is the genetic basis for FMPP. Activating LH/hCG receptor mutations can be sporadic or inherited in an autosomal dominant manner and selectively affects only boys.

REFERENCE/SOURCE

- Palmert MR, Chan YM, Dunkel L. Puberty and its disorders in the male. In: Sperling MA, Majzoub JA, Menon RK, Stratakis CA (Eds). Sperling Pediatric Endocrinology, 5th edition. Philadelphia, PA; Elsevier, Inc.; 2021. pp. 672-3.

11. A 10-month-old girl presented with breast development. Her bone age is normal for age, and she has normal growth velocity. What is the likely diagnosis?

A. Central precocious puberty
B. Peripheral precocious puberty
C. Primary hypothyroidism
D. Isolated premature thelarche

EXPLANATION

This girl has breast development in the absence of advancement of bone age and rapid growth velocity. This goes against central or peripheral PP. Primary hypothyroidism is not a common cause of sexual precocity at this age and is usually seen in older girls with acquired hypothyroidism. The most common cause of thelarche in infancy is isolated premature thelarche which presents with thelarche in the absence of excess growth or bone age advancement.

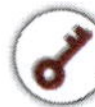

Key: D

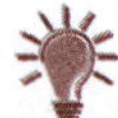

BOOST YOUR KNOWLEDGE

Premature thelarche denotes breast development before 8 years of age. In the first 2 years of life, the most common cause for this is a benign condition termed as isolated premature thelarche. Clinical and laboratory evaluation is needed to rule out central precocious puberty. In infants, this syndrome seems to be caused by a lag in inhibition of the transient activation of the hypothalamic-pituitary-gonadal (HPG) axis of the newborn.

REFERENCE/SOURCE

- Reselfield R, Cooke DW, Radovick S. Puberty in the female and its disorders. In: Sperling MA, Majzoub JA, Menon RK, Stratakis CA (Eds). Sperling Pediatric Endocrinology, 5th edition. Philadelphia, PA; Elsevier, Inc.; 2021. p. 560.

12. Which of the following is considered the cut-off for indicating the onset of puberty in a boy?

A. Testicular volume 3 mL
B. Testicular volume 4 mL
C. Testicular volume 5 mL
D. Testicular volume 6 mL

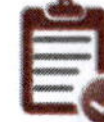

EXPLANATION

The first change of puberty in the male is increase of testicular volume. This can be measured with the help of an orchidometer. A testicular volume of 4 mL or more or testicular length of more than or equal to 2.5 cm indicates pubertal onset in males.

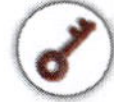

Key: B

BOOST YOUR KNOWLEDGE

In boys, pubertal growth spurt is evident in later part of puberty at genital stage 3–4, averaging about 9.5 cm/year.

REFERENCE/SOURCE

- Sharma R. Physiology of puberty. In: Desai M, Menon PSN, Bhatia V, Seth A (Eds). Pediatric Endocrine Disorders, 4th edition. Hyderabad, India: Universities Press; 2022. p. 135.

13. Which of the following best defines premature pubarche?

A. Onset of pubic hairs before 8 years of age in girls and boys
B. Onset of pubic hairs before 7 years of age in girls and 8 years in boys
C. Onset of pubic hairs before 8 years of age in girls and 9 years in boys
D. Onset of pubic hairs before 9 years of age in girls and boys

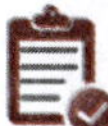

EXPLANATION

Premature pubarche is defined as onset of pubic hairs before 8 years of age in girls and 9 years in boys. Most commonly, it results from premature activation of adrenal androgens, known as premature adrenarche, an idiopathic condition characterized by clinical evidence of adrenal androgen action in the form of axillary/pubic hairs, acne, and adult type of body odor. Usually, the bone age is normal or slightly advanced and adult height potential is not compromised.

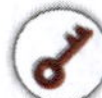

Key: C

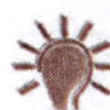

BOOST YOUR KNOWLEDGE

The differential diagnosis of premature pubarche includes premature adrenarche, nonclassic congenital adrenal hyperplasia, virilizing tumors of adrenal/gonadal origin, central precocious puberty, or exogenous androgen exposure.

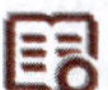

REFERENCE/SOURCE

- Rosenfeld R. Normal and premature adrenarche. Endocr Rev. 2021;42(6):783-814.

14. A boy with delayed puberty was noted to have bilateral ptosis and pectus carinatum deformity. What is the likely diagnosis?

A. Kallmann syndrome
B. Bardet-Biedl syndrome
C. CHARGE association
D. Noonan syndrome

EXPLANATION

Delayed puberty is seen in several syndromic conditions including all the conditions listed above. However, the features of ptosis and pectus carinatum suggest a diagnosis of Noonan syndrome in this child. Diagnostic features of other conditions listed include anosmia, synkinesia, unilateral renal agenesis (Kallmann syndrome), obesity, polydactyly, retinitis pigmentosa (Bardet–Biedl syndrome), and coloboma, heart defects, growth retardation and ear anomalies (CHARGE association).

Key: D

BOOST YOUR KNOWLEDGE

Noonan syndrome is a common condition with a prevalence of about 1:1,000–2,500. Short stature, typical facial features, and cardiac anomalies are typical features. Inheritance is predominantly autosomal dominant, and the most common underlying mutations are seen in *PTPN11* gene. Although puberty is delayed, it is not absent.

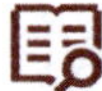

REFERENCE/SOURCE

- Dahlgren J, Noordam C. Growth, endocrine features, and growth hormone treatment in Noonan syndrome. J Clin Med. 2022;11(7):2034.

15. Parents of an otherwise healthy, 10-year-old boy are concerned about his penile length being small compared to his peers. He has stretched penile length (SPL) of 5 cm and bilaterally scrotal testes of 2 mL each. He weighs 65 kg and has a height of 140 cm. His luteinizing hormone (LH), follicle-stimulating hormone (FSH), and total testosterone values are prepubertal. What is the most usual diagnosis in this scenario?

A. Webbed penis
B. Buried penis
C. Micropenis due to hypogonadism
D. Trapped penis

EXPLANATION

The boy clinically is obese, and his SPL is normal for age. Since most boys of this age would be prepubertal, the low LH, FSH, and testosterone are age appropriate. The most common diagnosis in this child is obesity with buried penis.

Key: B

BOOST YOUR KNOWLEDGE

Webbed penis is when scrotal sac extends onto the ventral aspect of the penile shaft, giving the visual appearance of a small penis, but palpation of the corpora will reveal the true state. A trapped penis refers to a penis that has become entrapped by scar tissues or excessive excision of preputial or shaft skin following an intervention such as a circumcision. Often associated malformations such as chordee give an appearance of small penis. These conditions need to be ruled out in children presenting with concerns of micropenis. True micropenis is defined as stretched penile length <2.5 SD (2–2.5 cm) in infants.

REFERENCE/SOURCE

- Stancampiano MR, Suzuki K, O'Toole S, Russo G, Yamada G, Faisal Ahmed S. Congenital micropenis: etiology and management. J Endocr Soc. 2021;6(2):bvab172.

16. Which of the following is the most appropriate choice of pharmacological treatment in boys with constitutional delay of growth and puberty (CDGP)?

A. Low dose depot testosterone esters
B. Aromatase inhibitors
C. Human chorionic gonadotropin (hCG)
D. Long-acting testosterone undecanoate

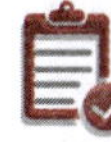

EXPLANATION

While in some cases of CDGP, reassurance and follow-up are all that is sufficient, often pharmacological treatment is needed for psychosocial reasons. Short-term treatment with low-dose (50–100 mg monthly) testosterone esters (testosterone enanthate, cypionate, or propionate) are most used. These have been shown to improve growth velocity and self-image without adversely impacting the bone age. Long-acting testosterone undecanoate is useful for testosterone replacement for hypogonadal men once a full dose has been reached. While aromatase inhibitors and hCG have been used for CDGP, the choice at present remains low-dose testosterone esters for a short term (3–6 months).

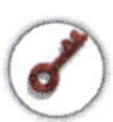

Key: A

BOOST YOUR KNOWLEDGE

Constitutional delay of growth and puberty is the most common cause of delayed puberty. It is diagnosis of exclusion after ruling out systemic, psychological, or endocrine disorders causing transient or permanent delay of puberty. Growth, bone age, and adrenarche is often delayed and family history of delayed puberty/growth spurt is common. Increase in the testicular volume spontaneously or after a short course of testosterone supports the diagnosis of CDGP. If spontaneous puberty is not seen by 18 years of age, a diagnosis of permanent hypogonadism is likely.

REFERENCE/SOURCE

- Styne DM. Physiology and disorders of puberty. In: Melmed S, Auchus RJ, Goldfine AB, Koenig RJ, Rosen CJ (Eds). Williams Textbook of Endocrinology, 14th edition. Philadelphia, PA: Elsevier, Inc.; 2020. pp. 1116-7.

17. Which of the following is *not* an essential criterion for the diagnosis of polycystic ovary syndrome in adolescent girls?

A. Clinical and/or biochemical hyperandrogenism
B. Persistent oligo/amenorrhea 3–4 years postmenarche
C. Ultrasound showing polycystic ovarian morphology
D. Exclusion of disorders which can cause similar presentation

EXPLANATION

Polycystic ovary syndrome (PCOS) is a common cause of hyperandrogenism in adolescent and young women. The diagnostic difficulty in adolescence is caused by features overlapping with normal adolescence such as acne and irregularity of menses in the first couple of years after menarche. In adults, as per the Rotterdam criteria, diagnosis of PCOS in made in women with any two of the features of clinical and/or hyperandrogenism, oligo/anovulation and PCO morphology on pelvic ultrasound, after ruling out conditions which can cause similar clinical picture. However, pelvic ultrasound is not useful for the diagnosis of PCOS. In adolescents, as there is a high incidence of multifollicular ovaries in normal girls in few years following menarche. Hence, ultrasonography (USG) is not recommended to diagnose PCOS in adolescents. USG is usually done to rule out adrenal/ovarian tumors in girls with hyperandrogenism.

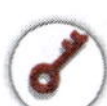

Key: C

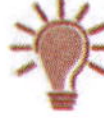

BOOST YOUR KNOWLEDGE

Other conditions which can cause hyperandrogenism in adolescents include exogenous exposure to androgens, nonclassic congenital adrenal hyperplasia, virilizing adrenal or gonadal tumors, Cushing syndrome, primary hypothyroidism, and hyperprolactinemia. These need to be ruled out on clinical examination and necessary laboratory testing. The diagnosis of nonclassic CAH is confirmed with cosyntropin stimulated 17-hydroxyprogesterone levels of >10 ng/mL.

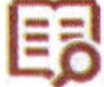

REFERENCE/SOURCE

- Peña AS, Witchel SF, Hoeger KM, Oberfield SE, Vogiatzi MG, Misso M, et al. Adolescent polycystic ovary syndrome according to the international evidence-based guideline. BMC Med. 2020;18(1):72.

18. Which of the following conditions (previously thought to be benign) is now known to be associated with long-term increased risk of endocrine and metabolic complications?

A. Isolated premature thelarche
B. Isolated scrotal/pubic hairs of infancy
C. Isolated premature adrenarche
D. Isolated premature menarche

EXPLANATION

The spectrum of pubertal disorders includes some variations of normal puberty in addition to extremes of progressive precocious puberty and pathological delayed puberty. Isolated premature adrenarche was thought to be a benign variation. However, several studies have now shown that isolated premature adrenarche is associated with later risk of PCOS and its related metabolic complications. Premature adrenarche can be an early symptom of PCOS and other hyperandrogenic conditions such as congenital adrenal hyperplasia and virilizing tumors. Isolated premature thelarche most often regresses by 2.5–3 years of life, however a 10–20% of these cases can go on to have central precocious puberty, hence it needs a careful follow-up. Isolated scrotal/pubic hairs of infancy are seen commonly after 6 months of life, can show some increase in size and distribution (usually not more than Tanner stage 3) and needs to be differentiated from other hyperandrogenic conditions such as congenital adrenal hyperplasia. Isolated premature menarche can be a presenting feature of conditions causing peripheral precocious puberty or local causes such as trauma or polyps.

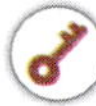

Key: C

BOOST YOUR KNOWLEDGE

Obesity and low birth weight are common risk factors for isolated premature adrenarche and subsequent PCOS. Premature adrenarche has no adverse effects on the onset and progression of gonadarche and final height but can have long-term metabolic consequences.

REFERENCE/SOURCE

- Witchel SF, Azziz R, Oberfield SE. History of polycystic ovary syndrome, premature adrenarche, and hyperandrogenism in pediatric endocrinology. Horm Res Paediatr. 2022;95(6):557-67.

CHAPTER

23.6 Adrenal Disorders

M Vijayakumar

1. **A 20-day-old boy presented with hyperpigmentation and dehydration. His serum electrolytes levels were altered (sodium 131 mEq/L and potassium 6.5 mEq/L). Genitalia were normal with both testes in the scrotal sac. His mother's brother was 15 years old and he was on hydrocortisone and fludrocortisone for "Addison's disease" and monthly injections of testosterone for delayed puberty. Identify this illness.**

A. Congenital adrenal hyperplasia (CAH; 21 hydroxylase deficiency—salt-losing variety)
B. Adrenal hypoplasia congenita (DAX1 mutation)
C. NR5A1 mutation
D. Lipoid adrenal hyperplasia

EXPLANATION

This boy has features of salt-losing crisis and hyperpigmentation. 95% of the cases are caused by CAH, of which 21-hydroxylase deficiencies are the most common. Important clue in this case is that his mother's brother is having (X-linked recessive) hypoadrenalism and testosterone deficiency, pointing toward an X-linked recessive disorder of adrenocortical hypofunction and hypogonadism. Hence, diagnosis is adrenal hypoplasia congenita (DAX1 mutation).

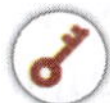

Key: B

BOOST YOUR KNOWLEDGE

Adrenal hypoplasia congenita is an X-linked disorder caused by mutations in NR0B1 (*DAX1* gene), which is expressed in the adrenal glands, hypothalamus, pituitary gland, and gonads. Affected neonates present just like salt-losing CAH, and older children with features similar to Addison disease and hypogonadotropic hypogonadism. NR5A1 mutation (*SF1* gene) produces adrenal hypoplasia with disorders of sex development (DSD; XY sex reversal).

Some genetic causes for primary adrenal insufficiency:

Name	*Genetics*	*Clinical features in addition to adrenal insufficiency*
Triple A syndrome (Allgrove syndrome)	AAAS mutation	Achalasia, alacrimia, cognitive defects, hyperkeratosis
Smith-Lemli-Opitz syndrome	DHCR7 mutation	Craniofacial malformations, developmental delay, cholesterol deficiency
Wolman disease	LIPA mutation	Bilateral adrenal calcification, hepatosplenomegaly
IMAGe syndrome	POLE mutation	Intrauterine growth restriction, metaphyseal dysplasia, genital abnormalities
Pallister Hall syndrome	GLI3 mutation	Hypothalamic hamartoma, hypopituitarism, imperforate anus, postaxial polydactyly

2. A 10-year-old boy on treatment for Addison disease for the past 3 years developed progressive defective vision and gait abnormalities. His speech has become incomprehensive recently. Name the investigation to confirm the diagnosis.

A. Blood for very-long-chain fatty acids (VLCFAs)
B. Magnetic resonance imaging (MRI) to assess neuronal loss
C. Abdominal ultrasound to look for adrenal calcifications
D. Visual evoked potential

EXPLANATION

The clinical condition is adrenoleukodystrophy (ALD), a peroxisomal disorder. Adrenal gland is involved in ALD and other peroxisomal disorders such as Refsum disease and Zellweger syndrome. ALD is an X-linked recessive disorder and *all boys presenting with features of primary adrenal insufficiency should be evaluated for ALD*. ALD is caused by mutations of *ABCD1* gene, which prevent normal transport of VLCFAs into peroxisomes, preventing oxidation of VLCFAs. Newborn screening is instituted for ALD in USA. Neuroimaging shows a garland of contrast enhancement near to the posterior hypodense lesions in periventricular white matter in the occipital and posterior parietal lobes.

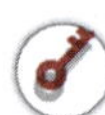

Key: A

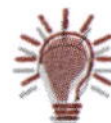

BOOST YOUR KNOWLEDGE

Adrenoleukodystrophy is the most common metabolic cause of adrenal failure. Adrenomyeloneuropathy is seen in adults. Newborn screening and early allogenic hematopoietic stem cell transplantation are now carried out as a treatment of choice. Lorenzo oil (4:1 mixture of glyceryl trioleate and glyceryl trierucate) is not very much effective in the established case.

3. A 10-year-old boy presented with hyperpigmentation and tiredness. Investigations revealed hyponatremia and hypoglycemia. Serum cortisol was found to be low and adrenocorticotropic hormone (ACTH) high suggestive of primary adrenal insufficiency. His serum calcium level was low (5.8 mg/dL) and phosphorous high 5.6 mg/dL. What is the likely diagnosis?

A. Addison disease
B. Multiple endocrine neoplasia
C. Autoimmune polyendocrinopathy syndrome 1
D. Autoimmune polyendocrinopathy syndrome 2

EXPLANATION

Approximately 50% of children with autoimmune adrenal insufficiency have autoimmune destruction of other endocrine glands. This combination is called autoimmune polyglandular syndrome (APS). APS1, also called autoimmune polyendocrinopathy-candidiasis-ectodermal dystrophy (APECED), is characterized by chronic mucocutaneous candidiasis (usually the initial manifestation), hypoparathyroidism, and adrenal insufficiency (which develops later). Other associated features include vitiligo, nail dystrophy, alopecia, enamel hypoplasia, and gonadal failure. Inheritance is autosomal recessive and genetic abnormality is the mutations in *AIRE* (autoimmune regulator) gene. Adrenal failure is a late manifestation and often the cause of death if not detected early. Hence all children having identified hypoparathyroidism should be closely monitored for possible adrenal insufficiency.

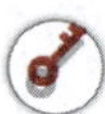

Key: C

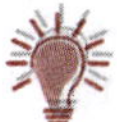

BOOST YOUR KNOWLEDGE

APS2, also known as Schmidt syndrome, is characterized by adrenal insufficiency and thyroiditis and Carpenter syndrome is associated with adrenal insufficiency and type 1 diabetes. Although it is much more common than APS1, presentations are often late (20–40 years).

4. A 10-year-old girl presented with tiredness, fatigability, and not gaining weight for the past few months. Her blood pressure (BP) was on the lower side (80/60 mm Hg) and had low random blood sugar (40 mg/dL) at the time of examination. Electrolytes showed Na 129 mEq/L and K 5.9 mEq/L. Which investigation will you do to confirm the clinical condition?

A. Morning cortisol followed by ACTH stimulation test
B. Cardiac evaluation to rule out myocarditis
C. Fasting and postprandial blood sugar and HbA1C
D. Sepsis screen

EXPLANATION

Features are suggestive of primary adrenal insufficiency. (Patients with central secondary adrenal insufficiency do not have mineralocorticoid deficiency). Clinical findings of untreated primary adrenal insufficiency are often nonspecific and include fatigue, nausea, and vomiting. Signs of mineralocorticoid deficiency include hypotension, dehydration, metabolic acidosis, and electrolyte abnormalities. Adrenal crisis results from acute adrenal insufficiency. They usually have features of both mineralocorticoid and glucocorticoid deficiency. This condition should be suspected in any child with shock if clinical features fail to respond even to vigorous fluid resuscitation and inotropic agents.

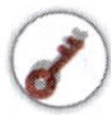

Key: A

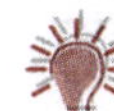

BOOST YOUR KNOWLEDGE

Measurement of basal cortisol in the morning (between 6.00 AM and 8.00 AM) is the initial screening step. If serum cortisol is very low (<3 μg/dL) and ACTH >100 pg/mL at 8.00 to 9.00 AM with classic clinical features, this test itself may be confirmatory. If basal cortisol is normal (>8 μg/dL), adrenal insufficiency is unlikely. In indeterminate cases, ACTH stimulation test is a must. Serum cortisol <18 μg/dL 30 or 60 minutes after IV injection of 250 μg of synthetic ACTH is confirmatory.

5. A 14-day-old boy presented with dehydration and hyperpigmentation around the genital area. His electrolyte levels were as follows: Serum sodium 129 mEq/L and potassium 4.9 mEq/L. He has lost almost 1 kg since birth. Mention the investigation of choice.

A. Serum 17-hydroxyprogesterone (17-OHP)
B. Serum 17-hydroxypregnenolone
C. Serum 11-deoxycorticosterone
D. Serum ACTH

EXPLANATION

Congenital adrenal hyperplasia is a group of disorders of cortisol biosynthesis, inherited in an autosomal recessive (AR) manner. Cortisol deficiency results in an increased production of ACTH, which stimulates the adrenals to produce intermediary metabolites. Most common form of CAH is 21-hydroxylase deficiency (CYP21), which constitutes 90% of all forms of CAH. The incidence of classic 21-hydroxylase deficiency is about 1 in 20,000 and 70% of which are salt-losing form and remaining constitute simple virilizing variety.

Classic salt-losing variety presents at age 10–14 days with dehydration, hyperpigmentation, hyperkalemia, hyponatremia, hypoglycemia, and metabolic acidosis. Blood level of 17-OHP is the diagnostic test, which will be very high. Girls will have features of virilization.

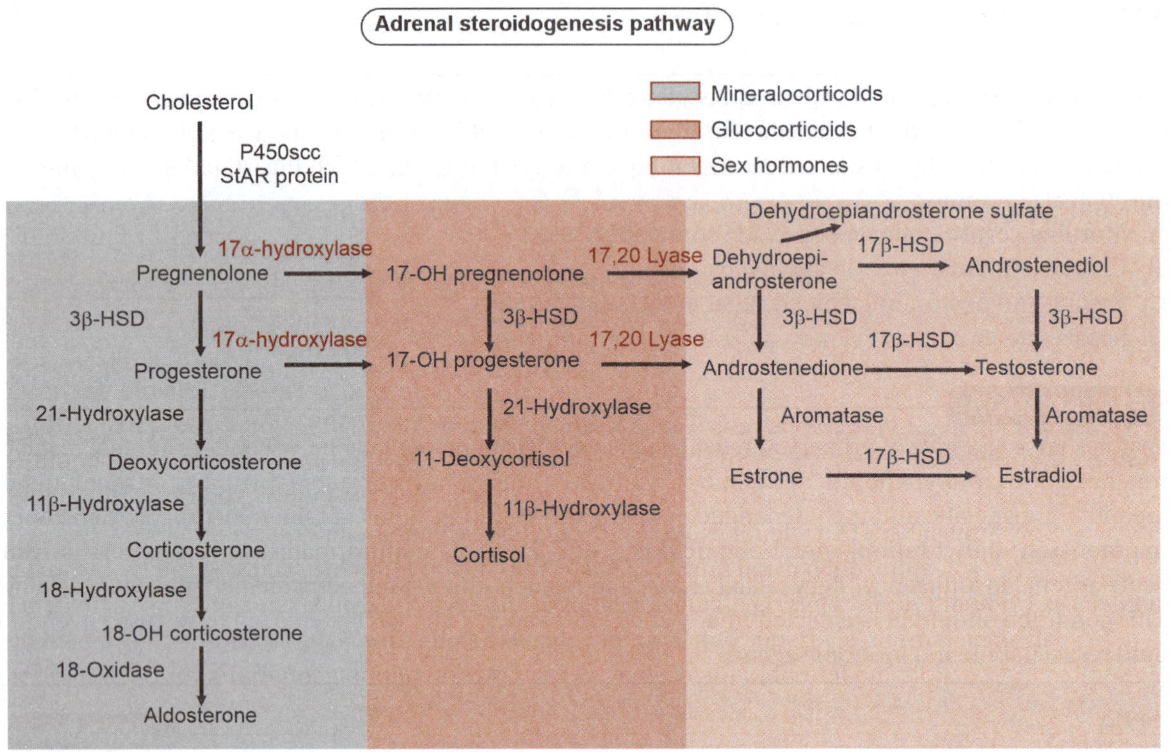

 **Key: A**

 **BOOST YOUR KNOWLEDGE**

21-hydroxylase enzyme deficiency is a spectrum of diseases in which salt-losing variety is having <1% of enzyme activity. Simple virilizing type has 1–2% enzyme activity and they will not manifest as an overt mineralocorticoid deficiency. Nonclassic form, with some enzymatic activity, will not manifest in the newborn period. They will have mild hyperandrogenism and present during adolescence with oligomenorrhea, hirsutism, or acne.

Affected neonates with classic CAH will have very high levels of 17-OHP (>3,500 ng/dL) with salt-losing variety having levels as high as >10,000 ng/dL. If a positive value is obtained in newborn screening (done between 2 and 4 days after birth), a confirmatory test should be done. A common method used in newborn screening is DELFIA (dissociation-enhanced lanthanide fluorescence immune assay). Most prefer liquid chromatography followed by tandem mass spectrometry for confirmation (second tier test), because assay by DELFIA may result in false positivity due to cross reaction with other steroid metabolites. Those with intermediate results should be confirmed by using ACTH stimulation tests.

6. A 1-month-old baby is admitted for evaluation of undescended testes. He is having palpable inguinal testes on both sides. Examination revealed skeletal abnormalities in the form of craniosynostosis, midface hypoplasia, and bowing of both femur bones. Newborn screening showed mild elevation of 17-OHP (1,000 ng/dL). Which type of CAH is more likely?

A. Classic 21-hydroxylase deficiency
B. 17-hydroxylase deficiency
C. P450 oxidoreductase (POR)
D. 3-beta-hydroxysteroid dehydrogenase

EXPLANATION

P450 oxidoreductase is essential for the function of cytochrome p450 enzymes, mainly 21-hydroxylase, 17-hydroxylase, and aromatase. Deficiency of 17-hydroxylase produces incomplete masculinization in males and 21-hydroxylase deficiency leads to virilization in females. Reduced aromatase activity in the placenta results in unopposed action of androgens produced by fetal adrenals leading to virilization in the mother. This condition is also associated with congenital anomalies, collectively called *Antley–Bixler syndrome*. Salient features include craniosynostosis, brachycephaly, midface hypoplasia, and bony abnormalities.

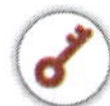

Key: C

BOOST YOUR KNOWLEDGE

P450 oxidoreductase is a rare form of CAH, mimicking classic 21-hydroxylase deficiency. This may be picked up in newborn screening because 17-OHP levels may be mildly elevated. Other conditions producing mild elevation in 17-OHP include 11-beta-hydroxylase deficiency and 3-beta-hydroxysteroid dehydrogenase deficiency.

- *Conditions producing false positive 17-OHP results in newborn screening:* Premature and sick infants
- *False negative results:* Administration of antenatal steroids such as betamethasone

7. Name the type of CAH producing hypertension and incomplete virilization in boys.

A. 11-beta-hydroxylase deficiency
B. 17-hydroxylase deficiency
C. Steroidogenic acute regulatory protein (StAR) deficiency
D. 21-hydroxylase deficiency

EXPLANATION

11-beta-hydroxylase deficiency and 17-hydroxylase deficiency produce hypertension, which will be prominent only after the neonatal period. As seen in the figure in the Question 5 explanation, 17-hydroxylase deficiency blocks conversion of pregnenolone to 17-hydroxypregnenolone as well as that of progesterone to 17-OHP. Aldosterone synthesis remains unaffected and pathway moves more in this direction producing more mineralocorticoids, explaining hypertension. Sex hormone production is diminished, hence resulting in undervirilized male babies. 11-beta-hydroxylase deficiency also produces hypertension, which is due to elevated levels of deoxycorticosterone, which has mineralocorticoid activity. But this condition produces features of androgen excess unlike 17-hydroxylase deficiency.

Key: B

BOOST YOUR KNOWLEDGE

Both 11-beta-hydroxylase (5%) and 17-hydroxylase deficiency (1%) are rare forms of CAH. But if a child with CAH develops hypertension, one must consider these rare possibilities.

8. A 14-day-old neonate presented with salt-losing crisis and hypoglycemia. Abdominal ultrasound revealed massive adrenal enlargement. Which among the following conditions is the most likely possibility?

A. StAR deficiency
B. 11-beta-hydroxylase deficiency
C. 17-hydroxylase deficiency
D. 21-hydroxylase deficiency

EXPLANATION

All forms of CAH produce enlargement of the adrenal gland in the imaging study, but this is not taken as a diagnostic criterion while evaluating CAH. StAR deficiency produces massive enlargement of the gland because of storage of cholesterol.

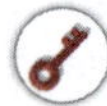

Key: A

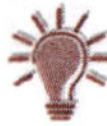

BOOST YOUR KNOWLEDGE

StAR deficiency is characterized by marked accumulation of cholesterol and lipids in the adrenal cortex and gonads. Conversion of cholesterol to pregnenolone is severely impaired, leading to severe impairment of all steroidogenesis. StAR helps in the movement of cholesterol from outer to inner membrane of mitochondria. Salt-losing features are evident in neonates. Males remain undervirilized.

9. A 6-month-old baby is being evaluated for developmental delay. He was born of a difficult labor and was extracted by vacuum. Abdominal ultrasound revealed bilateral adrenal calcifications. Which among the following is the most common to have such a finding?

A. Wolman disease
B. Neuroblastoma
C. Ganglioneuroma
D. Adrenal hemorrhage

EXPLANATION

Hemorrhage into the adrenal gland is the most common cause of adrenal calcification, often secondary to anoxia or trauma. Neuroblastoma, ganglioneuroma, adrenocortical carcinoma, pheochromocytoma, adrenal gland cysts, etc., can have adrenal calcification. Tuberculosis used to be a cause for adrenal calcification and Addison disease. Wolman disease is a lipid disorder producing bilateral calcifications.

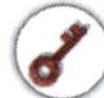

Key: D

BOOST YOUR KNOWLEDGE

All conditions causing adrenal gland calcification are not serious, careful evaluation is a must.

10. A 2-year-old girl presented with recently appeared pubic and axillary hairs. Examination revealed clitoromegaly. Investigation results showed very high levels of dehydroepiandrosterone sulfate (DHEAS) >1,000 μg/dL. Which is the most likely diagnosis?

A. CAH
B. Virilizing adrenal tumor
C. Exogenous administration of sex steroids
D. Pheochromocytoma

EXPLANATION

The majority of adrenocortical tumors produce signs of virilization, which almost mimic features of virilizing CAH. Accelerated growth velocity, muscle hypertrophy, acne, penile enlargement, and development of pubic and axillary hair are other features.

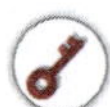

Key: B

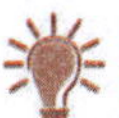

BOOST YOUR KNOWLEDGE

Feminizing tumors (10%) secrete high levels of estrogens, resulting in gynecomastia in boys and premature thelarche in girls. Tumors of adrenal medulla such as pheochromocytoma will not develop virilization. Serum levels of DHEA/DHEAS will be markedly elevated in adrenocortical tumors.

11. A 10-year-old boy presented with obesity and moon face. Examination revealed mild buffalo hump and white striae over abdomen. His morning (8.00 AM) serum cortisol level was 3 μg/dL. What is the provisional diagnosis?

A. Exogenous Cushing syndrome
B. Cushing disease
C. Cushing syndrome due to ectopic ACTH secreting tumor
D. Adrenocortical tumor

EXPLANATION

When any child presents with Cushingoid features, the first step is to rule out exogenous causes of corticosteroid exposure, such as intermittent oral steroids for asthma, rheumatologic illness, or malignancy. Morning cortisol (8.00 AM) gives a clue if you suspect Cushing syndrome, which will be low in exogenous steroid exposure.

Exogenous obesity also produces some buffalo hump and striae. Linear growth acceleration is the rule in exogenous obesity, but growth faltering is the characteristic feature in Cushing syndrome. Striae are seen in exogenous obesity also. Cushing syndrome is characterized by thick violaceous striae.

Key: A

BOOST YOUR KNOWLEDGE

Exposure to steroid medication (either oral, topical, or inhaled) is the most common cause of Cushing syndrome in children. Clinical features of hypercortisolism with low cortisol levels are suggestive of exogenous Cushing syndrome. A careful history of drug intake is a must before investigating for pathological causes.

12. A 5-year-old boy presented with headache, dizziness, and visual disturbances. Examination revealed that he was hypertensive (BP 240/150 mm Hg). He was not edematous or obese and not on chronic medications. Cardiac and renal evaluations were normal. Investigations revealed hypokalemia. Serum cortisol was normal. Plasma renin activity was suppressed. Which of the following is most likely?

A. Pheochromocytoma
B. Primary aldosteronism
C. Cushing syndrome
D. CAH—11-beta-hydroxylase deficiency

EXPLANATION

In this condition, the child did not have edema and other features of Cushing syndrome. 11-beta-hydroxylase deficiency will not produce severe hypokalemia. Hypokalemia and suppression of renin–angiotensin system points toward increased aldosterone secretion and primary hyperaldosteronism. Aldosterone-secreting adenomas are the most common one in children although very rare. Plasma levels of aldosterone and 24-hour urine aldosterone concentration are high. Plasma levels of renin are persistently low. Ratio of plasma aldosterone concentration and renin activity is always high (>30). Treatment is surgical removal of adenoma. Hyperaldosteronism because of bilateral adrenal hyperplasia is managed by mineralocorticoid antagonists such as spironolactone or eplerenone.

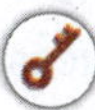

Key: B

BOOST YOUR KNOWLEDGE

Increased aldosterone effect should be looked for if a child presents with refractory hypertension and hypokalemia. Aldosterone is the prime regulator of sodium, potassium, and volume status. Look for rare genetic conditions if the child is hypertensive with low levels of aldosterone and renin. These diseases of mineralocorticoid excess include Liddle syndrome, pseudohypoaldosteronism, and syndrome of apparent mineralocorticoid excess. If the child is having features of catecholamine excess (headache, sweating, and tachycardia), evaluate for plasma and urine catecholamines.

13. A 10-year-old boy presented with headache and dizziness. He is having palpitation, dizziness, and sweating along with headache. The symptoms were exaggerated during exercise. He was on treatment for attention-deficit/hyperactive disorder (ADHD). Examination revealed an emaciated child with BP 200/120 mm Hg. His CBC, electrolytes, blood urea, creatinine, and urine analysis results were normal. Which of the following investigations is the most ideal?

A. Urinary excretion of vanillylmandelic acid (VMA)
B. Urinary excretion of metanephrine
C. Urinary excretion of homovanillic acid (HVA)
D. Urinary catecholamines

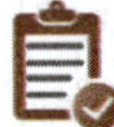

EXPLANATION

All these tests are intended for evaluating pheochromocytoma. Pheochromocytoma produces epinephrine and norepinephrine. The best provisional diagnostic test 24-hour urinary estimation of metanephrines (normetanephrine and metanephrine). Total urinary metanephrine excretion exceeds 300 µg/day. Although urinary excretion of VMA is also elevated, vanilla-containing substances in food can produce false elevation, hence not routinely done. Measurement of plasma normetanephrines is also an investigation of choice.

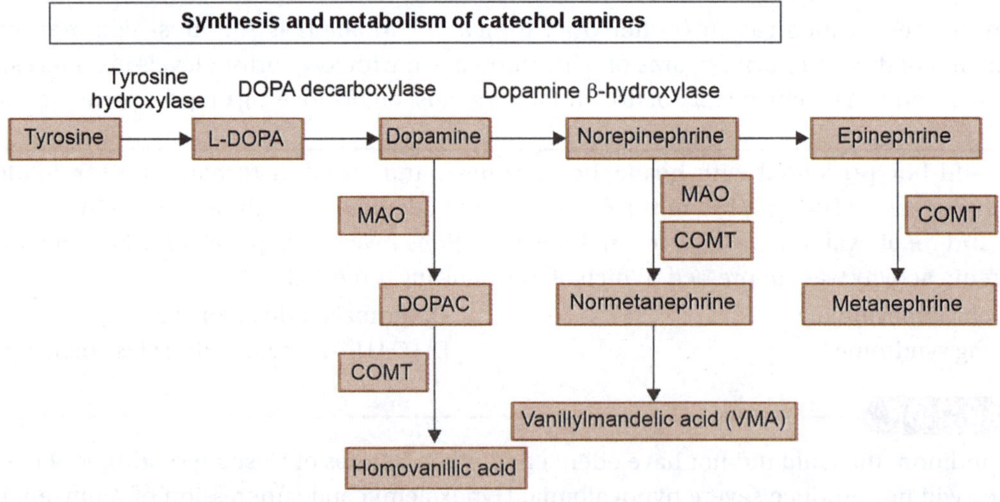

(COMT: catechol-O-methyltransferase; DOPAC: 3,4 dihydrophenyl acetic acid; MAO: mono amino oxidase)

Key: B

BOOST YOUR KNOWLEDGE

Pheochromocytomas and paragangliomas are rare causes of hypertension in children. Tumors of the adrenal medulla are called pheochromocytoma and those of extra-adrenal origins are called paragangliomas. They secrete catecholamines. Hypersecretion of norepinephrine, epinephrine, and dopamine from the tumor produces hypertension, tachycardia, sweating, and headache. High incidence of ADHD is reported in these children, often associated with multiple endocrine neoplasia (MEN) and Von Hippel Lindau (VHL) disease. All routine laboratory investigations for hypertension (CBC, electrolytes, urea, creatinine, and urine analysis) will be normal in these children. Measurement of 24-hour fractionated urinary metanephrines is the investigation of choice. Those with positive test should be further evaluated with imaging to confirm and localize the tumor.

14. An 8-year-old girl with type 1 diabetes was brought to you. Her parents have noticed weight loss for the past 3 months and frequent hypoglycemia and reduced insulin requirements. Which hormone deficiency we should anticipate?

A. Insulin
B. Glucagon
C. Thyroxine
D. Cortisol

EXPLANATION

Cortisol enhances gluconeogenesis and cortisol deficiency results in hypoglycemia. Type 1 diabetes is often associated with other autoimmune disorders such as Addison disease and hence if a child with type 1 diabetes is having weight loss and reduced insulin requirements, the possibility of associated cortisol deficiency should be thought of.

Key: D

BOOST YOUR KNOWLEDGE

Cortisol has many effects on growth and electrolyte homoeostasis. Cortisol deficiency inhibits growth by its action on growth plate, insulin-like growth factor 1 (IGF-1), and growth hormone (GH) action. It also reduces serum sodium level [arginine vasopressin (AVP) inhibition and reduced free water excretion] and induces hypocalcemia by impairing vitamin D activation.

15. A 28-day-old neonate is having prolonged jaundice. He is having midline cleft lip, palate, and micropenis. Investigation showed low free T4 and thyroid-stimulating hormone (TSH) levels and baby was put on thyroxine. But he collapsed 3 days after initiation of thyroxine and required fluid resuscitation. Which of the following may be the cause of sudden deterioration in his general condition?

A. Cortisol deficiency
B. AVP deficiency
C. GH deficiency
D. Gonadotropin deficiency

EXPLANATION

This neonate is having central hypothyroidism as a part of multiple pituitary hormone deficiency (panhypopituitarism), because he is having micropenis, midline cleft lip, and palate. Always rule out other pituitary hormone deficiencies before starting thyroxine especially ACTH deficiency leading to low cortisol level. Cortisol deficiency causes conjugated hyperbilirubinemia in the neonatal period.

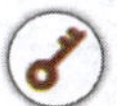

Key: A

BOOST YOUR KNOWLEDGE

Thyroxine increases body metabolism and enhances the conversion of cortisol to cortisone precipitating adrenal insufficiency. Hence cortisol deficiency should be identified and treatment should be initiated before starting GH or thyroxine.

16. Which of the following genetic defects produces isolated ACTH deficiency?

A. *SOX*
B. *HESX1*
C. *POMC*
D. *PROP1*

EXPLANATION

Isolated ACTH deficiency is seen in *POMC* gene defects. This condition is associated with ACTH deficiency, blond hair, and obesity. Proconvertase defects also produce obesity and ACTH deficiency. TPIT produces a severe neonatal form of ACTH deficiency. Many of the genetic defects resulting in ACTH deficiency also produce other pituitary hormone deficiencies and extrapituitary manifestations.

Key: C

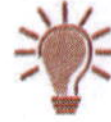

BOOST YOUR KNOWLEDGE

Common genetic forms of multiple pituitary hormone deficiency

Genetic forms	Deficient hormone and clinical features
POU1F1	GH, PRL, and TSH
PROP1	GH, PRL, TSH, FSH, LH, and ACTH
LHX3	GH, PRL, TSH, LH, FSH. Short neck, limited neck rotation, and sensorineural deafness
LHX4	GH, TSH, ACTH, small AP, EPP, Arnold–Chiari malformation, and cerebellar abnormalities
HESX1	GH, variable other pituitary hormone deficiencies, small AP, EPP, optic nerve hypoplasia, and septo-optic dysplasia
SHH	GH, single central incisor
SOX2	LH, FSH, GH, anophthalmia, microphthalmia, and sensorineural deafness

(ACTH: adrenocorticotropic hormone; AP: anterior pituitary; EPP: ectopic posterior pituitary; FSH: follicle-stimulating hormone; GH: growth hormone; LH: luteinizing hormone; PRL: prolactin; TSH: thyroid-stimulating hormone)

17. A 1-year-old boy presented with micropenis and right-sided inguinal hernia. His serum sodium levels were low (129 nmol/L). Examination revealed microcephaly and syndactyly. Investigations showed low serum cortisol 4 µg/dL. Which of the following is the likely lipid abnormality in this child?

A. High low-density lipoprotein (LDL)
B. High high-density lipoprotein (HDL)
C. High triglycerides
D. Low cholesterol

EXPLANATION

Most likely diagnosis is Smith-Lemli-Opitz syndrome (SLOS). Characteristic features include micropenis suggesting androgen deficiency, hyponatremia, and physical abnormalities such as microcephaly, upturned nares, and syndactyly. Low cholesterol level is the characteristic lipid profile abnormality in this condition. As the final step of cholesterol biosynthesis is affected in this condition, levels of 7-dehydrocholesterol are elevated in this condition.

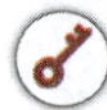

Key: D

BOOST YOUR KNOWLEDGE

Micropenis with salt wasting denotes associated testicular hormonal defects. High cholesterol level is associated with syndromes such as Wolman disease.

18. An 8-year-old boy is admitted to pediatric intensive care unit (PICU) with high fever and irritability. His condition suddenly deteriorated with poor peripheral circulation, cold extremities, and prolonged capillary filling time. His BP was low. Investigations revealed serum sodium 129 mmol/L and potassium 6.2 mmol/L. He was started on fluid bolus. Which emergency medication will be of help?

A. Adrenalin
B. Noradrenaline
C. Dopamine
D. Hydrocortisone

EXPLANATION

Features are suggestive of adrenal crisis, probably due to adrenal hemorrhage (Waterhouse–Friderichsen syndrome). Treatment of choice is intravenous hydrocortisone.

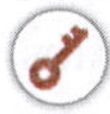

Key: D

BOOST YOUR KNOWLEDGE

Classical Waterhouse–Friedrichsen syndrome is described in meningococcal infection. Petechial rash will be diagnostic, which is most seen in the trunk and lower portions of the body.

19. A 3-month-old girl is admitted for evaluation of failure to thrive. She had persistent diarrhea. Clinical examination revealed abdominal distension and hepatosplenomegaly. She had hyperpigmentation around genitalia. Investigations showed low serum sodium (128 mmol/L), high potassium (6 mmol/L), and hypoglycemia. Serum cortisol level was 3 μg/dL. Which of the following conditions is the most likely diagnosis?

A. Tay–Sachs disease
B. Fabry disease
C. Krabbe disease
D. Wolman disease

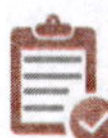

EXPLANATION

Wolman disease is characterized by primary adrenal insufficiency and calcifications in the adrenal glands. These children present with malabsorption, failure to gain weight, and hepatosplenomegaly. High cholesterol levels are usually seen in these children. These children usually die at infancy.

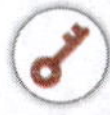

Key: D

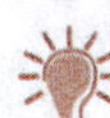

BOOST YOUR KNOWLEDGE

Wolman disease is inherited in autosomal recessive form and defective enzyme is lysosomal acid lipase (LAL), resulting in the accumulation of cholesteryl esters and triglycerides in visceral organs. Cholesterol ester storage defect is a less severe form of this illness. Drugs suppressing cholesterol synthesis, cholestyramine, and diet modifications are instituted as treatment. Recombinant lysosomal acid lipase, sebelipase-alfa is approved by the FDA recently.

20. A 7-year-old boy is diagnosed as having simple virilizing form of CAH. He is having rapid pubertal progression recently. His testicular volume was 6 mL on both sides. What investigation should be done and what is the treatment of choice?

A. 17-OHP and increase the dose of hydrocortisone
B. Plasma renin activity and start fludrocortisone
C. Gonadotropin-releasing hormone (GnRH) test and start GnRH analogs
D. Ultrasound of both testes and modify hydrocortisone treatment

EXPLANATION

In the case of CAH, rapid pubertal development indicates secondary central precocious puberty. In such cases, addition of GnRH analogs such as leuprolide is the treatment of choice.

Key: C

BOOST YOUR KNOWLEDGE

CAH, both salt losing and simple virilizing forms are the spectrum of same disease process and treatment is hydrocortisone and fludrocortisone. In simple virilizing form, addition of fludrocortisone in the treatment protocol reduces the requirement of hydrocortisone and hence its side effects. The dose of hydrocortisone should be titrated based on linear growth, development of side effects such as weight gain and cushingoid features, and 17-OHP measurements. Dose of fludrocortisone should be titrated based on BP, electrolyte levels, and plasma renin activity. If the child develops features of central precocious puberty, the child should be evaluated, and GnRH analogs should be initiated. Ultrasound of the testes is performed every year (after the age of 5 years) to look for testicular adrenal rest tumors.

REFERENCES/SOURCES

- Miller WL, Fluck CE, Breault DT, Feldman BJ. Adrenal cortex and its disorders. In: Sperling MA (Ed). Sperling Pediatric Endocrinology, 5th edition. Philadelphia: Elsevier; 2021. pp. 425-90.
- Vijayakumar M. Adrenal insufficiency and polyglandular syndromes. In: Gupta P, Menon PSN, Ramji S, Lodha R (Eds). PG Textbook of Pediatrics, 3rd edition. New Delhi: Jaypee Brothers Medical Publishers; 2022. pp. 2924-9.
- White PC. Disorders of adrenal gland. In: Kliegman RM, St Geme III JW (Eds). Nelson Textbook of Pediatrics, 21st edition. Elsevier; 2019. pp. 2954-86.

SECTION 24

Rheumatology

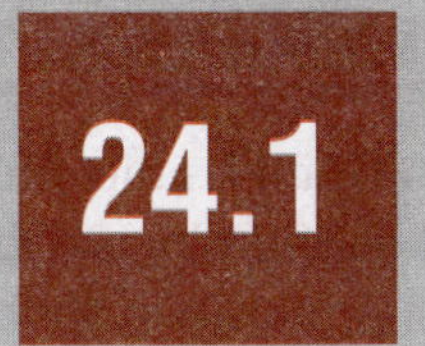

CHAPTER 24.1

Juvenile Idiopathic Arthritis and Systemic Lupus Erythematosus

Madhumita Nandi

1. A 7-year-old girl has fever for last 2 months, photosensitive rash, hypertension, hematuria, and bilateral pleural effusion. She has thrombocytopenia. C3 and C4 are low. Antinuclear antibody (ANA) and anti-dsDNA tests are positive (done by appropriate methods). What is the most likely pattern of joint involvement in this child?

A. Early symmetric polyarthritis of small joints
B. Late symmetric polyarthritis of large joints
C. Early symmetric polyarthritis of both small and large joints
D. Early oligoarthritis

EXPLANATION

From the clinical and laboratory features mentioned above, the most likely diagnosis is systemic lupus erythematosus (SLE) with nephritis. Arthritis of SLE is an early feature (within 1 year). So, this excludes option B. Also, it involves multiple joints. So that excludes option D. Now in between A and C, option C is more appropriate as both big and small joints may be involved.

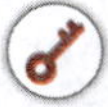

Key: C

BOOST YOUR KNOWLEDGE

Arthritis of SLE is most often present in the first year of diagnosis. Involvement of multiple joints, with or without pain with characteristic morning stiffness, is one of the clinical manifestations of SLE. Both small and large joints may be involved. Tenosynovitis is often present, but joint erosions or other radiographic changes are rare.

REFERENCE/SOURCE

- Sadun RE, Ardoin SP, Schanberg LE. Systemic lupus erythematosus. In: Kliegman RM, St Geme III JW, Blum NJ, Shah SS, Tasker RC, Wilson KM (Eds). Nelson Textbook of Pediatrics, 21st edition. Elsevier; 2019. pp. 1274-9.

2. An 8-year-old girl is prescribed combination antitubercular drugs under National Tuberculosis Elimination Programme (NTEP). About 6 weeks after that, she develops fever, arthralgia, and rashes on face. Examination reveals bilateral pleural effusion. Investigations show thrombocytopenia and leukopenia. Urine routine examination is normal. Which of the following is *true* regarding this condition?

A. She should be meticulously monitored for renal manifestations of the disease
B. Hepatitis is a rare finding in such cases
C. The manifestations will resolve after withdrawal antitubercular therapy (ATT)
D. AntiSm antibody is the most common antibody associated

EXPLANATION

This girl has most likely developed drug-induced lupus (isoniazid and/or rifampicin could be the offending drug). Drug-induced lupus does not show significant hypocomplementemia or renal or neurological disease, rather hepatitis is more common as compared to true SLE (excludes options A and B). Antihistone antibody is characteristically associated. The symptoms are often reversible on withdrawal of the offending drug.

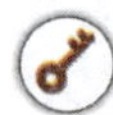

Key: C

BOOST YOUR KNOWLEDGE

Drug-induced lupus is triggered by exposure to specific medications, including hydralazine, minocycline, many anticonvulsants, sulfonamides, and antiarrhythmic agents. Though some of these agents may trigger true SLE in genetically predisposed individuals, more often these agents provoke a reversible lupus-like syndrome. Unlike SLE, drug-induced lupus affects males and females equally. A genetic predisposition toward slow drug acetylation may increase the risk of drug-induced lupus. Circulating antihistone antibodies are often present in drug-induced SLE (detected in only up to 20% of individuals with SLE). Hepatitis, which is rare in SLE, is more common in drug-induced lupus. Individuals with drug-induced lupus are less likely to demonstrate antibodies to dsDNA, hypocomplementemia, and significant renal or neurologic disease. In contrast to SLE, manifestations of drug-induced lupus typically resolve after withdrawal of the offending medication.

REFERENCE/SOURCE

- Sadun RE, Ardoin SP, Schanberg LE. Systemic lupus erythematosus. In: Kliegman RM, St Geme III JW, Blum NJ, Shah SS, Tasker RC, Wilson KM (Eds). Nelson Textbook of Pediatrics, 21st edition. Elsevier; 2019. pp. 1274-9.

3. A 10-year-old girl diagnosed with SLE with stage 4 nephritis, 1 year ago, was doing well on mycophenolate mofetil (MMF), low-dose prednisolone, and hydroxychloroquine (HCQ). Suddenly, she developed fever 3 days ago with some petechial spots on the trunk. On examination, she has pallor and mild icterus. Liver is just palpable and the tip of spleen is palpable. On investigations, Hb is 8 g/dL, total leukocyte count (TLC) of 6,000/mm^3, platelet 46,000/mm^3, serum glutamic-oxaloacetic transaminase (SGOT) 206 IU/dL, serum glutamic-pyruvic transaminase (SGPT) 160 IU/dL, erythrocyte sedimentation rate (ESR) 08/1st hour, and C-reactive protein (CRP) 66 mg/dL. What is the most likely diagnosis?

A. SLE disease flare
B. SLE complicated by systemic infection
C. SLE complicated by macrophage activation syndrome (MAS)
D. SLE flare with MAS

EXPLANATION

	Fever	Petechial spots	Enlarged liver	Enlarged spleen	Hb	TLC	Platelet	ESR	CRP	Liver enzymes
SLE disease flare	+	+	±	±	Low	±	Low	Normal	Normal	Mild rise
SLE complicated by systemic infection	+	±	±	+	May be low	High	High	Rise	High	May or may not rise
SLE complicated by MAS	+	+	±	++	Low	May be low	Low	Low or normal	High	Rise
SLE flare with MAS	+	+	±	++	Low	±	Low	Low/normal	High	Rise

(CRP: C-reactive protein; ESR: erythrocyte sedimentation rate; Hb: hemoglobin; MAS: macrophage activation syndrome; SLE: systemic lupus erythematosus; TLC: total leukocyte count)

From the above table, as there is anemia and thrombocytopenia, with raised liver enzymes and CRP, without any significant rise of ESR, MAS seems to be the most likely diagnosis here, that is, she is having MAS without disease flare or infections.

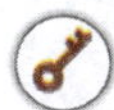

Key: C

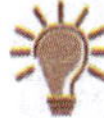

BOOST YOUR KNOWLEDGE

Broadly, SLE patients need to be monitored for some life-threatening complications such as disease flare, severe infections, and MAS. It is important to differentiate between these conditions clinically and by appropriate laboratory tests because immediate lifesaving treatment decisions need to be taken. Immunomodulators are needed for flares and MAS, which may aggravate infections, if present. On the other hand, infections need appropriate treatment with antibiotics.

Increased protein, red blood cell (RBC), cast in urine routine examination (R/E), reduced C3 and C4, and positive ds-DNA may give further clue to lupus nephritis flare. Cultures need to be sent for diagnosing suspected infections. For MAS, further tests such as ferritin, triglyceride, fibrinogen, and lactate dehydrogenase (LDH) need to be sent.

Simple rule of thumb:

- Patient well, counts decreasing or normal: Going into remission
- *Patient sick, counts decreasing:* Think of MAS (Next ESR can differentiate between these two conditions, ESR rises in flare but remains low or normal in MAS)
- *Patient sick, counts increasing:* Think of infection

REFERENCE/SOURCE

- Sadun RE, Ardoin SP, Schanberg LE. Systemic lupus erythematosus. Nelson Textbook of Pediatrics, 21st edition. Elsevier; 2019. pp. 1274-9.

4. A 12-year-old girl presents with fever, rash, facial puffiness, hematuria, and menorrhagia. After appropriate investigations and renal biopsy, she is diagnosed with stage III lupus nephritis with immune thrombocytopenia. She is given pulse methylprednisolone followed by oral steroids, MMF, and HCQ. What is the recommended maintenance dose of HCQ in SLE that is required to prevent disease flares?

A. 2–3 mg/kg
B. 4–5 mg/kg
C. 6–7 mg/kg
D. 10 mg/kg

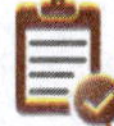

EXPLANATION

Hydroxychloroquine is recommended for all individuals with SLE. In addition to treating mild SLE manifestations such as rash and mild arthritis, HCQ prevents SLE flares and improves lipid profile. Given that risk factors for ocular toxicity include duration of use and dose, HCQ in SLE should never be prescribed at doses >6.5 mg/kg (maximum 400 mg daily), and newer ophthalmology guidelines recommend limiting maintenance dosing to 4–5 mg/kg.

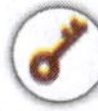

Key: B

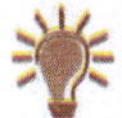

BOOST YOUR KNOWLEDGE

Potential toxicities of HCQ include retinal deposition and subsequent vision impairment; therefore, annual ophthalmology examinations are recommended for patients taking HCQ.

REFERENCES/SOURCES

- Fanouriakis A, Kostopoulou M, Alunno A, Aringer M, Bajema I, Boletis JN, et al. 2019 update of the EULAR recommendations for the management of systemic lupus erythematosus. Ann Rheum Dis. 2019;78(6):736-45.
- Sadun RE, Ardoin SP, Schanberg LE. Systemic lupus erythematosus. In: Kliegman RM, St Geme III JW, Blum NJ, Shah SS, Tasker RC, Wilson KM (Eds). Nelson Textbook of Pediatrics, 21st edition. Elsevier; 2019. pp. 1274-9.

5. This 6-month-old baby presented with a rash (as shown in the Figure) since 2 months of age. It has partially subsided after some medication from a local practitioner. Baby was born at term by normal vaginal delivery (NVD) to a healthy mother. But on probing she says that sometimes she gets some rashes after exposure to sunlight. Immediately this baby should be screened for which life-threatening serious condition.

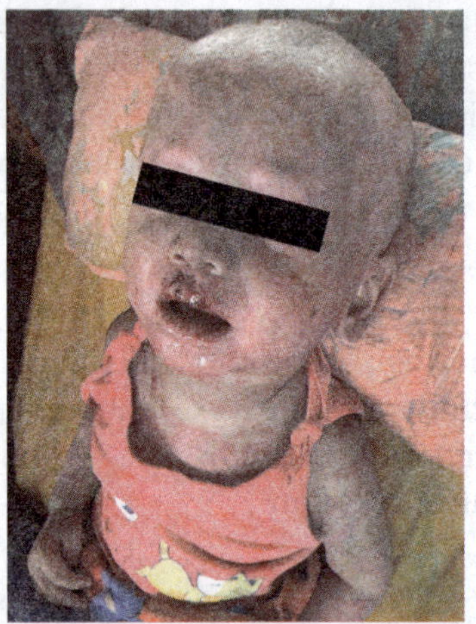

Courtesy: Professor Madhumita Nandi.

A. Acute liver failure
B. Congenital heart block
C. Sepsis and septic shock
D. Immune thrombocytopenia

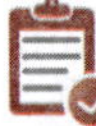

EXPLANATION

The age of onset of this macular rash along with mother's history of photosensitivity is a strong pointer to possibility of neonatal lupus. Congenital heart block is the most feared life-threatening condition. Positive titers of anti-Ro and anti-La antibodies are diagnostic. Though the baby may have some hepatitis and cytopenia also, this condition is generally self-limiting except the cardiac complications.

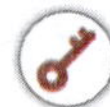

Key: B

BOOST YOUR KNOWLEDGE

Clinical manifestations of neonatal lupus include a characteristic annular or macular rash typically affecting the face (especially the periorbital area), trunk, and scalp. The rash can be present at birth but more often appears within the first 6–8 weeks of life, after exposure to ultraviolet (UV) light, and typically lasts 3–4 months. Infants may also have cytopenia and hepatitis, each occurring in approximately 25% of cases, but the most feared complication is congenital heart block. Mothers may be apparently asymptomatic and sometimes diagnosed to be anti-Ro/La positive after characteristic clinical features develop in the baby.

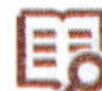

REFERENCE/SOURCE

- Sadun RE, Ardoin SP, Schanberg LE. Systemic lupus erythematosus. In: Kliegman RM, St Geme III JW, Blum NJ, Shah SS, Tasker RC, Wilson KM (Eds). Nelson Textbook of Pediatrics, 21st edition. Elsevier; 2019. pp. 1274-9.

6. An 8-year-old boy develops pain and swelling of both knee and ankle joints, which is additive in nature. He is advised to be tested for rheumatoid arthritis (RA) factor. Which of the following regarding this test is true?

A. It has a great diagnostic value in juvenile idiopathic arthritis (JIA)
B. It should be used to monitor the progress of the disease
C. RA positive patients are more likely to develop eye complications
D. It is IgM antibody

EXPLANATION

Rheumatoid factor (RA or RF) is a family of antibodies against Fc portion of IgG. It has only prognostic value in pJIA (polyarticular JIA; associated with more severe joint manifestations). ANA positivity, rather than RA positivity, is associated with anterior uveitis. RF positive polyarthritis is usually associated with uveitis.

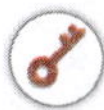

Key: C

BOOST YOUR KNOWLEDGE

The main role of RA in children lies in classifying a subset of JIA-RA positive polyarthritis, a variety usually characterized by prolonged and deforming arthritis, which may progress well into adulthood. For categorizing such, at least two samples should be positive at least 3 months apart. So, there is no role of repeating it if the first sample is negative. Also, once two samples at appropriate interval turn positive, there is no role of repeating it further for monitoring or follow-up.

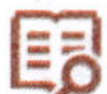

REFERENCE/SOURCE

- Gupta P, Menon PSN, Ramji S, Lodha R (Eds). PG Textbook of Pediatrics (Chapter 46.2), 3rd edition. New Delhi: Jaypee Brothers Medical Publishers; 2022.

7. This 12-year-old girl has had a history of fever, chest pain, and myalgia for last 2 months. She has this rash on face and this lesion on the palate. The palatal lesion is not painful but has irritating sensation while eating. Which of the following is the most appropriate initial serological test for this child?

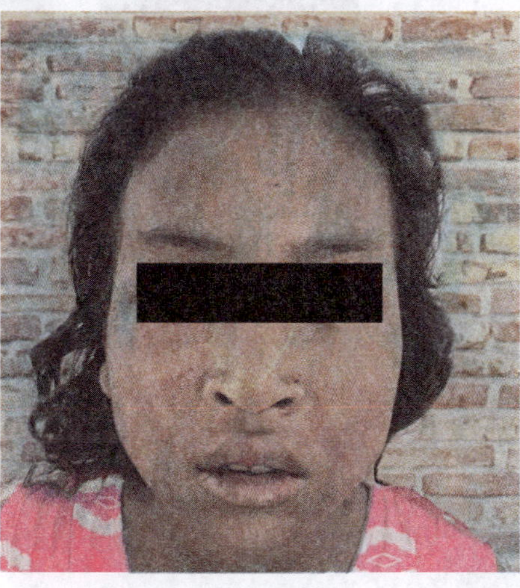

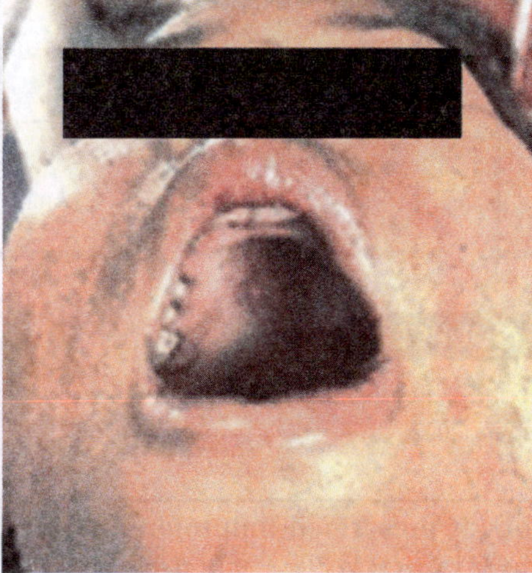

A. ANA by enzyme-linked immunosorbent assay (ELISA)
B. ANA by indirect immunofluorescence (IIF) using HEp-2 cells
C. Anti-dsDNA by IF using HeLa cells
D. Anti-dsDNA by direct IF using HEp-2 cells

EXPLANATION

Most specific test for ANA is IIF using HEp-2 cell line of human laryngeal epithelial carcinoma. ANA by ELISA is much less specific. It is no longer recommended. According to the European League Against Rheumatism (EULAR)/American College of Rheumatology (ACR) 2019 SLE criteria, ANA positivity at a titer of at least 1:80 by IF is mandatory entry level criteria.

Key: B

BOOST YOUR KNOWLEDGE

Apart from more specificity, IIF-ANA helps in delineating the pattern of staining, which helps further knowing the exact type of ANA.

The flowchart given below is explanatory.

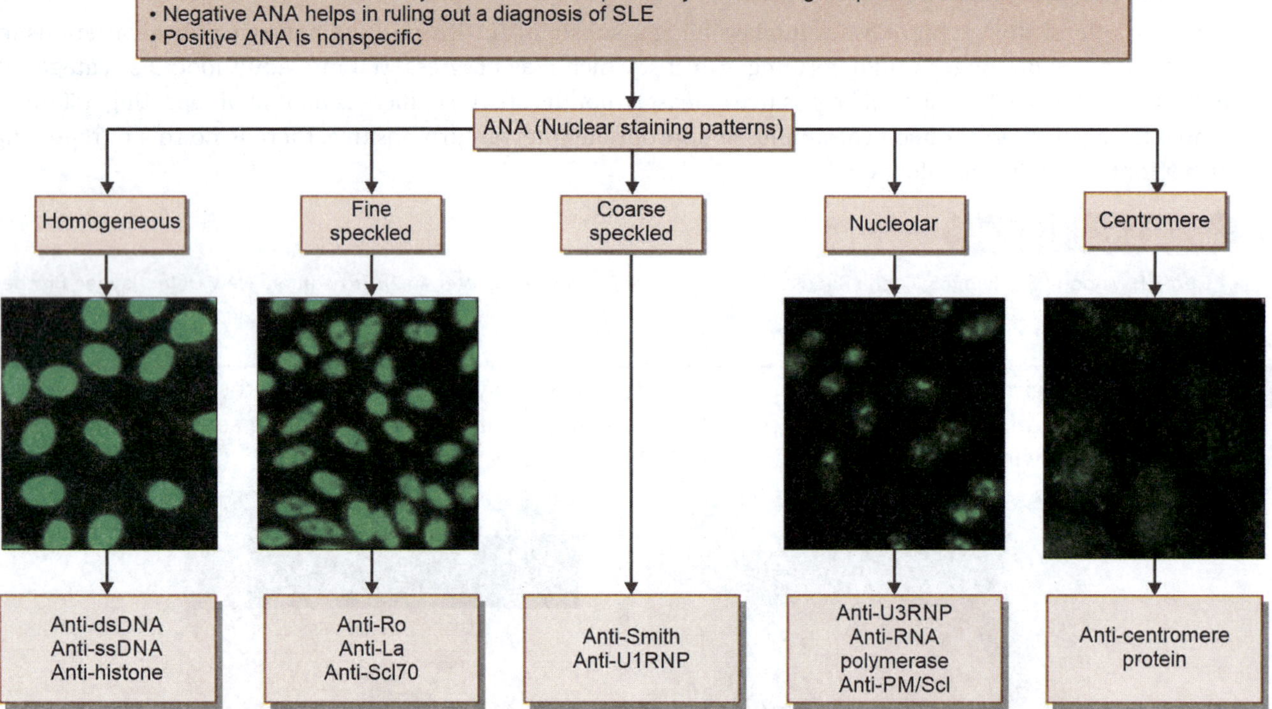

REFERENCE/SOURCE

- Gupta P, Menon PSN, Ramji S, Lodha R (Eds). PG Textbook of Pediatrics (Chapter 46.2), 3rd edition. New Delhi: Jaypee Brothers Medical Publishers; 2022.

8. A 9-year-old boy is prescribed ibuprofen and methotrexate (MTX) for JIA. Which of the following is TRUE regarding use of MTX in JIA?

A. It is most effective for systemic JIA
B. Therapeutic effects are achieved in 6–8 weeks
C. Needs renal function monitoring for possible renal toxicity
D. Folate @5 mg/week, which reduces its side effects, should be given on the same day of MTX

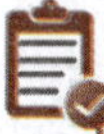

EXPLANATION

Methotrexate is effective in 60–70% of pJIA, but not very effective in systemic JIA (sJIA). One must wait for at least 6–8 weeks to see therapeutic effects have been achieved or not. Liver and hematological toxicities need to be monitored. Folate must be given, but not on the same day.

Key: B

BOOST YOUR KNOWLEDGE

Methotrexate is widely used disease-modifying antirheumatic drug (DMARD). It is a folic acid analog that inhibits several different enzymes in folate pathway by MTX polyglutamates and finally inhibits enzymes that catalyze the final steps of purine synthesis resulting in accumulation of adenosine. Adenosine has anti-inflammatory properties because it downregulates inflammatory cytokines such as tumor necrosis factor-alpha (TNF-α), interferon gamma (IFN-γ), interleukin-6 (IL-6), and IL-8, and also inhibits proliferation of synovial cells.

REFERENCE/SOURCE

- Gupta P, Menon PSN, Ramji S, Lodha R (Eds). PG Textbook of Pediatrics (Chapter 46.2), 3rd edition. New Delhi: Jaypee Brothers Medical Publishers; 2022.

9. A 12-year-old girl presents with alopecia, bilateral pleural effusion, and petechial rashes all over the body. She has anemia, thrombocytopenia, gross hematuria, and hypertension. ANA by IF is positive (1:360). C3 and C4 are low. Which of the following is least likely to occur in her?

A. Malar rash sparing the nasolabial folds
B. Nasal septal perforation
C. Oral ulcers that are painful when they encounter an irritant
D. Annular erythema over the forehead and scalp following sun exposure

EXPLANATION

Most likely diagnosis is SLE with nephritis. Photosensitivity, malar rash, and oral ulcers are typical mucocutaneus manifestations of SLE. All these were in the previous 11-point ACR classification criteria of SLE 1997. Nasal septal perforation is not typical of SLE, rather it may occur following necrotizing vasculitis typical of granulomatosis with polyangiitis (GIP) previously called Wegener granulomatosis.

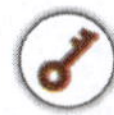

Key: B

BOOST YOUR KNOWLEDGE

Possible mucocutaneous manifestations of SLE are malar rash, discoid (annular) rash, photosensitive rash, cutaneous vasculitis (petechiae, palpable purpura, digit ulcers, gangrene, and urticaria), livedo reticularis, periungual capillary abnormalities, Raynaud phenomenon, alopecia, oral and nasal ulcers, panniculitis, and chilblains.

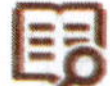

REFERENCE/SOURCE

- Sadun RE, Ardoin SP, Schanberg LE. Systemic lupus erythematosus. In: Kliegman RM, St Geme III JW, Blum NJ, Shah SS, Tasker RC, Wilson KM (Eds). Nelson Textbook of Pediatrics, 21st edition. Elsevier; 2019. pp. 1274-9.

10. A 10-year-old boy suffering from pJIA is given leflunomide as a DMARD. Which of the following regarding leflunomide is TRUE?

A. It is a pyrimidine synthesis inhibitor
B. It is a purine synthesis inhibitor
C. It is a calcineurin inhibitor
D. It is a dihydrofolate reductase (DHFR) inhibitor

EXPLANATION

Leflunomide is an immunomodulatory oral drug that gets metabolized in the body to its active form A77-1726, also known as teriflunomide. It acts by inhibiting the mitochondrial enzyme dihydro-orotate dehydrogenase, which prevents the synthesis of ribonucleotide uridine monophosphate pyrimidine (rUMP) and decreases rUMP levels, further activating P53. The activation of P53 restricts the progression of the G1 to S-phase in the cell cycle. This results in reduced proliferation of activated and autoimmune lymphocytes, thus promoting anti-inflammatory and immunomodulatory effects.

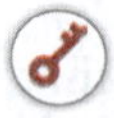

Key: A

BOOST YOUR KNOWLEDGE

Leflunomide is a DMARD approved for the treatment of RA that offers an alternative to MTX for treatment of JIA. Dosing is oral, once daily, and weight based: 10 mg for children 10–40 kg. Adverse reactions include paresthesia and peripheral neuropathy, gastrointestinal (GI) intolerance, elevated liver transaminases and hepatic failure, cytopenia, alopecia, and teratogenesis. Avoidance of pregnancy is essential. Laboratory tests [e.g., complete blood count (CBC) and liver function tests (LFTs)] are monitored every 4 weeks for the 1st 6 months of treatment, then every 8–12 weeks.

REFERENCES/SOURCES

- Dvergsten JA, Morgan E, Rabinovich CE. Treatment of rheumatic diseases. In: Kliegman RM, St Geme III JW, Blum NJ, Shah SS, Tasker RC, Wilson KM (Eds). Nelson Textbook of Pediatrics, 21st edition. Elsevier; 2019. pp. 1252-7.
- Goldenberg MM. Leflunomide, a novel immunomodulator for the treatment of active rheumatoid arthritis. Clin Ther. 1999; 21(11):1837-52.

11. This child (shown in figure) was diagnosed as oligoarticular JIA and some nonsteroidal anti-inflammatory drug (NSAID) was prescribed. He returned with vesiculobullous lesions, which subsequently healed to form small hypopigmented scars. What is the drug most likely to have been prescribed?

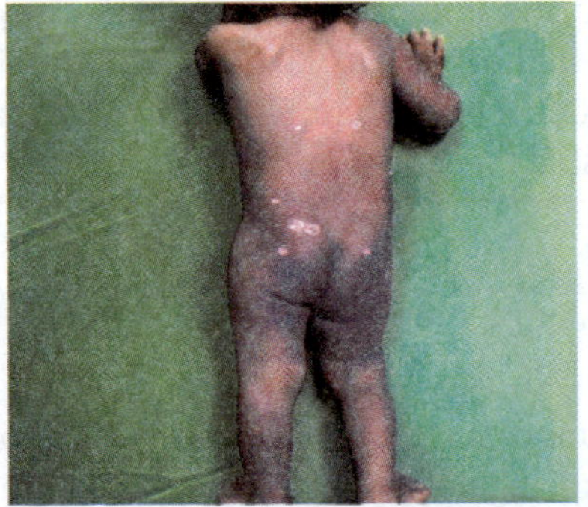

Courtesy: Professor Rakesh Mondal.

A. Naproxen
B. Ibuprofen
C. Celecoxib
D. Indomethacin

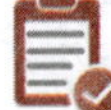

EXPLANATION

This is pseudoporphyria and the most likely culprit is naproxen. It is characterized by small, hypopigmented depressed scars. If pseudoporphyria develops, the inciting NSAID should be discontinued because scars can persist for years or may be permanent.

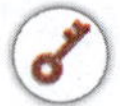

Key: A

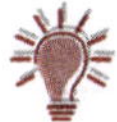

BOOST YOUR KNOWLEDGE

The most frequent adverse effects of NSAIDs in children are nausea, decreased appetite, and abdominal pain. Gastritis or ulceration occurs less frequently in children. Less common adverse effects (≤5% of children undergoing long-term NSAID therapy) include mood change, concentration difficulty that can simulate attention deficit disorder, sleepiness, irritability, headache, tinnitus, alopecia, anemia, elevated liver enzyme values, proteinuria, and hematuria. Additional rare NSAID-specific adverse reactions include aseptic meningitis associated with ibuprofen and pseudoporphyria associated with naproxen.

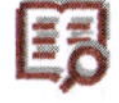

REFERENCE/SOURCE

- Dvergsten JA, Morgan E, Rabinovich CE. Treatment of rheumatic diseases. In: Kliegman RM, St Geme III JW, Blum NJ, Shah SS, Tasker RC, Wilson KM (Eds). Nelson Textbook of Pediatrics, 21st edition. Elsevier; 2019. pp. 1252-7.

12. A 10-year-old boy, suffering from fever, evanescent rash and pain, and gelling of multiple joints is given a diagnosis of sJIA. Poor prognosis of sJIA is related to all of the following, *except*:

A. Polyarthritis
B. Polyserositis
C. Fever >3 months
D. Increased inflammatory markers (ESR and platelet) >6 months

EXPLANATION

Prolonged fever, polyarthritis, and raised inflammatory markers are associated with poor prognosis. RA positive pJIA is associated with prolonged and debilitating course.

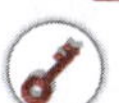

Key: B

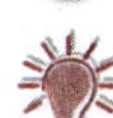

BOOST YOUR KNOWLEDGE

Although the course of JIA in an individual child is unpredictable, some prognostic generalizations can be made based on disease type and course. Children with persistent oligoarticular disease fare well, with a majority achieving disease remission. Those with extended oligoarticular disease have a poorer prognosis. Children with oligoarthritis, particularly girls who are ANA positive and with onset of arthritis before 6 years of age, are at the greatest risk for development of chronic uveitis. The child with pJIA often has a more prolonged course of active joint inflammation and requires early and aggressive therapy. Predictors of severe and persistent disease include young age at onset, RF seropositivity or rheumatoid nodules, presence of anticyclic citrullinated peptide (CCP) antibodies, and many affected joints. Disease involving the hip and hand/wrist is also associated with a poorer prognosis and may lead to significant functional impairment. sJIA is often the most difficult to control in terms of both articular inflammation and systemic manifestations. Poorer prognosis is related to polyarticular distribution of arthritis, fever lasting >3 months, and increased inflammatory markers, such as platelet count and ESR for >6 months.

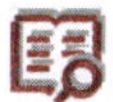

REFERENCE/SOURCE

- Dvergsten JA, Morgan E, Rabinovich CE. Treatment of rheumatic diseases. In: Kliegman RM, St Geme III JW, Blum NJ, Shah SS, Tasker RC, Wilson KM (Eds). Nelson Textbook of Pediatrics, 21st edition. Elsevier; 2019. pp. 1252-7.

13. A 10-year-old boy with JIA is given some biologic modifying agent after which he develops rash, petechial spots, hepatitis, and pleural effusion. He tests positive for antihistone antibody. Which is the most likely offending agent?

A. Etanercept
B. Anakinra
C. Rituximab
D. Tocilizumab

EXPLANATION

Tumor necrosis factor alpha (TNF-α) inhibitors, including etanercept, infliximab, and adalimumab, may be associated with lupus-like manifestations.

Key: A

BOOST YOUR KNOWLEDGE

Anti-TNF-α-induced lupus (ATIL) represents a major diagnostic and therapeutic challenge. Most cases of ATIL are caused by infliximab, followed by etanercept and adalimumab. Symptoms can range from common, mild cutaneous lesions to rare, serious pleural or pericardial effusions, deep venous thrombosis, life-threatening pneumonitis, and neuritis. Constitutional symptoms often present in association with positive autoantibody serology. Diagnosis can be considered if there is a temporal relationship between symptoms and anti-TNF-α therapy and at least one serologic and one nonserologic ACR criteria. The main approach in the treatment of ATIL is the withdrawal of the offending drug.

REFERENCE/SOURCE

- Dvergsten JA, Morgan E, Rabinovich CE. Treatment of rheumatic diseases. In: Kliegman RM, St Geme III JW, Blum NJ, Shah SS, Tasker RC, Wilson KM (Eds). Nelson Textbook of Pediatrics, 21st edition. Elsevier; 2019. pp. 1252-7.

14. A 14-year-old girl is given a diagnosis of SLE nephritis based on appropriate biochemical, histopathological, and serological tests after she presents with clinical features of facial puffiness, alopecia, and malar rash. Which of the following is the most frequent neuropsychiatric symptom she is likely to have?

A. Chorea
B. Seizures
C. Headache
D. Psychosis

EXPLANATION

Headache has been reported in up to 95% of patients of SLE during the course of the disease.

Key: C

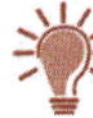

BOOST YOUR KNOWLEDGE

	1 year of diagnosis (%)	*Any time (%)*
Psychosis	5–12	8–18
Seizures	5–15	5–47
Headache	5–22	10–95
Cognitive dysfunction	6–15	12–55
Acute confusional state	5–15	8–35
Peripheral nerve involvement	<5	<5
Cardiovascular disease	5–30	25–60
Pericarditis	12–20	20–30

Headache reported in 95% of cases.

REFERENCE/SOURCE

- Sadun RE, Ardoin SP, Schanberg LE. Systemic lupus erythematosus. In: Kliegman RM, St Geme III JW, Blum NJ, Shah SS, Tasker RC, Wilson KM (Eds). Nelson Textbook of Pediatrics, 21st edition. Elsevier; 2019. pp. 1274-9.

15. **A 10-year-old boy has painful swelling of multiple joints, including big and small joints. Which of the following is the most likely indicator that it is probably not JIA?**

A. Morning stiffness
B. Joint erythema
C. Joint tenderness
D. Restriction of movement

EXPLANATION

Joint erythema is a sign of acute arthritis such as pyogenic arthritis. Involved joints in JIA are often swollen, warm to touch, and uncomfortable on movement or palpation with reduced range of motion (ROM), but usually are not erythematous.

Key: B

BOOST YOUR KNOWLEDGE

Arthritis must be present ≥6 weeks to make a diagnosis of any JIA subtype. Arthritis is defined by intra-articular swelling or the presence of ≥2 of the following signs: limitation in ROM, tenderness or pain on motion, and warmth. Initial symptoms may be subtle or acute and often include morning stiffness with a limp or gelling after inactivity.

REFERENCE/SOURCE

- Wu EY, Rabinovich CE. Juvenile idiopathic arthritis. In: Kliegman RM, St Geme III JW, Blum NJ, Shah SS, Tasker RC, Wilson KM (Eds). Nelson Textbook of Pediatrics, 21st edition. Elsevier; 2019. pp. 1258-67.

16. **A 4-year-old girl presents with pain and swelling of both knee joints. After examination, and exclusion of other possibilities by appropriate laboratory investigations, she is given a diagnosis of JIA. Which of the following is an indicator that she needs more meticulous screening for eye complications?**

A. RA seropositivity
B. ANA seropositivity
C. Anti-CCP seropositivity
D. Persistent thrombocytosis

EXPLANATION

Elevated ANA titers are present in 40–85% of children with oligoarticular or polyarticular JIA but are rare with sJIA. ANA seropositivity is associated with increased risk of chronic uveitis in JIA. Approximately 5–15% of patients with polyarticular JIA are seropositive for RF. Anti-CCP antibody and RF are markers of more aggressive disease. Thrombocytosis is a marker of inflammation and corelates with disease activity.

Key: B

BOOST YOUR KNOWLEDGE

Uveitis is a well-known threatening comorbid condition of JIA and affects around 10% of the patients depending on JIA subtype. Early age of JIA onset, oligoarticular subtype, and ANA reactivity are the main risk factors for the development of uveitis. The current management is to start early a steroid-sparing effective immunomodulatory systemic treatment. It is important to recognize and treat it early to prevent any visual damage that could impair visual acuity.

REFERENCE/SOURCE

- Wu EY, Rabinovich CE. Juvenile idiopathic arthritis. In: Kliegman RM, St Geme III JW, Blum NJ, Shah SS, Tasker RC, Wilson KM (Eds). Nelson Textbook of Pediatrics, 21st edition. Elsevier; 2019. pp. 1258-67.

17. A 13-year-old girl undergoes kidney biopsy on suspicion of lupus nephritis. Which of the following will be a marker of chronicity of the disease?

A. Fibrinoid necrosis
B. Hyaline deposits
C. Fibrous crescents
D. Interstitial inflammation

EXPLANATION

The National Institutes of Health (NIH) lupus nephritis activity and chronicity indices, comprises six activity scores (AI) and four chronicity scores (CI). As is evident from the accompanying table, AI can have a maximum score of 24/24 whereas the maximum CI could be 12/12. This score helps in prognosticating renal outcome and the need for more aggressive immunomodulator drugs. The more the AI, the more the chance that immunomodulators will be effective. Less AI and more CI means immunomodulators may not be so effective in reversing the pathology. In such cases, renal replacement therapy may be the only option. As per the Table below, fibrous crescents indicates chronicity.

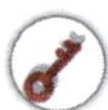

Key: C

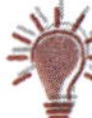

BOOST YOUR KNOWLEDGE

Index	*Score**
Modified activity indices:	
Endocapillary hypercellularity	0–3
Neutrophils/karyorrhexis	0–3
Fibrinoid necrosis	(0–3) × 2
Hyaline deposits	0–3
Cellular/fibrocellular crescents	(0–3) × 2
Interstitial inflammation	0–3
Modified chronicity indices:	
Total glomerulosclerosis† score	0–3
Fibrous crescents	0–3
Tubular atrophy	0–3
Interstitial fibrosis	0–3

*1, <25%; 2, 25–50%; 3, >50% glomeruli/tubules/cortical interstitium involved.
†Global and/or segmental sclerosis.

REFERENCES/SOURCES

- Choi SE, Fogo AB, Lim BJ. Histologic evaluation of activity and chronicity of lupus nephritis and its clinical significance. Kidney Res Clin Pract. 2023;42(2):166-73.
- Gupta P, Menon PSN, Ramji S, Lodha R (Eds). PG Textbook of Pediatrics (Chapter 46.2), 3rd edition. New Delhi: Jaypee Brothers Medical Publishers; 2022.

18. A 10-year-old has polyarthritis refractory to NSAID, MTX, and oral steroids. Which of the following biologic response modifier has recently been approved for usage in such children orally?

A. Tofacitinib, a JAK-STAT inhibitor
B. Tocilizumab, an anti-IL-6 agent
C. Abatacept, a T-cell costimulatory blocking agent
D. Rituximab, an anti-CD20 agent

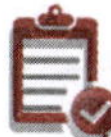

EXPLANATION

Biologic response modifiers (BRMs) have been a game changer in the management of JIA. But their only downside is their cost and need to be given parenterally. Tofacitinib is a synthetic JAK-STAT inhibitor that has been approved by the Food and Drug Administration (FDA) to be given orally.

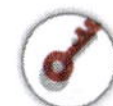

Key: A

BOOST YOUR KNOWLEDGE

The main research in the management of JIA is going on in the field of biologics. Western data show as many as 50–60% of patients need biologicals for optimum control of disease. In a resource-poor setting, their affordability often becomes the limiting factor. But the recent introduction of biosimilars has significantly reduced the cost of such therapy. Tofacitinib is a synthetic JAK-STAT inhibitor that has been approved by the FDA to be given orally.

REFERENCE/SOURCE

- Gupta P, Menon PSN, Ramji S, Lodha R (Eds). PG Textbook of Pediatrics (Chapter 46.2), 3rd edition. New Delhi: Jaypee Brothers Medical Publishers; 2022.

19. An 8-year-old child has pain and additive swelling of both ankles, knee joints, and several metacarpophalangeal joints of both hands. Which of the following is a predictor that his joint manifestations will be persistent and prolonged, probably even up to adulthood?

A. High serum ferritin level
B. RA positivity on two occasions
C. Older age at onset
D. Presence of rash

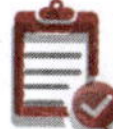

EXPLANATION

Rheumatoid arthritis factor, though not having any diagnostic value, if positive on two occasions >12 weeks apart is a strong predictor of severe and persistent joint disease, sometimes up to adulthood. Serum ferritin is an inflammatory marker and has no long-term predictability. The age of onset also has no role in predictability of disease course, except younger girls who are ANA positive have higher incidence of uveitis and so need more stringent ophthalmological monitoring. Similarly, the presence of rash is also not a predictor of prolonged illness.

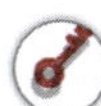

Key: B

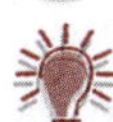

BOOST YOUR KNOWLEDGE

Neither ANA and RA nor serum ferritin have any diagnostic value in JIA. RA or RF is a family of antibodies against Fc portion of IgG. It has a prognostic value in pJIA (associated with more severe, deforming, and persisting joint manifestations). ANA positivity is associated with increased incidence uveitis. So, neither RA nor ANA should be repeated once positive. Serum ferritin is a marker of acute inflammation, and so is used to monitor disease activity. And serum ferritin of very high value is a predictor of possibility of complications such as MAS.

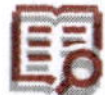

REFERENCE/SOURCE

- Sadun RE, Ardoin SP, Schanberg LE. Systemic lupus erythematosus. In: Kliegman RM, St Geme III JW, Blum NJ, Shah SS, Tasker RC, Wilson KM (Eds). Nelson Textbook of Pediatrics, 21st edition. Elsevier; 2019. pp. 1274-9.

20. Which among the following gets maximum weightage in the 2019 EULAR/ACR classification criteria for SLE?

A. Thrombocytopenia
B. Oral ulcers
C. Fever
D. Pericardial effusion

EXPLANATION

Domains	*Criteria*	*Weight*
Constitutional	Fever	2
Hematologic	Leukopenia	3
	Thrombocytopenia	4
	Autoimmune hemolysis	4
Neuropsychiatric	Delirium	2
	Psychosis	3
	Seizure	5
Mucocutaneous	Nonscarring alopecia	2
	Oral ulcers	2
	Subacute cutaneous or discoid lupus	4
	Acute cutaneous lupus	6
Serosal	Pleural or pericardial effusion	5
	Acute pericarditis	6
Musculoskeletal	Joint involvement	6
Renal	Proteinuria >0.5 g/24 hour	4
	Renal biopsy class II or V lupus nephritis	8
	Renal biopsy class III or IV lupus nephritis	10
Antiphospholipid Ab	Anti-cardiolipin Ab or Anti-β_2GP1 Ab or Lupus anticoagulant	2
Complement protein	Low C3 or low C4	3
	Low C3 and low C4	4
Systemic lupus erythematosus-specific Ab	Anti-dsDNA Ab or Anti-Sm Ab	6

Key: D

BOOST YOUR KNOWLEDGE

The 2019 EULAR/ACR SLE classification criteria make ANA positivity at ≥1:80 by HEp2 IF or an equivalent method an entry level mandatory criterion. Then it gives several clinical and laboratory criteria for weighted scoring. A total score of ≥10 in the presence of entry level criteria makes a diagnosis of SLE. While calculating the weighted scores, only one with maximum score is taken from each subcategory.

REFERENCE/SOURCE

- Gupta P, Menon PSN, Ramji S, Lodha R (Eds). PG Textbook of Pediatrics (Chapter 46.2), 3rd edition. New Delhi: Jaypee Brothers Medical Publishers; 2022.

CHAPTER 24.2

Vasculitis Disorders

Pavneet Kaur, Narendra Bagri

1. A 1-year-old boy presented to the outpatient department (OPD) with a history of high-grade fever for 8 days, without any other localizing symptoms. A primary care physician had treated him with antibiotics (amoxicillin) for suspected UTI [urine R/M: 15 pus cells/HPF (high power field)]. The examination was unremarkable except for marked irritability and a nappy rash. Investigations done on day 7 of illness reveal:

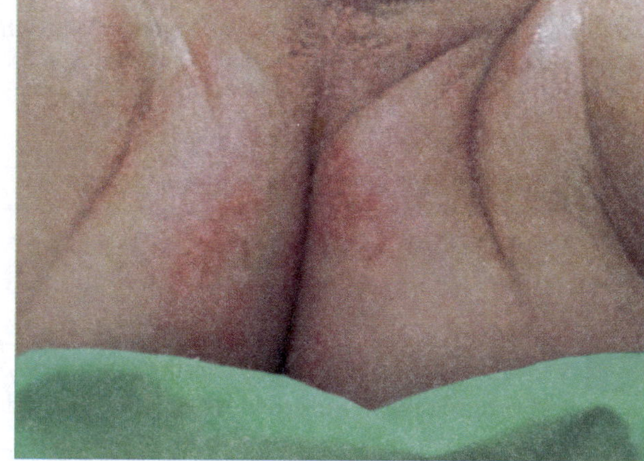

- *Urinalysis:* Leukocyte esterase, nitrate reductase negative, pus cells 13/HPF
- *Hb:* 9 g/dL, TLC 18,000/mm^3 (78% neutrophils), platelets 5,00,000/mm^3
- *ESR:* 50 mm/1st hour, CRP 30 mg/L
- *Blood and urine cultures:* Sterile
- *Dengue IgM and malaria rapid diagnostic test:* Negative
- Alanine aminotransaminase 2× ULN, serum albumin 3g/dL

What would be the next most appropriate treatment strategy?

A. Intravenous 3rd generation cephalosporins
B. Intravenous immunoglobulins
C. Intravenous methylprednisolone
D. Nonsteroidal anti-inflammatory drugs (NSAIDs)

EXPLANATION

Although this child does not fulfil the criteria for typical Kawasaki disease, the clinical features merit further investigation. An elevated CRP/ESR with ancillary laboratory parameters (anemia, leukocytosis, thrombocytosis, transaminitis, and sterile pyuria) supports the diagnosis of incomplete Kawasaki disease and prompt management. Intravenous immune globulin (IVIG) is the most appropriate treatment in this child.

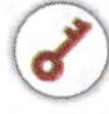

Key: B

BOOST YOUR KNOWLEDGE

Diagnosis of incomplete Kawasaki disease can be challenging. However, any child with clinically compatible features in the context of fever for five or more days should be investigated (CRP, ESR, CBC, RFT, urinalysis, and echocardiogram). A particularly higher index of suspicion is required for infants where investigations should be prompted by any fever of unknown origin lasting for >1 week. Since the diagnosis is primarily clinical, the child should be monitored for additional features. Re-evaluation should be undertaken as and when needed, for timely identification and treatment.

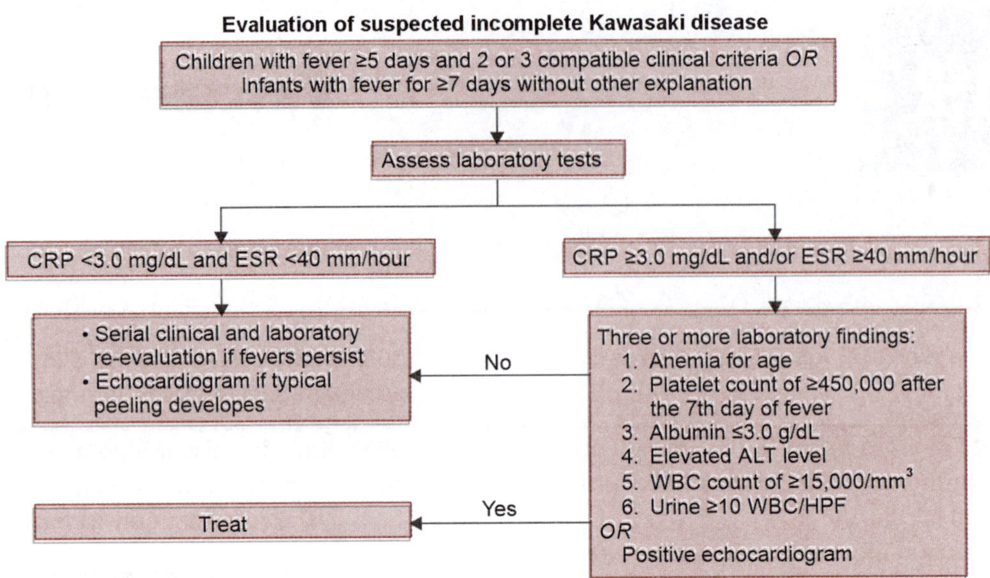

(ALT: alanine aminotransferase; CRP: C-reactive protein; ESR: erythrocyte sedimentation rate; WBC: white blood cell)

Source: McCrindle BW, Rowley AH, Newburger JW, Burns JC, Bolger AF, Gewitz M, et al. Diagnosis, treatment, and long-term management of Kawasaki disease: a scientific statement for health professionals from the American Heart Association. Circulation. 2017;135(17): e927-99.

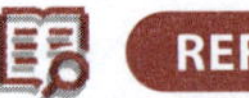

REFERENCE/SOURCE

- Kliegman RM, St Geme III JW. Nelson Textbook of Pediatrics, 21st edition. Elsevier; 2019. Chapter 191: Kawasaki disease. p. 1314.

2. A 14-year-old girl was brought to the emergency with a history of fever for 3 days and multiple loose stools, rashes and progressive breathlessness. The family had finished their coronavirus disease (COVID) quarantine 2 weeks back. She was found to be in hypotensive shock at triage and was resuscitated. Point-of-care echocardiography revealed myocardial dysfunction and elevated left main coronary artery Z scores (2.5). Laboratory investigations showed neutrophilic leukocytosis, platelet count of 90,000/mm^3, elevated D-dimers, and elevated CRP with normal PT/aPTT/fibrinogen levels. What is the likely diagnosis?

A. Kawasaki shock syndrome
B. Multisystem inflammatory syndrome in children (MIS-C)
C. Toxic shock syndrome
D. Acute severe acute respiratory syndrome (SARS) COVID-19 infection

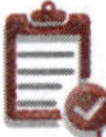

EXPLANATION

Older age group with fulminant multisystem presentation and a history of COVID-19 infection favors the diagnosis of multisystem inflammatory syndrome in children. The clinical and laboratory parameters further support the diagnosis of MIS-C.

Key: B

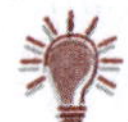

BOOST YOUR KNOWLEDGE

Fever, raised inflammatory markers, preceding evidence of COVID infection and presentation not attributable to sepsis are essential for the diagnosis of MIS-C.

World Health Organization (WHO) criteria

*World Health Organization case-definition of MIS-C**
0–19 years of age:
Fever ≥3 days
AND two of the following:
1. Rash or bilateral nonpurulent conjunctivitis or mucocutaneous inflammatory signs (oral, hands, or feet)
2. Hypotension or shock
3. Features of myocardial dysfunction, pericarditis, valvulitis, or coronary abnormalities (including ECHO findings or elevated Troponin/NT-proBNP)
4. Evidence of coagulopathy [by prolonged PT, partial thromboplastin time (PTT), elevated D-dimers]
5. Acute gastrointestinal symptoms (diarrhea, vomiting, or abdominal pain)

AND
Elevated markers of inflammation such as ESR, C-reactive protein, or procalcitonin
AND
No other obvious microbial cause of inflammation, including bacterial sepsis, staphylococcal or streptococcal shock syndromes
AND
Evidence of COVID-19 (RT-PCR antigen test or serology positive), or likely contact with patients with COVID-19

*Multisystem inflammatory syndrome (MIS) in children and adolescents temporally related to COVID-19.

Multisystem inflammatory syndrome in children is an entity distinct from Kawasaki disease. It also has a higher propensity for macrophage activation syndrome. The recommended treatment is—high-dose intravenous immunoglobulin (IVIG) at 2 g/kg and methylprednisolone at ~2 mg/kg/day in divided doses. Glucocorticoids have a favorable effect on the fever compared to IVIG monotherapy. Low-dose aspirin is also used (3–5 mg/kg, maximum 81 mg daily) unless thrombocytopenic or actively bleeding. Significant left ventricular dysfunction (EF < 35%) merits anticoagulation with enoxaparin.

Patients with severe clinical presentation (ICU admission, significant cardiovascular involvement, and evidence of macrophage activation syndrome) are treated with methylprednisolone pulses (30 mg/kg/day × 3 days) followed by oral prednisolone (~2 mg/kg/day in divided doses), tapered over 2–3 weeks in relatively uncomplicated cases, and tapered over 4–8 weeks in more complex cases. Refractory MIS-C cases are often treated with tumor necrosis factor (TNF)-alpha blockade, IL-6, or IL-1 receptor antagonists.

	MIS-C	*Kawasaki disease*
Presenting age	~10 years old	<5 years old
Race/ethnic predisposition	Black, hispanic	Asian
Gender	Males > females	Males > females
ICU admission/inotrope support	>50%	~5%
Presenting features	Fever, gastrointestinal symptoms (abdominal pain, vomiting, and diarrhea)	Rash, conjunctivitis, and oral mucosal changes
Cardiovascular involvement	Myocarditis, left ventricular dysfunction, and coronary artery aneurysms (uncommon)	Coronary artery aneurysms

Source: Patel JM. Multisystem inflammatory syndrome in children (MIS-C). Curr Allergy Asthma Rep. 2022;22(5):53-60.

Also, when compared with COVID-19, Kawasaki disease (KD), and toxic shock syndrome (TSS), patients with MIS-C had significantly higher prevalence of cardiac complications, elevated markers of inflammation and cardiac damage, thrombocytopenia, and lymphopenia.

REFERENCE/SOURCE

- Godfred-Cato S, Abrams JY, Balachandran N, Jaggi P, Jones K, Rostad CA, et al. Distinguishing multisystem inflammatory syndrome in children from COVID-19, Kawasaki disease and toxic shock syndrome. Pediatr Infect Dis J. 2022;41(4):315-23.

3. Which of the following regarding Kawasaki disease pathology is correct?

A. Its pathogenesis involves a triphasic process that may last weeks to years
B. Involves coronaries but spares mesenteric arteries
C. Clinical inflammatory process and markers resolve with defervescence of fever
D. Causes fusiform aneurysms in the acute phase and saccular aneurysms in the late phase

EXPLANATION

- In addition to coronaries, it may involve mesenteric, femoral, and brachial arteries.
- The inflammatory process may continue despite the resolution of fever.
- It causes saccular aneurysms in the acute phase and fusiform aneurysms in the late phase.

Key: A

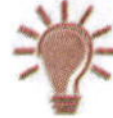

BOOST YOUR KNOWLEDGE

The 1st phase is neutrophilic necrotizing arteritis occurring in the first 2 weeks of illness that involves the endothelium and then out to the coronary wall—giving rise to saccular aneurysms. The 2nd phase of subacute/chronic vasculitis driven by lymphocytes, plasma cells, and eosinophils, may last weeks to years—resulting in fusiform aneurysms. The vessels then develop smooth muscle cell myofibroblasts, leading to progressive stenosis in the 3rd phase. Thrombi may form in the lumen and obstruct blood flow.

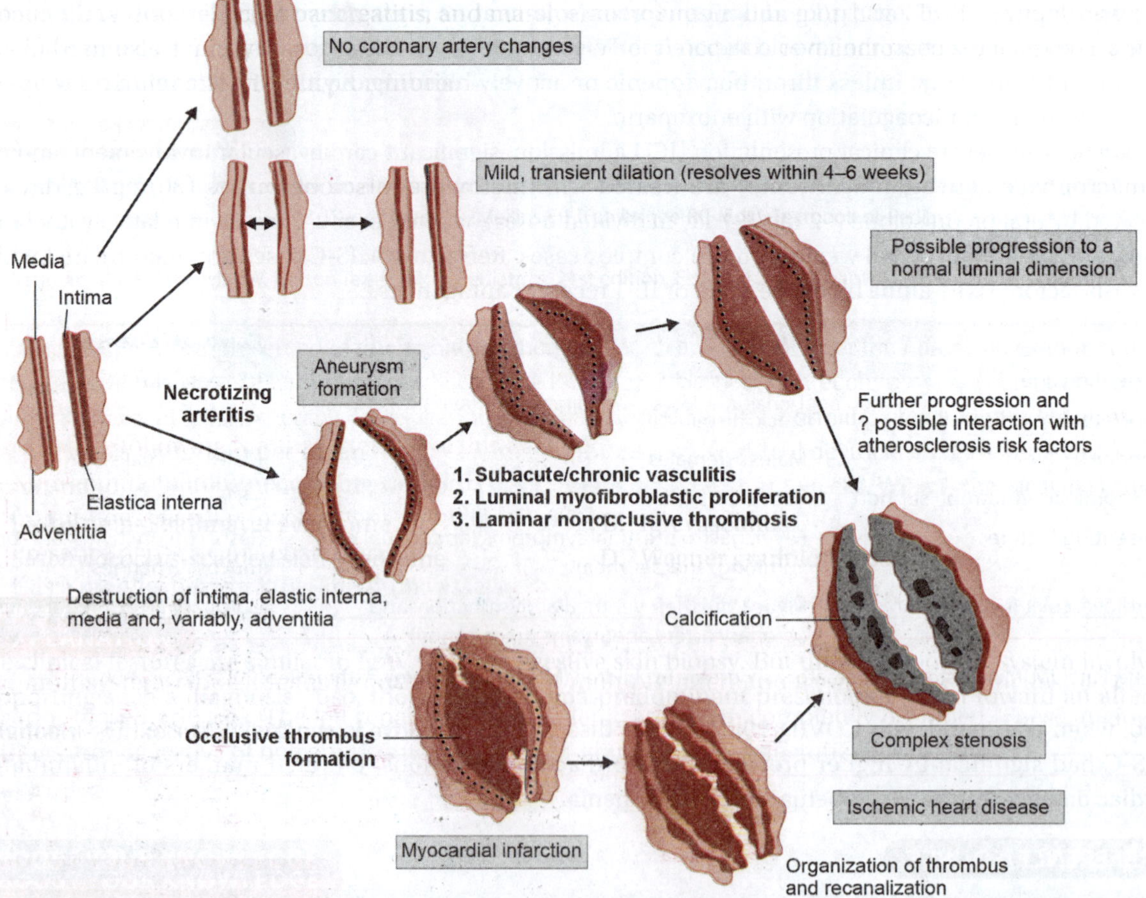

Source: Modified from Kato H. Cardiovascular complications in Kawasaki disease: coronary artery lumen and long-term consequences, Prog Pediatr Cardiol. 2004;19:137-45.

REFERENCE/SOURCE

- Nelson Textbook of Pediatrics, 21st edition. Elsevier; 2019. Chapter 191: Kawasaki disease. p. 1310.

4. Which of the following is a predictor of IVIg unresponsiveness in Kawasaki disease?

A. Serum sodium >150 mmol/L days
B. Age >36 months
C. Platelet count <30 × 10^4/mm^3
D. CRP <1 mg/L

EXPLANATION

All of these are components of the Kobayashi criteria—validated for prediction of IVIg unresponsiveness as detailed below.

Multivariable predictors of IVIG unresponsiveness in a Simple Scoring Model

	Logistic coefficient (β)	*SE*	*Odds ratio*	*95% CI*		*Score points*
				Lower	*Upper*	
Sodium ≤133 mmol/L	1.47	0.23	4.34	2.75	6.87	2
Days of illness at initial treatment ≤4	1.31	0.25	3.70	2.29	6.00	2
AST ≥100 IU/L	1.27	0.25	3.57	2.21	5.77	2
Neutrophil ≥80%	1.21	0.27	3.34	1.99	5.62	2
CRP ≥10 mg/dL	0.81	0.24	2.25	1.39	3.63	1
Age ≤12 months	0.79	0.28	2.20	1.26	3.83	1
Platelet count ≤30.0 × 10^4/mm^3	0.72	0.23	2.06	1.31	3.25	1

Key: C

BOOST YOUR KNOWLEDGE

This large multicenter study (n = 546 in the development dataset, and 204 in validation dataset) showed that high AST, CRP, and neutrophils; low age in months, sodium, and platelet count; and administration of IVIG early in the course of illness were independent risk factors for IVIG unresponsiveness. Each of these variables has also been reported to be a risk factor for coronary artery abnormalities (CAA). This criterion is based on an Asian cohort and hence may not perform as well in the non-Asian populations.

Other scores in use are the Egami and Sano scores.

	Sensitivity	*Specificity*	*Positive predictive value*	*Negative predictive value*
Kobayashi score ≥5	0.70	0.68	0.37	0.89
Egami score ≥3	0.56	0.71	0.34	0.86
Sano score ≥2	0.45	0.81	0.39	0.85

REFERENCES/SOURCES

- Kobayashi T, Inoue Y, Takeuchi K, Okada Y, Tamura K, Tomomasa T, et al. Prediction of intravenous immunoglobulin unresponsiveness in patients with Kawasaki disease. Circulation. 2006;113(22):2606-12.
- Takeshita S, Kanai T, Kawamura Y, Yoshida Y, Nonoyama S. A comparison of the predictive validity of the combination of the neutrophil-to-lymphocyte ratio and platelet-to-lymphocyte ratio and other risk scoring systems for intravenous immunoglobulin (IVIG)-resistance in Kawasaki disease. PLoS One. 2017;12(5):e0176957.

5. Which of the following is *not* a therapeutic option for Kawasaki disease?

A. Anakinra
B. Cyclosporine
C. Secukinumab
D. Infliximab

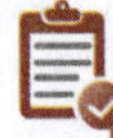

EXPLANATION

Apart from secukinumab, all of these biologicals have been explored in trials in the context of Kawasaki disease.

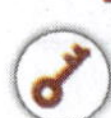

Key: C

BOOST YOUR KNOWLEDGE

As TNF-α is markedly increased in children with KD, especially in case of coronary artery lesions, infliximab has been trialed both as rescue therapy and a primary therapy.

Etanercept has also been studied as primary therapy in a double-blind multicenter trial. Although there was a decrease in IVIG resistance in subgroups of children >1 year of age and of African American ethnicity, there was also no overall difference in coronary outcomes between the etanercept and placebo groups, but less progression of dilation in patients with baseline coronary artery dilation was noticed.

Data regarding the potential role of T-cells in KD have led to the use of cyclosporine. Coronary artery Z-scores were similar in the treatment groups at 12 weeks, and the incidence of moderate or greater aneurysms in this study was very low. No adverse events were reported with the use of cyclosporine.

The potential role of cyclophosphamide in KD is extremely limited, but it may be useful in cases with persistent active disease unresponsive to conventional therapy.

A dramatic response to plasmapheresis in refractory cases of KD also has been reported, but is impeded by technical limitations. It should be reserved for children with active inflammation who have failed all available medical interventions.

Studies from the animal model of KD and whole blood gene expression profiles from KD children have highlighted the role of IL-1β in disease pathogenesis. Current trials are testing IL-1 blockade with anakinra alone and in combination with atorvastatin to block endothelial-to-mesenchymal transition.

REFERENCE/SOURCE

- Son MBF, Burns JC, Newburger JW. Kawasaki disease (Chapter 35). In: Petty RE, Laxer RM, Lindsley CB, Wedderburn LR, Mellins ED, Fuhlbrigge RC (Eds). Textbook of Pediatric Rheumatology, 8th edition. Elsevier; 2021.

6. A 3-year-old boy was presented with fever for 8 days, associated with irritability, swelling of the hands and feet, redness of the whites of the eyes, swellings in the neck, and irritation and inflammation of the mouth, lips, and throat. There were no other localizing signs/symptoms. Which of the following is *not* characteristic of this condition?

A. It is the leading cause of acquired heart disease in children

B. Genome-wide association studies (GWAS) have found a genetic basis for predisposition including single nucleotide polymorphisms (SNPs) in the human leukocyte antigen class II region-HLA-DQB2 and HLA-DOB

C. 70–80% of untreated children develop coronary artery abnormalities (CAA) including aneurysms

D. <5% of children treated with intravenous immune globulin (IVIG) develop CAA

EXPLANATION

In Kawasaki disease, approximately 20–25% of untreated children develop CAA including aneurysms, whereas <5% of children treated with IVIG develop CAA.

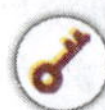

Key: C

BOOST YOUR KNOWLEDGE

Kawasaki disease is the leading cause of acquired heart disease in children in most developed countries, including the United States and Japan.

A genetic role in the pathogenesis of KD seems likely, as evidenced by the higher risk of KD in Asian children regardless of country of residence and in siblings and children of individuals with a history of KD. Furthermore, linkage studies and genome-wide association studies (GWAS) have identified significant potential associations between polymorphisms in the *ITPKC* gene, a T-cell regulator, with increased susceptibility to KD and more severe disease. Other candidate genes for KD identified by GWAS include *CASP3*, *BLK*, and *FCGR2A*. Lastly, associations of SNPs in the human leukocyte antigen class II region (HLA-DQB2 and HLA-DOB) with KD have been reported. The concordance rate among identical twins, however, is approximately 13%.

REFERENCE/SOURCE

- Kliegman RM, St Geme III JW. Nelson Textbook of Pediatrics, 21st edition. Elsevier; 2019. Chapter 191: Kawasaki disease.

7. A 4-year-old boy, presented to the OPD with a violaceous palpable rash on the buttocks and legs for 2 weeks. There was an associated history of bilateral knee pain and swelling, along with intermittent colicky abdominal pain. Which of the following immunoglobulin deposits on histopathology is hallmark of underlying disease?

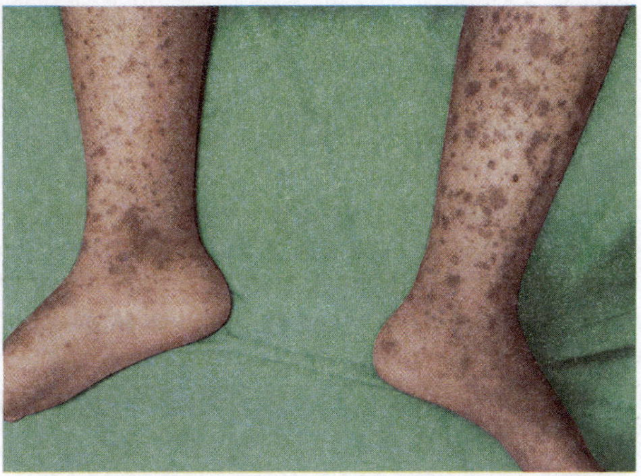

A. IgA
B. IgD
C. IgG
D. IgG4

EXPLANATION

Palpable purpura with arthritis and characteristic abdominal pain point toward a diagnosis of IgA vasculitis as per EULAR/PRINTO/PRES classification criteria.

Criterion	*Definition*	*Sensitivity*	*Specificity*
Purpura (mandatory)	Purpura* (palpable, in crops) or petechiae, with lower limb predominance	89%	86%
And at least one out of four of the following:			
Abdominal pain	Diffuse, acute, colicky pain; may include intussusception and gastrointestinal bleeding	61%	64%
Histopathology	Leukocytoclastic vasculitis with predominant IgA deposits; or proliferative glomerulonephritis with predominant IgA deposits	93%	89%
Arthritis, arthralgias	• *Arthritis*: Acute joint swelling or pain with limitation of motion • *Arthralgia:* Acute joint pain without joint swelling or limitation of motion	78%	42%
Renal involvement	• *Proteinuria:* >0.3 g/24 hour; spot urine albumin to creatinine ratio >30 mmol/mg; or ≥2+ on dipstick • *Hematuria:* Red cell casts; urine sediment showing >5 red cells per high-power field or red cell casts	33%	70%

*Not related to thrombocytopenia

Nephritis, orchitis, posterior reversible encephalopathy syndrome (PRES), ataxia, Guillain–Barré syndrome, neuropathy although rare, are all recognized disease-related complications but papular-purpuric glove-and-sock syndrome is a differential (associated with parvovirus B19 infection).

Key: A

BOOST YOUR KNOWLEDGE

Palpable purpura or petechiae (not related to thrombocytopenia) is a mandatory criterion for diagnosis of IgA vasculitis, not a complication. Also, there is no single diagnostic test. Hence, diagnosis depends on clinical features supported by laboratory parameters (e.g., urinalysis, histopathology), which differentiate it from other vasculitis [anti-neutrophil cytoplasmic antibody (ANCA)-associated post-streptococcal glomerulonephritis and lupus nephritis].

REFERENCE/SOURCE

- Brogan P, Nott KA. Immune complex small-vessel vasculitis: IgA vasculitis (Henoch–Schönlein) and hypersensitivity vasculitis (Chapter 33). In: Petty RE, Laxer RM, Lindsley CB, Wedderburn LR, Mellins ED, Fuhlbrigge RC (Eds). Textbook of Pediatric Rheumatology, 8th edition. Elsevier; 2021.

8. Which of the following is a risk factor for renal involvement in Henoch–Schönlein purpura?

A. Older age (>10 years)
B. Absence of GI symptoms
C. Normal C3
D. Thrombocytopenia

EXPLANATION

Older age group is more predisposed to renal involvement, not younger. Hence, they should be actively monitored for renal involvement.

Key: A

BOOST YOUR KNOWLEDGE

Glomerulonephritis affects up to one-third of children with IgA vasculitis but is serious and potentially life-threatening in <10%. The onset is generally within 4–6 weeks of the onset of the rash. However, certain characteristics such as male gender, older age (>10 years), severe gastrointestinal symptoms, arthritis/arthralgia, persistent purpura, relapse, raised leukocyte and/or platelet counts, elevated antistreptolysin titer, low complement C3 and presence of microscopic dermal edema with direct immunofluorescence (DIF) showing perivascular C3 deposition may be predictive of renal disease. Such children must be monitored, especially for the initial 6 months for timely identification and treatment of renal involvement.

REFERENCE/SOURCE

- Brogan P, Nott KA. Immune complex small-vessel vasculitis: IgA vasculitis (Henoch–Schönlein) and hypersensitivity vasculitis (Chapter 33). In: Petty RE, Laxer RM, Lindsley CB, Wedderburn LR, Mellins ED, Fuhlbrigge RC (Eds). Textbook of Pediatric Rheumatology, 8th edition. Elsevier; 2021.

9. In Henoch–Schönlein purpura (HSP), if urinalysis reveals microscopic hematuria and, nephritic range proteinuria; clinical evidence of acute deterioration of renal function within days. What therapy should be considered?

A. Prednisolone, concomitant therapy with angiotensin-converting enzyme (ACE)/angiotensin receptor blockers (ARBs)
B. Corticosteroids and methotrexate
C. Tapering corticosteroids over 2 years
D. IV methylprednisolone pulse with IV cyclophosphamide induction

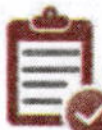

EXPLANATION

The above features suggest rapidly progressive glomerulonephritis. This necessitates urgent immunomodulation with IV pulse steroid and cyclophosphamide to address disease activity.

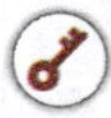

Key: D

BOOST YOUR KNOWLEDGE

Indications for renal biopsy in IgA vasculitis:

- Nephrotic or nephritic syndrome at presentation; rapidly progressive glomerulonephritis
- *Severe proteinuria:* Protein—creatinine ratio >2 mg/mg; 3+/4+ proteinuria on dipstick on 2 or more occasions
- *Persistent mild-to-moderate proteinuria:* Protein—creatinine ratio 0.2–2 mg/mg; 1+/2+ proteinuria on dipstick for >2 weeks
- Impaired glomerular filtration rate (GFR) <60 mL/min/1.73 m^2
- Persistent microscopic hematuria without proteinuria (protein—creatinine <0.2) for >4 weeks

Treatment: Treatment of immunoglobulin-A vasculitis (IgAV) is predominantly supportive. However, organ and/or life-threatening complications require glucocorticoid as well as cytotoxic therapy (cyclophosphamide). In the absence of organ and/or life-threatening complications, glucocorticoids can still be considered for severe manifestations to decrease the disease severity and duration.

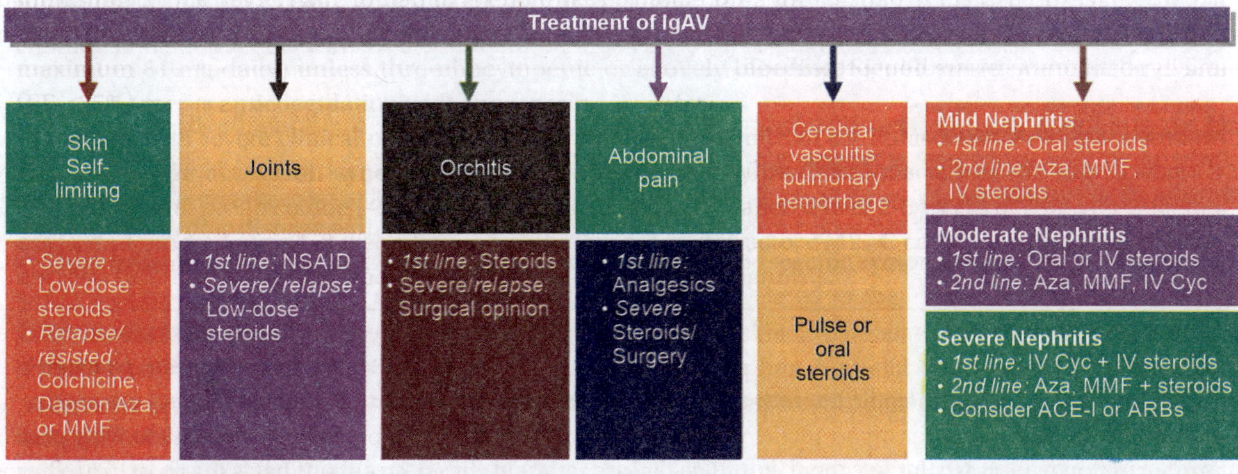

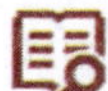

REFERENCE/SOURCE

- Abu-Zaid MH, Salah S, Lotfy HM, El Gaafary M, Abdulhady H, Tabra SAA, et al. Consensus evidence-based recommendations for treat-to-target management of immunoglobulin A vasculitis. Ther Adv Musculoskelet Dis. 2021;13.

10. Which of the following is one of the classification criteria for IgA vasculitis?

A. Acute colicky abdominal pain
B. Proteinuria >1 g/24 hours
C. Thrombocytopenia <1,00,000/mm^3
D. Biopsy showing predominant C3 deposition on IF

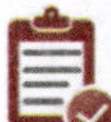

EXPLANATION

Diffuse acute colicky pain is a key feature for clinical diagnosis. Nonthrombocytopenic purpura is an essential criterion for diagnosis. For renal involvement nephritic features are sufficient. Tissue should reflect IgA deposition predominantly.

Classification criteria for Henoch–Schönlein Purpura*
European League Against Rheumatism/Pediatric Rheumatology European Society Criteria†
Palpable purpura (in absence of coagulopathy or thrombocytopenia) and one or more of the following criteria must be present: • Abdominal pain (acute, diffuse, and colicky pain) • Arthritis or arthralgia • Biopsy of affected tissue demonstrating predominant IgA deposition • Renal involvement (proteinuria >0.3 g/24 hours), hematuria or red cell casts

*Classification criteria are developed for use in research and not validated for clinical diagnosis.

†Developed for use in pediatric populations only.

Source: Adapted from Ozen S, Pistorio A, Iusan SM, Bakkaloglu A, Herlin T, Brik R, et al. EULAR/PRINTO/PRES criteria for Henoch–Schönlein purpura, childhood polyarteritis nodosa, childhood Wegener granulomatosis and childhood Takayasu arteritis: Ankara 2008. Part II. Final classification criteria. Ann Rheum Dis. 2010;69(5):798-806.

Key: A

BOOST YOUR KNOWLEDGE

Gastrointestinal manifestations occur in approximately 50–60% of children, usually within a week after appearance of rash to 30 days. In around 15% it may precede other manifestations. The small bowel is the most frequently involved gastrointestinal tract because of its predilection toward ischemic injury. Bowel wall vasculitis can lead to intussusception, gangrene, or overt perforation, obstruction and stricture formation, protein-losing enteropathy, hepatobiliary disease, acute pancreatitis, and massive gastrointestinal hemorrhage. Even asymptomatic patients may have mucosal injury as suggested by the presence of fecal occult blood, increased stool alpha-1-antitrypsin, and hypoalbuminemia without proteinuria.

REFERENCES/SOURCES

- Brogan P, Nott KA. Immune complex small-vessel vasculitis: IgA vasculitis (Henoch–Schönlein) and hypersensitivity vasculitis (Chapter 33). In: Petty RE, Laxer RM, Lindsley CB, Wedderburn LR, Mellins ED, Fuhlbrigge RC (Eds). Textbook of Pediatric Rheumatology, 8th edition. Elsevier; 2021.
- Kliegman RM, St Geme III JW. Nelson Textbook of Pediatrics, 21st edition. Elsevier; 2019. Chapter 192: Vasculitis syndromes.

11. A boy aged 14 months presented to the pediatric emergency with a history of fever for 7 days. On examination, he was noted to have tender orofacial, limb, and scrotal edema interspersed with ecchymoses. These persisted despite appropriate antimicrobial therapy. Investigations revealed sterile cultures, normal platelet counts, echocardiography, and urinalysis with no other organ involvement. Skin biopsy showed leukocytoclastic vasculitis with occasional demonstration of perivascular IgA deposition. The disease remitted within 2 weeks. What is the most likely diagnosis?

A. Finkelstein–Seidlmayer syndrome
B. IgA vasculitis
C. *Staphylococcus*-scalded skin syndrome
D. Wegner granulomatosis

EXPLANATION

The clinical features are similar to IgAV with a suggestive skin biopsy. But there is no organ-system involvement supporting such a diagnosis. Also, the age and edema-predominant presentation point toward an alternative diagnosis—Finkelstein–Seidlmayer syndrome.

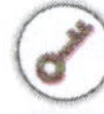

Key: A

BOOST YOUR KNOWLEDGE

Infantile acute hemorrhagic edema (Finkelstein–Seidlmayer syndrome) affects infants between 4 and 24 months of age with acute onset of fever, purpura, ecchymoses, and inflammatory edema of the limbs, ears, and face. It has a benign course with spontaneous remission in 1–3 weeks but may recur. Internal organ involvement (kidneys, gastrointestinal tract) is rare. Histopathology shows leukocytoclastic vasculitis with occasional demonstration of perivascular IgA deposition. It is unclear whether this condition is truly a separate entity from IgAV. A cohort study from Israel, describing 26 patients under the age of 2 years, found a frequent presence of arthralgia/arthritis (35%) and gastrointestinal symptoms (35%), although renal involvement was rare. Since, it is a self-limiting condition, the treatment is supportive. However, all efforts should be made to distinguish from IgAV by diligent follow-up.

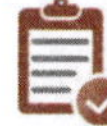

REFERENCES/SOURCES

- Brogan P, Nott KA. Immune complex small-vessel vasculitis: IgA vasculitis (Henoch–Schönlein) and hypersensitivity vasculitis (Chapter 33). In: Petty RE, Laxer RM, Lindsley CB, Wedderburn LR, Mellins ED, Fuhlbrigge RC (Eds). Textbook of Pediatric Rheumatology, 8th edition. Elsevier; 2021.
- Kliegman RM, St Geme III JW. Nelson Textbook of Pediatrics, 21st edition. Elsevier; 2019. Chapter 192: Vasculitis syndromes.

12. Which HLA locus is associated with increased susceptibility to IgA nephritis?

A. HLA B10
B. HLA B34
C. HLADRB1*07
D. HLA D27

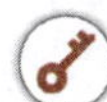

EXPLANATION

HLA-B34 and HLA-DRB1*01 alleles have been positively and negatively linked to nephritis respectively.

Key: B

BOOST YOUR KNOWLEDGE

Immunoglobulin-A vasculitis occasionally clusters in families, suggesting a genetic component.

When comparing genetic variants between healthy and IgAV patients, the biggest difference was found in human leukocyte antigen (*HLA*) genes. Variants HLA-DRB1*01 and HLA-DRB1*11 was associated with IgAV susceptibility, whereas HLA-DRB1*07 was negatively associated with IgAV. HLA-B*4102 was found to be a susceptibility marker for IgAV development irrespective of HLA-DRB1 status.

REFERENCES/SOURCES

- Brogan P, Nott KA. Immune complex small-vessel vasculitis: IgA vasculitis (Henoch–Schönlein) and hypersensitivity vasculitis (Chapter 33). In: Petty RE, Laxer RM, Lindsley CB, Wedderburn LR, Mellins ED, Fuhlbrigge RC (Eds). Textbook of Pediatric Rheumatology, 8th edition. Elsevier; 2021.
- Kliegman RM, St Geme III JW. Nelson Textbook of Pediatrics, 21st edition. Elsevier; 2019. Chapter 192: Vasculitis syndromes.

13. As per the United Network of Organ Sharing database, what is the approximate 10-year post-transplant graft loss from recurrent disease following transplant in IgA vasculitis nephritis?

A. 04%
B. 14%
C. 34%
D. 64%

EXPLANATION

Post-transplant renal graft survival is 80% at 5 years and 58.8% at 10 years; with graft loss from recurrent disease occurring in 13.6%.

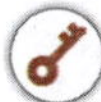

Key: B

BOOST YOUR KNOWLEDGE

Immunoglobulin-A vasculitis can be organ-threatening and even progress to end-stage-renal disease. In such cases, renal transplantation can be considered. However, appropriate counseling must be done to explain the possibility of recurrence (35% at 5 years post-transplant) and subsequent risk of graft loss despite appropriate immunosuppression.

A retrospective cohort study of 339 adult patients with IgAV using the United Network of Organ Sharing database observed a graft survival of 80% at 5 years and 58.8% at 10 years; graft loss from recurrent disease occurred in 13.6%.

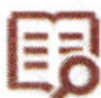

REFERENCE/SOURCE

- Brogan P, Nott KA. Immune complex small-vessel vasculitis: IgA vasculitis (Henoch–Schönlein) and hypersensitivity vasculitis (Chapter 33). In: Petty RE, Laxer RM, Lindsley CB, Wedderburn LR, Mellins ED, Fuhlbrigge RC (Eds). Textbook of Pediatric Rheumatology, 8th edition. Elsevier; 2021.

14. An 8-year-old boy presented to his physician with a history of fever for 4 weeks, diffuse abdominal pain and generalized body aches for 10 days, with discoloration of fingertips for 2 days. Examination revealed pallor, generalized muscle tenderness and a lace-like rash. Systemic examination was unremarkable except for mild generalized abdominal tenderness. Lab investigations showed: Hemoglobin: 6.7 g/dL, Leukocyte count: 35,890/mm^3 (Neutrophils: 88%), ESR: 29 mm/hr, CRP: 46 mg/L

Blood and urine cultures were sterile.

Further diagnostic evaluation showed a normal echocardiogram. Serum ANA was negative with normal C3 and C4 levels. However, the CECT abdomen showed a splenic and renal infarct with angiographic abnormalities. The digital subtraction angiography showed the findings in given image:

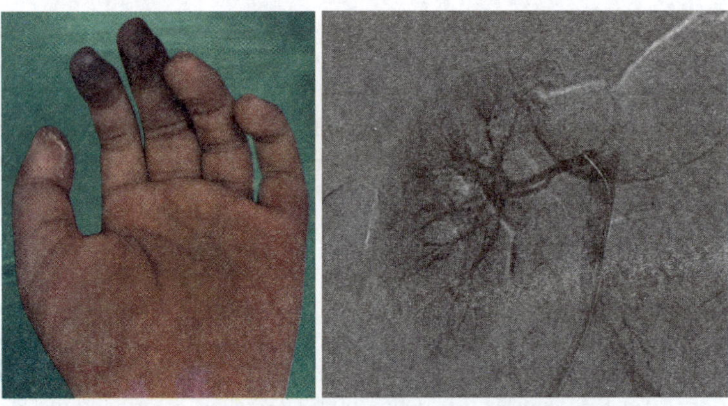

Courtesy: Dr Priyanka Naranjee, Professor Manisha Jana.

Which of the following is a characteristic of this disease?

A. Non-granulomatous necrotizing vasculitis
B. Continuous vascular involvement throughout vessel extent
C. Presence of p-ANCA is characteristic
D. Has a predilection for large-medium vessels

EXPLANATION

The multisystem clinical features with evidence of multiple microaneurysms in the branches of celiac and superior mesenteric axis. The left renal artery and splenic artery are completely occluded. These angiographic findings are suggestive of polyarteritis nodosa—a non-granulomatous necrotizing vasculitis.

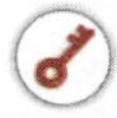

Key: A

BOOST YOUR KNOWLEDGE

Biopsies in polyarteritis nodosa (PAN) show necrotizing vasculitis with granulocytes and monocytes infiltrating the walls of small and medium-sized arteries. Involvement is usually segmental and tends to occur at vessel bifurcations. Granulomatous inflammation is absent, and deposition of complement and immune complexes is rarely observed. Serology for ANCA is negative.

REFERENCE/SOURCE

- Eleftheriou D, Dusser P, Koné-Paut I. Polyarteritis nodosa (Chapter 34). In: Petty RE, Laxer RM, Lindsley CB, Wedderburn LR, Mellins ED, Fuhlbrigge RC (Eds). Textbook of Pediatric Rheumatology, 8th edition. Elsevier; 2021.

15. Which of the following is a known poor prognostic factor in polyarteritis nodosa?

A. Absence of gastrointestinal involvement
B. Digital gangrene
C. Cardiomyopathy
D. Vasculitic ulcers

EXPLANATION

Although a part of classification criteria, cutaneous involvement does not have prognostic value. Poor prognostic factors in PAN include elevated serum creatinine, proteinuria, severe GI involvement, cardiomyopathy, and central nervous system (CNS) involvement.

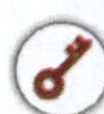

Key: C

BOOST YOUR KNOWLEDGE

The course of PAN varies from mild disease with few complications to a severe, multiorgan disease with high morbidity and mortality. Identification of poor prognostic factors in PAN aids prioritization of early and aggressive immunosuppressive therapy, which increases the likelihood of clinical remission.

REFERENCE/SOURCE

- Kliegman RM, St Geme III JW. Nelson Textbook of Pediatrics, 21st edition. Elsevier; 2019. Chapter 192.3.

16. Which of the following is *not* a component of the classification criteria for childhood polyarteritis nodosa?

A. Gastrointestinal involvement—mesenteric/bowel ischemia
B. Muscle involvement—myalgia/tenderness
C. Peripheral neuropathy
D. Skin involvement—livedo reticularis, skin nodules, or infarcts

EXPLANATION

Although a frequently involved organ system, GI involvement is not a part of the classification criteria.

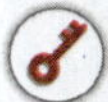

Key: A

BOOST YOUR KNOWLEDGE

Imaging or histopathological evidence of characteristic vasculitis is sine qua non for diagnosis. Clinically skin, musculoskeletal, renal, and neural involvement are added systemic criteria. Notably, hypertension is a distinct criterion from renal involvement.

Evidence of necrotizing vasculitis in medium or small arteries or an angiographic abnormality showing aneurysm, stenosis, or occlusion of a medium- or small-sized artery (histopathology or angiography mandatory), plus one out of five of the following criteria:

1. Skin involvement (livedo reticularis, skin nodules, or infarcts)
2. Myalgia or muscle tenderness
3. Hypertension (systolic/diastolic blood pressure >95th percentile for height)

4. Peripheral neuropathy (sensory peripheral neuropathy or motor mononeuritis multiplex)
5. Renal involvement [proteinuria >0.3 g/24 hours or >30 mmol/mg of urine albumin : creatinine ratio on a spot morning sample; hematuria or red blood cell casts, >5 red blood cells/high-power field, red blood cell casts in the urinary sediment, or equal to 2+ on dipstick; or impaired renal function, measured or calculated glomerular filtration rate (Schwartz formula) <50% normal]

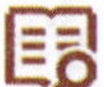

REFERENCE/SOURCE

- Eleftheriou D, Dusser P, Koné-Paut I. Polyarteritis nodosa (Chapter 34). In: Petty RE, Laxer RM, Lindsley CB, Wedderburn LR, Mellins ED, Fuhlbrigge RC (Eds). Textbook of Pediatric Rheumatology, 8th edition. Elsevier; 2021.

17. Which of the following genetic aberration is expected in the case of a monogenic polyarteritis nodosa?

A. Gain of function in *ADA2* gene, autosomal recessive inheritance
B. Loss of function in *ADA2* gene, autosomal dominant inheritance
C. Gain of function in *STING* gene, autosomal dominant inheritance
D. Loss of function in *STING* gene, autosomal dominant inheritance

EXPLANATION

STimulator of INterferon Gene (*STING*)-associated vasculopathy with onset in infancy (SAVI) is caused by a gain of function in STINGs, autosomal dominant inheritance.

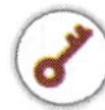

Key: C

BOOST YOUR KNOWLEDGE

Necrotizing vasculitis can also be associated with primary immunodeficiencies, e.g., deficiency in recombination activating gene 1 and 2 (*RAG1* and *RAG2*) or transporter associated with antigen processing (TAP). It can be observed in some autoinflammatory monogenic diseases such as DADA2, STING-associated vasculopathy with onset in infancy (SAVI), and the proteasome-associated autoinflammatory disease. Monogenic PAN has treatment implications:

Disease	*Age of onset*	*Genetics*	*General symptoms*	*Neuro-logical*	*Musculo-skeletal*	*Skin*	*Immuno-deficiency*	*Other*	*Treatment*
DADA2	Any	Homozygous loss of function mutations in *ADA2* gene; autosomal recessive	Fever	Intracranial hemorrhage; neuropathy; vision loss; ischemic strokes	Myalgia, arthralgia, arthritis	Livedo racemosa; subcutaneous nodules; petechiae/ purpura; necrosis	Humoral immunodeficiency; cytopenias including pure red cell aplasia	Central retinal artery occlusion, optic nerve atrophy; uveitis	TNF-α blockade therapy; corticosteroids; hematopoietic stem cell transplantation
SAVI	Infancy	Heterozygous gain of function mutations in *STING* gene; autosomal dominant	Recurrent low-grade fevers	Not reported	Myositis, arthritis	Ulcerative lesions with eschar formation and tissue infarction; scarring of the ear cartilage; perforation of the nasal septum; livedo reticularis	Leukopenia	Interstitial lung disease; failure to thrive; anemia, thrombocytosis	Janus kinase inhibition, corticosteroids

REFERENCE/SOURCE

- Eleftheriou D, Dusser P, Koné-Paut I. Polyarteritis nodosa (Chapter 34). In: Petty RE, Laxer RM, Lindsley CB, Wedderburn LR, Mellins ED, Fuhlbrigge RC (Eds). Textbook of Pediatric Rheumatology, 8th edition. Elsevier; 2021.

18. Which of the following drugs were evaluated in the MYPAN randomized controlled trial for induction of remission in childhood-onset polyarteritis nodosa?

A. Mycophenolate mofetil and anakinra
B. Mycophenolate mofetil and cyclophosphamide
C. Mycophenolate mofetil and infliximab
D. Mycophenolate mofetil and methylprednisolone pulse

EXPLANATION

Considering the possible benefit of the less toxic mycophenolate mofetil for, induction of remission in childhood onset PAN, an international, open-label, Bayesian RCT was undertaken to investigate the relative effectiveness compared to cyclophosphamide (CYC).

Key: B

BOOST YOUR KNOWLEDGE

Eleven patients with newly diagnosed childhood PAN were randomized (1:1) to receive mycophenolate mofetil (MMF) or intravenous CYC; all patients received the same glucocorticoid regimen. The primary endpoint was remission within 6 months while compliant with glucocorticoid taper.

Baseline disease activity and features were similar between the two treatment groups. The primary endpoint was met in four of six patients (67%) in the MMF group and four of five patients (80%) in the CYC group. Time to remission was shorter in the MMF group compared to the CYC group (median 7.1 weeks vs. 17.6 weeks). No relapses occurred in either group within 18 months. Two serious infections were found to be likely linked to MMF treatment. Physical and psychosocial quality-of-life scores were superior in the MMF group compared to the CYC group at 6 months and 18 months. Combining the prior expert opinion with results from the present study provided posterior estimates of remission of 71% for MMF [90% credibility interval (90% CrI) 51, 83] and 75% for CYC (90% CrI 57, 86).

Although with a small sample only, the trial results indicated that rates of remission induction in childhood PAN are similar with MMF treatment and CYC treatment, and MMF treatment might be associated with better health-related quality of life than CYC treatment.

REFERENCE/SOURCE

- Paul A. Brogan, Barbara Arch, Helen Hickey, Jordi Anton, Este Iglesias, Eileen Baildam, et al. Mycophenolate mofetil versus cyclophosphamide for remission induction in childhood polyarteritis nodosa: an open-label, randomized, Bayesian noninferiority trial. Arthritis Rheumatol. 2021;73(9):1673-82.

19. A 13-year-old girl presented to a pediatric emergency with an excruciating headache. History revealed fever, malaise, and weight loss for 8 weeks. She was persistently symptomatic despite being on anti-tuberculosis treatment (ATT) started based on a positive Mantoux test. On examination, she was (stage 2) hypertensive, with asymmetrical radial pulse volumes and a blood pressure difference of 20 mm Hg in the lower and upper limbs. On auscultation, an epigastric bruit was audible.

I. What is the likely diagnosis?

A. Takayasu arteritis type I
B. Takayasu arteritis type I, II, III
C. Takayasu arteritis type II, III, IV
D. Takayasu arteritis type III, IV, V

EXPLANATION

A hypertensive adolescent girl with constitutional symptoms, asymmetric pulses, abdominal bruit, and positive tuberculin test raises the suspicion of Takayasu arteritis. Considering the renal vascular involvement—the infradiaphragmatic subtype of disease seems most likely.

Classification of vessel type involvement in Takayasu arteritis (TA)

Vessel type involvement:

I. Branches from the aortic arch
IIa. Ascending aorta, aortic arch and its branches
IIb. Ascending aorta, aortic arch and its branches, thoracic descending aorta
III. Thoracic descending aorta, abdominal aorta, and/or renal arteries
IV. Abdominal aorta and/or renal arteries
V. Combined features of type IIb and IV

Key: D

BOOST YOUR KNOWLEDGE

The frequency of positive tuberculin test associated with TA was found to be as high as 43–44%. The association with tuberculosis is very rare in developed countries. The causality of TB and TA however has not been established. It is theorized that the immune response in TA could be a result of cross-reaction between homologous protein present in the vascular wall of the host and the mycobacterial heat shock 65-kD.

REFERENCES/SOURCES

- Hashkes PJ. Takayasu arteritis and other vasculitides (Chapter 37). In: Petty RE, Laxer RM, Lindsley CB, Wedderburn LR, Mellins ED, Fuhlbrigge RC (Eds). Textbook of Pediatric Rheumatology, 8th edition. Elsevier; 2021.
- Magar MT, Kafle S, Poudel A, Patel P, Cancarevic I. Takayasu's arteritis and its association with *Mycobacterium tuberculosis*: a systematic review. Cureus. 2021;13(8):e16927.

II. Which investigation would help diagnose this condition?

A. p-ANCA
B. MR angiogram
C. Endovascular ultrasound
D. pro-BNP

EXPLANATION

Imaging evidence of characteristic lesions is mandatory for diagnosis. Either CT/MR angiography can be undertaken.

Classification criteria (PRES/EULAR) for pediatric Takayasu arteritis:

These criteria are based on the comparison of 87 patients with Takayasu arteritis to 1,096 patients with other types of pediatric vasculitis. The sensitivity of these criteria was 100% and specificity was 99.9%.

Mandatory criterion:

Angiographic abnormalities [demonstrated by conventional angiography, computed tomography (CT) or magnetic resonance imaging (MRI)] pull one of the five following criteria:

1. Pulse deficit or claudication
2. Blood pressure discrepancy >10 mm Hg between the four limbs
3. Bruits over the major arteries
4. Hypertension
5. Elevated acute phase reactant (erythrocyte sedimentation rate or co-reactive protein)

Key: B

BOOST YOUR KNOWLEDGE

The diagnosis of TA in children is most based on the clinical triad of constitutional symptoms, hypertension, and elevated acute phase reactants with angiographic demonstration of stenosis of the aorta and its major branches.

One of the most difficult issues is differentiating it in the "burned-out" phase, from anatomical variants, particularly fibromuscular dysplasia (FMD) in which proximal stenosis of the large vessels can be found. This problem may be exacerbated in children where FMD is more often manifested as the middle aortic syndrome compared with adults. Conversely, patients diagnosed with FMD may have TA.

An important aid in differentiating the two entities is the finding of dilatations and aneurysms in TA. In FMD, dilatations are limited to post-stenotic segments.

Vessel wall imaging can determine TA with findings characteristics of wall edema, concentric wall thickening, and contrast enhancement not found in FMD and the middle aortic syndrome. Serial imaging and 18-fluorodeoxyglucose positron emission tomography (18FDG-PET) scans can also help differentiate these conditions.

REFERENCE/SOURCE

- Hashkes PJ. Takayasu arteritis and other vasculitides (Chapter 37). In: Petty RE, Laxer RM, Lindsley CB, Wedderburn LR, Mellins ED, Fuhlbrigge RC (Eds). Textbook of Pediatric Rheumatology, 8th edition. Elsevier; 2021.

III. What is *true* about the long-term disease course?

A. Undulant biphasic course with rare relapses
B. Risk of accelerated atherosclerosis present
C. 50% 5-year mortality rate
D. Poorly amenable to surgical intervention

EXPLANATION

Takayasu arteritis is usually a relapsing chronic disease. Given the chronic endothelial insult and inflammation, children and adolescents with TA are probably at high risk for accelerated atherosclerosis.

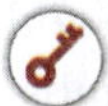

Key: B

BOOST YOUR KNOWLEDGE

A relapsing chronic disease with a triphasic disease course:

- Early inflammatory disease characterized by constitutional nonspecific symptoms
- Chronic/relapsing stenotic/aneurysmal phase—symptoms related to the effect of blood vessel changes on various organs, and
- Burned-out phase with fibrotic changes

Now, we know that these phases are not sequential but often occur simultaneously. The disease is monophasic in 20–25% of patients.

Causes of death in TA include aortic dissection, cardiomyopathy, heart failure, hypertensive crises, myocardial infarction, stroke, and renal failure. Risk factors for mortality were younger age at onset and higher damage score but not a delayed time to diagnosis, cardiac involvement, nor the need for surgical intervention. The overall 5-year survival in adults is 70–90%. Among pediatric TA, especially from developing countries, mortality was as high as 22–35% after 10–15 years of follow-up.

Surgical management: In children with inactive TA but with significant arterial stenosis or aneurysms, surgical, and endovascular procedures may be necessary, especially in patients with difficult-to-control hypertension, abdominal angina, and/or claudication. It is preferable and safer to perform these procedures when the disease is quiescent. The proportion of children who underwent surgical procedures in cohorts of pediatric TA since 2010 was nearly 50% (range 16–90%) with a varied success rate for treatment of hypertension (range 50–83%).

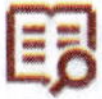

REFERENCE/SOURCE

- Hashkes PJ. Takayasu arteritis and other vasculitides (Chapter 37). In: Petty RE, Laxer RM, Lindsley CB, Wedderburn LR, Mellins ED, Fuhlbrigge RC (Eds). Textbook of Pediatric Rheumatology, 8th edition. Elsevier; 2021.

20. Which of the following are associated with Takayasu arteritis?

A. Antinuclear antibodies
B. Antineutrophil cytoplasmic antibodies
C. Anti-endothelial antibodies
D. Anti-myoglobin antibodies

EXPLANATION

Takayasu arteritis is large vessel vasculitis with frequent seropositivity for anti-endothelial antibodies.

Key: C

BOOST YOUR KNOWLEDGE

Autoimmunity, particularly B cell-mediated autoimmunity, is implicated in TA. B cells also play a role in TA by promoting endothelial cell activation through the secretion of anti-endothelial cell antibodies. Anti-aorta and anti-endothelial cell antibodies (AECAs) have been detected in patients with TA. AECAs target endothelial proteins, such as the endothelial protein C receptor and scavenger receptor class B type 1, which act as negative regulators of endothelial activation. Blockade of these regulatory receptors by AECAs leads to a proinflammatory phenotype.

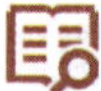

REFERENCE/SOURCE

- Bhandari S, Butt SRR, Ishfaq A, Attaallah MH, Ekhator C, Halappa Nagaraj R, et al. Pathophysiology, Diagnosis, and Management of Takayasu Arteritis: A Review of Current Advances. Cureus. 2023;15(7):e42667.

21. A 14-year-old girl presented to the emergency with epistaxis. A review of history revealed a 2-month history of fever, lassitude, recalcitrant sinusitis, and hemoptysis. On examination, she was noted to have a saddle nose and bilateral pulmonary infiltrates. Investigations revealed the ANCA pattern as shown in Figure. Which is the most common organ system involved in this condition?

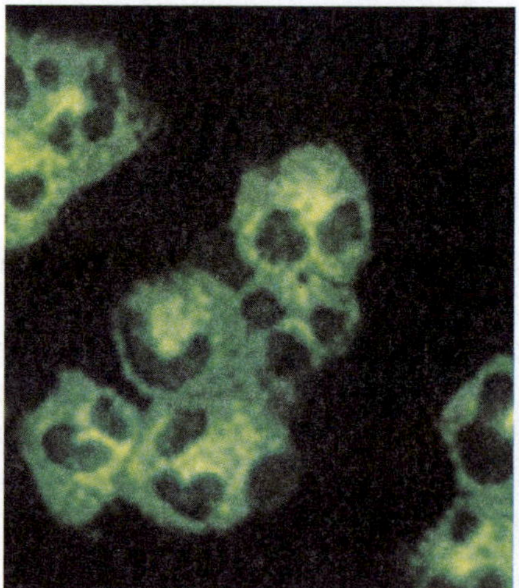

A. Gastrointestinal
B. Central nervous system
C. Renal
D. Pulmonary

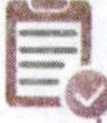

EXPLANATION

These clinical features and c-ANCA pattern are suggestive of granulomatosis with polyangiitis. The most common organ involvement in this small vessel vasculitis is renal.

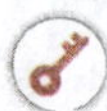

Key: B

BOOST YOUR KNOWLEDGE

In granulomatosis with polyangiitis, the frequencies of organ system involvement throughout the disease course follow respiratory tract 74%; kidneys 83%; joints 65%; eyes 43%; skin 47%; sinuses 70%, and nervous system 20%.

Upper airway involvement can manifest as sinusitis, nasal ulceration, epistaxis, otitis media, and hearing loss. Lower respiratory tract symptoms include cough, wheezing, dyspnea, subglottic stenosis, hemoptysis, and pulmonary hemorrhage. Compared with adults, childhood granulomatosis with polyangiitis (GPA) is more frequently complicated by inflammation-induced damage to the nasal cartilage can produce a saddle nose deformity. Ophthalmic involvement includes conjunctivitis, scleritis, uveitis, optic neuritis, and invasive orbital pseudotumor (causing proptosis). Perineural vasculitis or direct compression on nerves by granulomatous lesions can cause cranial and peripheral neuropathies. Hematuria, proteinuria, and hypertension in GPA signal renal disease. Cutaneous lesions include palpable purpura and ulcers. Venous thromboembolism is a rare but potentially fatal complication of GPA.

REFERENCE/SOURCE

- Cabral DA, Morishita KA. Antineutrophil cytoplasmic antibody associated vasculitis (Chapter 36). In: Petty RE, Laxer RM, Lindsley CB, Wedderburn LR, Mellins ED, Fuhlbrigge RC (Eds). Textbook of Pediatric Rheumatology, 8th edition. Elsevier; 2021.

22. Which of the following features best differentiates microscopic polyangiitis from granulomatous polyangiitis?

A. Lack of ANCA positivity
B. Cartilage destruction less common
C. Renal involvement
D. Poor response to glucocorticoid therapy

EXPLANATION

The clinical presentation of MPA closely resembles that of GPA. However, sinus disease with cartilaginous destruction is characteristic of GPA. Systemic features such as fever, weight loss, myalgias, and arthralgias predominate in MPA. Peripheral neuropathy has been reported in both these conditions.

Key: B

BOOST YOUR KNOWLEDGE

Although the ANCA-associated vasculitides have overlapping manifestations, sinus disease with destructive symptoms is more prevalent in granulomatosis with polyangiitis. Upper and lower respiratory tract inflammation is also seen in eosinophilic granulomatosis with polyangiitis, but cartilage destruction is rare.

Presenting manifestations (reported as percentages) in children:

Clinical Feature	***GPA (n = 183)***	***MPA (n = 48)***
Constitutional/General	88	85
Renal	83	75
Pulmonary	74	44
Ear, Nose, Throat:	70	4
Nasal involvement	53	0
Sinusitis	39	0
Subglottic involvement	10	0
Hearing loss	10	0
Oral ulcers	15	4

Source: Adapted from Petty RE, et al. Textbook of Pediatric Rheumatology, 8th edition. Elsevier: OHCE 2020, Chapter 36, Table 36.2.

REFERENCE/SOURCE

- Cabral DA, Morishita KA. Antineutrophil cytoplasmic antibody associated vasculitis (Chapter 36). In: Petty RE, Laxer RM, Lindsley CB, Wedderburn LR, Mellins ED, Fuhlbrigge RC (Eds). Textbook of Pediatric Rheumatology, 8th edition. Elsevier; 2021.

23. **A 14-year-old was referred from the asthma clinic considering difficult-to-treat asthma. She had poor control despite appropriate steroid therapy and compliance. Her serial chest X-rays revealed bilateral persistent pulmonary infiltrates. There was no evidence of any comorbid infection. Here urinalysis was normal and blood counts showed eosinophilia of 10%.**

What is the expected pattern of ANCA on immunofluorescence?

A. 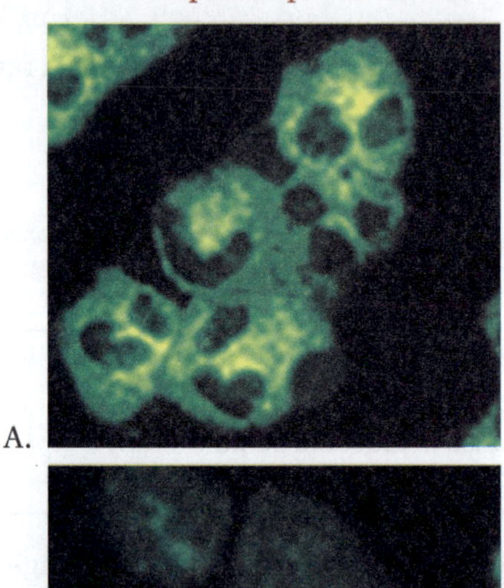

B. 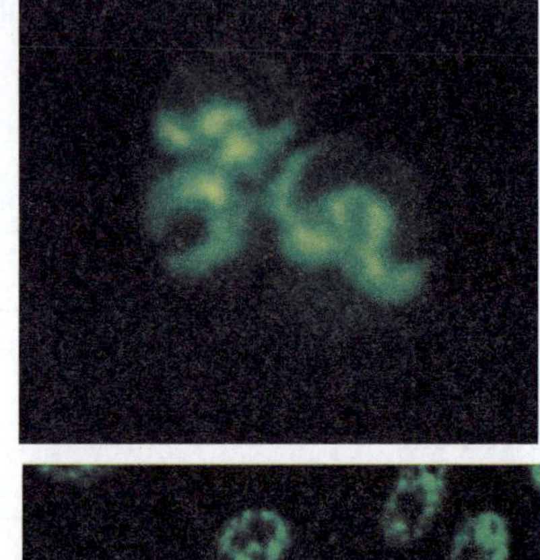

C. 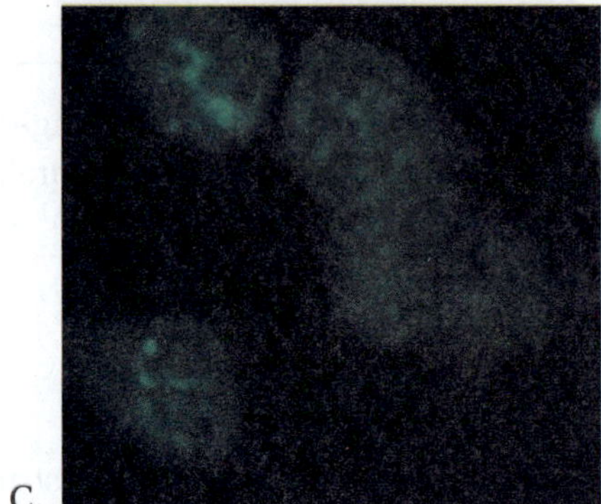

D. 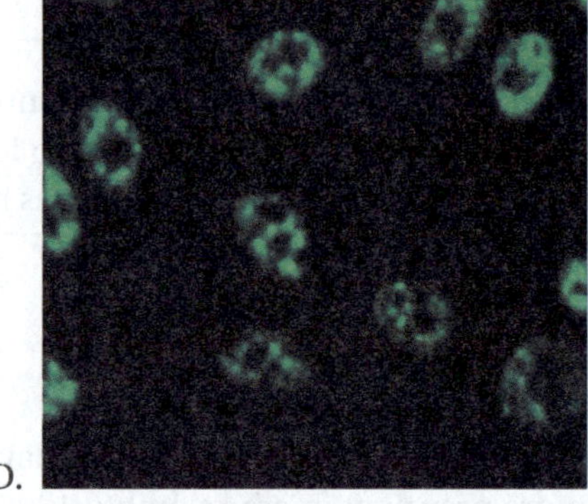

EXPLANATION

The history is suggestive of eosinophilic granulomatosis with polyangiitis—a necrotizing ANCA-associated small vessel vasculitis. It is mostly associated with anti-MPO type of ANCA (pANCA), is seen in 1/3rd of pediatric EGPA.

Sample A shows a cytoplasmic ANCA pattern while B shows a perinuclear ANCA pattern. Sample C is negative for ANCA, and D shows a speckled pattern of ANA.

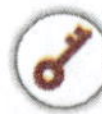

Key: B

BOOST YOUR KNOWLEDGE

As opposed to PAN, EGPA involves predominantly small rather than medium-sized vessels. Asthma, peripheral blood eosinophilia, and systemic vasculitis in two or more extrapulmonary sites are required to make a diagnosis. It is a triphasic disease with a protracted prodrome, making it difficult to distinguish from allergic entities at the outset. Difficult-to-treat asthma with multisystem involvement generally prompt suspicion and investigation. Histopathologically, the angiitis may be granulomatous or nongranulomatous. It is important to rule out parasitic infections, drug reactions, acute and chronic eosinophilic pneumonia, allergic bronchopulmonary aspergillosis, eosinophilic leukemia, and idiopathic hypereosinophilic syndrome (HES). Unlike EGPA, HES has no evidence of vasculitis.

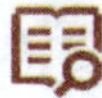

REFERENCE/SOURCE

- Cabral DA, Morishita KA. Antineutrophil cytoplasmic antibody associated vasculitis (Chapter 36). In: Petty RE, Laxer RM, Lindsley CB, Wedderburn LR, Mellins ED, Fuhlbrigge RC (Eds). Textbook of Pediatric Rheumatology, 8th edition. Elsevier; 2021.

24. A 15-year-old boy presented to an ophthalmologist with progressive acute deterioration in vision. Examination revealed posterior uveitis and thrombophlebitis. He had a history of recurrent episodic oral blister-ulceration and acne since 6 months back.

Which of the following is a minor criterion for the diagnosis of this entity?

A. Positive pathergy test
B. Ocular lesions
C. Genital aphthosis
D. Oral aphthosis

EXPLANATION

The history of oral ulceration, posterior uveitis, and thrombophlebitis points towards a vasculitic' pathology fulfilling criteria for Behçet's disease. Although a known phenomenon, thrombophlebitis does not contribute to the diagnostic criteria.

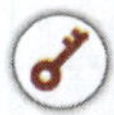

Key: A

BOOST YOUR KNOWLEDGE

Oral or genital aphthosis and ocular lesions are major criteria (each equally weighted) for diagnosis of Behçet's disease. Ancillary features supporting diagnosis include pathergy test, skin, neurologic, and vascular lesions. The vasculitis of Behçet's disease involves both the arterial and venous systems and vessels of any size, i.e., "variable vessel vasculitis". It is characteristically associated with arterial or venous thromboses and aneurysms. Superficial or deep venous thromboses are common in adults but occur only in 5–15% of children. Most thromboses are venous (lower extremities). Albeit rare, pulmonary artery thrombosis is among the most severe features of the disease—with high morbidity and mortality. Patients who develop superficial thrombophlebitis are more likely to develop major venous occlusions.

Diagnostic criteria for Behçet's disease

International Study Group for Behçet's disease	***International criteria for Behçet's diseases***
Diagnosis established by presence of one major and two minor criteria in absence of other clinical's	Diagnosis established by score ≥4
Major criterion: • Recurrent oral ulceration (herpetiform ulceration or minor or major aphthous ulcer recurring ≥3 times in one 12-month period)	*Two points each:* • Oral aphthosis • Genital aphthosis • Ocular lesions
Minor criteria: • Recurrent genital ulceration (aphthous ulceration or scarring) • Eye lesions (anterior uveitis, posterior uveitis, and retinal vasculitis) • Skin lesions (erythema nodosum, pseudofolliculitis, papulopustular lesions, and acneiform nodules post-adolescent patients) • Positive pathergy test	*One point each:* • Skin lesions • Neurologic manifestations • Vascular manifestations • Positive pathergy test

REFERENCE/SOURCE

- Ozen S. Behçet disease (Chapter 38). In: Petty RE, Laxer RM, Lindsley CB, Wedderburn LR, Mellins ED, Fuhlbrigge RC (Eds). Textbook of Pediatric Rheumatology, 8th edition. Elsevier; 2021.

CHAPTER

24.3 Juvenile Dermatomyositis, Antiphospholipid Syndrome, and Scleroderma

Priyankar Pal, Ravali Pratima Goud

1. What is the most common visceral manifestation of systemic sclerosis in children?

A. Pulmonary disease
B. Renal artery disease
C. Gastrointestinal disease
D. Cardiac fibrosis

EXPLANATION

Pulmonary disease is the most common visceral manifestation of systemic sclerosis and includes both vascular and interstitial involvement.

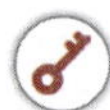

Key: A

BOOST YOUR KNOWLEDGE

Symptoms range from asymptomatic disease to exercise intolerance, dyspnea at rest, and right-sided heart failure. Pulmonary arterial hypertension is a poor prognostic sign, developing because of lung disease or independently as part of the vasculopathy. Clinical manifestations of pulmonary arterial hypertension in children appear late in the course, are subtle, and include cough and dyspnea on exertion. Pulmonary evaluation should include pulmonary function tests (PFTs) such as diffusion capacity of carbon monoxide (DLCO), bronchoalveolar lavage (BAL), and high-resolution computed tomography (HRCT) of the chest. PFTs reveal decreased vital capacity and decreased DLCO, whereas neutrophilia or eosinophilia on BAL suggest active alveolitis. Chest CT is much more sensitive than chest radiographs, which are often normal, showing typical basilar ground-glass abnormalities, reticular linear opacities, nodules, honeycombing, and mediastinal adenopathy.

REFERENCE/SOURCE

- Van Mater HA, Rabinovich CE. Scleroderma and Raynaud phenomenon. Kliegman RM, St Geme III JW (Eds). Nelson Textbook of Pediatrics, 21st edition. Elsevier; 2019. p. 1287.

2. A 5-year-old child presented with the following lesion on the scalp extending into forehead. Which of the following is *not* associated with this condition?

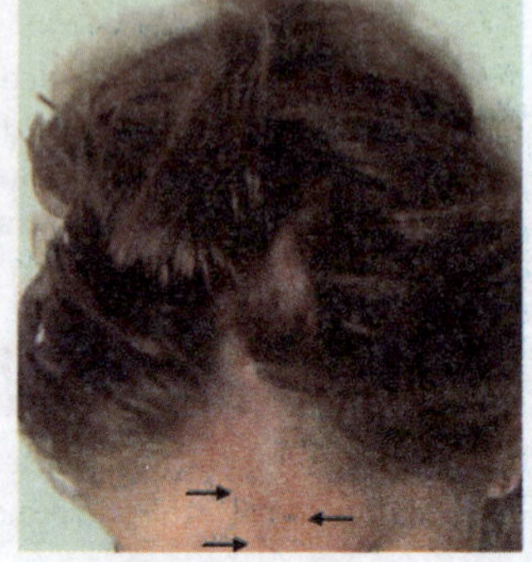

A. Seizures
B. Hemifacial atrophy
C. Contralateral uveitis
D. Learning and behavioral changes

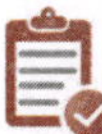

EXPLANATION

The given picture depicts *en coup de sabre* lesion of localized scleroderma. It is associated with ipsilateral uveitis.

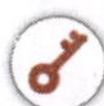

Key: C

BOOST YOUR KNOWLEDGE

Children with *en coup de sabre* may have symptoms unique to central nervous system (CNS) involvement, such as seizures, hemifacial atrophy, ipsilateral uveitis, and learning and behavioral changes.

REFERENCE/SOURCE

- Van Mater HA, Rabinovich CE. Scleroderma and Raynaud phenomenon. Kliegman RM, St Geme III JW (Eds). Nelson Textbook of Pediatrics, 21st edition. Elsevier; 2019. p.1286.

3. A 10-year-old girl was diagnosed with systemic sclerosis, presented with multiple episodes of Raynaud phenomena requiring vasodilators. Finger to palm distance on flexion is 1–1.9 cm, with distal esophageal hypoperistalsis, left ventricular ejection fraction being 45% on echocardiogram. What is the score of this child on Medsger severity scale?

A. Mild
B. Moderate
C. Severe
D. End Stage

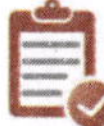

EXPLANATION

Medsger severity scale is used in systemic sclerosis to grade the organ involvement. The child with the above parameters has mild score.

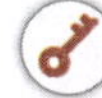

Key: A

BOOST YOUR KNOWLEDGE

Medsger Systemic Sclerosis Severity Scale

Organ system	*0 (Normal)*	*1 (Mild)*	*2 (Moderate)*	*3 (Severe)*	*4 (End stage)*
General	• Weight loss <5% • Hct 37% • Hb 12.3 g/dL	• Weight loss 5–10% • Hct 33–37% • Hb 11.0–12.2 g/dL	• Weight loss 10–15% • Hct 29–33% • Hb 9.7–10.9 g/dL	• Weight loss 15–20% • Hct 25–29% • Hb 8.3–9.6 g/dL	• Weight loss 20%+ • Hct 25% • Hb <8.3 g/dL
Peripheral vascular	No RP; RP not requiring vasodilators	RP requiring vasodilators	Digital pitting scars	Digital tip ulcerations	Digital gangrene
Skin	TSS 0	TSS 1–14	TSS 15–29	TSS 30–39	TSS 40+
Joint/tendon	FTP 0–0.9 cm	FTP 1.0–1.9 cm	FTP 2.0–3.9 cm	FTP 4.0–4.9 cm	FTP 5.0+ cm
Muscle	Normal proximal muscle strength	Proximal weakness, mild	Proximal weakness, moderate	Proximal weakness, severe	Ambulation aids required
Gastro-intestinal tract	Normal esophagogram; normal small bowel series	Distal esophageal hypoperistalsis; small bowel series abnormal	Antibiotics required for bacterial overgrowth	Malabsorption syndrome; episodes of pseudo-obstruction	Hyperalimentation required

Contd...

Contd...

Organ system	0 (Normal)	1 (Mild)	2 (Moderate)	3 (Severe)	4 (End stage)
Lung	• DLCO 80%+ • FVC 80%+ • No fibrosis on radiograph • sPAP <35 mm Hg	• DLCO 70–79% • FVC 70–79% • Basilar rales; fibrosis on radiograph • sPAP 35–49 mm Hg	• DLCO 50–69% • FVC 50–69% • sPAP 50–64 mm Hg	• DLCO <50% • FVC <50% • sPAP 65+ mm Hg	Oxygen required
Heart	ECG normal LVEF 50%+	• ECG conduction defect • LVEF 45–49%	• ECG arrhythmia • LVEF 40–44%	• ECG arrhythmia requiring therapy • LVEF 30–40%	CHF LVEF <30%
Kidney	No history of SRC with serum creatinine <1.3 mg/dL	History of SRC with serum creatinine <1.5 mg/dL	History of SRC with serum creatinine 1.5–2.4 mg/dL	History of SRC with serum creatinine 2.5–5.0 mg/dL	History of SRC with serum creatinine >5.0 mg/dL or dialysis required

(CHF: congestive heart failure; DLCO: diffusing capacity of the lungs for carbon monoxide; ECG: electrocardiogram; FTP: finger to palm; FVC: forced vital capacity; Hct: hematocrit; LVEF: left ventricular ejection fraction; RP: Raynaud phenomenon; sPAP: systolic pulmonary artery pressure; SRC: scleroderma renal crisis; TSS: total skin thickness score)

REFERENCE/SOURCE

- Van Mater HA, Rabinovich CE. Scleroderma and Raynaud phenomenon. Kliegman RM, St Geme III JW (Eds). Nelson Textbook of Pediatrics, 21st edition. Elsevier; 2019. p. 1287.

4. A 13-year-old girl presented with complaints of her hands turning pale and then bluish on exposure to cold. She also had excessive firmness and thickening of her skin in the last year. What is the chief cytokine involved in pathogenesis of her condition?

A. Tumor necrosis factor (TNF)-alpha
B. Transforming growth factor (TGF)-beta
C. Interleukin 1
D. Interferon-alpha

EXPLANATION

The above patient has systemic sclerosis. TGF-beta is the chief cytokine involved in pathogenesis.

Key: B

BOOST YOUR KNOWLEDGE

TGF-beta stimulates tissue fibrosis via increased collagen production and endothelial cell damage via influence of adhesion molecules.

REFERENCE/SOURCE

- Torok KS, Stevens AM. Juvenile systemic sclerosis. In: Petty RE, Laxer RM, Lindsley CB, Wedderburn L, Fuhlbrigge RC, Mellins ED (Eds). Textbook of Pediatric Rheumatology, 8th edition. US: Elsevier Health Sciences; 2020. p. 379.

5. A 3-year-old girl presented with loss of buccal pad of fat. There is a history of refusal to climb staircases. On examination, her anthropometry was within normal limits, there were flat red papulosquamous rashes over her knuckles, elbows, and knees. What is your diagnosis?

A. Juvenile dermatomyositis (JDM)
B. Marasmus
C. Psoriasis
D. Eczema

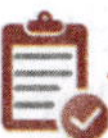

EXPLANATION

The above child has history of proximal muscle weakness, with Gottron papules and lipodystrophy involving the cheeks seen in JDM.

Key: A

BOOST YOUR KNOWLEDGE

Gottron papules are flat-topped, erythematous, popular, or papulosquamous lesions over the metacarpophalangeal, interphalangeal joints, extensor aspect of the elbows, knees, and medial malleoli. Lipodystrophy is reported in 3–10% of patients. Lipodystrophy is characterized by a progressive partial or generalized loss of subcutaneous fat. Symmetric proximal muscle weakness is usually the earliest symptom in JDM.

REFERENCE/SOURCE

- Pilkington CA, Feldman BM, Sontichai W. Juvenile dermatomyositis and other inflammatory muscle diseases. In: Petty RE, Laxer RM, Lindsley CB, Wedderburn L, Fuhlbrigge RC, Mellins ED (Eds). Textbook of Pediatric Rheumatology, 8th edition. US: Elsevier Health Sciences; 2020. p. 362.

6. A 3-year-old girl presented with difficulty in climbing the staircase, combing hair over last 6 months with the nail findings as shown in figure. What is your diagnosis?

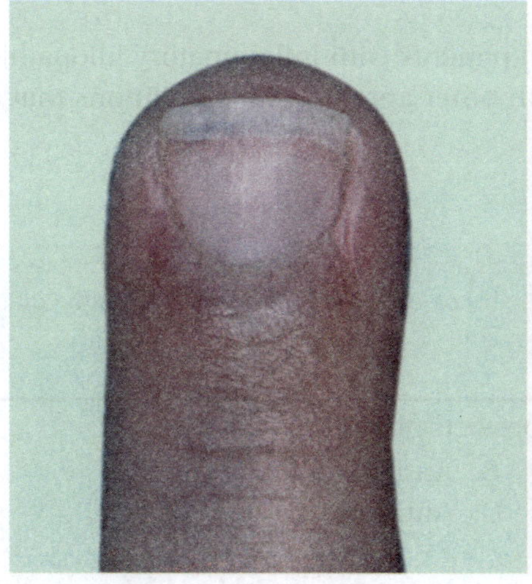

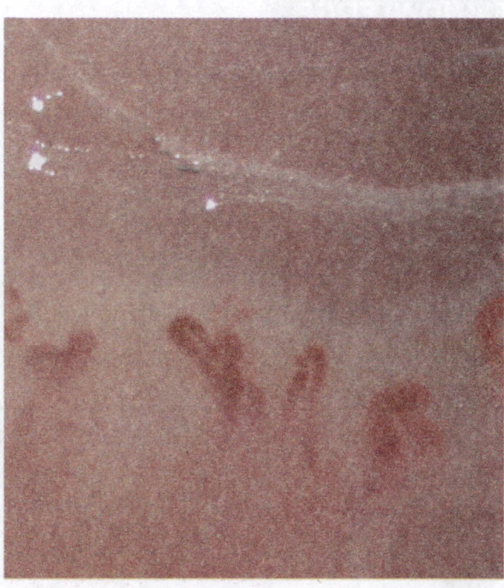

A. Psoriasis
B. Onychomycosis
C. Peripheral neuropathy
D. JDM

EXPLANATION

This child has proximal muscle weakness with abnormal nailfold capillary pattern with the classic changes of dermatomyositis. Nailfold capillaroscopy reveals capillary dropout and enlarged and tortuous capillaries.

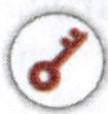

Key: D

BOOST YOUR KNOWLEDGE

Nailfold capillary changes reflect small-vessel vasculopathy in JDM. Nailfold capillaroscopy is a noninvasive and inexpensive technique to visualize the capillary network directly and assess abnormalities of microcirculation. In the area just proximal to the nail, capillaries from the subpapillary venous plexus run parallel to the skin surface.

In JDM, the changes seen include capillary dropout, enlarged, and elongated capillaries (sometimes becoming "giant capillaries"), bushy capillaries, and areas of hemorrhage—all of which result in a reduced nailfold capillary density.

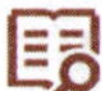

REFERENCE/SOURCE

- Pilkington CA, Feldman BM, Sontichai W. Juvenile dermatomyositis and other inflammatory muscle diseases. In: Petty RE, Laxer RM, Lindsley CB, Wedderburn L, Fuhlbrigge RC, Mellins ED (Eds). Textbook of Pediatric Rheumatology, 8th edition. US: Elsevier Health Sciences; 2020. p. 363.

7. Which of the following is *not* a myositis specific antibody?

A. Anti-PM-Scl antibody
B. Anti-Mi2 antibody
C. Anti-NXP2 antibody
D. Anti-p155/140 antibody

EXPLANATION

Anti-PM-Scl antibody is seen in myositis scleroderma overlap disease.

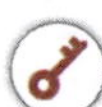

Key: A

BOOST YOUR KNOWLEDGE

Myositis-specific antibodies are present specifically in patients with inflammatory idiopathic myositis, whereas myosotis-associated antibodies occur in patients with other autoimmune conditions that are associated with myositis.

REFERENCE/SOURCE

- Pilkington CA, Feldman BM, Sontichai W. Juvenile dermatomyositis and other inflammatory muscle diseases. In: Petty RE, Laxer RM, Lindsley CB, Wedderburn L, Fuhlbrigge RC, Mellins ED (Eds). Textbook of Pediatric Rheumatology, 8th edition. US: Elsevier Health Sciences; 2020. p. 367.

8. Presence of which of the following antibodies in JDM predicts poor prognosis?

A. Anti-p155/140 antibody
B. Anti MJ antibody
C. Anti-MDA5 antibody
D. Anti-Mi-2

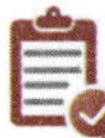

EXPLANATION

Anti MJ antibody predicts poor prognosis in JDM.

Key: B

BOOST YOUR KNOWLEDGE

Presence of anti MJ antibody predicts poor prognosis with frequent muscle cramps, atrophy, joint contractures, and dysphonia; gastrointestinal ulcerations; and bleeding.

REFERENCE/SOURCE

- Pilkington CA, Feldman BM, Sontichai W. Juvenile dermatomyositis and other inflammatory muscle diseases. In: Petty RE, Laxer RM, Lindsley CB, Wedderburn L, Fuhlbrigge RC, Mellins ED (Eds). Textbook of Pediatric Rheumatology, 8th edition. US: Elsevier Health Sciences; 2020. p. 367.

9. At what temperature would you store the sample for testing antiphospholipid antibody assay?

A. 25–28°C B. <10°C
C. -6°C D. <4°C

EXPLANATION

Sample for testing antiphospholipid antibody should be stored below 4°C.

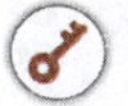

Key: D

BOOST YOUR KNOWLEDGE

The plasma may be tested immediately or frozen at –70°C as quickly as possible and stored. Repeated freezing and thawing is to be avoided. Thawing is to be done at 37°C for 5 min to avoid formation of cryoprecipitate. Serum or double-centrifuged platelet poor plasma is be suitable for ELISA tests for ACA and aβ2GP1 antibodies. Samples can be stored at 2–8°C for 2–3 days or at –20°C or below for longer durations.

REFERENCE/SOURCE

- Laffan M, Manning R. Investigation of a thrombotic tendency. In: Bain BJ, Bates I, Laffan MA, Lewis SM (Eds). Dacie and Lewis Practical Haematology, 11th edition. China: Churchill Livingstone; 2011. p. 448.

10. Which of the following dermatological manifestations is associated with antiphospholipid antibody syndrome?

A. Livedo reticularis B. Lichen planus
C. Lichen atrophicus D. Pemphigus vegetans

EXPLANATION

Livedo reticularis is associated with antiphospholipid antibody (APLA) syndrome.

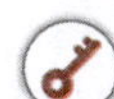

Key: A

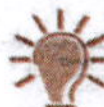

BOOST YOUR KNOWLEDGE

Skin manifestations associated with APLA syndrome include livedo reticularis, chronic leg ulcers, and superficial thrombophlebitis.

REFERENCE/SOURCE

- Avcin T, O'Neil KM. Antiphospholipid syndrome. In: Petty RE, Laxer RM, Lindsley CB, Wedderburn L, Fuhlbrigge RC, Mellins ED (Eds). Textbook of Pediatric Rheumatology, 8th edition. US: Elsevier Health Sciences; 2020. p. 336.

When contrast reaches the dilated small bowel loops, there are filling defects with a "soap bubble appearance in the loop in the midline. These imaging findings are suggestive of meconium ileus. Most patients with meconium ileus have cystic fibrosis.

- Differential diagnosis for a microcolon includes ileal atresia; however, contrast does not reflux into the dilated bowel that lies proximal to the atresia.
- Total colonic aganglionosis/Hirschsprung disease may also present with microcolon, but the filling defects in the dilated small bowel may not be present, and the transition zone may be more distally in the proximal colon.
- Meconium plug syndrome is typically characterized by small caliber of descending colon with dilated proximal colon with filling defects from meconium plugs scattered in the colon. Colonic atresia is another cause of [illegible]

A. Duodenal atresia

B. Duodenal atresia and esophageal atresia

C. Esophageal atresia

D. Normal bowel gas pattern for a neonate

SECTION 25

Specialities

CHAPTER 25.1 Pediatric Radiology

Gayathri Sreedhar

1. A term newborn presents with respiratory distress at birth. Following support lines placements (endotracheal tube, enteric tube, umbilical arterial, and venous catheters), a babygram was obtained (shown in given Figure). Which of the following is associated with poor prognosis in this condition?

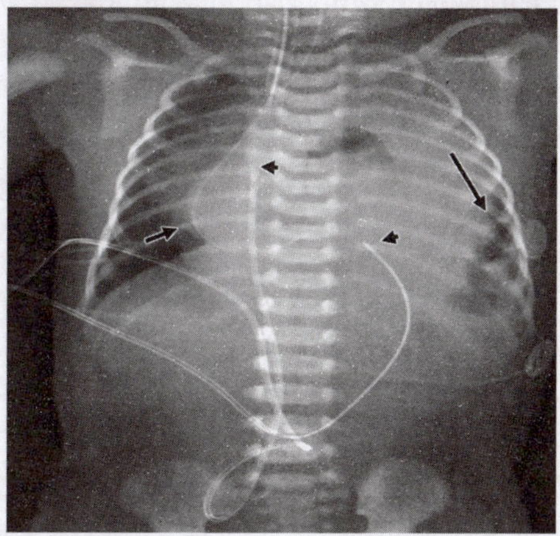

A. Splenic herniation into the chest
B. Bowel malrotation
C. Pulmonary hypoplasia
D. Presence of hernia sac

EXPLANATION

Image demonstrates bubbly, round, and tubular air-filled lucencies in the chest (long arrow) displacing the heart and mediastinum. Additionally, there is a paucity of bowel gases in the abdomen. The enteric tube is distorted in its course and reaches the intrathoracic stomach. The umbilical venous and arterial lines (short arrows) have an unusual course about the spine as well. The course of the umbilical venous line suggests a degree of liver herniation into the chest. These findings suggest a diagnosis of congenital diaphragmatic hernia. Early surgical repair is needed for survival. Factors that portend a poor prognosis include the degree of pulmonary hypoplasia measured on fetal ultrasound and fetal magnetic resonance imaging (MRI), pulmonary arterial hypertension, degree of liver herniation, absence of a hernia sac (fused peritoneum and serosal layer of pleura), and associated anomalies, particularly congenital heart disease.

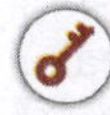

Key: C

BOOST YOUR KNOWLEDGE

Diaphragmatic hernias can occur posteriorly and laterally through patent pleuroperitoneal canal, aka Bochdalek hernias, during fetal development. These are more common on the left side. Beyond neonatal period, anterior and medial diaphragmatic hernias through foramen of Morgagni are more common. This may contain liver or bowel and is more common on the right side.

Imaging differentials for congenital diaphragmatic hernia include congenital pulmonary airway malformation in which a multicystic gas-filled appearance of the cysts can mimic bowel loops. There is less distortion of the support lines and tubes seen with congenital diaphragmatic hernias and the abdomen is normal in appearance. Prenatal imaging, when available, often provides valuable information for the right diagnosis.

REFERENCES/SOURCES

- Mehollin-Ray AR. Congenital diaphragmatic hernia. Pediatr Radiol. 2020;50(13):1855-71.
- Slovis TL, Caffey J. Abdominal wall and its abnormalities. In: Kaste SC (Ed). Caffey's Pediatric Diagnostic Imaging, 11th edition. Philadelphia, PA: Mosby/Elsevier; 2008.

2. **A 1-year-old girl presented with recent onset drooling. She was playing with some electronic toys a few hours before the onset of symptoms. The frontal view of the chest is shown in given Figure. What is the most dreaded complication of this foreign body?**

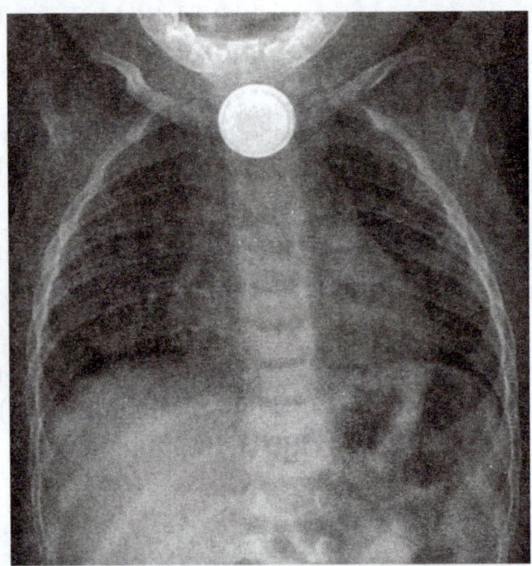

A. Metabolic alkalosis and subsequent hypoventilation
B. Aortic injury with aortoesophageal fistula
C. Advancing to the stomach and distal intestines with perforation
D. Aspiration pneumonia

EXPLANATION

Ingestion of a disc-shaped metallic foreign body is seen on the frontal radiograph with a double halo/ring enface appearance. It is highly suggestive of a button battery. Batteries that measure 20 mm or more in diameter increase the risk of complications. The North American Society for Pediatric Gastroenterology, Hepatology, and Nutrition (NASPGHAN) releases guidelines for their management based on location, size, clinical stability, and patient age.

Lithium cell batteries cause caustic injury to the esophagus, particularly at the negative pole. Unwitnessed ingestion is the major cause of fatalities. Major complications include tracheoesophageal fistula, esophageal perforation, esophageal stricture, and vocal cord paralysis.

- Aortoenteric fistula, which can happen even after battery removal, is a catastrophic cause of fatality and the most feared complication. Aspiration can be seen with esophageal foreign bodies and is not specific to button battery.

- A button battery that has advanced to and beyond the stomach may still have caused esophageal injury prior to advancement. However, in older kids, this may be an indication to consider observation only. Younger kids with battery in the stomach may benefit from endoscopic removal.
- Metabolic alkalosis is not a feared complication, as the caustic injury is local to the esophagus in impacted button batteries.

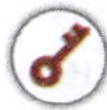
Key: B

BOOST YOUR KNOWLEDGE

Thoracic inlet, mid-esophagus at aortic arch, and lower esophageal sphincter are the common sites of impaction of button batteries. Computed tomography angiography (CTA) and MRI are the preferred modalities to evaluate for aortic injury and distance of inflammation from aorta. When an esophageal injury is seen at endoscopy, CTA or MRI assessment is suggested by the NASPGHAN algorithm. On radiographs, the step-off/beveled edge is seen on a true lateral view. The small side is the negative pole and the side most likely to cause severe injury. Edema surrounding the injury may lead to tracheal narrowing and mediastinal widening. Rarely, two coins of different sizes lodged at the same level may mimic a button battery on radiographs.

REFERENCES/SOURCES

- Grey NEO, Malone LJ, Miller AL, Carroll HF, Khalaf RT, Kramer RE, et al. Magnetic resonance imaging findings following button battery ingestion. Pediatr Radiol. 2021;51(10):1856-66.
- Leinwand K, Brumbaugh DE, Kramer RE. Button battery ingestion in children: a paradigm for management of severe pediatric foreign body ingestions. Gastrointest Endosc Clin N Am. 2016;26(1):99-118.

3. A newborn presented with delayed passage of meconium. An abdominal radiograph is shown in the given Figure. A contrast enema done subsequently is also presented. Which of the following is the cause of microcolon in this patient?

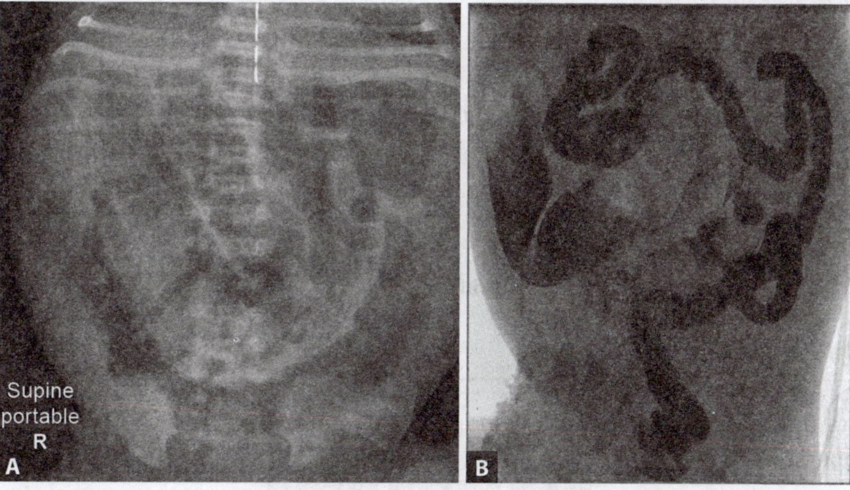

A. Meconium ileus related to cystic fibrosis
B. Total colonic Hirschsprung disease
C. Distal ileal atresia
D. Meconium plug syndrome

EXPLANATION

Frontal view of the abdomen demonstrates abnormally dilated bowel loops. The contrast enema performed subsequently demonstrates a markedly narrowed caliber of the colon with the cecum in the right upper quadrant.

When contrast reaches the dilated small bowel loops, there are large filling defects with a few regions of soap bubble appearance in the loop in the midline. These imaging findings are suggestive of meconium ileus. Most patients with meconium ileus have cystic fibrosis.

- Differential diagnosis for a microcolon includes ileal atresia, however, contrast does not reflux into the dilated bowel that lies proximal to the atresia.
- Total colonic aganglionosis/Hirschsprung disease may also present with microcolon, however, the filling defects in the dilated small bowel may not be present, and the transition zone may lie more distally in the proximal colon.
- Meconium plug syndrome is typically characterized by small caliber of descending colon with dilated proximal colon with filling defects from meconium plugs scattered in the colon. Colonic atresia is another cause of microcolon, seen distal to the atretic segment.

Key: A

BOOST YOUR KNOWLEDGE

About 10–20% of patients with cystic fibrosis will present with meconium ileus at birth. Cystic fibrosis is caused by a mutation in the *CFTR* gene. Bowel obstruction caused by thick and tenacious meconium occluding distal ileum can be further complicated by perforation, meconium psuedocyst, volvulus, or atresia. Leak of meconium leads to meconium peritonitis which may later calcify and lead to a walled off pseudocyst formation. Water soluble contrast agent that is hyperosmolar to plasma is preferred when meconium ileus is suspected as it draws water into the lumen of the bowel, thereby aiding in disimpaction. Attention to patient's baseline hydration is necessary.

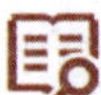

REFERENCES/SOURCES

- Maxfield CM, Bartz BH, Shaffer JL. A pattern-based approach to bowel obstruction in the newborn. Pediatr Radiol. 2013;43(3): 318-29.
- Ngo AV, Stanescu AL, Phillips GL. Neonatal bowel disorders: practical imaging algorithm for trainees and general radiologists. Am J Roentgenol. 2018;210(5):976-88.

4. Find given X-ray of a 34-week-preterm for whom a nasogastric tube was unable to be advanced to the stomach. Which of the following is the top differential consideration?

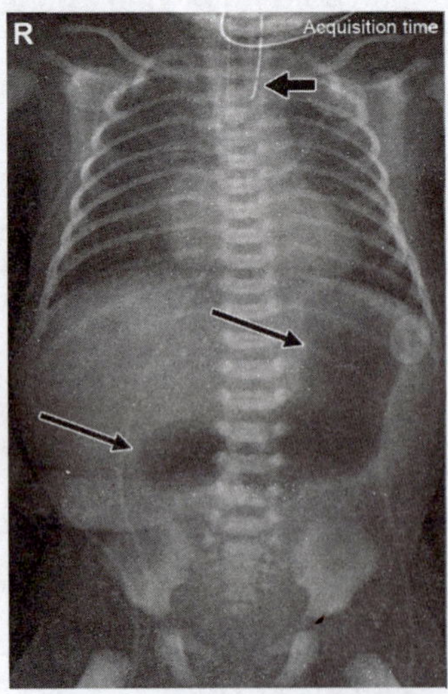

A. Duodenal atresia
B. Duodenal atresia and esophageal atresia
C. Esophageal atresia
D. Normal bowel gas pattern for a neonate

EXPLANATION

The radiograph demonstrates the classic double bubble appearance with a gas distended stomach and proximal duodenum (thin black oblique arrows). There is absence of distal gas. Double-bubble appearance can be seen with duodenal atresia, duodenal stenosis or web, jejunal atresia, midgut volvulus, and annular pancreas. The absence of distal gas makes duodenal atresia more plausible than the other etiologies. In addition, the chest portion of the X-ray demonstrates that the nasogastric tube could not be advanced beyond the midthoracic esophagus level (thick black arrow). This raises the suspicion of esophageal atresia. The endotracheal tube is seen to the right of this enteric tube.

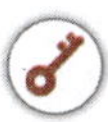

Key: B

BOOST YOUR KNOWLEDGE

More than half of patients with duodenal atresia have associated anomalies. Trisomy 21/Down's syndrome is a common association. Malrotation, annular pancreas, biliary anomalies, and esophageal atresia are other associated anomalies. Cardiac, renal, and anorectal anomalies can also be seen. Prenatal diagnosis can be made when the double-bubble sign is seen in fetal ultrasound and MRI. In cases where distal bowel gas is present, an emergent upper gastrointestinal (GI) study to rule out malrotation with volvulus is considered necessary. True duodenal atresia is treated surgically with a duodenoduodenostomy.

REFERENCES/SOURCES

- Bishop, Juliet C, Johnson CT, Miller JMM, Jelin E, Blakemore K, et al. The double bubble sign: duodenal atresia and associated genetic etiologies. Fetal Diagn Ther. 2020;47(2):98-103.
- Maxfield CM, Bartz BH, Shaffer JL. A pattern-based approach to bowel obstruction in the newborn. Pediatr Radiol. 2013;43(3):318-29.

5. An 11-year-old boy presented with a right frontal swelling. Radiographs revealed a lytic lesion of the right frontal bone. A CT scan with intravenous (IV) contrast demonstrated a soft tissue mass with underlying bony destruction (Figures B and C). A 3D reconstruction of the bony lesion is shown as well (Figure D). Which of the following is *not* an imaging differential for this lesion?

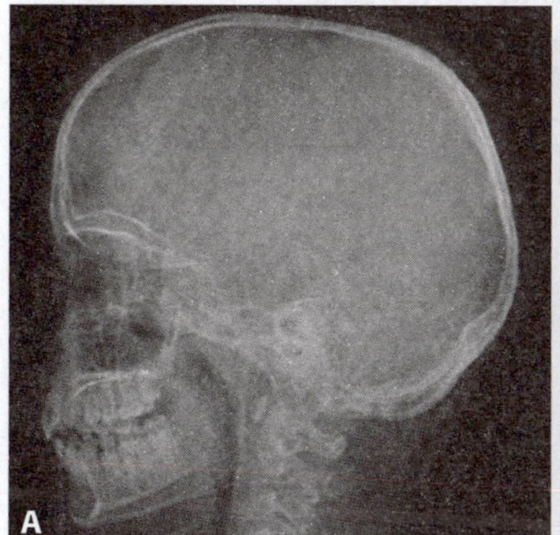

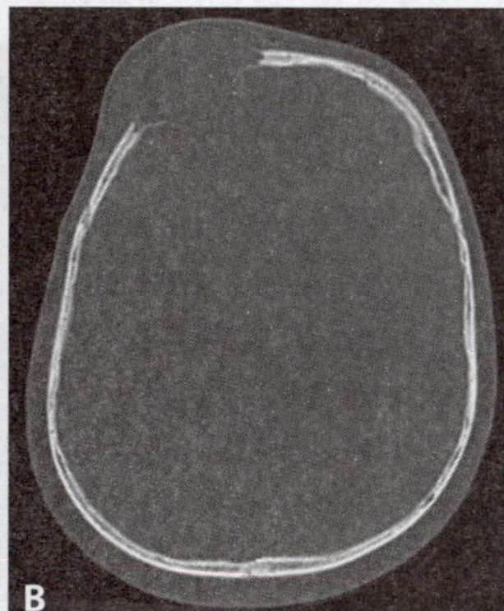

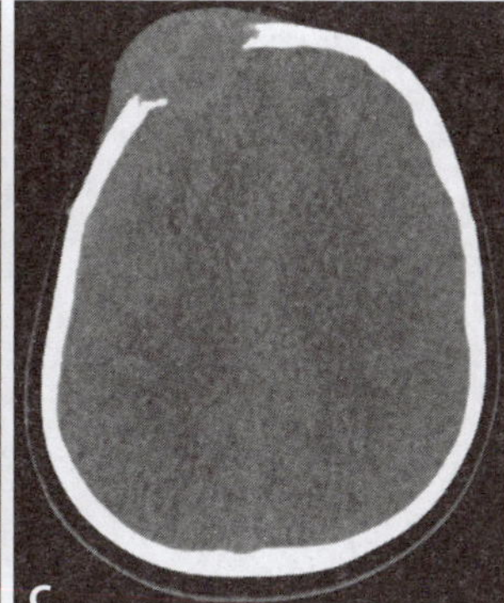

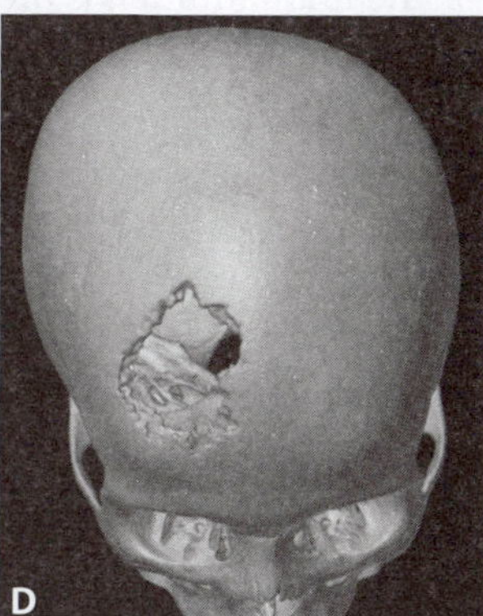

A. Langerhans cell histiocytosis
B. Metastatic neuroblastoma
C. Ewing's sarcoma
D. Fibrous dysplasia

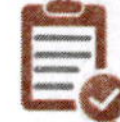

EXPLANATION

Lateral view of the skull demonstrates a geographic lytic lesion with overlying soft tissue swelling, which is better seen on the CT. The margins of this lytic lesion have beveled edges with asymmetric involvement of the inner versus outer table of the calvarium. This beveling is even better seen on the 3D reformats of the calvarium.

There is no periosteal reaction or sclerotic bony margin. No additional calvarial lesions are seen. The findings are most compatible with Langerhans cell histiocytosis (LCH). Metastatic neuroblastoma is more commonly seen in younger children, and skull lesions can be seen. These demonstrate a spiculated radiating appearance on bone windows. Ewing's sarcoma is another differential with lytic lesions but is likely to be associated with periosteal reaction and permeative bone destruction pattern. Fibrous dysplasia can be sclerotic or cystic/lytic in appearance, however, soft tissue mass is not associated with fibrous dysplasia. Expansion of the marrow with the lesion can be seen with fibrous dysplasia.

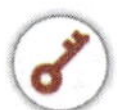

Key: D

BOOST YOUR KNOWLEDGE

Well defined punched out lytic skull lesions are the typical lesions seen in LCH. The skull is a very common location for bony lesions of LCH. LCH can be either a single system or multisystem disease. Bone is the most involved organ. Liver, spleen, thymus, skin, lungs, central nervous system, hemopoeitic system/bone marrow, GI tract, and lymph nodes are other commonly involved organs. Clonal proliferation of dendritic Langerhans cells is seen on pathology and confirms the diagnosis. Whole body MRI, skeletal survey of the whole body and fluorodeoxyglucose (FDG) positron emission tomography (PET) are the modalities used to diagnose multisystem involvement. While single bony lesions may regress spontaneously, this patient underwent resection and cranioplasty of the resected bony site. Multifocal disease typically warrants chemotherapy.

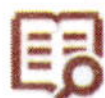

REFERENCES/SOURCES

- Kilborn TN, Teh J, Goodman TR. Paediatric manifestations of Langerhans cell histiocytosis: a review of the clinical and radiological findings. Clini Radiol. 2003;58(4):269-78.
- Schmidt S, Eich G, Hanquinet S, Tschäppeler H, Waibel P, Gudinchet F. Extra-osseous involvement of Langerhans' cell histiocytosis in children. Pediatr Radiol. 2004;34(4):313-21.

6. A 12-year-old boy fell over the bike handle following an accident during downhill biking. Patient complains of diffuse abdominal pain. CT of the abdomen with intravenous contrast was obtained. Single axial image through the midabdomen is presented in given Figure. Which of the following describes the abnormality?

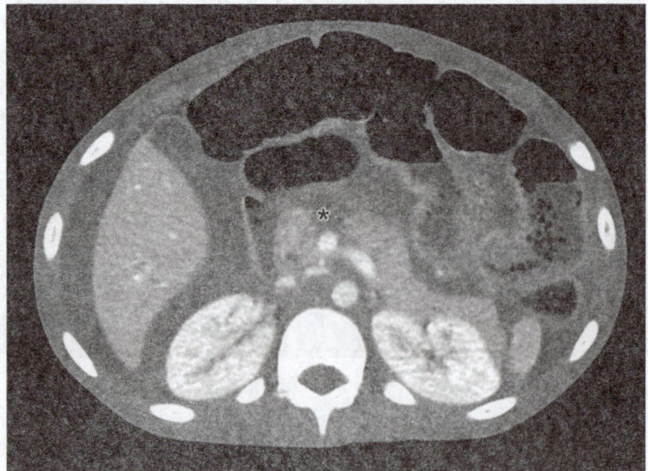

A. Pancreatic laceration with severe ascites and bowel wall thickening
B. Bowel wall thickening and ascites with right renal hilar laceration
C. Severe ascites with hepatic laceration at the gallbladder fossa
D. Bowel wall pneumatosis with severe ascites suggestive of pneumatosis intestinalis

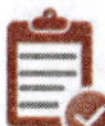

EXPLANATION

Axial image through the abdomen demonstrates severe ascites surrounding the liver, and between the bowel loops and anterior to the pancreas. There is bowel wall thickening, however, there is no nondependent bowel wall air collection to suggest pneumatosis. In the setting of trauma, the bowel wall thickening raises suspicion for a bowel injury. The kidneys are imaged near their hila. There is no laceration transecting parenchyma in the kidneys or the liver. However, there is a focal fluid collection in the neck of the pancreas with disruption of the continuity of the head and body of the pancreas (black star). This is consistent with pancreatic laceration with ductal disruption.

Key: A

BOOST YOUR KNOWLEDGE

Blunt pancreatic injuries occur from anterior-posterior (AP) compression force to abdomen. They are most commonly seen in the pancreatic body where it is fixed anterior to the spine. Liver, duodenum, and vascular injuries may be associated with a pancreatic injury. The American Association for Surgery in Trauma (AAST) grading system is used to guide management. Complete transection of the gland with pancreatic duct injury may require surgical intervention with options including percutaneous drainage, ductal stenting, distal pancreatectomy, and Whipple procedure in severe cases.

REFERENCES/SOURCES

- Biyyam DR, Hwang S, Patel MC, Bardo DME, Bailey SS, Youssfi M. CT findings of pediatric handlebar injuries. Radiographics. 2020;40(3):815-26.
- Søreide K, Weiser TG, Parks RW. Clinical update on management of pancreatic trauma. HPB (Oxford). 2018;20(12):1099-08.

7. A 2.5-year-old girl presented with pain in the left leg following a trip to the trampoline park. She is refusing to bear weight on the left leg. A frontal and lateral view of the knee was obtained on the day of injury (Figures A and B). A follow-up lateral view was obtained after 4 weeks (Figure C). What is the type of injury seen here?

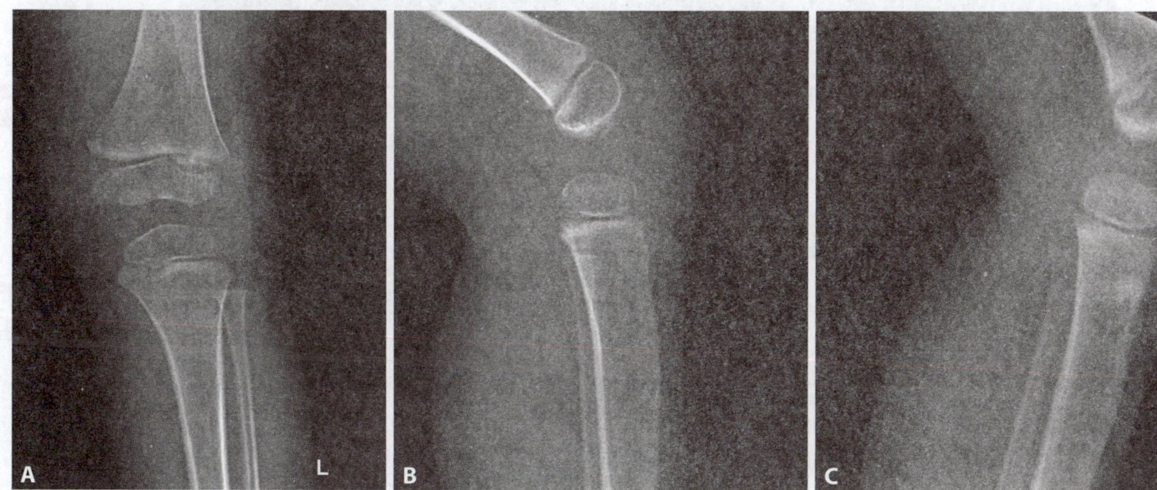

A. Patellar fracture
B. Salter-Harris type II fracture of proximal tibia
C. Toddler's fracture
D. Proximal tibial horizontal buckle fracture

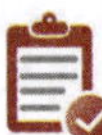

EXPLANATION

Lateral view of the tibia demonstrates a subtle buckle fracture of the anterior proximal tibial metaphyseal cortex (Figure B). The frontal view is normal, reiterating the need for two views to demonstrate fractures—an adage in radiology aka "one view is no view". The follow-up lateral radiograph of the tibia demonstrates healing of this fracture with sclerosis (Figure C). The patellar ossification centers are not fully ossified and the appearance is normal for age. The tibial physis demonstrates a normal appearance with no fracture line reaching physis in this case to suggest a Salter-Harris type fracture. A Toddler's fracture in the tibia is typically seen in the mid to distal shaft as a spiral fracture line and may also be difficult to spot in initial imaging. It heals with sclerosis and periosteal reaction on follow-up radiographs.

Key: D

BOOST YOUR KNOWLEDGE

Trampoline-related proximal tibial fractures typically occur in younger children between 2 and 5 years of age and are more likely to occur when jumping with a heavier person on the trampoline or inflatable castles. They can occur in the absence of a collision or fall and are thought to arise from the load of the upward recoiling surface during downward descent of the child. These are generally either buckle or transverse fractures of the proximal metaphysis of the tibia. Severe fractures may demonstrate a fracture line coursing towards the physis, aka Salter-Harris type II fractures.

REFERENCES/SOURCES

- Boyer RS, Jaffe RB, Nixon GW, Condon VR. Trampoline fracture of the proximal tibia in children. Am J Roentgenol. 1986;146(1): 83-5.
- Jeong C, Lee SU, Kim HG, Joo SY. Trampoline-related fractures of the proximal tibia in children. J Orthop Surg Res. 2021;16(1):551.

8. A 4-month-old boy presented with fall from couch/sofa. Parents brought in the child for lethargy and decreased responsiveness after the incident. Chest radiograph and head CT were obtained. Other highly specific findings with this entity include the following *except*?

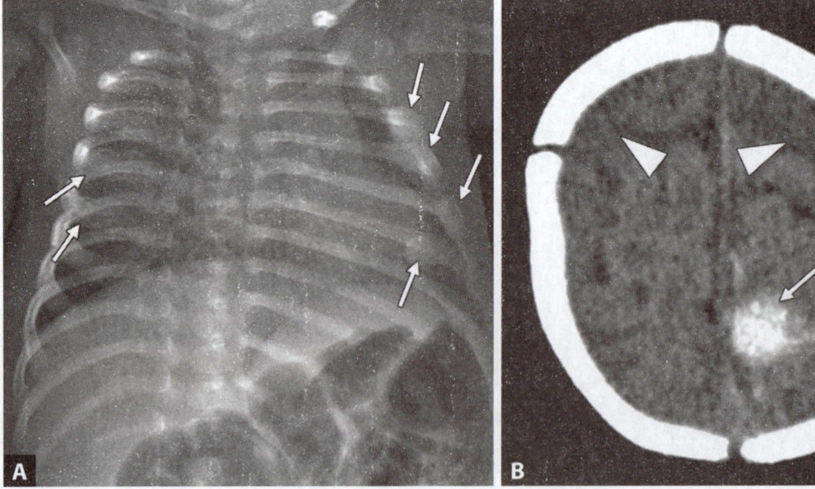

A. Corner metaphyseal fractures
B. Vertebral compression fractures
C. Clavicular fractures
D. Scapular acromion fracture

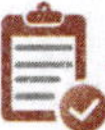

EXPLANATION

The findings of multiple healing rib fractures with calluses (arrows on Figure A) and bilateral subdural hemorrhages (arrowheads on Figure B) with an additional hyperdense hemorrhage (arrow on Figure B) leading to "mixed density subdural hemorrhage" are findings highly suggestive of nonaccidental trauma. Some fractures have a high specificity of being associated with nonaccidental trauma and include corner/classic metaphyseal fractures and posterior rib fractures. Scapular fractures of the mid acromion, spinous process fractures, vertebral compression fractures, and epiphyseal separation of the distal humerus are less common but highly specific for nonaccidental trauma or child abuse as well. Long bone fractures and clavicular fractures can often be seen with child abuse, however, they have a relatively lower specificity.

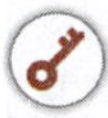

Key: C

BOOST YOUR KNOWLEDGE

Fatal head injuries in children <2 years of age are most commonly related to child abuse. The work-up of child abuse includes careful physical examination, retinal examination, neuroimaging to look for intracranial and spinal abnormalities, and a skeletal survey to look for acute and healing fractures. Inconsistency between the presenting history and the severity of imaging findings is a common theme in the presentation of nonaccidental trauma patients. MRI of the brain and spine are better at fully documenting the extent of the subdural hemorrhages, parenchymal damage, and spinal ligament as well as cord damage. A follow-up skeletal survey done after 2 weeks of initial presentation may sometimes demonstrate healing fractures that were previously too subtle on imaging.

REFERENCES/SOURCES

- Choudhary AK, Servaes S, Slovis TL, Palusci VJ, Hedlund GL, Narang SK, et al. Consensus statement on abusive head trauma in infants and young children. Pediatr Radiol. 2018;48(8):1048-65.
- Kemp AM, Dunstan F, Harrison S, Morris S, Mann M, Rolfe K, et al. Patterns of skeletal fractures in child abuse: systematic review. BMJ. 2008;337:a1518.
- Walters MM, Forbes PW, Buonomo C, Kleinman PK. Healing patterns of clavicular birth injuries as a guide to fracture dating in cases of possible infant abuse. Pediatr Radiol. 2014;44(10):1224-9.

9. **A 10-year-old boy presented with pain and swelling of the knee for last 1 week. AP and lateral view of the knee were obtained. Which of the following is *true* for this entity?**

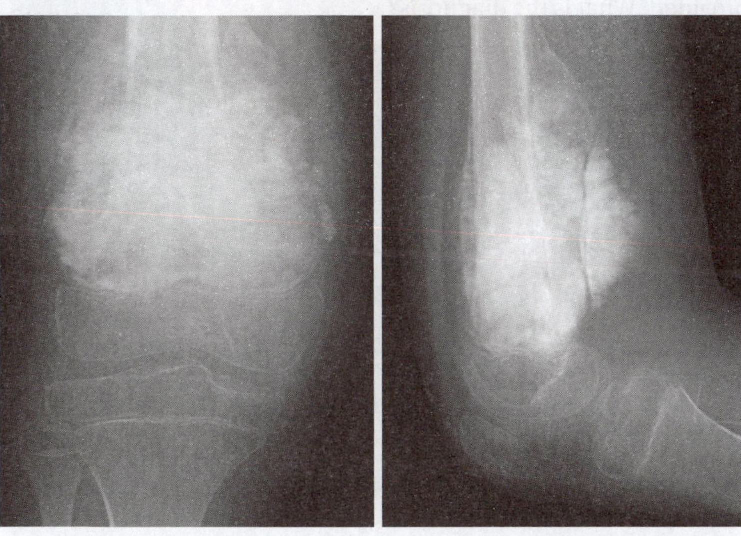

A. It is the most common malignant primary bone tumor in children
B. Only 10% cases are seen in the bones around the knee
C. There is no periosteal reaction
D. Radiographs are inadequate for early diagnosis

EXPLANATION

Images demonstrate a distal femoral metaphyseal lesion with moth eaten pattern of destruction from a sclerotic lesion. There are indistinct borders of transition with a cloud-like osteoid matrix. There is aggressive periosteal reaction with a sunburst appearance. These findings are seen with classic osteosarcoma. Bone production within the tumor is responsible for the sclerotic densities. Metaphyseal location is the most common with more than half of the cases occurring in the distal femoral or proximal tibial metaphysis. Radiographs are highly suggestive in most cases. MRI evaluates the full extent of the lesion and demonstrates early skip metastases in the long bones.

Key: A

BOOST YOUR KNOWLEDGE

Osteosarcoma occurrence has a bimodal age distribution with 10–30 years and above 60 years of age. Up to 20% of tumors have metastatic disease at diagnosis. Most common metastases is to lungs. Treatment involves neoadjuvant chemotherapy for tumor necrosis, followed by surgical resection and follow-up chemotherapy. Limb salvage surgical procedures are preferred, if possible. Joint-to-joint imaging with MRI when there is long bone involvement is crucial to rule out skip metastases. Metastatic evaluation with chest CT is preferred where, calcified as well as noncalcified metastatic nodules may be seen.

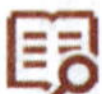

REFERENCES/SOURCES

- Harrison DJ, Geller DS, Gill JD, Lewis VO, Gorlick R. Current and future therapeutic approaches for osteosarcoma. Expert Rev Anticancer Ther. 2018;18(1):39-50.
- Kaste SC. Imaging pediatric bone sarcomas. Radiol Clin North Am. 2016;49(4):749–vii.

10. A 15-year-old boy underwent contrast enhanced CT of the neck and chest for neck and pleuritic pain. Axial (Figure A) and coronal (Figure B) CT images through the neck are provided. An additional axial image (Figure C) through the lungs is provided. What is the diagnosis?

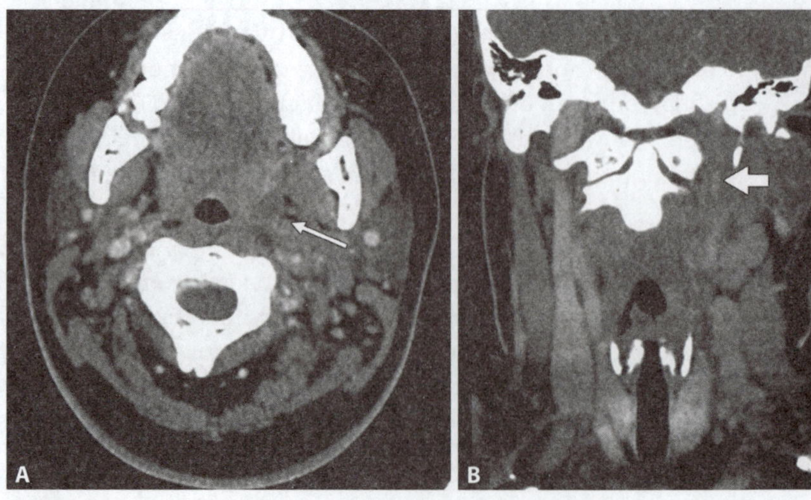

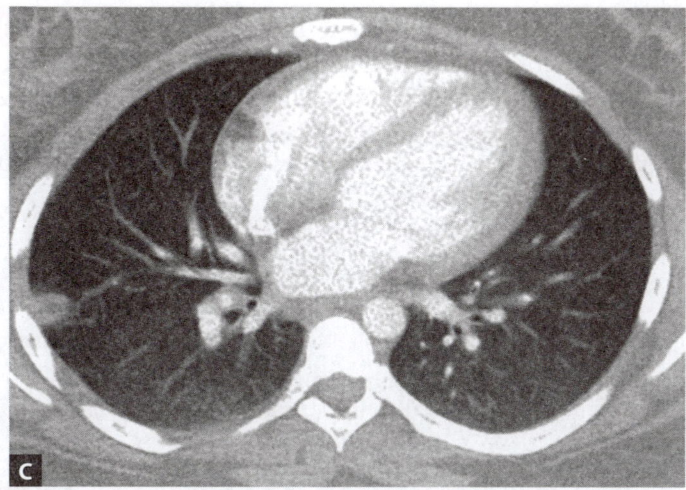

A. Retropharyngeal abscess
B. Lemierre syndrome
C. Metastases from neck tumor
D. Pneumonia

EXPLANATION

Contrast-enhanced axial images through the neck demonstrate a rim enhancing lesion near the left tonsil consistent with a peritonsillar abscess. Coronal images through the neck demonstrate absence of any flow through the left jugular vein with inflammatory soft tissue in the left carotid space (surrounding the left internal carotid artery). Axial lung window images through the chest demonstrate a pleural based right upper lobe consolidation/nodule. This constellation of finding is termed Lemierre syndrome and comprises of the classic triad of head and neck infection, neck vein thrombosis, and septic emboli (lung nodules in the case). The retropharyngeal space is normal, and the prevertebral muscles appear symmetric as well. Pneumonia as an isolated condition, is not expected to have the neck findings seen in this case. Metastases from a tumor in the neck should not cause thrombophlebitis of the jugular vein that does not lie in contiguity with the lesion itself.

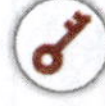

Key: B

BOOST YOUR KNOWLEDGE

Lemierre syndrome or postpharyngitic anaerobic sepsis with venous thrombosis is most caused by *Fusobacterium necrophorum* (an oral anaerobic gram-negative bacillus—an oral commensal bacterium). Other bacterial agents and polymicrobial etiology is possible. Sore throat, fever, tender swollen neck, and constitutional symptoms can be seen at the presentation. It is seen in the adolescent and young adult age group with a 2:1 male:female preponderance. Mortality is high and infection may spread to distant organs. Imaging may be the first clue to diagnosis. If intracranial spread is suspected, consider MRI evaluation.

REFERENCES/SOURCES

- Gore MR. Lemierre syndrome: a meta-analysis. Int Arch Otorhinolaryngol. 2020;24(3):e379-85.
- Valerio L, Corsi G, Sebastian T, Barco S. Lemierre syndrome: current evidence and rationale of the Bacteria-Associated Thrombosis, Thrombophlebitis and LEmierre syndrome (BATTLE) registry. Thromb Res. 2020;196:494-9.

11. A 3-month-old boy with bilious vomiting presents to the emergency room. Ultrasound through the upper abdomen (Figures A and B) was performed. Subsequently, an upper GI examination with oral administration of water-soluble contrast (Isovue-200) was performed (Figure C). What is the diagnosis?

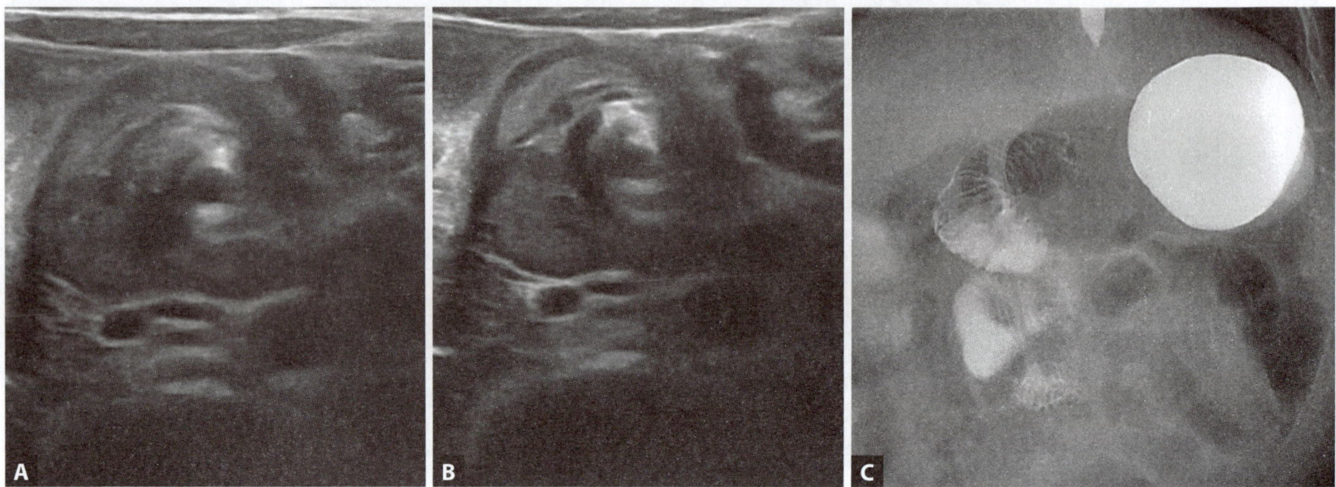

A. Intussusception
B. Duodenal web
C. Midgut volvulus
D. Pyloric stenosis

EXPLANATION

Two consecutive ultrasound transverse images coursing superior to inferior in the upper abdomen demonstrate the clockwise rotation of branches of superior mesenteric vein around the superior mesenteric artery, along with twisting of the bowel. This "whirlpool" sign is better seen on real-time sonography with color Doppler evaluation. Traditional contrast upper GI examination demonstrates dilated duodenum with spiral/corkscrew appearance inferiorly. Duodenum does not have the normal configuration where in the duodenojejunal junction lies to the left of the spine at the level of the pylorus. These findings are classically seen with midgut volvulus. Pyloric stenosis typically does not cause bilious emesis, and demonstrates a thickened pyloric muscle on ultrasound and gastric outlet obstruction on upper GI examination. Intussusception, typically seen in an older age group, demonstrates a bowel-in-bowel appearance that volvulus can mimic. However, color Doppler is useful in demonstrating the swirling of mesenteric vessels, and upper GI examination will be normal in that case. Bilious emesis is not a typical feature of intussusception. Duodenal web on an upper GI examination demonstrates a dilated duodenum on ultrasound and either obstruction at the second portion of duodenum or the classic Windsock deformity later in life where the web-balloons distally in the duodenum.

Key: C

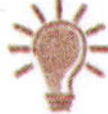

BOOST YOUR KNOWLEDGE

Midgut volvulus is caused by abnormal fixation of the small bowel with a short mesenteric root that predisposes to twisting of small bowel around superior mesenteric artery leading to devastating small bowel ischemia and necrosis in the absence of urgent surgical intervention. Most cases present in the first few months of life. Increasingly in dedicated pediatric hospitals, ultrasound is being considered as a first-line modality to diagnose volvulus. Traditionally, upper GI fluoroscopy has been the imaging modality of choice for diagnosis. Both have a very high sensitivity for diagnosis of midgut volvulus. The sensitivity for diagnosis of malrotation without midgut volvulus is lower for ultrasound than fluoroscopy.

REFERENCES/SOURCES

- Long FR, Kramer SS, Markowitz RI, Taylor GE. Radiographic patterns of intestinal malrotation in children. Radiographics. 1996;16(3):547-56.
- Nguyen HN, Sammer MBK, Ditzler MG, Carlson LS, Somcio RJ, Orth RC, et al. Transition to ultrasound as the first-line imaging modality for midgut volvulus: keys to a successful roll-out. Pediatr Radiol. 2021;51(4):506-15.

12. **A 17-year-old girl with arm twitches that are concerning for seizures on initial evaluation presents in the clinic. Initial CT demonstrates an area of encephalomalacia. Subsequently, an MRI of the brain with MR angiography is performed (Figures A to C). Traditional four vessel cerebral angiogram is performed to confirm the diagnosis (Figures D and E). What is the diagnosis?**

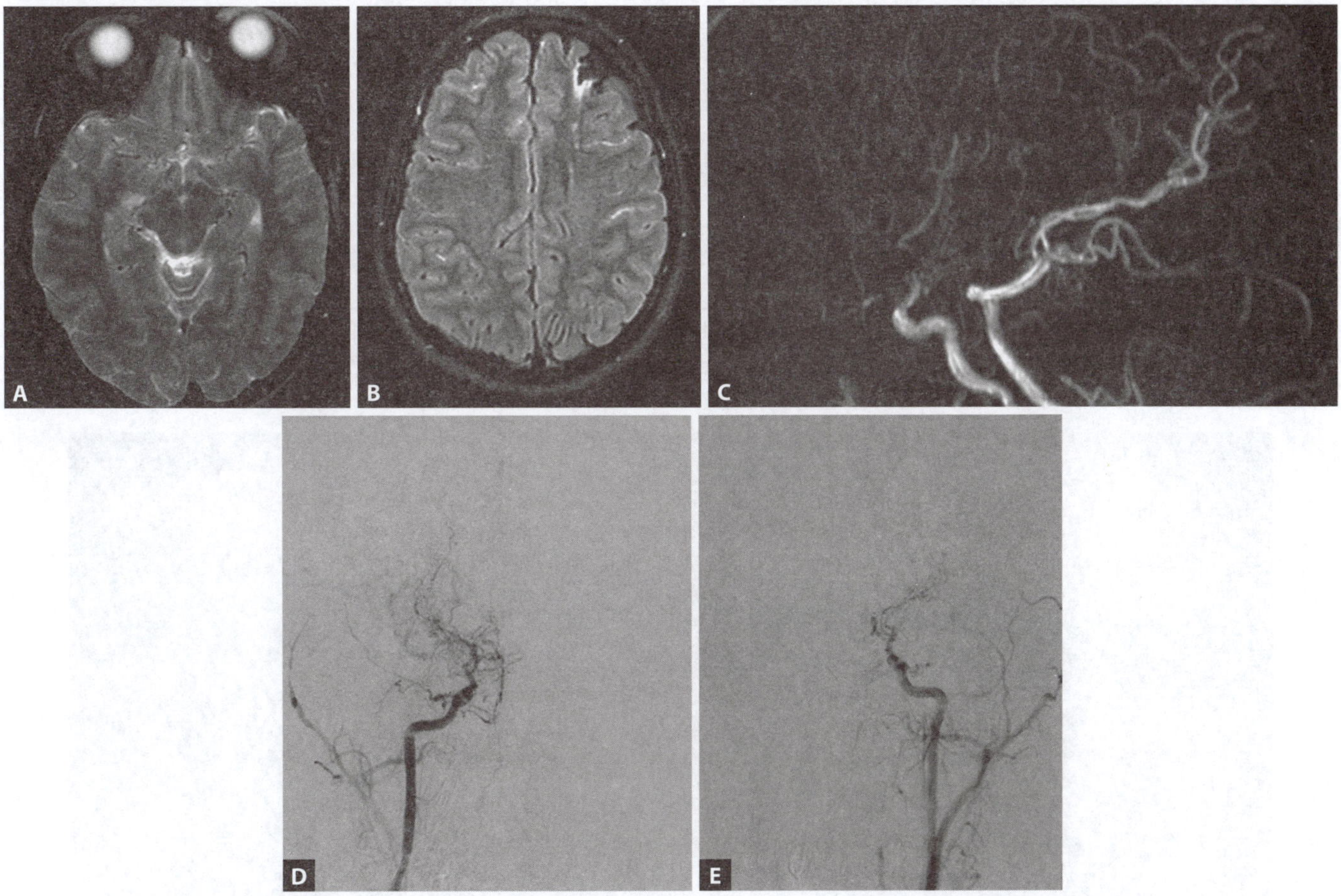

A B C D E

A. Reversible cerebral vasoconstriction syndrome
B. Vasculitis
C. Meningitis
D. Moyamoya disease

EXPLANATION

Axial T2-weighted image (Figure A) demonstrates absence of the flow voids at the terminal internal carotid artery region with multiple small vessels/collaterals. Axial T2 FLAIR image (Figure B) demonstrates "ivy sign" of leptomeningeal FLAIR hyperintense engorged pial collateral vessels. An old left frontal gliotic region is seen.

Maximum intensity projection image of a magnetic resonance angiography (MRA) (Figure C) demonstrates occluded distal internal carotid arteries on both sides. Right and left common carotid artery injections (Figures D and E) on conventional angiography demonstrate the lenticulostriate collaterals on both sides aka "Puff of smoke". Constellation of findings is seen with Moyamoya disease.

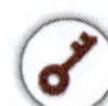

Key: D

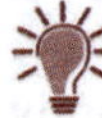

BOOST YOUR KNOWLEDGE

Progressive narrowing of the terminus of internal carotid arteries with appearance of several collateral vessels is characteristic of Moyamoya disease. Patients may present with ischemic infarction, transient ischemic attacks, headache, and a variety of neurological deficits as a result. Moyamoya like arteriopathy (Moyamoya syndrome) as a secondary Moyamoya can be seen with sickle cell disease, neurofibromatosis type 1, trisomy 21, and a variety of additional etiologies. In later stages, posterior cerebral circulation may be involved as well.

REFERENCES/SOURCES

- Currie S, Raghavan A, Batty R, Connolly DJ, Griffiths PD. Childhood moyamoya disease and moyamoya syndrome: a pictorial review. Pediatr Neurol. 2011;44(6):401-13.
- Kaseka ML, Slim M, Muthusami P, Dirks PB, Westmacott R, Kassner A, et al. Distinct clinical and radiographic phenotypes in pediatric patients with Moyamoya. Pediatr Neurol. 2021;120:18-26.

13. A 3-year-old child presented with left hip pain and limping. There is a history of fall from tricycle 3 months ago. Frontal radiograph of the pelvis was obtained in neutral and frog leg projections (Figures A and B). Which of the following is *correct* about this disease?

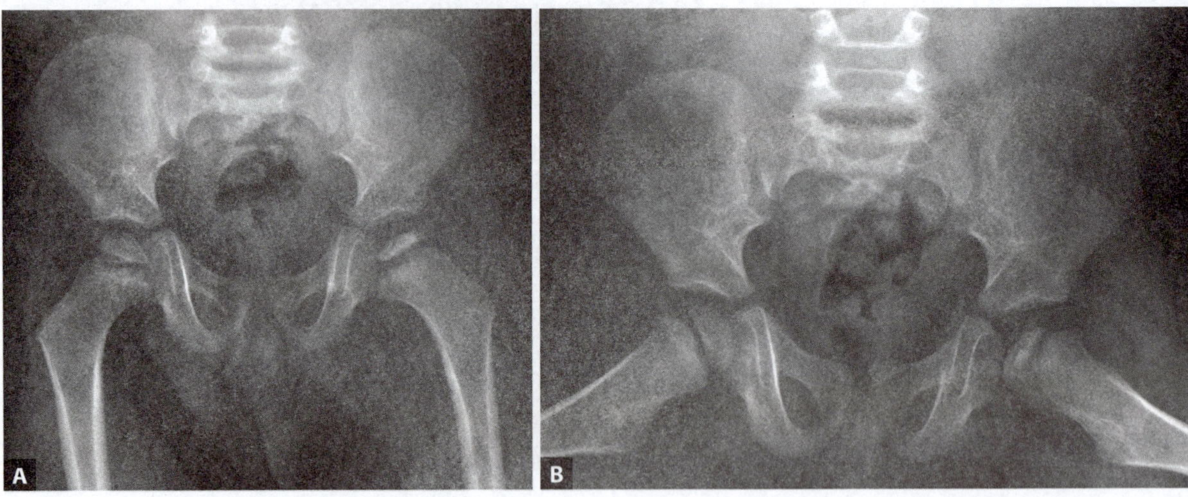

A. More common in males versus female
B. Obesity is a predisposing factor
C. Trauma and infection are the most common causes
D. Hyperperfusion of femoral head is seen on bone scan early in disease

EXPLANATION

Radiographs demonstrate sclerosis, subchondral lucency/fracture, and fragmentation of the femoral head on the left side. There is flattening of the left femoral epiphysis and relative widening of the metaphysis. These findings are suggestive of Legg–Calvé–Perthes disease. It is four to five times more common in males than females and occurs in the 4–10-year-old period most commonly. Trauma and infection are differential diagnoses of hip pain in a child; however, these imaging findings are not seen with either. Infection presents with septic joint effusion or lytic femoral metaphyseal lesions from osteomyelitis. Obesity and adolescent age group are associated with slipped capital femoral epiphysis and not Perthes disease. The femoral head demonstrates decreased perfusion on nuclear medicine bone scan in early disease, followed by increased perfusion in the delayed revascularization phase.

Key: A

BOOST YOUR KNOWLEDGE

Perthes disease is an idiopathic avascular necrosis of the femoral epiphysis. The aim of treatment is to maintain the rounded nature of the femoral head. Asymmetrical and incongruent femoral head leads to early onset osteoarthritis. Both MRI and nuclear medicine scans demonstrate the ischemia associated with acute onset Perthes disease in the femoral head. During the healing phase of Perthes disease, there is enlargement of femoral head with incongruent hip joint contour. Asynchronous, but bilateral, disease is seen in up to 20% of patients.

REFERENCES/SOURCES

- Divi SN, Bielski RJ. Legg-Calvé-Perthes Disease. Pediatr Ann. 2016;45(4):e144-9.
- Hitesh H. Perthes disease: evaluation and management. Orthop Clin North Am. 2014;45(1):87-97.

14. A 5-week-old child was brought with a left-sided hip click on clinical examination. An X-ray of the pelvis obtained at 1.5 years of age is presented. What is the diagnosis?

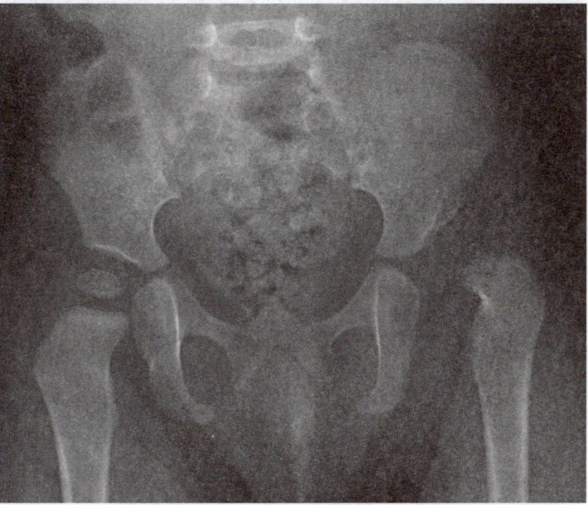

A. Developmental hip dysplasia
B. Legg-Calvé-Perthes diseases
C. Scurvy
D. Vitamin D deficiency rickets

EXPLANATION

Developmental hip dysplasia is characterized by a shallow acetabulum that allows for subluxation of the femoral head. This is best seen on ultrasound in the first 6 months of life due to the cartilaginous nature of the femoral head that is not visible on radiographs. The abnormal location predisposes to abnormal growth at the hip. Once femoral head ossifies, radiographs are more useful.

Key: A

BOOST YOUR KNOWLEDGE

Displacement of femoral head from acetabulum can be seen during real time imaging during Barlow test. Ultrasound is most useful after 4 weeks of age, when physiological immaturity of the hip is expected to resolve. Limb shortening, and secondary hip osteoarthritis or a pseudoacetabulum formation are some of the issues associated with uncorrected developmental hip dysplasia. Treatment with Pavlik harness is first tried conservatively. In case of failure of conservative management open reduction with spica cast and in later cases femoral and acetabular osteotomies for reconstruction may be needed.

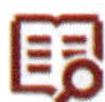

REFERENCES/SOURCES

- Barrera CA, Cohen SA, Sankar WN, Ho-Fung VM, Sze RW, Nguyen JC. Imaging of developmental dysplasia of the hip: ultrasound, radiography and magnetic resonance imaging. Pediatr Radiol. 2019;49(12):1652-68.
- Collins-Sawaragi YC, Jain K. How to use… Hip examination and ultrasound in newborns. Arch Dis Child Educ Pract Ed. 2018;103(1): 34-40.

15. A 5-day-old child presented with a vascular lesion in the lower midline back. Screening ultrasound of the spine demonstrated an echogenic mass overlying the distal cord/conus which terminates at L3/L4 disc space level. Sagittal T1-weighted MR image of the lumbar spine is slow provided. Which of the following is the diagnosis?

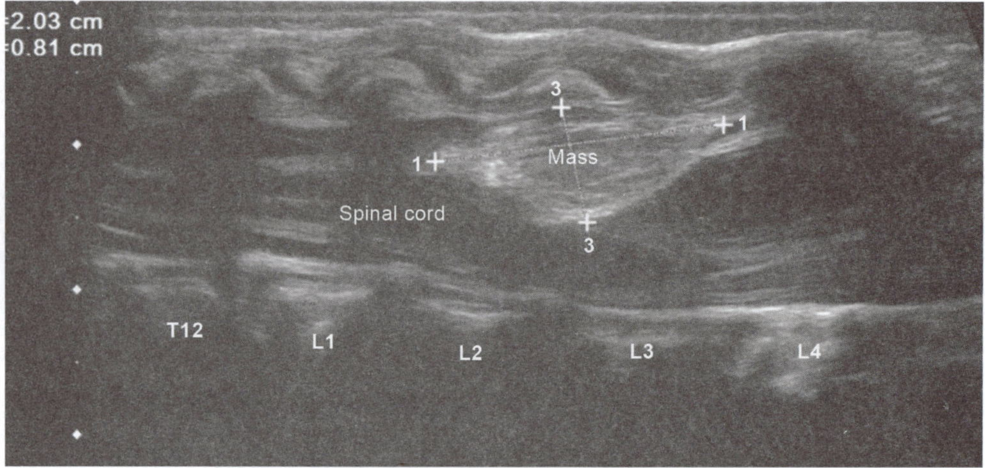

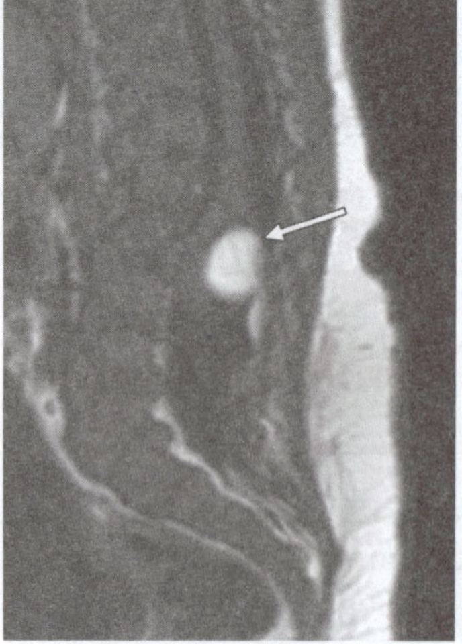

A. Meningomyelocele
B. Filum fibrolipoma
C. Instraspinal lipoma
D. Terminal myelocystocele

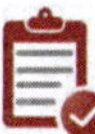

EXPLANATION

Ultrasound demonstrates a low-lying conus. Normal conus terminates above L2 lower border in a term infant. The echogenic mass seen on ultrasound demonstrates T1 hyperintensity on the MRI (typically fat signal). Hence, this is a spinal lipoma. Meningomyelocele is an open neural tube defect seen prenatally or at birth and is characterized by deficient skin and exposed meninges. Filum fibrolipoma refers to fatty infiltration of the filum terminale, which extends from the tip of the conus to the dorsal canal at S2. Terminal myelocystocele refers to cystic enlargement of the distal spinal central canal and its protrusion beneath the skin.

Key: C

BOOST YOUR KNOWLEDGE

By term gestation, the conus medullaris ascends to the level above L2–L3 disc space. Ultrasound is used as a screening examination when cutaneous stigmata associated with tethered cord or closed spinal dysraphism are seen. These include subcutaneous lipoma, hair tuft hemangioma, dermal sinus, or nevi. A fatty mass associated with the spinal cord without any connection to the subcutaneous fat is consistent with an intradural lipoma.

REFERENCES/SOURCES

- Hertzler DA 2nd, DePowell JJ, Stevenson CB, Mangano FT. Tethered cord syndrome: a review of the literature from embryology to adult presentation. Neurosurg Focus. 2010;29(1):E1.
- Rhodes RH. Congenital spinal lipomatous malformations. Part 1. Spinal lipomas, lipomyeloceles, and lipomyelomeningoceles. Fetal Pediatr Pathol. 2020;39(3):194-245.

16. A 4-year-old girl presents with abdominal pain, nausea, and constipation about 6 weeks after bone marrow transplant. Abdominal radiograph and subsequent CT (axial lung window image through midabdomen) was done. Which of the following is implicated in causation of this condition?

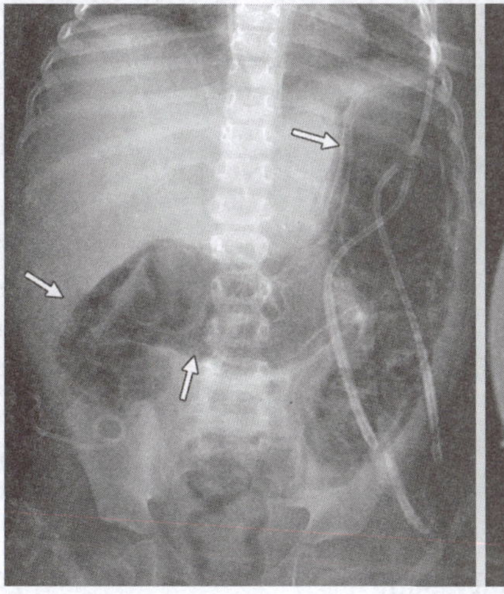

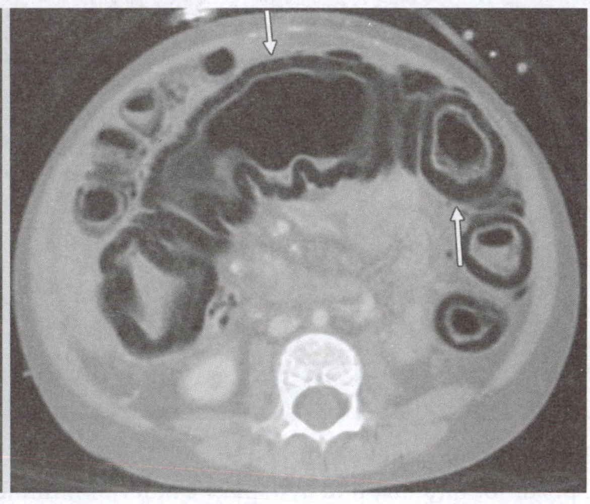

A. IV fluids
B. Radiation therapy
C. Steroid therapy
D. History of surgical resection

EXPLANATION

The frontal view of the abdomen demonstrates curvilinear air pockets outlining bowel wall. The bowel is dilated and follows mostly the colonic contour. An axial CT image confirms the presence of circumferential air in the colonic wall (arrows) outside of the lumen. Findings are typical for pneumatosis intestinalis.

There are some benign and some worrisome causes of pneumatosis. Corticosteroids, some chemotherapeutic agents, stem cells, and solid organ transplants (with or without graft vs. host disease) and vasculitis can cause benign pneumatosis. Alternatively, enterocolitis, bowel obstruction, trauma, and ischemic bowel disease can lead to pneumatosis as well.

Key: C

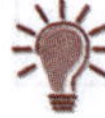

BOOST YOUR KNOWLEDGE

Pneumatosis intestinalis outside of the neonatal period is more commonly due to benign conditions that can be managed conservatively with bowel rest. When worrisome for an alternative cause, surgical exploration and more aggressive therapies may be needed. The gas seen on imaging exists in the submucosal and subserosal layers of the bowel wall. Free intraperitoneal air/pneumoperitoneum may accompany severe cases, and management does not differ when small amounts of pneumoperitoneum are encountered. Colon is the most commonly affected portion of the bowel. Bowel wall thickening, ascites, disease confined to small bowel, mesenteric fat stranding, and portal venous air are some factors more commonly associated with worrisome causes of pneumatosis.

REFERENCES/SOURCES

- Korhonen K, Lovvorn HN 3rd, Koyama T, Koehler E, Calder C, Manes B, et al. Incidence, risk factors, and outcome of pneumatosis intestinalis in pediatric stem cell transplant recipients. Pediatr Blood Cancer. 2012;58(4):616-20.
- Lee KS, Hwang S, Hurtado Rúa SM, Janjigian YY, Gollub MJ. Distinguishing benign and life-threatening pneumatosis intestinalis in patients with cancer by CT imaging features. Am J Roentgenol. 2013;200(5):1042-7.

17. A 15-year-old girl presented with headache and growth hormone deficiency. MRI with MR venography of the brain demonstrated the following findings (Figures A to C). What is the diagnosis?

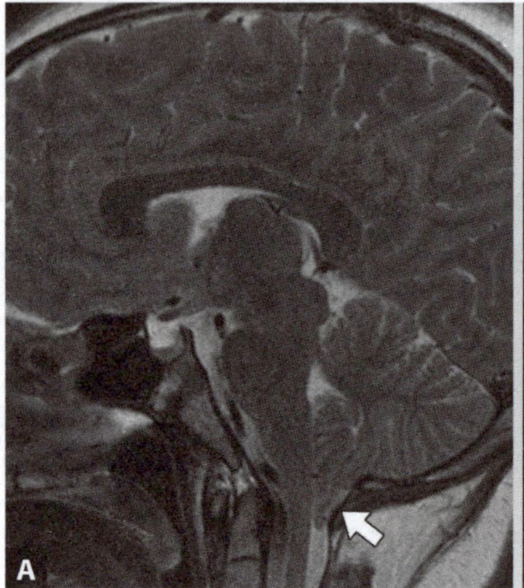

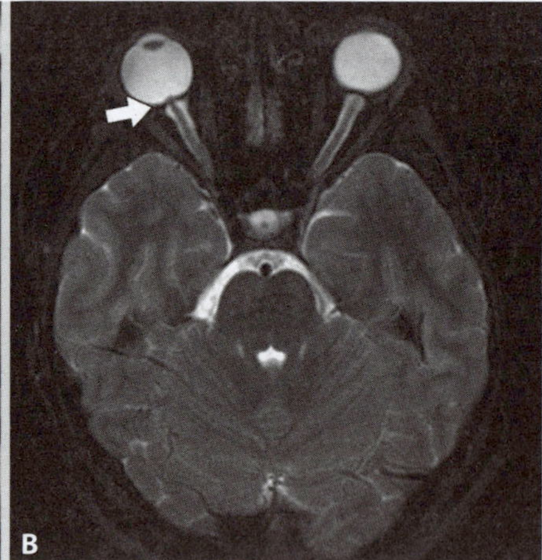

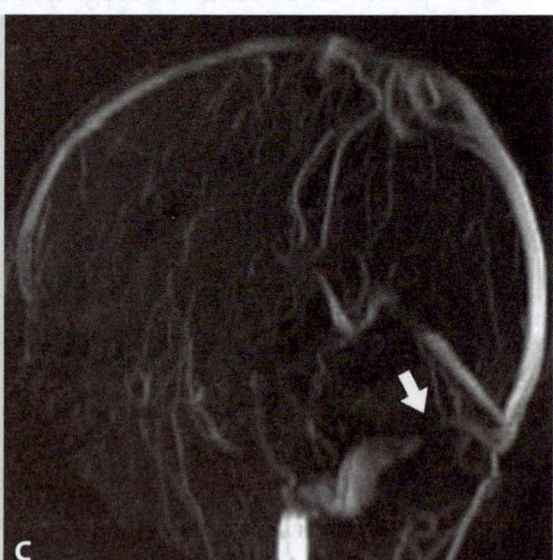

A. Chiari 1 malformation/deformity
B. Ectopic posterior pituitary and hypoplastic anterior pituitary gland
C. Idiopathic intracranial hypertension
D. Dural venous sinus thrombosis

EXPLANATION

Images demonstrate downward displacement of the cerebellar tonsils (arrow in Figure A). There is dilatation of the optic nerve sheath with intraocular protrusion of the optic nerve head and posterior flattening of the globe (arrow in Figure B). There is stenosis of the transverse sinuses in their lateral course before the sigmoid sinus (arrow in Figure C). This constellation of finding can be seen with idiopathic intracranial hypertension (IIH). There is patency of the dural venous sinuses on MR venography image. The given set of images does not demonstrate the pituitary region well (pituitary imaging was normal in this patient). Chiari 1 malformation and deformity as the cause of cerebellar tonsillar ectopia is seen as an isolated finding with small posterior fossa. This is a close mimicker.

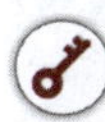

Key: C

BOOST YOUR KNOWLEDGE

Idiopathic intracranial hypertension most commonly presents with headache. Visual symptoms, vertigo, and pituitary dysfunction are occasionally associated symptoms. All patients demonstrate papilledema on eye exam. Most pediatric cases are females in their second decade, with higher prevalence in obese individuals. Symptomatic relief and prevention of visual loss are the goals of therapy. Medical management can be supplemented by cerebrospinal fluid (CSF) drainage techniques, both temporary and permanent. Venous stent placement in the transverse sinuses is a controversial treatment and assumes causality of sinus stenosis in IIH.

REFERENCES/SOURCES

- Boyter E. Idiopathic intracranial hypertension. JAAPA. 2019;32(5):30-35.
- Sivasankar R, Pant R, Indrajit IK, Negi RS, Sahu S, Hashim PI, et al. Imaging and interventions in idiopathic intracranial hypertension: a pictorial essay. Indian J Radiol Imaging. 2015;25(4):439-44.

18. An 18-year-old girl presented with right lower extremity swelling, pain, and difficulty in ambulation for last 2 days, and hip pain for last 2 weeks. There was no history of trauma. There is a recent history of starting birth control pills (3 months ago). Family history of early onset stroke was present in paternal grandfather. Doppler ultrasound of the right lower extremity and midabdomen were done (Figures A to C). Subsequently, interventional radiology was contacted and an image from the procedure is shown. What is the procedure shown in Figure D?

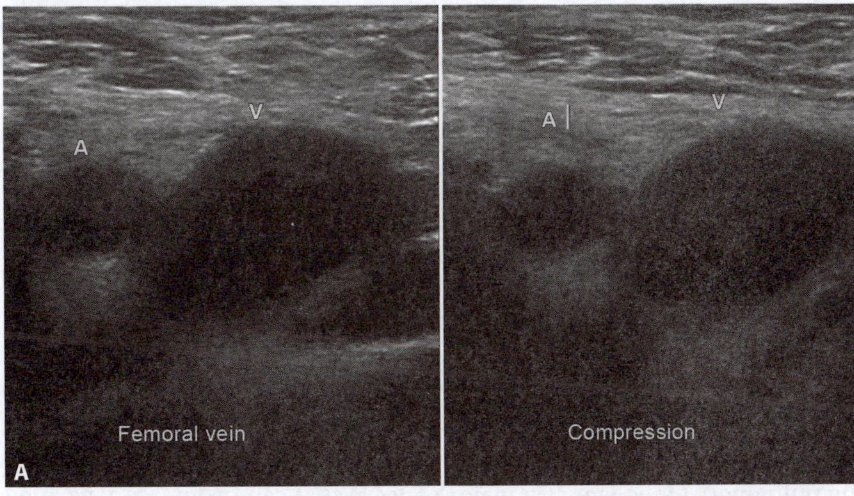

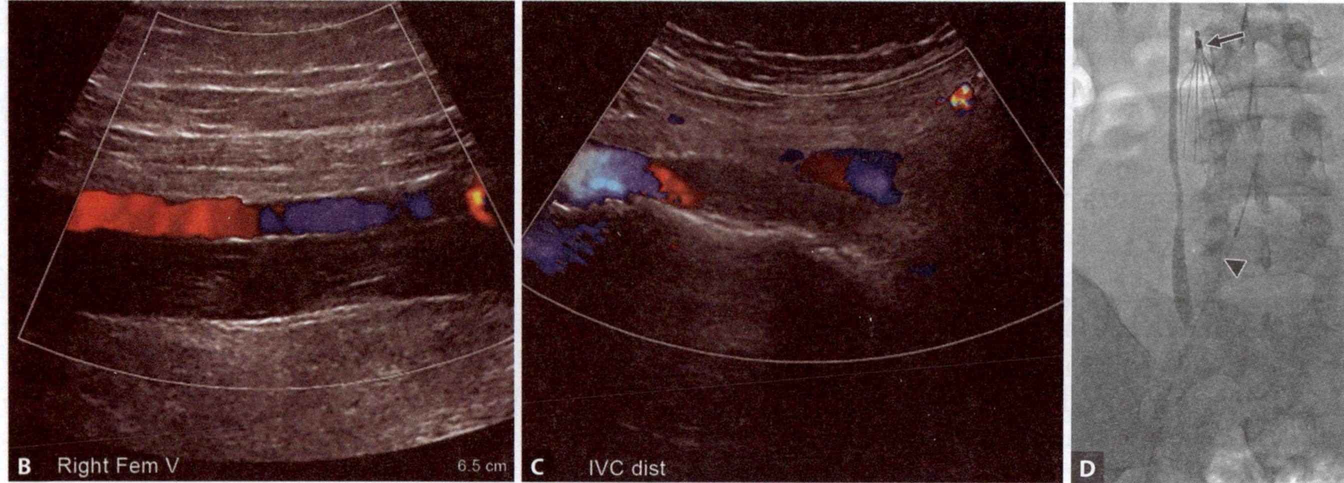

A. Abdominal angiography demonstrating patency of inferior vena cava (IVC) following thrombolysis
B. Removal of a migrated intrauterine device as the cause of thrombosis
C. IVC filter placement with thrombolysis catheter in place
D. Arterial stent in the aorta following angioplasty for aortic thrombosis

EXPLANATION

Ultrasound images demonstrate noncompressibility of the femoral vein in the upper thigh (Figure A), absence of color flow on Doppler imaging in the femoral vein (Figure B), and absence of flow in the distal abdominal IVC (Figure C). These findings confirm a long segment thrombosis of the right femoral vein, reaching up to the intra-abdominal IVC. This thrombus was treated with the introduction of an IVC filter via the jugular approach. The deployed IVC filter with a conical design comprising of several legs and a superior retrieval hook is shown in Figure D (arrow). Following placement of IVC, filter patient underwent digital subtraction angiography of the right lower extremity veins. An AngioJet (R) catheter was advanced over a glidewire in the common iliac vein (arrowhead in Figure D). These catheters are capable of infusing tissue plasminogen activator (tPA) as well as are amenable to mechanical thrombectomy. Overnight infusion of tPA and heparin lead to significant improvement in the thrombus burden. Follow-up imaging demonstrated recanalization of the veins. The contrast filled structure to the right of the IVC filter is contrast in the ureter and not a vein. Intravenous contrast is used for guiding placement of the filter as well as during the venography for mechanical thrombectomy. Aortic stents and intrauterine devices have a different image profile and shape compared to the IVC filters.

Key: C

BOOST YOUR KNOWLEDGE

Deep vein thrombosis (DVT) increases in incidence with age. Thrombosis of smaller deep veins, such as tibial and peroneal veins, may sometimes resolve spontaneously. The possibility of thrombus extension or travel into the lungs, causing pulmonary embolism, is a major concern that can be fatal. Above knee DVT is an indication for anticoagulation therapy. IVC filter placement should be considered in patients with IVC thrombosis or patients who may not be candidates for anticoagulation. Thrombolysis should be considered where there is extensive iliofemoral disease, as in this case. This does carry a higher risk of major bleeding and must be used judiciously.

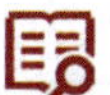

REFERENCES/SOURCES

- Kaufman JA, Barnes GD, Chaer RA, Cuschieri J, Eberhardt RT, Johnson MS, et al. Society of Interventional Radiology Clinical Practice Guideline for inferior vena cava filters in the treatment of patients with venous thromboembolic disease: developed in collaboration with the American College of Cardiology, American College of Chest Physicians, American College of Surgeons Committee on Trauma, American Heart Association, Society for Vascular Surgery, and Society for Vascular Medicine. J Vasc Interv Radiol. 2020;31(10):1529-44.
- White RH. The epidemiology of venous thromboembolism. Circulation. 2003;107(23 Suppl 1):I4-8.

19. A 1-year-old boy presented with vague abdominal pain and constipation. Abdominal radiograph demonstrates a vague density in the right upper abdomen with possible punctate calcification (Figure A). Subsequent abdominal CT demonstrates a large abdominal mass with solid-cystic composition and punctate calcifications (Figures B to D). Which of the following is *correct* about the staging system for this tumor?

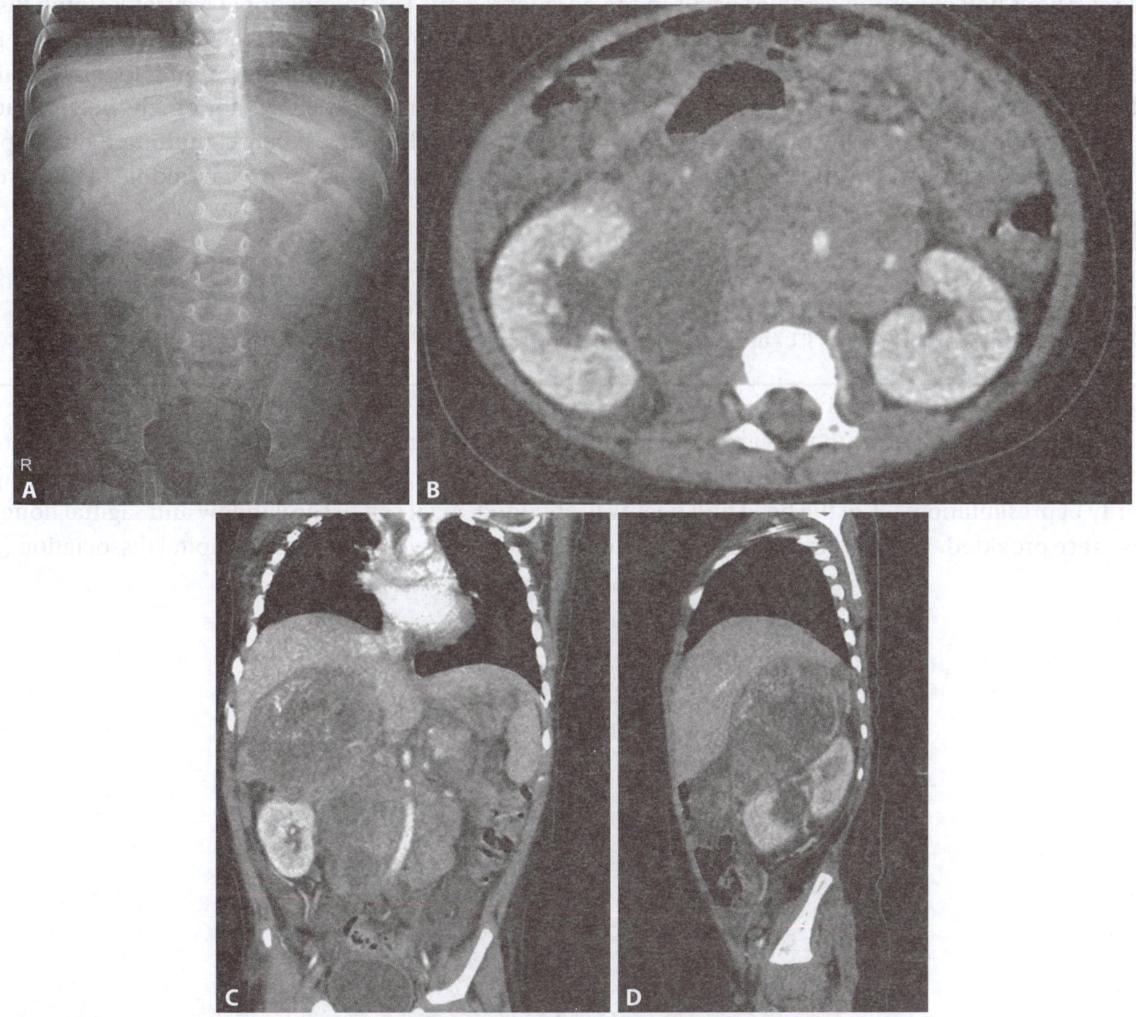

A. Risk group staging system puts children into "risk" categories
B. Presence of tumor thrombus in the IVC is an important staging finding
C. Pretreatment extent of tumor system (PRETEXT) groups the tumor with further annotations for tumor involvement of vasculature, tumor rupture, multifocality, metastases, etc.
D. PET/CT is utilized to stage disease extent based on extension below and above the diaphragm

EXPLANATION

Images demonstrate a large retroperitoneal mass centered in the right adrenal region with punctate calcifications. There is no claw sign with kidneys to suggest renal origin. The liver is displaced and does not appear involved. The aorta is elevated away from the vertebral column. There is narrowing of the IVC. There is no enlargement of the IVC with tumor, however, the tumor crosses midline to reach the left side. These findings suggest neuroblastoma as the likely etiology, and help to differentiate it from Wilms tumor and hepatoblastoma, which are the other common pediatric solid abdominal malignancies.

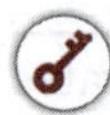

Key: A

BOOST YOUR KNOWLEDGE

Neuroblastoma is the second most common solid malignancy of childhood following cranial nervous system tumors. About half of neuroblastomas occur in the adrenal region. The International Neuroblastoma Risk Group Staging System, developed in 2009, includes image-defined risk factors (IDRFs) to categorize disease into four stages: Localized (L1, L2) and metastatic (M, MS). The IDRFs are critical in determining locoregional spread, and a list of IDRFs is based on the location of the primary tumor (neck, chest, abdomen, pelvis, paraspinal, etc.). Metastatic disease mostly occurs in marrow, bone, and lymph nodes, involves multimodality approach to diagnosis, and includes CT, MRI, and nuclear medicine whole body metaiodobenzylguanidine (MIBG) scan.

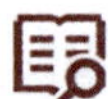

REFERENCES/SOURCES

- Morin CE, Artunduaga M, Schooler GR, Brennan RC, Khanna G. Imaging for staging of pediatric abdominal tumors: an update, from the *AJR* special series on cancer staging. Am J Roentgenol. 2021;217(4):786-99.
- Newman EA, Abdessalam S, Aldrink JH, Austin M, Heaton TE, Bruny J, et al. Update on neuroblastoma. J Pediatr Surg. 2019;54(3):383-9.

20. A 7-year-old boy was involved in a motor vehicle accident. Child was sitting unrestrained in the back seat of a car, when a truck collided with the car. The patient needed resuscitation in the trauma bay and was emergently intubated before any imaging. Radiographs were deemed nondiagnostic. Based on mechanism of injury and severity of presentation, CT of the head and neck was obtained. Axial soft tissue window and sagittal bone window images are provided. Which of the following has the highest specificity for atlanto-occipital dissociation (AOD)?

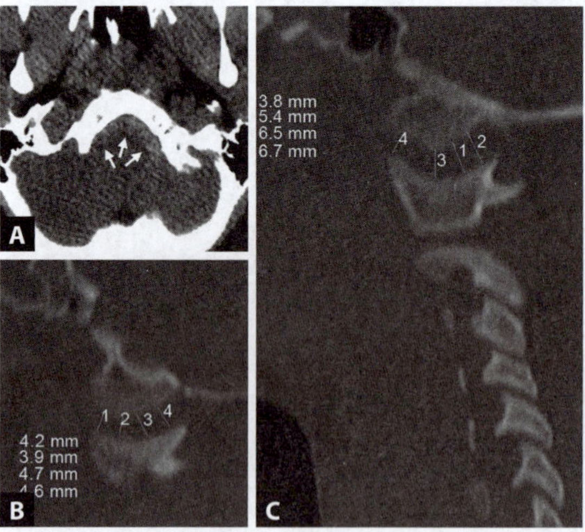

A. Basion-dens interval above 12 mm
B. Occipital condyle to C1 arch interval (average) above 4 mm
C. Ratio of interspinous distance between C1-2/C2-3 >2.5
D. Powers ratio above 1 (Basion to C1 posterior arch/opisthion to anterior C1 arch)

EXPLANATION

The images demonstrate retroclival hemorrhage at the foramen magnum (arrows in Figure A), right (Figure B), and left (Figure C) sagittal bone window images demonstrate consistently increased occipital condyle to C1 arch interval (CCI). CCI above 4 mm in children is considered abnormal and has the highest sensitivity and specificity for severe AOD. Basion-dens interval may be difficult to measure in children and may be falsely elevated before the dens ossifies. Opisthion is difficult to visualize on sagittal cervical spine radiographs, and makes Powers ratio difficult to calculate. Despite many additional proposed measurements to evaluate for craniocervical junction injuries, most are insensitive for mild injuries, and a high clinical suspicion should mandate additional imaging, including MRI and MRA or CTA.

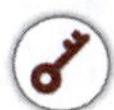

Key: B

BOOST YOUR KNOWLEDGE

Atlanto-occipital dissociation is the most feared and devastating cervical injury. It is caused by disruption of ligaments between the occiput and C1, AOD leads to cord injury ranging from stretching to frank transection at the craniocervical junction. The dissociation can result in the skull being displaced superiorly, anteriorly, or posteriorly with respect to the C1. Radiographs are generally inadequate for evaluation as measurements are difficult to make, and no measurement criteria is 100% sensitive. A Basion-dens distance of <12 mm is considered by some to be normal. The value is lower in adults as the dens is completely ossified in adulthood. On CT scan, the CCI measured as the average of four measurements on sagittal and coronal images above 4 mm has a very high specificity for AOD. A CCI 2.5 mm has a higher sensitivity with lower specificity. Age specific change in CCI has been demonstrated as well. The presence of subarachnoid hemorrhage at the craniocervical junction or retroclival hemorrhage on CT are both associated with AOD. Ultimately, MR imaging may be necessary in the pediatric age group for diagnosis of ligamentous disruption and cord injury. Tectorial membrane disruption, hemorrhage, widening of joints, and cord injury can all be seen on MRI. Evaluation for vertebral artery injury can be done on MRA or CTA.

REFERENCES/SOURCES

- Corcoran B, Linscott LL, Leach JL, Vadivelu S. Application of normative occipital condyle-C1 interval measurements to detect atlanto-occipital injury in children. Am J Neuroradiol. 2016;37(5):958-62.
- Steinmetz MP, Lechner RM, Anderson JS. Atlantooccipital dislocation in children: presentation, diagnosis, and management. Neurosurg Focus. 2003;14(2):ecp1.

CHAPTER 25.2

Pediatric Dermatology

Payal

1. A 2-year-old child presents with progressive neurological deterioration, he has silvery gray hair, light skin, and history of recurrent pyogenic infection. His investigations point towards hypogammaglobulinemia and defective cell-mediated immunity (CMI). On peripheral smear examination, neutrophils lack giant intracytoplasmic granules. What is the most likely diagnosis?

A. Elejalde syndrome
B. Griscelli syndrome
C. Chédiak-Higashi syndrome
D. Hermansky–Pudlak syndrome

EXPLANATION

Griscelli syndrome has silvery hair, defective CMI and compromised humoral immunity. However, it lacks the giant granules in neutrophils unlike Chédiak-Higashi syndrome. Elejalde syndrome lacks defects in CMI.

Key: B

BOOST YOUR KNOWLEDGE

Silvery hair disorders

Features	*Griscelli syndrome*	*Chédiak-Higashi syndrome*	*Elejalde syndrome*
Neurological deterioration	Present, less severe	Present, less severe	Very severe
Defects in CMI and humoral immunity	Present	Present	Absent
Neutrophil giant intracytoplasmic granules	Absent	Present	Absent

REFERENCE/SOURCE

- Palit A, Inamdar AC, Raghunatha S. Textbook of Pediatric Dermatology, 2nd edition. New Delhi: Jaypee Brothers Medical Publishers; 2014. p. 332.

2. A 2-year-old child presents with widespread large blisters and erosions for 1 day. On examination, purulent conjunctivitis is noted, the child is febrile, irritable but hemodynamically stable, the skin is tender, with sheet-like peeling of the skin on slight pressure, the mucosae are unaffected. Gram stain from the blister is sterile. What is the next best step in management of this child?

A. Promptly start oral steroids
B. Promptly start oral cyclosporine
C. Promptly start intravenous immunoglobulin (IVIG)
D. Promptly start antistaphylococcal antibiotics

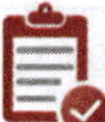

EXPLANATION

The child is suffering from Staphylococcal-scalded Skin Syndrome (SSSS). Pointers towards diagnosis are large blisters and sheet-like erosions with sparing of mucosae. The child can have preceding infection of conjunctiva, throat, and nares. Gram's stain from blister is sterile as the disease is toxin mediated.

Key: D

BOOST YOUR KNOWLEDGE

The closest differential diagnoses of SSSS are Stevens–Johnson syndrome-toxic epidermal necrolysis (SJS-TEN) and pemphigus vulgaris.

- TEN is a severe adverse cutaneous drug reaction, also presents with sheet-like peeling of skin, but the child is sick. Mucosae are always and severely involved with blistering, and hemorrhagic crusts.
- Pemphigus vulgaris is very rare in childhood. It presents with blisters, but sheet-like peeling is usually not seen, mucosal involvement is predominant.

REFERENCE/SOURCE

- Hoeger PH, Kinsler V, Yan AC, Bodemer C, Larralde M, Luk D, et al. Harper's Textbook of Pediatric Dermatology, Volume 1, 4th edition. Hoboken, New Jersey: Wiley-Blackwell; 2019. pp. 54.8-54.9.

3. Identify the *correct* statement about neonatal lupus erythematosus (NLE).

A. Cardiomyopathy is the most common cardiac disorder
B. Conduction defect of NLE is reversible
C. Cutaneous and cardiac manifestations coexist in 90% cases
D. Risk of recurrence of NLE in subsequent pregnancies is as high as 25%

EXPLANATION

All the statements apart from option D are false. The most common cardiac defect is conduction defect, mostly complete heart block (CHB), which once established is irreversible. Cutaneous and cardiac manifestations coexist in about 10% of cases.

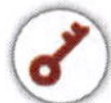

Key: D

BOOST YOUR KNOWLEDGE

NLE occurs due to transplacental transfer of maternal autoantibodies [Immunoglobulin G (IgG)]. Most patients (90%) present with cutaneous manifestation, which may be present at birth (two-thirds). "Raccoon eye" or "Owl eye" appearance is described for the classical periorbital NLE lesions. Skin lesions are transient and heal without scarring. Cardiac involvement is seen in 60% of cases of NLE. CHB is the most common cardiac lesion, and may start intrauterine, bradycardia can be detected by fetal heart rate monitoring and echocardiography. CHB is irreversible. Other cardiac defects are cardiomyopathy, atrial septal defect (ASD), and patent ductus arteriosus (PDA).

REFERENCE/SOURCE

- Palit A, Inamdar AC, Raghunatha S. Textbook of Pediatric Dermatology, 2nd edition. New Delhi: Jaypee Brothers Medical Publishers; 2014. p. 583.

4. A 2-year-old child presents with fever, joint pain, and palpable purpura on both legs for 3 days. Skin biopsy shows features of leukocytoclastic vasculitis with predominant immunoglobulin A (IgA) immune complex deposition around the vessels. Which of the following statements is *true* regarding the course of this disease in children?

A. Has a protracted course with frequent recurrences in younger children
B. Renal involvement is less common in older children as compared to younger children
C. Headache is the most common central nervous system (CNS) manifestation
D. Systemic steroids are the first line treatment for isolated cutaneous disease

EXPLANATION

The condition in the given scenario is Henoch-Schönlein purpura (HSP). It is the most common small vessel vasculitis in children. It has a self-limiting course in children especially <2-year-old. The younger children have a lower risk of renal complication (25% in <2-year-old, 50% in older). Headache is the most common CNS manifestation. Systemic steroids are not the first-line treatment for isolated cutaneous lesions, symptomatic management or dapsone can be given.

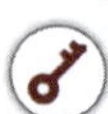

Key: C

BOOST YOUR KNOWLEDGE

Henoch-Schönlein purpura is a small vessel vasculitis with IgA dominant immune complex deposition, especially in skin, gastrointestinal (GI) tract, and glomeruli. 75% cases are seen within 2–11 years of age. Cutaneous features aid in clinical diagnosis as dependent palpable purpura is a mandatory criterion for HSP, usually in lower limbs, buttocks, and occasionally upper limbs. In infants, edema of the face, ears, and extremities can occur. Recurrent crops of skin lesions can occur for a few weeks to months. Arthralgia and arthritis can be seen in 60–84 % cases, GI symptoms can range from mild abdominal pain to acute abdomen due to intussusception.

REFERENCE/SOURCE

- Palit A, Inamdar AC, Raghunatha S. Textbook of Pediatric Dermatology, 2nd edition. New Delhi: Jaypee Brothers Medical Publishers; 2014. p. 602.

5. A 7-month-old, recently weaned infant presents with diarrhea, periorificial erosions, and brownish thin crusts. The child is afebrile but irritable. Her serum zinc levels were normal. However, the child improved markedly with oral zinc therapy. Which other test can help in making the diagnosis in such a case?

A. Serum albumin
B. Serum calcium
C. Serum gamma-glutamyl transferase (GGT)
D. Serum alkaline phosphatase (ALP)

EXPLANATION

The above scenario is typical of acrodermatitis enteropathica (AE). The diagnosis is mostly clinical and can be confirmed by low serum zinc level (<50 mg/dL). Estimation of serum ALP level may give an approximate idea of serum zinc, as it is a zinc dependent enzyme. It is low in zinc deficiency. Some cases of AE may have normal zinc levels; in such cases serum ALP level is especially helpful.

Key: D

BOOST YOUR KNOWLEDGE

Acrodermatitis enteropathica is an autosomal recessive (AR) disorder with unclear pathogenesis. Mutation of *SLC39A* gene which encodes zinc binding ligand (ZIP4 protein) causes poor intestinal absorption of zinc.

Clinical features are multisystemic, with the classic triad of symptoms: diarrhea, periorificial dermatitis, and alopecia. In the acute phase, there is oozy dermatitis involving periorificial areas which can progress to necrosis and eschar formation. Diffuse alopecia of scalp, eyebrows, and eyelashes with photophobia and irritability, can also be seen. Differential diagnosis (D/D) includes biotin deficiency and heritable organic acidurias. Diagnosis is mostly clinical, confirmed by low serum zinc levels.

REFERENCE/SOURCE

- Palit A, Inamdar AC, Raghunatha S. Textbook of Pediatric Dermatology, 2nd edition. New Delhi: Jaypee Brothers Medical Publishers; 2014. p. 626.

6. A full term, healthy neonate develops blotchy erythematous macules with central yellow white papules and pustules over the face, trunk and extremities on 3rd day of life. Palms and soles are spared. Microscopic examination of the pustule contents reveals only eosinophils. What is the most likely diagnosis?

A. Transient neonatal pustular melanosis
B. Miliaria rubra
C. Miliaria crystallina
D. Erythema toxicum neonatorum

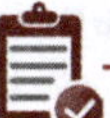

EXPLANATION

Erythema toxicum neonatorum is benign, self-limiting condition, seen in full term neonates. It can occur anytime from birth to up to 2 weeks of age, most commonly in the first 4 days of birth. The eruption is characterized by papules, vesicles, or pustules on an erythematous background. Palms and soles are spared. Microscopic examination from the lesions reveals only eosinophils.

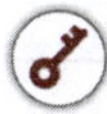

Key: D

BOOST YOUR KNOWLEDGE

Transient neonatal pustular melanosis: It is also a benign condition seen in term babies, with pustules or vesicles on normal looking skin. The lesions are present at birth and resolve with hyperpigmentation. Microscopic examination of pustules reveals neutrophils.

Miliaria crystallina and miliaria rubra: Common conditions in hot humid weathers, occur due to transient obstruction of eccrine sweat glands. Miliaria crystallina is characterized by asymptomatic, superficial, noninflammatory, and pinpoint clear vesicles. Miliaria rubra is characterized by erythematous papules. Usually appear after the first week of life.

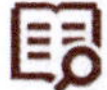

REFERENCE/SOURCE

- Palit A, Inamdar AC, Raghunatha S. Textbook of Pediatric Dermatology, 2nd edition. New Delhi: Jaypee Brothers Medical Publishers; 2014. pp. 16-17.

7. A 4-year-old child presents with high grade fever for 5 days. He has cervical lymphadenopathy, nonpurulent conjunctivitis, polymorphous exanthem, palmar erythema, and edema. Which of the following statement is *true* about the course of this disease?

A. In the acute phase, the dominant cardiac manifestation is myocarditis
B. In the acute phase, there is highest risk of coronary artery aneurysm formation
C. Thrombocytopenia is marked in subacute phase of this disease
D. In patients with previously normal echocardiogram, aneurysm can frequently develop after 8 weeks of illness

EXPLANATION

The scenario is of Kawasaki disease (KD). The clinical course of Kawasaki disease is divided into three phases. The acute phase lasts up to 7–14 days, where myocarditis is the dominant cardiac manifestation. The risk of coronary artery aneurysm formation is highest in subacute phase, and thrombocytosis is seen in this phase. Aneurysms are unusual after 8 weeks of the disease.

Key: A

BOOST YOUR KNOWLEDGE

Kawasaki disease or mucocutaneous lymph node syndrome is an acute systemic inflammatory vasculitis, seen mostly in infants and children <5 years of age.

Diagnostic guidelines: High grade fever >5 days *plus* any four out of the five from the following:
(1) Acute nonpurulent cervical lymphadenopathy, (2) Bilateral (B/L) nonpurulent conjunctivitis, (3) Palmoplantar erythema and edema or desquamation in convalescence, (4) Polymorphous exanthem, and (5) Strawberry tongue, reddening of lips, and diffuse enanthem.

D/D: Scarlet fever, toxic shock syndrome (TSS), SSSS, measles, adenovirus infection, Rocky Mountain spotted fever (RMSF), SJS-TEN. The treatment is IVIG plus aspirin.

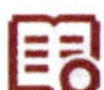

REFERENCE/SOURCE

- Hoeger PH, Kinsler V, Yan AC, Bodemer C, Larralde M, Luk D, et al. Harper's Textbook of Pediatric Dermatology, Volume 2, 4th edition. Hoboken, New Jersey: Wiley-Blackwell; 2019. pp. 168.5.

8. Which of the following statements *best* describes neonatal herpes infection?

A. It is a severe, often fatal infection of the neonates, which requires immediate treatment
B. Herpes simplex virus type 1 (HSV-1) accounts for 75–80% cases of neonatal herpes infection
C. CNS and other systemic involvement are not seen in neonatal herpes
D. No active treatment is required

EXPLANATION

Neonatal herpes is a severe, often fatal infection, caused by vertical transmission of HSV during vaginal delivery. Herpes simplex virus type 2 (HSV-2) accounts for 75–80% cases. CNS can be involved and disseminated multisystem infection is also seen. Immediate treatment with intravenous (IV) acyclovir is recommended.

Key: A

BOOST YOUR KNOWLEDGE

Neonatal herpes usually manifests within the first 4 weeks, mostly within the 1st week. Genital HSV in the mother (active or latent), poses a great risk to neonate. Three clinical presentations are seen: (1) Skin, eye, and mouth (SEM), (2) CNS, and (3) Disseminated. Those affected with SEM disease should also be evaluated for CNS and disseminated infection. Disseminated disease has mortality up to 50%.

REFERENCE/SOURCE

- Palit A, Inamdar AC, Raghunatha S. Textbook of Pediatric Dermatology, 2nd edition. New Delhi: Jaypee Brothers Medical Publishers; 2014. p. 183.

9. A healthy, full term 1-month-old neonate was brought with nodular induration of the upper back, and buttocks. He is afebrile and appears active. A diagnosis of subcutaneous fat necrosis is made based on the clinical findings. What is the most important investigation in this patient?

A. Skin biopsy
B. Magnetic resonance imaging (MRI)
C. Serum calcium levels
D. Ultrasonography (USG)

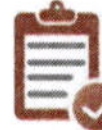

EXPLANATION

Subcutaneous fat necrosis, although benign and self-limiting, can be complicated by hypercalcemia, hence, serum calcium levels need to be checked and hypercalcemia has to be managed.

Key: C

BOOST YOUR KNOWLEDGE

Subcutaneous fat necrosis commonly occurs in the first 4 weeks of life in-term or post-term infants. Usual presentation is firm to rubbery, erythematous to skin-colored nodules, usually on upper back, buttocks, cheek, or proximal extremities. History of fetal distress, birth asphyxia, and meconium aspiration is common. It is generally a mild disease, but can cause hypoglycemia, thrombocytopenia, hypertriglyceridemia, lactic acidosis, and life-threatening hypercalcemia. The skin lesions resolve spontaneously by 3 months.

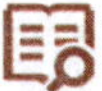

REFERENCE/SOURCE

- James WD, Berger TG, Elston DM. Andrew's Diseases of the Skin, 12th edition. Philadelphia, PA: Elsevier; 2016. p. 484.

10. A 9-month-old child presents with itchy excoriated papules in the finger webs, abdomen, back, palms, and soles. The mother also complained of nocturnal itching. Which statement correctly describes the treatment of the infant in this case?

A. Permethrin 1% cream is the treatment of choice
B. Permethrin 5% cream is the treatment of choice
C. Oral ivermectin is the treatment of choice
D. Gamma benzene hexachloride is the treatment of choice.

EXPLANATION

The scenario describes scabies in an infant. Treatment of choice in infants is by overnight application of permethrin 5% cream, which is to be repeated after 7 days. GBHC is not used for children <2 years of age. Oral ivermectin is also not recommended in infants.

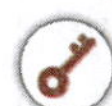

Key: B

BOOST YOUR KNOWLEDGE

Scabies is a common ectoparasite infestation caused by *Sarcoptes scabiei var hominis.* Intense itching with nocturnal exacerbation is the usual complaint. The cutaneous lesions include papules, papulovesicles, burrows, and excoriations. Palms and soles are usually involved in infants, which are usually not seen in older children. The condition is contagious; hence, treatment of the entire family is essential.

REFERENCE/SOURCE

- Palit A, Inamdar AC, Raghunatha S. Textbook of Pediatric Dermatology, 2nd edition. New Delhi: Jaypee Brothers Medical Publishers; 2014. pp. 286-7.

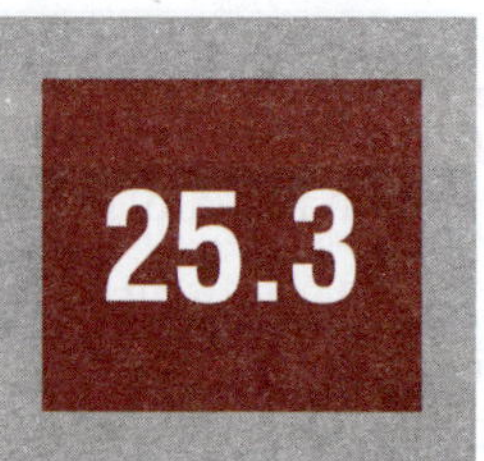

CHAPTER 25.3 Pediatric Ophthalmology

Payal Gupta

1. An otherwise healthy 5-month-old girl is brought in your outpatient department (OPD). The mother complaints that the child does not seem to respond to visual stimuli like switching on the lights in room, moving objects and toys, and does not seem to recognize her. The most important preliminary ophthalmic evaluation by you before referring to an ophthalmologist would be:

A. Ocular examination using a bright torch light
B. Assessment of extraocular movements
C. Distant direct ophthalmoscopy
D. Assessment of visual acuity

EXPLANATION

The clinical scenario presented indicates bilateral visual impairment. The aim of preliminary examination here is to rule out any media opacities that need urgent attention to prevent permanent blindness.

- Distant direct ophthalmoscopy (DDO), done using a pocket direct ophthalmoscope at a distance of 25–30 cm, assesses the red reflex. Presence of a normal red reflex rules out any media opacity at the level of cornea, anterior chamber, lens, vitreous, or retina.
- Absence of red reflex (also called as leukocoria or white reflex) warrants urgent ophthalmology referral.
- Ocular examination using a bright torch light confirms the mother's history of not responding to switching on of lights, and a gross idea of external appearance of eye including cornea and pupil.
- Extraocular movements in this case can be assessed with sound stimuli only, as a visually impaired baby will not respond to visual stimulus.
- Visual acuity assessment in infants need dedicated charts or equipment and are better suited to pediatric ophthalmology OPD setup.

Therefore, in suspected visual impairment in an infant as presented in the clinical scenario above, DDO should be done as the preliminary ophthalmic evaluation of choice.

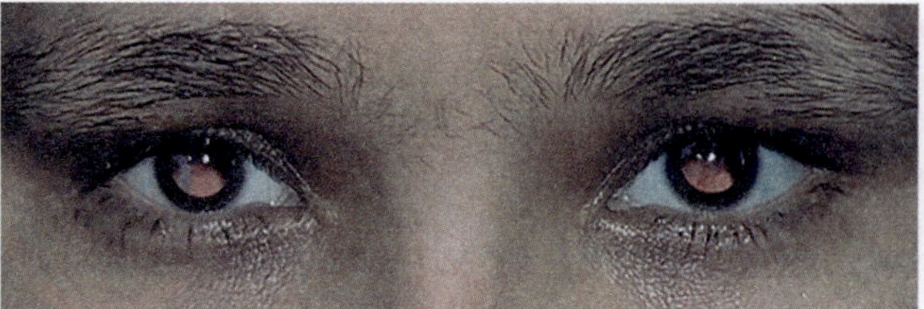

Red reflex

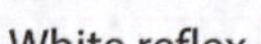

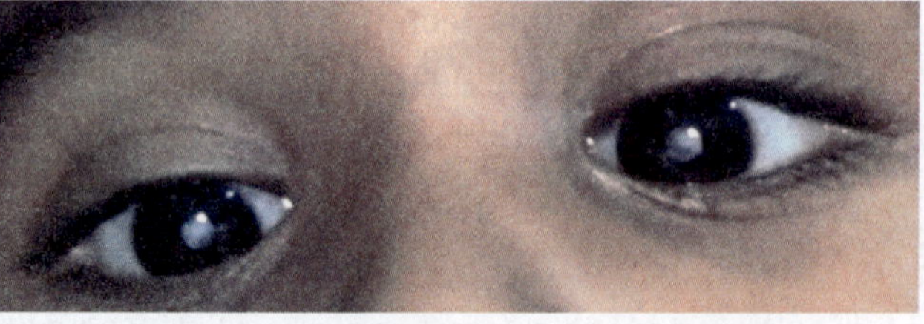

White reflex

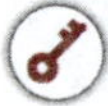

Key: C

BOOST YOUR KNOWLEDGE

Causes of Leukocoria

1. *Congenital:*
   - Cataract
   - Persistent hyperplastic primary vitreous
   - Coats' disease
   - Choroidal coloboma
   - Retinal detachment
   - *Vitreoretinal dysplasias:* Norrie disease, incontinentia pigmenti, Walker–Warburg syndrome
2. *Inflammatory:*
   - Cyclitic membrane
   - Endophthalmitis
   - Toxocariasis
   - Retinal detachment
3. *Neoplastic:*
   - Retinoblastoma
   - Retinocytoma
   - Retinal astrocytoma
4. *Traumatic:*
   - Cataract
   - Retinal detachment
5. *Others:*
   - Retinopathy of prematurity (ROP)

REFERENCE/SOURCE

- Gupta P. Examination of the Eye. In: Gupta P (Ed). Clinical Methods in Pediatrics, 5th edition. New Delhi: CBS Publishers and Distributors (P) Ltd; 2021. p. 429.

2. Hydrostatic sac massage is advised as first line of treatment in congenital nasolacrimal duct obstruction. When done adequately, it is effective in over 95% of cases. If not effective, surgical intervention with syringing and therapeutic probing can be done after the age of:

A. 1 month B. 4 months
C. 1 year D. 4 years

EXPLANATION

Sac massage is highly effective when done timely and adequately. In cases not responding to this conservative management, syringing and therapeutic probing is attempted. Although exact time is controversial, it is recommended to be done after at least 9 months of age. If even probing fails, it can be repeated till 3–4 years of age. After 4 years of age, neither sac massage nor probing helps, as the bony structure around the sac and nasolacrimal duct is well developed at this age. Recommended procedure in such cases is dacryocystorhinostomy with intubation.

Key: C

BOOST YOUR KNOWLEDGE

Congenital nasolacrimal duct obstruction is the most common cause of childhood epiphora (watering from eye), caused by a membranous block of valve of Hasner.

Next figure is a diagram of schematic diagram of lacrimal drainage (measurements correspond to adult dimensions of fully formed lacrimal system).

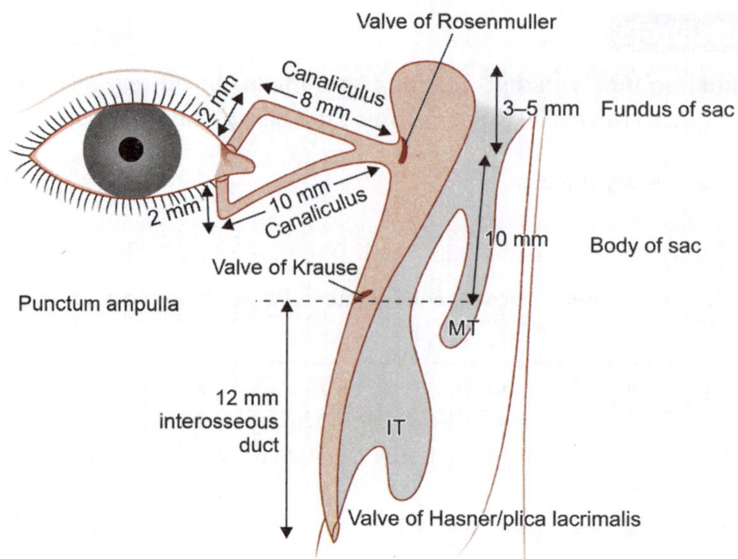

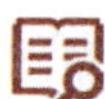

REFERENCES/SOURCES

- Chaudhuri Z, Vanathi M. Postgraduate Ophthalmology, Volume 2, 2nd edition. New Delhi: Jaypee Brothers Medical Publishers; 2021. p. 1700.
- Gupta P. Examination of the Eye. In: Gupta P (Ed). Clinical Methods in Pediatrics, 5th edition. New Delhi: CBS Publishers and Distributors (P) Ltd; 2021. pp. 438-9.

3. A mother of a 9-month-old boy complains that her child has been having watering from both eyes and prefers to keep his head buried on her chest or shoulders. On torch-light examination, you appreciate epiphora and confirm severe photophobia. Which other ocular feature of this triad is suggestive of primary congenital/infantile glaucoma?

A. Leukocoria
B. Megalocornea
C. Blepharospasm
D. Corneal edema

EXPLANATION

The classical triad of primary infantile/congenital glaucoma is *epiphora, photophobia, and blepharospasm.* Other variable features depending on the severity could be megalocornea, corneal edema appreciated as bluish discoloration or haziness of cornea, and raised intraocular pressure. Leukocoria or white reflex is not a feature of primary childhood glaucoma.

Key: C

BOOST YOUR KNOWLEDGE

- *Causes of epiphora in infants are:*
  - Congenital glaucoma
  - Congenital nasolacrimal duct obstruction
  - Ophthalmia neonatorum
  - Keratomalacia
- *Megalocornea is defined as corneal diameter of:*
  - >11 mm in neonates
  - >12 mm in infants
  - >13 mm at any age

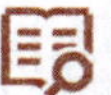

REFERENCE/SOURCE

- Gupta P. Common eye abnormalities. In: Gupta P, Menon PSN, Ramji S, Lodha R (Eds). PG Textbook of Pediatrics, Volume 3, 3rd edition. New Delhi: Jaypee Brothers Medical Publishers; 2022. p. 3248.

4. A 4-year-old child with a renal disease on conservative management, has been advised regular ophthalmic follow-up for screening of acquired cataract. What is the likely diagnosis?

A. Wilms' tumor
B. Lowe syndrome
C. Nephrotic syndrome
D. Polycystic kidney disease

EXPLANATION

All four options are renal diseases. Options (B), (C), and (D) can be managed conservatively, while surgical intervention is treatment of choice in (A).

- Wilms' tumor and Lowe syndrome are associated with congenital/developmental cataract.
- Oral steroids are first line of therapy in conservative management of nephrotic syndrome. Most common ocular side effect of systemic steroids is development of cataract.
- Polycystic kidney disease unless complicated to chronic kidney disease, is very rarely associated with acquired cataracts.

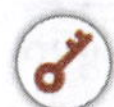

Key: C

BOOST YOUR KNOWLEDGE

Ocular associations of the following are:

- *Wilms' tumor:* Ptosis, nystagmus, congenital cataract, congenital aniridia, corneal opacity, and raised increased intraocular pressure (IOP) with secondary glaucoma.
- *Lowe syndrome:* Nystagmus, congenital cataract, infantile glaucoma, and corneal or conjunctival keloids.

Causes of acquired cataract in children:

- Trauma
- Long-term (~3 months) systemic/topical steroid use and even short-term use in steroid responders.
- Complicated cataract because of uveitis.
- Cataracts secondary to chronic retinal detachment, intraocular tumor, intraocular foreign body, or post-laser therapy for ROP.

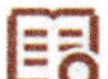

REFERENCE/SOURCE

- Chaudhuri Z, Vanathi M. Pediatric lenticular abnormalities. In: Chaudhuri Z, Vanathi M (Eds). Postgraduate Ophthalmology, Volume 2, 2nd edition. New Delhi: Jaypee Brothers Medical Publishers; 2021. p. 2144.

5. Parents of a 2-week-old neonate with congenital rubella syndrome come to you with already diagnosed bilateral congenital cataract, seeking guidance to delay the surgical procedure in view of systemic issues. What will be the right age for surgery?

A. Before 4 weeks of age
B. Between 6 and 10 weeks of age
C. After attaining 6 months of age
D. Anytime between 1 and 6 years of age

EXPLANATION

Prompt surgical intervention is needed in visually significant cataracts.

- In case of bilateral cataracts, surgery should be done *within 6 weeks preferably* and *latest by 10 weeks*, to prevent permanent visual impairment resulting from stimulus deprivation amblyopia. Care should be taken that the fellow eye is also operated within 1–2 weeks.
- In unilateral dense cataracts, probability of developing amblyopia soon is higher. In such instances, it is advisable to operate at 4–6 weeks.
- In either case, considering systemic involvement, anesthesia related risks, and higher rates of postoperative complications, one should operate at least *after* 4 weeks of life.

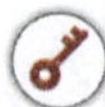

Key: B

BOOST YOUR KNOWLEDGE

Clinical features associated with dense congenital cataracts:

- Poor fixing and following
- White reflex
- Nystagmus
- Strabismus
- Microcornea

6. A 28-week-preterm with birth weight 1,200 g is admitted in your neonatal intensive care unit (NICU) on oxygen supplementation. When should the child be referred for ROP screening?

A. At birth
B. Within 1 week of birth
C. At 3–4 weeks of chronological age
D. After attaining 34 weeks of gestational age

EXPLANATION

The ROP screening should be done before discharging the baby or 30 days of age, whichever is sooner.

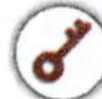

Key: C

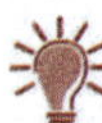

BOOST YOUR KNOWLEDGE

Criteria for ROP screening:

- All infants born at 34 weeks or less gestational age
- All infants weighing 2,000 g or less at birth
- All infants born at >34 weeks gestational age with associated risk factors
- Other preterm infants based on the discretion of the pediatrician or neonatologist.

Risk factors for ROP:

- Cardiorespiratory support
- Prolonged oxygen requirement
- Respiratory distress syndrome
- Chronic lung disease
- Fetal hemorrhage
- Blood transfusion
- Sepsis
- Exchange transfusion

- Interventricular hemorrhage
- Apnea
- Poor postnatal weight gain

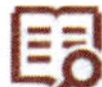

REFERENCES/SOURCES

- IIPH, Hyderabad. (2019). Project Operational Guidelines—Prevention of Blindness from Retinopathy of Prematurity in Neonatal Care Unit. [online] Available from https://phfi.org/wp-content/uploads/2019/05/2018-ROP-operational-guidelines.pdf. [Last accessed July, 2024].
- Shukla R, Murthy GVS, Gilbert C, Vidyadhar B, Mukpalkar S. Operational Guidelines for ROP in India: A summary. Indian J Ophthalmol. 2020;68(Suppl 1):S108-14.

7. An 8-year-old girl with penetrating injury to left eye with bow and arrow presents in emergency. On examination, there is visible protrusion of uveal tissue through a large corneoscleral tear. The emergency setup you are working at has no ophthalmic backup. Primary management before referring to a higher center for ophthalmic care would be:

A. Patch and bandage the eye tightly using sterile gauze piece
B. Patch and bandage the eye lightly using a plastic eye shield
C. Do not patch the eye at all and start antibiotic ointment
D. Wash the eye thoroughly with 500 mL normal saline

EXPLANATION

In cases of suspected penetrating eye injury (open globe trauma), following things need to be taken care of before ophthalmology referral.

- No pressure on eyelids (prevents extrusion of ocular contents)
- No attempt to remove any protruding matter or foreign body from the eye
- No eye drops or ointments to be given
- Do not pressure patch to avoid sticking of ocular contents to the dressing
- Place an eye shield covering, but not touching the surface of the open globe
- Check tetanus immunization status, repeat if needed
- Start broad spectrum systemic antibiotics
- Urgently consult an ophthalmologist

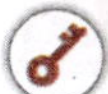

Key: B

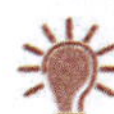

BOOST YOUR KNOWLEDGE

Washing the eye with saline is recommended first line of therapy in chemical/thermal injuries with closed globe.

REFERENCE/SOURCE

- Gupta P. Ocular emergencies. In: Gupta P, et al. (Eds): Principles of Pediatric Neonatal Emergencies, 4th edition. New Delhi: Jaypee Brothers Medical Publishers; 2020. p. 848.

8. A 12-year-old girl has been referred to you with history of recurrent anterior uveitis and no systemic complaints at present. Baseline investigations with complete blood counts, liver and renal function tests, chest X-ray, and Mantoux test, as advised by the ophthalmologist were within normal limits. Erythrocyte sedimentation rate (ESR) and C-reactive protein (CRP) counts were both slightly elevated. Which of these investigations could be recommended to rule out the most common cause of uveitis in this age group?

A. Rheumatoid (RA) factor
B. Human leukocyte antigen B27 (HLA-B 27)
C. Antinuclear antibody (ANA) profile
D. Serum angiotensin-converting enzyme (ACE) levels

EXPLANATION

Juvenile idiopathic arthritis (JIA) is the *most common cause* of uveitis in children <16 years.

- *ANA:* children without JIA can also test positive for ANA
- *RA factor:* Though rarely present in children with JIA, if present, it confirms diagnosis of RA factor positive polyarticular JIA.
- *HLA B27:* Not all who test positive have, or will ever develop the disease (Behçet's disease).
- *Serum ACE:* Increased in sarcoidosis, another common cause of uveitis in children.

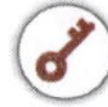

Key: A

BOOST YOUR KNOWLEDGE

Symptoms of acute anterior uveitis:

- Painful red eye
- Blurry vision
- Mild upper and lower lid swelling
- Photophobia

Signs (needs slit-lamp evaluation):

- Circumcorneal congestion
- Cells and flare in anterior chamber
- Sluggish pupillary reaction
- Poor glow because of media haze

REFERENCE/SOURCE

- Gupta P, Menon PSN, Ramji S, Lodha R (Eds). PG Textbook of Pediatrics, Volume 3, 3rd edition. New Delhi: Jaypee Brothers Medical Publishers; 2022. p. 3233 Box 1.

9. A 9-year-old girl with facial features presented in the given picture is planned for frontalis sling surgery under general anesthesia. The ophthalmologist has referred the patient to a pediatrician to rule out any systemic illnesses. You examine the child and find no systemic anomalies. However, knowing the systemic association of this eye disease, you would counsel her mother for the following possibility.

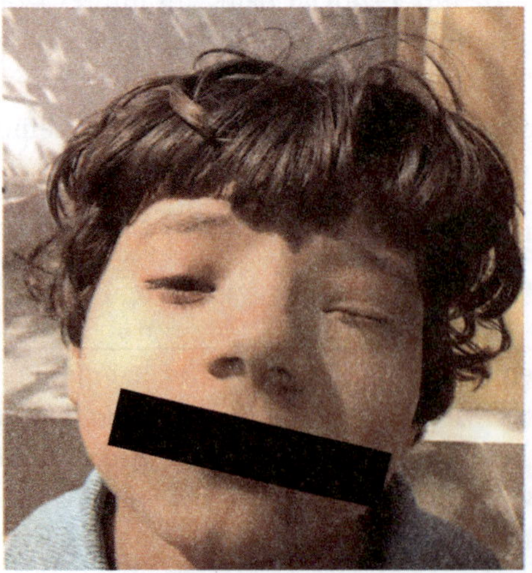

A. Menorrhagia
B. Primary amenorrhea
C. Severe dysmenorrhea
D. Secondary amenorrhea

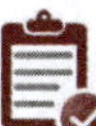

EXPLANATION

The girl in the figure has *blepharophimosis* (short palpebral fissure width), *ptosis* (drooping of eyelid), *Epicanthus inversus* (inverted epicanthal fold), and *telecanthus* (broad nasal bridge); blepharophimosis syndrome (BPES) is an inherited eyelid disease.

Blepharophimosis syndrome type I includes these four major features along with primary ovarian insufficiency, whereas BPES type II includes only the four major features. In cases of primary ovarian failure, menarche is usually normal but is followed by oligomenorrhea and secondary amenorrhea.

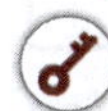

Key: D

BOOST YOUR KNOWLEDGE

BPES may occur as an autosomal dominant trait or sporadically and is linked to 3q23, and mutation in the *FOXL2* gene. Moreover, it is also accompanied by poorly developed nasal bridge and hypoplasia of the superior orbital rim. These patients may also have poorly developed nasal bridge and hypoplasia of superior orbital rim. They are also at an increased risk of developing refractive error, strabismus, lacrimal abnormalities and amblyopia. Systemic abnormalities like mental retardation and gonadal atrophy with infertility may coexist with BPES.

REFERENCE/SOURCE

- Bhattacharjee K, Bhattacharjee H, Kuri G, Shah ZT, Deori N. Single stage surgery for blepharophimosis syndrome. Indian J Ophthalmol. 2012;60(3):195-201.

10. Which of these systemic diseases, does not need sophisticated equipment for ocular examination and can be easily examined in a bedside referral by an ophthalmologist of basic setup to rule out its ocular association?

A. Wilson disease
B. Bacterial endocarditis
C. Sturge–Weber syndrome
D. Juvenile idiopathic arthritis

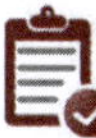

EXPLANATION

	Ocular association	*Examination*	*Equipment*
Wilson disease	Kayser–Fleischer ring	Golden, brown ring in the peripheral cornea	Slit lamp
Bacterial endocarditis	Roth spots	White-centered retinal hemorrhage	Ophthalmoscope
Sturge–Weber syndrome	Glaucoma	• Raised intraocular pressure • Angle malformation • Neovascularization	Tonometer, gonio-mirror, slit lamp
JIA	Anterior uveitis	Cells and flare in anterior chamber	Slit lamp

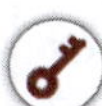

Key: B

BOOST YOUR KNOWLEDGE

- A fundoscopy for retinal evaluation can be easily done bedside using a direct or an indirect ophthalmoscope, which are easy to carry and mostly available in all basic ophthalmic setups.
- Slit lamp biomicroscope is also usually available in ophthalmic OPD setups, but is not easily portable. Examination with tonometer and gonio-mirror also require use of slit lamp.
- Handheld slit lamp and tonometer are also an option, but due to financial constraints may not be available at many establishments.

REFERENCE/SOURCE

- Gupta P, Basu S, Gupta P. Ophthalmic disorders. In: Gupta P (Ed). UG Textbook of Pediatrics. New Delhi: Jaypee Brothers Medical Publishers; 2023.

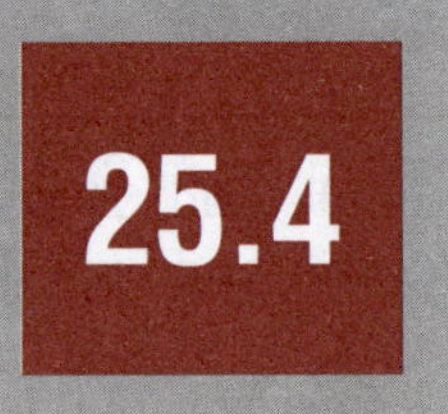

CHAPTER 25.4 Pediatric Psychiatry

Janaki Rajagopalan

1. A 15-year-old girl is brought to the *emergency*, after she fainted in school assembly. This is the third time this has happened in the last week. Her mother reports that she has lost >10 kg in the last 4 months, and she has been restricting her eating, eating only vegan food and small portions. She has also been exercising excessively by running and spending up to 2 hours in the apartment gym everyday. The girl herself says that she was often called fat by her friends and losing weight has made her feel more confident. Her current body mass index (BMI) is 16, and despite the doctor telling her that she is underweight, she says that she wants to lose another 4 kg to reach a weight of 41 kg (her height is 168 cm). Her bloods reveal low sodium and potassium levels, rest normal. Her electrocardiogram (ECG) shows bradycardia. She denies using any laxatives or purging. What is the diagnosis and what is the next step in the management of this young girl?

A. *Anorexia nervosa (AN) restrictive type:* Advice admission to start refeeding as patient medically compromised and lacks insight

B. *Anorexia nervosa restrictive type:* Treat on outpatient basis and recommend seeing a psychiatrist

C. *Avoidant/restrictive food intake disorder (ARFID):* Treat on outpatient basis and recommend seeing a psychiatrist

D. *Avoidant/restrictive food intake disorder (ARFID):* Advice admission to start refeeding as patient is medically compromised and lacks insight

EXPLANATION

The criteria for AN restrictive type are met and as per the hierarchy of diagnoses, the diagnosis of AN precedes ARFID diagnosis. In this case, the child lacks insight into her illness and wants to lose weight, which is a risk to self. Sodium and potassium are low and she has bradycardia which increases the risk of arrhythmias. A common cause of mortality in AN is due to cardiac arrhythmias and QTc prolongation. Hence, the child requires admission for medical compromise and feeding.

Key: A

BOOST YOUR KNOWLEDGE

Anorexia nervosa is classified as a feeding and eating disorder in the Diagnostic and Statistical Manual of Disorders, fifth edition (DSM-5). The criteria of amenorrhea have been removed from the diagnostic criteria. ARFID as a category has been included to incorporate the feeding and eating disorders which were not fitting into AN or bulimia nervosa (BN) to improve the sensitivity of the criteria.

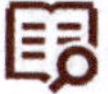

REFERENCES/SOURCES

- American Psychiatric Association. Diagnostic and Statistical Manual of Mental Disorders, 5th edition (DSM-5). Washington, DC: American Psychiatric Association; 2013.
- American Psychiatric Association. Treatment of patients with eating disorders, 3rd edition. American Psychiatric Association. Am J Psychiatry. 2006;163:4-54.
- Sadock BJ, Sadock VA. Chapter 22. In: Sadock BJ, Sadock VA, Ruiz P (Eds). Kaplan and Sadock's Comprehensive Textbook of Psychiatry, Volume 1, 10th edition. Philadelphia, PA: Wolters Kluwer; 2017. p. 2065.
- Sadock BJ, Sadock VA. Chapter 47. In: Sadock BJ, Sadock VA, Ruiz P (Eds). Kaplan and Sadock's Comprehensive Textbook of Psychiatry, Volume 2, 10th edition. Philadelphia, PA: Wolters Kluwer; 2017. p. 3622.

2. A developmentally normal young boy is going on a boat ride with his parents and asks them "mommy when does the ocean stop and take rest?". According to Jean Piaget, which stage of cognitive development is the child in?

A. Concrete operational stage
B. Preoperational stage
C. Formal operational stage
D. Sensorimotor stage

EXPLANATION

The boy is attributing human like qualities to an inanimate object like the ocean, a feature of a flaw in thinking called egocentrism. Giving animate qualities to inanimate objects is part of this flaw, and is called animism. These flaws are present in the preoperational stage of cognitive development, which persists from ages 2-7.

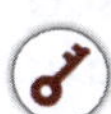

Key: B

BOOST YOUR KNOWLEDGE

Jean Piaget proposed that children's thought processes go through a series of four major stages:

1. *The sensorimotor period (birth to age 2):* The major development during the sensorimotor stage is the acquisition of the concept of object permanence between 4 and 18 months of age.
2. *The preoperational period (ages 2-7):* There are flaws in thinking in the stage which include centration, irreversibility, and egocentrism. Egocentrism in thinking is characterized by a limited ability to share another person's viewpoint. For example, if you ask a preoperational girl whether her sister has a sister, she will probably say "no" if they are the only two girls in the family. Animism—the belief that all things are living, just like oneself.
3. *The concrete operational period (ages 7-11):* Children can perform operations only on images of tangible objects and actual events and they master reversibility and decentration.
4. *The formal operational period (age 11 onward):* Children begin to apply their operations to abstract concepts in addition to concrete objects. During this stage, youngsters come to enjoy the contemplation of abstract concepts.

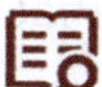

REFERENCES/SOURCES

- Sadock BJ, Sadock VA. Chapter 35. In: Sadock BJ, Sadock VA, Ruiz P (Eds). Kaplan and Sadock's Comprehensive Textbook of Psychiatry, Volume 2, 10th edition. Philadelphia, PA: Wolters Kluwer; 2017. p. 3359.
- Weiten W. Human development across the lifespan (Chapter 10). In: Weiten W (Ed). Psychology Themes and Variations, 10th edition. Belmont, USA: Wadsworth, Cengage Learning; 2012. p. 351.

3. **A 4-year-old girl presents with abnormal hand movements. The child was developing normally until 3 years ago, when her development seemed to regress with deceleration in head growth, gait abnormalities, loss of purposeful hand movements, repetitive stereotypical movement (hand-wringing), loss of speech, and breathing abnormalities. On physical examination, there is a lack of coordination, and speech is slurred. What is the mode of inheritance of the described disorder?**

A. Autosomal dominant
B. X-linked dominant
C. X-linked recessive
D. Autosomal recessive

EXPLANATION

The history is suggestive of Rett syndrome (RTT), which is classified as a pervasive developmental disorder. RTT is an X-linked dominant condition with lethal consequences in hemizygous males. Mutations in *MECP2* are found in the majority of classic RTT cases; recent studies found two additional genes, cyclin-dependent kinase-like 5 (*CDKL5*) and forkhead box G1 (*FOXG1*) involved in the pathogenesis of RTT.

Key: B

BOOST YOUR KNOWLEDGE

In RTT, there is apparently normal psychomotor development during the first 6–18 months of life, followed by a rapid regression in language and motor skills. The hallmark is loss of purposeful hand use and replaced by repetitive stereotypical hand movements. Head growth may begin decelerating as early as at age 3 months. Seizures occur in about 90% of females, mostly with generalized tonic-clonic seizures and partial complex seizures. They may have screaming fits and inconsolable crying by age 18–24 months. Additional characteristics include autistic features, panic-like attacks, bruxism, episodic apnea and/or hyperpnoea, seizures, gait ataxia and apraxia, and tremors. After rapid deterioration, the neurologic manifestations become relatively stable. Other features including failure to thrive, may be partially related to oropharyngeal and gastroesophageal incoordination, resulting in poor dietary intake. Constipation is also very common in RTT. More than 80% of patients have scoliosis. About 70% of patients also have osteopenia which increases the risk of fractures. One of the most life-threatening problems in RTT is cardiac arrhythmia that includes prolonged QT interval, T-wave abnormalities, and reduced heart rate variability, which may account for some cases of sudden death in RTT. Epidemiology—1/10,000 live female births. It is one of the common causes of mental retardation in females.

REFERENCES/SOURCES

- Neul JL, Kaufmann WE, Glaze DG, Christodoulou J, Clarke AJ, Bahi-Buisson N, et al. Rett syndrome: revised diagnostic criteria and nomenclature. Ann Neurol. 2010;68(6):944-50.
- Sadock BJ, Sadock VA. Chapter 35. In: Sadock BJ, Sadock VA, Ruiz P (Eds). Kaplan and Sadock's Comprehensive Textbook of Psychiatry, Volume 2, 10th edition. Philadelphia, PA: Wolters Kluwer; 2017. p. 4609.
- Thapar A, Scott S, Leckman J, Snowling MJ, Pine DS, Taylor EA (Eds). Rutter's Child and Adolescent Psychiatry, 6th edition. Wiley-Blackwell; 2015. p. 726 (Table).

4. **An adolescent with autism spectrum disorder (ASD) tends to repeat the last few words of the sentence that anyone says to him. This speech disorder that is seen in ASD is called:**

A. Echopraxia
B. Phonological inhibition
C. Echolalia
D. Grapheme dysfunction

EXPLANATION

Echopraxia is the repetition of action (praxis) which may occur in ASD, but is not a speech disorder; Phonological inhibition is the inability to form words or sounds; Grapheme dysfunction occurs in learning disorders such as dyslexia, where the identification of sounds and letters may be affected. Echolalia is the repetition of what a person hears. This is often seen as repetition of last few words of what someone says to them.

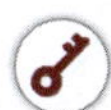
Key: C

BOOST YOUR KNOWLEDGE

The DSM-5 has made substantial changes to ASD. The new criteria include: (1) Persistent and pervasive deficits in social communication and social interaction, and (2) Restricted, repetitive patterns of behavior, interests, and activities. As now defined, ASD can be subcategorized by the presence or absence of intellectual impairment and/or an associated medical condition. In addition, the identification of three severity levels helps clarify the need for additional social or occupational services. For example, a patient requiring "very substantial support" might display extreme behavioral inflexibility or might possess 20 words of intelligible speech.

REFERENCES/SOURCES

- Rutter M. Chapter 51. In: Thapar A, Scott S, Leckman J, Snowling MJ, Pine DS, Taylor EA (Eds). Rutter's Child and Adolescent Psychiatry, 6th edition. Wiley-Blackwell; 2015. p. 665 (Table).
- Sadock BJ, Sadock VA. Chapter 44. In: Sadock BJ, Sadock VA, Ruiz P (Eds). Kaplan and Sadock's Comprehensive Textbook of Psychiatry, Volume 2, 10th edition. Philadelphia, PA: Wolters Kluwer; 2017. p. 3571.

5. A 16-year-old boy is brought to the emergency by his parents, after he hurt his younger brother. Due to aggressive behavior towards the staff in emergency department (ED), he is given 10 mg intramuscular (IMI) haloperidol and 25 mg IMI promethazine. He is sedated for some time but develops stiffness of his neck and inability to swallow. What is the diagnosis and what treatment should be given?

A. Extrapyramidal symptoms due to IMI antipsychotic use; intravenous (IV) benztropine 1–2 mg to be repeated 1–2 hourly, until symptoms settle up to maximum of 6 mg
B. Extrapyramidal symptoms due to IMI antipsychotic use; Wait and watch
C. Oculogyric crisis; Diazepam 10 mg orally
D. Akathisia; Benztropine 2 mg orally

EXPLANATION

As the adolescent is drug naïve and has been given IMI haloperidol, this is likely to be extrapyramidal side effects (EPSE)—dystonia due to antipsychotic use. If a patient is experiencing acute onset of EPSE, particularly dystonia, emergency airway intervention may be required, as laryngeal and pharyngeal dystonic reactions may increase the risk of imminent respiratory arrest. IV benztropine must be administered at this point to decrease this risk.

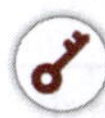
Key: A

BOOST YOUR KNOWLEDGE

Antipsychotics especially first generation such as haloperidol and chlorpromazine may cause EPSE. The common EPSEs are:

- *Dystonia:* Involuntary muscle contractions resulting in abnormal posturing or repetitive movements. Onset—within 48 hours of drug exposure in 50% of cases, and within 5 days in 90% of cases. May affect different body parts—back and extremities (opisthotonus), neck (torticollis), jaw (trismus), eyes (oculogyric crisis), abdominal wall, and pelvic muscles (tortipelvic crisis), and facial and tongue muscles (buccolingual crisis).
- *Akathisia:* Subjective feeling of internal restlessness and a compelling urge to move, leading to the objective observation of repetitive movements shifting from one foot to another. Onset—within 4 weeks of starting or increasing the dosage of medication. Risk of increase in suicidal ideation, self-harm, and harm to others.

- *Drug-induced parkinsonism:* Tremor, rigidity, and slowing of motor function in the truncal region and extremities. Appears as masked facies, stooped posture, and a slow shuffling gait.
- *Tardive dyskinesia:* Involuntary choreoathetoid movements affecting orofacial and tongue muscles, and less commonly the truncal region and extremities. Long-term side effect of use of antipsychotics.

REFERENCES/SOURCES

- Grover S, Avasthi A. Clinical Practice Guidelines for the Management of Schizophrenia in Children and Adolescents. Indian J Psychiatry. 2019;61(Suppl 2):277-93.
- Sadock BJ, Sadock VA, Ruiz P (Eds). Kaplan and Sadock's Comprehensive Textbook of Psychiatry, 10th edition. Philadelphia, PA: Wolters Kluwer; 2017. pp. 1497, 1526, 1528.

6. What is the approximate percentage prevalence of schizophrenia in biological siblings as against the general population prevalence of 1%?

A. 2% B. 5%
C. 10% D. 20%

EXPLANATION

Schizophrenia is a highly heritable condition. Percentage of morbidity varies according to the degree of relationship. For siblings, it is 10%.

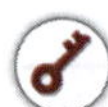

Key: C

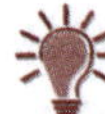

BOOST YOUR KNOWLEDGE

Different types of studies were done to determine the heritability of schizophrenic illnesses, mainly twin studies, and adoption studies. The percentages of morbidity quoted in family studies are as follows:

- Siblings—10%
- Parents—5%
- Children—13%
- Siblings, if one parent schizophrenic—16.7%
- Children, if both parents are schizophrenic—46%
- Identical twin—50%

REFERENCES/SOURCES

- Sadock BJ, Sadock VA. Chapter 12.4. In: Sadock BJ, Sadock VA, Ruiz P (Eds). Kaplan and Sadock's Comprehensive Textbook of Psychiatry, 10th edition. Philadelphia, PA: Wolters Kluwer; 2017. p. 1439.
- Thapar A, Scott S, Leckman J, Snowling MJ, Pine DS, Taylor EA (Eds). Rutter's Child and Adolescent Psychiatry, 6th edition. Wiley-Blackwell; 2015. pp. 777-8.

7. In the Strange Situation Experiment, a 12-month-old child throws all the toys in her reach on her mother's exit, and on her mother's return, she turns around and does not look at her, pushing her mother away when she tries to approach her. This attachment pattern of alternate aggression and withdrawal is:

A. Anxious-ambivalent B. Disorganized
C. Secure D. Avoidant

EXPLANATION

Attachment is an evolutionary biological mechanism in which infants are biologically programmed to emit behavior (smiling, cooing, clinging, and so on) that triggers an affectionate, protective response from adults. The different patterns of attachment are: *Secure attachment*—Infants play and explore comfortably with their mother present, become visibly upset when she leaves, and are quickly calmed by her return; *Anxious-ambivalent attachment* (also called resistant attachment)—Infants appear anxious even when their mothers are near and protest excessively when she leaves, but they are not particularly comforted when she returns; *Avoidant attachment*—Children seek little contact with their mothers and often are not distressed when she leaves; and *Disorganized attachment*—Child is unpredictable in their behavior alternating between aggression, clinging, and withdrawal.

 **Key: B**

BOOST YOUR KNOWLEDGE

John Bowlby was interested in Harry Harlow's wire monkey experiment and proposed the evolutionary theory of attachment. Mary Ainsworth and her colleagues (1978) found that attachments fall into three categories. Most infants develop a secure attachment. The category of disorganized attachment was added later. Child abuse and trauma victims may form this kind of attachment.

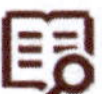

REFERENCES/SOURCES

- Sadock BJ, Sadock VA, Ruiz P (Eds). Kaplan and Sadock's Comprehensive Textbook of Psychiatry, Volume 2, 10th edition. Philadelphia, PA: Wolters Kluwer; 2017. p. 4543.
- Weiten W. Human development across the lifespan (Chapter 10). In: Weiten W (Ed). Psychology Themes and Variations, 10th edition. Belmont, USA: Wadsworth, Cengage Learning; 2012. p. 346.

8. A 16-year-old boy is brought to the emergency with a history of 4 days of not sleeping >2 hours a night, pacing around at night, claiming to be talking to God, and being a messenger of God. He says to doctor that he owns the hospital, and that God has told him that he is going to get the Nobel prize in medicine next year. His affect is elated with increased psychomotor activity. There is family history of bipolar affective disorder in a first degree relative and no history suggestive of drug use or organicity. What is the next step in management?

A. Admit and do baseline investigations including thyroid function test (TFT), urine drug screen, and computed tomography (CT) scan brain plain. Take a detailed collateral history. Start lithium/olanzapine/sodium valproate as a mood stabilizer

B. Wait and watch. If patient's situation worsens, then family can bring back to hospital

C. Ask the family to take the patient to a psychiatrist in the outpatient setting

D. Admit and start on lorazepam 1 mg TDS

EXPLANATION

The boy is an adolescent who is in the age range for the onset of bipolar affective disorder (15–25 years, 1st peak of onset). With a positive family history, no drug use or organicity evident, it is likely that this is a first episode mania—symptoms are suggestive of a "classic euphoric mania". In such a situation where the young boy is having grandiose delusions and possible auditory hallucinations, decreased sleep and increased energy levels, there is a risk of further deterioration and risk to reputation. Hence, admission should be advised. Blood tests such as complete blood count, liver and kidney functions, TFT, electrolytes, urine routine microscopy, ECG, and CT scan brain should be done to rule out organicity and also a baseline to start mood stabilizer. In this case, lithium is preferable due to family history, no substance use and "classic euphoric mania". Wait and watch may be a dangerous strategy, as patient's mental health may deteriorate rapidly. The outpatient setting will not suit for a patient who is so unwell. Any delay in treatment with mood stabilizer is unwarranted as the diagnosis is clear, hence, giving only benzodiazepines will not be adequate.

 **Key: A**

BOOST YOUR KNOWLEDGE

Pharmacotherapy is the mainstay of treatment for children and adolescents with bipolar disorder. Choice of drug should be based on:

- Evidence of effectiveness
- Phase of illness
- Subtype of disorder (psychosis, mixed episode, and rapid cycling)
- Adverse effect profile with respect to the patient
- Patient's history of medication response
- Possibly, also a family member's history of medication response.

REFERENCES/SOURCES

- American Psychiatric Association. Diagnostic and Statistical Manual of Mental Disorders, 5th edition (DSM-5). Washington, DC: American Psychiatric Association; 2013.
- Sadock BJ, Sadock VA. Chapter 51.2. In: Sadock BJ, Sadock VA, Ruiz P (Eds). Kaplan and Sadock's Comprehensive Textbook of Psychiatry, Volume 2, 10th edition. Philadelphia, PA: Wolters Kluwer; 2017. p. 3686.
- Stahl MS. Stahl's essential psychopharmacology: prescriber's guide, 5th edition. New York, NY: Cambridge University Press; 2014.

9. A 6-year-old girl has difficulty sitting in one place in class, runs around all the time, fidgets with things, and keeps moving about. She is unable to concentrate in class and is often in trouble for interrupting the teacher and asking questions. She speaks fast and does not allow others to speak in a group. She finds it difficult to wait for her turn. She has had several accidents and tends to be clumsy. She loses stationery all the time. She has these symptoms at home and at school, and has been noted to have them since she attended preschool (3 years of age). Her height and weight are around 50th percentile. What is this child's most likely diagnosis, and what is the preferred medication choice for her?

A. Bipolar affective disorder (BPAD), mood stabilizer such as lithium
B. Generalized anxiety disorder (GAD), selective serotonin reuptake inhibitor (SSRI) such as sertraline
C. Attention deficit hyperactivity disorder (ADHD), stimulant such as methylphenidate
D. Obsessive compulsive disorder (OCD), SSRI such as sertraline

EXPLANATION

The symptoms are present since 3 years of age and are persistent in all environments (home and school). There is no mention of mood symptoms and though speaking fast may be a symptom of mania, the other symptoms of interrupting and talking over others, difficulty in waiting for her turn, and the nonepisodic course of illness are indicative of ADHD. There are no symptoms suggestive of GAD or OCD. Hence, the most likely diagnosis is ADHD, and the preferred medication choice is a stimulant such as methylphenidate.

Key: C

BOOST YOUR KNOWLEDGE

The ADHD is one of the most common childhood psychiatric disorders. ADHD affects around 5–7% of school-aged children. It is more common in male children than in female children (2:1 ratio). 6 out of 9 criteria for attention deficit and/or hyperactivity impulsivity must be met in order to meet the cutoff for the diagnosis of ADHD. Some symptoms should have started prior to age 12 and the symptoms should be present in more than one environment. Diagnosis is made by a detailed history and psychological testing. Based on symptoms, ADHD is categorized as:

- *Combined presentation:* If enough symptoms of both criteria, inattention and hyperactivity-impulsivity, were present for the past 6 months.

- *Predominantly inattentive presentation:* If enough symptoms of inattention, but not hyperactivity-impulsivity, were present for the past 6 months.
- *Predominantly hyperactive-impulsive presentation:* If enough symptoms of hyperactivity-impulsivity, but not inattention, were present for the past 6 months.

The treatment is multimodal with psychotherapy, family therapy, modification of environment, social situation change/ input, etc., and pharmacotherapy.

REFERENCES/SOURCES

- American Psychiatric Association. Diagnostic and Statistical Manual of Mental Disorders, 5th edition (DSM-5). Washington, DC: American Psychiatric Publishing; 2013.
- Sadock BJ, Sadock VA. Chapter 45.1. In: Sadock BJ, Sadock VA, Ruiz P (Eds). Kaplan and Sadock's Comprehensive Textbook of Psychiatry, Volume 2, 10th edition. Philadelphia, PA: Wolters Kluwer; 2017. p. 3587.
- Shah R, Grover S, Avasthi A. Clinical practice guidelines for the assessment and management of attention-deficit/hyperactivity disorder. Indian J Psychiatry. 2019;61(Suppl 2):176-93.

10. An 11-year-old child is brought to the psychiatric outpatient department on the advice of his pediatrician. His mother reports that he has been spending about an hour in the toilet in the morning for past 3–4 months, whereas earlier he used to spend only 20 minutes. She says, he washes his hands if he touches anything, and asks others not to touch him. Lately, he has been asking his mother to wash her hands 7 times before she starts cooking, and gets very upset if she does not count aloud. When they go out for get-togethers, he does not eat citing some reasons. When questioned, he says that he has to wash his hands 7 times to get the "just right" feeling, and feels anxious if he does not do so. He fears his family or he may contract some deadly illness, if he does not do it "right". He knows that this is absurd but cannot stop himself as he feels anxious. He denies hearing any voices or having any other fears. He sleeps well. What is the likely diagnosis and what is the first line of management?

A. Bipolar affective disorder; start mood stabilizer
B. Generalized anxiety disorder; start cognitive behavioral therapy (CBT) and consider SSRI
C. Brief psychotic disorder; start antipsychotic
D. OCD; start CBT and consider SSRI

EXPLANATION

Mood symptoms are not evident in the history neither has any generalized worries been mentioned. It is clear from history that there are no psychotic symptoms and the child has insight into his symptoms. The symptoms are repetitive compulsive rituals which are associated with magical thinking (if he does not wash his hands 7 times then something may happen to his family). This is also associated with the obsessive thinking that it has to be "just right". As the child is only 11 years old, starting with CBT and then going on to medications is recommended.

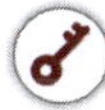

Key: D

BOOST YOUR KNOWLEDGE

The OCD prevalence is about 1–4%. There is male preponderance in child and adolescents (3:2), but there is slight female preponderance among patients with adult-onset OCD. Nearly half of adults with OCD have their first symptom before 11 years, and nearly one-fourth have their first symptom between 11 and 18 years of age. Evidence from family, linkage, twin, and segregation studies have shown that OCD has a genetic component of risk; heritability ranges from 45 to 65%. In childhood-onset OCD, family history of OCD or obsessive-compulsive spectrum disorder is more often present when compared to adult-onset OCD.

Childhood-onset OCD have more evidence of perinatal risk factors, subclinical OCD symptoms, the presence of comorbid conditions in three-fourths of cases, neuropsychological deficits, covert symptoms, the significant role of environmental triggers with high family accommodation (like in the above case mother takes part in child's rituals) and less insight. The world health organization (WHO) lists OCD among the group of the highest disabling conditions.

REFERENCES/SOURCES

- Avasthi A, Sharma A, Grover S. Indian Clinical Practice Guidelines for the Management of Obsessive-Compulsive Disorder in Children and Adolescents. J Psychiatry. 2019;61(Suppl 2):306-16.
- Sadock BJ, Sadock VA. Chapter 52.1. In: Sadock BJ, Sadock VA, Ruiz P (Eds). Kaplan and Sadock's Comprehensive Textbook of Psychiatry, Volume 2, 10th edition. Philadelphia, PA: Wolters Kluwer; 2017. p. 3695.

Index

A

B

C

D

E

F

H

I

J

K

L

M

N

O

P

Q

R

S

T

U

W

X

Y

Z